NEURAL BLOCKADE
in Clinical Anesthesia
and Management of Pain

NEURAL BLOCKADE
in Clinical Anesthesia and Management of Pain

edited by

Michael J. Cousins, M.B., B.S., M.D. (SYD.), F.F.A.R.A.C.S., F.F.A.R.C.S.
Professor and Chairman
Department of Anaesthesia and Intensive Care and
Chairman, Pain Management Unit
Flinders Medical Centre
The Flinders University of South Australia
Adelaide, Australia

Phillip O. Bridenbaugh, M.D.
Professor and Chairman
Department of Anesthesia
University of Cincinnati Medical Center
College of Medicine
Cincinnati, Ohio

With 39 Contributors

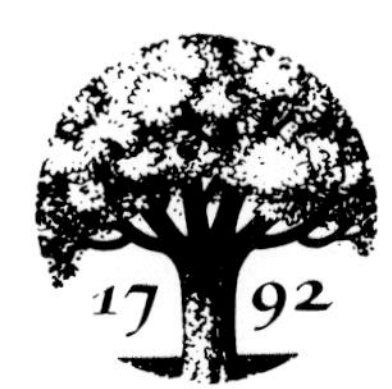

J. B. Lippincott Company
Philadelphia · Toronto

 Printed in the United States of America. For information address J. B. Lippincott Company, East Washington Square, Philadelphia, Penna. 19105

6 5 4 3

Library of Congress Cataloging in Publication Data

Main entry under title:

Neural blockade in clinical anesthesia and management of pain.

Bibliography
Includes index
1. Nerve block. 2. Nerves—Drug effects.
3. Pain—Physiological aspects. I. Cousins, Michael J.
II. Bridenbaugh, Phillip O. DNLM: 1. Nerve block.
2. Pain—Therapy. W0300 N494
RD84.N48 617′.966 79-23787
ISBN 0-397-50439-X

The authors and publisher have exerted every effort to ensure that drug selection and dosage set forth in this text are in accord with current recommendations and practice at the time of publication. However, in view of ongoing research, changes in government regulations, and the constant flow of information relating to drug therapy and drug reactions, the reader is urged to check the package insert for each drug for any change in indications and dosage and for added warnings and precautions. This is particularly important when the recommended agent is a new or infrequently employed drug.

To patients with acute or chronic pain

The theoretical and practical information in this text is dedicated to more enlightened and effective use of neural blockade for the management of all types of pain and for prevention of the harmful sequelae of severe unrelieved pain.

Contributors

Søren S. Barner, M.D., M.D.O.S.
Assistant Professor, Institute for Experimental Research in Surgery, University of Copenhagen; and, Senior Registrar, Eye Department, Gentofte Hospital, Copenhagen, Denmark

F. R. Berry, M.B., B.S., (Syd.), F.F.A.R.A.C.S.
Head of Emergency Centre, Royal Perth Hospital, Perth, Australia

Jørn Boberg–Ans, M.D., Ph.D. in Ophthalmology (Copenhagen)
Eye surgeon
Head, Charlottenlund Ophthalmological Clinic, Charlottenlund, Denmark

David E. Bresler, Ph.D.
Director, Pain Control Unit, University of California at Los Angeles Hospital and Clinics; and, Adjutant Assistant Professor of Anesthesiology, Gnathology and Occlusion, and Psychology, University of Los Angeles, Schools of Medicine, Dentistry and the College of Letters and Sciences, Los Angeles, California

L. Donald Bridenbaugh, M.D.
Director, Department of Anesthesiology, The Mason Clinic; and, Clinical Professor of Anesthesiology, University of Washington, School of Medicine, Seattle, Washington

Phillip O. Bridenbaugh, M.D.
Professor and Chairman, Department of Anesthesia, University of Cincinnati Medical Center, College of Medicine, Cincinnati, Ohio

Peter Brownridge, M.B., Ch.B., D.R.C.O.G., F.F.A.R.C.S.
Senior Specialist in Charge of Obstetric Anaesthesia, Department of Anaesthesia and Intensive Care, Flinders Medical Centre, The Flinders University of South Australia, Adelaide, Australia

F. Peter Buckley, M.B., B.S., F.F.A.R.C.S.
Assistant Professor, Department of Anesthesiology, University of Washington, School of Medicine, Seattle, Washington

Michael J. Cousins, M.B., B.S., M.D. (Syd.), F.F.A.R.A.C.S., F.F.A.R.C.S.
Professor and Chairman, Department of Anaesthesia and Intensive Care; and, Chairman, Pain Management Unit, Flinders Medical Centre, The Flinders University of South Australia, Adelaide, Australia

Rudolph H. de Jong, M.D.
Richard Saltonstall Professor for Research in Anesthesia, Tufts University, School of Medicine, Boston, Massachusetts

Brian Dwyer, M.B., B.S. (Sydney), F.F.A.R.C.S., F.F.A.R.A.C.S.
Director of Anaesthetics and Director of Pain Clinic, St. Vincent's Hospital; and, Member of the Board of Faculty of Anaesthetists, Royal Australisian College of Surgeons, Sydney, N.S.W., Australia

B. Raymond Fink, M.D.
Professor, Department of Anesthesiology, University of Washington, School of Medicine, Seattle, Washington

Jeffrey G. Garber, D.M.D.
Assistant Professor of Anesthesia, University of Pennsylvania, School of Medicine; and, Assistant Professor of Pharmacology and Oral Surgery, University of Pennsylvania, School of Dental Medicine, Philadelphia, Pennsylvania

David Gibb, M.B., B.S. (Sydney), M.Sc. (Med)., F.F.A.R.C.S., F.F.A.R.A.C.S.
Staff Specialist, St. Vincent's Hospital; and, Senior Lecturer, School of Physiology and Pharmacology, University of New South Wales, Sydney, N.S.W., Australia

C. J. Glynn, M.B., B.S., M.Sc. (Oxon), F.F.A.R.C.S.
Clinical Coordinator/Lecturer, Pain Unit, Department of Anaesthesia and Intensive Care, Flinders Medical Centre, The Flinders University of South Australia, Adelaide, Australia

Dr. C. McK. Holmes, M.B., Ch.B., F.F.A.R.C.S., F.F.A.R.A.C.S.
Specialist Anaesthetist, Dunedin Hospital; and, Senior Lecturer in Anaesthesia, University of Otago, Dunedin, New Zealand

Jon William Joseph, M.D.
Fellow, American College of Anesthesia; and, Diplomat, American Board of Anesthesia; and, Staff Anesthesiologist, Methodist Hospital, St. Louis Park, Minnesota

Jordan Katz, M.D.
Professor and Vice Chairman, Department of Anesthesiology, University of California Medical School, San Diego; and, Chief, Anesthesiology Service, U.S. Veteran's Administration Medical Center, La Jolla, California

Ronald L. Katz, M.D.
Professor and Chairman, Department of Anesthesiology, University of California at Los Angeles, School of Medicine, Los Angeles, California

William F. Kennedy, Jr., M.D.
Professor, Department of Anesthesiology, University of Washington, School of Medicine; and, Attending Anesthesiologist, University of Washington, Affiliated Hospitals, Seattle, Washington

Leo A. Keoshian, M.D., F.A.C.S
Clinical Associate Professor, Department of Surgery, Stanford University, School of Medicine, Stanford, California

Jorgen A. Kirchhoff, M.D.
Chief of Section, Department of Anesthesia, University Hospital, Rigshopitalet, Copenhagen, Denmark

Sampson Lipton, F.F.A.R.C.S.
Director, Centre for Pain Relief, Department of Medical and Surgical Neurology, Walton Hospital, Liverpool; and Clinical Lecturer in Anaesthesia, Liverpool University Medical School; and, Visiting Fellow, Bioengineering Unit, University of Salford, Lancashire, United Kingdom

J. W. Lloyd, M.A. (Oxon) D.A., F.F.A.R.C.S.
Consultant Anaesthetist, Nuffield Department of Anaesthetics, Radcliffe Infirmary; and, Director, Oxford Regional Pain Relief Unit, Abingdon, Oxford, United Kingdom

J. Bertil Löfström, M.D., Ph.D.
Professor, Department of Anesthesiology, Linköping University at the University Hospital, Linköping, Sweden

Kevin McCaul, M.B.E., E.D., F.F.A., R.A.C.S., F.F.A.R.C.S., R.C.S.I. (Hon)
Honorary Consultant Anaesthetist, Royal Women's Hospital, Melbourne; and, Chairman, Anaesthetic Mortality and Morbidity Committee, Government of Victoria, Carlton, Victoria, Australia

James E. McLennan, M.D.
Assistant Professor of Surgery (Neurosurgery), University of Cincinnati, College of Medicine, Cincinnati, Ohio

Laurence E. Mather, Ph.D.
Senior Lecturer, Department of Anaesthesia and Intensive Care, Flinders Medical Centre, The Flinders University of South Australia, Adelaide, Australia

Ronald D. Miller, M.D.
Professor of Anesthesia and Pharmacology, Medical School, University of California, San Francisco, San Francisco, California

William L. Munger, M.D.
Assistant Professor in Residence, Department of Anesthesia, University of California, San Francisco, San Francisco, California

Terence M. Murphy, M.B., Ch.B., F.F.A.R.C.S
Associate Professor, Anesthesiology; and, Acting Director, Pain Clinic, University of Washington, School of Medicine, Seattle, Washington

Patrick Edward Powell, M.D.
Staff Anesthesiologist, St. Rose Hospital, Hayward, California

David H. Ralston, M.D.
Assistant Professor and Director, Division of Obstetric Anesthesia; and, Affiliate, Child Development and Mental Retardation Center, Department of Anesthesiology, University of Washington, Seattle, Washington

Ottheinz Schulte-Steinberg, M.D.D.A. (McGill)
Chief of Department of Anaesthesia, Kreiskrankenhaus Starnberg, Academic Teaching Hospital of The Ludwig-Maximilians-University Munich, Starnberg, Germany

D.B. Scott, M.D., F.R.C.P.E., F.F.A.R.C.S.
Consultant Anaesthetist, Royal Infirmary; and, Senior Lecturer, Department of Anaesthetics, University of Edinburgh, Edinburgh, Scotland

Bernard Roy Simpson, M.D., D.Phil. (OXON), F.F.A.R.C.S.
Chief, Department of Anesthesiology; and, Medical Director, Anesthesia Services, Baylor University Medical Center; and, Clinical Professor of Anesthesiology, Southwestern Medical School, University of Texas, Dallas; and, Honorary Consultant Anaesthetist, Royal Prince Alfred Hospital Sydney, N.S.W., Australia

Mark Swerdlow, M.D., M.Sc., F.F.A.R.C.S., D.A.
Director, North West Regional Pain Relief Centre, Hope Hospital; and, University of Manchester, School of Medicine, Honorary Lecturer in Anaesthesia, Salford, United Kingdom

Gordon Taylor, M.B., B.S., L.R.C.P., M.R.C.S., F.F.A.R.C.S.
Clinical Associate Professor of Anesthesia, Department of Anesthesia, Stanford University, School of Medicine, Stanford; and, Anesthesiologist, Carson-Tahoe Hospital, Carson City, Nevada

Gale E. Thompson, M.D.
Anesthesiologist, The Mason Clinic, Seattle, Washington

Geoffrey T. Tucker, B.Pharm., Ph.D.
Senior Lecturer in Clinical Pharmacology and Therapeutics, University of Sheffield, Department of Therapeutics, Hallamshire Hospital, Sheffield, United Kingdom

Peter R. Wilson, M.B., B.S., Ph.D., F.F.A.R.A.C.S.
Senior Lecturer and Senior Specialist, Pain Management Unit, Department of Anaesthesia and Intensive Care, Flinders Medical Centre, The Flinders University of South Australia, Adelaide, Australia

Foreword

Neural Blockade in Clinical Anesthesia and Management of Pain must be the most ambitious project of its kind ever undertaken. Aimed primarily at the relief of pain during surgery, this book ranges from a consideration of the physiology, pharmacology, and toxicology of the local analgesic agents in common use to a number of the less orthodox methods of relieving suffering of various origins. The book is indeed encyclopedic in its coverage and, like encyclopedias in other sciences, each section has been entrusted to a recognized world authority in his own special field. No book on local analgesia could have a sounder pedigree.

There are situations in which, manifestly, local anesthesia is preferable to general. Apart from these, improved sedation and longer-acting analgesic drugs have improved patient acceptance; but the practitioner still has to acquire the necessary "know-how" to deposit the solution with reasonable accuracy for it to be effective. Both the editors are renowned for their practical teaching, which should be a sound guarantee that both the expert and the tyro can turn to this book for guidance and profit.

Neural blockade offers far more to the patient than merely analgesia during surgery. Rapid growth in application of neural blockade to postoperative, post-traumatic, and obstetric pain management is extensively covered in this text. Even more extensive is the breadth and depth of scientific information and clinical application of neural blockade in chronic pain; this is presented as completely and concisely as possible.

SIR ROBERT MACINTOSH,
D.M., F.R.C.S. (EDIN),
HON F.F.A.R.C.S., England,
Ireland, and Australasia.
Emeritus Nuffield Professor
of Anaesthetics, University of Oxford

Preface

". . . I would recommend trying cocaine as a local anesthetic . . ." *Von Anrep (1880)*

It is now exactly 100 years since the first thorough pharmacologic investigation of cocaine and the discovery of its local anesthetic properties by Von Anrep (as noted in the engrossing historical account in Chap. 1 by Professor B. Raymond Fink). Perhaps as a result of Von Anrep's lack of enthusiasm for his results, almost 4 years elapsed before Koller used cocaine for local anesthesia in humans; then, progress in the development of techniques was relatively rapid between 1884 and the 1940s. However, detailed pharmacologic and physiologic studies of neural blockade did not begin in earnest until the 1950s. The major contributions to current knowledge date back only 25 years, with some of the most significant being delayed until the application of modern techniques of pharmacology and physiology in the last 10 to 15 years.

This relatively recent coming of age of pharmacologic and physiologic knowledge about neural blockade posed a clear challenge to the editors to present in *Neural Blockade in Clinical Anesthesia and Management of Pain* the latest data, together with more established anatomical and technical knowledge. Also, the rapid development of the use of neural blockade in postoperative and post-traumatic pain, obstetric pain, and other forms of acute pain called for documentation of efficacy and safety in these settings. The ineffectual management of persistent (or chronic) pain by the majority of the medical profession has suddenly given way to a much needed wave of interest and activity. Here again, it was seen to be important to document what is currently known of the place and proven benefits of neural blockade in pain diagnosis and management and to indicate areas where controlled data are not yet available.

The physiologic basis of local anesthetic action and central nervous system toxicity has only come into focus in the last decade, and Professor de Jong was asked to distill his definitive contributions in Chapter 2. Even more recent has been the vital knowledge of local anesthetic pharmacokinetics (Chap. 3); G. T. Tucker and L. E. Mather were chosen to present this material because of their extensive publications of fundamental data in this area over the past 6 to 8 years. Of equal importance to the safe use of neural blockade were definitive studies in humans by D. B. Scott (Chap. 4) and others on toxic blood concentrations of the various modern local anesthetics and their relationship to blood concentrations usually achieved during neural blockade.

Detailed physiologic and pharmacologic studies of central neural blockade gained great impetus in the 1960s from the work of Bromage in Montreal, Bonica's group at the University of Washington, and Moore's group at the Mason Clinic in Seattle. One of the editors, (M. J. C.) had early associations with Bromage's group and the other (P. O. B.) was Director of Anesthesia at the Mason Clinic. Representatives from these institutions have been assembled to present this contribution to the scientific basis of neural blockade (Professor W. F. Kennedy, Dr. F. P. Buckley, and Dr. D. H. Ralston; Dr. G. E. Thompson, Dr. L. D. Bridenbaugh, and Professor P. O. Bridenbaugh; and Professor M. J. Cousins).

". . . Since whom, science has control of pain . . ."
Epitaph for W. H. G. Morton, 1819–1868

Unfortunately this encouraging epitaph, referring to the discovery of anesthesia, did not apply to acute postoperative and post-traumatic pain and even less to chronic pain. The explosive increase in knowledge of pain transmission now provides an opportunity to improve the current situation in which postoperative pain still ranks highest in patient complaints following surgery, while chronic pain imposes a heavy toll in human suffering, with an annual cost in the United States, alone, of over $50 billion.

Exciting and unprecedented progress in knowledge of spinal cord and brain mechanisms of pain have emanated from a number of groups throughout the world. The Mayo Clinic group (Professor F. W. L. Kerr, Dr. T. L. Yaksh, *et al.*) have been prominent among those defining a whole new range of possibilities for interruption of pain conduction at the spinal cord level. Dr. Peter Wilson participated in this work at the Mayo Clinic and continues to pursue this promising expansion of the scope of neural blockade as presented in Neurologic Mechanisms of Pain (Chap. 24). New clinical applications of this work developed by the Flinders group, plus some recent data describing the nature of chronic pain and use of neural blockade as developed at the Oxford Pain Relief Unit by Dr. J. Lloyd and Dr. C. J. Glynn, are presented in Chapter 31 by Dr. C. J. Glynn. In Chapter 28, Dr. D. Bressler and Professor R. Katz explore less invasive methods of manipulating pain conduction and the pain "experience" in comparison to neural blockade.

Clinical uses of neural blockade are now being carefully evaluated and their proper contribution to clinical care is reflected by those units that have incorporated various techniques as a routine in their management of surgical, obstetrical, and "pain" patients.

One of the goals of *Neural Blockade in Clinical Anesthesia and Management of Pain* is to make this experience available to other centers throughout the world in the hope that some current inconsistencies in the application of the full range of benefits of neural blockade will be overcome. Thus, authors in the clinical application sections of the book are drawn from many states of the United States and Australia, from a number of centers in the United Kingdom, from Scandinavia and Germany, and from New Zealand. A number of the contributors have pioneered the applications described or have played a major part in their modern use, for example: Dr. Mack Holmes (intravenous neural blockade); Professor Bertil Löfström (lumbar sympathetic blockade); Dr. Kevin McCaul (caudal blockade); Professor Roy Simpson (postoperative pain management); and Dr. Sam Lipton (percutaneous cordotomy). Dr. Brian Dwyer, Dr. Mark Swerdlow, Dr. Sam Lipton, and Dr. John Lloyd were some of the earliest to apply the collaborative approach to pain management, while Professor Jordon Katz, Associate Professor Terence Murphy, Dr. Donald Bridenbaugh, and Professor Ronald Katz were prominent in the first wave of anesthesiologists in the United States to be encouraged by the early pioneering stimulus of John J. Bonica and Daniel C. Moore.

A very critical evaluation of the current status of local anesthetic blockade in chronic pain diagnosis and management was desired for Chapter 26; to this end a clinician with interest and experience in pain management, but also with an established reputation in other areas of anesthesia research, was chosen, Professor Ronald Miller. On the other side of the clinical profile, a frank coverage of the complications of neural blockade seemed an appropriate task for a clinician with one of the most long-standing and ongoing commitments to pain diagnosis and management, Dr. Mark Swerdlow.

Authors were included from clinical units with major continuing use of neural blockade in special settings: Dr. J. G. Garber (dental); Dr. J. Boberg–Ans and Dr. S. S. Barner (eye); Associate Professor G. Taylor, Dr. D. H. Ralston, and Dr. P. Brownridge (obstetrics); Dr. Leo Keoshian (plastic surgery); Dr. F. R. Berry and Dr. J. A. Kirchoff (outpatient surgery); Dr. O. Schulte–Steinberg (pediatrics); Dr. F. P. Buckley (postoperative); Dr. D. Gibb, Professor J. Katz, Dr. W. Munger, Professor R. Katz, Dr. D. Bressler, Associate Professor T. M. Murphy, and Dr. C. J. Glynn (chronic pain).

The editors have both had a longstanding interest and regard for the contribution neural blockade has to offer to clinical care of patients in the settings presented in this text. Both have trained in research outside their own country and in other fields in addition to being trained in the practices of neural blockade. They feel strongly that the scientific data on the clinical use of neural blockade should be presented in a manner which can be scrutinized by clinicians and basic scientists who do not have a particular enthusiasm for local anesthesia or who have previously not had access to this field. Also, neural blockade should be seen in the context of other approaches to pain management, as discussed in Chapters 27 and 28.

The early development of *Neural Blockade in Clinical Anesthesia and Management of Pain* was greatly helped by a major International Symposium on Neural Blockade and Pain held in Sydney, Australia, in 1975, at which the majority of contributors presented material that had been developed in outline over the previous year. From criticisms and discussions of this material, the text was developed and refined. The complete editing process involved two prolonged visits to the United States by one editor and two to Australia by the other.

They hope that readers find the text useful whatever their field of medicine and that at the least it will encourage the effective and safe use of neural blockade in the wide range of situations in which improved relief of human suffering is possible. It is also their sincere wish that some will be stimulated to extend knowledge in which deficiencies currently exist, as indicated in the text.

MICHAEL J. COUSINS, M.B., B.S., M.D.
PHILLIP O. BRIDENBAUGH, M.D.

Acknowledgments

A work of the magnitude of *Neural Blockade in Clinical Anesthesia and Management of Pain* is never achieved without a high cost to the families and professional associates of the editors. Both editors were appointed to Chairs of Anesthesiology during the gestation period of the book, thus greatly compounding the usual challenge of a major editorial task. The editors wish to express their deep appreciation of the support and understanding of their families who made bearable the sometimes unbearable task of "two jobs." In recognition of their professional colleagues in the Department of Anaesthesia and Intensive Care, Flinders University of South Australia and Flinders Medical Centre, and the Department of Anesthesia, University of Cincinnati, the editors wish to note that they remain mindful of the assistance they received and the willingness of their staffs to persevere because they believed this project to be worthwhile.

To their teachers the editors owe their early interest in neural blockade and application of scientific method to improved clinical care: Professor Philip Bromage and Professor Lloyd McLean at McGill University, Montreal; and Professor Richard Mazze, Professor John P. Bunker, Professor Ellis Cohen, and Professor C. Philip Larson, Jr., at Stanford University (M.J.C.); Dr. L. D. Bridenbaugh and Dr. Daniel C. Moore at the Mason Clinic, Seattle; Sir Robert MacIntosh at Oxford University; and Professor Benjamin Covino at Harvard University (P.O.B.).

The authors also express their thanks to the institutions that supported the preparation of this text by providing facilities during the editing process: The Mason Clinic, Seattle; the University of Cincinnati, Ohio; Stanford University; the Royal North Shore Hospital of Sydney, Australia; and the Flinders University of South Australia and Flinders Medical Centre, Adelaide, Australia.

Color illustrations are now almost prohibitively expensive, however, a text relying partly on anatomical clarity requires such a medium. The use of color was supported by Astra Chemicals, U.S.A. and Astra Chemicals, Australia; Roche, Australia; Glaxo Group of Companies, Australia, Ciba Geigy, Australia, and Spembly Ltd., England.

Many of the illustrations in the text were prepared in the medical illustration departments of the various authors' institutions. However, a number required redrawing to preserve uniformity of style and a considerable number of original illustrations were drawn in the Medical Illustration and Media Department, Flinders Medical Centre, Flinders University of South Australia, Adelaide, Australia. The authors are very grateful for the high quality of these figures and wish to express their particular thanks to Mr. Alan Bentley for his artistic skill while preserving anatomical integrity and his willingness to persevere with the editors' attempts to explain the practical points they wished to clarify.

Many authors and publishers gave permission for their work to be quoted or reproduced and due acknowledgment has been made in the text.

The text was originally planned by Professor M. J. Cousins and nursed through its early stages by the then Editor-in-Chief of Medical Books, J. B. Lippincott Company, Mr. Lewis Reines. Professor Phillip Bridenbaugh commenced work on the text early in 1976, and both editors rapidly came to appreciate the benefits of a running partner. Soon after this time, J. Stuart Freeman, Jr., became Editor-in-Chief of Medical Books, J. B. Lippincott, and the editors express their thanks to him and to Laura Dabundo of the Copy Editorial Department for guiding the text to its present form.

Both editors had considerable secretarial support that extended far beyond the onerus task of typing and retyping a massive manuscript: at Flinders University of South Australia, Flinders Medical Centre, Miss Josephine O'Grady and Mrs. Lyn Arman and at the University of Cincinnati Medical Center, Mrs. Glenda Jones. Also, the following figures are original art produced in the Department of Medical Illustrations and Media at the Flinders

Medical Center, Adelaide, Australia: Figs. 4-1, 4-2, 4-3, 7-7, 7-8, 7-9, 7-15, 8-2, 8-7, 8-11, 8-30, 8-31, 8-32, 8-35, 10-5, 10-7, 10-8, 10-9, 10-11, 10-13, 10-14, 10-16, 11-10, 12-10, 13-1, 13-12, 13-18, 15-10, 18-4, and 31-3. Finally but by no means least the editors thank Michele Cousins who proofread all text and checked the references.

Particular thanks are also due to Sir Robert Macintosh and E. & S. Livingstone, Edinburgh, for granting permission to redraw or modify a number of illustrations from Sir Robert's classic monographs—'Local Analgesia, Abdominal Surgery' (1962); 'Local Analgesia, Head and Neck,' 2nd Edition (1955) and Sir Robert Macintosh's 'Lumber Puncture and Spinal Analgesia' eds. Lee, J. A. and Atkinson, R. S. (1978).

Many helped with proofreading and made suggestions for text modification. In particular the staffs of the Department of Anesthesiology, University of Cincinnati and Flinders Medical Centre made large contributions.

In addition the editors would like to thank Noel Cass, Colin Shanks, Kester Brown, Bill Crosby, Ken Hardy, John Rigg, Mark Swerdlow, Brian Dwyer, David Gibb, Fred Berry and Prithvi Raj.

Contents

Section E: Specialized Surgical Applications

Section F: Complications of Neural Blockade

Part Three: Neural Blockade in the Management of Pain

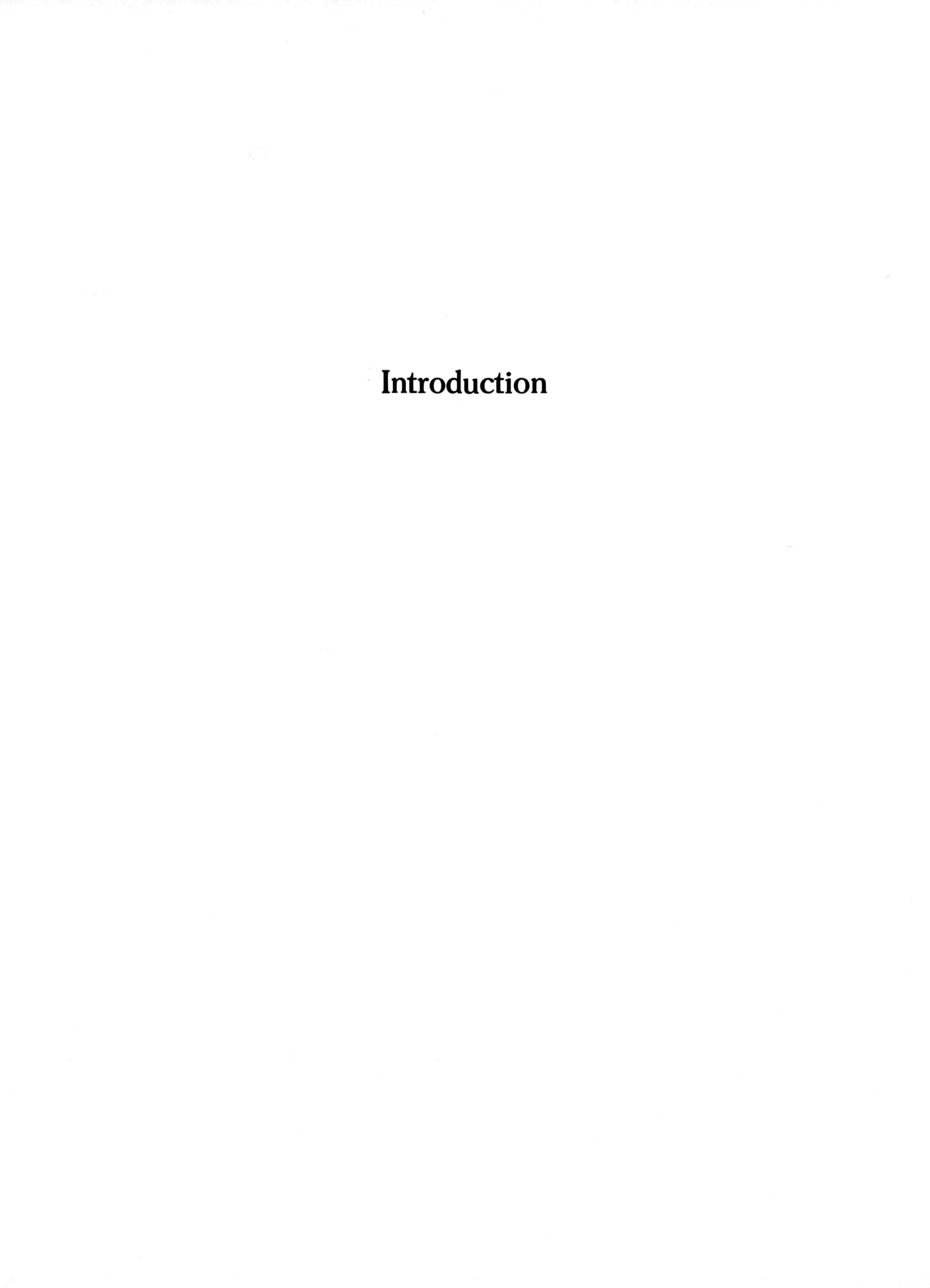

Introduction

1 History of Local Anesthesia

B. Raymond Fink

COCAINE ANESTHESIA

Koller's demonstration in 1884 of ocular surface anesthesia with cocaine had antecedents almost as lengthy as those of general anesthesia 40 years earlier (Fig. 1-1).[44] Albert Niemann's success in isolating and naming the alkaloid from the leaves of *Erythroxylon coca* was recorded in 1860 in a report, signed W. (for H. Wöhler), which also related the passionate chewing of the leaves and the deleterious mental effects this had on the Coqueros of Peru.[55] A thorough pharmacologic investigation of the properties of the alkaloid in frogs was presented by von Anrep in 1880 in a 35-page report, which ended as follows: "the animal experiments have no practical application; nevertheless I would recommend trying cocaine as a local anesthetic in persons of melancholy disposition."[73] Plainly, von Anrep was most impressed by the stimulating properties of cocaine, and these seem also to have been uppermost in the mind of Sigmund Freud when he suggested a study of the drug to Koller.

Freud wanted to know more about the analeptic action of cocaine, which he hoped might be useful in curing one of his great friends of addiction to morphine. This friend was a pathologist and had developed an unbearably painful thenar neuroma after accidentally cutting himself while performing an autopsy. Freud obtained a supply of cocaine from the manufacturing firm of Merck and shared it with Koller, who was to help him investigate its effects on the nervous system. Koller was a junior intern in the Ophthalmological Clinic at the University of Vienna and longed to obtain the coveted appointment of assistant in the clinic, on the strength of a worthy piece of research. But there was local opposition and though the research proved worthy enough, it did not secure him the appointment. Deeply disappointed, he moved to the Netherlands and, 2 years later, emigrated to the United States.

Koller's discovery was no accident for he was keenly aware of the limitations of general anesthesia in ophthalmological surgery. He had delved into the literature and presumably read von Anrep's suggestion about local anesthesia and taken it seriously enough to try it experimentally. After making some dramatic tests on animals, Koller tried it on himself and performed an operation for glaucoma with cocaine topical anesthesia on September 11, 1884, 4 days before the Congress of Ophthalmology was due to meet in Heidelberg. Koller immediately wrote a paper for the Congress, but, being an impecunious intern, he could not afford the train fare to Heidelberg so he gave the paper to a visiting ophthalmologist from Trieste, Dr. Brettauer, who had stopped in Vienna on his way to the Congress. Brettauer's news from Heidelberg reached New York in a letter from H. D. Noyes, an American ophthalmologist who had attended the Heidelberg Congress.[56]

The late 1800s were a period of ferment in science and technology in Europe and the United States. Pravaz in Lyon and Wood in Edinburgh in the early 1850s together invented the glass syringe and hypodermic hollow needle.[59,77] Pravaz was introducing ferric chloride into aneurysms through a trocar to make them clot, but Wood had in mind the injection of drugs in the neighborhood of nerve trunks for the purpose of relieving neuralgic pain, an idea that earns him the title of "father in lore of nerve block." Eulenberg apparently used this technique on the superior laryngeal nerve in 1864. Wood is credited with the invention of the hollow needle, but a hollow needle is not mentioned as such in his report. He does mention the attempted use and failure of acupuncture needles for the introduction of morphine and its successful introduction with an "elegant little syringe." Six years after Darwin's epochal book, Lister, in 1865, opened a new era in surgery by applying Pasteur's proof of nonspontaneous generation to the elimination of sepsis. Pflüger showed that the seat of respiration was in the tissues and not in the blood, and Ringer in 1882 dem-

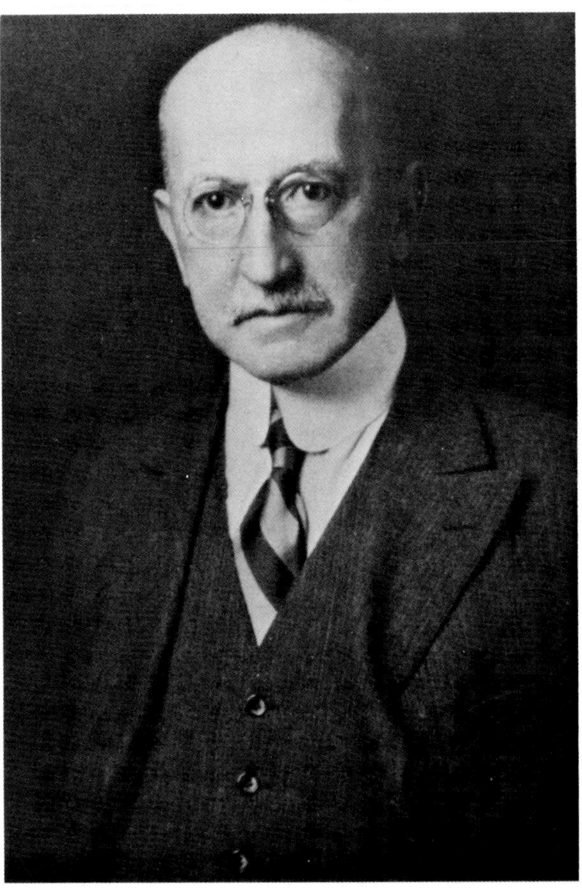

Fig. 1-1. Carl Koller, M.D.

onstrated the need for calcium and potassium salts to maintain the excitability of the heart, the same year that produced the world's first electrical power station (in New York). The establishment of the coal tar industry in Germany led to large-scale production of pharmaceuticals, of which the marketing of cocaine by Merck was one result. 1886 saw the introduction of steam sterilization of dressings by von Bergmann, and 1890, the use of surgical rubber gloves, initially to protect the hands of Halsted's instrument nurse from the disinfectant.

Noyes's letter to the New York Medical Record excited numerous readers to test the new wonder drug and many of them rushed into print with astounding experiences. The very first note to appear was published within 5 weeks of Noyes's letter. It was written by N. J. Hepburn, a New York ophthalmologist.[39] There were no standards for drug trials in those days, and the tradition of self-experimentation was inviolate. If a researcher or physician wanted to know whether a drug was safe, he tried it on himself. Hepburn describes how on October 16, 1884, he experimented with a 2-per-cent solution of cocaine, giving himself a series of subcutaneous injections of 0.4 ml (8 mg) at intervals of 5 minutes. He noted that by the time of the eighth injection, the agreeable stimulating effects of the drug—rapid respiration and pulse, a feeling of warmth, pleasant hallucinations—had reached a point that he felt it best to stop. For reasons that Hepburn does not state, he repeated the performance 2 days later, and then found it possible to carry the number of 0.4 ml injections to 16 before the general disturbance persuaded him to cease. Four days later, he records, he was at it again, and this time he tried a larger unit volume and amount (10 mg), and was able to tolerate 16 of those. It seems clear that Hepburn was addicted. Otherwise, why would he have increased the size of the injections?

By November 29, 1884, the ophthalmologist Bull was able to report that he had used the drug to produce anesthesia of the cornea and conjunctiva in more than 150 cases.[14] He gave sound reasons for his enthusiasm: he saved the time required for complete etherization and avoided the enormous engorgement of the ocular blood vessels produced by the ether, the danger of vomiting, and the disadvantage that results because almost any apparatus for producing anesthesia by inhalation is a physical interference for the operator.

Conduction Anesthesia

After the publication of Noyes's letter, the idea of injecting cocaine directly into tissues in order to render them insensible occurred, simultaneously, to several American surgeons. W. B. Burke injected five minims (drops) of 2-per-cent solution close to a metacarpal branch of the ulnar nerve and extracted a bullet painlessly from the base of his patient's little finger.[15] But it was Halsted and his associates who most clearly saw the great possibilities of conduction block. The term was introduced by Franck 7 years later, though he may well have borrowed part of it from Corning, for in 1886 Corning was writing that "the thought of producing anaesthesia by abolishing conduction in sensory nerves, by suitable means, should have been rife in the minds of progressive physicians." Corning himself quite possibly got the idea from Halsted, for Halsted later attested that Corning was a frequent observer at the Roosevelt Hospital, New York, where Halsted, assisted by Hall, performed his teaching. In 1884 Hall described how he blocked a cutaneous branch of the ulnar nerve in his own forearm.[35] He and Halsted made injections into the musculocutaneous nerve of the leg and the ulnar nerve. Hall noted the appearance of marked constitutional symptoms, giddiness, severe nausea, cold perspiration, and dilated pupils, but this did not daunt these bold pioneers, and the same evening Halsted blocked Hall's supratrochlear nerve and removed an adjoining congenital cystic tumor. He also induced Nash, a dental surgeon, to tend to Hall's own upper incisor tooth after injection of cocaine into the infraorbital nerve at the infraorbital foramen, and Halsted thereafter performed an inferior dental nerve block on a medical student volunteer, and later did the same to Hall. Hall's report was quite explicit in predicting that, once the limits of safety had been determined, this mode of administration would find very wide application in the Outpatient Department.

The daring experimenters at the Roosevelt Hospital unfortunately became addicted to the new drug, and no more was heard from them about its use in surgery. But that Hall and Halsted were the true fathers of conduction anesthesia can scarcely be doubted.[37]

The great advantage of local anesthesia with cocaine was, of course, that it anesthetized only the part of the body on which the operation was to be performed. However, a price was paid in toxicity and time. Rapid absorption limited the safe quantity to 30 mg and the useful duration of anesthesia to 10 or 15 minutes. In 1885 Corning sought a means of prolonging the local anesthetic effects for surgical and other purposes, although he was primarily interested in the application of the drug to the therapeutics of neurologic disease.[18] His notion of pharmacokinetics was that after the introduction of cocaine beneath the skin, a certain period of time elapses during which the anesthetic agent is diffused throughout the surrounding tissue, the capillary circulation having a dual effect, first as a distributor, and afterward as a dilutor and rapid remover of the anesthetic substance. In his first article of 1885, Corning describes how he experimentally injected 0.3 ml of a 4-per-cent solution of cocaine into the lateral antebrachial nerve and obtained immediate anesthesia of the skin supplied by this nerve as far as the wrist.[18] He found that simple arrest of the circulation in the involved part by compression or constriction proximal to the point of injection intensified the anesthesia and prolonged it indefinitely. He used an Esmarch bandage for this purpose and pointed out that the method was readily applicable to surgery of all the extremities. The Riva-Rocci cuff tourniquet had not yet been invented. Esmarch had introduced his elastic bandage in 1874 for the purpose of producing a bloodless field in major amputations.[28]

As has briefly been mentioned previously, François-Franck first applied the term *blocking* to the infiltration of a nerve trunk in any part.[31] He found that the effect of the blocking drug is not limited to the purely sensory fibers because it paralyzes all nerves, whether motor or sensory, and that the sensory anesthesia is much more promptly manifested than the motor paralysis, a confirmation of von Anrep's observation of 1879. François-Franck spoke of the action of cocaine as a "physiological section," transitory and noninjurious.

Corning's principle of prolonging the local anesthetic action of cocaine by arresting the circulation in the anesthetized area inspired Braun in 1903 to dispense with the elastic tourniquet and substitute epinephrine, a "chemical tourniquet" as he called it.[11] Epinephrine had become available in pure form after Abel isolated it from the suprarenal medulla in 1897.[1]

The suggestion for this use of epinephrine came from ophthalmologic practice, in which it had been introduced to limit hemorrhage and to render the conjuctiva bloodless, as well as to treat certain diseases, notably glaucoma, and in which it was noticed that it prolonged the local effect of other drugs in general and of cocaine in particular. This observation had been confirmed by rhinologists and had enabled them to reduce the concentration and dose of cocaine and correspondingly to limit the hazard of toxicity.[54] Initially, in Braun's solution, the epinephrine was present in concentrations from 1:10,000 to 1:100,000. The first experiments to determine the dosage to be injected subcutaneously were made by Braun on himself. He found his limit of tolerance was 0.5 mg (0.5 ml of 1:1000 solution), after which general symptoms occurred and he had to lie down.

Braun introduced the term *conduction anesthesia* and felt that the use of epinephrine rendered conduction anesthesia in other parts of the body as effective as that in an extremity. In 1905 Braun published a textbook on local anesthesia, giving detailed descriptions of the technique for every region.[12]

Infiltration Anesthesia

Some 10 years earlier, a different approach, termed *infiltration anesthesia,* had been advocated by Schleich.[64] Schleich applied the principle that pure water has a weak anesthetic effect but is painful on injection, whereas physiologic saline is not.

The observation that subcutaneous injection of water produces local anesthesia was apparently first made by Potain, in 1869. Halsted, in a short letter to the editor of the New York Medical Journal, dated September 19, 1885, baldly asserted that[36]: the skin can be completely anesthetized to any extent by cutaneous injections of water; he had of late used water instead of cocaine in skin incisions; and the anesthesia did not always vanish just as soon as hyperemia supervenes.

Schleich believed that there must be a solution of such concentration between "normal" (0.6% salt solution) and pure water that would not provoke pain on injection and yet be usefully anesthetic, and he thought it was a 0.2-per-cent solution of sodium chloride. To this, he added cocaine to a concentration of 0.02 per-cent and employed it to produce a field of cutaneous anesthesia in the surgery of hydrocele, sebaceous cyst, hemorrhoids, and small abscesses.

The reason why Schleich's hypotonic solutions produced impairment of sensation does not appear to have been explained. In light of later work, it seems likely that loss of electrolyte from nerve fibers was involved.

Braun dismissed Schleich's solutions as unphysiologic and insisted that injections into the tissues for whatever purpose must be composed of fluids of the same osmotic tension as the body fluids. Inasmuch as most local anesthetic solutions are hypotonic, a corresponding amount of an indifferent salt, such as sodium chloride, must be added to prevent any injurious action upon the tissue.

Nevertheless, Schleich's infiltration technique was an important advance in that it extended the field of a small quantity of anesthetic. For the idea of using a weak solution of cocaine to avoid toxic reactions and fatalities, Schleich was probably indebted to Paul Reclus. Enthusiasm for local anesthesia diminished as the experimentation had led to casualties. Reclus clearly understood that the basic cause of accidental deaths was overdose because of the use of unnecessarily high concentrations.[61] He realized that undue absorption was avoidable by using lower concentrations, and he eventually reduced the strength of his cocaine solutions to 0.5-per-cent.

The toxicity of cocaine, coupled with its vast potential for usefulness in surgery, led to an intensive search for less toxic substitutes. But decreased toxicity without increased irritancy—or impractically brief effectiveness—proved elusive until the synthesis of procaine (Novocain) by Einhorn in 1904.

Intravenous Regional Anesthesia

In 1908 Bier devised a very effective method of bringing about complete anesthesia and motor paralysis of a limb.[9] He injected a solution of Novocain into one of the subcutaneous veins, exposed between two constricting bands in a space that had previously been rendered bloodless by an elastic rubber bandage carried from fingers or toes. The injected solution permeated the entire section of the limb very quickly, producing what Bier called *direct vein anesthesia* in 5 to 15 minutes. The anesthesia lasted as long as the upper constricting band was kept in place. After it was removed, sensation returned in a few minutes.

SPINAL ANESTHESIA

Somewhat paradoxically, the first spinal anesthesia occurred 5 years before the first lumbar puncture. The term *spinal anesthesia* was introduced by Corning in his famous second paper of 1885.[19] It was the fruit of a brilliant yet erroneous idea, for what he had in mind was neither spinal nor epidural anesthesia as presently understood. Corning was under the mistaken impression that the interspinal blood vessels communicated with those of the spinal cord, and his intention was to inject cocaine into the minute interspinal vessels and have it carried by communicating vessels into the spinal cord, where it would produce the same effect as a transverse myelitis. Doubtless, it was for this reason he performed his injection in the lower thoracic region. He makes no mention of the cerebrospinal fluid, nor of how far he introduced the needle.

His objective was clearly expressed by the title of the article, "Spinal Anaesthesia and Local Medication of the Cord with Cocaine." There is no doubt that Corning was quite literally aiming directly at the spinal cord, as he introduced a hypodermic needle—he does not say of what size—between the spinal processes of the T11 and T12. He wrote, "I reasoned that it was highly probable that, if the anesthetic was placed between the spinous processes of the vertebrae, it would be rapidly transported by the blood to the substance of the cord and would give rise to anaesthesia of the sensory and perhaps also of the motor tracts of the same. To be more explicit, I hoped to produce artificially a temporary condition of things analogous in its physiological consequences to the effects observed in transverse myelitis or after total section of the cords." Corning's report was based on a series of two: one dog and one man. In the case of the man he injected a total of 120 mg of cocaine in a period of 5 minutes, about four times the potentially lethal dose. Corning implies that he was using the procedure partly as a treatment for masturbation. What he achieved in the man was probably what is now called *epidural* or *extradural anesthesia,* and, in the dog, which received 13 mg, *spinal anesthesia,* as judged by the rates of onset. Corning certainly did have an original idea, as he was at no small pains to indicate, but the results were a lucky accident because the experiment could easily have been fatal and was conceived on the basis of an entirely erroneous notion of the local circulation. There is, of course, no direct communication between the extradural blood vessels and those of the spinal cord so it is rather difficult to understand on what Corning based his expectations.

Gray's Anatomy, at least as early as 1870, had a section on the meninges, including the subarachnoid space and cerebrospinal fluid,[33] but Corning did not report seeing the cerebrospinal fluid drip from the needle and evidently did not expect to see that. Although the anatomy books in English at the time clearly delineate the spinal meninges and cerebrospinal fluid, the contemporary German and French language textbooks do not. Corning had a long line of New England ancestors, but he received his medical education in Europe at the University of Wurtzburg[4], and so possibly never learned the basic facts of meningeal anatomy. In any case, how he got the idea that the venous channels between the spinal processes of the vertebrae were a direct avenue into the spinal cord remains unclear. Perhaps he invented it. Certainly, he did not check his understanding in *Gray's Anatomy,* and reading his scientific articles conveys the impression that scholarship was not his strong point. His articles are rather opinionated and do not name any colleagues, although it is known, as has been mentioned, that he attended the demonstration of Hall and Halsted at the Roosevelt Hospital, where the first explorations of the use of cocaine for regional nerve block took place.

Lumbar Puncture

Corning was a neurologist and not a surgeon, and he thought of his use of cocaine as a new means of managing neurologic disorders, but he did foresee that it would probably find application as a substitute for etherization in genitourinary or other branches of surgery. However, nothing came of his suggestion until 14 years later, perhaps partly because his logic was faulty and his technique wrongly conceived. At that time, the procedure of lumbar puncture had not yet been invented, let alone standardized. It fell to Quincke to do this, by basing his approach on the anatomical ground that the subarachnoid spaces of the brain and spinal cord were continuous and ended in the adult at the level of S2, whereas the spinal cord extended only to L2.[60] Thus, a puncture effected between the third or fourth lumbar intervertebral space would not damage the spinal cord.

Lumbar puncture, as the title of Quincke's article indicated, was invented as a treatment for hydrocephalus. Quincke acknowledged in his communication that he followed in the steps of Essex Wynter, who 6 months earlier had described the use of a Southey's tube and trocar for a similar purpose.[78] This device was originally designed to drain edema fluid in cases of dropsy. Wynter introduced the tube between the lumbar vertebrae, after making a small incision in the skin, for the purpose of instituting drainage of the fluid in two cases of tuberculous meningitis. Quincke's method was a vast improvement and became the standard technique, thanks to a detailed description that is still up-to-date. Quincke prescribed bed rest for the 24 hours following the puncture. Quincke's needles had an internal diameter of from 0.5 to 1.2 mm, and only the larger ones were equipped with a stylet. It is interesting to note that he entered the skin 5 to 10 mm from the midline. Thus, the paramedian approach is and has always been the classic one, and not the median approach as is sometimes taught.

It took 8 years for Quincke's technique to be applied to the production of what is now called *spinal anesthesia.* No doubt, great courage was required to introduce a drug as toxic as cocaine directly into the nervous system as Corning had done in 1885.

Unfortunately, Corning's audacity had no direct sequel unless the title of Bier's paper is taken as an implied tribute to Corning. (Bier does not mention him by name.) August Bier published his epoch-making paper on spinal anesthesia in 1899, under the title *Versuche über Cocainisirung des Ruckenmarkes* (Researches on cocainisation of the spinal cord).[8] Apparently, Bier, too, assumed that intrathecal injection of cocaine produced anesthesia by a direct action on the spinal cord. Bier had a certain amount of luck on his side; he worked at the same institution as Quincke and would have been familiar with his technique and might even have borrowed his needles.

Bier, of course, was a surgeon, and it is noticeable that for many years virtually all the extensions of technique in the use of local anesthetics were developed by surgeons. They first performed the block and then performed the operation. This makes Corning's interest in cocaine all the more remarkable because he was genuinely an outsider in the field and may well have been viewed as such. He seems to have eluded the hazard to which several of the American surgical pioneers of regional anesthesia fell victim when conscientious zeal led them to experiment on themselves befoe trying their ideas on patients.

Bier wanted to apply cocaine anesthesia for major operations and saw spinal anesthesia as a way of safely producing a maximum area of anesthesia with a minimum amount of drug. It was his opinion that the spectacular insensitivity to pain evoked by small amounts of cocaine injected into the dural sac resulted from its spread in the cerebrospinal fluid and that it acted not only on the surface of the spinal cord but especially on the unsheathed nerves that traverse the intramembranous space. However, this understanding was not conclusive. The extent of the anesthesia produced was somewhat unpredictable, so Bier decided to obtain a better understanding by experimenting on himself. His assistant, Hildebrandt, performed the lumbar puncture on Bier, but when the time came to attach the syringe to the needle, a crisis developed; the needle did not fit. A considerable amount of cerebrospinal fluid and most of the cocaine dripped onto the floor. To save the experiment, Hildebrandt volunteered his own body. This time there was a good fit and complete success.

However, the success was not unqualified. The experimenters celebrated with wine and cigars, and the next day Bier suffered an oppressive headache that took 9 days to go away. Hildebrandt's hangover developed even before the night was over. Moreover, while he was anesthetized, Hildebrandt had been unscientifically kicked in the shins to demonstrate the depth of the analgesia, and in the aftermath he duly developed painful bruises in the places where no pain had been.

As Bier emphasized in his paper, his cases proved that by the injection of extraordinarily small amounts of cocaine (5 mg) into the dural sac, about two-thirds of the entire body could be made insensible enough for the painless performance of major operations. Complete loss of sensation lasted about 45 minutes. Bier decided that the escape of a considerable amount of cerebrospinal fluid was probably responsible for the aftereffects. He believed that in his own case some type of circulatory disturbance was present, because he felt absolutely well in a supine position but had a sensation of very strong pressure in the head and felt dizzy only if he sat up. Bier concluded that the escape of cerebrospinal fluid should be avoided if possible, and strict rest in bed should be observed. Bier said that the size of the needle should be very fine and that, after the dural sac had been entered, the stylet should be withdrawn and the opening immediately closed with a finger so that as little cerebrospinal fluid as possible escaped.

Halsted introduced the use of rubber gloves at operations in the winter of 1889 to 1890, but not with the intention of avoiding wound infection. That consequence was actually serendipitous. His motive was to spare the hands of his operating room nurse, who had developed a dermatitis from mercurous chloride. Soon the operators took to wearing them as well, but out of convenience. It was not until 1894 that the wearing of gloves was recommended as part of aseptic technique.[38] It surely is a fortunate coincidence that Bier did not start his work on spinal anesthesia until after this important prophylactic measure had become generally available.

The news of Bier's work in April 1899 spread quickly, and his method of subarachnoid spinal anesthesia was soon brought into prominence by a report of 125 cases by Tuffier.[71] In the summer of 1900, Tuffier enunciated the rule "never inject the cocaine solution until the cerebrospinal fluid is distinctly recognized." The sensation caused by Tuffier's demonstrations is well-conveyed by Hopkins, who wrote: "To be able to converse with a patient during the performance of a hysterectomy, the patient all the while evincing not the slightest indication of pain (and even being unable to tell where the knife was being applied) was certainly a marvel, and was well worth crossing the Atlantic to see."[41]

In the United States, spinal anesthesia was adopted for obstetrics by Marx and for general surgery by a number of surgeons, most prominently, Matas.[51,52] Matas's article begins with an extensive historical review of older methods of local and regional anesthesia. In his description of spinal anesthesia, cocaine hydrochloride, in the amount of 10 to 20 mg, was dissolved in distilled water. The solution instilled was therefore clearly hypotonic. Fowler preferred to have his patients in the sitting position for the injection and—not surprisingly—was often astonished by rapid and complete anesthesia.[30] Gravity methods were not yet understood.

Aseptic precautions were strictly observed, and E. W. Lee mentions that the injection he used consisted of 12 to 20 minims of a 2-per-cent sterilized solution prepared in hermetically sealed tubes by Truax, Green and Company of Chicago.[47] This is the earliest reference I have found to this method of packaging. It was an important advance because previously it was necessary for the surgeon to prepare his own solution from tablets and sterilize it.

In 1912, Gray and Parsons of Birmingham, England, undertook an extensive study of variations in blood pressure associated with the induction of spinal anesthesia.[34] They concluded that the bulk of the fall in arterial blood pressure during the high spinal anesthesia is attributable to the diminished negative intrathoracic pressure during inspiration, which is dependent on abdominal and lower thoracic paralysis. They noted that when the negative pressure in the thorax is increased, the arterial blood pressure rises.

It was by then quite clear that one of the principal dangers of spinal anesthesia is the lowering of the blood pressure. Believing this to be the primary hindrance to its more universal adoption among urologists, Smith, working with Porter, reported in 1915 the results of 50 experiments on cats.[68] They found that the quantity of anesthetic solution was more important for diffusion than its concentration, dilute solutions usually spreading farther than concentrated ones. The introduction of procaine beneath the dura in the region in which the splanchnic nerves arise caused as profound a fall in blood pressure as was caused by complete resection of the cord in the upper thoracic region. This, they thought, proved that the fall in blood pressure was not due to toxicity of the drug or to paralysis of the bulbar vasomotor center but to paralysis of the vasomotor fibers that regulate the tonus of the blood vessels in the splanchnic area. Since these nerve roots originate between T2 and T7, the main clinical objective, they believed, was to prevent cephalad diffusion of the drug from reaching this height and paralyzing these nerve roots.

In 1927 to 1928, Labat emphasized that the danger of spinal anesthesia was not from the fall in blood pressure as such but from the associated cerebral anemia, both being attributable to the increased volume of blood in the viscera, due to splanchnic paralysis and vasomotor collapse. He expressed the belief that this cerebral anemia can be avoided by placing the patient in the Trendelenburg position immediately following the intraspinal injection and that, by this procedure, the brain will be kept amply supplied with blood, and irremediable respiratory failure will be avoided.

To ensure that the blood pressure will not drop during spinal anesthesia, the practice of administering ephedrine subcutaneously was introduced.

The idea of making the injected solution hyperbaric with glucose, in order to obtain control over the intrathecal spread of the solution, originated with Barker.[6] Barker employed stovaine, a substance named for the English translation of its inventor, Fourneau.[23] Stovaine was less toxic than cocaine but slightly irritating and was eventually superseded by procaine (Novocain), synthetized by Einhorn in 1904. Barker's stovaine came directly from the laboratory of Billon in Paris, where it was made up in 5-per-cent glucose especially for Barker and packaged in sterile ampules. Barker was a professor of surgery at the University of London, and his article is exceedingly thoughtful, based on some 80 cases. He describes experiments with a glass model of the spinal canal, conforming to the shape seen in a mesial section of a cadaver and bearing a T-junction in the lumbar region to simulate the injection site.

Years later, Pitkin, in 1928, and Etherington-Wilson, in 1934, experimented with a similar apparatus but without acknowledging any debt to Barker.[29,58] Their goal was the opposite of Barker's, to obtain control over the rate of ascent of the drug by making the injected solution hypobaric. Control was achieved by varying the time the patient was kept sitting upright after the injection. Pitkin did this by mixing alcohol with the Novocain solutions, a mixture he called *spinocaine,* but he categorically warned against the sitting position. He controlled level by tilting the table and illustrated this with a figure showing an "altimeter" attachment.

Barker stressed such points of technique as raising the head on pillows; whenever he injected a heavy fluid intradurally, he kept the level of analgesia below the transverse nipple line. At times, he seated the patient on the edge of the table with the feet on a low chair to make the fluid run into the sacral end of the dural sac, where it quickly affected the root of the nerves supplying the anus and the perineum.

Barker advocated puncture in the midline as being easier and allowing more even spread of the injected fluid than the paramedian approach. He, too, emphasized that in no case should the analgesic compound be injected unless the cerebrospinal fluid runs satisfactorily. Perfect asepsis in the entire procedure was, above all else, absolutely necessary. Moreover, no trace of germicides should be left on the skin, because they could be conveyed by the needle into the spinal canal, where their irritating qualities are particularly undesirable. Barker enjoined that all needles, syringes, and other instruments for the procedure were to be kept apart for this sole use, including the little sterilizer in which they were boiled. Billon's sterilized, sealed ampules were to be opened only a moment before use.

Barker's rational approach to the use of a hyperbaric solution for spinal anesthesia was apparently forgotten when stovaine was replaced by improved drugs and had to be rediscovered after quasi-isobaric solutions of each new drug repeatedly led to unsatisfactory control of level. The lessons of the past were ignored, forgotten by surgeons, and not yet learned by anesthesiologists. Indeed, there were few anesthesiologists to learn. In 1920, Hepburn continued Barker's experience with stovaine, and Sise, an anesthesiologist at the Lahey Clinic, applied Barker's method to novocaine in 1928 and to tetracaine in 1935.[40,66,67]

To this day, no ready-made, combined solution of tetracaine and glucose is on the market, at least not in the United States. Sise revived the use of glucose in order to weight his spinal solution of tetracaine. Tetracaine's great advantage as a spinal anesthetic was its relatively prolonged duration of action without undue toxic effects, but this advantage was partially negated by the vagaries of its segmental spread which resulted from its being used in an approximately isobaric solution. Sise, therefore, mixed the solution with an equal or greater volume of 10-per-cent glucose, and the patient lay on his side with his head down and the table tilted to a 10° angle. The patient was then turned on his back and a good-sized pillow inserted under his head and shoulder to give as marked a bend upward as possible at this point. The slant was adjusted for the next few minutes as dictated by the level of analgesia.

A refinement of this technique was the saddle-block method described in detail by Adriani and Roman-Vega.[3] Anesthesia deliberately confined to the perineal area was obtained by performing the lumbar puncture and injection with the patient sitting on the operating table and remaining so for 35 to 40 seconds after the injection.

An article that announced a hypobaric solution and the associated modifications in the technique of spinal anesthesia was published by Babcock in 1912.[5] He dissolved 80 mg of stovaine in 2 ml of 10-per-cent alcohol, thus obtaining a solution whose specific gravity was less than 1.000, well below that of cerebral spinal fluid, which he took to be 1.0065. The anesthesia was chiefly a nerve root anesthesia and not the "true spinal cord anesthesia" obtained with the standard solutions. Babcock said that its lightness will cause this particular anesthetic solution to rise rapidly within the cavity of the arachnoid. He stressed that the patient should promptly have the head and shoulders lowered after the injection, but he rather perversely insisted that during the injection the patient should be sitting upon the operating table, the legs hanging over the side of the table. He further notes that "in most cases spinal anesthesia enables me to operate entirely free from the worry and watchfulness associated with etherization by an untrained assistant. . . . I have thus been able to operate successfully upon the neck, face, and even the cranium . . ." But let us not fail to note that Babcock also promulgated the following dictum: "*Death from spinal anesthesia usually indicates inefficient or insufficiently prolonged methods of resuscitation.*" The emphasis is his.

A method for continuous spinal anesthesia was described by W. T. Lemmon in 1940.[48] It was performed with a special mattress, a malleable needle, and special tubing, and was proposed for long operations that required abdominal relaxation. The equipment was original but not the idea. In 1907, Dean wrote of having so arranged the exploring needle that it can be left *in situ* during the operation, so that at any moment another dose can be injected without moving the patient beyond a slight degree.[22] Dean furthermore conceived the notion of treating postoperative pain by additional injections, since he believed it was quite possible that a recurrence of pain or abdominal distention might be treated in this manner. Whether anything ever came of the proposal, he did not say. Lemmon's ponderous technique was quickly simplified by Tuohy.[72] He performed continuous spinal anesthesia by means of a ureteral catheter introduced in the subarachnoid space through a needle with a Huber point.

EPIDURAL ANESTHESIA

The feasibility of injecting a local anesthetic by the caudal route was demonstrated by the French urologist Cathelin in 1901. Cathelin based his approach on a careful anatomical study of the sacral canal and its contents.[16] He found that fluids injected into the extradural space through the sacral hiatus rise to a height proportional to the amount and speed of injection. His objective was to develop a method that would be less dangerous but just as effective as subarachnoid lumbar anesthesia. He was successful in reducing the danger, but his efforts to demonstrate the efficiency of the caudal injection for surgical operations were disappointing, and indeed Cathelin himself thought its principal sphere of usefulness lay in the treatment of bladder incontinence and of enuresis in children.

Reflecting on the similarities in the innervation of

the bladder and uterus, the gynecologist Stoeckel thought that if the pain of childbirth was largely uterine in origin, as seemed probable, the caudal epidural method of Cathelin offered an ideal approach to painless obstetrics.[69] Cathelin himself had considered pregnancy a contraindication to epidural injection because of the hazard of toxic absorption of cocaine. Stoeckel, however, had begun to use Novocain and considered the reduced toxicity of the new drug acceptable. Stoeckel described this experience with caudal anesthesia in the management of labor in 1909. He wrote that various concentrations of Novocain and epinephrine produced predictably varying degrees of success for the single injection. Pain relief averaged 1 to 1-1/2 hours in duration, but, warned Stoeckel, the greater the analgesic effect, the greater the hazard of impairing the forces of labor. These reservations, of course, would not apply to its use for surgical operations, and Läwen, in 1910, described how he used Stoeckel's experience and Cathelin's ideas to perform a variety of interventions in the vicinity of the perineum.[45]

Läwen gave the method careful study. He injected colored fluids into the sacral canal of cadavers and demonstrated that the fluid never appeared in the spinal canal, showing that the spinal canal was completely separated from the sacral canal by the dura mater. Gros, in the pharmacology laboratory, had established that procaine penetrated the nerve sheaths more rapidly if sodium bicarbonate was added. Läwen at once exploited this discovery, and, by using a greater amount of an alkaline solution of stronger concentration (20–25 cc of a 1.5- to 2-% solution), produced anesthesia in the gluteal region, rectum, anus, skin of the scrotum, penis, upper and inner parts of the thigh, and the vulva and vagina. He performed all the common operations on these parts and, hence, was the first to employ sacral anesthesia for operative work, reporting 47 cases with an incidence of failure of 15 per cent.

Pauchet, in 1914, was credited with overcoming this incidence of failure by injecting the sacral nerves individually through the posterior sacral foramina, a method which has become known as *transsacral anesthesia*.

The duration of satisfactory anesthesia from a single peridural injection is limited to a few hours. After Lemmon's demonstration of continuous spinal anesthesia in 1940, it was not long before the continuous technique was transferred to obstetrical delivery by Edwards and Hingson, in which it had an important sphere of usefulness.[27] This was a rational development, since Cleland had determined that all the sensory fibers that supply the uterus, cervix, and perineum could be blocked by a sacral peridural injection of local anesthetic.[17] Edwards and Hingson realized that the continuous method enabled them to start the anesthesia in the early stages of labor and to continue it for however long was necessary to the completion of labor and repair of an episiotomy or laceration, 5 or 6 hours on the average.

Continuous caudal block in obstetrics was also announced by Manalan in 1942, independently of Hingson's group.[49] Manalan's technique was the simpler of the two. He introduced a No. 4 ureteral silk catheter through the lumen of a 14-gauge needle and then withdrew the needle, leaving the catheter in place. Later, he substituted a nylon catheter for the silk catheter because the nylon one could more easily be sterilized. Block and Ruchberg substituted a continuous gravity drip for the intermittent injections, primarily out of convenience for the anesthetist.[10]

However, the earliest intimation of continuous regional anesthesia in the practice of obstetrics came from Eugen Aburel of Rumania.[2] For repeating the injections without discomfort to the patient, Aburel had a special combination of catheter and needle made by the firm Maupiac: He introduced the needle paravertebrally into the lumbosacral plexus, injected 30 ml of 0.05-per-cent dibucaine solution (erroneously), and then introduced an elastic silk catheter similar to a ureteral catheter through the needle, before withdrawing the needle and fixing the catheter with adhesive tape. Repeated injections were given through the catheter, which was "tolerated well, during a rather long period of time." The results, however, were apparently not very satisfactory.

Paravertebral Conduction Anesthesia

Matas, the eminent American pioneer and historian of regional anesthesia, recorded that Sellheim, injecting close to the posterior roots of T8 to T12, in addition to the ilioinguinal and iliohypogastric nerves, was able to perform abdominal operations successfully.[53] Sellheim is, therefore, credited by Matas as being the originator of the paravertebral method of anesthesia.

It was 6 years later, Kappis having in the meantime greatly improved on Sellheim's technique, that the method was first used in urologic surgery. According to Kappis, success with conduction anesthesia of the trigeminal nerve led him to seek an anatomically reliable approach to conduction anesthesia of the spinal nerves at their exit from between the vertebrae.[42] In his paper, he described posterior approaches to the lower seven cervical nerves for the purposes of cervical and brachial plexus block. He had cautioned against blocking C4 bilaterally at the same time. He made up his own solution of Novocain-adrenalin and let it stand for an hour because he believed this improved its effectiveness. The method for paravertebral block of the thoracic nerves and the first four lumbar nerves was given in this same paper, and was used in a great many upper abdominal operations. Finally, Kappis pointed out that these techniques could also be used to treat acute and chronic pain with procaine, or even with alcohol if motor function could be neglected. Two years later, Kappis described his posterior approach to the splanchnic plexus.[43]

In 1922, Läwen found unilateral paravertebral block of selected spinal nerves useful in the differential diagnosis of intra-abdominal disease.[46] For example, he observed that a 10-ml injection of 2-per-cent procaine at T10 could completely relieve the pain of a severe biliary colic for 3 hours. The use of segmental paravertebral block for the differential diagnosis of painful conditions was an original idea of Läwen's. At the suggestion of Pal, it was then tried as a therapeutic measure in the hope of obtaining pain relief in acute cholecystitis, but without significant success, by Brunn and Mandl in 1924.[13] Kappis had treated a case of angina pectoris in this manner in 1923, and von Gaza used 0.5-per-cent Novocain diagnostically prior to resection of the affected paravertebral nerves.[74]

In 1925, Mandl reported 16 cases of angina pectoris in which he injected Novocain, 0.5 per-cent, paravertebrally with excellent results.[50] The next year Swetlow attempted to destroy the afferent sensory fibers altogether by substituting 85-per-cent alcohol for the procaine and for the most part obtained satisfactory relief of pain for several months.[70]

The pioneer of alcohol injection for the purpose of producing a long-lasting interruption of neural conduction was Schloesser.[65] Schloesser presented the method as a means of managing convulsive facial tic, and he obtained paralysis that lasted from days to months, according to the quantity of alcohol injected. He suggested that the method would also be useful for supraorbital neuralgia and tic douloureux. Like many a pioneer, he was too far ahead of his time.

Segmental peridural anesthesia, under the name of *metameric anesthesia* was used for the first time 1921 by Fidel Pagés, a Spanish military surgeon.[57] To Dogliotti, however, belongs the credit for systematizing and popularizing the peridural principle to produce what he termed *segmental peridural spinal anesthesia*.[24] In the light of later theory, which requires that three consecutive internodes be blocked to prevent saltatory conduction, it is interesting to see Dogliotti's iteration of the need to bathe a sufficient length of the spinal nerves. He emphasized that, if the anesthetic solution is injected in sufficient quantity (50–60 ml) and under adequate pressure, it will be quite easy to subject the spinal nerves to the action of the injected fluid throughout their length in the spinal canal, the intervertebral foramina, and even beyond.[24] Dogliotti's method was easier and, without question, simpler than paravertebral regional block, since only one puncture was needed. He stressed the sudden loss of resistance when the point of the needle, having pierced the ligamentum flavum, entered the epidural space.[26] The usefulness of this technique was extended further when Curbelo decided to apply the Tuohy armamentarium for continuous spinal anesthesia to continuous segmental peridural anesthesia.[20] In one case, he left the catheter in place for as long as 4 days and administered a total of 10 injections of 15 ml of 2-per-cent procaine solution for the production of a continuous sympathetic lumbar block.

Diagnostic Procaine Block

The pioneer in the use of procaine for determining the pathways of obscure pain was von Gaza.[74] Mandl, following his examples, described the effect of paravertebral injection of local anesthetic in relieving angina pectoris.[50] But it was left to White to discover and demonstrate the wide diagnostic usefulness of procaine block of sensory or sympathetic nerves, as the case may be, in determining the pathways of peripheral pain.[76] White emphasized the advantage to the surgeon and the patient of knowing exactly how much relief of suffering or improvement of circulation might be expected from an operation.

Conceptually, it was but a short step from diagnostic block to therapeutic block, and indeed the step was taken by von Gaza and by Brunn and Mandl in 1924 in the management of visceral pain. In the same year, Royle in Australia demonstrated that relief of deforming contractions and spastic paralyses (Little's disease) could be obtained by cutting off the sympathetic nerve supply to the musculature of the affected parts.[62] Long-term pain relief by neurolytic injection of alcohol was developed by Swetlow for the interruption of cardiac afferent inflow and subsequently applied to paravertebral sympathetic block in the treatment of severe intractable pain, particularly the pain of malignant disease.[70]

In 1930, Dogliotti took the bold step of injecting absolute alcohol into the subarachnoid space, hoping to produce by simple chemical means a posterior rhizotomy like that previously attainable only by surgery.[25] At the opposite end of the local anesthetic spectrum, Sarnoff and Arrowood exploited the continuous subarachnoid injection of dilute procaine (0.2 %) to obtain a differential block limited to efferent sympathetic fibers and afferent fibers subserving pain.[63] As far as they were concerned, this was a physiologic experiment. Others subsequently adapted it to the differential diagnosis of chronic low back pain.

Wertheim and Rovenstine, anesthesiologists at the New York University College of Medicine, devised and described a technique of suprascapular nerve block in the treatment of intractable shoulder pain, such as subacromial bursitis.[75] They reported that the analgesic effect of a 2-per-cent procaine injection may continue for 4 to 6 weeks.

ANESTHESIOLOGY

One of the more noticeable and surprising features in the history of the first 50 years of local anesthesia is the almost total uninvolvement of anesthesiologists. Virtually all the developments were devised by surgeons and basic scientists. Also surprising is the miniscule nature of the contribution from Britain, the country of Snow and Lister and pioneering investigation in general. There is no easy explanation. In most of the medical world, the practice of anesthesia was a poor relation, comparatively unhonored and unskilled, without opportunity or incentive for innovative work. In the British quarter of the globe, general anesthesia was administered by physicians and perhaps generated a certain sense of security and a tendency to leave well enough alone. Everywhere, if local anesthesia was the choice, the surgeon did both the choosing and the injecting. It was not until nerve block began to be perceived as an independent diagnostic and therapeutic tool that a demand arose for regional anesthetic skill independent of surgical operation. This period saw the beginnings in the United States of anesthesiology as an individual specialty, welcomed by forward-looking surgeons such as Mayo, who established Labat, one of the first regional anesthesiologists, as a lecturer at his renowned clinic in Minnesota.

Not least of the services rendered by the development of regional anesthesia was the stimulation of a higher level of vigilance and physiologic awareness in anesthetic practice as a whole. No better proof of this trend could be desired than what is provided by anesthesia records. Charted records of the vital signs during an operation were apparently being kept by Dr. Codman at the Massachusetts General Hospital at the close of the 19th century, stimulated by the recommendations of Cushing.[7] It must be remembered that a convenient method of measuring the blood pressure was not available until Riva-Rocci invented the arm cuff in 1896, and that 10 years were to elapse before Korotkoff, a Russian army surgeon, discovered the auscultatory method. Thus, the first analgesia charts of Goldan showed only the pulse rate, and when blood pressure was added, only the systolic pressure. Cushing's insistence on charted records was of a piece with other aspects of his greatness as a medical scientist and surgeon. Following the lead of Crile, he sought to combat shock in major amputations by cocainizing

NOVEMBER 3, 1900]

Sol. cocain ....% How and when prepared ....
Site of punct .... Quantity injected ....
Time of " .... Needle removed ....
First symptom ....
Complete anesthesia at .... Ended at ....
Operation ....

BEGIN ....
ENDED .... Operator ....

Every 10 minutes.

Pupil																		
Pulse																		
Resp.																		

Nausea .... Vomiting ....
Subj. symptoms ....
Obj. symptoms ....
Headache ....
Untoward symp. and treatment ....
Extent of anesthesia; how determined ....
Reac. to heat ....
" " cold ....
" " pressure ....
Reverse for remarks.

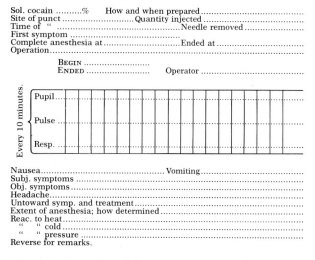

Fig. 1-2. Facsimile of Goldan's chart, the earliest published anesthesia chart. (Goldan, S.O.: Intraspinal cocanization for surgical anesthesia. Philadelphia Med. J., 6:850, 1900)

the large nerve trunks before dividing them and kept graphic track of the patient's condition by having the vital signs measured every 5 minutes.[21]

The first written record, however, of the progress of a patient during anesthesia was published by Goldan in the Philadelphia Medical Journal, November 3, 1900.[32] It was a chart designed specifically for registering the course of "intraspinal cocainization" and provided for the recording of three vital signs, pupil, pulse, and respiration, every 10 minutes (Fig. 1-2). Goldan's paper has a further title to scholarly distinction; it seems to have been the earliest paper in the literature of local anesthesia to include a list of bibliographic citations. Historically, Goldan's paper is also of interest for his concluding remark: ". . . . a remedy for the headache may be found not in simple analgesics, but drugs exerting their influences upon the circulation . . . Increasing the blood-pressure favors an increased secretion of cerebrospinal fluid with an increased tension in the veins retarding absorption." Goldan gave full details of 16 cases of spinal anesthesia, a large series for that time, and explicitly described himself as an anesthetist. It thus seems incontrovertible that the practice of careful record keeping in the operating room, an indispensable foundation to the progress of anesthesiology, was a fundamental original contribution by a practicing specialist in regional anesthesia.*

REFERENCES

1. Abel, J.J.: On the blood-pressure-raising constituent of the suprarenal capsule. Johns Hopkins Hosp. Bull., *8*:151, 1897.
2. Aburel, E.: L'anesthésie locale continue (prolongée) en obstétrique. Bull. Soc. Obstet. Gynécol., *20*:85, 1931.
3. Adriani, J., and Roman-Vega, D.: Saddle block anesthesia. Am. J. Surg., *71*:12, 1946.
4. Anonymous: Biographical sketch of Doctor James Leonard Corning, of New York City, and his recent remarkable discoveries in local anesthesia. Va. Med. Mon., *12*:713, 1886.
5. Babcock, W.W.: Spinal anesthaesia; with report of surgical clinics. Surg. Gynecol. Obstet., *15*:606, 1912.
6. Barker, A.E.: Clinical experiences with spinal analgesia in 100 cases and some reflections on the procedure. Br. Med. J., *1*:665, 1907.
7. Beecher, H.K.: The first anesthesia records (Codman, Cushing). Surg. Gynecol. Obstet., *71*:789, 1940.
8. Bier A.: Versuche über Cocainisirung des Rückenmarkes. Dtsch. Z. Chir., *51*:361, 1899.

* Dr. R. A. Gordon has recently drawn attention to an anesthetic chart for use in hospital practice, arranged by Dr. C. R. 'Reilly and published in Lancet *34*:636, 1901.

9. ———: Ueber einen neuen Weg Localanästhesie an den Gliedmassen zu erzeugen. Arch. Klin. Chir., *86*:1007, 1908.
10. Block, N., and Rochberg, S.: Continuous caudal anesthesia in obstetrics. Am. J. Obstet. Gynecol., *45*:645, 1943.
11. Braun, H.: Ueber den Einfluss der Vitalität der Gewebe auf die örtlichen und allgemeinen Giftwirkungen localanästhesirender Mittel und über die Bedeutung des Adrenalins für die Localanästhesie. Arch. Klin. Chir., *69*:541, 1903.
12. ———: Local Anesthesia Its Scientific Basis and Practical Use. Ed. 3., Philadelphia, Lea & Febiger, 1914.
13. Brunn, F., and Mandl, F.: Die paravertebrale Injektion zur Bekämpfung visceraler Schmerzen Wien. Klin. Wochenschr., *37*:511, 1924.
14. Bull, C.S.: The hydrochlorate of cocaine as a local anaesthetic in ophthalmic surgery. N. Y. Med. J., *40*:609, 1884.
15. Burke, W.C., Jr.: Hydrochlorate of cocaine in minor surgery. N. Y. Med. J., *40*:616, 1884.
16. Cathelin F.: Une nouvelle voie d'injection rachidienne. Méthodes des injections épidurales par le procédé du canal sacré. Applications à l'homme. C.R. Soc. Biol. (Paris), *53*:452, 1901.
17. Cleland, J.G.P.: Paravertebral anesthesia in obstetrics. Surg. Gynecol. Obstet., *57*:57, 1938.
18. Corning, J.L.: On the prolongation of the anaesthetic effect of the hydrochlorate of cocaine, when subcutaneously injected. An experimental study. N. Y. Med. J., *42*:317, 1885.
19. ———: Spinal anaesthesia and local medication of the cord. N. Y. Med. J., *42*:483, 1885.
20. Curbelo, M.M.: Continuous peridural segmental anesthesia by means of a ureteral catheter. Anesth. Analg. (Cleve.), *28*:13, 1949.
21. Cushing, H.: On the avoidance of shock in major amputations by cocainization of large nerve-trunks preliminary to their division. Ann. Surg., *36*:321, 1902.
22. Dean, H.P.: Relative value of inhalation and injection methods of inducing anaesthesia. Br. Med. J., *2*:869, 1907.
23. De Lapersonne, F.: Un nouvel anesthésique local, la stovaine. Presse Méd. *12*:233, 1904.
24. Dogliotti, A.M.: Eine neue Methode der regionären Anästhesie: "Die peridurale segmentäre Anästhesie." Zentralbl. Chir., *58*:3141, 1931.
25. ———: Proposta di un nuovo metodo di cura delle algie periferiche. L'alcoolizzazione sottomeningea delle radici posteriori. Considerazioni sulle prime 30 osservazione cliniche. Minerva Med., *1*:536, 1931.
26. ———: A new method of block anesthesia. Segmental peridural spinal anesthesia. Am. J. Surg., *20*:107, 1933.
27. Edwards, W.B., and Hingson, R.A.: Continuous caudal anesthesia in obstetrics. Am. J. Surg., *57*:459, 1942.
28. Esmarch, F.: Ueber künstliche Blutleere. Arch. Klin. Chir., *17*:292, 1874.
29. Etherington-Wilson, E.: Intrathecal nerve root block. Some contributions and a new technique. Proc. R. Soc. Med., *27*:325, 1934.
30. Fowler, R.G.: Cocain analgesia from subarachnoid injection, with a report of forty-four cases together with a report of a case in which antipyrin was used. Philadelphia Med. J., *6*:843, 1900.
31. Francois-Franck, C.A.: Action paralysante locale de la cocaine sur les nerfs et les centres nerveux. Applications à la technique expérimentale. Arch. Physiol. Norm. Pathol., *24*:562, 1892.
32. Goldan, S.O.: Intraspinal cocainization for surgical anesthesia. Philadelphia Med. J., *6*:850, 1900.

33. Gray, H.: Anatomy Descriptive and Surgical. ed. 5. pp. 572–574. Philadelphia, Henry C. Lea, 1870.
34. Gray, H.T., and Parsons, L.: Blood pressure variations associated with lumbar puncture and the induction of spinal anesthesia. Q. J. Med., *5*:339, 1912.
35. Hall, R.J.: Hydrochlorate of cocaine. N. Y. Med. J., *40*:643, 1884.
36. Halsted, W.S.: Water as a local anesthetic. N. Y. Med. J., *42*:327, 1885.
37. ———: Practical comments on the use and abuse of cocaine; suggested by its invariably successful employment in more than a thousand minor surgical operations. N. Y. Med. J., *42*:294, 1885.
38. ———: Surgical Papers by William Stewart Halsted. vol. 1, pp. 37–39. Baltimore, Johns Hopkins Press, 1924.
39. Hepburn, N.J.: Some notes on hydrochlorate of cocaine. Medical Record, *26*:534, 1884.
40. Hepburn, W.G.: Stovain spinal analgesia. Am. J. Surg., *34*:87, 1920.
41. Hopkins, G.S.: Anesthesia by cocainization of the spinal cord. Philadelphia Med. J., *6*:864, 1900.
42. Kappis, M.: Ueber Leitungsanästhesie an Bauch, Brust, Arm und Hals durch Injektion ans Foramen intervertebrale. Münch. Med. Wochenschr., *1*:794, 1912.
43. ———: Erfahrungen mit Lokalanästhesie bei Bauchoperationen. Ver. Dtsch. Ges. Chir., *43*:87, 1914.
44. Koller, C.: On the use of cocaine for producing anaesthesia on the eye. Lancet, *2*:990, 1884.
45. Läwen A.: Über die Verwertung der Sakralanästhesie für chirurgische Operationen. Zentralbl. Chir., *37*:708, 1910.
46. ———: Ueber segmentäre Schmerzaufhebung durch paravertebrale Novokaininjektionen zur Differentiäldiagnose intra-abdominaler Erkrankungen. Med. Wochenschr., *69*:1423, 1922.
47. Lee, E.W.: Subarachnoidean injections of cocain as a substitute for general anesthesia in operations below the diaphragm, with report of seven cases. Philadelphia Med. J., *6*:865, 1900.
48. Lemmon, W.T.: A method for continuous spinal anesthesia. Ann. Surg., *111*:141, 1940.
49. Manalan, S.A.: Caudal block anesthesia in obstetrics. J. Indiana State Med. Assoc., *35*:564, 1942.
50. Mandl, F.: Die Wirkung der paravertebralen Injektion bei "Angina pectoris." Arch. Klin. Chir., *136*:495, 1925.
51. Marx, S.: Analgesia in obstetrics produced by medullary injections of cocain. Philadelphia Med. J., *6*:857, 1900.
52. Matas, R.: Local and regional anesthesia with cocain and other analgesic drugs, including the subarachnoid method, as applied in general surgical practice. Philadelphia Med. J., *6*:820, 1900.
53. ———: Local and regional anesthesia: a retrospect and prospect. Am. J. Surg., *25*:189, 1934.
54. Mayer, E.: Clinical experience with adrenaline. Philadelphia Med. J., *7*:819, 1901.
55. Niemann, A.: Ueber eine organische Base in der Coca. Annalen Chemie, *114*:213, 1860.
56. Noyes, H.D.: The ophthalmological congress in Heidelberg. Medical Record, *26*:417, 1884.
57 Pagés, F.: Anestesia metamerica. Rev. Sanid. Milit. Argent., *11*:351-365.
58. Pitkin, G.P.: Controllable spinal anesthesia. Am. J. Surg., *5*:537, 1928.
59. Pravaz, C.G.: Sur un nouveau moyen d'opérer la coagulation du sang dans les artères, applicable à la guérison des anévrismes. C.R. Acad. Sci. (Paris), *36*:88, 1853.
60. Quincke, H.: Die Lumbalpunction des Hydrocephalus. Ber. Klin. Wochenschr., *28*:929, 1891.
61. Reclus P.: Analgésie locale par la cocaïne. Rev. Chir., *9*:913, 1889.
62. Royle, N.D.: A new operative procedure in the treatment of spastic paralysis and its experimental basis. Med. J. Aust., *1*:77, 1924.
63. Sarnoff, S.J., and Arrowood, J.G.: Differential spinal block. Surgery, *20*:150, 1946.
64. Schleich, C.L.: Zur Infiltrationsanästhesie. Therapeutische Monathefte, *8*:429, 1894.
65. Schloesser: Heilung periphärer Reizzustände sensibler und motorischer Nerven. Klin. Monatsbl. Augenheilkd., *41*:244, 1903.
66. Sise, L.F.: Spinal anesthesia for upper and lower abdominal operations. N. Engl. J. Med., *199*:61, 1928.
67. ———: Pontocain-glucose for spinal anesthesia. Surg. Clin. North Am., *15*:1501, 1935.
68. Smith, G.S., and Porter, W.T.: Spinal anesthesia in the cat. Am. J. Physiol., *38*:108, 1915.
69. Stoeckel, W.: Über sakrale Anästhesie. Zentralbl. Gynaekol., *33*:1, 1909.
70. Swetlow, G.I.: Paravertebral alcohol block in cardiac pain. Am. Heart J., *1*:393, 1926.
71. Tuffier, T.: Analgésie chirurgicale par l'injection sous-arachnoïdienne lombaire de cocaïne. C.R. Soc. Biol., *1 II Series*:882, 1899.
72. Tuohy, E.B.: Continuous spinal anesthesia: its usefulness and technic involved. Anesthesiology. *5*:142, 1944.
73. Von Anrep, B.: Ueber die physiologische Wirkung des Cocain. Pflüger's Arch., *21*:38, 1879.
74. von Gaza, W.: Die Resektion der paravertebralen Nerven und die isolierte Durchschneidung des Ramus communicans. Arch. Klin. Chir., *133*:479, 1924.
75. Wertheim, H.M., and Rovenstine, E.A.: Suprascapular nerve block. Anesthesiology, *2*:541, 1941.
76. White, J.C.: Diagnostic novocaine block of the sensory and sympathetic nerves. A method of estimating the results which can be obtained by their permanent interruption. Am. J. Surg., *9*:264, 1930.
77. Wood, A.: New method of treating neuralgia by the direct application of opiates to the painful points. Edinburgh Med. Surg. J., *82*:265, 1855.
78. Wynter, W.E.: Four cases of tuberculosus meningitis in which paracentesis of the theca vertebralis was performed for the relief of fluid pressure. Lancet, *1*:981, 1891.

APPENDIX 1A: CHRONOLOGY OF LOCAL ANESTHESIA

1564 Pare (France)
Local anesthesia by nerve compression

1600 Valverdi (Italy)
Regional anesthesia by compression of nerves and blood vessels supplying operative area

1646 Severino (Italy)
Refrigeration anesthesia by use of freezing mixtures of snow and ice

1656 Wren (England)
First experiments with intravenous injection

1784 Moore (England)
Local anesthesia of extremity by compression of nerve trunks

1839 **Taylor and Washington (USA)**
Hypodermic injection
1843 **Wood (Scotland)**
Morphine injection (Published 1855)
1845 **Rynd (Dublin)**
Hypodermic Needle
1853 **Pravaz (France)**
Hypodermic Syringe
1855 **Gaedicke (Germany)**
Isolation of alkaloid from leaves of cocoa plant
1860 **Niemann (Germany)**
Purification and naming of cocaine
1873 **Bennett (Scotland)**
Anesthetic properties of cocaine
1878 **von Anrep (Germany)**
Pharmacologic effects of cocaine (Published 1879–1880)
1884 **Koller (Austria)**
First topical use of cocaine (eye surgery)
Halstead and Hall (USA)
Neural blockade with cocaine (in each other)
Burke (USA)
Removal of bullet from finger under nerve block with cocaine
1885 **Corning (USA)**
"Spinal anesthesia" (Actually injected epidurally)
1890 **Reclus (France)**
Early use of infiltration anesthesia
1891 **Quinke (Germany)**
Lumbar puncture technique
1892 **Schleich (Germany)**
Introduced infiltration anesthesia
François-Franck
Coined term nerve *blocking*
1897 **Braun (Germany)**
Cocaine toxicity related to absorption; advocated use of epinephrine
1898 **Bier (Germany)**
First planned spinal anesthetic
1899 **Tuffier (France)**
Report of 125 spinal anesthetics
Tait and Caglieri (USA)
First use of spinal anesthesia in USA (". . . never inject . . . until csf. . . . recognized")
1900 **Tait and Caglieri (USA)**
Detailed studies of subarachnoid space and spinal anesthesia in animals and humans
1901 **Cathelin and Sicard (France)**
Independently discovered caudal epidural block using cocaine
1902 **Braun (Germany)**
Use of epinephrine in nerve blocking. —term *conduction anesthesia*
1904 **Einhorn (Germany)**
Synthesis of procaine (Novocaine)
1905 **Braun (Germany)**
Text *Local Anesthesia*
1907 **Barker (UK)**
Introduction of hyperbaric spinal anesthetic solutions
1908 **Crile (USA)**
Anociassociation: regional block plus light general anesthesia
1912 **Gray and Parsons (UK)**
1915 **Smith and Porter (USA)**
Blood pressure changes during spinal anesthesia
1922 **Labat (USA)**
Text "Regional Anesthesia: Its Technique and Clinical Application"
Founded American Society of Regional Anesthesia (1923)
1942 **Allen (USA)**
Refrigeration anesthesia for amputation
Edwards and Hingson (USA)
Continuous caudal anesthesia in obstetrics

APPENDIX 2A: CHRONOLOGY OF LOCAL ANESTHETIC AGENTS

Cocaine
1860 Purification and naming by Niemann (Germany)
1884 First clinical use, topical (Koller; Germany)
First clinical use, nerve block (Halsted; USA)
Procaine
1904 Synthesis by Einhorn (Germany)
1905 Clinical introduction (Braun; in Germany)
Stovaine*
1904 Synthesis by Fourneau (France)
Cinchocaine (Nupercaine, dibucaine)
1925 Synthesis by Meischer
1930 Clinical introduction (Uhlmann)
Amethocaine (Pontocaine, Tetracaine)
1928 Synthesis by Eisleb
1932 Clinical introduction
Lignocaine (Lidocaine)
1943 Synthesis by Lofgren and Lundqvist
1947 Clinical introduction (Gordh)
Mepivacaine
1956 Synthesis by Ekstam and Egner
1957 Clinical introduction (Dhunér)
Prilocaine
1959 Synthesis by Lofgren and Tegner
1960 Clinical introduction (Wielding)
Bupivacaine
1957 Synthesis by Ekstam
1963 Clinical introduction (Widman)
Etidocaine
1971 Synthesis by Takman
1972 Clinical introduction (Lund)

* Discarded, too toxic.

APPENDIX 3A: CHRONOLOGY OF INDIVIDUAL NEURAL BLOCKADE TECHNIQUES

Spinal analgesia

1898 Bier (Germany)
First use for surgery in humans

1940 Lemmon (USA)
Continuous spinal anesthesia

1946 Adriani and Roman-Vega (USA)
Saddle block spinal

Lumbar epidural analgesia

1921 Pagés (Spain)
First use for surgery

1931 Dogliotti (Italy)
Popularized surgical use

1949 Curbelo
Used Tuohy equipment for continuous blockade

Caudal epidural analgesia

1901 Sicard, Cathelin (France)
First use for surgery

1909 Stoeckel
Use in obstetrical pain

1910 Läwen (Germany)
Popularized surgical use

1913 Danis (Belgium)
Transsacral approach

1942 Edwards and Hingson (USA), Manalan
Continuous caudal

"Continuous" regional techniques

1931 Aburel (Rumania)
Continuous paravertebral lumbosacral plexus block

Paravertebral somatic block

1906 Sellheim
Thoracic paravertebral block

1912 Kappis
Paravertebral block for surgery and also for pain relief

1922 Läwen
Use in diagnosis of abdominal disease

Celiac block

1906 Braun
Anterior surgical approach

1914 Kappis
Posterior approach

Paravertebral lumbar sympathetic block

1926 Mandl

Stellate Ganglion (Cervicothoracic sympathetic) block

1930 Labat
Posterior approach

1934 Leriche and Fontaine
Anterior approach (used for cerebrovascular accidents)

1948 Apgar
Anterior approach

1954 Moore
Paratracheal approach

Brachial plexus block

1884 Halstead
Injection under direct vision

1897 Crile

1911 Hirschel
"Blind" axillary injection
Kulenkampff
Supraclavicular technique

1940 Patrick
Basis of current supraclavicular technique

1958 Burnham
Axillary perivascular technique

1964 Winnie and Collins
Subclavian

1970 Winnie
Interscalene

Cervical plexus block

1939 Rovenstine and Wertheim

Intravenous regional anesthesia

1908 Bier
Injection between two cuffs

1963 Holmes
Injection below a single cuff after exsanguination

Intra-arterial regional anesthesia

1912 Goyanes (Spain)
Arterial injection below a cuff

Diagnostic blockade in pain management

1924 von Gaza
Procaine blockade in investigation of pain pathways

1930 Mandl
Paravertebral procaine block in diagnosis of angina pectoris

1930 White
Blockade of sensory and sympathetic nerves in pain diagnosis

Therapeutic nerve block in pain management

1899 Tuffier
Spinal cocaine for pain of sarcoma of leg

1901 Cushing
Regional anesthesia used to describe pain relief by nerve block

1903 Schloesser
Trigeminal alcohol block

1924 von Gaza, Braun, Mandl
Local anesthetic neural blockade for management of visceral pain

1924 Royle
Surgical sympathectomy for pain of spastic paralysis

1926 Swetlow
Neurolytic sympathetic block with alcohol for angina pectoris and abdominal pain

1930 Dogliotti
Neurolytic subarachnoid alcohol block

1941 Wertheim and Rovenstine
Suprascapular local anesthetic nerve block for shoulder pain.

APPENDIX 4A: CHRONOLOGY OF THE STUDY OF COMPLICATIONS OF NEURAL BLOCKADE

1884 Halstead and Associates (USA)
Cocaine addiction

1889 Reclus (France)
Toxicity due to systemic absorption defined
Bier and colleagues (Germany)
Severe postlumbar puncture headache

1900 Goldan (USA)
Development of anesthetic record of "intraspinal" cocainization

1901 Dandois (Belgium)
Paraplegia after subarachnoid cocaine

1906 Koenig (USA)
Permanent neurologic sequelae in several patients following spinal cocaine

1907 Barker (UK)
Recognition of need to control level of block

1912 Gray and Parsons (UK)
Recognition of vascular pooling due to sympathetic blockade

1927–1928 Labat (USA)
Emphasis on maintenance of cerebral perfusion

1952 Sancetta and colleagues
Cardiovascular effects of "low and high" spinal anesthesia

1953 Gillies (UK)
Studies of cardiovascular effects

1953– Greene (USA)
Studies of physiologic effects of spinal anesthesia

1954 Dripps and Vandam (USA)
Long-term follow-up of 10,098 spinal anesthetics; failure to discover major neurologic sequelae
Importance of meticulous technique and safe handling of drugs stressed

1960– Bromage and colleagues (Canada)
Studies of physiology and pharmacology of epidural blockade

1965– Braid and Scott (UK); Tucker and Mather (USA); Boyes and Covino (USA); Harrison and colleagues (USA); De Jong and colleagues (USA)
Studies of pharmacokinetics and toxicity of local anesthetics

1970– Bonica and colleagues (USA)
Studies of cardiovascular effects of central neural blockade

PART ONE

Basic Pharmacology and Physiology of Neural Blockade

2 Clinical Physiology of Local Anesthetic Action

Rudolph H. de Jong

NEURAL SITE OF ACTION

Local anesthetics belong to a surprisingly homogeneous family of drugs that temporarily halt impulse traffic along nerves in a predictable and reversible manner. Because of that quality, local anesthetics are widely used to suppress the centralward flow of pain-related impulses during surgical procedures. Since the mechanisms by which these drugs block impulse conduction are becoming better known, many responses to nerve block can nowadays be interpreted in physiologic terms.

Such basic understanding is important to the clinician, especially when his block is only partly successful or when complications arise. To understand how local anesthetics block peripheral nerves or spinal roots, attention must first be focused on events in single axons—the fundamental impulse-transmitting unit.

Nerve Membrane

In essence, a nerve fiber (axon) is a cylinder of axoplasm, encased in a membrane that separates it from the extracellular fluid. Functionally, the membrane is the most important part of the nerve fiber. This was ingeniously demonstrated by an experiment wherein axoplasm of a giant axon was replaced with a potassium-containing solution. Removal of the axoplasm did not significantly alter the impulse-conducting properties of the remaining membrane shell.

The nerve membrane may be viewed as a semipermeable structure separating a potassium-rich ionic solution, on the inside, from a sodium-rich ionic solution on the outside. The large ionic gradients across the membrane give rise to an electrochemical resting potential on the order of -70 to -90 mV (about the equilibrium potential for potassium). A membrane with this potential across it is said to be *polarized* (Fig. 2-1), analogous to a loaded pistol ready to be fired by a light pull on the cocked trigger.

The nerve membrane consists of a double-layered framework of lipid molecules with discrete globs of protein molecules spaced throughout it. Through this lipid skeleton run channels (pores) with a diameter approximating that of small ions. Passage through these pores is quarded by "gates" that open and close under the influence of electrical fields, while selectivity for preferred ions is conveyed by fixed aperture "filters" that bar oversized ions.

Disregarding more detailed associated information[15,33] we may consider the pore width in the resting nerve membrane to be such that potassium ions can pass freely back and forth through their specialized channels, whereas sodium ions are essentially barred passage through their channels (Fig. 2-2). Selective exclusion of sodium from the nerve interior means that the (resting) membrane's voltage is generated by the ionic potassium battery. Such a charged resting membrane is said to be *polarized*.

Depolarization. When the membrane is triggered by an electrical impulse, a number of changes take place in rapid order. Initially, the gates that earlier locked the sodium channels now swing open. Sodium ions, driven by the combined forces of concentration gradient and electrostatic attraction, avalanche inward. The inward sodium rush is so massive that the membrane potential is not just neutralized but overshoots the mark, causing a brief swing to polarity reversal (Fig. 2-3).

Soon thereafter, potassium ions start to leave the axon interior down their (outward) concentration gradient, and "shutters" in the sodium channel begin to close, stemming the inrush of sodium ions. Clearly, a relatively weak and brief electrical field may trigger profound voltage changes that approach and often exceed 100 mV. The rapid change in membrane permeability to sodium ions, and the corresponding voltage changes, are called *depolarization* (Fig. 2-4); the activity is manifested by an

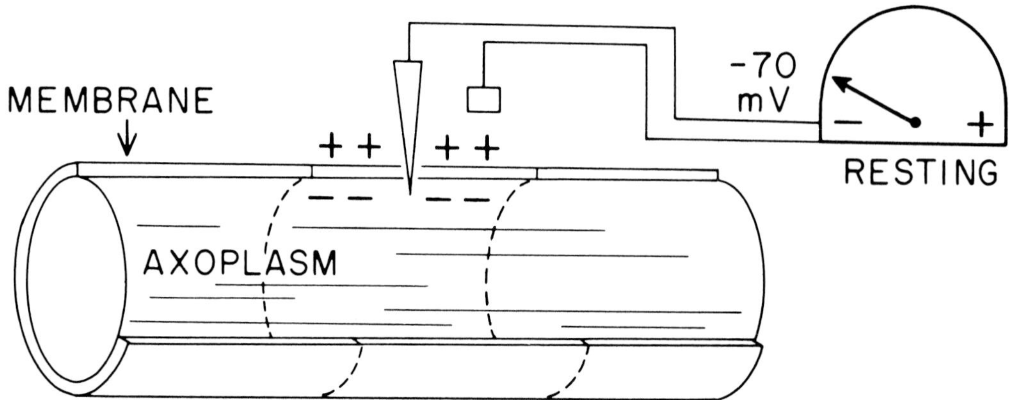

Fig. 2-1. Resting potential. A microelectrode penetrating the membrane of a resting (inactive) giant axon records a transmembrane resting potential of about −70 mV. The axon interior is negatively charged with respect to the exterior. (de Jong, R.H.: Physiology and Pharmacology of Local Anesthesia. Springfield, Charles C Thomas, 1970)

action potential or *impulse*. An apt analogy is the loaded pistol; a light pull on the trigger sets off powerful forces that exceed the triggering force manyfold.

The disturbance in the electrical status quo initiated by depolarization of a small region of the membrane sets up electrical fields that extend several millimeters along the axon. These fields induce small current flows in adjacent areas, thereby initiating depolarization at the new site. Current flowing to and from the new site, in turn, sets up fields that induce depolarization at ever more distant sites along the axon. Depolarization thus is a self-regenerative process that, once initiated, travels by spreading depolarization along the length of the axon.

The traveling voltage pulse is the nerve's fundamental information unit. A useful comparison is with a powder fuse (as used to ignite a remote stick of dynamite); once the fuse is lit, the spark travels along it, heat generated at one area being sufficient to ignite the next stretch, and so on. Plainly, if the process of depolarization is interrupted somewhere along the nerve fiber, an impulse can no longer be transmitted, and the nerve becomes unexcited. That is to say, the nerve is blocked. To return to the

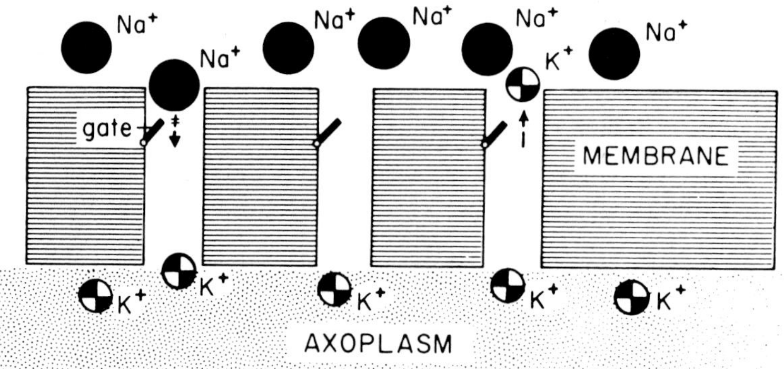

Fig. 2-2. Ionic segregation. Greatly simplified representation of transmembrane ionic channels. At rest, gates block sodium passage, whereas potassium ions (represented as smaller spheres) freely traverse the membrane. (de Jong, R.H.: Physiology and Pharmacology of Local Anesthesia. Springfield, Charles C Thomas, 1970)

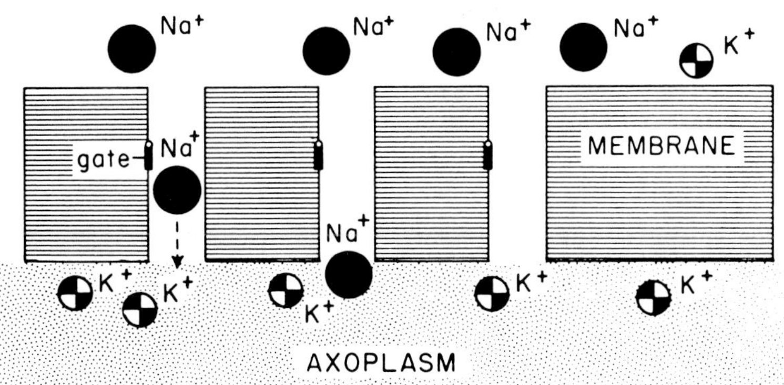

Fig. 2-3. Depolarization. Electrical fields accompanying an impulse swing the sodium channel's gates open. Whipped inward by the push of the concentration gradient and the pull of the electrostatic gradient, the sodium avalanche briefly reverses the membrane potential. (de Jong, R.H.: Physiology and Pharmacology of Local Anesthesia. Springfield, Charles C Thomas, 1970)

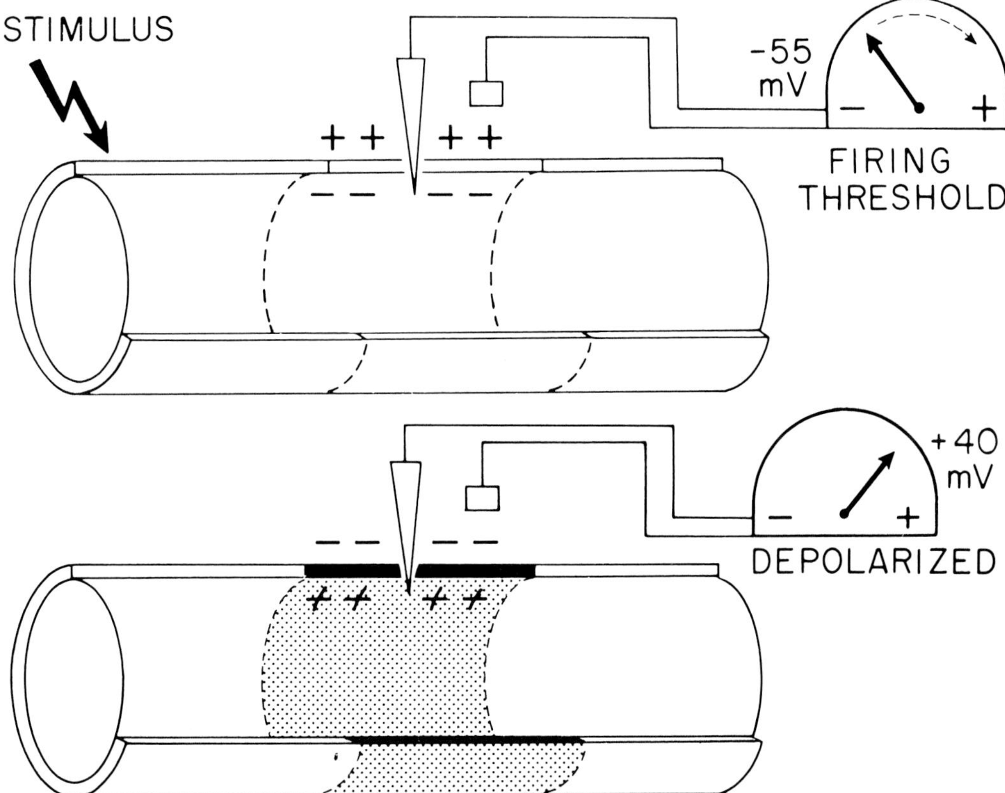

Fig. 2-4. Action potential. The giant axon's microelectrode records the inward sodium current as a reversal of membrane potential; the membrane interior is now positively charged. The large voltage swing is registered as the action potential. As the depolarized membrane patch assumes a charge opposite that of neighboring patches, currents will begin to flow. (de Jong, R.H.: Physiology and Pharmacology of Local Anesthesia. Springfield, Charles C Thomas, 1970)

foregoing analogy, if a patch of the powder fuse is moistened, the traveling spark, on arrival, will sputter, then die out—its progress is halted.

Repolarization. Normal membrane polarization is soon restored following depolarization. As the electrical field that surrounds the impulse fades away in the distance, the sodium channels shutter down, once again to bar sodium entrance to the axon interior. Meanwhile, potassium ions continue their outward trek till the push of the potassium concentration gradient is matched once more by the inward pull of the electrostatic gradient. Steady state returns; the membrane has *repolarized* to its former resting potential, ready to be activated by a fresh impulse. Repolarization permits up to a thousand impulses per second to travel along a nerve.

Thus, each depolarization sequence dumps sodium into the nerve and bleeds potassium from it. Eventually, both the sodium and the potassium ionic gradients would be wiped out, and the nerve would become unexcited. This potential defect is corrected by a continually active transport mechanism (the so-called sodium pump) that extrudes invading sodium ions from the axon and returns wayward potassium ions. (Worth noting at this stage is that local anesthetics do not impede the sodium pump.)

Nerve

The preceding description of impulse conduction—with the signal propagated by spreading electrical fields—strictly applies only to nonmyelinated axons (C fibers). In these axons, impulse velocity is slow, though the thicker the axon, the faster the impulse travels. With evolution of more complex ner-

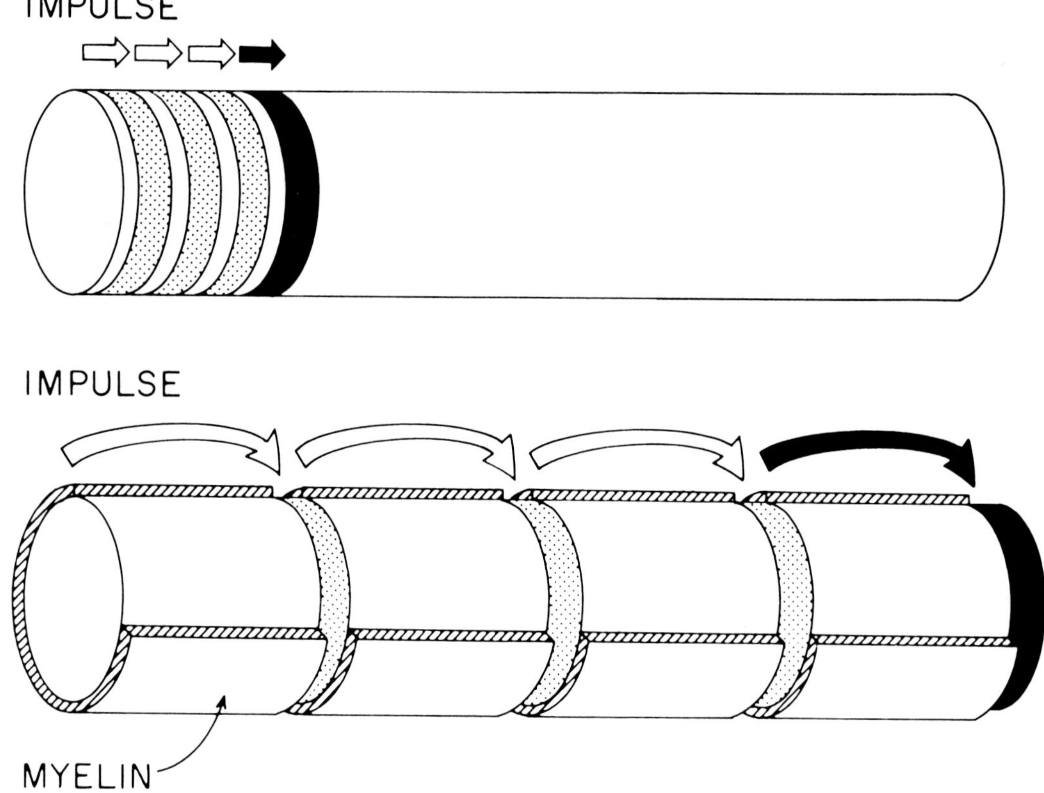

Fig. 2-5. Impulse propagation. Nonmyelinated (*upper*) and myelinated (*lower*) axons of equal diameter are here contrasted. In the former, the impulse creeps forward by a process of sequential depolarization of neighboring membrane patches; in the myelinated axon the impulse jumps forward by skipping from one node to the next. Note how much farther ahead four depolarizations have moved the impulse in the myelinated axon. (de Jong, R.H.: Physiology and Pharmacology of Local Anesthesia. Springfield, Charles C Thomas, 1970)

vous systems, much of the animal's size would have to be given over to an inordinately large neural cable system to convey messages quickly from one end to the other.

Nature has solved this limitation by depositing *myelin* (a lipid-insulating material) around the axon, thereby greatly reducing current wastage and improving electrical efficiency. At regular intervals, which are the farther apart the thicker the axon, the myelin is lacking. At these *nodes of Ranvier,* the membrane of myelinated axons contacts the extracellular fluid directly. These nodes, being more excitable than the rest of the membrane, permit an impulse to skip rapidly from node to node, instead of slowly crawling forward along the surface of unmyelinated nerve (Fig. 2-5). *Saltatory* (by jumps) impulse conduction notably speeds conduction. In humans, for example, fast alpha fibers conduct impulses at rates up to 100 m per sec while their C fibers conduct at a bare 1 or 2 m per sec.

MECHANISMS OF ACTION

Local anesthetics have the remarkable property of blocking impulse conduction in nerve fibers. While many other substances (phenol or alcohol, for example) share this property, local anesthetics are unique in that their action is reversible. Local anesthetics block a nerve without damaging it.

Even so, striking changes in nerve function herald the onset of blockade. Local anesthetics progressively lower the amplitude of the compound action potential, retard its rate of rise, elevate the firing threshold, slow the velocity of impulse conduction, and lengthen the refractory period. These changes progress until the ever smaller local currents drop below the ever rising firing threshold; the nerve is rendered unexcited or, as generally said, is *blocked.*

Conclusive evidence indicates that local anesthetics impede sodium ion access to the axon interior, probably by physically occluding the transmembrane sodium channels. With sodium entrance denied, depolarization cannot take place; the axon thus remains polarized. A local anesthetic block is a *nondepolarization block,* resembling in some ways the action of curare at the neuromuscular junction.

The insulating properties of myelin limit local anesthetic access to the nerve membrane; everywhere, that is, except at the nodes. Since so little membrane is exposed, and since much of the local anesthetic will be absorbed by the myelin, a relatively greater density (*i.e.*, higher concentration) of local anesthetic is required to produce conduction block in myelinated than in nonmyelinated fibers.

Further, as impulses can skip over one or two consecutive blocked (*i.e.,* unexcited) nodes, it follows that at least 5 or 6 mm of nerve must be bathed in anesthetic solution. In fact, taking irregular diffusion into whole myelinated or unmyelinated nerve into account, a minimum of perhaps 8 to 10 mm of nerve must be covered by anesthetic solution to ensure thorough blockade.[30]

There is little doubt that local anesthetics block impulse conduction by interfering with the process fundamental to generation of the action potential; that is, the transient rise in membrane permeability to sodium ions. Much more difficult to answer is how local anesthetics alter the membrane's configuration to stem the invasion by sodium ions. The place to look, evidently, is at or near the sodium channel; for it is the voltage-dependent gating function that is somehow impeded by local anesthetic molecules.

An external site of membrane attachment of local anesthetics, based mainly on their rapid action, has long been suggested. Recent evidence, however, inexorably points to the sodium channel's internal (axoplasmic) mouth as the likely site of local anesthetic action.[10,58] That local anesthetics are effective too when applied externally must therefore be attributed to their diffusion through the membrane.[31] In fact, nondiffusable local anesthetic cation is virtually inactive when it is applied externally, yet produces instant block when it is perfused internally through an axon.[44] In this regard, alone, local anesthetics differ fundamentally from marine toxins such as tetrodotoxin, which plug the sodium channel by occluding the pore's external entrance.[50]

Manipulating the external sodium concentration —and thus the transmembrane sodium gradient— further demonstrates that local anesthetics impede the influx of sodium. When a nerve is placed in a weak anesthetic solution, the action potential grows smaller and begins later, exactly as if the nerve were bathed in a sodium-poor solution. Exposure to a local anesthetic, in other words, is equivalent to reducing the sodium concentration gradient across the membrane.[45] Then, too, a nerve operating in a low sodium environment is blocked by a lower than normal concentration of local anesthetic. In contrast, a much higher than normal anesthetic concentration is necessary to block conduction in a nerve bathed in a sodium-rich medium. In fact, impulse conduction in a local anesthetic-blocked nerve can be restored by bathing it in a sodium-rich solution.

Local anesthetics do not block the passage of the

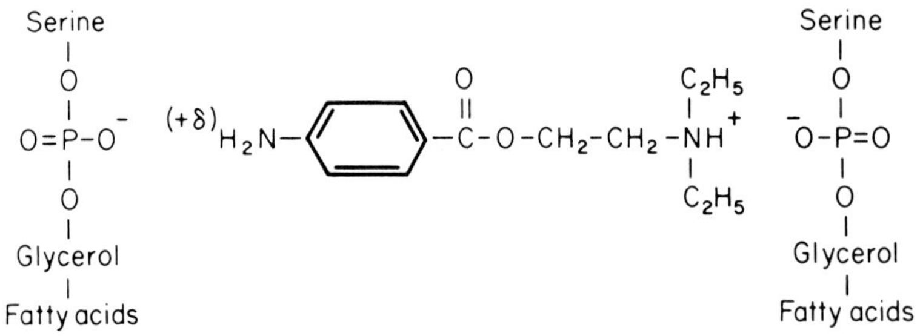

Serine – O – $O{=}P{-}O^-$ – O – Glycerol – Fatty acids

$(+\delta)\ H_2N-C_6H_4-C(=O)-O-CH_2-CH_2-NH^+(C_2H_5)_2$

Serine – O – $^-O{-}P{=}O$ – O – Glycerol – Fatty acids

Fig. 2-6. Bridge complex formation between one local anesthetic molecule (procaine) and two phospholipid molecules. Procaine's polar aromatic amine and aliphatic amine groups are shown oriented toward the oppositely charged phosphate groups. (de Jong, R.H.: Physiology and Pharmacology of Local Anesthesia. Springfield, Charles C Thomas, 1970)

sodium ion *per se* but rather the ionic traffic through sodium channels. A nerve bathed in a sodium-substitute solution is blocked just as readily by local anesthetics as it would be in a sodium-containing medium.[9]

Whereas the exact locus of a local anesthetic's channel-blocking action is as yet uncertain, its attachment to phospholipid membrane components is well documented. This, in turn, is linked to the important function of phospholipids in excitability; an artificial membrane that lacks phospholipid is nonexcitable.[6] The negatively charged phosphate tails of the phospholipid molecule, in particular, are essential to excitability. Local anesthetics, having two positively charged ends, attach to (and so bridge) two phosphate groups, one molecule thereby stabilizing two anionic phosphate tails (Fig. 2-6). The electrostatically stable complex so formed may be responsible for firmly gluing the gating structures together, so preventing their opening; however, it is not yet clear if local anesthetics do indeed prevent gating changes in the sodium channels.

A current working hypothesis for the sequence of events in normal nerve conduction and in the presence of neural blockade is shown in Figure 2-7.

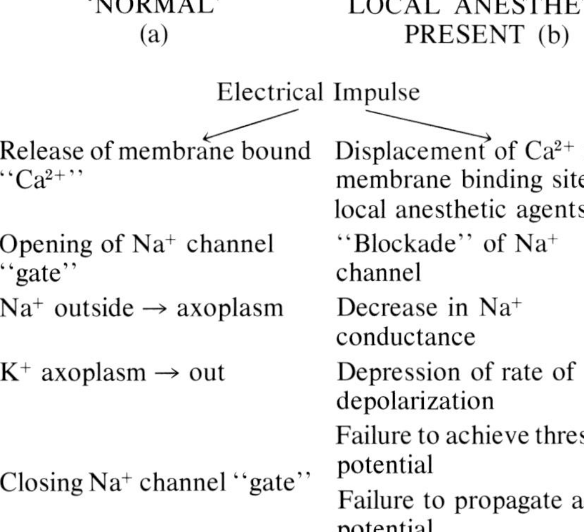

Fig. 2-7. Sequence of events in neural blockade.

PHYSIOLOGY OF ACTION

The diameter of a nerve fiber has turned out to be a most important physical factor to which nerve function, conduction velocity, excitability, and modality—as well as sensitivity to local anesthetics—are related. A thick fiber is less readily blocked by local anesthetics than a thin one. In other words, the thicker a nerve fiber, the greater the concentration of local anesthetic required to block conduction. This may be attributable in part to changes in the surface-area-to-volume relationship as diameter increases, and in part to the greater internodal distance of thick nerve fibers.[30]

Preganglionic autonomic B fibers are an exception to the rule.[32] These fibers, though myelinated, are more readily blocked than any other fiber group, even the nonmyelinated C fibers. This laboratory observation is borne out clinically; sympathetic blockade after a subarachnoid or peridural block extends several segments beyond the cutaneous dermatomic level. One explanation for this wayward behavior may be that mammalian C fibers are bunched together in so-called Remak bundles whose Schwann cells hamper diffusion and so hinder ready drug access.

Fiber Size and Function

The diameter and myelinization of a nerve fiber determine (to a degree) its sensitivity to local anesthetics as well as its message-carrying function. To simplify description, nerve fibers have been categorized into three major classes. Myelinated somatic nerves are called *A fibers;* myelinated preganglionic autonomic nerves, *B fibers;* and nonmyelinated axons, *C fibers*. The B and C fibers are of relatively similar size; whereas the A fibers vary in diameter from 4 to 20 μm approximately (see Table 3-2).[15]

Accordingly, A fibers are further divided into four groups according to decreasing size: alpha, beta, gamma, and delta. Largest are the alpha fibers, related to motor function, proprioception, and reflex activity. Beta fibers also innervate muscle and transmit touch and pressure sensations, while gamma fibers control muscle spindle tone. The thinnest A fibers—the delta group—subserve pain and temperature functions and signal tissue damage.

The thinly myelinated B fibers are preganglionic autonomic axons that innervate vascular smooth muscle, among others; B fibers thus assume cardinal importance during spinal or peridural anesthesia. The nonmyelinated C fibers, like the myelinated delta fibers, subserve pain and temperature transmission, as well as postganglionic autonomic functions. C fibers are thinner than myelinated fibers (about 1 μm) and have a much lower conduction velocity than even A-delta fibers.

It is evident from this summary that humans are equipped with two separate conducting systems that convey pain-related messages: one system relaying signals rapidly and comprising myelinated A-delta fibers, the other comprising slowly conducting nonmyelinated C fibers.

Minimum Blocking Concentration (C_m)

The minimum blocking concentration (C_m) is defined as the lowest concentration of local anesthetic *in vitro* that will block a given nerve within a reasonable period of time (commonly 10 min). The C_m of a local anesthetic is thus comparable to the minimum alveolar anesthetic concentration (MAC) of a general anesthetic. Another similarity with inhalation agents is the necessity to administer initially a highter concentration of drug to achieve an effective concentration at the site of action in the nervous system; that is, MAC in the brain for inhalation agents, or C_m in the axon for local anesthetics. (It should be understood that C_m has been determined *in vitro;* thus for blockade of mixed somatic nerve function an administered concentration of 1% lidocaine appears to be necessary to achieve the C_m of approximately 0.07% lidocaine at the axon.) The concept is important clinically, for only drug concentrations greater than C_m will solidly anesthetize a nerve. As the pharmacologic potency of local anesthetics varies greatly, each agent has a unique C_m.

As described above, the thicker a nerve fiber the greater the concentration of local anesthetic required to block it; a thick axon thus has a greater C_m than a thin one. As a yardstick, the C_m of A-alpha motor fibers is approximately twice that of A-delta sensory fibers. As mentioned above, B fibers have the lowest C_m of mammalian axons.

The C_m of an axon with given diameter is the same whether it runs in a peripheral nerve or in a spinal rootlet. The local anesthetic pool, however, is subject to numerous influences that act to reduce the final anesthetic concentration reaching the nerve membrane. Dilution by tissue fluid, fibrous tissue barriers, absorption, destruction, and scatter are examples. The final concentration of drug eventually arriving at the axon depends on the magnitude of these factors and on the length of exposure to them. For instance, much less local anesthetic is needed for subarachnoid than for peridural block, not because the C_m changes when an axon traverses the vertebral canal, but because spinal roots are flimsily protected in the subarachnoid space. Additionally, the drug is absorbed faster into the bloodstream from the vascular extradural than from the marginally perfused intradural space.

Differential Nerve Block

Because thick nerve fibers are less readily blocked by local anesthetics than thin ones, it might happen that the thin fibers of a nerve trunk would be blocked, while the thicker fibers would remain unblocked. For instance, it is often noted when anesthetizing a peripheral nerve that pain is obtunded completely (A-delta and C fibers are blocked) but that motor function and touch (alpha and beta fibers) are unaffected. Without forewarning, the patient's retention of muscle control might be disconcerting to a surgeon accustomed to equating anesthesia with limp muscles. Further, as large fibers convey touch and light pressure sensations, an anxious patient might misinterpret the perception of incision and tissue manipulation as pain. This situation is called a *differential block* (Fig. 2-8).

If motor block is to accompany sensory blockade—desirable when setting a fracture, for instance—a more concentrated local anesthetic solution is employed. This ensures that the C_m of even the larger motor fibers is reached. Further, during the block's induction phase the intraneural anesthetic concentration rises with time. Thus, merely waiting a few more minutes may yet raise the anesthetic concentration above the C_m for motor nerves, and so build up toward full motor blockade after all.

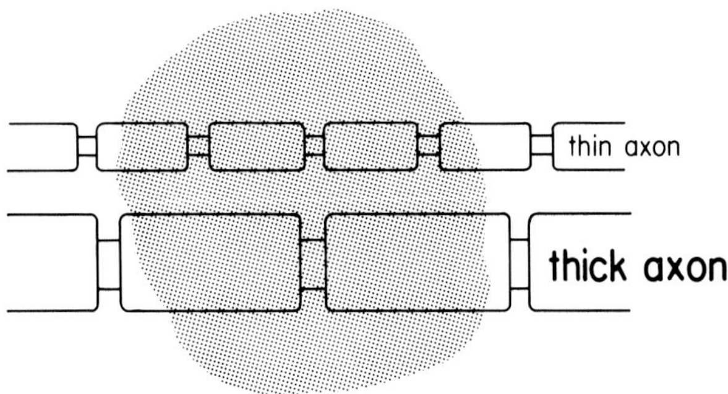

Fig. 2-8. Differential nerve block. Internodal distance is proportional to axon diameter. While three sequential nodes of the thin axon (*top*) are securely coated, the local anesthetic pool coats only one node of the thick axon (*bottom*). As impulses can skip over one and even two anesthetized nodes, neural traffic along the thick axon continues unimpeded, whereas the thin axon is solidly blocked.

Threshold (Wedensky) Block

As described above, differential block refers to complete blockade of one nerve modality (*e.g.*, sympathetic) with partial blockade of other modalities (*e.g.*, sensory and motor). Within one modality, it is possible to produce a blockade that may be ineffective under the following circumstances. When the C_m for a particular nerve and local anesthetic combination has just been reached, the nerve (by definition) no longer conducts a single impulse. A seeming inconsistency of the resultant threshold state of the nerve is that every second or third member of a train of impulses may breach the block. Such a threshold block, in effect, divides the frequency of a train of impulses by one-half or one-third.

This so-called Wedensky block has traditionally been explained on the basis that the nonconducted impulse (which precedes the conducted impulse) briefly lowers the firing threshold of the nerve; another impulse arriving during this period of facilitation was thought to induce just sufficiently more depolarization to trigger the membrane. However, an alternative explanation of *frequency-dependent blockade* implies that each new impulse intensifies local anesthetic block. Thus, following the passage of an action potential, a nerve with a low concentration of local anesthetic remains super-refractory to further stimulation for a period of time. This results in the dropping out of every second or third impulse from a train of stimuli.[11]

Whatever the underlying mechanism, the reduced ability of a marginally blocked axon to transmit fast trains of impulses becomes more pronounced the thinner the axon.[30] As impulses generated by noxious stimuli generally occur in high frequency barrages and are conducted along thin axons, the perception of pain is particularly vulnerable to threshold block phenomena.

When the anesthetic concentration at the nerve membrane rises beyond C_m, blockade becomes increasingly more profound, and progressively fewer of a train of impulses are conducted. Because the local anesthetic concentrations that are used clinically far exceed the C_m, the threshold phase ordinarily is traversed swiftly. This phase is most easily demonstrated during recovery from a block when the concentration gradients are shallower, and changes, correspondingly slower.

Even so, threshold block is encountered clinically. For instance, a patient may be insensitive to a pinprick stimulus when he is tested following nerve block, yet he might still discern a high-intensity stimulus such as a surgical incision. To be sure, the incisional pain is much less intense than it would have been without the block; the burning component of pain, in particular, seems to be attenuated.

Threshold block often (though incorrectly) is referred to as *breakthrough* of a local anesthetic block. Threshold block may be converted to total blockade either by waiting for more local anesthetic to reach the nerve or, by adding more local anesthetic. Either way, the objective is to raise the anesthetic concentration well above C_m.

Frequency-Dependent Conduction Block

Another consideration of local anesthetic action is that isolated axons are more sensitive to local anesthetic blockade if the frequency of impulse traffic in the nerve is increased.[11,30] Thus, an axon only partially blocked with a low concentration of local anesthetic is completely blocked when the frequency of impulses is increased.

Though all of the local anesthetics in common use show this effect, the more lipid-soluble agents (bupivacaine, tetracaine, and etidocaine) show a greater degree of enhanced block, and the duration of enhancement is more prolonged (Fig. 2-9).[11] The implications of these findings for clinical practice remain to be determined, however.

*p*H Effects on Nerve Blockade

The pure synthetic local anesthetic is a weakly basic amine, soluble in lipids but poorly soluble in water. Salts of the local anesthetic base, in contrast, are readily soluble and stable in aqueous solution. The usual local anesthetic solution contains a salt (commonly the hydrochloride) of the local anesthetic base. In this aqueous solution, the positively charged species of the local anesthetic (the *cation*) is in dissociation equilibrium with the uncharged local anesthetic *base* according to:

$$R{\equiv}NH^+ \leftrightarrows R{\equiv}N + H^+$$
$$\text{CATION} \leftrightarrows \text{BASE} + \text{PROTON}$$

water ← *lipid*
soluble → *soluble*

It is apparent from this dissociation reaction that the relative concentrations of cation and base vary with the hydrogen ion concentration of the solution. When the pH of the solution equals the local anesthetic's pK_a (negative logarithm of the dissociation constant), equal amounts of cation and base exist in the solution. Since the pK_a of most local anesthetics ranges between 7.5 and 9 (see Tabe 3-2), the solution contains considerably more anesthetic cation than base at tissue pH. The proportion of the concentrations of cation and base in solution is derived from this equation:

$$\log \frac{[\text{cation}]}{[\text{base}]} = \text{pK}_a - \text{pH}$$

where [cation] and [base] denote concentration of the local anesthetic cation and base, respectively.

The Specific Receptor Theory describes the mechanism of action of most local anesthetics.[13] The cation (*i.e.*, the positively charged species) is the form of the drug that binds to oppositely charged membrane receptors and plugs the sodium channels, so rendering the nerve unexcited. Hence, the cation concentration determines blockade of impulse conduction (Fig. 2-10). The concentration of local anesthetic base, in contrast, determines drug penetration, and thereby the quantity of local anesthetic to reach nerve membrane receptors.

The proportion of base is increased by raising the pH of the solution; alkalinizing a local anesthetic solution accordingly enhances drug penetrance. On the other hand, an acidified solution is less effective clinically than the same solution at body pH, as fewer local anesthetic molecules reach the neural target.

One immediate result of local anesthetic dissociation is the common observation that local anesthetics are ineffective when they are injected into an infected area, such as when an abscess is lanced. Dentists, in particular, encounter this disappointment frequently; even with a perfect mandibular block, the pulpitis-affected tooth (which the dentist wishes to drain) may be nearly as tender after the block as before. Because the pH of injected tissue is lowered by the formation of lactic and other acids, less local anesthetic base dissociates. While much cation is formed, it is virtually inaccessible, for (being electrically charged) the cation cannot migrate to the neural target without assistance from the uncharged anesthetic base, and that is in short supply.

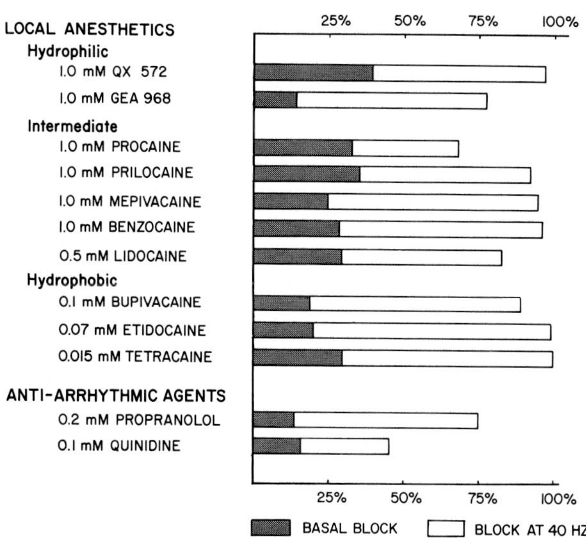

Fig. 2-9. Frequency-dependent conduction block. Local anesthetics are arranged in order of increasing potency and (roughly) increasing lipid solubility; quinidine and propranolol are grouped separately. Bars represent an average of two to three nerves with each agent. The shaded area represents basal block, the clear area, the additional block produced by 40-Hz stimulation.

Another consequence of dissociation is the reduced anesthetic potency that certain additives may impart. For instance, commercial local anesthetic solutions that contain epinephrine have 0.05 to 0.1 percent sodium bisulfite added to lower the pH to 4.2 (compared to 6.8 for the plain solutions) to minimize catecholamine oxidation.[16] These acid solutions would be expected to dissociate less lipid-soluble base than the nearly neutral untreated local anesthetic solution. Hence, the recommendation that epinephrine be added to the local anesthetic solution shortly before injection is logically sound, though definitive clinical data are lacking.

Membrane Expansion Theory. Although this explanation of the mechanism of action of commonly

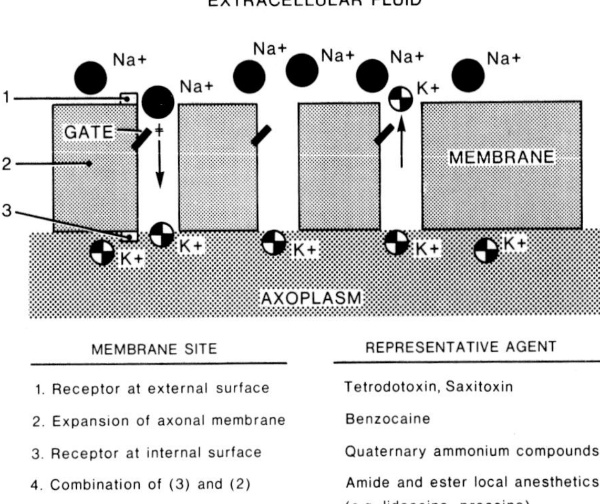

EXTRACELLULAR FLUID
Na+
GATE
MEMBRANE
K+
AXOPLASM
1
2
3
MEMBRANE SITE
REPRESENTATIVE AGENT
1. Receptor at external surface
Tetrodotoxin, Saxitoxin
2. Expansion of axonal membrane
Benzocaine
3. Receptor at internal surface
Quaternary ammonium compounds
4. Combination of (3) and (2)
Amide and ester local anesthetics (e.g. lidocaine, procaine)

Fig. 2-10. Possible sites of local anesthetic action (see text).

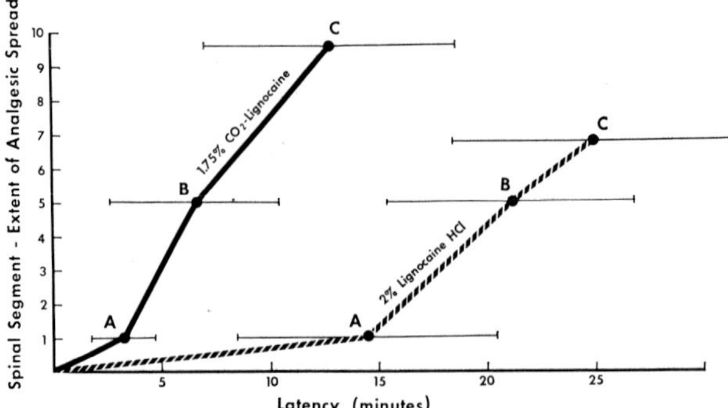

Fig. 2-11. Effect of carbon dioxide on local anesthetic action. Latency of onset and spread of analgesia for hydrochloride and carbonated base salts of 2-per-cent lidocaine; mean times (min) ± SD. (Cousins, M.J., and Bromage, P.R.: A comparison of the hydrochloride and carbonated salts of lignocaine for candal analgesia in outpatients. Br. J. Anaesth., *43*:1149, 1971)

used local anesthetics is useful, it does not fully account for anesthetic activity. Some drugs with significant local anesthetic action (*e.g.*, benzocaine) are incapable of forming cations at physiologic *p*H. According to the membrane expansion theory, these agents act by entry of the nonionized drug into the nerve membrane with resultant "swelling" and, perhaps, closure of the sodium channel. Possibly, some of the activity of commonly used local anesthetics with high-lipid solubility (*e.g.*, etidocaine) might also be explained by this mechanism (Fig. 2-10).

Biotoxins, such as tetrodotoxin and saxitoxin, have yet another mode of action. These substances, the most powerful local anesthetic agents known, do not penetrate nerve membrane at all but bind specifically to pores at the external surface of the sodium channel.

Since there is considerable controversy about the mechanism or mechanisms of action of local anesthetics, a summary of some of the data on the three main theories is presented in Table 2-1.

Carbonated Local Anesthetic Salts. Another demonstration of the effect of *p*H on local anesthetic dissociation is provided by the carbon dioxide salts of local anesthetics. As discussed in Chapter 3, a carbonate salt of lidocaine is formed by adding carbon dioxide to the local anesthetic base at 2 atmospheres pressure. The resultant salt is buffered to a *p*H of 6.5 and, thus, has a fairly high proportion of lipid-soluble base to penetrate lipid barriers, including the axonal membrane. On injection, carbon dioxide diffuses out of solution with a resultant local increase in *p*H to 7.5 and further facilitation of transport of lipid-soluble base. The released carbon dioxide rapidly diffuses into the axon interior, and here the *p*H falls, which forces dissociation of the local anesthetic to the cationic active form. This effect results in "ion-trapping," similar to that seen in the kidney, further favoring the rapid movement of the local anesthetic into the axon.

In support of this theory, it has been shown *in vitro* that exposure of axons to equal amounts of carbonate or hydrochloride lidocaine resulted in a tenfold increase in the degree of blockade for the carbonate salt compared to the hydrochloride salt.[8] The effect of carbon dioxide on local anesthetic action *in vitro* depends on at least three mechanisms: a direct depressant effect of carbon dioxide on axons, diffusion trapping, and conversion of the local anesthetic base to active cation inside the axon.[8] Clinically, indeed, carbon dioxide salts have a more rapid onset and more extensive spread of analgesia compared to hydrochloride salts when used for epidural or caudal block (Fig. 2-11).[12]

Cyclization. A new approach to providing optimal proportions of local anesthetic base and cation derives from a clever chemical trick. By juggling interatomic distances, a molecule can be synthesized with a tendency to curl its aminoalkyl tail around and onto itself, so forming a ringlike structure. Such cyclization of an uncharged (base) local anesthetic molecule yields a quaternary amine (cation) with the usual impulse-blocking properties.[52]

Table 2-1. Theories on Mechanisms of Local Anesthetics*

Theory	*Premises Concerning the Resting State*	*Action of Agent*	*Outcome*	*Comments*
Surface charge theory	High density of fixed-charge Transmembrane potential (total) ≠ resting potential (ionic)	Lipophilic (benzene ring) end of agent binds to membrane Hydrophilic (cationic) end in solution	Net-charge wholly or partially neutralized Action currents from neighboring unanesthetized nerve insufficient to reduce membrane potential to threshold level Conduction block	Sparsely supported from nerve fiber studies; well supported from model experiments on phospholipid bilayer membranes and liposomes; decrease in cationic permeability observed in both systems
Membrane expansion theory	Nerve membrane impermeable to ions except at specific channels, which are permeable during action potential	Anesthetic agents increase freedom of movement of lipid molecules—especially at aqueous lipid interface Some part of membrane critical for conduction in an expanded state	Expanded state (or conformational change) leads to constriction of ion channels and prevention of ion flow No action potential generated → conduction block	Satisfactory evidence for anesthetic agents increasing freedom of movement of lipid molecules; conduction blockade by a variety of general anesthetic agents can be reversed by applying pressure (*pressure reversal*) but that of clinically-used local anesthetic cannot (Type 4, Fig. 2-10)
	Clinically useful agents have relatively narrow range of pK_a values Charged cationic form (conjugate acid; BH^+) important to conduction block Relationship between (B) and (BH^+) is given by Henderson-Hasselbach equation $\left(pH = pK_a + \log\frac{(B)}{(BH^+)}\right)$	B responsible for penetration to the site of action B and BH^+ equilibrate in axoplasm in accordance with pH	Degree of blockade proportional to (BH^+) in axoplasm Quaternary ammonium derivatives also effective in axoplasm (Type 3, Fig. 2-10)	Satisfactory evidence for local anesthetic receptor being at or near the sodium channel; some degree of stereospecificity from studies with enantiomeric pairs

* Mather, L. E., and Cousins, M. J.: Drugs *18*:185–205, 1979.

Since this cyclization is independent of *p*H, a solution composed of predominantly anesthetic base can be injected and allowed to diffuse into the nerve. Once in the nerve, cyclization takes place, the anesthetically active cation is formed, and block ensues. This class of drugs is all the more attractive because the cation (being charged) cannot easily diffuse outward. The anesthetic drug is thereby trapped, and very long-lasting anesthesia is the result.

As has been mentioned, the marine toxins also offer a new approach to providing very potent local anesthesia. Currently, these agents have eluded synthesis and are far too toxic systemically; thus they are at a developmental stage only.

PHYSIOLOGY OF NEURAL BLOCKADE

At this point, the experimental evidence for local anesthetic action, based on knowledge of events in single axons, must be applied to the nerve, the complex structure with which anesthesiologists deal.

Intraneural injection is prone to damage axons and their blood vessels by compression. This is because the nerve's tough outer sheath acts as a physical barrier that traps intraneural fluid. At the very least, intraneural injection is uncomfortable to the patient; for that reason alone local anesthetic is always placed near—rather than inside—a nerve. How much drug eventually reaches the nerve (and how much is "wasted") depends to a large extent on the anesthetist's anatomical knowledge and clinical skill, and on the various factors that affect vascular absorption of local anesthetics.

Delivery Phase

Since the local anesthetic is generally injected into the fluid medium surrounding a nerve, the drug's molecules must diffuse through many layers of fibrous and other tissue barriers before they ultimately reach indivdual axons. The density of non-neural tissue components in a peripheral nerve varies. Much fibrous tissue, and even some fat, is found in the sciatic nerve; considerably less in other peripheral nerves. An exception to this is spinal rootlets, floating nearly naked in the subarachnoid compartment's fluid; drug diffusion and penetration accordingly are rapid, so that just a small amount of local anesthetic produces swift and solid blockade.

The first step in moving the anesthetic to its neural target site is mass movement (spread) of the injected solution. A large volume spreads farther and exposes more nerves to the anesthetic (but, of course, also increases the vascular absorption surface). Mass movement is particularly important in subarachnoid (spinal) anesthesia, with the drug's spreading upward and downward in the spinal fluid, according to the baricity of the fluid that contains the local anesthetic.

Diffusion, the movement of drug molecules away from the site of injection, is governed by gradients. Molecules move from an area of dense population (high concentration) to one of low concentration, the rate of diffusion being greater the steeper the concentration gradient. Since diffusion is a relatively slow process, the local anesthetic solution is inexorably diluted with tissue fluid. At the same time, drug is continuously absorbed by vascular and lymphatic channels. In addition, a substantial portion of the supply of available anesthetic is bound to non-neural tissue elements encountered along the diffusion path; generally, the more lipophilic the agent, the slower the onset of block. Clearly, to produce solid anesthesia, the blocking solution must be deposited as near to the nerve as possible.

However, though proximity to the nerve is important, blockade can be further enhanced by limiting local vascular drug absorption. Absorption is most successfully slowed, and the block correspondingly prolonged, by incorporating a vasoconstrictor into the local anesthetic solution. The vasoconstrictor (with epinephrine still considered most efficacious) restricts the local circulation so that the rate of local anesthetic absorption is reduced.[4] Similarly, drug injected into vigorously perfused tissue (*e.g.*, peridural space) is absorbed much faster than is drug injected into a marginally perfused region, such as the lumbar subarachnoid space.[7] Highly fat-soluble local anesthetics, such as etidocaine and bupivacaine, are extensively bound to local tissue depots and also to plasma proteins. Vascular uptake appears to be less affected by the addition of epinephrine to solutions of these local anesthetics, and thus is less of an influence on the amount of drug available for action on the nerve.

Concentration Effect. Early reports implied that the more concentrated the anesthetic solution, the faster is the absorption and the higher the blood level. Recent clinical studies, however, fail to demonstrate an important rise in blood level when the same net dose of local anesthetic is injected in more concentrated form (mepivacaine being one exception; see Chap. 3). This intuitively makes sense;

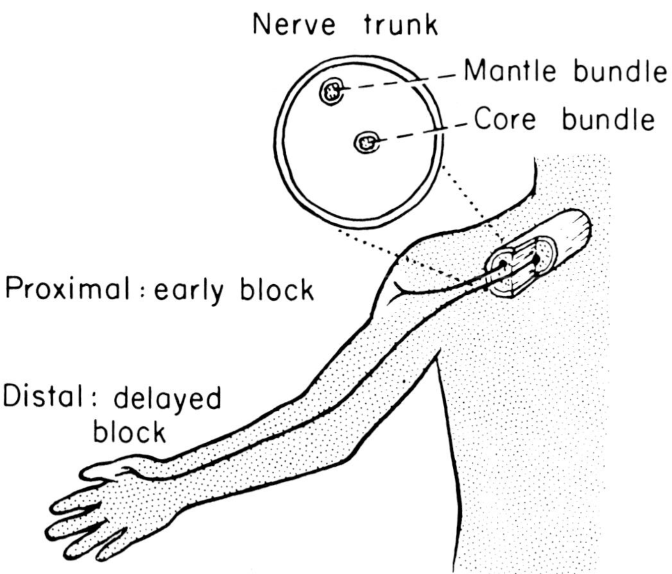

Fig. 2-12. Somatotopic distribution. Axons in large peripheral nerve trunks (*e.g.*, axillary terminus of brachial plexus) are arranged so that the outer (mantle) fibers innervate the more proximal structures, and the inner (core) fibers, the more distal parts of a limb. With the local anesthetic diffusing inward down the mantle-to-core gradient, the analgesia salient sweeps down the limb in proximal-to-distal fashion. (de Jong, R.H.: Physiology and Pharmacology of Local Anesthesia. Springfield, Charles C Thomas, 1970)

while drug is absorbed more slowly from a dilute than from a concentrated solution, a greater volume of the weaker solution must be injected to reach the same total drug mass, thereby spreading absorption over a larger capillary surface area. The net rate of drug absorption, accordingly, remains nearly constant.[56]

The limiting condition probably is tissue-binding capacity. If unoccupied tissue-binding sites remain, the ratio of free to bound drug is independent of concentration. If, however, tissue-binding sites become saturated, then proportionately more free (unbound) drug becomes available; the diffusion gradient steepens, and more drug is absorbed into the circulation. Saturation of tissue-binding sites probably explains why mepivacaine blood levels tend to rise with increasing concentration.[60]

It has been said that topical application, with a high concentration of local anesthetic produces even higher blood concentrations. This seems to be the case with cocaine, but it certainly does not apply for topically used lidocaine.[34,63]

Induction Phase

After the local anesthetic has been deposited near a nerve trunk, it diffuses from the nerve's outer surface toward the nerve's center. Accordingly, axons that reside in the outer layers of the nerve (*mantle fibers*) are anesthetized well before axons that course through the nerve's inner layers (*core fibers*). Topographically, the fibers in a nerve trunk are arrayed in concentric layers. Fibers that innervate a limb's distal parts assume a central position in the nerve's core, whereas those that innervate the limb's proximal parts lie in the nerve's mantle.

As the local anesthetic diffuses through a nerve trunk from mantle to core, anesthesia tends to spread along the limb in a proximal to distal direction.[15] This can easily be observed during axillary block; the subject first notes that the upper arm becomes numb, analgesia spreading from there down the arm to reach the fingers last (Fig. 2-12).

Excellent demonstration of concentric somatotopic innervation within a nerve derives from clinical experiments with intravenous regional anesthesia. (Local anesthetic solution is injected into an extremity vein, while inflow and outflow of blood are halted by a proximally applied occlusive tourniquet.) On cross-section, the nerve's core is more densely vascularized than the mantle region. Engorged with a backflow of local anesthetic, these veins transform into an anesthetic source centered in the core. Under these conditions, blockade progresses in a distal-to-proximal direction, as the drug now diffuses from core to mantle.[48] By the same principle, when the trunks of the brachial plexus are blocked as a result of the supraclavicular approach, paresis precedes analgesia because axons that innervate the shoulder-girdle muscles inhabit the mantle position high in the neck.[66]

The rapidity of onset of nerve block is (roughly) proportional to the logarithm of the concentration

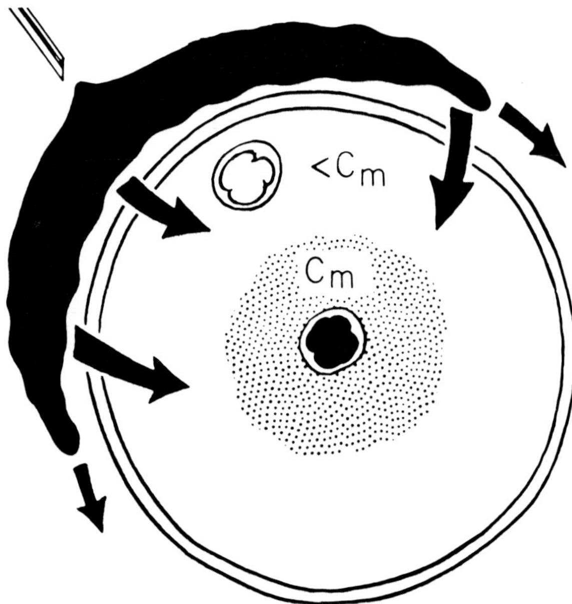

Fig. 2-13. Reinjection sequence. Fresh anesthetic solution is injected when blockade just begins to wane. As the mantle fibers lie closest to the newly injected anesthetic puddle, their C_m is rapidly restored; the entire innervated territory is quickly reanesthetized. (de Jong, R.H.: Physiology and Pharmacology of Local Anesthesia. Springfield, Charles C Thomas, 1970)

of the drug. This means that doubling the drug concentration will only modestly hasten the onset of block, although, of course, the more concentrated solution will block thicker fibers, too. Concentrated anesthetic solutions increase nerve penetration and the size of the fiber that is blocked; they have a lessened effect on the speed of onset of block.

Recovery Phase

During recovery from nerve block, the diffusion gradient is reversed. The nerve's core retains a higher anesthetic concentration than the exposed mantle, which, bathed in extracellular fluid, loses drug more readily than the well-shielded core. Accordingly, regression of analgesia takes place initially in territory innervated by mantle fibers and lastly in that supplied by core fibers, so that normal sensation returns initially to the proximal and lastly to the distal parts of the limb. The assumption that there is an avascular core may not hold true close to the origin of the brachial plexus, where recovery patterns following supraclavicular block suggest faster absorption from the core than from the mantle.[66]

Diffusion from the nerve and absorption into the vascular bed mainly account for termination of blockade. It has been found empirically that the duration of the block is related linearly to the logarithm of the anesthetic concentration. Thus, repeated doubling of the anesthetic concentration will have progressively less effect on duration. More important is the lipoprotein solubility of the individual local anesthetic agents; for example, agents with high lipoprotein solubility, such as bupivacaine and etidocaine, dislodge slowly from neural tissue, and blockade therefore persists for a long time (see Chap. 3).

Periodic ("Continuous") Nerve Block

A lengthy operation or prolonged labor might easily outlast the duration of a single anesthetic blockade and thus would require repeated administration to keep the patient pain-free. To facilitate reinjection, a catheter often is placed in the vicinity of the nerves to be blocked. Local anesthetic solution can thereby be replenished on an as-needed basis, a technique widely (though imprecisely) known as *continuous nerve block*.

Events during initial injection through the catheter are no different from those discussed above, progressing through induction, equilibrium, and regression. They deviate, however, when the block starts to wear off and the patient begins to sense some vague discomfort. At this moment, the mantle fibers (being closest to the external environment) have suffered the greatest anesthetic loss through outward diffusion and have dropped their anesthetic content below C_m. It is this restoration of neural traffic in mantle fibers that the patient senses, and it is at this moment that anesthetic replenishment normally is instituted.

At this time, however, the core's anesthetic concentration still is comfortably above C_m, by virtue of its remoteness from the external environment. Thus, freshly injected anesthetic has to travel a much shorter distance since only the outer shell's anesthetic supply must be replenished. The C_m is thus quickly reestablished throughout the nerve's entire innervation territory; accordingly, solid conduction blockade is quickly restored (Fig. 2-13).

Further setting the second (and subsequent) injections apart from the original injection is that a considerable anesthetic residual remains lodged in the mantle fibers. This is because anesthetic concentrations below C_m, though falling short of supplying a sufficient mass of blocking molecules to plug all sodium channels, nevertheless leave some channels occupied. Hence, to block all sodium channels again, fewer local anesthetic molecules are needed the next time; conduction block thus is reestablished not only sooner but also with less anesthetic than originally required.

By the same token, since the non-neural components also retain absorbed anesthetic, less drug is taken up for nonblocking purposes, leaving more anesthetic molecules free to attach to neural receptors. Hence, the quality ("depth") of the block, especially of the thicker, more resistant motor fibers, seems to improve during a continuous nerve block—a phenomenon called *augmentation*. Augmentation can also be observed clinically in epidural block if a small, repeated dose (3–4 ml) of local anesthetic is injected approximately 20 minutes after the first dose. There is no increase in the level of blockade; however, within the segments blocked, there is a more solid blockade of the entire range of fiber sizes. Presumably, the fibers with only partial blockade take up additional local anesthetic and thereby achieve the C_m.

Tachyphylaxis, a drug's declining effectiveness when it is given repeatedly, is often observed when a continuous nerve block is employed over a long period of time. It is less liable to occur if a blocking agent is reinjected; soon after the first signs of returning sensation; in fact, the aforementioned augmentation of blockade is more likely to occur than not under these conditions.[5] When the block is allowed to lapse, however (as when attempting to provide postoperative pain relief), tachyphylaxis frequently occurs. Hallmarks of tachyphylaxis are ever shorter duration of action, fading anesthetic potency, and shrinking analgesic field. Timing evidently is a prime consideration that determines whether augmentation or tachyphylaxis follow reinjection.[5]

Tachyphylaxis may well prove to be the result of several unrelated clinical factors. (In the laboratory, for instance, nerve block does not seem to lessen with time.) Important in this regard are anatomical causes such as perineural edema, microhemorrhage, or miniclots that may result from irritation by the catheter or from the anesthetic solution. Each, singly or combined, tends physically to shield the nerve from total contact with the anesthetic. Too, the nerve's epineurium itself may become swollen. Other plausible causes are hypernatremia (from the anesthetic solution's saline carrier) and, last but not least, acidosis from anesthetic solutions at *p*Hs well below 7.

Though the mechanism may not exactly be known, the effect seems to be clear. To take advantage of augmentation, the local anesthetic solution should be reinjected soon after the patient senses discomfort, topping-up with a dose that is from one-fourth to one-third less than the original "priming" dose. If a delay of 10 or more minutes is unavoidable, then more drug must be given to offset tachyphylaxis, on the order of one-fourth to one-third more than the priming dose.[5] Also, commercial solutions that contain epinephrine and acid antioxidants, such as sodium metabisulfite (which lowers the *p*H of the solution and so increases the likelihood of tachyphylaxis), should be avoided.

SYSTEMIC ACTIONS OF LOCAL ANESTHETIC AGENTS

The reaction of distant organs to circulating local anesthetic is critically important because it is primarily their limits of endurance that determine the maxiumum allowable ("safe") drug dosage. Especially critical in this regard are the reaction patterns of the central nervous system (CNS).

In regional block procedures, the local anesthetic is deposited near a peripheral nerve or spinal root. Eventually, however, the drug enters the bloodstream, either by absorption from the injection site or by inadvertent intravascular injection. The resultant concentration of local anesthetic in the blood—hereafter called the *blood level*—is governed by how much local anesthetic is administered and by how fast it is absorbed, as well as by how quickly the anesthetic is removed from the blood through tissue uptake, metabolism, and excretion. With blood acting as the initial drug carrier, it should not be surprising that local anesthetic toxicity is closely linked to blood level; the higher the local anesthetic concentration in the blood, the greater the chance of toxic symptoms, and the longer they last.

Though the peripheral neural effects of local anesthetics are dose-related—that is, the larger the dose, the more profound and longer-lasting the block—the CNS effects are more complex. Paradoxically, local anesthetics are potent anticonvulsants at low blood levels, whereas at high blood levels they act as convulsants. In between these extremes lies a broad spectrum of CNS responses that range from drowsiness to irrational behavior, and from tingling of the tongue or lips to twitching of the limbs. Intriguing as the anticonvulsant properties may be, it is the threat of convulsions that most concerns clinicians.

Any measure that either lowers the anesthetic's blood level or raises the brain's seizure threshold *pari passu* reduces the risk of reactions. Such measures thus provide additional safety at higher doses within the recommended dose range. One way of lowering the blood level, already discussed, is to slow intravascular absorption by localized vasoconstriction with epinephrine.

Preconvulsant Manifestations

As has been shown, perineurally injected local anesthetic eventually appears in the bloodstream. When the blood level is low, seizure protection is provided; when it is high, generalized convulsions ensue. In an ill-defined range between these two extremes are blood levels that give rise to telltale symptoms that proclaim the presence of high concentrations of local anesthetic in the brain's blood supply.

The earliest known records of CNS responses to local anesthetics describe the euphoric and stimulant qualities of cocaine. Such excitement may be seen with procaine, too. The new amide-linked local anesthetics, on the other hand, induce sedation and amnesia rather than euphoria. Otherwise, local anesthetics (whether of the ester or amide family) evoke remarkably similar experiences in humans.

Commonly reported symptoms of a rising local anesthetic blood level may be any combination of headache, lightheadedness (different, it is said, from that produced by alcohol), numbness and tingling of lips or tongue, ringing in the ears, drowsiness, blurring of vision along with difficulty in focusing, and often either a flushed or chilled sensation. Objectively, confusion, slurred speech, nystagmus, and muscle tremors or twitches may be observed (see Chap. 4).

Disappointingly few electrical clues of imminent toxic disturbance are registerd at the brain's cortical surface by standard electroencephalography (EEG). By contrast, profound alterations may be recorded from neural structures buried deep within the brain. Components of the limbic system—the amygdala and hippocampus, in particular—develop self-sustaining spike or spike-and-wave spindle bursts that coincide with the onset of behavioral reactions in laboratory animals; such patterns are considered representative of a focal seizure generator.[51,61,64]

Local anesthetic-induced focal limbic seizures have been recorded in humans, too. Patients under investigation for refractory epilepsy have developed characteristic spindle bursts at deep temporal lobe electrode sites, accompanied by a typical aura, when they were challenged with lidocaine.[23] Clinically, too, the symptom complex of mild local anesthetic toxicity bears striking resemblance to that of psychomotor or temporal lobe epilepsy.[14,23,35]

Local Anesthetic Seizures

Certainly the most dramatic (and potentially the most hazardous) complication of local anesthetic administration is the sudden onset of generalized tonic-clonic convulsions. Local anesthetic-induced convulsions (local anesthetic seizures, for short) differ in several key aspects from organic convulsive disorders. The two react oppositely, for instance, to hyperventilation. Unless otherwise specified, the convulsions (seizures, fits) mentioned in this chapter are induced by local anesthetics.

The greater part of our still-limited understanding of seizure mechanisms is derived from studies in experimental animals. Laboratory work, reinforced by clinical observation, suggests that the initial reaction setting off a local anesthetic seizure differs in several fundamental respects from grand mal epilepsy, even though the ultimate external manifestations of both are identical. It is because of this fundamental difference that some aspects of prophylaxis and therapy of local anesthetic-induced convulsions deviate from those of epilepsy.

Though total local anesthetic dosage is a convenient guide for use in most cases, it is all too apparent that rate, mode, and site of administration are important determinants of toxicity as well. This is, of course, because the brain reacts to the concentration of anesthetic delivered to it by the bloodstream, regardless of how the drug got into the blood. Thus, the local anesthetic blood level is the ultimate guide to the toxic threshold.

Warning Signs. At subseizure blood levels, the signs and symptoms of early CNS toxicity soon fade. But, occasionally, these symptoms progress to the point of seizures. It is important, then, to recognize the danger signals that foreshadow an imminent convulsion.

The data derive from observations of animals, there being few controlled observations of humans. In monkeys, drowsiness and nystagmus preceded lidocaine or mepivacaine convulsions. These portents were accompanied by recognizable preseizure EEG patterns of slow waves and irregular spike-and-wave complexes at (arterial) blood levels of 12 to 16 μg per ml.[40] Other agents—bupivacaine and etidocaine, in particular—do not cause sleepiness, so that the transition from the alert to the convulsing monkey is quite sudden.[41] Similar observations have been made in cats, and seem to apply to humans, as well.[27,56]

Seizure Incidence. An estimate of how commonly seizures are encountered in daily clinical practice can be obtained from several large series, though the special conditions that surround each series must be kept in mind. In some 36,000 patients to whom regional anesthesia was administered, 1.5 per cent had some kind of drug reaction, though convulsions accounted for only 0.3 per cent.[37] In a large-scale survey of peridural anesthesia, the incidence of convulsions varied from 0.7 to 4.4 per 1,000 administrations[38]; while a survey of the morbidity associated with intrapartum local anesthesia uncovered 3.5 to 4.1 convulsions per 1,000 procedures.[3]

Hazards. Of great concern to patient, family, and clinician alike is whether convulsions following a local anesthetic misadventure imply an immediate (or latent) threat to health. Undeniably, morbidity and mortality have followed an overdose of a local anesthetic, so it is important to consider instances when the seizure episode was properly managed. Drug-induced convulsions need not cause irreparable damage, as is evident from one successful case in which more than four times the limiting dose of mepivacaine (12.2 mg/kg) was inadvertently injected, with nothing worse than headache and muscle pains afterwards.[39]

Survival. By itself, a convulsion is not necessarily fatal. Nonetheless, the death rate from local anesthetic seizures can be considerable in untreated animals. Over 60 per cent of untreated rats succumbed to supraconvulsant doses of local anesthetic, for instance.[2,57] Four of six dogs that suffered procaine convulsions and were left untreated soon died; the two survivors had frequent and prolonged seizure spasms during which they became cyanotic.[36]

The duration of a spell of seizures is clearly an important factor that determines the ultimate harm. Brief seizures in spontaneously breathing cats, some made to convulse once or twice weekly for 6 months or more, caused no neurologic or behavioral changes, whereas cats made to convulse for hours on end suffered irreversible brain damage.[17,28,64]

The margin of safety between convulsant and lethal doses is considerably widened if elementary cardiorespiratory resuscitation is practiced. Properly ventilated dogs survived four procaine seizures, initiated at 7-day intervals, seemingly none the worse for the experience several months later.[36] The same obtained in cats furnished ventilatory assistance as needed.[17] This is because the convulsing brain compensates itself (up to a point) for its greatly elevated oxygen demand.[53] Though respiratory and circulatory support undoubtedly enhance survival chances, there is no question that a reduction in seizure frequency and duration is of additional benefit.[2,29,43]

Adverse Effects in Humans. Clear evidence that patients have been adversely affected by seizures, is difficult to find. However, the cardiovascular depression caused by the high anesthetic blood level, and the respiratory impediment caused by uncoordinated muscle spasms, may indirectly affect brain function through reduced cerebral blood flow and hypoxemia.

Parenthetically, the rising oxygen demand of the hyperactive brain and the metabolic demands of violently contracting muscles in patients paralyzed for electroconvulsive therapy could be satisfactorily met by proper ventilation.[46]

Locus of Action. Experimental inquiries suggest that local anesthetic seizures arise neither from cortical nor from brain stem sites but rather from subcortical regions. In animals with recording electrodes permanently implanted in the brain, Eidelberg and coworkers observed that cocaine induced spindle bursts were confined to the nuclear complex of the amygdala.[24] Subsequent laboratory research has extended this work, which demonstrates that the initial CNS reaction to any bloodborne anesthetic often is a series of spindle bursts or spike discharges that originate in the amygdala.

In humans, the amygdala (Latin for *almond*) is a modest cluster of nuclei situated centrally in the ventral temporal lobe, just anterior and superior to the tip of the lateral ventricle's inferior horn (Fig. 2-14). The amygdala forms part of the limbic complex, comprising the hippocampus and other less distinct nuclear masses that encircle the base of the brain. Fundamentally, an intact amygdala appears to be essential for the performance of survival-related behavioral patterns, such as food collection and self-defense, and in the overall integration of sensory input.[49] Rather than being a command post, the amygdala serves as a modulator and processor of more complex CNS functions.

The electrical changes recorded from permanently implanted electrodes appear generally to be characteristic for local anesthetics. The most striking finding is that blood-borne subconvulsant doses of local anesthetics produce significant disturbances confined to the amygdala. The first suggestion of a tempest in the amygdala appears within seconds of intravenous injection, when initial slowing and in-

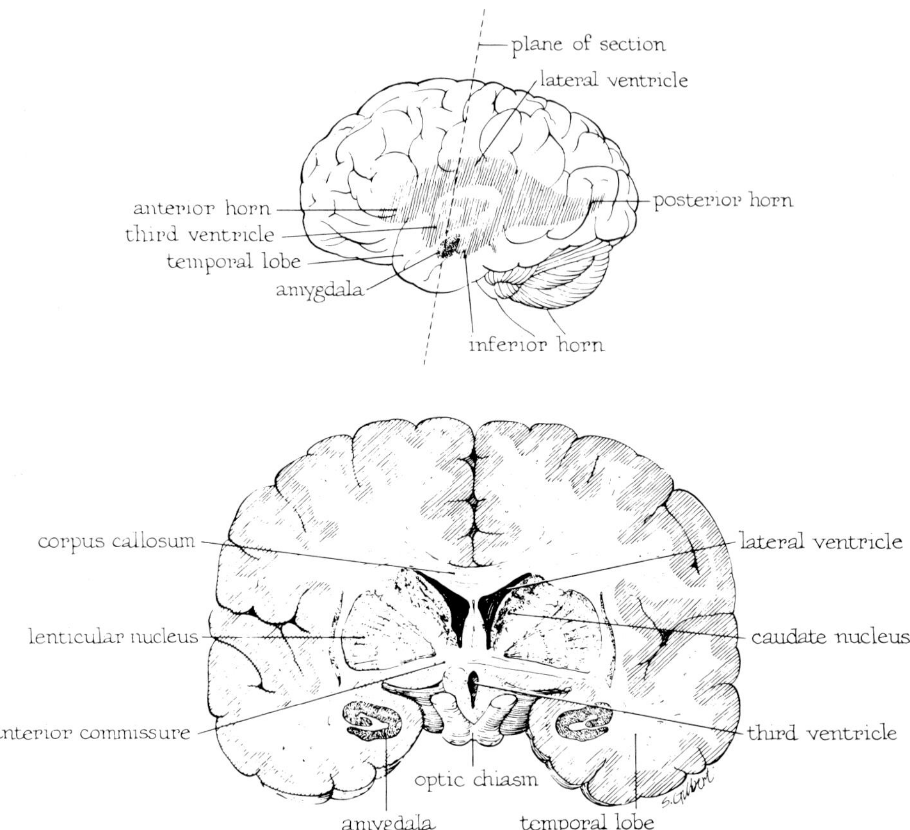

Fig. 2-14. Human amygdala is situated at the forward tip of the lateral ventricle's inferior horn (top). Its location deep in the temporal lobe is well shown in the crossectional view (*bottom*). (de Jong, R.H.: Physiology and Pharmacology of Local Anesthesia. Springfield, Charles C Thomas, 1970)

creased amplitude of ongoing electrical activity are followed shortly by paroxysmal discharges of spike or spindle bursts.[26,47,62,64]

While there is no doubt that focal amygdaloid discharges have not been observed in nonhuman primates infused slowly with lidocaine, mepivacaine, prilocaine, bupivacaine, or etidocaine, it seems reasonable to regard the nonconvulsant phenomena observed in humans as expressions of selective local anesthetic action on subcortical portions of the brain.[40,41] The limbic system is a particularly attractive candidate for this site because the CNS manifestations of a local anesthetic reaction resemble those of a temporal lobe seizure. In humans, epigastric, auditory, visual, or olfactory sensations; apprehension; changes in level of consciousness; confusion; staring; salivation; and so forth have been observed upon infusing lidocaine and have been likened to petit mal seizures.[14,23]

Seizure-Modifying Factors. The threshold blood level of anesthetic that determines synchronous epileptiform discharge activity can be modified by a variety of factors that point the way to improved prophylaxis and therapy. The brain's seizure threshold is influenced by acid-base status, by the presence of other drugs, by cerebral circulation and metabolism, and by a host of lesser known modifiers.[15]

The arterial carbon dioxide tension (Pa_{CO_2}) evidently affects the convulsant dose of local anesthetics. In acute studies on cats and dogs, it was found that the higher the Pa_{CO_2}, the less local anesthetic was required to precipitate generalized seizures.[22,25] In contrast, the lower the Pa_{CO_2}, the more drug was required to produce seizures (Fig. 2-15). Thus lowering the Pa_{CO_2} by hyperventilation, for example, raises the cortical seizure threshold to local anesthetics and lessens the chance that the drug will

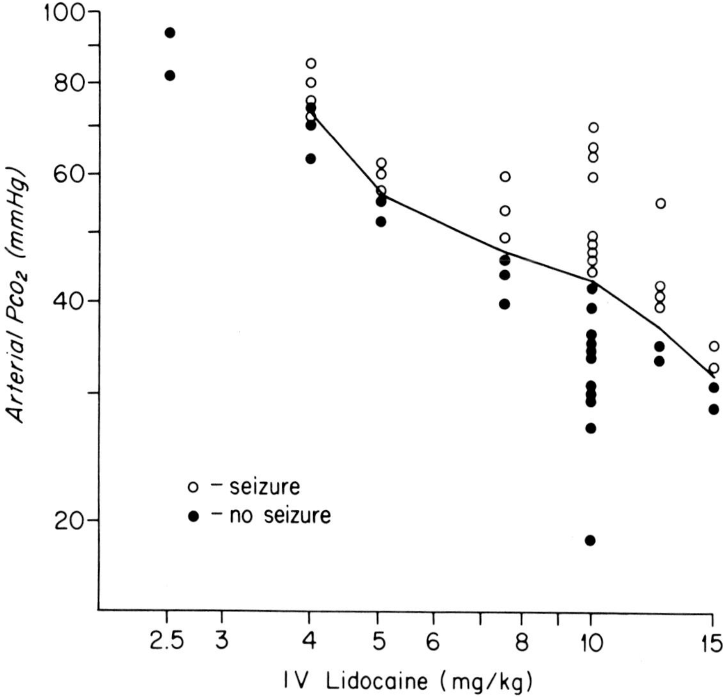

Fig. 2-15. Hypercarbia renders the cat's brain more susceptible to local anesthetic-induced convulsions. Reducing the arterial carbon dioxide level (as with hyperventilation), in contrast, renders the brain more resistant to anesthetic overdose. The line connects the boundary between convulsant (*open circles*) and nonconvulsant (*filled circles*) doses of lidocaine. (de Jong, R.H.: Physiology and Pharmacology of Local Anesthesia. Springfield, Charles C Thomas, 1970)

cause convulsions. In monkeys, which develop a marked respiratory and metabolic acidosis during their prolonged convulsions, increasing the inspired carbon dioxide concentration has less spectacular effect; it is mainly the metabolic acidosis that governs toxicity in this species.[41,42]

Why respiratory and metabolic acidosis, singly or combined, should boost local anesthetic toxicity has been the source of more speculative writing than substantive research. At first, it would appear that acidosis, with its lower than normal *p*H, would favor dissociation in the direction of the cation, which, being charged, would not cross the blood-brain barrier—hence less drug would enter the brain and the toxicity would be lower. Yet, the opposite is true. Perhaps the most plausible point is the high brain to blood partition coefficient for local anesthetics that tends to buffer ionic shifts in the blood compartment.[27] That is to say, the brain's large stores of local anesthetic would suffer little dislocation from external *p*H changes. Intraneuronally, however, there is a marked effect. As carbon dioxide rapidly diffuses from blood into brain cells, active cation species dissociate locally, thereby enhancing the anesthetic's apparent CNS toxicity.

Anticovulsants

Experimental convulsions from cocaine overdose were first described in 1868. While less toxic synthetic substitutes have become available since then, local anesthetics still retain cocaine's propensity to induce convulsions in all mammals, including humans. As a result, pharmacologists have searched ceaselessly for drugs that would lessen the toxic hazards of local anesthetics. Not surprisingly, standard antiepileptic drugs were early and prime candidates for this role. However, these drugs are not just ineffective, some are countereffective—an important point for consultants to remember.

The current pharmacologic approach to preventing and treating local anesthetic-induced convulsions stems from the classic work by Hofvendahl, who investigated a variety of cortical depressants in 1921. Most effective in controlling experimental cocaine convulsions was barbital (Veronal), a barbituric acid derivative. Tatum and colleagues, using similar reasoning, independently arrived at the same conclusion in 1925, noting that barbiturates prevent as well as arrest cocaine-induced seizures.

Based on these venerable experiments, barbiturates are frequently administered prophylactically prior to local anesthetic injection. Rarely, in the intervening 50 years has it been appreciated that the usual 1 to 2 mg per kg prophylactic dose of barbiturate is a homeopathic shadow of the necessary 70 mg per kg of intravenous barbital; clinical experience certainly bears out the relative impotence of routine barbiturate premedication.[1]

Because barbiturate dosage must be pushed up into the CNS depressant range, little improvement in reducing morbidity and mortality is to be expected. Thus, though phenobarbital (70 mg/kg, IP) completely prevented cocaine convulsions in mice, it did not reduce the anesthetic's mortality rate.[54] Pentobarbital (20 mg/kg, IP) lowered the incidence of procaine (200 mg/kg, IP) seizures in mice from 90 to 20 per cent, and double that dose completely suppressed seizures, but neither barbiturate reduced the incidence of mortality.[54]

So matters stood for nearly half a century, until the peculiarly selective stimulation of the amygdala by local anesthetics was recognized. This suddenly narrowed the search to anticovulsants that exert a selective quieting effect on limbic brain structures. Benzodiazepines met that stipulation particularly well. Of several compounds tested, diazepam (Valium) proved to be especially effective, combining minimal undesirable side-effects with optimal seizure suppression.[17,29,65]

In untreated cats, the median convulsant dose (CD_{50}) of lidocaine is 8.4 mg per kg. Yet 1 hour after diazepam injection (0.25 mg/kg, IM), none of the cats convulsed when 8.4 mg per kg lidocaine was given intravenously.[17] In fact, the lidocaine CD_{50} was doubled (to 16.8 mg/kg) by diazepam premedication. Similar elevation of the lidocaine CD_{50} (12.8 to 21.1 mg/kg) was obtained by diazepam prophylaxis in monkeys. In this species, 17.8 mg per kg lidocaine caused six of six untreated monkeys to convulse, whereas 1 hour after diazepam (0.25 mg/kg, IM), only one of these six monkeys convulsed.[20]

Diazepam stops ongoing convulsions as competently as it prevents them. In monkeys, in which local anesthetic-induced seizures tend to be particularly protracted, intravenous diazepam (0.1 mg/kg) halted convulsions within a minute, as rapidly as a rapid-acting barbiturate, like thiopental.[29,41,43] Even less diazepam (0.05 mg/kg) was 100 per cent successful in aborting convulsions in monkeys given 20 mg/kg lidocaine.[20] This small dose was just on the brink of efficacy, however, as four of six monkeys that received just a little more lidocaine (25 mg/kg) continued to convulse—albeit with considerable attentuation of intensity and duration. In this series, too, 0.1 mg per kg diazepam (IV) was consistently successful in halting convulsions from large doses of lidocaine.

Barbiturates for premedication have served as the benchmark of prophylaxis for more than 50 years; any competing agent will have to prove its superiority. In equally suppressive doses, barbiturate-treated animals slept longer, recovered later, and suffered more cardiorespiratory mishaps from lidocaine injection than their diazepam-treated mates.[18,65] In rats given median lethal doses (LD_{50}) of procaine, lidocaine, or tetracaine, none convulsed and none died after diazepam pretreatment.[2] Thiopental, administered until ataxia resulted, was less impressive on both counts, lowering the overall seizure incidence from 78 to 6l per cent, and the mortality rate from 50 to 33 per cent. Poorest performer of all was pentobarbital; it reduced neither the overall incidence of convulsions nor that of deaths.

Side-Effects. As far as can be determined experimentally, diazepam at standard therapeutic doses does not add to the cardiovascular depression from lidocaine overdose. In fully monitored monkeys in which local anesthetic seizures were arrested with diazepam, no cardiorespiratory depressant effects of the treatment were noted; in fact, diazepam hastened recovery two- to threefold over untreated convulsing controls.[43]

Duration of Action. In animal experiments, diazepam absorption has been shown to be rapid, with elevation of threshold to lidocaine seizures already well established (at a respectable 50% above control) 15 minutes after intramuscular injection.[19] Between 30 and 120 minutes, seizure prophylaxis is maximal (at 2 or more times the control seizure threshold), then declines slowly to a residual 50 per cent elevation 5 hours later. Diazepam's anticonvulsant effects in humans appear to be even longer-lasting; not for lack of rapid metabolism, but rather because pharmacologically active metabolites (desmethyldiazepam and oxazepam) are formed that are comparable in anticonvulsant potency to diazepam itself.[55]

Diazepam's poor water solubility occasionally causes erratic absorption after intramuscular injection and precipitation when added to an intravenous infusion. For these reasons, a water-soluble benzodiazepine such as chlordiazepoxide (Librium) may be preferable in conjunction with local anesthetics, since oral administration would infrequently be necessary. Longer-acting (and more potent) benzodiazepines such as clonazepam (Clonopin) may be attractive when prolonged exposure to the local anesthetic is anticipated.

MANAGEMENT OF CENTRAL NERVOUS SYSTEM REACTIONS

There are two aspects to consider in the management of CNS reactions. One is how to prevent a reaction from occurring in the first place. The other is what to do when suddenly faced with a reaction.

Easily the most conspicuous clinical manifestation of local anesthetic toxicity is a generalized convulsion. During a convulsion, respiration is impaired or impossible because of violent and uncoordinated contractions of airway, chest, and abdominal muscles. A less conspicuous, but equally vital sign is when circulation is impaired owing to local anesthetic-induced cardiovascular depression. Convulsions thus pose an immediate threat to brain and heart, a threat that becomes increasingly critical the longer the seizures last. The abrupt onset and the possibly serious consequences of local anesthetic seizures make imperative that anyone who administers a local anesthetic know how to manage CNS reactions.

Prevention of Seizures

Convulsions do not occur unless the blood level of the local anesthetic exceeds a certain minimum threshold. Accordingly, the surest way of preventing seizures is to limit the total anesthetic dose. With local or regional anesthesia, a vasoconstrictor (*e.g.*, epinephrine) should be incorporated into the anesthetic solution whenever possible to slow vascular absorption; longer-lasting anesthesia is an added bonus. It is important, of course, to guard against inadvertent intravascular injection and, as an extra precaution, to administer a test dose before proceeding with the full therapeutic dose (see Chap. 3). It is worth stressing at this point that high blood levels may occur immediately after accidental intravascular injection, or up to 20 to 30 minutes following tissue injection. To take advantage of "premonitory signs," it is essential to monitor and to keep continued verbal contact with the patient during the first 20 to 30 minutes following injection.

Premonitory signs usually warn of an impending convulsion. Should warning signs such as anxiety, sudden somnolence, muscle twitching, and so forth be observed during induction, the drug injection should be stopped, and preventive measures instituted. The protective effect of hyperventilation, which raises the cortical seizure threshold to local anesthetics, may be used to advantage at this stage. Often, administering oxygen and asking the patient to breathe deeply suffice. Should a seizure develop later, some nitrogen washout has been accomplished, and the replacement with oxygen would safeguard cerebral and cardiac oxygenation.

A common hospital and office routine is to precede local anesthetic administration with a nondepressant dose of barbiturate (on the order of 1–2 mg/kg) in hopes of minimizing CNS reactions. This is a false hope; seizure protection is slight unless near-anesthetic doses of barbiturate are administered. Fortunately, if experimental work is any indication, effective prophylaxis is attainable with diazepam (Valium) and related benzodiazepines. The great advantage of the benzodiazepines over barbiturates is that they combine maximal seizure protection with minimal physiologic disturbance. However, this advantage should not be taken as a justification for exceeding recommended safe dosages of local anesthetics.

Without controlled clinical studies it is difficult to recommend dosage schedules for diazepam that provide optimal prophylaxis with the fewest side-effects. Laboratory evidence suggests that as little diazepam as 0.1 mg/kg raises the seizure threshold, with additional drug providing increasingly more protection. This amount (7 mg for a 70-kg person) is well below the 10 mg (about 1.5 mg/kg) intramuscular dose commonly employed as preanesthetic medication in many centers; thus, it seems to be a suitably conservative guide.

Treatment of Seizures

Preventive measures notwithstanding, convulsions occasionally do result from accidental intravascular injection, unusually rapid absorption, or simple overdose. Local anesthetic seizures ordinarily are brief because the human blood level quickly falls during the early phases of rapid dilution and distribution. Rarely does a cluster of seizures last more than a minute (though it may seem like an eternity to the hapless clinician). Local anesthetic seizures should not cause morbidity if appropriate resuscitation equipment is at hand, the patient is properly prepared (see Chap. 4), and the person administering the regional block is well-versed in the treatment of seizures. Regional block of any type should not be performed without these precautions.

Important in treatment is protecting the patient from physical injury during the seizure, perhaps by padding him with pillows. Oxygen may be started (if on hand) while encouraging the patient to hyperventilate between fits. If the patient is unresponsive, the clinician should institute manual ventilation to oxygenate the blood and to wash out carbon dioxide. If there are no mechanical devices available, mouth-to-mouth respiration should be instituted, if need be. As a rule, vigorous spontaneous respiration resumes soon after the seizure ends.

Though the brain normally regulates itself for its suddenly increased oxygen demand, the cardiovascular depression that accompanies local anesthetic overdose may thwart the natural mechanism. A simple way to increase cerebral perfusion is to raise the feet. These measures should suffice until the overriding priority for oxygenation has been met.

Thiopental (Pentothal), 50 to 100 mg given intravenously, is widely recommended as an effective anticonvulsant. The clinician should resist the temptation to use too much thiopental (or any other rapidly acting barbiturate), because respiratory and cerebral depression may ensue. New studies in nonhuman primates have demonstrated the efficacy of small amounts (0.05–0.1 mg/kg) of intravenous diazepam. Seizures have now been arrested in humans with intravenous doses of diazepam as low as 2.5 to 5 mg. Controlled clinical studies have not yet compared diazepam and thiopental treatment of local anesthetic convulsions, however.

Short-acting neuromuscular blocking agents like succinylcholine have been advocated to stop the convulsive muscle spasms of a seizure. While these drugs may be perfectly safe when experienced personnel administer them, the hazards of muscle paralysis should be kept in mind, especially because the paralyzing agent does not arrest the brain's electrical seizure discharges—it merely arrests their external muscular manifestations.

On the other hand, when prolonged seizures threaten effective ventilation, muscle relaxants may well be drugs of choice, particulary because hyperventilation raises the brain's seizure threshold to local anesthetics. Indications for paralyzing agents are the inability to ventilate a convulsing patient adequately, and recurrent convulsions refractory to incremental doses of a barbiturate or benzodiazepine.

Overtreatment

In the flush of excitment that follows an unexpected reaction, overtreatment may all too easily result. Barbiturates and benzodiazepines both are CNS depressants; thus they may delay recovery of full consciousness if too much of either is given. Also, there are hazards associated with neuromuscular blocking agents—though these agents are safe in the hands of personnel trained in artificial ventilation—when they are used outside the operating room where help and equipment seldom are readily available.

The time for vigorous intravenous therapy is when simpler measures have failed. By abolishing the visual clues of a seizure, drugs may give a false aura of therapeutic accomplishment, for none are wholly innocuous.

REFERENCES

1. Adriani, J.: Barbiturates combined with local anesthetics (Editorial) Anesthesiology, *29*:405, 1968.
2. Aldrete, J.A., and Daniel, W.: Evalution of premedicants as protective agents against convulsive (LD_{50}) doses of local anesthetic agents in rats. Anesth. Analg., *50*:127, 1971.
3. Berger, G.S.., Tyler, C.W., and Harrod, E.K.: Maternal deaths associated with paracervical block anesthesia. Am. J. Obstet. Gynecol., *118*:1142, 1974.
4. Bonica, J.J., Akamatsu, T.J., Berges, P.U., Morikawa, K.I., and Kennedy, W.F.: Circulatory effects of peridural block: II. Effects of ephinephrine. Anesthesiology, *34*:514, 1971.
5. Bromage, P.R., Pettigrew, R. T., and Crowell, D.E.: Tachyphylaxis in epidural analgesia: I. Augmentation and decay of local anesthesia. J. Clin. Pharmacol., *9*:30, 1969.
6. Büchi, J., and Perlia, X.: Structure-activity relations and physico-chemical properties of local anesthetics. Intern. Encycl. Pharmacol. Ther. (Local Anesth.), Section 8: Vol. 1, Chapter 2, 1971.
7. Burfoot, M.F., and Bromage, P.R.: The effects of epinephrine on mepivacaine absorption from the spinal epidural space. Anesthesiology, *35*:488, 1971.
8. Catchlove, R.F.H.: The influence of CO_2 and *p*H on local anesthetic action. J. Pharmacol. Exp. Ther., *181*:298, 1972.
9. Condouris, G.A.: Conduction block by cocaine in sodium-depleted nerves with activity maintained by lithium, hydrazinium or guanidinium ions. J. Pharmacol. Exp. Ther., *141*:253, 1963.

10. Courtney, K.R.: Mechanism of frequency-dependent inhibition of sodium currents in frog myelinated nerve by the lidocaine derivative GEA 968. J. Pharmacol. Exp. Ther., *195*:225, 1975.
11. Courtney. K.R., Kendig, J.J., and Cohen, E.N.: Frequency-dependent conduction block: The role of nerve impulse pattern in local anesthetic potency. Anesthesiology,*48*:111, 1978.
12. Cousins, M.J., and Bromage, P.R.: A comparison of the hydrochloride and carbonated salts of lignocaine for caudal analgesia in outpatients. Br. J. Anaesth., *43*:1149, 1971.
13. Covino, B.G., and Vassalo, H.G.: Local Anesthetics: Mechanisms of Action and Clinical Use. New York, Grune Stratton, 1976.
14. Crampton, R.S., and Oriscello, R.G.: Petit and grand mal convulsions during lidocaine hydrochloride treatment of ventricular tachycardia. J.A.M.A., *204*:201, 1968.
15. de Jong, R.H.: Local Anesthetics. Springfield, Charles C Thomas, 1977.
16. de Jong, R.H., and Cullen, S.C.: Buffer demand and *p*H of local anesthetic solutions containing epinephrine. Anesthesiology, *24*:801, 1963.
17. de Jong, R.H., and Heavner, J.E.: Diazepam prevents local anesthetic seizures. Anesthesiology, *34*:523, 1971.
18. ———: Local anesthetic seizure prevention: Diazepam versus pentobarbital. Anesthesiology, *36*:449, 1972.
19. ———: Convulsions induced by local anaesthetic: Time course of diazepam prophylaxis. Can. Anaesth. Soc. J., *21*:153, 1974.
20. ———: Diazepam prevents and aborts lidocaine convulsions in monkeys. Anesthesiology, *41*:226, 1974.
21. ———: Lidocaine's CNS toxicity is species dependent. Abstr. Sci. Papers A.S.A. 1974 meeting, p. 165, 1974.
22. de Jong, R.H., Wagman, I.H., and Prince, D.A.: Effect of carbon dioxide on the cortical seizure threshold to lidocaine. Exp. Neurol., *17*:221, 1967.
23. de Jong, R.H., and Walts, L.F.: Lidocaine-induced psychomotor seizures in man. Acta. Anaesthesiol. Scand. *23* (*Suppl.*): 598, 1966.
24. Eidelberg, E., Lesse, H., and Gault, F.P.: An experimental model of temporal lobe epilepsy *In* G.H. Glaser, (ed.): Studies of the Convulsant Properties of Cocaine. 1963.
25. Englesson, S.: The influence of acid-base changes on central nervous system toxicity of local anaesthetic agents. I. Acta Anaesthesiol. Scand., *18*:79, 1974.
26. ———: The influence of acid-base changes on central nervous system toxicity of local anaesthetic agents, II. Acta Anaesthesiol. Scand., *18*:88, 1974.
27. Englesson, S., and Matousek, M.: Central nervous system effects of local anaesthetic agents. Br. J. Anaesth., *47*:241, 1975.
28. Epstein, M.H., and O'Connor, J.S.: Destructive effects of prolonged status epilepticus. J. Neurol. Neurosurg. Psychiatry, *29*:251, 1966.
29. Feinstein, M.B., Lenard, W., and Mathias, J.: The antagonism of local anesthetic induced convulsions by the benzodiazepine derivative diazepam. Arch. Int. Pharmacodyn. Ther., *187*:144, 1970.
30. Franz, D.N., and Perry, R.S.: Mechanisms for differential block among single myelinated and non-myelinated axons by procaine. J. Physiol., *235*:193, 1974.
31. Frazier, D.T., Narchashi, T., and Yamada, M.: The site of action and active form of local anesthetics. II. Experiments with quaternary ammonium compounds. J. Pharmacol. Exp. Ther., *171*:45, 1970.
32. Heavner, J.E., and de Jong, R.H.: Lidocaine blocking concentrations for B- and C- nerve fibers. Anesthesiology, *40*:228, 1974.
33. Hille, B.: Ionic basis of resting and action potential, *In* Handbook of the Nervous System. vol. 1. Handbook of Physiology Series. Baltimore, Williams and Wilkins, 1976.
34. Karvonen, S., *et al.*: Blood lidocaine concentrations after arterial and venous local anesthesia of the respiratory tract using an ultrasonic nebulizer. Acta Anaesthesiol. Scand. *20*:156, 1976.
35. La Gruta, V., Amato, G., and Zagami, M.T.: The importance of the caudate nucleus in the control of convulsive activity Electroencephalogr. Clin. Neurophysiol., *31*:57, 1971.
36. Mark, L.C., Brand, L., and Goldensohn, E.S.: Recovery after procaine-induced seizures in dogs. Electroencephalogr. Clin. Neurophysiol. *16*:280, 1964.
37. Moore, D.C., and Bridenbaugh, L.D.: Oxygen: The antidote for systemic toxic reactions from local anesthetic drugs. J.A.M.A., *174*:842, 1960.
38. Moore, D.C., Bridenbaugh, L.D., Bridenbaugh, P.O., Thompson, G.E., and Tucker, G.T.: Does compounding of local anesthetic agents increase their toxicity in humans? Anesth. Analg., *51*:422, 1972.
39. Munson, E.S. (ed.): Case history number 72. Mepivacaine overdose in a child. Anesth. Analg., *52*:422, 1973.
40. Munson, E.S., Gutnick, M.J., and Wagman, I.H.: Local anesthetic drug-induced seizures in rhesus monkeys. Anesth. Analg., *49*:986, 1970.
41. Munson, E.S., Tucker, W.K., Ausinisch, B., and Malagodi, H.: Etidocaine, Bupivacaine, and lidocaine seizure thresholds in monkeys. Anesthesiology, *42*:471, 1975.
42. Munson, E.S., and Wagman, I.H.: Acid-base changes during lidocaine induced seizures in *Macaca Mulatta*. Arch. Neurol., *20*:406, 1969.
43. ———: Diazepam treatment of local anesthetic-induced seizures. Anesthesiology, *37*:523, 1972.
44. Narahashi, T., Frazier, D.T., and Yamada, M.: The site of action and active form of local anesthetics. I. Theory and *p*H experiments with tertiary compounds. J. Pharmacol. Exp. Ther., *171*:32, 1970.
45. Nathan, P.W., and Sears, T.A.: Differential nerve block by sodium-free and sodium-deficient solutions, J. Physiol. (Lond.),*164*:375, 1962.
46. Posner, J.B., Plum, F., and Van Poznak, A.: Cerebal metabolism during electrically induced seizures in man. Arch. Neurol., *20*:388, 1969.
47. Prince, D.A., and Wagman, I.H.: Activation of limbic system epileptogenic foci with intravenous lidocaine. Electroencephalogr. Clin. Neurophysiol., *21*:416, 1966.
48. Raj, P.P., Garcia, C.E., Burleson, J.W., and Jenkins, M.T.: The site of action of intravenous regional anesthesia. Anesth. Analg., *51*:776, 1972.
49. Richardson, J.S.: The amygdala: Historical and functional analysis. Acta Neurobiol. Exp. Warsz. *33*:623, 1973.
50. Ritchie, J.M.: Mechanism of action of local anaesthetic agents and biotoxins. Br. J. Anaesth., *47*:191, 1975.
51. Robinson, W.M., and Jenkins, L.C.: Central nervous system effects of bupivacaine. Can. Anaesth. Soc. J., *22*:358, 1975.
52. Ross, S.B., and Akerman, S.B.A.: Cyclization of three N-haloalkyl-N-methylaminoaceto-2, 6-xylidide derivatives in relation to their local anesthetic effect *in vitro* and *in vivo*. J. Pharmacol. Exp. Ther., *182*:351, 1972.
53. Sakabe, T., Maekawa, T., Ishikawa, T., and Takeshita, H.: The effects of lidocaine on canine cerebral metabolism and circulation related to the electroencephalogram. Anesthesiology, *40*:433, 1974.

54. Sanders, H.D.: A comparison of the convulsant activity of procaine and pentylenetetrazol. Arch. Int. Pharmacodyn. Ther., *170*:165, 1967.
55. Schallek, W., Schlosser, W., and Randall, L.C.: Recent developments in the pharmacology of the benzodiazephines. Adv. Pharmacol. Chemother., *10*:119, 1972.
56. Scott, D.B.: Evaluation of the toxicity of local anaesthetic agents in man. Br. J. Anaesth., *47*:56, 1975.
57. Staniweski, J.A., and Aldrete, J.A.: The effects of inhalation anaesthetic agents on convulsant (LD_{50}) doses of local anaesthetics in the rat. Can. Anaesth. Soc. J., *17*:602, 1970.
58. Strichartz, G.: Molecular mechanisms of nerve block by local anesthetics. Anesthesiology, *45*:421, 1976.
59. Truant, A.P., and Takman, B.: Differential physical-chemical and neuropharmacologic properties of local anesthetic agents. Anesth. Analg., *38*:478, 1959.
60. Tucker, G.T., Moore, D.C., Bridenbaugh, P.O., Bridenbaugh, L.D., and Thompson, G.E.: Systemic absorption of mepivacaine in commonly used regional block procedures. Anesthesiology, *37*:277, 1972.
61. Tuttle. W.W., and Elliot, H.W.: Electrographic and behavioral study of convulsants in the cat. Anesthesiology, *30*:48, 1969.
62. Tuttle, W.W., and Riblet, L.A.: Investigation of the amygdaloid and olfactory electrographic response in the cat after toxic dosage of lidocaine. Electroencephalogr. Clin. Neurophysiol., *28*:601, 1970.
63. Van Dyke, C., *et al.:* Cocaine: Plasma concentrations after intranasal application in man. Science, *191*:859, 1976.
64. Wagman, I.H., de Jong, R.H., and Prince, D.A.: Effects of lidocaine on the central nervous system. Anesthesiology, *28*:155, 1967.
65. Wesseling, H., Bovenhorst, G.H., and Wiers, J.W.: Effects of diazepam and pentobarbitone on convulsions induced by local anesthetics in mice. Eur. J. Pharmacol., *13*:150, 1971.
66. Winnie, A.P., La Vallee, D.A., Pesosa, B., and Masud, Z.K.: Clinical pharmacokinetics of local anaesthetics. Can. Anaesth. Soc. J., *24*:252, 1977.

3 Absorption and Disposition of Local Anesthetics: Pharmacokinetics

Geoffrey T. Tucker and Laurence E. Mather

The use of regional anesthesia requires administering sufficient local anesthetic to be effective but not so much that toxicity develops. Just as the anesthesiologist must have a thorough knowledge of the anatomical and physical landmarks, he must also appreciate local anesthetic action through knowledge of the individual characteristics and limitations of each of the range of local anesthetic molecules. He must also be familiar with the kinetics of absorption and disposition of the local anesthetics in the body—their rates of distribution between blood and tissues and eventual metabolism and elimination by the kidney.

In reviewing the absorption and disposition of local anesthetics, it is important to examine the relationship between the physicochemical properties of the agents and their fate in the body and to delineate the role of local anesthetic pharmacokinetics in the overall response to regional anesthesia. This response is a complex function of pharmacokinetics-pharmacodynamics, the physiologic consequences of neural blockade, and the pathophysiologic status of the patient. Each of these factors can influence the others.

STRUCTURE AND PHYSICOCHEMICAL PROPERTIES OF LOCAL ANESTHETICS

Structure: The Family Album (Fig. 3.1–3.5)

"Ester Caines." Cocaine was the first local anesthetic recognized and studied both scientifically and medically. It was found naturally-occurring in South America by German scientists during the 1850's and first introduced into clinical medicine in the latter part of the 19th century. By studying its structure, German chemists synthesized procaine which was used widely in World War I. After this war, many ester-caines were developed from procaine. These include tetracaine and chloroprocaine which remain popular today.

"Amide Caines." The first of the amides was a carbamoyl quinoline derivative, dibucaine, which was much sturdier than the "ester caines" but was too toxic for use other than in spinal anesthesia (Fig. 3-4).

The next important development occurred in Sweden where some significant mutations resulted in a new, hardy breed of "amide" or "anilide caines." Thus, the labile ester linkage was replaced by the chemically sturdier amide grouping (Fig. 3-5). Lidocaine was the first of these, followed shortly by mepivacaine and prilocaine. Unlike the other agents, the aromatic moiety in prilocaine is o-toluidine (2-methylaniline) rather than 2,6-xylidine (2-6-xylidine-2,6-dimethylaniline), and this has important metabolic consequences. Also, the aliphatic amino group is secondary, in contrast to most other local anesthetics in which it is tertiary. Bupivacaine and etidocaine are the most recently developed "amide caines."

Mepivacaine, prilocaine, bupivacaine, and etidocaine, but not lidocaine, all have an asymmetric carbon atom (*asymmetric* because it has bonded to it 4 different functional groups; the structures are mirror images and are therefore not superimposable and may differ in physicochemical and pharmacologic properties). Consequently, although the racemates are used clinically, these agents can exist in two stereoisomeric forms.

Physicochemical Properties

There are essentially three mechanisms involved in the movement of local anesthetic molecules within the body. The first is *bulk flow* of the injected solution at the site of administration; the second is *diffusion* into and through aqueous and lipoprotein barriers; and the third is *vascular transport*. Of these, diffusion is most directly dependent upon the physicochemical properties of the agent (see Chap. 2).

According to Fick's law, the rate of passive diffu-

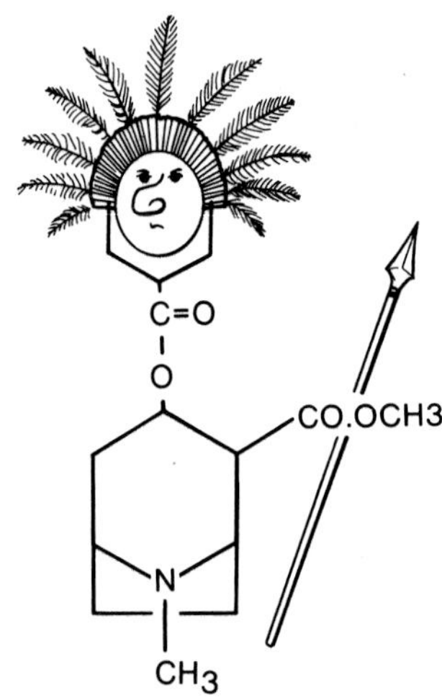

'Co' Sth. America (1850)

Fig. 3-1. Cocaine. (Tucker, G.T.: transformation and toxicity of local anaesthetics. Acta Anaesthesiol. Belg., *26*[*Suppl.*]:123, 1975)

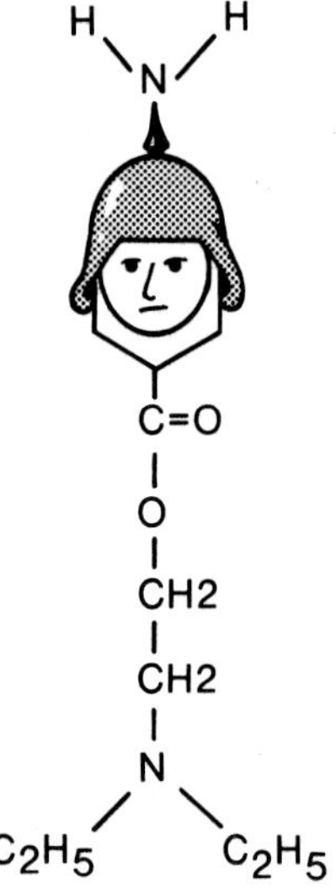

'Pro' Germany (1905)

Fig. 3-2. Procaine. (Tucker, G.T.: Biotransformation and toxicity of local anaesthetics. Acta Anaesthesiol. Belg., *26*[*Suppl.*]:123, 1975)

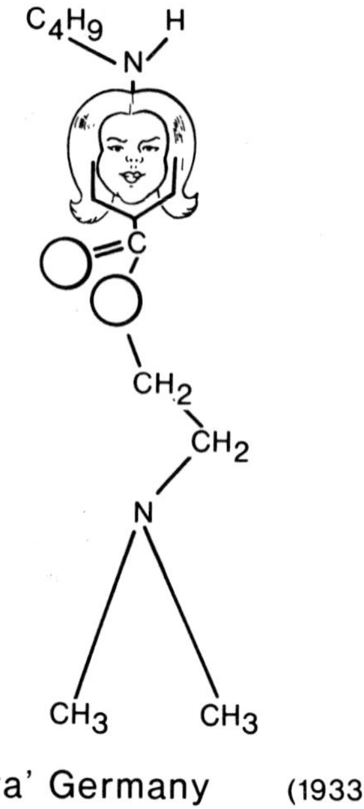

'Tetra' Germany (1933)

Fig. 3-3. Tetracaine. (Tucker, G.T.: Biotransformation and toxicity of local anaesthetics. Acta Anaesthesiol. Belg., *26*[*Suppl.*]:123, 1975)

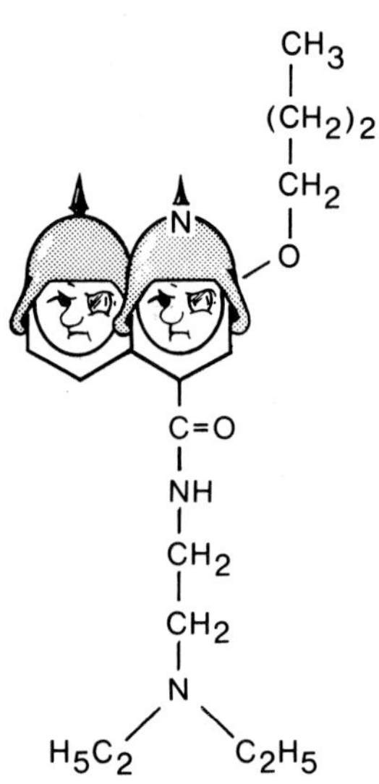

'Dibu' Germany (1932)

Fig. 3-4. Dibucaine.

sion (dQ/dt) of a drug through a biologic membrane at steady state may be approximated by equation 1, in which D is the diffusion coefficient of the drug in the membrane; A and δ are, respectively, the area and thickness of the membrane; K is the partition coefficient of drug between the aqueous and membrane phases; and Δc is the concentration gradient.

$$1.\ \frac{dQ}{dt} = \frac{-DK\Delta cA}{\delta}$$

Inasmuch as they determine D,K, and Δc, physicochemical properties will clearly influence the rate of transfer of local anesthetic at the membrane level, and potentially, therefore, the time-course of anesthetic and pharmacologic effects. By influencing the *equilibrium* distribution of the drugs between fluids and tissues, physicochemical properties also modulate activity and overall drug movement in the bloodstream.

Fick's law contains terms that are not amenable to study. But there exist a number of physicochemical properties that do elucidate the biologic behavior of these drugs.

Some physicochemical properties of a selection of the "caines" are given in Table 3-1.

Features Common to Most Local Anesthetics

Weak Bases with $pK_a > 7.4$. (Free base poorly water-soluble)

Thus dispensed as acidic solution, hydrochloride salts, (pH 4–7), which are more highly ionized and thus water-soluble

Exist in solution as equilibrium mixture of nonionized, lipid-soluble (free base) and ionized, water-soluble (cationic) forms

Body buffers raise pH and therefore increase amount of free base present

Lipid-soluble (free base) form crosses axonal membrane

Water-soluble (cationic) form is active blocker for most agents

---

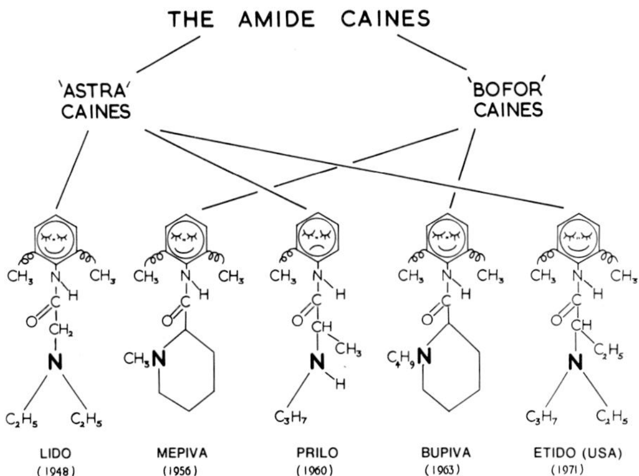

Fig. 3-5. The "amide caines." (*left to right*) lidocaine, mepivacaine, prilocaine, bupivacaine, and etidocaine. (Tucker, G.T.: Biotransformation and toxicity of local anaesthetics. Acta Anaesthesiol. Belg., *26*[*Suppl.*]:123, 1975)

As the table shows, quite small chemical changes in the aromatic portion of ester or amine portion of amide local anesthetic agents markedly alter physical properties such as lipid/water partition coefficients and protein binding. These, in turn, have marked effects on potency and various clinical features such as onset time and duration of anesthesia. For example, addition of a four-carbon butyl group to the lipophilic aromatic amino end with subtractions of two carbons from the hydrophilic amino end of the ester procaine gives tetracaine and results in more than a 100-fold increase in lipid solubility, a ten-fold increase in protein binding, and a marked increase in potency. With the amide mepivacaine, substitution of a four-carbon butyl group for the one-carbon methyl group on its hydrophilic amine end gives bupivacaine with a 35-fold increase in partition coefficient and increased protein binding and potency. Similarly, substitution in the lidocaine molecule of a propyl for an ethyl group at the amine end and addition of an ethyl group at the alpha carbon in the intermediate chain yield etidocaine. This results in a 50-fold increase in partition coefficient, increased protein binding and potency, and a duration of local anesthetic action at least twice that of lidocaine (see Chap. 4).

Molecular Weight. The diffusion coefficient of a compound is partly determined by its shape and its molecular weight (more accurately, molecular volume). Smaller molecules diffuse faster. However, since the molecular weights of the common local anesthetics are within a narrow range, this factor should not contribute significantly to differences in their kinetics (Table 3-1).

Aqueous and Lipid Solubility. The partition coefficients of drugs determined in aqueous/organic solvent systems *in vitro* are often used to indicate their relative *in vivo* partition characteristics or degree of lipid solubility. The higher values for the long-acting agents tetracaine, bupivacaine, and etidocaine suggest more extensive entry into body membranes

(*Text continues on p. 50.*)

Table 3-1. Physiochemical Properties of Local Anesthetics

	Chemical Configuration			*Physicochemical Properties*				*Biologic Properties*		
Agent	*Aromatic Lipophilic*	*Intermediate Chain*	*Amine Hydrophilic*	*Molecular Weight (base)*	pK_a* *(25° C)*	*Partition Coefficient*‡	*Per Cent Protein Binding*	*Equieffective*† *Anesthetic Concentration*	*Approximate Anesthetic Duration (min)*†	*Site of Metabolism*
Esters										
Procaine	H—N(H)—C_6H_4—	$COOCH_2CH_2$	—$N(C_2H_5)_2$	236	8.9	0.02	5.8§	2	50	Plasma
Chloroprocaine	N_2N—$C_6H_3(Cl)$—	$COOCH_2CH_2$	$N(C_2H_5)_2$	271	8.7	0.14		2	45	Plasma
Tetracaine	$H_9C_4N(H)$—C_6H_4—	$COOCH_2CH_2$	—$N(CH_3)_2$	264	8.5	4.1	75.6§	0.25	175	Plasma
Amides										
Prilocaine	CH_3—C_6H_4—	NHCOCH(CH_3)	—N(H)(C_3H_7)	220	7.9	0.9	55 approx.	1	100	Liver, lung

Mepivacaine	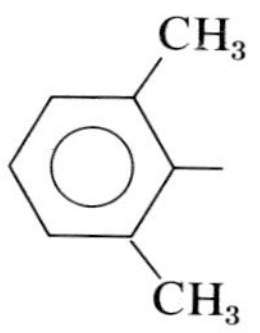 (2,6-dimethylphenyl: CH_3, CH_3)	NHCO	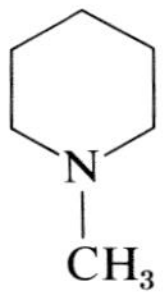 piperidyl, N—CH_3	246	7.6	0.8	77.5[‖]	1	100	Liver
Lidocaine		$NHCOCH_2$	—N(C_2H_5)(C_2H_5)	234	7.9	2.9	64.3[‖]	1	100	Liver
Bupivacaine		NHCO	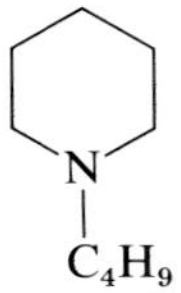 piperidyl, N—C_4H_9	288	8.1	27.5	95.6[‖]	0.25	175	Liver
Etidocaine		NHCOCH(C_2H_5)	—N(C_2H_5)(C_3H_7)	276	7.7	141	94[‖]	0.25	200	Liver

* pH corresponds to 50 per cent ionization
† Data derived from rat sciatic nerve blocking procedure
‡ n-heptane/*p*H 7.4 buffer
§ nerve homogenate binding
‖ plasma protein binding—2μg/ml
(Data from Ekenstam, B.: The effect of the structural variation on the local analgetic properties of the most commonly used groups of substances. Acta Anaesthesiol. Scand., *25* [*Suppl.*]:10, 1966; Truant, A. P., and Takman, B.: Differential physical–chemical and neuropharmacologic properties of local anesthetic agents. Anesth. Analg. (Cleve.), *38*:478, 1959; Tucker, G. T.: Biotransformation and toxicity of local anaesthetics. Int. Anesthesiol. Clin., *13*:33, 1975; Mather, L. E.: unpublished data)

and tissues as a result of greater hydrophobicity, and higher rates of diffusion (see Equation 1). A short time to reach equilibrium distribution will not necessarily result from a high partition coefficient since a higher rate of diffusion is offset by a greater capacity for membrane or tissue to bind drug. Also, aqueous solubility diminishes as lipid solubility increases. If a local anesthetic has too high a degree of lipid solubility, the correspondingly low aqueous solubility will place an upper limit on the amount of drug available for transport and activity.

Ionization. The inclusion of the amino group in the structure of most local anesthetics confers upon them the "split personality" of a weak base. This means that they exist in solution as an equilibrium mixture of the nonionized (free base) and the ionized (cationic) form (conjugate acid; Equation 2).

$$2.\quad \underset{\text{nonionized base}}{\overset{|}{\underset{/\ \backslash}{N:}}} + H^+ \overset{K_a}{\rightleftharpoons} \underset{\text{ionized cation (conjugate acid)}}{\overset{|}{\underset{/\ \backslash}{NH^+}}}$$

The position of equilibrium depends upon the dissociation constant (K_a) of the conjugate acid and on the local hydrogen ion concentration (Equation 3). Thus,

$$3.\ K_a = \frac{[H^+][\text{base}]}{[\text{conjugate acid}]}$$

where the square brackets indicate concentration or, more properly, activity. By rearranging and taking logarithms the familiar Henderson–Hasselbalch equation (Equation 4) can be obtained.

$$4.\ pK_a = pH - \log\frac{[\text{base}]}{[\text{conjugate acid}]}$$

where pK_a is defined, by analogy to pH, as the negative logarithm of the acid dissociation constant. Inspection of Equation 4 will also show that the pK_a is equal to the pH at which the local anesthetic is 50 per cent ionized.

The pK_a values of the common local anesthetics are all greater than physiological pH values, which means that the drugs will exist in the body predominantly in the ionized form (see Table 3-1). Procaine has the highest pK_a (8.9) and thus has a very small percentage of lipid-soluble, nonionized form present at physiological pH, which probably explains its poor spreading qualities. Tetracaine (pK_a, 8.5) has similarly poor ability to penetrate lipid barriers and is completely effective, in safe concentration, only when it is used by subarachnoid injection or very close to neural tissue.

Ionization is important to the solubility and activity of local anesthetics and their equilibrium distribution in various body compartments. Since the ionized forms are more water soluble than the free bases, the drugs are dispensed as their hydrochloride salts in acidic solutions. In contrast, since the free base forms are more lipid soluble, the nonionized fraction becomes essential for the passage of the agents through lipoprotein diffusion barriers to the site of action on the nerve membrane. Decreasing ionization by alkalization will effectively raise the initial concentration gradient of diffusible drug, thereby increasing rate of drug transfer and decreasing the latent period of a nerve block. Once at the nerve membrane, ionization is again necessary for complete anesthetic activity.[182] The aqueous phases on either side of many body membranes differ in their values of pH. Consequently, although nonionized drug concentrations in these phases will be the same at equilibrium, more or less ionized, and therefore total drug, will be present on one side, depending upon the pH gradient. For a weak base, the equilibrium ratio (R) of total drug concentration across the membrane is given by Equation 5. Thus,

$$5.\ R = \frac{1 + 10^{pK_a - pH_1}}{1 + 10^{pK_a - pH_2}}$$

where the subscripts 1 and 2 refer to the two aqueous compartments. Total drug concentration will be greater in the compartment having the lower pH. Thus, for example, lowered pH due to infection in tissues that surround a nerve results in less nonionized drug, which is the form capable of crossing the axonal membrane (see also Chap. 2).

Protein-Binding. Besides being more lipid soluble, the longer-acting local anesthetics also exhibit higher degrees of protein binding (Table 3-1). This suggests that the binding forces are predominantly hydrophobic. However, since a consistent relationship between partition coefficient and binding is not apparent, electronic or steric features might also contribute to differences in binding (Table 3-1).

Adsorption of local anesthetics to binding sites within membranes or tissues, while producing relatively high apparent partition coefficients, may also result in slower penetration rates. This may be considered either as a reduction in diffusion coefficient or as a decrease in Δc, the effective concentration gradient of diffusible drug. However, it should be remembered that some local anesthetic action (*e.g.*, that of benzocaine) may be due to "membrane expansion" following entry of local anesthetic into the axonal membrane. Binding of the drugs to proteins associated with the aqueous phases on either side of a membrane will affect the transfer and equilibrium distribution of total drug, analogously to ionization. Only the unbound drug will readily diffuse, and, again, this will modify net drug transfer rate by an influence on Δc.

At equilibrium, the concentration of unbound, nonionized drug will be the same on either side of the membrane, but total drug concentrations will differ, depending upon the relative capacities of the binding sites associated with the two aqueous phases and the *p*H values of these phases.[191]

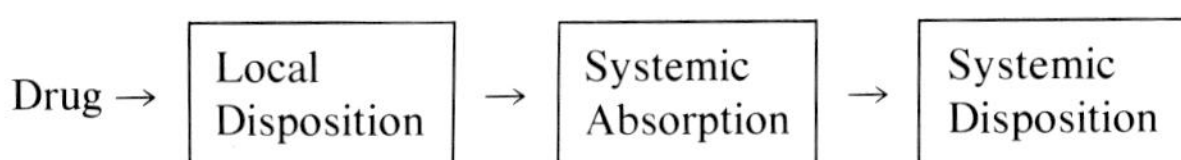

On the basis of understanding the different structures and physicochemical properties of important local anesthetics and some of the expected consequences of these differences, it is possible to inquire more specifically into their absorption and disposition in the various parts of the body. In doing so, the fate of the agents is best divided into a consideration of their *local disposition,* their *systemic absorption,* and their *systemic disposition.* The term *disposition* has a special meaning; it collectively refers to the processes of drug distribution into and out of tissues and drug elimination by excretion and metabolism, while specifically excluding the process of absorption into the bloodstream.

LOCAL DISPOSITION

In contrast to many drugs, the primary effects of local anesthetics at both a pharmacologic level (neural blockade) and at the clinical level (analgesia and anesthesia) can be measured fairly objectively. The anesthesiologist is particularly concerned with the onset, spread, quality, and duration of nerve block. Ultimately, however, these variables are dependent upon the distribution and dissipation of the drugs at the site of injection. Therefore, it would be valuable to have chemical measurements of the agents at these sites as a function of time in order to establish relationships between dose and effects. Regrettably, such data are quite sparse, even from animals. Therefore, knowledge of the local disposition, or neurokinetics, of local anesthetics remains largely theoretical and on the basis of spatiotemporal changes in anesthetic effect rather than direct measurements of intra- and perineural drug concentrations.

Factors that affect local disposition of local anesthetics include dispersion by bulk flow of the injected solution, diffusion, and binding of the agent. Metabolic breakdown seems less important. Local blood supply is also extremely critical, but this will be discussed in the context of systemic absorption. The relative importance of these factors varies with the actual site of local anesthetic injection. At present, most data on local disposition concern epidural block and brachial plexus block (see Chaps. 8 and 10).

BULK FLOW

The extent of spread of the injected solution might be expected to depend upon its volume, the force (speed) with which it is injected, the size of the injected space, and the physical resistance offered by tissues and fluids.

Bulk flow of local anesthetic solutions has been assessed, at least following peridural injection, using peridurograms and by external counting techniques.[46,53,147] Evaluation of the spread of analgesia may also indicate the extent of bulk flow. However, spread and bulk flow are not necessarily synonymous because spread of effect is also dependent on diffusion and, possibly, local perfusion.

Using peridurograms, Burn and colleagues showed that cervical or upper thoracic spread of solution was more likely with 40-ml than 20-ml lumbar epidural injections.[53] Hence the injection of a large volume of solution would be expected to result in a greater spread of analgesia and a more diffuse, less profound nerve block than the same dose injected in a smaller volume. This has been confirmed for epidural block by Erdemir and colleagues, who showed that an injection of 30 ml of 1 per cent lidocaine produced a significantly higher block than did 10 ml of a 3 per cent solution.[73] However, with concentrations above 1 per cent, the relationship becomes more complex. Bromage has found that the spread and intensity of block become independent of volume, when the concentration is between 2 and 5 per cent (same mass of drug), such that the mass of drug required per spinal segment is constant.[46] This suggests that, below a limiting volume and by discounting other variables, important dispersion of the agent is not influenced by initial bulk flow of the injected solution and probably occurs outside the peridural space.

Neither Burn and associates nor Nishimura and associates could demonstrate any effect of the rate of injection on spread of solutions in the epidural

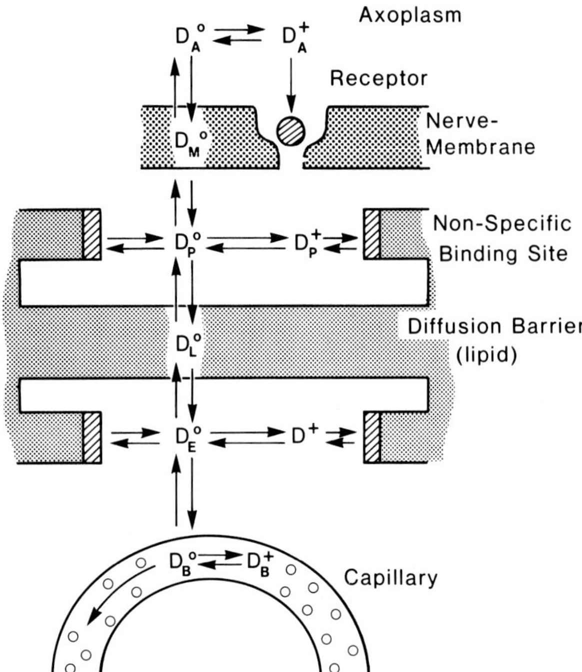

Fig. 3-6. This flowchart depicts the equilibria determining local anesthetic distribution near the site of action. ^{0} indicates uncharged drug; $^+$ indicates charged drug; D_A is drug in axoplasm; D_M is drug in membrane; D_P is drug in the vicinity of the membrane; D_L is drug in diffusion barrier; D_E is drug in extraneural fluid; D_B is drug in blood. (Tucker, G.T., Boyes, R.N., Bridenbaugh, P.O., and Moore, D.C.: Binding of anilide-type local anesthetics in human plasma I. Relationships between binding, physiochemical properties and anesthetic activity. Anesthesiology, *33*:287, 1970)

space.[53,147] In contrast, Erdemir and associates showed that an epidural injection of 20 ml of 2 per cent lidocaine at the rate of 1 ml per second produced a slightly higher spread of analgesia and a 14 per cent shorter duration of motor block than the same solution injected at 1 ml per 3 seconds. The more rapid injection was also accompanied by a greater incidence of incomplete analgesia and more discomfort to the patient.

Increases in the duration and longitudinal spread of epidural anesthesia with increasing age have been assigned to reduced lateral leakage of solution, owing to progressive sclerotic closure of the paravertebral foramina.[46] This is supported by the finding of increased residual peridural pressure after injection in older people, evidence from perildurograms, and more extensive cephalad spread shown by an external counting method.[46,147] However, the data of Burn and colleagues suggest that factors other than bulk flow are also responsible for enhanced vertical spread of analgesia in the elderly.[53] Although using 20 ml lumbar injections, they found evidence of reduced lateral spread of solution with age, this was not seen with 40 ml of solution, and when there was less lateral spread, it was not necessarily accompanied by greater longitudinal flow.

DIFFUSION

Once the local anesthetic has been deposited and physically spread in the extraneural fluids, it finds its way to sites of action in and on the nerve membrane by the process of diffusion. At various points along the way, nonspecific binding sites and *p*H differences will alter the rate and extent of this progression (Fig. 3-6). Specific factors involved depend upon physiologic aspects and upon drug-related characteristics, such as concentration, solution *p*H, and physicochemical properties.

Physiologic Factors

Inspection of Figure 3-6 shows that physiologic factors can be considered as diffusion to and from the nerve (extraneural), diffusion in and out of the nerve (neural), and diffusion within the nerve fiber (axonal).

Extraneural Diffusion. In most peripheral nerve block procedures and in subarachnoid block, the pathway taken by the local anesthetic to the neural surface is relatively short and uncomplicated. However, in epidural block, intradural spinal roots and spinal nerves in the paravertebral spaces are readily contacted (by leakage through the foramina), while translocation of drug by other routes to more remote sites also contributes to the block (see Chap. 8).

Binding Sites. Much of the dose of local anesthetic may be temporarily sequestered in extraneural tissues at the site of injection. The extent of this non-neural "binding," which may involve adsorption on proteins or simple solution in lipids, will depend upon the route of administration.

The "naked" nerves in the subarchnoid space contrast with the "overcoats" of fat provided for them in the epidural space. Binding may have two effects. By reducing the amount of agent free to diffuse onto the nerves, it effectively lowers clinical potency. On the other hand, by providing depots from which drug is slowly dissociated to maintain anesthetic concentrations in the nerve, it could prolong duration of block. High tissue binding also offers protection against systemic toxicity.

Neural Diffusion. Once at the surface of the nerve, there are a number of intraneural diffusion barriers before the local anesthetic can reach the individual nerve fibers. These barriers are broadly related to the anatomical layers of the nerve. The size of the nerve and the distribution of its fiber bundles are also critical factors (see Chap. 2).

Barriers. In peripheral nerve, Kristerson and colleagues showed that the epineural sheath is not a significant obstacle to the entry of radiolabeled mepivacaine and, presumably therfore, of other agents.[103] Removal of the sheath increases the potency of lidocaine, but this is probably due to the release of the tightly packed epineurium, which is normally a more formidable barrier.[106,160] The presence of fatty tissues in the epineurium of some nerves (*e.g.*, the sciatic nerve) may have an effect similar to that of extraneural binding sites. A greater proportion of connective tissue in the nerves of elderly people may also serve a depot function and contribute to the greater duration of neural blockade in the elderly, although other factors are probably of greater significance.[46,82] Capillaries and lymphatics in the epineurium presumably assist in removing drug from the nerve.

The fibroelastic perineurium and particularly the perilemma seem to constitute the main barrier to diffusion of drugs in the nerve.[103,106]

Spinal nerve roots differ from peripheral nerves in that they lack perineurium and much of the fibrous support provided by the epineurium and sheath. Consequently, onset of anesthesia is particularly rapid, and patients usually report an immediate feeling of warmth after subarachnoid injection of local anesthetics. The nerve coverings, missing from the roots, appear again as the dura which continues peripherally as the epineurium of the spinal nerves and the pia arachnoid, which is continuous with the perilemma of peripheral nerves.

The mechanism of epidural block involves translocation of local anesthetic along neural pathways. Thus, there are various routes for drug transfer from the epidural to the subarachnoid space to produce block of the spinal roots and the periphery of the cord: by direct diffusion across the dura, by diffusion and bulk flow through the arachnoid villi at the dural root sleeves, and by centripetal subperineural and subpial spread from the remote paravertebral nerve trunks. The evidence for the involvement of each of these routes has been reviewed by Bromage and is considered in detail in Chapter 8.[43,46]

Nerve Diameter and Distribution of Fibers. In vitro experiments with frog sciatic nerve indicate that the time until onset of block increases with an increase in nerve diameter.[22] It may be presumed, therefore, that diffusion from mantle to core takes longer in nerves of larger diameter. This probably explains, for example, why the relatively large S1 root is difficult to block after epidural injection, and delay of onset of block is observed in the corresponding dermatome.[46,82] Recovery from block should also be more rapid in thicker nerves. Clearly, mantle fibers will be blocked more readily and rapidly than those in the core of the nerve. Mantle fibers also innervate more proximal regions, which accounts for the observed outward progression of certain peripheral nerve blocks; hence, following injection of local anesthetic into the brachial plexus, the block proceeds from upper arm to hand and then to fingers.[62] In order to explain why the onset of motor block often precedes that of sensory loss after brachial plexus injection, Winnie and colleagues have suggested that the effect of the larger diameter of the motor fibers is offset by their more peripheral location in the median nerve, compared to sensory fibers.[208] According to the classical view, the sequence of recovery should be the same as that of onset, namely, arm first, then hand and fingers.[62] This follows if the concentration gradient within the nerve now becomes reversed, decreasing from core to mantle. However, this has been challenged by Winnie and associates, who observed the reverse order of recovery with significant motor block that outlasted sensory block.[209] To account for these findings, it was proposed that a more rapid vascular uptake of agent occurs near the more distally innervating sensory fibers located in the core of the nerve. As intraneural blood vessels pass from mantle to core, they become increasingly branched, exposing a progressively larger surface area for absorption. Hence, vascular absorption will be faster from the vicinity of sensory fibers than from that of more peripheral motor fibers.

Axonal Diffusion. The facility with which local anesthetic molecules hit their ultimate targets on the nerve membrane is dependent upon the distribution, density, and accessibility of the sodium channels along and around the nerve fibers. Important physical factors include the diameter of the axon, its degree of myelinization, and the internodal distances.

It is reasoned that if the number of ion transfers per unit volume of axon is constant and since the ratio of volume to surface area increases with fiber diameter, then a higher concentration of anesthetic should be required to block the greater number of

Table 3-2. Classification and Physiologic Characteristics of Nerve Fibers

Class	*A-alpha*	*A-beta*	*A-gamma*	*A-delta*	*B*	*C*
Function	Motor	Touch/pressure	Proprioception	Pain/temperature	Preganglionic autonomic (sympathetic)	Pain/temperature
Myelin	+++	++	++	++	+	–
Diameter (μ)	12–20	5–12	5–12	1–4	1–3	0.5–1
Conduction speed (m/sec)	70–120	30–70	30–70	12–30	14.8*	1.2
Onset time	0 ←	0 ←	0 ←	0 ←	0 →	0
Regression	Reverse of onset time (note some exceptions with long-acting agents, *e.g.*, etidocaine sympathetic block offset before sensory)†					
C_m (Parallels onset time)		Highest			Lowest	

Key. +++: heavily-myelinated ++: moderately-myelinated +: lightly-myelinated –: nonmyelinated
* Faster onset than smaller C fibers because C fibers are grouped together in less accessible "Remak bundles."
† Data from Bromage, P. R.: Physiology and pharmacology of epidural analgesia. Anesthesiology, *28*:592, 1967.
(Data from de Jong, R. H., and Nace, R. A.: Nerve impulse conduction during intravenous lidocaine injection. Anesthesiology, *29*:22, 1968; Heavner, J. E., and de Jong, R. H.: Lidocaine blocking concentrations for B- and C-nerve fibers. Anesthesiology, *40*:228, 1974; Scurlock, J. E., Heavner, J. E., and de Jong, R. H.: Differential B and C fibre block by an amide- and an ester-linked local anaesthetic. Br. J. Anaesth., *47*:1135, 1975).

sodium channels per unit surface area of a larger nerve fiber.

Myelinization increases fiber diameter and the length of the diffusion pathway to the membrane and probably serves as a nonspecific binding site for local anesthetic molecules. It is also associated with a nodal concentration of the sodium channels. Furthermore, since internodal distances increase with axon diameter, the probability of any single local anesthetic molecule (in a given concentration and volume of solution) finding a receptor is smaller with a large myelinated fiber (see Fig. 2-5).

Although some experimental evidence does suggest a direct relationship between minimal anesthetic concentration (C_m) and fiber size and myelinization, the relative resistance to blockade of the small, nonmyelinated postganglionic C fibers is anomalous in this respect (Table 3-2).[89,141,167] However, these fibers are grouped together in so-called Remak bundles, which make them less readily accessible.

The data in Table 3-2 have several clinical implications. Increased skin temperature may be the first clinical sign of onset of epidural or spinal blockade (B fibers), and this is followed by loss of pain/temperature sensation (A-delta, then C). However, at this stage A-gamma fibers (proprioception) may still be unblocked, and the appreciation of movement may be interpreted as discomfort. Certainly, touch and pressure (A-beta) are often not completely blocked, and some patients are unhappy about feeling any sensation.

Most of the short-acting agents (*e.g.*, lidocaine, mepivacaine) progressively block sympathetic, sensory, and motor fibers after epidural or spinal injection.

In contrast, some of the long acting agents (notably bupivacaine, and etidocaine) may show sensory-motor dissociation.[108] Bupivacaine usually behaves as expected; the highest concentrations are required to produce adequate motor block. On the other hand, etidocaine is capable of blocking motor fibers (A-alpha) at quite low concentrations, while pain fibers (A-beta) remain incompletely blocked.

Drug Factors

Concentration. As represented by Fick's law (Equation 1), diffusion simplifies to a first-order process. This means that at any given time the rate

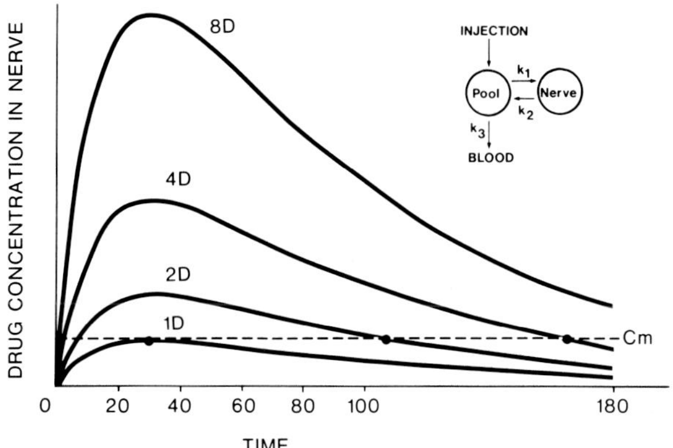

Fig. 3-7. Theoretical concentrations of local anesthetic in a nerve as a function of dose, assuming the agent enters and leaves the nerve by simple diffusion and that the minimum blocking concentration (C_m) is independent of dose (*k* terms are first-order rate constants; 1D is unit dose; 2D is twice unit dose, etc.).

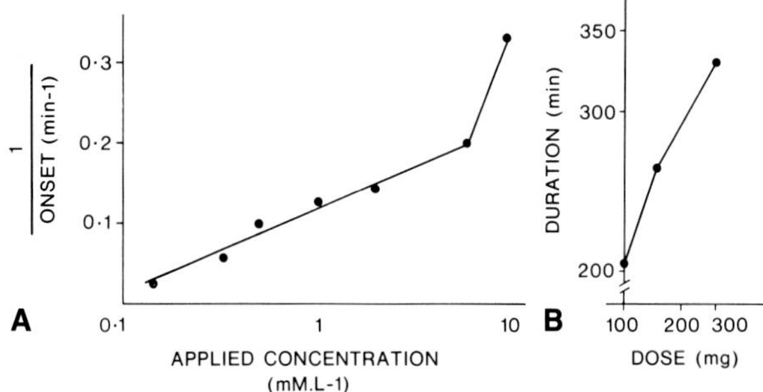

Fig. 3-9. (*A*) Observed relationship between time to 99 per cent disappearance of the A-alpha potential of frog sciatic nerve and applied concentration of lidocaine base. (Data from Rud, J.: Local Anaesthetics: An electrophysiological investigation of local anaesthesia of peripheral nerves, with special reference to lidocaine. Acta Physiol. Scand., *51*[*Suppl. 178*]:7, 1961; and de Jong, R.: Physiology and Pharmacology of Local Anesthesia. Springfield, Il., Charles C Thomas, 1970) (*B*) Observed relationship between duration of peridural block in humans and dose of etidocaine. (Lund, P.C., and Cwik, J.C., and Gannon, R.T.: Etidocaine (Duranest): A clinical and laboratory evaluation. Acta Anesthesiol. Scand., *18*:176, 1974)

of change of drug concentration in a "compartment", (*e.g.*, a nerve) is proportional to the concentration in that compartment. Thus, a simple model of diffusion of local anesthetics in and out of the nerve can be devised, as shown in Figure 3-7. By defining a C_m above which conduction is completely blocked, theoretical relationships between onset and duration of block and dose or applied concentration can be evaluated.

The onset time of blockade is usually much shorter than duration of anesthesia because initial concentration gradients are greater, and binding delays egress of drug from the nerve (*i.e.*, $k_1 > k_2$ in Fig. 3-7).

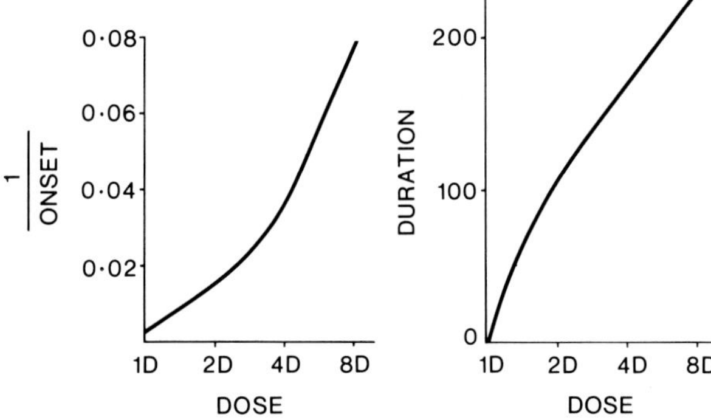

Fig. 3-8. The theoretical relationships between time to complete block and duration of nerve block and dose of local anesthetic. (Derived from intercepts of concentration-time profiles with the C_m value shown in Fig. 3-7.)

As shown in Figure 3-8, the model predicts that at higher doses the reciprocal of onset time becomes directly proportional to the logarithm of dose. Experimental data consistent with this profile are plotted in Figure 3-9. As dose is increased, a linear relationship develops between duration of anesthesia and logarithm of dose (Fig. 3-8). The dose-dependency of epidural block produced by etidocaine in humans agrees with the theoretical relationship, although other factors (saturation binding and vasomotor effects) not considered in the simple model may also be involved (Fig. 3-9).

Figure 3-10 shows the duration of anesthesia predicted by the model for a multiple-dose regimen, each dose being the same and given at the time when the neural drug concentration has returned to the C_m value. The relationship observed experimentally is more complex, however, since a form of tachyphylaxis may develop with progressive dosage.[50]

Physicochemical Properties. Among the agents in clinical use, increases in lipid solubility and affinity for neural and extraneural tissues are associated with prolongation of the duration of nerve block at equiactive concentrations both *in vitro* and *in vivo* (Table 3-1). This probably reflects the diminished concentration gradient out of the nerve that accompanies a greater tissue solubility. Thus, observed differences in the concentrations of etidocaine and

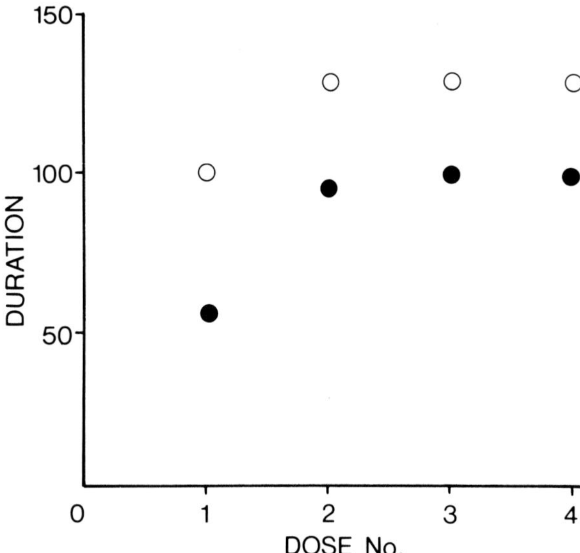

Fig. 3-10. Theoretical relationship between duration of anesthesia after successive equal doses given when blockade has regressed completely. (Constructed from the 2D dose profile of Fig. 3-7, assuming the same C_m [●] and a C_m 1.7 times higher [○])

lidocaine in the epidural fat and neural tissues of sheep at 12 hours after epidural injection of the agents are entirely consistent with differences in their physicochemical properties and duration of action (Fig. 3-11). Factors other than physicochemical characteristics may also be important, however, as indicated by studies of the action of the stereoisomers of the experimental agent RAD 109 on isolated nerves. Although the isomers have similar physicochemical properties and rates of washout from the nerve, the rates of return of action potential are quite different for each isomer.[9]

Physicochemical properties and the onset of clinical anesthesia are not necessarily related. A high lipid solubility and tissue affinity might be expected to retard diffusion onto nerve receptor sites by the impedance offered by nonspecific binding. This, together with low dosage, could explain the relatively slow onset of bupivacaine and tetracaine.[44,48] In contrast to these agents, etidocaine is rapidly acting yet has an even greater lipid solubility (Table 3-1).

A similar anomaly occurs with the phenomenon of sensory-motor dissociation. Etidocaine and tetracaine appear to be more effective than bupivacaine in blocking motor function, whereas the reverse is true for the relief of pain.[46] These differences have been explained on the basis of differences in the relative affinities of the drugs for motor and sensory nerve fibers.[108] However, experimental evidence for this is lacking. An alternative explanation may come from recent evidence of frequency-dependent conduction block (see Chap. 2 and 4).

The loss of lower limb reflexes in patients who receive high thoracic epidural blocks with etidocaine led Bromage to suggest that penetration of the cord and interference with long descending pathways contribute to the profound motor blockade seen with this agent.[45] Thus, he suggested that agents with high lipid solubilities will penetrate to greater depths and produce more profound block. However, as stated, this hypothesis is inadequate since both bupivacaine and etidocaine are highly lipid soluble. Furthermore, the sensory-motor dissociation seen with these agents is also manifest after peripheral nerve block procedures in which penetration of the cord is not a factor.[108,152]

pH Effects. Any factor that creates local extracellular acidosis will retard net diffusion of local anesthetic to the nerve by increasing drug ionization (see Equation 4). A low *p*H may be preexisting, for example, as a result of infection, or it may be induced by injection of the anesthetic solution. Likely effects of the injection on local *p*H have been reviewed by Rowland, and the mechanisms suggested are indicated in the following list.

Mechanisms for Lowering Local Extracellular *p*H by Local Anesthetic Solutions

Movement of intracellular carbon dioxide into solutions deficient in carbon dioxide

Dilution of local bicarbonate stores by large volumes of solution

Use of acidic solutions
- To dissolve agents as their salts (*p*H 5–7)
- To stabilize ester-type agents
- To stabilize added epinephrine with addition of sodium bisulfite (*p*H 3–4)

Effect of added epinephrine, causing local ischemia and increased cellular metabolism

(Data from Rowland, M: Local anesthetic absorption, distribution and elimination. *In* Eger, E. (ed.): Anesthetic Uptake and Action. pp. 332–366. Baltimore, Williams and Wilkins, 1974)

Of these, movement of carbon dioxide is probably fleeting; dilution of local bicarbonate stores is readily avoided; acidic solutions are rapidly counteracted by the buffer capacity of most tissues; and stabilizers may be circumvented by adding concen-

Table 3-3. **pH *of Cerebrospinal Fluid Following Subarachnoid Injection of Local Anesthetic Solutions in the Dog***

Time After Injection (min)	*10% Dextrose in Saline Control* (p*H, 5.5*)	*5% Lidocaine Hydrochloride + 7.5% Dextrose* (p*H, 4.5*)	*0.75% Etidocaine Hydrochloride + 5% Dextrose* (p*H, 4.2*)	*2% Procaine Hydrochloride* (p*H, 4.2*)	*4% Tetracaine Hydrochloride* (p*H, 4.2*)
0	7.41	7.34	7.40	7.36	7.37
2	7.26	6.10	6.20	6.40	6.80
5	7.36	6.40	6.89	6.74	6.93
15		6.90	7.24	7.23	7.10
30		7.10	7.27	7.32	7.21

(Based on unpublished data from Mather, L. E., Pavlin, E., and Middaugh, M., 1975)

trated epinephrine prior to the injection, rather than using a premixed acidic solution. The importance of vasoconstrictor and metabolic effects of epinephrine is indicated by the observation that whereas injection of a local anesthetic solution of *p*H of 3 lowers tissue *p*H below 7 for 45 minutes, a solution of the same *p*H, containing epinephrine (1:40,000), may maintain this level of tissue acidosis for 150 to 250 minutes. Despite these considerations, however, the literature contains little evidence to suggest that the addition of epinephrine significantly prolongs the onset of clinical nerve block. In fact, when epinephrine is added to etidocaine solutions at the time of injection, the opposite is true.[41,142]

Cohen and colleagues have suggested that acidosis could explain the development of tachyphylaxis to local anesthetics during multidose subarachnoid and epidural block.[59] They showed that repeated spinal injections of local anesthetic solutions in the dog resulted in a progressive fall in the *p*H of poorly buffered cerebrospinal fluid from 7.4 to 6.8. This has been confirmed by others after single doses and would be accompanied by a reduction in the fraction of nonionized agent and hence should decrease access of drug to the site of action (Table 3-3).

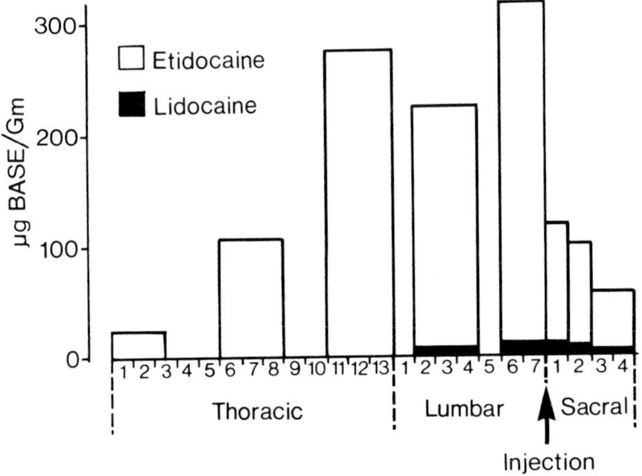

Fig. 3-11. Mean local anesthetic concentrations in peridural fat of sheep at 12 hours after peridural injection. Dose is 80 mg etidocaine hydrochloride and 50 mg lidocaine hydrochloride and 50 μg epinephrine; n is 6. (Unpublished data from Lebeaux, M., and Tucker, G.T.)

However, other data on *p*H effects suggest some contradictions. In sheep, duration of motor block after subarachnoid injections of lidocaine was longer when the *p*H of the solution was decreased from 6.5 to 4.5, although sensory blockade showed the expected opposite trend.[5]

Replacement of the hydrochloride salt solution of local anesthetic by carbonated solutions should obviate movement of carbon dioxide out of the nerve. In contrast, rapid penetration of carbon dioxide into the nerve to cause a lowering of intraneural *p*H could promote a more rapid production of active ionized drug species at the point where it is needed. Clinically, carbonated solutions of local anesthetics have indeed provided a more rapid and more profound block than comparable hydrochloride solutions (see Chap. 2).[13,47,163]

METABOLISM

When procaine is incubated with nerve tissue, it is hydrolyzed only to the extent of 1.2- to 4 per cent per hour, which can largely be accounted for by nonenzymatic breakdown.[148,172] Hydrolysis of ester-type agents in the vicinity of the nerve also seems to be slow since addition of a cholinesterase inhibitor to chloroprocaine solution did not prolong blockade.[109] Significant local metabolic alteration of the amide-type agents is even more unlikely because they are susceptible to the mixed-function oxidase system found predominantly in the liver (see below). The evidence suggests, therefore, that local metabolism has a negligible influence on the neurokinetics of local anesthetics and the time-course of conduction blockade.

SYSTEMIC ABSORPTION

A knowledge of the rates of systemic absorption of local anesthetics helps to set confidence limits on the likelihood of systemic toxic reactions following the various block procedures. Indirectly, these rates also suggest the relationship between blockade and the amount of drug remaining at the site of injection.

In humans, measurement of drug concentration-time profiles in the peripheral circulation has been widely used to assess the systemic uptake of the different agents. Since these profiles are the net result of both systemic absorption and disposition processes, they are mainly of value in determining relative changes in systemic drug uptake (*e.g.*, as a result of variation in dose, in route of injection, in concentration and volume of solution, and in kind and concentration of added vasoconstrictor, etc). These variables are usually assumed not to influence disposition kinetics. If blood drug concentration-time profiles are also available for intravenous administration, it then becomes possible to calculate absolute drug absorption rates with the aid of various techniques of pharmacokinetic analysis.[192,196] Measurement of the drug content of venous

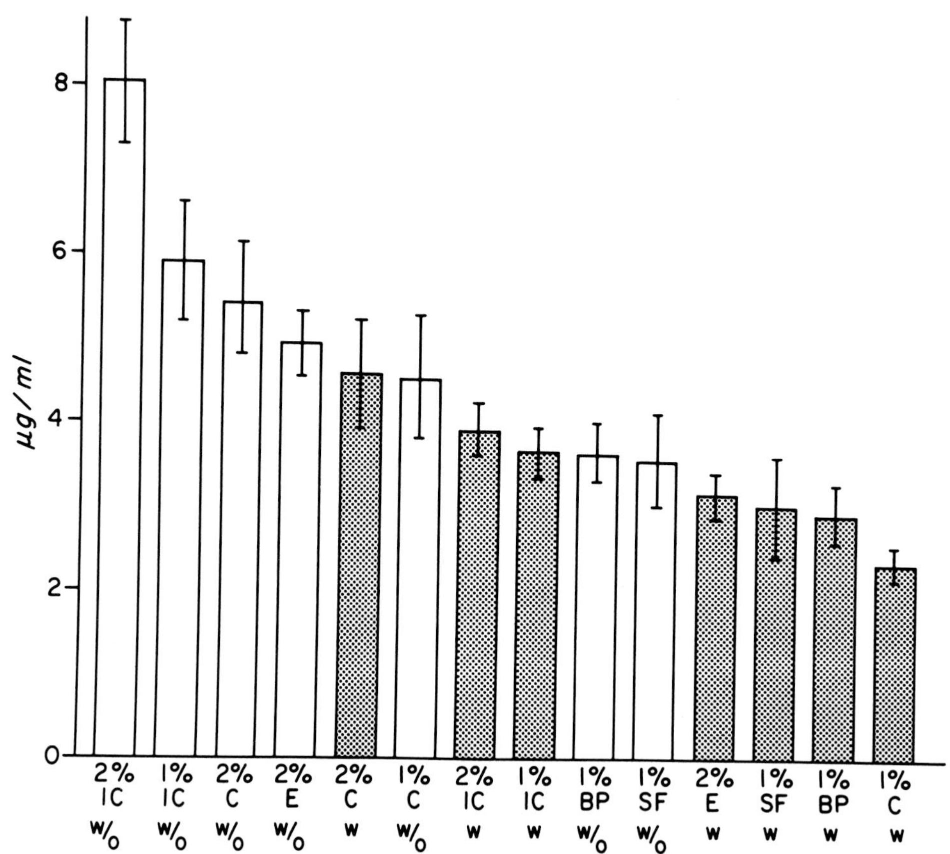

Fig. 3-12. Systemic absorption of mepivacaine in humans after various regional block procedures and the mean maximum plasma drug concentrations. (± S.E.M.) IC is intercostal block; C is caudal block; E is peridural block; BP is brachial plexus block; SF is sciatic/femoral block; w/o is solution without epinephrine; w is plus epinephrine, 1:200,000 (stippled blocks). (Tucker, G.T., Moore, D.C., Bridenbaugh, P.O., Bridenbaugh, L.D., and Thompson, G.E.: Systemic absorption of mepivacaine in commonly used regional block procedures. Anesthesiology, *37*:277, 1972)

blood draining away from the site of injection also has been used to provide estimates of absolute absorption rates.[52,75]

The mechanism of vascular uptake of local anesthetics involves diffusion across the capillary endothelium. It follows, therefore, that absorption will be more rapid if capillary density is high and if capillary diameter is large, since both factors increase the surface area available for transfer (see Equation 1). The increased blood volume in a dilated capillary, as well as factors that affect capillary permeability, will also promote net diffusion by increasing the drug concentration gradient across the membrane. Because diffusion of local anesthetics across the endothelium is probably rapid, uptake will be highly dependent on local blood flow. It will also be promoted if the agent has a high blood/tissue partition coefficient. Specific features of the injection site, of the agent, of the nerve block, and of the pathophysiology of the patient that influence these factors will be of prime importance in determining the absorption rates of local anesthetics.

Site of Injection

Using the same total dose in solution without epinephrine, Tucker and colleagues showed that the absorption rate of mepivacaine after various nerve block procedures decreased in the following order: intercostal block, caudal block, lumbar epidural block, brachial plexus and sciatic-femoral block (Fig. 3-12). Addition of epinephrine complicates this issue, however, and will be discussed below. Nevertheless, regardless of the presence of epinephrine, faster absorption following intercostal injection compared to epidural injection confirmed earlier studies with lidocaine and prilocaine and was substantiated by later studies with etidocaine.[40,165] This difference may be explained partly on the basis of sequestration of drug in epidural fat (producing a relatively low blood/tissue partition coefficient), and by the fact that although the epidural space is highly vascular compared to the intercostal area, most of the vessels traverse it rather than drain it (Fig. 3-11).[35]

Special concern has been expressed over the absorption rate of local anesthetics following cuff release after intravenous regional anesthesia. It has been suggested that cardiovascular collapse following this procedure may be related to sudden washout of a large amount of anesthetic from the blocked arm.[67] However, pharmacokinetic analysis has shown that, if the cuff is correctly inflated for at least 10 minutes after injection, only about 20 to 30 per cent of a dose of lidocaine enters the systemic

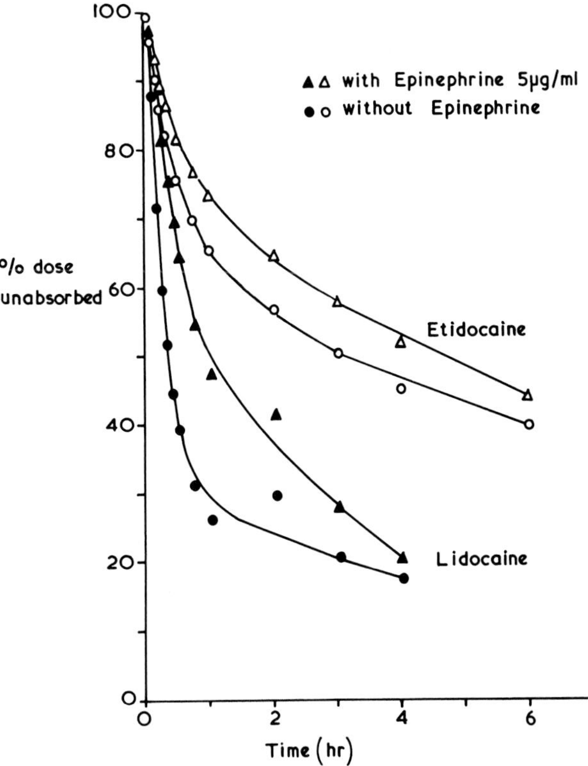

Fig. 3-13. Systemic absorption of etidocaine and lidocaine after peridural injection in humans. (Tucker, G.T., and Mather, L.E.: Pharmacokinetics of local anaesthetic agents. Br. J. Anaesth., *47*:213, 1975)

circulation during the first minute after cuff release, the rest emerging rather slowly with about 50 per cent of the dose still remaining in the arm after 30 minutes. Longer application of the cuff was also shown to result in a slower drug washout after release.[192]

Drug Factors

Physicochemical Properties. It would be reasonable to expect that the greater retention of more lipid-soluble, highly protein-bound agents such as etidocaine and bupivacaine in the fat and tissues of the epidural space should result in slower net systemic absorption compared to agents like lidocaine because they have lower blood/tissue partition coefficients (Fig. 3-11). This has been confirmed in humans by pharmacokinetic analysis of blood drug level data. Thus, Tucker and Mather have shown that the systemic uptake of amide-type agents after epidural injection is a biphasic process (Fig. 3-13).[196] The contribution of the initial rapid phase

Table 3-4. Epidural Doses of Local Anesthetics for Surgical Anesthesia and Maximum Whole Blood Concentrations in Relation to Toxic Threshold Concentrations

Agent	*Concentration (%)*	*Epinephrine (+, added; −, without)*	*Dose**	*Average C_{Max} (blood in µg/ml)*	*Approximate C_{Tox}† (blood in µg/ml)*	$\frac{C_{Tox}}{C_{Max}}$
Lidocaine	2	−	400	2.9	5–6	1.9
		+	500	2.4	5–6	2.3
Mepivacaine	2	−	400	3.5	5–6	1.6
		+	500	3.4	5–6	1.7
Bupivacaine	0.5–0.75	{+ / −	150‡	0.7	1.6	2.3
Etidocaine	1	{+ / −	200	0.6	2	3.3

* Usual maximum dose in premedicated but conscious patients
† Approximate threshold for moderate effects (intravenous infusion); blood concentrations refer to venous data
‡ Recent studies indicate that higher doses of bupivacaine (225 mg) may be used, provided direct vascular injection is carefully avoided.
(Tucker, G. T., and Mather, L. E.: Pharmacokinetics of local anesthetic agents. Br. J. Anaesth., *47*:213, 1975)

to overall absorption is greater with lidocaine than with the long-acting analogues.[121,177]

Slower net absorption of etidocaine and bupivacaine is of considerable significance for systemic safety of the agents. Differences in average maximum blood concentrations of etidocaine and bupivacaine compared to those of lidocaine and mepivacaine after usual epidural doses are greater than the differences in dosage (Table 3-4). This is due largely to differences in absorption rate and means that in relation to blood concentrations associated with toxicity, the margins of systemic safety of the long-acting, agents are certainly no worse than those of the short-acting drugs (as indicated by C_{Tox}/C_{Max} values in Table 3-4).

Vascular Activity. Although differences in absorption rates of various local anesthetics can be related to local binding influenced by physicochemical properties, an additional factor must be considered, namely, their effects on local blood flow. Local anesthetics are capable of modifying local perfusion, and hence their own absorption, by direct action on blood vessels at the site of injection and also indirectly, once absorbed, by causing changes in cardiovascular dynamics.

At a local level, the agents appear to have ambivalent effects, that may be concentration-dependent.[14] Vasodilatation is readily demonstrated, for example, by the increase in limb blood flow following intra-arterial injection (Table 3-5).[27] On this basis, bupivacaine and etidocaine are seen to produce more profound and prolonged effects than anesthetically less potent analogues. However, Aberg and Dhuner have shown that this vasodilatory effect may be converted to a vasoconstriction in some vascular beds, particularly in the presence of a low tone of the vascular smooth muscle.[3] Direct vasoconstrictor effects have also been demonstrated with isolated vessel preparations. For example, Blair has shown that the ability to produce a contractile response on isolated rat portal vein decreases in the following order: mepivacaine, prilocaine, procaine, lidocaine, tetracaine, bupivacaine, and etidocaine.[27] In contrast, and in agreement with

Table 3-5. Mean Percentage Increase in Femoral Artery Blood Flow in Dogs after Intra-arterial Injection of Local Anesthetics

*Agent**	*Minutes After Injection* 1	5
Bupivacaine	45.4	30.0
Etidocaine	44.3	26.6
Prilocaine	42.1	6.3
Tetracaine	37.6	14.0
Mepivacaine	35.7	9.5
Lidocaine	25.8	7.5

* Each agent injected rapidly in a dose of 1 mg in 0.1 ml of saline
(Data from Blair, M. R.: Cardiovascular pharmacology of local anaesthetics. Br. J. Anaesth., *47* [*Suppl.*]:247, 1975)

Table 3-6. Effect of Epinephrine on Maximum Plasma or Blood Concentrations of Local Anesthetics in Patients After Various Nerve Block Procedures

Agent	Block	Dose	Concentration (%)	Epinephrine Concentration ($\mu g/ml$)	Maximum Plasma or Blood Concentration ($\mu g/base/ml$)		Per Cent Reduction by Epinephrine	Sample Source (V, venous plasma, A, arterial plasma)
					Without Epinephrine	With Epinephrine		
Lidocaine	Epidural[35,36,165]	400 mg	2	12.5	4.3	3.1	28	V
	Epidural[35]	400 mg	2	5	4.3	2.9	31	V
	Epidural[166]	400 mg	2	5	3.2	2.1	34	A
	Intercostal[166]	400 mg	2	12.5	6.5	4.9	25	A
	Intercostal[166]	400 mg	2	5	6.5	5.3	19	A
Prilocaine	Epidural[166]	400 mg	2	12.5	2.7	2.2	16	A
	Epidural[166]	400 mg	2	5	2.7	2.2	17	A
	Epidural[166]	600 mg	2	5	4.9	2.4	50	A
	Epidural[112]	600 mg	2, 3	5	4.1	1.7	57	V
	Epidural[112]	900 mg	2, 3	5	5.2	3.2	38	V
	Intercostal[35,36,165]	400 mg	2	12.5	4.5	2.8	37	V
	Intercostal[165]	400 mg	2	5	4.5	3.6	19	V
Mepivacaine	Epidural[123]	6 mg/kg	2	5	1.3	1.3	3	V
	Brachial plexus[123]	6 mg/kg	2	5	2.1	1.5	28	V
	Brachial plexus[65]	5 mg/kg	2	5	1.99	1.61	19	V
Bupivacaine	Epidural[206]	150 mg	0.5	5	1.3	1.1	9	V
	Epidural[1]	100 mg	0.5	5	0.8	0.7	12	V
	Paracervical[92,93]	100 mg	0.5	5	0.7	0.2	70	V
	Paracervical[19]	50 mg	0.25	5	1.1	0.5	50	V
Etidocaine	Epidural[40,41,114]	200 mg	1	5	1.5	1.3	17	V
	Epidural[1,114]	200 mg	1	5	1.0	0.7	30	V
	Epidural[110]	300 mg	1	5	1.3	1.2	10	V
	Intercostal[40,41]	300 mg	1	5	2.7	2.3	15	A
	Intercostal[66]	100 mg	0.5	5	0.8	0.6	25	V

the results of limb blood flow experiments, etidocaine and bupivacaine were the most potent of these agents in relaxing norepinephrine-contracted veins.[27] Extrapolation of these findings to the response of blood vessels at sites of regional block is difficult. However, the evidence does suggest that of the available agents, bupivacaine and etidocaine are most likely to produce vasodilatation, and mepivacaine and prilocaine are most likely to produce a vasoconstriction. If this is so, the relatively prolonged absorption of the long-acting agents after epidural injection must more likely be a function of their local binding than of their vascular activity (Fig. 3-13).

Although differences in vascular activity do not necessarily account for differences in the relative absorption of agents, this activity has been shown to be of absolute importance as a determinant of drug uptake and duration of effect, particularly after local infiltration. The evidence for this comes largely from studies with optical isomers. For example, L(+)-prilocaine, D(+)-mepivacaine, and L(−)-bupivacaine exhibit considerably longer durations of action in some systems *in vivo* than their enantiomorphs or the DL-forms.[2,4,8,11] The fact that this phenomenon is not seen in isolated nerve preparations and that differences in systemic uptake of isomers is less marked when blood flow is stopped indicates that the vascular activity of the agents is stereoselective. For clinical purposes, the effect of tissue binding and vascular reactivity on peak plasma concentrations depends on the agent employed. Thus, vascular regulation of absorption may be a more important factor for the short-acting agents such as lidocaine and prilocaine. For the long-acting agents such as bupivacaine, tissue binding has predominance (Table 3-6).

Changes in local perfusion pressure caused by systemically mediated effects of local anesthetics may also influence their absorption. Below a threshold associated with convulsions and myocardial depression, which would decrease local perfusion, the systemic presence of local anesthetics causes an increase in cardiac output and mean arterial pressure, which might improve local perfusion.[27,31,95] The mechanism of these cardiovascular effects is probably a combination of an evoked increase in sympathetic activity in the central nervous system (CNS) and the direct venoconstrictor action mentioned previously.

Concentration and Volume. If dosage is kept constant, does changing the volume and concentration of the injected solution make any difference to drug absorption rates? The answer to this depends upon the agent and the volume and concentration employed. Inspection of Figure 3-12 shows that maximum plasma concentrations of mepivacaine are higher after caudal and intercostal injections of 25 ml of 2-per-cent solutions than after injection of 50 ml of 1-per-cent solutions.

In contrast, epidural injection of 400 mg of lidocaine as 20 ml of 2-per-cent or 40 ml of 1-per-cent solution produced identical maximum plasma drug levels, although decreasing the volume to 10 ml (4%) did result in significantly higher levels.[35] Lund and colleagues found no significant difference between plasma levels of etidocaine after epidural administration of 150 mg as 30 ml of 0.5-per-cent solution or as 20 ml of 0.75-per-cent solution. When 20 ml of 1.5-per-cent solution was used, proportionately higher maximum levels were achieved compared to the use of 30 ml of 1-per-cent solution.[110] This second difference was not, however, observed by others.[40] Initial plasma concentrations of lidocaine following cuff release after intravenous regional anesthesia were greater when 20 ml of 1-per-cent solution was used than when 40 ml of 0.5-per-cent solution was used.[192]

These data suggest that up to a point the greater surface area available for absorption that results from more extensive spread of a dilute solution is counteracted by the higher concentration gradient offered for absorption by a more concentrated solution. One explanation for the greater absorption rate seen when concentration is increased is that local binding sites become progressively more saturated, making a disproportionately greater amount of drug available for absorption and disproportionately less available for anesthetic activity. Alternatively, greater vasodilatation produced by more concentrated solutions could account for enhanced uptake. Both of these mechanisms should also result in disproportionate increases in plasma drug levels when concentration and mass of drug are increased but volume is kept constant. Unfortunately, the plasma drug level data available on this point are limited. Plasma concentrations increase linearly with dose, up to a 300 mg epidural dose (constant volume) of etidocaine, but beyond this, concentrations do indeed become disproportionately higher.[40,110]

Speed of Injection. Scott and colleagues showed that epidural injection of 20 ml of 2-per cent lidocaine over 15 seconds produced slightly higher maximum plasma drug levels than when injected over 60 seconds.[35,165] Although the difference was not statistically significant, it is consistent with the effects of speed of injection on depth and duration

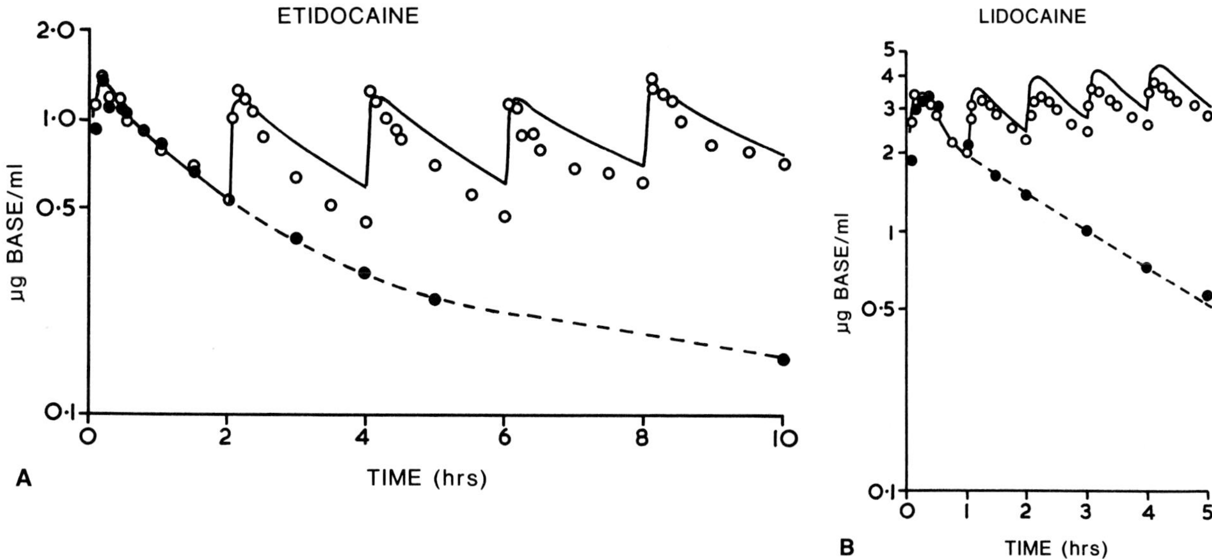

Fig. 3-14. Observed (○) and predicted (–) plasma concentrations following repeated peridural administration of (*A*) etidocaine and (*B*) lidocaine. (Data from Tucker, G.T., and Mather, L.E.: Pharmacokinetics of local anaesthetic agents. Br. J. Anaesth., *47*:213, 1975) Observed (●) plasma concentrations following single peridural injection. (Data from Tucker, G.T., *et al.*: Observed and predicted accumulation of local anaesthetic agent during continuous extradural analgesia. Br. J. Anaesth., *49*:237, 1977)

of anesthesia, as discussed previously. Furthermore, while speed of injection is of little importance to systemic safety provided that the injection is given correctly—should the needle enter an epidural vein, a more rapid injection could have considerably more serious consequences.

Number and Frequency of Injections. Based upon a simulation of the kinetics of local anesthetics after single epidural injections, we predicted the systemic and local accumulation of the agents during continuous epidural block procedures.[196] These predictions indicated that during multiple-dose regimens, systemic accumulation will tend to occur more rapidly with short-acting agents, whereas, despite an extended dosage interval, local accumulation should be more extensive with the long-acting drugs. Tucker and colleagues subsequently reported a close agreement between observed and predicted plasma concentrations of both lidocaine and etidocaine during multidose epidural injections for postoperative pain relief (Figs. 3-14 and 3-15).[195] Satisfactory agreement was also found between predicted and experimental lidocaine blood levels produced by a continuous lumbar epidural infusion (Fig. 3-16).[196]

Extensive local accumulation of local anesthetics, indicated by pharmacokinetic analysis,

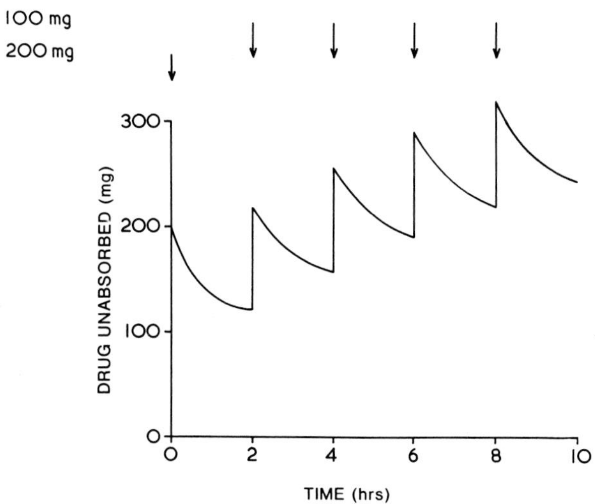

Fig. 3-15. Predicted local accumulation of etidocaine during repeated peridural injections. 200 ml given initially followed by 100 ml at 2-hour intervals. (Tucker, G.T., *et al.:* Observed and predicted accumulation of local anaesthetic agent during continuous extradural analgesia. Br. J. Anaesth., *49*:237, 1977)

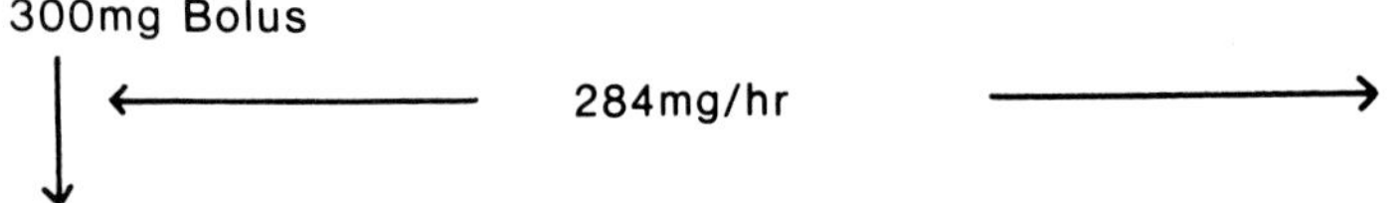

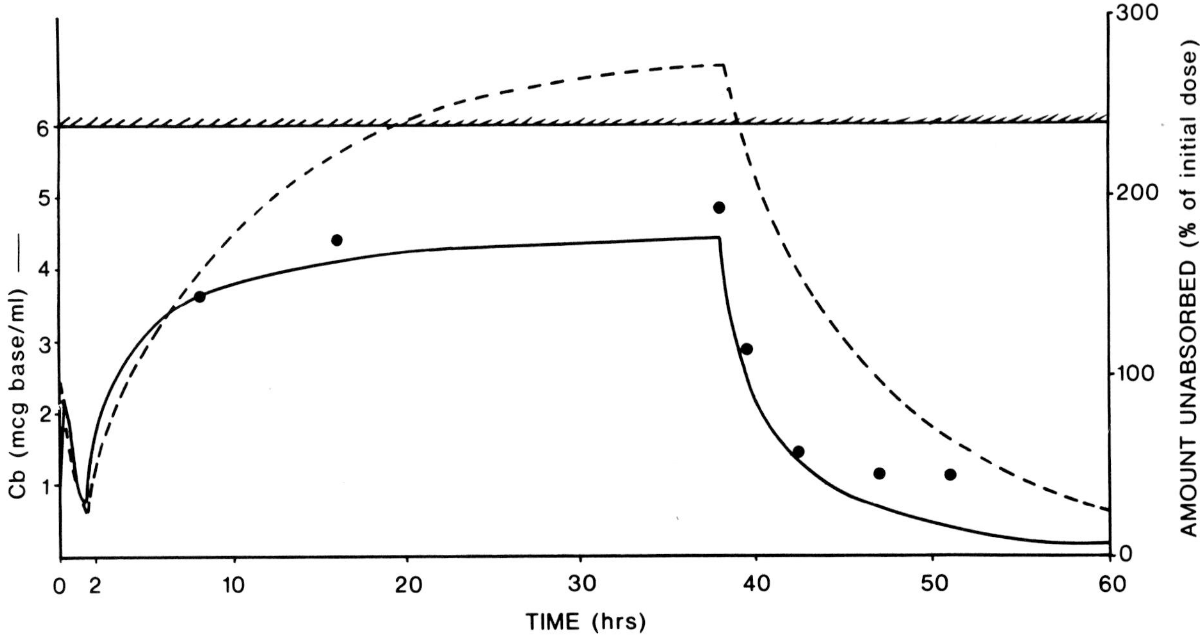

Fig. 3-16. Predicted local and systemic accumulation of lidocaine following a bolus peridural injection for surgical anesthesia and during a continuous peridural infusion for postoperative pain relief. (Hatching indicates minimal toxic blood drug concentrations; ● is experimental blood drug concentrations. (From Holmdahl, M.H., Sjögren, S., Strom, G., and Wright, B.: Clinical aspects of continuous epidural blockade for postoperative pain relief. Ups. J. Med. Sci., *77*:47, 1972; and Tucker, G.T., and Mather, L.E.: Pharmacokinetics of local anaesthetic agents. Br. J. Anaesth., *47*:213, 1975)

poses further questions about the mechanism of anesthesia and the possibility of local neurotoxicity of the agents (Fig. 3-15). Progressive local accumulation appears not to be associated with a concomitant decrease in anesthetic dose requirement nor with any increase in dosage interval.[128,175] In part, this may reflect the fact that the accumulation plateau of drug in the nerves is attained before it reaches a steady state of equilibrium in epidural fat or other tissue. However, at least with lidocaine and mepivacaine, local accumulation may be associated with an actual increase in the maintenance dose required to preserve adequate sensory blockade. This tachyphylaxis is well-documented clinically and is independent of the severity of pain.[50,59] Either there is a genuine reduction in effect at the receptor level or with successive injections the proportion of the dose reaching the receptors declines drastically. The latter may be explained on the basis of *p*H changes, as mentioned previously. Alternatively, local drug binding or the integrity of the epidural space may be altered on repeated injection, resulting in a different local distribution or increased systemic uptake of drug. The data shown in Figure 3-14 appear to exclude the second possibility in humans, but studies in dogs indicate reduced duration of block and increased systemic uptake of drug after successive daily epidural injections of lidocaine.[105]

Whether the accumulation and persistence of local anesthetics in the epidural space during continuous block procedures has any toxicologic significance is debatable. Animal studies and studies *in vitro* have demonstrated muscle necrosis following intramuscular injection of local anesthetics, impaired mitochondrial metabolism, and axonal transport of proteins following direct application to axons.[23,56,76,88] However, local neurotoxicity of local anesthetics is not recognized as a limiting factor in clinical practice. Neurologic sequelae have been documented with an approximated frequency of 1:10,000 following major conduction block, and there are a number of etiological factors that appear more important than the local anesthetic agent (see Chap. 8).[200]

Addition of Vasoconstrictors. In order to counteract increases in local blood flow that result from vasomotor blockade and the direct vasodilator action of local anesthetics, vasoconstrictor agents are often added to local anesthetic solutions. The degree to which the desired effects of a decrease in systemic absorption rate of local anesthetic and a prolongation of anesthesia are achieved is a complex function of the type, dose, and concentration of both local anesthetic and vasoconstrictor and of the characteristics of the site of injection.

Although epinephrine is the most commonly used vasoconstrictor, like many local anesthetics, it does have a dual action on blood vessels.[30] Skin and cutaneous vessels are always constricted, but muscle vessels may be constricted or dilated, which may explain why the addition of epinephrine decreases the absorption rate of mepivacaine to a greater extent after subcutaneous than after intramuscular injection. Epinephrine (1:200,000) added to mepivacaine solutions for various block procedures prolongs the time during which maximum arterial plasma drug concentrations occur. Maximum plasma drug concentrations are also reduced following all blocks, but the greatest effect, a 50 per cent decrease, was seen with intercostal block with a 2-per-cent solution (Fig. 3-12). Table 3-6 summarizes additional data on the effect of epinephrine on maximum plasma or blood concentrations of local anesthetics. Results with lidocaine and prilocaine suggest that the use of epinephrine concentrations greater than 1:200,000 produces only marginally greater decreases in maximum local anesthetic levels and should, therefore, be avoided, in view of side-effects associated with excessive systemic levels of epinephrine.[64] The importance of the dose of local anesthetic is also illustrated by results of studies with prilocaine. While epinephrine had little influence on a 400 mg epidural dose, the effect was significantly greater at 600 and 900 mg. Local anesthetic pharmacokinetics after paracervical injection appear to be particularly sensitive to the effects of epinephrine, as indicated by the results of studies with bupivacaine. However, for other routes the data suggest that addition of epinephrine reduces the absorption rates of the long-acting agents somewhat less effectively than those of the short-acting analogues.[131,133] This is also seen in calculated absorption-time profiles and is presumably due to greater competition for available drug by tissue-binding sites (Fig. 3-13). Although these studies have documented a lowering of local anesthetic plasma levels by epinephrine, such findings cannot necessarily be equated directly with its local vasoconstrictor effect. To do so supposes that epinephrine has no influence on the systemic disposition of local anesthetics. Thus, once epinephrine is absorbed into the circulation, it is potentially capable of increasing hepatic clearance of local anesthetics by elevation of hepatic blood flow. It may also modify perfusion at the site of blood sampling because although epidural injections of lidocaine without epinephrine cause an increase in leg blood flow and a decrease in arm blood flow, epinephrine-containing solutions have been reported to increase blood flow in both extremities. Accordingly, peripheral venous plasma levels of local anesthetics may reflect local hemodynamic changes, in addition to systemic absorption of the agents. Systemic cardiovascular effects of epinephrine may also interact with the local vasoconstrictor effects in modulating uptake of local anesthetic from sites of injection.[196]

Other vasopressor agents that have been advocated as alternatives to epinephrine include synthetic polypeptides related to vasopressin, such as octapressin, and the pure alpha-adrenoceptor agonist phenylephrine.[101] Addition of 50 μg per ml of phenylephrine to lidocaine solution was less effective than 5 μg per ml of epinephrine in reducing blood drug levels, although, as expected, its use was not associated with an elevation of cardiac output.[176]

Carbonation. The use of carbonated bupivacaine for epidural analgesia has been shown to be associated with significantly more rapid drug absorption than use of bupivacaine hydrochloride solution with and without added epinephrine (Fig. 3-17).[13] The difference between carbonated and plain solutions presumably is due to the vasodilating effect of the carbon dioxide and the rapid release of bupivacaine base from the carbonated solution.

Factors Related to Nerve Block

The hypotension that often results from epidural anesthesia may prolong the duration of blockade, owing to reduced perfusion of the epidural space and a slower systemic uptake of local anesthetic.

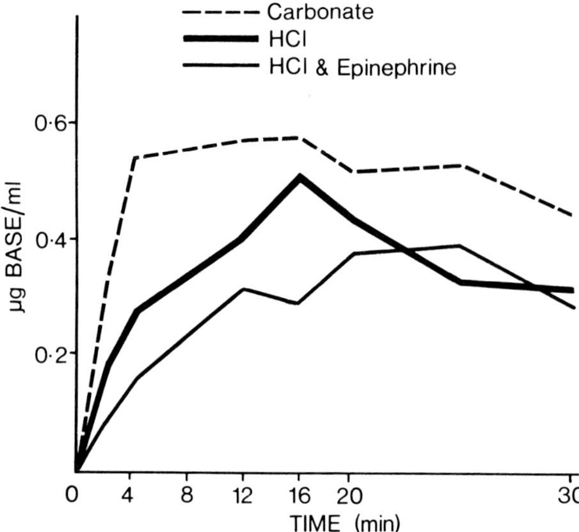

Fig. 3-17. The comparison of bupivacaine blood concentrations after peridural injection of 1.5 mg per kg bupivacaine in 0.5-per-cent solution. (Adapted from Appleyard, T.N., Witt, A., Atkinson, R.E., and Nicholas, R.D.G.: Bupivacaine carbonate and bupivacaine hydrochloride: A comparison of blood concentrations during epidural blockade for vaginal surgery. Br. J. Anaesth., *48*:1171, 1976)

Although this theory has yet to be examined rigorously, it is supported by the observation that prophylactic subcutaneous or intravenous injection of ephedrine results in shorter durations of anesthesia and elevated blood concentrations of some local anesthetic agents.[70,122]

Physical and Pathophysiologic Factors

Weight. Although negative correlations have been observed between maximum plasma concentrations of local anesthetics and body weight (surface area and lean body mass), the relationships are not strong enough to justify injection of these agents on a weight basis.[165,198] This does not necessarily apply for young children, although objective guidelines are lacking (see Chap. 4).

Age. Decreased vascular perfusion in the elderly might account, in part, for the observed increase in spread and duration of epidural anesthesia with age. If so, this does not appear to be accompanied by lower plasma concentrations of local anesthetics.[165,198]

Pregnancy. Epidural dosage requirements are reduced in pregnant women and, in part, this might be explained by an increased systemic drug absorption rate resulting from a hyperkinetic circulation.[46] However, no significant differences were observed between the kinetics of etidocaine in pregnant women at term and a group of older nonpregnant patients.[133]

Disease. Changes in local perfusion associated with altered hemodynamics in certain disease states or as a result of operative conditions can modify absorption of local anesthetics and, hence, duration of anesthesia. For example, acute hypovolemia has been shown to slow the absorption of lidocaine after epidural injection in dogs and to prolong anesthesia in patients undergoing thoracotomy with regional block.[135,151] On the other hand, the hyperkinetic circulation that may be associated with renal disease might partially account for the decreased duration of brachial plexus block observed in patients with chronic renal failure.[49]

SYSTEMIC DISPOSITION

After absorption from sundry sites of administration, local anesthetics are distributed by the blood-

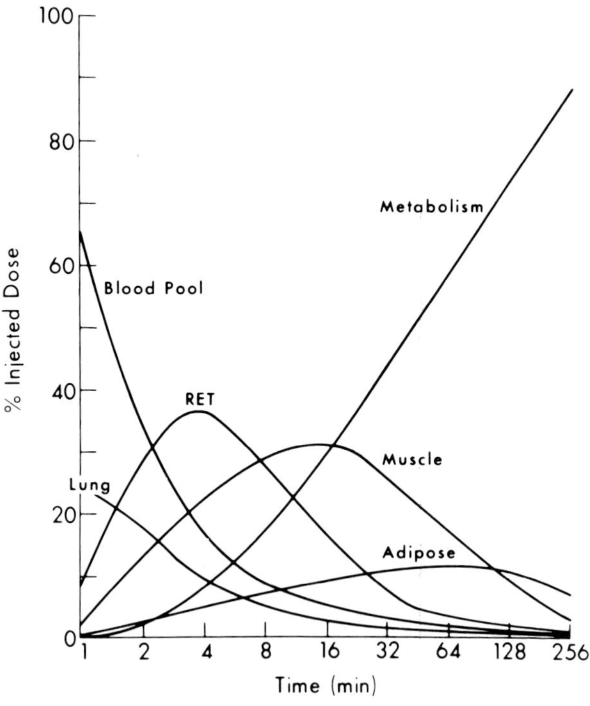

Fig. 3-18. A perfusion model of the distribution of lidocaine in various tissues and its elimination from humans following an intravenous infusion for 1 minute (RET = rapidly equilibrating tissues). Note the use of a logarithmic time scale to show more clearly the rapid changes immediately following injection. (Data from Benowitz, N., Forsyth, R.P., and Melmon, K.L.: Lidocaine disposition kinetics in monkey and man I. Prediction by a perfusion model. Clin. Pharmacol. Ther., *16*:99, 1974)

stream to the organs and tissues of the body and cleared, mostly by metabolism and to a small extent by renal excretion.

A physiologic model useful in describing the time-course of these processes has been elaborated recently by Benowitz and associates.[25] This perfusion model (it assumes no diffusion limitations) is based upon an extrapolation of equilibrium tissue/blood partition coefficients of lidocaine from monkeys to humans and estimates of normal cardiac output, regional blood flows, and hepatic extraction. It simulates the duration of the agent in various tissues, and its validity is supported by a close prediction of the arterial blood concentration-time curve of lidocaine after intravenous injection (Fig. 3-18).[192] Similar curves are obtained experimentally with the other amide-type agents, and it may be presumed that the model is general for these compounds (Fig. 3-19). Ester-type agents are probably distributed in the same way, but they are set apart from the amide group by the site and rate of their metabolism.

Distribution

The first organ to be exposed to local anesthetic once it has entered the systemic circulation is the lung. This organ provides the important buffer function of temporary sequestration of a large quantity of drug owing to a high lung/blood partition coefficient. Hence, the arterial blood drug concentration for toxicity which hits the target organs, the brain and heart (via the coronary circulation) is considerably attenuated compared to the drug concentration in the pulmonary artery (Fig. 3-20). Inadvertent injection of local anesthetic directly into the carotid or vertebral artery during stellate ganglion or interscalene block will of course bypass the lung, resulting in a high probability of CNS toxicity. Also, rapid injection into branches of the external carotid artery can result in retrograde flow into the cerebral circulation with similar consequences.

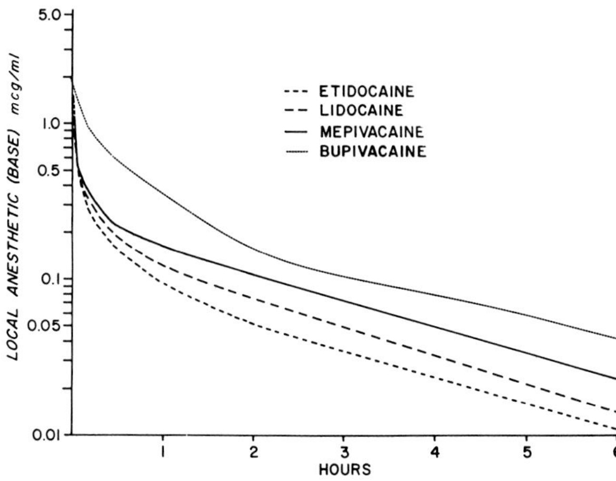

Fig. 3-19. Mean arterial whole blood concentrations of local anesthetics after intravenous infusion of 44.16 base equivalent of each drug at a constant rate over 10 minutes. (Tucker, G.T., and Mather, L.E.: Pharmacokinetics of local anaesthetic agents. Br. J. Anaesth., *47*:213, 1975)

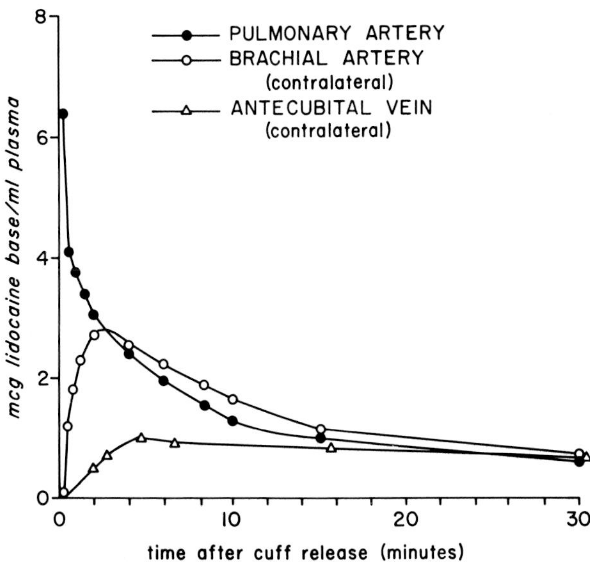

Fig. 3-20. Plasma lidocaine levels in a subject following cuff release after intravenous regional anesthesia with 3 mg kg^{-1} lidocaine hydrochloride (0.5% solution; 45 minutes cuff time; Tucker, G.T., and Boas, R.A.: Pharmacokinetic aspects of intravenous regional anesthesia. Anesthesiology, *34*:538, 1971)

After the lung, local anesthetic is distributed to other organs according to the proportion of the cardiac output that they receive. The time taken to achieve equilibrium distribution in each organ (*i.e.*, when incoming arterial drug concentration equals outgoing venous concentration) is directly proportional to its capacity for drug uptake (mass × tissue/blood partition coefficient) and inversely proportional to its blood flow. Thus, drug successively equilibrates in and redistributes from the small vessel-rich organs, the muscles, and finally the fat, where it is relatively highly soluble (Fig. 3-18). This progression, together with the process of drug elimination, accounts for the shape of the blood drug concentration-time profile, which is readily simulated by empirical, multiexponential equation (Fig. 3-19).[192,196]

Predominant factors that determine the tissue/blood partition coefficients of the various

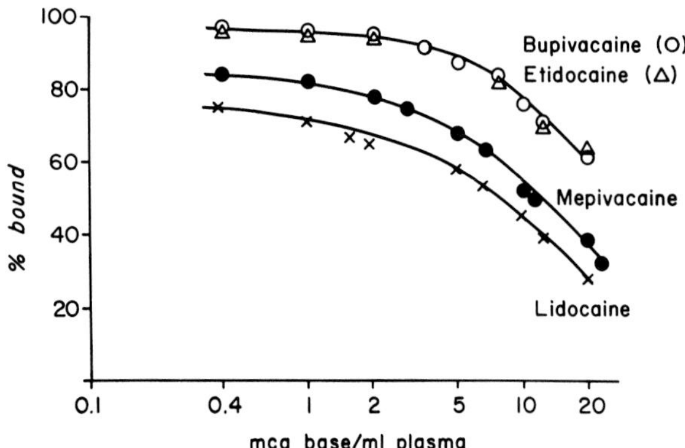

Fig. 3-21. Plasma binding of amide-type local anesthetics. (Tucker, G.T., and Mather, L.E.: Pharmacokinetics of local anaesthetic agents. Br. J. Anaesth., *47*:213, 1975)

agents in different tissues are plasma, erythrocyte, and tissue binding and the *p*H gradient between plasma and extravascular water spaces.

The long-acting amides are significantly more bound in plasma than the short-acting agents (Table 3-1). An important feature of this binding is that it approaches saturation—that is, the unbound fraction increases—as the total plasma drug concentration extends into the toxic range (Fig. 3-21). Albumin is not responsible for the majority of the binding as it is for many other drugs; instead, binding is largely the result of interaction with low-capacity–high affinity sites on lipid-rich alpha$_1$-globulins.[117,120,193]

Attachment of the agents to binding sites in or on the erythrocyte is of similar order to plasma binding.[193] However, in the presence of plasma proteins, plasma binding competes with binding to the erythrocytes. Hence blood/plasma drug concentration ratios are inversely related to plasma binding (Table 3-7). An assessment of overall drug distribution in the body is given by the steady state volume of distribution, (V_{Dss}).[196] This is determined with reference to total drug concentration in the blood and, under certain circumstances, is useful in comparing the distribution of related agents. The values of V_{Dss} for the amides vary over a relatively narrow range, which is another way of saying that they have similar tissue/blood partition coefficients (Table 3-7). The reason for this becomes apparent if the volume of distribution is calculated on the basis of unbound drug in blood. This gives a new term, V_{Dssf}, which, although it still includes the contribution of blood binding, affords an approximate indication of relative mean tissue affinities of the compounds. Clearly, the agents that are highly bound in the blood (low f_b values) are also highly associated with tissue-binding sites (high V_{Dssf}; Table 3-7). Consequently, the two factors tend to cancel, resulting in similar tissue/blood partition coefficients across the series of agents. This finding is not in conflict with the previous suggestion that blood/tissue partition coefficients of the agents differ widely at the site of injection since, in that case, blood-binding sites would tend to be saturated by the larger drug concentrations involved.

The relative acidity of intracellular water, CSF,

Table 3-7. Mean Values of Pharmacokinetic Parameters for the Disposition of Anilide-Type Local Anesthetics After Intravenous Injection in Humans

Parameter	*Mepivacaine*	*Lidocaine*	*Etidocaine*	*Bupivacaine*
λ	0.92	0.84	0.58	0.73
V_{Dss}(L)	84	91	133	72
T/2 (hr)	1.9	1.6	2.6	3.5
CL (L.min^{-1})	0.78	0.99	1.22	0.47
E	0.52	0.63	0.81	0.31
f_p	0.20	0.30	0.05	0.05
f_b	0.22	0.36	0.09	0.07
V_{Dssf}(L)	382	253	1478	1028

Key: λ, blood/plasma drug concentration ratio; V_{Dss}, steady state volume of distribution; T/2, half-life of terminal decay phase; CL, mean total body clearance; E, estimated hepatic extraction ratio assuming a normal liver blood flow of 1.5 L.min^{-1}; f_p, free fraction of drug in plasma in the clinical range of levels; f_b, free fraction of drug in blood, given by f_p/λ; V_{Dssf}, volume of distribution of free drug at steady state

(Data from Tucker, G. T., and Mather, L. E.: Pharmacokinetics of local anesthetic agents. Br. J. Anaesth., *47*:213, 1977)

and other body fluids compared to plasma water will cause extravascular ion-trapping of local anesthetics, according to Equation 5. For example, lung water with a pH of 6.7 is particularly acidic, and this probably contributes to the high tissue/blood partition coefficient of local anesthetics and other basic drugs in this organ.[68]

Excretion

Renal excretion of unchanged local anesthetics is a minor route of elimination, accounting for less than 6 per cent of the dose under normal conditions.[7,20,98,120,156,199] Acidification of the urine to about pH 5 increases this proportion up to 20 per cent, depending upon the agent, which is consistent with the hypothesis that less tubular reabsorption of drug occurs at lower pH owing to a greater degree of ionization. However, this increase in net excretion is not sufficient to warrant acidification of the urine as a means of speeding the elimination of local anesthetics in patients with toxic symptoms. Estimation of the renal clearances of the amide-type agents indicates that they enter the tubular fluid as a result of both glomerular filtration and tubular secretion.[74]

Secretion of unchanged local anesthetics down the pH gradient between blood and gastric juice is also a potential route of excretion. However, most of the drug that appears in the stomach contents subsequently passes into the intestine and is absorbed into the portal circulation.[98] High hepatic extraction en route further depletes the amount recycled into the systemic circulation (see later). Although the use of a stomach pump has been advocated for treatment of local anesthetic toxicity, especially in newborns, it is unlikely that this is of any value.[61] Gastric juice/blood drug concentration ratios may be quite high, but the proportion of the dose recycled by way of the stomach is unlikely to be significant.

Metabolism

Local anesthetics are largely eliminated by metabolic conversion to more polar compounds that are more easily removed by the kidney. Although the metabolism of these drugs is generally considered to be an inactivation or detoxification process, the possibility that the products may retain some of the activity of the parent drug or, indeed, have quite different pharmacologic effects should not be ignored. A knowledge of both the nature of the metabolic products and of the rate of metabolism of the parent drug is important.

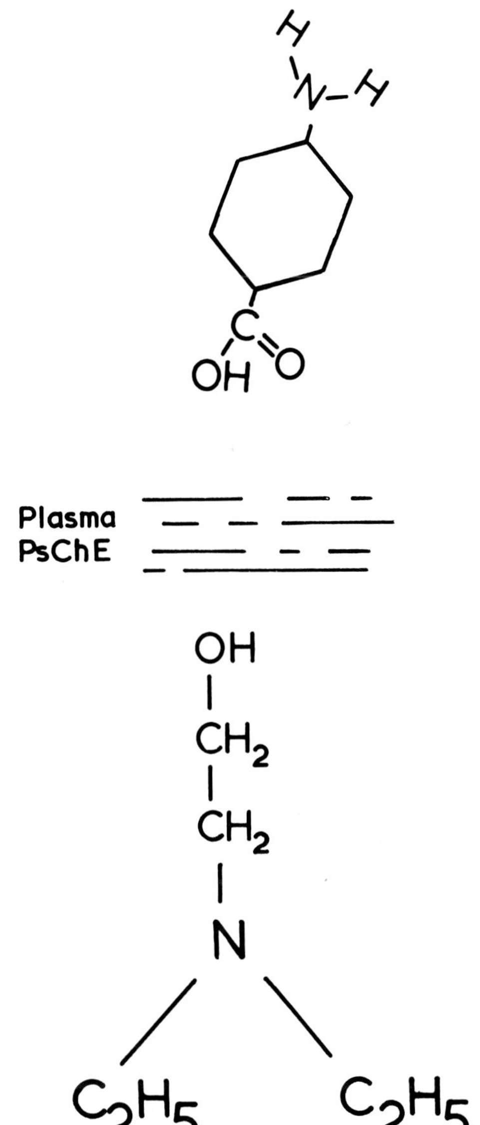

Fig. 3-22. Hydrolysis of procaine. (Tucker, G.T.: Biotransformation and toxicity of local anaesthetics. Acta Anaesthesiol. Belg., *26*[*Suppl.*]:123, 1975)

Esters. Cocaine is effectively detoxified by hydrolysis of the two ester groups (Fig. 3-1). The methyl ester is dissociated to produce benzoylecgonine; the benzoyl group is removed to give ecgonine methyl ester; and removal of both features leaves ecgonine. Further mutilation of cocaine by N-demethylation may give rise to an analogous set of nor-metabolites.[179,210] Pseudocholinesterase mediates benzoyl hydrolysis in human plasma, but the other metabolites are presumably formed in the liver. The intravenous plasma half-life of cocaine in humans is about 2.5 hours to 1 to 21 per cent of the dose is excreted unchanged in the urine and about 40 per cent as benzoylecgonine.[79,102]

The procaine derivatives are also detoxified by ester hydrolysis, partly in plasma by pseudocholinesterase and partly in the liver.[42,85,96] Procaine itself is cleaved to diethylaminoethanol and para-aminobenzoic acid (Fig. 3-22). The latter may be responsible for the allergic reactions sometimes associated with procaine administration.

A striking feature of the hydrolysis of the procaine-type agents is its rapidity, especially in human plasma, even though differences *in vitro* in the rates of breakdown of different ester agents can be demonstrated. For example, chloroprocaine is hydrolyzed four times faster than procaine, which is hydrolyzed four times faster than tetracaine (Fig. 3-23). It is difficult to detect even traces of these drugs in human blood after normal doses for regional block,[78,129] although some authors claim to have done so.[153] The clinical implications of this are clear. If a toxic level is attained, for example, following inadvertent intravenous injection, the ensuing systemic reaction should be relatively short-lived.[80]

On the other hand, if the esterase becomes saturated or substrate-inhibited because of a very high concentration of drug or if the enzyme is genetically atypical, then toxic reactions will be prolonged.[80,96] A number of recent reports have advocated renewed use of chloroprocaine for regional block, in part because of its very high margin of systemic safety, resulting from rapid hydrolysis.[78,81]

Amides. In contrast to the ester-agents, the amides are metabolized predominantly in the liver. Total body clearances (CL) of the drugs, calculated from blood drug concentration-time curves after intravenous injection, decrease in the following order: etidocaine, lidocaine, mepivacaine, bupivacaine (Table 3-7).[196] If metabolism is assumed to be confined to the liver, mean hepatic extraction ratios (E) may be calculated from the quotient of mean clearance and normal hepatic blood flow. The values of E obtained in this manner agree well with those determined by direct measurements of drug extraction across the liver by means of hepatic vein catheterization.[199] They also indicate that appreciable amounts of each drug are removed from the blood in transit through the liver and, therefore, that their clearances will depend significantly upon hepatic perfusion. Furthermore, it is evident that elimination is not restricted to the unbound drug in the circulation since E values are well in excess of the fractions of free drug in blood (f_b; Table 3-7).[118,196] Extraction is a function of total drug in blood. The implication of this is that in patients with lower blood-binding capacities, the rate of delivery of drug to the liver will be reduced. Hence, the elimination rate of both total and unbound (active) drug should be slower, and this may be associated with a prolongation of systemic drug effects.[197]

The relatively high clearance and extensive volume of distribution of etidocaine probably contribute to a greater systemic safety margin than those of bupivacaine.[116,164]

Prilocaine appears to have a pharmacokinetic

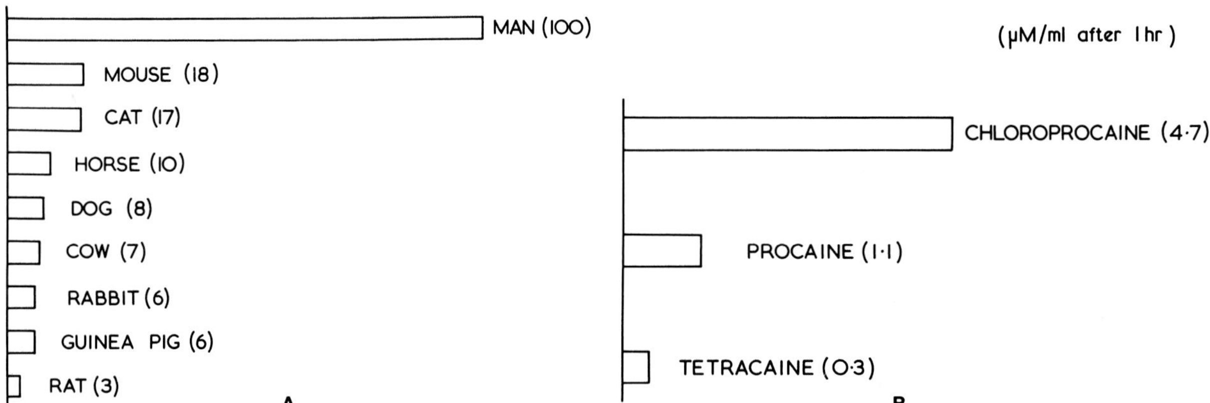

Fig. 3-23. (*A*) Relative rates of procaine hydrolysis in plasma of different mammalian species. (Aven, M.H., Light, A., and Foldes, F.F.: Hydrolysis of procaine in various mammalian plasmas. Fed. Proc., *12*(Abst. 986):299, 1953); (*B*) Hydrolysis rates of esters in pooled human plasma. (Data from Foldes, F.F., Davidson, G.N., Duncalf, D., and Kuwabarra, S.: The intravenous toxicity of local anesthetic agents in man. Clin. Pharmacol. Ther., *6*:328, 1965)

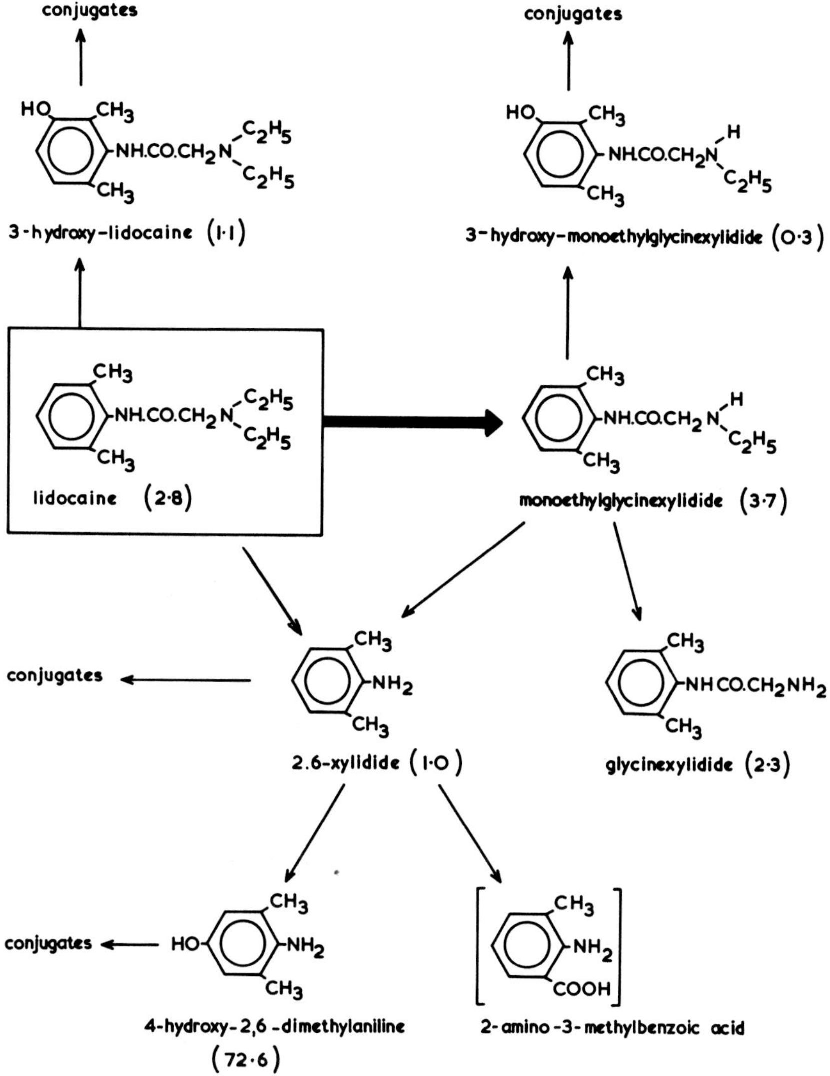

Fig. 3-24. Pathways for the biotransformation of lidocaine in humans. Values in parentheses indicate percentages of dose found in urine. (Boyes, R.N., A review of the metabolism of amide local anaesthetic agents. Br. J. Anaesth., *47*:225, 1975; and Keenaghan, J.B., and Boyes, R.N.: The tissue distribution, metabolism and excretion of lidocaine in rats, guinea pigs, dogs, and man. J. Pharmacol. Exp. Ther., *180*:454, 1972)

profile similar to that of etidocaine and therefore shares the same advantages in this respect as lidocaine and mepivacaine. Prilocaine has higher clearance, which may be explained by a greater hepatic extraction, in addition to the possibility, suggested from animal studies, that it is also metabolized in the lung.[10,111] Although experiments *in vitro* indicate that prilocaine binds more extensively to brain tissue than lidocaine, greater brain concentrations in animals are associated with less central toxicity than with lidocaine.[10]

Lidocaine Metabolism. Considerable efforts have been made over the past few years to characterize the metabolites of lidocaine and to determine whether they contribute materially to systemic activity and toxicity. Figure 3-24 is a scheme for the biotransformation of lidocaine in humans. Hydroxylation in the 3′-position is a minor path-

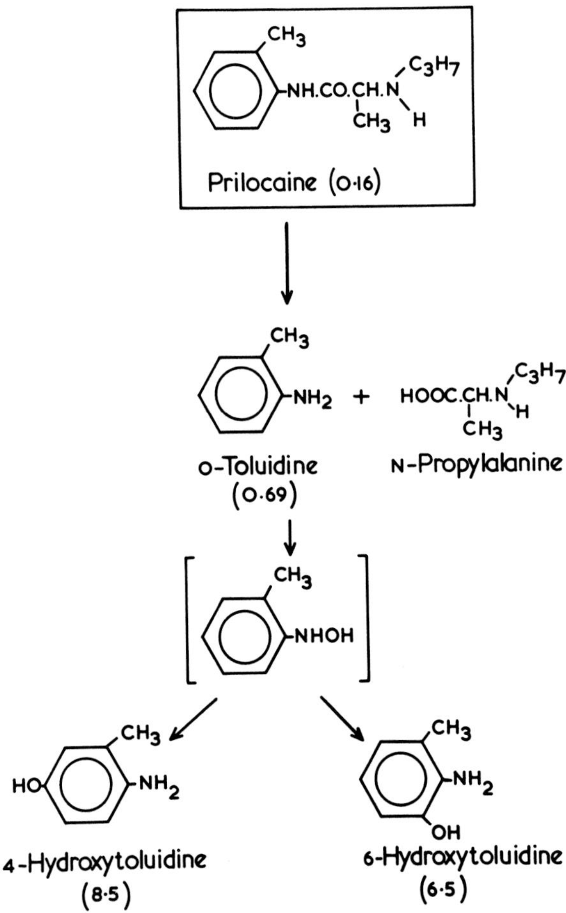

Fig. 3-25. Pathways for the biotransformation of prilocaine in humans. Values in parentheses indicate percentages of dose found in urine. (From Akerman, B., Astrom, A., Ross, S., and Telc, A.: Studies on the absorption, distribution and metabolism of labelled prilocaine and lidocaine in some animal species. Acta Pharmacol. Toxicol. (Kbh.), *24*:389, 1966)

way. While direct amide hydrolysis of lidocaine can occur, much of the dose is initially N-deethylated to monoethylglycinexylidide (MEGX), which, in turn, is either 3′-hydroxylated or is further N-deethylated to glycinexylidide (GX), but most is split at the amide link to give 2,6-xylidine. This is then hydroxylated in the 4-position so that most of the dose appears in the urine as 4-hydroxy-2,6-xylidine.[32,98,145] Other metabolites have been proposed, but their existence is more controversial. A novel cyclic metabolite initially claimed to be excreted in human urine was subsequently shown to be largely an artefact arising from the reaction of MEGX with trace amounts of acetaldehyde in solvents used in isolation procedures.[38,144] Nevertheless, experiments in monkeys suggested that it may be formed *in vivo* if a patient receiving lidocaine has also ingested alcohol and has an elevated body burden of acetaldehyde.[144] Mather and Thomas presented indirect evidence for the urinary excretion of the amide N-hydroxyderivatives of lidocaine and MEGX.[119] However, the presence of these compounds in urine could not be verified by others, although this fact does not preclude their transient existence as intermediates in the formation of other metabolites.[146] The significance of these amide N-hydroxy derivatives is that they or their possible conjugates may be potentially carcinogenic, mutagenic, and antigenic.[202]

In rodents, estimates of the lethality of MEGX are between 68 to 100 per cent, compared to lidocaine; values for the dose that produced convulsions in 50 per cent of the tested animal population (CD_{50}) indicate that it is 88 per cent as convulsant; while on the basis of plasma levels it appears to be equitoxic.[29,173] GX was found to be less toxic than MEGX and completely devoid of convulsant activity, death being entirely due to respiratory arrest.[180] These two metabolites have also been shown to have antiarrhythmic activity in animals. It is estimated that MEGX has between 33 and 83 per cent of the activity of lidocaine and that GX has 10 to 42 per cent of the activity, depending upon the experimental model used.[16,29,55,173,180] On the basis of plasma levels in rats, MEGX has 99 per cent and GX has 26 per cent of the activity of lidocaine.[180]

How do these animal data translate into clinical terms? Several groups have reported plasma or blood levels of MEGX, GX, and 4-hydroxyxylidine in patients who receive either intravenous infusions or epidural injections of lidocaine.[1,28,86,143,150,181] Average ratios of MEGX:lidocaine levels ranged from 0.23 to 0.46, and indeed in some patients MEGX probably contributes to the activity and toxicity of the parent drug. GX levels are generally quite low compared to lidocaine levels, at least at steady state, but occasionally much higher GX:lidocaine ratios have been observed. Direct intravenous injection of GX in two volunteers did not reproduce any of the major toxic effects associated with lidocaine.[180] There was a complete lack of any cardiovascular toxicity, but there was some impairment of mental concentration.

There is at present some information available about the pharmacokinetics of MEGX and GX in humans. MEGX has a relatively short half-life, slightly longer than that of lidocaine itself.[86,143] It is primarily eliminated by further metabolism; only about 12 per cent of the dose is excreted unchanged in the urine. GX has a much longer half-life (about 10 hours), and 50 per cent of a dose is excreted unchanged.[180] Its potential for cumulation, particularly in patients with renal disease, is therefore, relatively high.[60]

Prilocaine Metabolism. Prilocaine is split at the amide linkage to yield o-toluidine, which in turn is converted to 4- and 6-hydroxytoluidine, probably by rearrangement of an amide *N*-hydroxy intermediate (Fig. 3-25). 6-Hydroxytoluidine is held responsible for the methemoglobinemia seen when the dose of prilocaine exceeds about 600 mg.[100] Unlike single-side-chain o-toluidine, two-chain 2,6-xylidine which is present in the other amide caines does not produce significant methemoglobinemia (Fig. 3-5).[115]

Mepivacaine Metabolism. The structures of various mepivacaine metabolites found in human urine are shown in Figure 3-26.[125,126,186] Approximately 1 per cent of an oral dose is recovered as the N-demethylated derivative 2,6-pipecoloxylidide (PPX). A further 15 to 20 per cent appears as conjugates of the 3′-hydroxy compound (Fig. 3-26*b*), probably formed by an epoxide intermediate; 10 to 14 per cent as conjugates of the 4′-hydroxy compound (Fig. 3-26*c*), possibly formed by an amide N-hydroxy intermediate; and 10 per cent as various neutral lactams (Fig. 3-26 *d–f*). Animal data indicate that PPX and the 4′-hydroxy metabolite are, respectively, 68 per cent and 36 per cent as toxic as mepivacaine.[87] However, measurements of PPX plasma levels in human maternal and cord blood at delivery indicate very low values, PPX:mepivacaine ratios being generally less than 0.1.[124]

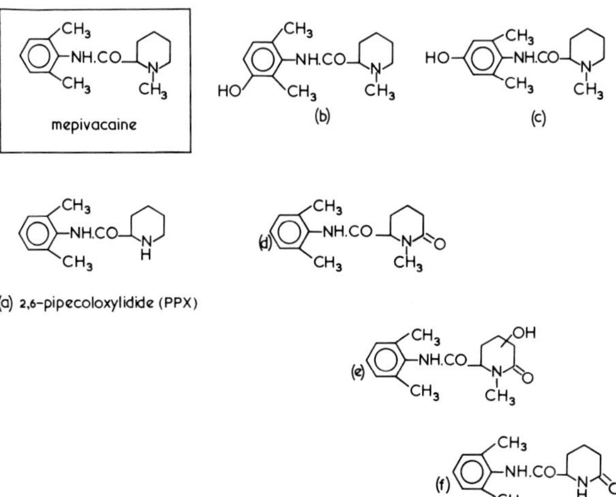

Fig. 3-26. Biotransformation products of mepivacaine in humans.

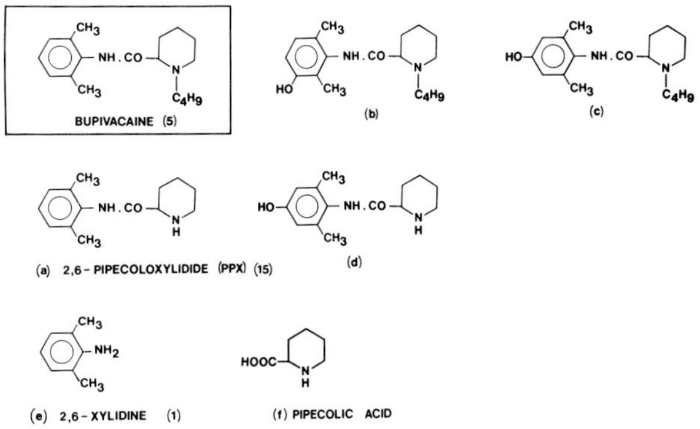

Fig. 3-27. Biotransformation products of bupivacaine.

Bupivacaine Metabolism. Routes of metabolism of bupivacaine in humans and their clinical significance are poorly characterized. In the rat, a large proportion of a dose is excreted as conjugates of the 3′ and 4′-hydroxy derivates, whereas the monkey excretes over 50 per cent as the hydrolysis product pipecolic acid.[57,84] Data in humans suggest that the amide hydrolysis pathway may be less important, at least, by the N-debutylated product (PPX), since only 5 per cent of a dose is excreted as PPX, whereas direct administration of PPX results in a 50 per cent recovery in the urine.[156] Some metabolites of bupivacaine are shown in Figure 3-27.

Etidocaine metabolism in humans has been extensively studied. However, although 20 compounds have been identified in urine (some of which are shown in Fig. 3-28), these account for only 40 per cent of the dose, and their toxicology is unknown.[134,187,201]

In humans, as well as the guinea pig, recovery of secondary amines and of 2,6-xylidine-related metabolites is considerably less than recovery of those of lidocaine.[32]

A comparison of the data available from studies in humans of the amide-type agents leads to the following, tentative conclusions:[190] First, amide hydrolysis is less facile when the amine nitrogen is contained within a piperidine ring (mepivacaine and bupivacaine) than when it is in an alkyl chain (lidocaine); in contrast, aromatic hydroxylation may be easier. Second, removal of an N-butyl group (bupivacaine) is easier than N-demethylation (mepivacaine). Third, alkyl branching (etidocaine, prilocaine) may direct metabolism through routes different than those observed to date for straight chain (lidocaine) and cyclic (mepivacaine, bupivacaine) analogues.

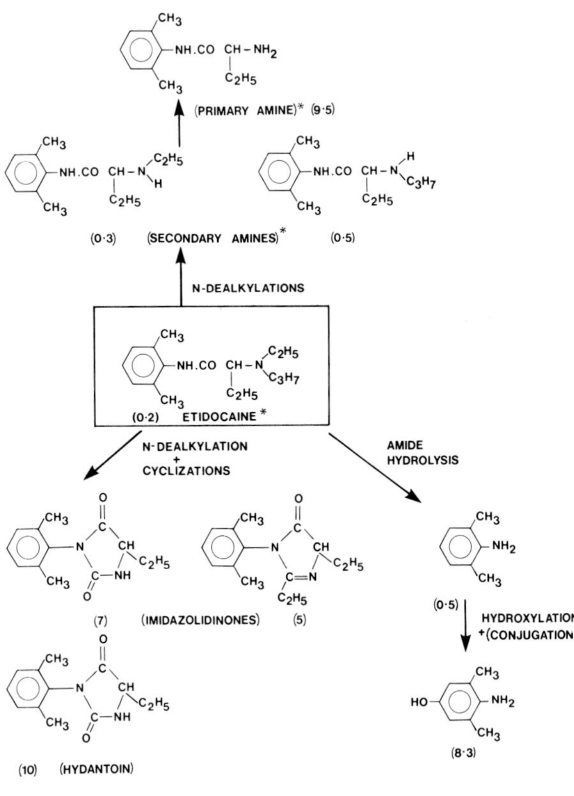

Fig. 3-28. Biotransformation products of etidocaine in humans. Values in parentheses indicate percentages of dose found in urine.

Physical and Pathophysiologic Factors

Weight. Limited data on amide-type agents indicate a poor correlation among body weight, surface area and lean body mass, and drug disposition kinetics in young male volunteers with normal height: weight ratios.[159,196] However, relationships in a wider range of body somatotypes have not been investigated.

Age. No differences in the disposition kinetics of lidocaine were found between young (24–34 years) and older (52–57 years) normal subjects.[159] In geriatric patients (61–71 years), lidocaine half-life and volume of distribution were both increased by about 70 per cent over a control group (22–26 years). Total body clearance, however, was the same in both groups.[143]

Sympathetic Blockade. High epidural block in normal humans is associated with a 20 per cent reduction in hepatic blood flow.[99] It is not known whether this significantly decreases the systemic clearance of the local anesthetic used. However, blockade to T6–7 with epidural tetracaine was shown to have no influence on the disposition kinetics of intravenous etidocaine in volunteers.[196]

Although differences in overall distribution of local anesthetic may not be apparent in the presence of sympathetic blockade, local distribution of the agent may be altered. Thus,large arteriovenous (A-V) differences in local anesthetic concentration across the arm compared to much smaller differences across the leg appear to be related to compensatory vasoconstriction in the upper limbs as a result of vasodilatation in the lower limbs produced by lumbar sympathetic block.[196] Presumably, the differences in A-V gradient mirror differences in the rate of tissue uptake of drug and in the degree of cutaneous shunting of blood and drug.[169,196]

Cardiovascular Disease. Lidocaine blood concentrations after intravenous injection in patients with congestive heart failure are approximately double those achieved in the control group, who received the same dose.[188] Blood levels of MEGX, formed from lidocaine, may also be elevated in heart failure.[86] These findings are a manifestation of a reduced volume of distribution and clearance of the agents (Table 3-8). The reduced volume of distribution appears to result from the autoregulatory redistribution of blood away from the periphery to support circulation in the heart and brain, which are then perfused with blood that contains higher than normal concentrations of drug. Changes in tissue/blood partition coefficients may also be responsible. The reduced clearance appears to be associated with diminished hepatic blood flow secondary to a low cardiac output or impaired hepatic extraction secondary to hepatocellular dysfunction or intrahepatic shunting.[26,188] Impaired extraction was shown to be the major factor reducing lidocaine clearance in hypovolemic monkeys.[26]

Following the use of local anesthetics for regional anesthesia in patients with circulatory depression or

Table 3-8. Lidocaine Disposition in Various Groups of Patients

	T/2 (*hr*)	V_{Dss} (*L/kg*)	*CL* (*ml/kg/min*)
Normal	1.8	1.32	10.0
Heart Failure	1.9	0.88	6.3
Liver Disease	4.9	2.31	6.0
Renal Disease	1.3	1.2	13.7

(Data from Thompson, P., *et al.*: Lidocaine pharmacokinetics in advanced heart failure, liver disease, and renal failure in humans. Ann. Intern. Med., *78*:499, 1973.) See Table 3.7 for definitions.

diminished cardiac output, abnormally elevated blood drug levels may not be observed, owing to diminished peripheral perfusion and slower uptake of drug from the site of injection.[135] Also, autoregulatory vasoconstriction may be impaired by extensive sympathetic blockade with concomitant effects on the volume of distribution of the drug.

Liver Disease. Although the hydrolysis of ester-type agents in plasma is prolonged significantly in patients with liver disease, presumably owing to decreased synthesis of pseudocholinesterase, the breakdown of these agents is still, in absolute terms, very rapid (Fig. 3-29).[155]

The clinical significance of altered disposition of the amides as a result of liver disease is probably greater than that of the esters. With lidocaine, for example, there are considerable increases in its half-life and volume of distribution and a decrease in its clearance in patients with cirrhosis (Table 3-8). The mechanism of the distribution change may be related to alterations in plasma or tissue binding or both, but this has not been investigated. Clearly, systemic accumulation of the amides will be more extensive and prolonged in patients with cirrhosis and the regression of systemic effects will be slower.[6] The acute phase of viral hepatitis is associated with an elevated volume of distribution and half-life, while a tendency toward decreased clearance occurs. No differences in plasma binding are apparent in the acute phase as compared to the recovery phase.[207]

Renal Disease. As might be expected for drugs that are eliminated almost entirely by the liver, disposition kinetics of the amides are unaffected by renal disease (Table 3-8). If anything, the elevation in cardiac output associated with impaired renal function in some patients might even promote drug clearance by a concomitant increase in hepatic blood flow.

In contrast to the parent drugs, polar metabolites of local anesthetics predominantly cleared by the kidneys will tend to accumulate in patients with renal disease. This is true of GX, formed from lidocaine, although the evidence suggests that the plasma levels reached are not likely to cause major toxicity.[60] Procaine hydrolysis in sera from patients with impaired renal function is slowed in proportion to the patient's blood urea nitrogen value.[155] A decreased pseudocholinesterase activity rather than competitive enzyme inhibition by other components of uremic serum appears to be responsible for this effect. As in patients with liver disease, the reduction in hydrolysis rate may be of little clinical significance.

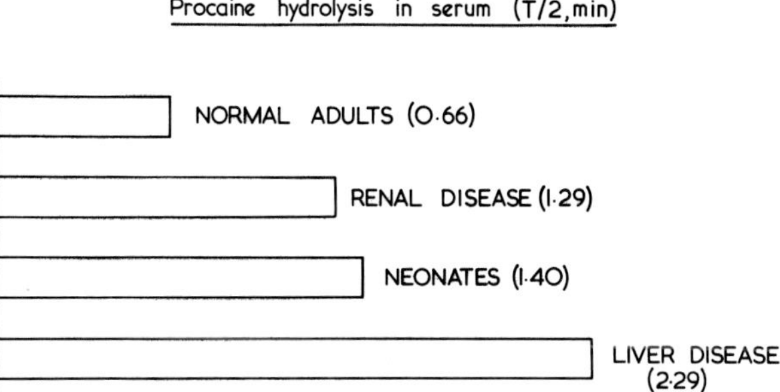

Fig. 3-29. Hydrolysis rates of procaine in serum of normal subjects, neonates and diseased patients. (Data from Reidenberg, M.M., James, M., and Dring, L.G.: The rate of procaine hydrolysis in serum of normal subjects and diseased patients. Clin. Pharmacol. Ther., *13*:279, 1972)

Pulmonary Disease. Despite the fact that compromised pulmonary function is one of the indications for regional anesthesia, the understanding of relationships between the disposition and toxicity of local anesthetics and pulmonary disease is far from complete. Currently, it is possible to speculate only on the effects of lung pathology and hypoxia, although the influence of acid-base imbalance, which will be discussed separately below, has been studied in some detail.

Any compromise in pulmonary perfusion, especially if shunting occurs, or alteration of the integrity of lung tissue could allow local anesthetic to escape early lung uptake and deliver excessive drug concentrations to the heart and brain.[192] The clinical significance of this possibility remains to be evaluated.

The influence of hypoxia on drug metabolism is not well defined. However, in animals acute hypoxia is associated with substantial reductions in total hepatic blood flow, and this may have consequences for the clearance of flow-dependent drugs, such as the local anesthetics.[157]

Acid-Base Imbalance. Englesson and colleagues have demonstrated a marked dependence of the dose of local anesthetic that produces CNS effects in cats on both Pa_{CO_2} and pH. Respiratory acidosis induced by carbon dioxide rebreathing was always accompanied by enhanced toxicity, but the increase was greater when there was an underlying metabolic acidosis rather than a normal or alkalotic state. Although these findings may be explained by an altered electrolyte balance or other mechanism that causes an increase in target organ "sensitivity," they can also be explained on the basis of altered drug disposition.

Because the values for pK_a are generally quite

close to the physiologic *p*H range, the ionization of local anesthetics and, hence, their distribution should be very sensitive to small changes in blood and tissue *p*H (Table 3-1). If the local anesthetic cation is responsible for effects in the brain, as it is at the nerve membrane, then a lowering of brain *p*H will increase the ionized: nonionized drug concentration ratio and lead to increased toxicity. This is so, of course, only if the absolute concentration of ionized drug in the brain increases also. The dynamic factors that determine this are complex and involve a consideration of a greater increase of ionized drug in blood (since extracellular *p*H changes are more dramatic than intracellular changes), increased drug ionization in other tissues tending to reduce access of drug to the brain, redistribution of drug from lipid stores to maintain concentrations of nonionized drug, decreased plasma drug binding and access of drug to the erythroctyes, and any effects of acidosis on hepatic blood flow and drug extraction.[170,191] Sjöstrand and Widman showed that the intravenous infusion of tritiated bupivacaine over 20 minutes into acidotic rabbits produced significantly higher blood and lung levels of radioactivity than in controls.[170] Total brain radioactivity was slightly but not significantly higher. These studies are not conclusive but give some support to the hypothesis that ionized concentrations of local anesthetics in the brain are elevated during acidosis.

Drug Actions and Interactions

Local Anesthetics. The disposition of local anesthetics may be modified by intrinsic factors—their dose and concentration-dependent effects on the cardiovascular system. Wiklund has shown that intravenous infusions of lidocaine (4 mg/min), bupivacaine and etidocaine (2 mg/min) are associated with a 25 to 30 per cent increase in liver blood flow, which in theory should increase the hepatic clearance of the agents.[199,203,204]

Increased toxicity as a result of competition for plasma- and tissue-binding sites or for access to metabolic enzymes is a possibility when local anesthetics are compounded in the same patient, particularly when two amides are used.[129] However, no differences in plasma concentration-time profiles of etidocaine were observed when intercostal block was performed with etidocaine alone and when it was given with bupivacaine for bilateral block.[39,40] Furthermore, although competition for plasma binding between the amides has been demonstrated *in vitro*, this appears to be significant only at excessive plasma levels of the individual agents.[194] There is evidence *in vitro* that plasma concentrations of etidocaine and bupivacaine in the clinical range may inhibit the plasma hydrolysis of chloroprocaine by 10 to 40 per cent, but the clinical significance of this observation is not known.[104]

General Anesthetics. Although general anesthesia is often combined with regional anesthesia which elevates the threshold for local-anesthetic-induced convulsions, the effects, if any, on the disposition kinetics of local anesthetics are not well defined.

We found only minimal differences in arterial concentration-time profiles of amide agents following epidural injection in conscious volunteers and in patients receiving methohexital by drip and light nitrous oxide and oxygen anesthesia.[196] In dogs, hepatic clearance of lidocaine was significantly reduced under halothane anesthesia, compared to nitrous oxide anesthesia.[54]

Premedicants. Arteriovenous concentration differences of amide local anesthetics measured in the arm were found to be significantly less in premedicated patients than in volunteers who received similar epidural injections. Therefore, it was suggested that administration of premedicants (*e.g.*, meperidine) to patients caused a generalized vasodilatation and opening of cutaneous shunts, which antagonized the compensatory vasoconstriction in the upper limbs produced by lumbar sympathetic blockade.[196] This theory has been subsequently confirmed by experiment. In addition, peak arterial concentrations of lidocaine following epidural injection were reduced by about 50 per cent in meperidine-premedicated subjects.* Morphine, by increasing cerebral blood flow, could increase the delivery of local anesthetic to the brain and predispose the patient to early CNS toxicity.[24] Diazepam, shown to raise the dose threshold to lidocaine-induced seizures in monkeys, also raises the convulsive plasma concentration of local anesthetic by a similar factor (see Chaps. 2 and 4).[17]

Sympathomimetic Agents. Benowitz and colleagues have documented the effects of norepinephrine (alpha-adrenoceptor stimulation) and of isoproterenol (beta-adrenoceptor stimulation) on the disposition kinetics of lidocaine in monkeys.[26] The former significantly increased half-life, decreased initial volume of distribution, and decreased clearance by a reduction in hepatic blood flow; the latter produced exactly the opposite effects. Accordingly, appropriate adjustments are indicated in the intravenous dosage of lidocaine in patients with ventric-

* Mather, L. E., Zachariah, P., and Murphy, T. M.: Unpublished data.

ular arrhythmias who also require these or other sympathomimetic agents. In the presence of norepinephrine, lidocaine dosage may need to be decreased; in the presence of isoproterenol, the reverse may be true. Both epinephrine and ephedrine are reported to increase total hepatic blood flow in humans, and, although this effect has been associated with a corresponding increase in lidocaine clearance, any influence of epinephrine added to solutions for nerve block on systemic disposition of local anesthetics remains to be studied.[205]

Beta-Blocking Agents. Branch and associates showed that the beta-blocking agent propranolol reduces the clearance of lidocaine in dogs.[37] The mechanism of this interaction was related to beta-blockade, causing a decrease in cardiac output and hepatic blood flow, hence reducing the rate of delivery of lidocaine to the liver.

Enzyme-Inducing Agents. A slightly greater clearance of lidocaine has been reported in epileptic patients compared to a group of controls.[90] This difference was not magnified by prior administration of phenobarbital to the epileptic patients, which suggest that established antiepileptic therapy might already have produced a maximal induction of microsomal enzymes and a maximal increase in the perfused mass of liver.

Other Therapeutic Agents. Administration of procainamide or diphenylhydantoin was shown to have no influence on steady state plasma lidocaine levels during continuous intravenous infusion in both patients and in dogs.[97]

On the basis of studies *in vitro* using relatively high concentrations of bupivacaine, Ghoneim and Pandya have claimed that considerable displacement of this agent from plasma-binding sites may occur in patients receiving diphenylhydantoin, quinidine, desipramine, or meperidine.[83] We have subsequently criticized this work, pointing out that the plasma concentrations of the displacing drugs used were well in excess of those encountered during clinical use.[197]

Placental Transfer and Neonatal Disposition

The importance of an understanding of placental transfer and neonatal disposition in the pharmacokinetics of local anesthetics is underlined by the continued appearance of reports that implicate these agents in the etiology of both acute CNS and cardiovascular changes in fetal function and, more recently, in long-term neurobehavioral deficits in the newborn.[15,33,34,154,161,174] This is not to say, however, that a case against the drugs has been established unequivocally except in reports of inadvertent injection of excessive dose directly into the fetus.

Some of the most convincing evidence for a depressant effect of local anesthetics on the fetal myocardium comes from studies of Andersson and associates, who showed that the addition of clinically realistic concentrations of mepivacaine to the solution perfusing isolated human fetal hearts produced dose-dependent deterioration in cardiac performance, especially in the presence of acidosis.[12] Heymann and associates have been able to reproduce the clinical picture of fetal cardiovascular and CNS depression, which sometimes follows obstetric regional anesthesia, by using intravenous infusion of local anesthetics into maternal sheep and fetal lambs.[91] Clinical studies by Shnider and colleagues and by Teramo have implicated the local anesthetic agent as the cause of fetal bradycardia after paracervical block on the basis that the incidence of this complication is agent- and dose-dependent and that it is associated with fetal blood drug concentrations higher than maternal levels.[15,183,184] This phenomenon was explained by the hypothesis that drug diffuses rapidly into the uterine arteries close to the site of injection, resulting in the delivery of high drug concentrations directly to the placenta.[15,178] In contrast to these findings, others have found fetal bradycardia after paracervical block to be associated with fetal : maternal drug concentration ratios of less than unity and lower than those observed when the heart rate was not depressed.[107,183]

Thus, Liston and associates proposed that the problem is not related to a direct toxic effect of the local anesthetic upon the fetus but to some factor that causes a reduction in placental perfusion, thereby reducing both fetal oxygen supply and the amount of drug transfer.[107] However, even if the local anesthetic is not the primary cause of fetal hypoxia and acidosis, the studies of Englesson, which were discussed previously, strongly suggest that the fetus will be more susceptible to the effects of local anesthetics under these conditions.[72]

A number of studies have suggested that local anesthetics might contribute to impaired neurobehavioral response in newborns. In some of these, the experimental design has been inadequate to distinguish between effects of maternal neural blockade *per se* and any influence of the local anesthetic (effectively, spinal versus epidural); interpretation is also complicated by the coadministration of narcotic analgesics.[34,174] However, the reports of Scanlon and colleagues stand out as indicating that babies whose mothers had received epidural lidocaine or mepivacaine had greater deficits than those whose mothers had received epidural bupivacaine or those who were delivered without epidural anesthesia.[34,154,174]

Placental Transfer. As a result of their rapid hydrolysis in maternal blood, local anesthetics of the ester-type do not appear to reach the fetus in significant quantities. Thus, the use of chloroprocaine in obstetrics has recently been readvocated to minimize fetal morbidity, especially following paracervical block.[78,81] In contrast to the esters, the amides rapidly appear in the fetal circulation after the mother has been injected. The concentrations obtained will depend upon the route of injection and are generally proportional to the concentrations achieved in maternal blood. However, measurement of cord/maternal plasma drug concentration ratios (U/M) also reveal significant differences in the transplacental distribution of the various agents. Considerably lower ratios are observed for bupivacaine and etidocaine than for mepivacaine and lidocaine, while prilocaine levels in cord samples may even exceed maternal levels (see following list).

U/M Ratios for Amides

Prilocaine, 1.0–1.1
Lidocaine, 0.5–0.7
Mepivacaine, 0.7
Bupivacaine, 0.2–0.4
Etidocaine, 0.2–0.3

Since there is a strong inverse relationship between average U/M ratios and the degree of plasma binding of the agents, it might be assumed that the differences are explained by a retarding effect of binding on transplacental drug equilibration. However, in itself, this does not seem likely in view of the probability that placental transfer of these small lipid-soluble molecules is perfusion-limited. Also, an alternative factor must be invoked to account for the rapid establishment of the ratios and for their relative stability with time. A reason for this becomes apparent when the binding of the agents is compared in maternal and cord plasma. At similar total plasma drug concentrations, the percentage of drug bound in cord plasma is only one-third to two-thirds of that bound in maternal plasma, and this appears to result from a relative lack of alpha$_1$-globulin in the fetus.[120] Accordingly, equilibrium distribution of total drug across the placenta will favor the maternal side since this has the greater binding capacity (Fig. 3-30). This effect may, however, be partially offset by ion-trapping of local anesthetic in fetal blood, which is relatively more acidic than maternal blood, especially if the fetus is distressed.[183,194] Impaired placental perfusion in acidotic and asphyxiated fetuses may also comprise transfer of local anesthetic back from the fetus to the mother.[138,139]

Although total drug concentrations differ on either side of the placenta, it should be stressed that normally there appears to be no barrier to the transfer of unbound drug. Since pharmacologic activity is generally related to free drug concentration in

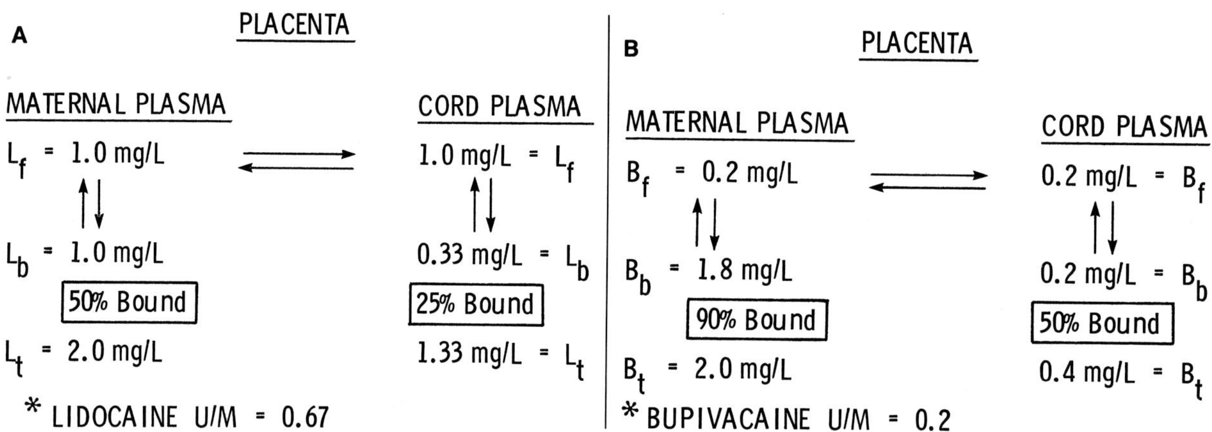

Fig. 3-30. This schematic shows how transplacental distribution of local anesthetics may be predicted from differences in binding of the drugs in maternal and cord plasma. (*A*) Lidocaine, (*B*) Bupivacaine. f, b, t, represent free, bound, and total drug concentrations, respectively.

plasma water, a low U/M ratio for total drug does not in itself signify a reduced risk of fetal or neonatal toxicity. At equilibrium, unbound drug concentations are generally similar in mother and fetus (Fig. 3-30). This possibly explains why a total blood drug concentration of 3 μg per ml of lidocaine or mepivacaine appears to be the maximum tolerated level in the fetus, compared to about 6 μg/ml in the adult.[136] These levels correspond to similar concentrations of unbound drug.

A low U/M ratio, signifying a reduced rate of total drug delivery to the fetus, may be an advantage if this significantly slows the rate at which the drug distribution equilibrium occurs in vital fetal tissues. However, the observation that fetal scalp capillary:maternal blood concentration ratios of both lidocaine and bupivacaine are relatively stable after about 20 minutes indicates that this may be of importance only when delivery occurs quite soon after injection.[21,211] Similar umbilical artery:umbilical vein concentration ratios observed with the various agents also suggest that their equilibration rates in the fetus are comparable, although the relevance of this measurement may be obscured by a considerable shunting of fetal blood by way of the foramen ovale and the ductus arteriosus.[194]

Metabolites of local anesthetics, namely MEGX, parahydroxyxylidine, PPX, PABX, and EABX have been determined in fetal blood after injection of parent drugs into the mother.[28,133] However, the significance of this in relation to fetal toxicity is not known.

Neonatal Drug Disposition. Having left the womb, the newborn can no longer rely on the placenta as a means of returning local anesthetic from whence it came. Clearance of the drugs now depends upon the ability of immature hepatic and renal systems to handle them.

Any investigation of the kinetics of local anesthetics in the newborn following neural blockade in the mother is handicapped by the difficulty of knowing how much of a dose the patient received. Furthermore, when drug metabolites are detected, it is difficult to separate the quantity manufactured by the infant from the contribution donated *in utero* by the mother. Despite these problems, studies have indicated that fetal liver is less able to metabolize local anesthetics than the adult organ, with the implication that the fetal kidney may play a more prominent role in net drug elimination.

Thus, Meffin and colleagues showed that the human neonate has a very limited capacity for aromatic hydroxylation of mepivacaine, an observation subsequently confirmed by Moore who studied disposition of the drug after direct subcutaneous injection into newborns.[124,*] Moore also recovered 50 per cent of the dose as unchanged drug in neonatal urine, compared to a recovery of 5 per cent in the adult. An enhanced role of renal excretion in the neonate is also indicated by studies in which lidocaine was injected into fetal and neonatal lambs and adult sheep. The average proportion of the dose excreted after 4 hours in the urine of each was 1.6 per cent, 16.4 per cent, 1.4 per cent, respectively.[137] These data suggest that there may be some justification for using forced diuresis to promote local anesthetic elimination in intoxicated babies.

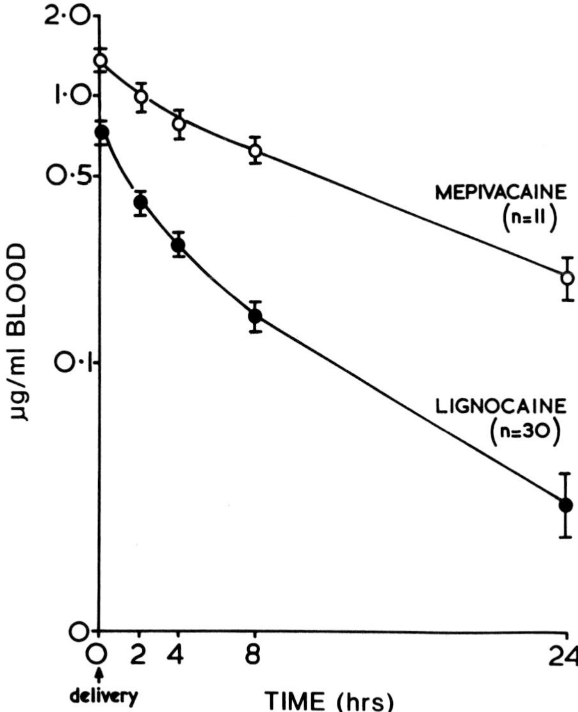

Fig. 3-31. Postnatal, neonatal blood concentrations of local anesthetic after peridural injection into their mothers. (Brown, W.U., *et al.:* Newborn blood levels of lidocaine and mepivacaine in the first postnatal day following epidural anesthesia. Anesthesiology, *42*:698, 1975)

Several studies suggest that the rates of elimination of local anesthetics are considerably slower in neonates than in adults. Plasma elimination half-lives are variously quoted as 3 to 3.5 hours and 5 to 7 hours for lidocaine, 9 to 11 hours for mepivacaine,

* Moore, G.M.: Ph.D. Thesis, University of Sydney, 1975. See Eur. J. Clin. Pharm., *14*:203, 1978.

and around 18 to 25 hours for bupivacaine.[51,58,127,*] In part, these relatively high values probably reflect reduced blood drug binding in the neonate, resulting in a reduced rate of total drug delivery to the organs of elimination. This would be compatible with Moore's observation of greater apparent volumes of distribution (per kg of body weight) of lidocaine and mepivacaine in the neonate than in the adult. Total clearances (per kg of body weight) of lidocaine was similar in neonate and adult, but for mepivacaine neonatal clearances were half of those in the adult. If animal studies reliably provide guidance, the disappearance rate may be reduced further during hypothermia associated with acidosis and hypertension.[140]

Clinical implications of the data accumulated on placental transfer and neonatal disposition of local anesthetics are currently thought to favor the use of either rapidly metabolized chloroprocaine or bupivacaine because of the lack of effect on neurobehavioral response.[154] Mepivacaine appears less desirable than lidocaine, owing to its longer elimination half-life in the newborn, while prilocaine tends to be avoided because of the possibility of inducing methemoglobinemia, especially in an already hypoxic fetus.

REFERENCES

1. Abdel-Salam, A.R., Vonwiller, J.B., and Scott, D.B.: Evaluation of etidocaine in extradural block. Br. J. Anaesth., *47*:1081, 1975.
2. Aberg, G.: Toxicological and local anaesthetic effects of optically active isomers of two local anaesthetic compounds. Acta Pharmacol. Toxicol. (Kbh.), *31*:273, 1972.
3. Aberg, G., and Dhuner, K.G.: Effects of mepivacaine (Carbocaine) on femoral blood flow in the dog. Acta Pharmacol. Toxicol. (Kbh.), *31*:267, 1972.
4. Aberg, G., and Wahlstrom, B.: Vascular effects of mepivacaine. Acta Physiol. Scand., *330*[*Suppl.*]:71, 1969.
5. Adams, H.J.: Effect of *p*H on spinal anesthesia with lidocaine in sheep. Pharmacol. Res. Comm., *7*:551, 1975.
6. Adjepon-Yamoah, K.K., Nimmo, J., and Prescott, L.F.: Gross impairment on hepatic drug metabolism in a patient with chronic liver disease. Br. Med. J., *4*:387, 1974.
7. Adjepon-Yamoah, K.K., and Prescott, L.F.: Lignocaine metabolism in man. Br. J. Pharmacol., *47*:672, 1973.
8. Adler, R., Adler, G., and Aberg, G.: Effects of optically active isomers and racemate of mepivacaine (Carbocaine) in dental anaesthesia. Sven. Tandlak. Tidskr., *62*:501, 1969.
9. Akerman, B.: Uptake and retention of the enantiomers of a local anaesthetic in isolated nerve in relation to different degrees of blocking of nervous conduction. Acta Pharmacol. Toxicol. (Kbh.), *32*:225, 1973.
10. Akerman, B., Astrom, A., Ross, S., and Telc, A.: Studies on the absorption, distribution and metabolism of labelled prilocaine and lidocaine in some animal species. Acta Pharmacol. Toxicol. (Kbh.), *24*:389, 1966.
11. Akerman, B., Persson, N.H. and Tegner, C.: Local anaesthetic properties of the optically active isomers of prilocaine (Citanest). Acta Pharmacol. Toxicol. (Kbh.) *25*:233, 1967.
12. Andersson, K.E., Gennser, G., and Nilsson, E.: Influence of mepivacaine on isolated human foetal hearts at normal and low *p*H. Acta Physiol. Scand., *353*[*Suppl.*]:34, 1970.
13. Appleyard, T.N., Witt, A., Atkinson, R.E., and Nicholas, R.D.G.: Bupivacaine carbonate and bupivacaine hydrochloride: A comparison of blood concentrations during epidural blockade for vaginal surgery. Br. J. Anaesth., *46*:530, 1974.
14. Aps, C., and Reynolds, F.: The effect of concentration in vasoactivity of bupivacaine and lignocaine. Br. J. Anaesth., *48*:1171, 1976.
15. Asling, J.H., Shnider, S.M., Margolis, A.J., Wilkinson, G.R., and Way, E.L.: Paracervical block in obstetrics.II: Etiology of fetal bradycardia following paracervical block anesthesia. Am. J. Obstet. Gynecol., *107*:626, 1970.
16. Astrom, A.: General pharmacology and toxicology of lidocaine. *In* Scott, D.B., and Julian, D.V. (eds.): Lidocaine in the Treatment of Ventricular Arrhythmias. Pp. 128–138. Baltimore, Williams & Wilkens, 1971.
17. Ausinsch, B., Malagodi, M.H., and Munson, E.S.: Diazepam in the prophylaxis of lignocaine seizures. Br. J. Anaesth., *48*:309, 1976.
18. Aven, M.H., Light, A., and Foldes, F.F.: Hydrolysis of procaine in various mammalian plasmas. Fed. Proc., *12*:986, 1953.
19. Beazley, J.M., Taylor, G., and Reynolds, F.: Placental transfer of bupivacaine after paracervical block. Obstet. Gynecol., *39*:2, 1972.
20. Beckett, A.H., Boyes, R.N., and Appleton, P.J.: The metabolism and excretion of lignocaine in man. J. Pharm. Pharmacol., *18*:76s, 1966.
21. Belfrage, P., Raabe, N., and Berlin, A.: Lumbar epidural analgesia with bupivacaine in labour. Am. J. Obstet. Gynecol., *121*:360, 1975.
22. Bennett, A.L., Wagner, J.C., and McIntyre, A.R.: The determination of local anesthetic potency by observation of nerve action potential. J. Pharmacol. Exp. Ther., *75*:125, 1942.
23. Benoit, P.W., and Belt, W.D.: Some effects of local anaesthetic agents on skeletal muscle. Exp. Neurol., *34*:264, 1972.
24. Benowitz, N.: Clinical applications of the pharmacokinetics of lidocaine. *In* Melmon, K.L. (ed.): Cardiovascular Drug Therapy. Philadelphia, F.A. Davis, 1975.
25. Benowitz, N., Forsyth, R.P., and Melmon, K.L.: Lidocaine disposition kinetics in monkey and man I. Prediction by a perfusion model. Clin. Pharmacol. Ther., *16*:87, 1974.
26. Benowitz, N., Forsyth, R.P., Melmon, K.L., and Rowland, M.: Lidocaine disposition kinetics in monkey and man II. Effects of hemorrhage and sympathomimetic drug administration. Clin. Pharmacol. Ther., *16*:99, 1974.
27. Blair, M.R.: Cardiovascular pharmacology of local anaesthetics. Br. J. Anaesth., *47*[*Suppl.*]:247, 1975.
28. Blankenbaker, W.L., DiFazio, C.A., and Berry, F.A.: Lidocaine and its metabolites in the newborn. Anesthesiology, *42*:325, 1975.

* The estimate of bupivacaine half-life contrasts markedly with a mean value of 5 ± 2 (SD) hours calculated from data provided by Dr. G.W. Stephen, University of London. (See Arch. Dis. Child., *52*:638, 1977.)

29. Blumer, J., Strong, J.M., and Atkinson, A.J.: The convulsant potency of lidocaine and its N-dealkylated metabolites. J. Pharmacol. Exp. Ther., *186*:31, 1973.
30. Bonica, J.J., Akamatsu, T.J., Berges, P.U., Morikawa, K., and Kennedy, W.F.: Circulatory effects of peridural block II: Effects of epinephrine. Anesthesiology, *34*:514, 1971.
31. Bonica, J.J., Berges, P.U., and Morikawa, K.I.: Circulatory effects of peridural block: I. Effects of levels of analgesia and dose of lidocaine. Anesthesiology, *33*:619, 1970.
32. Boyes, R.N.: A review of the metabolism of amide local anaesthetic agents. Br. J. Anaesth., *47*:225, 1975.
33. Brackbill, Y.: Psychophysiological measures of pharmacological toxicity in infants: Perinatal and postnatal effects. *In* Morselli, P.L., Garattini, S., and Serini, F. (eds.): Basic and Therapeutic Aspects of Perinatal Pharmacology. Pp. 21–28. New York, Raven Press, 1975.
34. Brackbill, Y., Kane, J., Manniello, R.L., and Abramson, D.: Obstetric meperidine usage and assessment of neonatal status. Anesthesiology, *40*:116, 1974.
35. Braid, D.P., and Scott, D.B.: The systemic absorption of local analgesic drugs. Br. J. Anaesth., *37*:394, 1965.
36. ______: The effect of adrenaline on the systemic absorption of local anaesthetic drugs. Acta Anaesthesiol. Scand., *23* [*Suppl.*]:334, 1966.
37. Branch, R.A., Shand, D.G., Wilkinson, G.R., and Nies, A.S.: The reduction of lidocaine clearance by DL-propranolol: An example of hemodynamic drug interaction. J. Pharmacol. Exp. Ther., *184*:515, 1973.
38. Breck, G.D., and Trager, W.F.: Oxidative N-dealkylation: A Mannich intermediate in the formation of a new metabolite of lidocaine in man. Science, *173*:544, 1971.
39. Bridenbaugh, P.O.: Intercostal nerve blockade for evaluation of local anaesthetic agents. Br. J. Anaesth., *47*:306, 1975.
40. Bridenbaugh, P.O., Tucker, G.T., Moore, D.C., Bridenbaugh, L.D., and Thompson, G.E.: Preliminary clinical evaluation of etidocaine (Duranest): A new long-acting local anesthetic agent. Acta Anaesthesiol. Scand., *18*:165, 1974.
41. Bridenbaugh, P.O., et al.: Role of epinephrine in regional block anesthesia with etidocaine: A double-blind study. Anesth. Analg. (Cleve.), *53*:430, 1974.
42. Brodie, B.B., Lief, P.A., and Poet, R.: The fate of procaine in man following its intravenous administration and methods for the estimation of procaine and diethylaminoethanol. J. Pharmacol. Exp. Ther., *94*:359, 1948.
43. Bromage, P.R.: Physiology and pharmacology of epidural analgesia. Anesthesiology, *28*:592, 1967.
44. Bromage, P.R.: A comparison of bupivacaine and tetracaine in epidural analgesia for surgery. Can. Anaesth. Soc. J., *16*:37, 1969.
45. ______: Lower limb reflex changes in segmental epidural analgesia. Br. J. Anaesth., *46*:504, 1974.
46. ______: Mechanism of action of extradural analgesia. Br. J. Anaesth., *47*[Suppl.]:199, 1975.
47. Bromage, P.R., Burfoot, M.E., Crowell, D.E., and Truant, A.P.: Quality of epidural blockade. III: Carbonated local anaesthetic solutions. Br. J. Anaesth., *39*:197, 1967.
48. Bromage, P.R., and Gertel, M.: An evaluation of two new local anaesthetics for major conduction blockade. Can. Anaesth. Soc. J., *17*:557, 1970.
49. ______: Brachial plexus anesthesia in chronic renal failure. Anesthesiology, *36*:488, 1972.
50. Bromage, P.R., Pettigrew, R.T., and Crowell, D.E.: Tachyphylaxis in epidural analgesia: I. Augmentation and decay of local anesthesia. J. Clin. Pharmacol., *9*:30, 1969.
51. Brown, W.U., *et al.*: Newborn blood levels of lidocaine and mepivacaine in the first postnatal day following maternal epidural anesthesia. Anesthesiology, *42*:698, 1975.
52. Burfoot, M.F., and Bromage, P.R.: The effects of epinephrine on mepivacaine absorption from the spinal epidural space. Anesthesiology, *35*:488, 1971.
53. Burn, J.M., Guyer, P.B., and Langdon, L.: The spread of solutions injected into the epidural space. A study using epidurograms in patients with the lumbosciatic syndrome. Br. J. Anaesth., *45*:338, 1973.
54. Burney, R.G., and DiFazio, C.A.: Hepatic clearance of lidocaine during N_2O anesthesia in dogs. Anesth. Analg. (Cleve.), *55*:322, 1976.
55. Burney, R.G., DiFazio, C.A., Peach, M.J., Petrie, K.A., and Sylvester, M.J.: Anti-arrhythmic effects of lidocaine metabolites. Am. Heart. J., *88*:65, 1974.
56. Byers, M.R., Fink, B.R., Kennedy, R.D., Middaugh, M.E., and Hendrikson, A.E.: Effects of lidocaine on axonal morphology, microtubules and rapid transport in rabbit vagus nerve *in vitro*. J. Neurobiol., *4*:125, 1973.
57. Caldwell, J., Notarianni, L.J., Smith, R.L., and Sneddon, W.: The metabolism of bupivacaine in the rat. Br. J. Pharmacol., *61*:135P, 1977.
58. Caldwell, J., *et al.*: Pharmacokinetics of bupivacaine administered epidurally during childbirth. Br. J. Clin. Pharmacol., *3*:956P, 1976.
59. Cohen, E.N., Levine, D.A., Colliss, J.E., and Gunther, R.E.: The role of *p*H in the development of tachyphylaxis to local anesthetic agents. Anesthesiology, *29*:994, 1968.
60. Collinsworth, K.A., *et al.*: Pharmacokinetics and metabolism of lidocaine in patients with renal failure. Clin. Pharmacol. Ther., *18*:59, 1975.
61. Datta, S., Houle, G.L., and Fox, G.S.: Concentration of lidocaine hydrochloride in newborn gastric fluid after elective caesarian section and vaginal delivery with epidural analgesia. Can. Anaesth. Soc. J., *22*:79, 1975.
62. de Jong, R.: Physiology and Pharmacology of Local Anesthesia. Springfield, Il., Charles C Thomas, 1970.
63. de Jong, R.H., and Nace, R.A.: Nerve impulse conduction during intravenous lidocaine injection. Anesthesiology, *29*:22, 1968.
64. Dhuner, K.G.: Frequency of general side reactions after regional anaesthesia with mepivacaine with and without vasoconstrictors. Acta Anaesthesiol. Scand., *48*[*Suppl.*]:23, 1972.
65. Dhuner, K.G., Harthon, J.G.L., Herbring, B.G., and Lie, T.: Blood levels of mepivacaine after regional anaesthesia. Br. J. Anaesth., *37*:746, 1965.
66. Dhuner, K.G., and Lund, N.: Intercostal blocks with etidocaine. Acta Anaesthesiol. Scand., *60[Suppl.]*:39, 1975.
67. Editorial: J.A.M.A., *193*:300, 1965.
68. Effros, R.M., and Chinard, F.P.: The *in vivo p*H of the extravascular space of the lung. J. Clin. Invest., *48*:1963, 1969.
69. Ekenstam, B.: The effect of the structural variation on the local analgetic properties of the most commonly used groups of substances. Acta Anaesthesiol. Scand., *25 [Suppl.]*:10, 1966.
70. Engberg, G., Holmdahl, M.H., and Edstrom, H.H.: A comparison of the local anesthetic properties of bupivacaine and two new long-acting agents, HS 37 and etidocaine, in epidural analgesia. Acta Anaesthesiol. Scand., *18*:277, 1974.
71. Englesson, S.: The influence of acid-base changes on central nervous system toxicity of local anaesthetic agents I. An

experimental study in cats. Acta Anaesthesiol. Scand., *18*:79, 1974.

72. Englesson, S., and Grevsten, S.: The influence of acid-base changes on central nervous system toxicity of local anaesthetic agents II. Acta Anaesthesiol. Scand., *18*:88, 1974.
73. Erdemir, H.A., Soper, L.E., and Sweet, R.E.: Studies of factors affecting peridural anesthesia. Anesth. Analg. (Cleve.), *44*:400, 1966.
74. Erikssson, E.: Prilocaine, an experimental study in man of a new local anaesthetic with special regards to efficacy, toxicity, and excretion. Acta Chir. Scand., *358*[*Suppl.*]:55, 1966.
75. Evans, C.J., Dewar, J.A., Boyes, R.N., and Scott, D.B.: Residual nerve block following intravenous regional anaesthesia. Br. J. Anaesth., *46*:668, 1974.
76. Fink, B.R.: Acute and chronic toxicity of local anaesthetics. Can. Anaesth. Soc. J., *20*:5, 1973.
77. Fink, B.R., Aasheim, G., Kish, S.J., and Croley, T.S.: Neurokinetics of lidocaine in the infraorbital nerve of the rat *in vivo:* Relation to sensory block. Anesthesiology, *42*:731, 1975.
78. Finster, M., Perel, J.M., Hinsvark, O.N., and O'Brien, J.E.: Reassessment of the metabolism of 2-chloroprocaine hydrochloride (Nesacaine). *In* Abstracts of Scientific Papers—Annual Meeting, San Francisco. Chicago, American Society of Anesthesiologists, 1973.
79. Fish, F., and Wilson, W.D.C.: Excretion of cocaine and its metabolites in man. J. Pharm. Pharmacol., *21*:135s, 1969.
80. Foldes, F.F., Davidson, G.N., Duncalf, D., and Kuwabarra, S.: The intravenous toxicity of local anesthetic agents in man. Clin. Pharmacol. Ther., *6*:328, 1965.
81. Freeman, D.W., and Arnold, N.I.: Paracervical block with low doses of chloroprocaine. J.A.M.A., *231*:56, 1975.
82. Galindo, A., Hernandez, J., Benavides, O., Ortegon de Munoz, S., and Bonica, J.J.: Quality of spinal extradural anaesthesia: The influence of spinal nerve root diameter. Br. J. Anaesth., *47*:41, 1975.
83. Ghoneim, M.M., and Pandya, H.: Plasma protein binding of bupivacaine and its interaction with other drugs in man. Br. J. Anaesth., *46*:435, 1974.
84. Goehl, T.J., Davenport, J.B., and Stanley, M.J.: Distribution, biotransformation and excretion of bupivacaine in the rat and the monkey. Xenobiotica, *3*:761, 1973.
85. Greene, N.M.: The metabolism of drugs employed in anesthesia. Anesthesiology, *29*:327, 1968.
86. Halkin, H., Meffin, P., Melmon, K.L., and Rowland, M.: Influence of congestive heart failure on blood levels of lidocaine and its active monodeethylated metabolite. Clin. Pharmacol. Ther., *17*:669, 1975.
87. Hansson, E., Hoffmann, P., and Kristerson, L.: Fate of mepivacaine in the body: II. Excretion and biotransformation. Acta Pharmacol. Toxicol. (Kbh.), *22*:213, 1965.
88. Haschke, R.H., and Fink, B.R.: Lidocaine effects on brain mitochondrial metabolism *in vitro*. Anesthesiology, *42*:737, 1975.
89. Heavner, J.E., and de Jong, R.H.: Lidocaine blocking concentrations for B- and C-nerve fibers. Anesthesiology, *40*:228, 1974.
90. Heinonen, J., Takki, S., and Jarho, L.: Plasma lidocaine levels in patients treated with potential inducers of microsomal enzymes. Acta Anaesthesiol. Scand., *14*:89, 1970.
91. Heymann, M.A., Teramo, K.A.W., and Rudolph, A.M.: Effects of local anesthetic agents on fetal circulation. *In* Morselli, P.L., Garattini, S., and Serini, F. (eds.): Basic and Therapeutic Aspects of Perinatal Pharmacology. Pp. 97–106. New York, Raven Press, 1975.
92. Hollmen, A., Korhonen, M., and Ojala, A.: Bupivacaine in paracervical block: Plasma levels and changes in maternal and foetal acid-base balance. Br. J. Anaesth., *41*:603, 1969.
93. Hollmen, A., Ojala, A., and Korhonen, M.: Paracervical block with Marcaine/adrenaline. Acta Anaesthesiol. Scand. *13*:1, 1969.
94. Holmdahl, M.H., Sjögren, S., Strom, G., and Wright, B.: Clinical aspects of continuous epidural blockade for postoperative pain relief. Ups. J. Med. Sci., *77*:47, 1972.
95. Jorfeldt, L., *et al.:* The effect of local anaesthetics on the central circulation and respiration in man and dog. Acta Anaesthesiol. Scand., *12*:153, 1968.
96. Kalow, W.: Hydrolysis of local anesthetics by human serum cholinesterase. J. Pharmacol. Exp. Ther., *104*:122, 1952.
97. Karlsson, E., Collste, P., and Rawlins, M.D.: Plasma levels of lidocaine during combined treatment with phenytoin and procainamide. Eur. J. Clin. Pharmacol., *7*:455, 1974.
98. Keenaghan, J.B., and Boyes, R.N.: The tissue distribution, metabolism and excretion of lidocaine in rats, guinea pigs, dogs and man. J. Pharmacol. Exp. Ther., *180*:454, 1972.
99. Kennedy, W.F., Everett, G.B., Cobb, L.A., and Allen, G.D.: Simultaneous systemic and hepatic hemodynamic measurements during high peridural anesthesia in normal men. Anesth. Analg. (Cleve.), *50*:1069, 1971.
100. Kiese, M.: Relationship of drug metabolism to methemoglobin formation. Ann. N. Y. Acad. Sci., *123*:141, 1965.
101. Klingenstrom, P., Nylen, B., and Westermark, L.: A clinical comparison between adrenaline and octapressin as vasoconstrictors in local anaesthesia. Acta Anaesth. Scand., *11*:35, 1967.
102. Kogan, M.J., Verebey, K.G., Depace, A.C., Resnick, R.B., and Mule, S.J.: Quantitative determination of benzoylecgonine and cocaine in human biofluids by gas-liquid chromatography. Analyt. Chem., *49*:1965, 1977.
103. Kristerson, L., Nordenram, A., and Nordqvist, P.: Penetration of radioactive local anaesthetic into peripheral nerve. Arch. Int. Pharmacodyn. Ther., *157:*148, 1965.
103. Kristerson, L., Nordenram, A., and Nordqvist, P.: Penetration of radioactive local anaesthetic into peripheral nerve. Arch. Int. Pharmacodyn. Ther., *157:*148, 1965.
104. Lalka, D., *et al.:* Bupivacaine and other amide local anesthetics inhibit hydrolysis of chloroprocaine by human serum. Anesth. Analg. (Cleve.) *57*:534, 1978.
105. Lebaux, M.: Experimental epidural anaesthesia in the dog with lignocaine and bupivacaine. Br. J. Anaesth., *45*:549, 1973.
106. Levy, A.A., Wallace, D.N., and Dobkin, A.B.: Uptake of local anaesthetics: Movement of ethanol into frog sciatic nerve. Can. Anaesth. Soc. J., *22*:186, 1975.
107. Liston, W.A., Adjepon–Yamoah, K.K., and Scott, D.B.: Foetal and maternal lignocaine levels after paracervical block. Br. J. Anaesth., *45*:750, 1973.
108. Lofstrom, B.: Blocking characteristics of etidocaine (Duranest). Acta Anaesthesiol. Scand. *60*[*Suppl.*]:21, 1975.
109. Luduena, F.P.: Duration of local anesthesia. Annu. Rev. Pharmacol., *9*:503, 1969.
110. Lund, P.C., Bush, D.F., and Covino, B.G.: Determinants of etidocaine concentration in the blood. Anesthesiology, *42*:497, 1975.
111. Lund, P.C., and Covino, B.G.: Distribution of local anesthetics in man following peridural anesthesia. J. Clin. Pharmacol., *7*:324, 1967.
112. Lund, P.C., and Cwik, J.C.: Citanest: A clinical and laboratory study. Anesth. Analg. (Cleve.), *44*:623, 1965.

113. Lund, P.C., Cwik, J.C., and Gannon, R.T.: Etidocaine (Duranest): A clinical and laboratory evaluation. Acta Anaesthesiol. Scand., *18*:176, 1974.
114. Lund, P.C., Cwik, J.C., and Pagdanganan, R.T.: Etidocaine: A new long-acting local anesthetic agent. Anesth. Analg. (Cleve.), *52*:482, 1973.
115. McLean, S., Starmer, G.A., and Thomas, J.: Methaemoglobin formation by aromatic amines. J. Pharm. Pharmacol., *21*:441, 1969.
116. Malogodi, M.H., Munson, E.S., and Embro, M.J.: Relation of etidocaine and bupivacaine toxicity to rate of infusion in rhesus monkeys. Br. J. Anaesth., *49*:121, 1977.
117. Mather, L.E., Long, G.J., and Thomas, J.: The binding of bupivacaine to maternal and foetal plasma proteins. J. Pharm. Pharmacol., *23*:359, 1971.
118. ______: The intravenous toxicity and clearance of bupivacaine in man. Clin. Pharmacol. Ther., *12*:935, 1971.
119. Mather, L.E., and Thomas, J.: Metabolism of lidocaine in man. Life Sci., *11*:915, 1972.
120. ______: Bupivacaine binding to plasma protein fractions. J. Pharm. Pharmacol., *30*:653, 1978.
121. Mather, L.E., Tucker, G.T., Murphy, T.M., Stanton-Hicks, M., and Bonica, J.J.: Effect of adding adrenaline to etidocaine and lignocaine in extradural anaesthesia II: Pharmacokinetics. Br. J. Anaesth., *48*:989, 1976.
122. ______: Haemodynamic drug interaction: Peridural lignocaine and intravenous ephedrine. Acta Anaesthesiol. Scand., *20*:207, 1976.
123. Matthes, H., and Schabert, P.: Vergleichende Undersuchungen über Blutspiegel von mepivacain nach Resorption aus verscheidenen geweben. Acta Anaesthesiol. Scand. *23* [*Suppl.*]:371, 1966.
124. Meffin, P., Long, G.J., and Thomas, J.: Clearance and metabolism of mepivacaine in the human neonate. Clin. Pharmacol. Ther., *14*:218, 1973.
125. Meffin, P., Robertson, A.V., Thomas, J., and Winkler, J.: Neutral metabolites of mepivacaine in humans. Xenobiotica, *3*:191, 1973.
126. Meffin, P., and Thomas, P.: The relative rates of formation of the phenolic metabolites of mepivacaine in man. Xenobiotica, *3*:625, 1973.
127. Mihaly, G.W., *et al.*: The pharmacokinetics of the anilide local anaesthetics in neonates. I. Lignocaine. Eur. J. Clin. Pharmacol., *13*:143, 1978.
128. Moir, D.D.: Recent advances in pain relief in childbirth II: Regional anaesthesia. Br. J. Anaesth., *43*:849, 1971.
129. Moore, D.C., Bridenbaugh, L.D., Bridenbaugh, P.O., Thompson, G. E., and Tucker, G.T.: Does compounding of local anesthetic agents increase their toxicity in humans? Anesth. Analg. (Cleve.), *51*:579, 1972.
130. Moore, D.C., Bridenbaugh, L.D., Bridenbaugh, P.O., and Tucker, G.T.: Bupivacaine hydrochloride: Laboratory and clinical studies. Anesthesiology, *32*:78, 1970.
131. Moore, D.C., *et al.*: Arterial and venous plasma levels of bupivacaine (Marcaine) following epidural and intercostal nerve blocks. Anesthesiology, *45*:39, 1976.
132. Moore, D.C., *et al.*: Bupivacaine (Marcaine): An evaluation of its tissue and systemic toxicity in humans. Acta Anaesthesiol. Scand., *21*:109, 1977.
133. Morgan, D.J., Cousins, M.J., McQuillan, D., and Thomas, J.: Disposition and placental transfer of etidocaine in pregnancy. Eur. J. Clin. Pharmacol., *12*:359, 1977.
134. Morgan, D.J., Smyth, M.P., Thomas, J., and Vine, J.: Cyclic metabolites of etidocane in humans. Xenobiotica, *7*:365, 1977.
135. Morikawa, K.I., Bonica, J.J., Tucker, G.T., and Murphy, T.M.: Effect of acute hypovolaemia on lignocaine absorption and cardiovascular response following epidural block in dogs. Br. J. Anaesth., *46*:631, 1974.
136. Morishima, H.O., Daniel, S.S., Finster, M., Poppers, P.J., and James, L.S.: Transmission of mepivacaine hydrochloride (Carbocaine) across the human placenta. Anesthesiology, *27*:147, 1966.
137. Morishima, H.O., *et al.*: Renal excretion of lidocaine in fetal and neonatal lambs and adult sheep. *In* Abstracts of scientific Papers—Annual Meeting, Chicago. Chicago, American Society of Anesthesiologists, 1975.
138. Morishima, H.O., Heymann, M.A., and Rudolph, A.M.: Transfer of lidocaine across the sheep placenta to the fetus. Am. J. Obstet. Gynecol., *122*:581, 1975.
139. Morishima, H.O., Heymann, M.A., Rudolph, A.M., and Barrett, C.T.: Toxicity of lidocaine in the fetal and newborn lamb and its relationship to asphyxia. Am. J. Obstet. Gynecol., *112*:72, 1972.
140. Morishima, H.O., Mueller-Heubach, E., and Shnider, S.M.: Body temperature and disappearance of lidocaine in newborn puppies. Anesth. Analg. (Cleve.), *50*:938, 1971.
141. Murphy, T.M., Mather, L.E., Stanton-Hicks, M., and Bonica, J.J.: The duration of sympathetic blockade following peridural anesthesia with different local anesthetic agents. Proc. First Meeting, International Association for the Study of Pain, Florence, Italy, 1975.
142. Murphy, T.M., Mather, L.E., Stanton-Hicks, M.d'A., Bonica, J.J., and Tucker, G.T.: Effects of adding adrenaline to etidocaine and lignocaine in extradural anaesthesia. I: Block characteristics and cardiovascular effects. Br. J. Anaesth., *48*:893, 1976.
143. Nation, R.L., Triggs, E.J., and Selig, M.: Lignocaine kinetics in cardiac patients and aged subjects. Br. J. Clin. Pharmacol., *4*:439, 1977.
144. Nelson, S.D., Breck, G.D., and Trager, W.F.: *in vivo* metabolite condensations. Formation of N1-ethyl-2-methyl-N3-(2, 6-dimethylphenyl)-4-imidazolinone from the reaction of a metabolite of alcohol with a metabolite of lidocaine. J. Med. Chem., *16*:1106, 1973.
145. Nelson, S.D., Garland, W.A., Breck, G.D., and Trager, W.F.: Quantification of lidocaine and several metabolites utilizing chemical-ionization mass spectrometry and stable isotope labelling. J. Pharm. Sci., *66*:1180, 1977.
146. Nelson, S.D., Garland, W.A., and Trager, W.F.: Lack of evidence for the formation of N-hydroxyamide metabolites of lidocaine in man. Res. Commun. Chem. Pathol. Pharmacol., *8*:45, 1974.
147. Nishimura, N., Kitahara, T., and Kusakabo, T.: The spread of lidocaine and I-131 solution in the epidural space. Anesthesiology, *20*:785, 1959.
148. Nordqvist, P.: The occurrence of procaine esterase in peripheral nerve and its influence on procaine block. Acta Pharmacol. Toxicol. (Kbh.), *8*:217, 1952.
149. Poppers, P., Covino, B.G., and Boyes, R.N.: Epidural block with etidocaine for labor and delivery. Acta Anaesthesiol. Scand. *160*[*Suppl.*]:89, 1975.
150. Prescott, L.F., Adjepon–Yamoah, K.K., and Talbot, R.G.: Impaired lignocaine metabolism in patients with myocardial infarction and cardiac failure. Br. Med. J., *1*:939, 1976.
151. Quimby, C.W.: Influence of blood loss on the duration of regional anesthesia. Anesth. Analg. (Cleve.), *44*:387, 1965.
152. Radtke, H., Nolte, H., Fruhstorfer, H., and Zenz, M.: A comparative study between etidocaine and bupivacaine in ulnar nerve block. Acta Anaesthesiol. Scand. *60* [*Suppl.*]:17, 1975.

153. Raj, P.P., Rosenblatt, R., Miller, J., Katz, R.L., and Carden, E.: Dynamics of local anesthetic compounds in regional anesthesia. Anesth. Analg. (Cleve.), *56*:110, 1977.
154. Ralston, D.H., and Shnider, S.M.: The fetal and neonatal effects of regional anesthesia in obstetrics. Anesthesiology, *48*:34, 1978.
155. Reidenberg, M.M., James, M., and Dring, L.G.: The rate of procaine hydrolysis in serum of normal subjects and diseased patients. Clin. Pharmacol. Ther., *13*:279, 1972.
156. Reynolds, F.: Metabolism and excretion of bupivacaine in man: A comparison with mepivacaine. Br. J. Anaesth., *43*:33, 1971.
157. Roth, R.A., and Rubin, R.J.: Role of blood flow in carbon monoxide and hypoxic hypoxia-induced alerations in hexobarbital metabolism in rats. Drug Metab. & Dispos., *5*:460, 1976.
158. Rowland, M.: Local anesthetic absorption, distribution and elimination. *In* Eger, E., II.(ed.): Anesthetic Uptake and Action Pp. 332–366. Baltimore, Williams & Wilkins, 1974.
159. Rowland, M., Thomson, P., Guichard, A., and Melmon, K.L.: Disposition kinetics of lidocaine in normal subjects. Ann. N. Y. Acad. Sci., *179*:383, 1971.
160. Rud, J.: Local anaesthetics: An electrophysiological investigation of local anaesthesia of peripheral nerves, with special reference to lidocaine. Acta Physiol. Scand., *51* [*Suppl. 178*]:7, 1961.
161. Scanlon, J.W., Brown, W.U., Weiss, J.B., and Alper, M.H.: Neurobehavioural responses of newborn infants after maternal epidural anesthesia. Anesthesiology, *40*:121, 1974.
162. Scanlon, J.W., *et al.*: Neurobehavioral responses and drug concentration in newborns after maternal epidural anesthesia with bupivacaine. Anesthesiology, *45*:400, 1976.
163. Schulte-Steinberg, O., Hartmuth, L., and Shutt, L.: Carbon dioxide salts of lignocaine in brachial plexus block. Anaesthesia, *25*:191, 1970.
164. Scott, D.B.: Evaluation of the toxicity of local anaesthetic agents in man. Br. J. Anaesth., *47*:56, 1975.
165. Scott, D.B., Jebson, P.J.R., Braid, D.P., Ortengren, B., and Frisch, P.: Factors affecting plasma levels of lignocaine and prilocaine. Br. J. Anaesth., *44*:1040, 1972.
166. Scott, D.B., Littlewood, D.G., Drummond, G.B., Buckley, P.F., and Covino, B.G.: Modification of the circulatory effects of extradural block combined with general anaesthesia by the addition of adrenaline to lignocaine solutions. Br. J. Anaesth., *49*:917, 1977.
167. Scurlock, J.E., Heavner, J.E., and de Jong, R.H.: Differential B and C fibre block by an amide- and an ester-linked Br. J. Anaesth., *47*:1135, 1975.
168. Shnider, S.M., and Gildea, J.: Paracervical block anesthesia in obstetrics, III, Choice of drug: Fetal bradycardia following administration of lidocaine, mepivacaine, and prilocaine. Am. J. Obstet. Gynecol., *116*:320, 1973.
169. Sivarajan, M., Amory, D.W., Lindbloom, L.E., and Schwettmann, R.S.: Systemic and regional blood-flow changes during spinal anesthesia in the rhesus monkey. Anesthesiology, *43*:78, 1975.
170. Sjöstrand, U., and Widman, B.: Distribution of bupivacaine in the rabbit under normal and acidotic conditions. Acta Anaesthesiol. Scand., *50*:1, 1973.
171. Sjögren, S., and Wright. B.: Blood concentration of lidocaine during continuous epidural blockade. Acta Anaesthesiol. Scand., *16* [*Suppl. 46*]:51, 1972.
172. Skou, J.C.: Local anaesthetics.III. Distribution of local anaesthetics between the solid phase/aqueous phase of peripheral nerves. Acta Pharmacol. Toxicol. (Kbh.), *10*:297, 1954.
173. Smith, E.R., and Duce, B.R.: The acute antiarrhythmic and toxic effects in mice and dogs of 2-ethylamino-2′, 6′-acetoxylidine (L-86), a metabolite of lidocaine. J. Pharmacol. Exp. Ther., *179*:580, 1971.
174. Standley, K., Soule, A.B., Copans, S.A., and Duchowny, M.S.: Local-regional anesthesia during childbirth: Effect on newborn behaviour. Science, *186*:634, 1974.
175. Stanton-Hicks, M. D'A.: A study using bupivacaine for continuous peridural analgesia in patients undergoing surgery of the hip. Acta Anaesthesiol. Scand., *15*:97, 1971.
176. Stanton-Hicks, M. D'A. Berges, P.U., and Bonica, J.J.: Circulatory effects of peridural block. IV: Comparison of the effects of epinephrine and phenylephrine. Anesthesiology, *39*:308, 1973.
177. Stanton-Hicks, M., Murphy, T.M., Bonica, J.J., Mather, L.E., and Tucker, G.T.: Effects of extradural block: Comparison of the properties, circulatory effects and pharmacokinetics of etidocaine and bupivacaine. Br. J. Anaesth., *48*:575, 1976.
178. Steffenson, J.L., Shnider, S.M., and de Lorimer, A.A.: Transarterial diffusion of mepivacaine. Anesthesiology, *32*:459, 1970.
179. Stewart, D.J., Inaba, T., Tang, B.K., and Kalow, W.: Hydrolysis of cocaine in human plasma. Life Sci., *20*:1557, 1977.
180. Strong, J.M., *et al.*: Pharmacological activity, metabolism, and pharmacokinetics of glycinexylidide. Clin. Pharmacol. Ther., *17*:184, 1975.
181. Strong, J.M., Parker, M., and Atkinson, A.J.: Identification of glycinexylidide in patients treated with intravenous lidocaine. Clin. Pharmacol. Ther., *14*:67, 1973.
182. Takman, B.: The chemistry of local anaesthetic agents: Br. J. Anaesth., *47*:183, 1975.
183. Teramo, K., and Rajamaki, A.: Foetal and maternal plasma levels of mepivacaine and foetal acid-base balance and heart rate after paracervical blodk during labour. Br. J. Anaesth., *43*:300, 1971.
184. Teramo, K., and Widholm, G.: Studies of the effect of anaesthetics on the foetus. I. The effect of paracervical block with mepivacaine upon foetal acid-base values. Acta Obstet. Gynecol. Scand. *46* [*Suppl.*]:23, 1967.
185. Thomas, J., Long, G., Moore, G., and Morgan, D.: Plasma protein binding and placental transer of bupivacaine. Clin. Pharmacol. Ther., *19*:426, 1976.
186. Thomas, J., and Meffin, P.: Aromatic hydroxylation of lidocaine and mepivacaine in rats and humans. J. Med. Chem., *15*:1046, 1972.
187. Thomas, J., Morgan, D., and Vine, J.: Metabolism of etidocaine in man. Xenobiotica, *6*:39, 1976.
188. Thomson, P., *et al.*: Lidocaine pharmacokinetics in advanced heart failure, liver disease, and renal failure in humans. Ann. Intern. Med., *78*:499, 1973.
189. Truant, A.P., and Takman, B.: Differential physical-chemical and neuropharmacologic properties of local anesthetic agents. Anesth. Analg. (Cleve.), *38*:478, 1959.
190. Tucker, G.T.: Biotransformation and toxicity of local anaesthetics. Acta Anaesthesiol. Belg. *26* [*Suppl.*]:123, 1975.
191. ———: Plasma binding and disposition of local anesthetics. Int. Anesthesiol. Clin., *13*:33, 1975.
192. Tucker, G.T., and Boas, R.A.: Pharmacokinetic aspects of intravenous regional anesthesia. Anesthesiology, *34*:538, 1971.
193. Tucker, G.T., Boyes, R.N., Bridenbaugh, P.O., and

Moore, D.C.: Binding of anilide-type local anesthetics in human plasma I: Relationships between binding, physicochemical properties and anesthetic activity. Anesthesiology, *33*287, 1970.

194. ______: Binding of anilide type local anesthetics in human plasm. II Implications *in vivo* with special reference to transplacental distribution. Anesthesiology, *33*:304, 1970.

195. Tucker, G.T., *et al:* Observed and predicted accumulation of local anaesthetic agent during continuous extradural analgesia. Br. J. Anaesth., *49*:237, 1977.

196. Tucker, G.T., and Mather, L.E.: Pharmacokinetics of local anaesthetic agents. Br. J. Anaesth., *47*:213, 1975.

197. ______: Plasma protein binding of bupivacaine and its interaction with other drugs in man. Br. J. Anaesth., *47*:1029, 1975.

198. Tucker, G.T., Moore, D.C., Bridenbaugh, P.O., Bridenbaugh, L.D., and Thompson, G.E.: Systemic absorption of mepivacaine in commonly used regional block procedures. Anesthesiology, *37*:277, 1972.

199. Tucker, G.T., Wiklund, L., Berlin, A., and Mather, L.E.: Hepatic clearance of local anesthetics in man. J. Pharmacokinet. Biopharm., *5*:111, 1977.

200. Usubiaga, J.: Neurological complications following epidural anesthesia. Int. Anesthesiol. Clin., *13*:1, 1975.

201. Vine, J., Morgan, D., and Thomas, J.: The identification of eight hydroxylated metabolites of etidocaine by chemical ionization mass spectrometry. Xenobiotica. *8*:509, 1978.

202. Weisburger, J.H., and Weisburger, E.K.: Biochemical formation and pharmacological, toxicological, and pathological properties of hydroxylamines and hydroxamic acids. Pharmacol. Rev., *25*:1, 1973.

203. Wiklund, L.: Human hepatic blood flow and its relation to systemic circulation during intravenous infusion of lidocaine. Acta Anaesthesiol. Scand., *21*:148, 1977.

204. ______: Human hepatic blood flow and its relation to systemic circulation during intravenous infusion of bupivacaine or etidocaine. Acta Anaesthesiol. Scand., *21*:189, 1977.

205. Wiklund, L., Tucker, G.T., and Engberg, G.: Influence of intravenously administered epinephrine on splanchnic haemodynamics and clearance of lidocaine. Acta Anaesthesiol. Scand., *21*:275, 1977.

206. Wilkinson, G.R., and Lund, P.C.: Bupivacaine levels in plasma and cerebrospinal fluid following peridural administration. Anesthesiology, *33*:482, 1970.

207. Williams, R., Blaschke, T.F., Meffin, P.J., Melmon, K.L., and Rowland, M.: Influence of viral hepatitis on the disposition of two compounds with high hepatic clearance: Lidocaine and indocyanine green. Clin. Pharmacol. Ther., *20*:290, 1976.

208. Winnie, A.P., Lavallee, D.A., Sosa, B.P., and Masud, K.Z.: Clinical pharmacokinetics of local anaesthetics. Can. Anaesth. Soc. J., *24*:252, 1977.

209. Winnie, A.P., Tay, C-H., Patel, K.P., Ramamurthy, S., and Durrani, Z.: Pharmacokinetics of local anesthetics during plexus blocks. Anesth. Analg., *56*:852, 1977.

210. Woods, L.A., McMahon, F.G., and Seevers, M.H.: Distribution and metabolism of cocaine in the dog and rabbit. J. Pharmacol. Exp. Ther., *101*:200, 1951.

211. Zador, G., Englesson, S., and Nilsson, B.A.: Low dose intermittent epidural anaesthesia in labour. I. Clinical efficacy and lidocaine concentrations in maternal and foetal blood. Acta Obstet. Gynecol. Scand. *34*[*Suppl.*]:3,1974.

4 Clinical Pharmacology of Local Anesthetic Agents

D. B. Scott and Michael J. Cousins

In recent years there has been a resurgence of interest in local anesthesia. The realization that general anesthetic agents might not be as free from side-effects as was originally thought has led to an increased use of narcotic analgesics, often at a high dosage, in conjunction with muscle relaxants. The analgesia supplied by local anesthetic techniques, however, is usually much superior and is not associated with depression of the central nervous system (CNS). Such analgesia allows a pain-free emergence from anesthesia and may be continued well into the postoperative period. Abolition of the painful input to the CNS during and after an operation prevents or modifies the stress response to surgery, thus permitting a more rapid recovery.

Moreover, there has been a considerable increase in the basic information available on local anesthesia. Clarification of the anatomy of regional anesthesia and the physiologic effects of major nerve blocks and, perhaps most important, the flood of basic pharmacologic data about the agents used have allowed the performance of regional techniques with a maximum of effect and a minimum of toxicity. This chapter describes the wide range of agents and traces the early development of local anesthetics, when only one or two agents were known, to the present when many agents provide great versatility. It can now be said that a full knowledge of the clinical pharmacology of local anesthetics enables the achievement of effective and safe regional block for the entire range of local anesthetic techniques.

THE "SPECTRUM" OF LOCAL ANESTHETICS

The evolution, development, and popularity of regional anesthesia has, over the years, been closely related to the introduction, from time to time, of newer and more effective local anesthetic agents and an increasing knowledge of the clinical pharmacology of all local anesthetics.

The naturally occurring drug cocaine was the first to be used. Although it was isolated by Niemann in 1860, 24 years were to elapse before Koller realized its potential and used it to anesthetize the cornea in ophthalmic surgery. It was quickly realized that by injecting cocaine many operations could be performed without recourse to general anesthesia. Thus, the techniques of infiltration, nerve block, and spinal anesthesia were introduced. However, the high toxicity and habit-forming tendency of cocaine were soon recognized, and numerous fatalities were reported. This led to a search for synthetic alternatives with less toxicity (see also Chap. 1).

As a result of the knowledge of the structure of cocaine, several drugs with local anesthetic properties were synthesized, but each presented practical difficulties, either in manufacture or in clinical use. However, in 1905, Einhorn introduced procaine, which was to hold pride of place for the next half-century. Although it is a reasonably safe drug, procaine suffers from three major defects: namely, a limited spreading power, so that highly accurate placement of the drug is essential to success; a relative lack of potency, which led to imperfect results in large-nerve blockade; and a short duration of effect. In addition, because it is an ester, it is unstable in solution and cannot be autoclaved.

In 1932, while investigating antipyretics, Miescher discovered dibucaine, which is extremely potent and has a long duration of action. Its toxicity, however, made it unpopular when large doses were required, and it found its major role in spinal anesthesia, particularly in Great Britain and Australia. An important property of the drug is its stability in solution—owing to its being an amide rather than an ester. This simple fact, however, was apparently not appreciated at the time, and it was not until 1948, when Löfgren reported the local anesthetic properties of lidocaine, that the importance of the amide bond became fully apparent. Lidocaine, therefore, was, at last an agent with marked stability, good spreading power and potency, and a reasonable duration of effect. Since that time other drugs similar to lidocaine have been introduced, such as mepivacaine and prilocaine. The next important step, however, was the introduction of bupivacaine in the early 1960s and the recognition of its prolonged duration of action. This fact has considerable impact, particularly for the use of bupivacaine in extradural block with both single-dose and continuous techniques. The usefulness of long-acting agents is now well-recognized, and the latest drug in this field is etidocaine (Fig. 4-1).

Clinical Properties and Uses

Currently, the choice of agents is wide, and, although there will undoubtedly be future additions, it is now possible to select a drug that will fulfill most of the anesthetic requirements for all of the regional block techniques. The primary considerations when choosing among the agents are shown in Figure 4-1 and Table 4-1 and are discussed below.

As described in Chapter 3 and illustrated in Table 3-1, local anesthetics have certain common characteristics, but their physicochemical properties differ considerably. These differences in partition coefficient (oil/water solubility), protein binding, and pK_a play an important part in determining aspects of neural blockade, such as latency and duration of action, potential toxicity, and ability to cross lipid barriers.

Effectiveness. An agent must be effective for the required block, but its effectiveness depends upon the type of nerve fibers to be blocked: motor, sensory, or autonomic. It has become clear that certain drugs can preferentially affect one of these functions; for example, bupivacaine may often produce intense analgesia without marked motor paralysis, whereas etidocaine provides analgesia that is much more frequently accompanied by motor blockade. Blockade of sensory and motor fibers is required for surgical procedures, whereas obstetric analgesia may be obtained by autonomic blockade alone.

Speed of Onset (Latency). A long period of latency may not be a disadvantage if the operation is not urgent, but a short period of latency would be essential in an emergency. Thus, lidocaine and chloroprocaine have advantages for the latter situation whereas bupivacaine may be satisfactory in the former. Onset time is considerably affected by the concentration of solution, stronger solutions being more rapid in their effect (Table 4-2).[57]

Spreading Power. Most agents now in common use have the ability to spread along tissue planes. This property is of considerable importance to the success rate of a nerve block. Procaine requires great accuracy in needle placement and consequently has a substantial failure rate, much greater than that seen with an agent such as lidocaine.

Duration of Action. Some agents, such as chloroprocaine, have a brief duration of action, which would be useful if the rapid return of normal function is desirable. Other agents, such as bupivacaine and etidocaine, might be preferred for their long duration of action if the surgical procedure was lengthy or for postoperative pain relief. Duration of action also depends on the dose and concentration of the drug and epinephrine used (Table 4-2).[19] Thus bupivacaine in weak solution without epinephrine lasts no longer than lidocaine with epinephrine (see Table 4-4).[57]

Toxicity. While it is generally desirable to use drugs of the lowest possible toxicity, toxicity may not be of concern if the dose to be used is small. Thus, although dibucaine and tetracaine are relatively toxic compounds, their use in spinal anesthesia, which only requires low dosage, is not contraindicated. In contrast, for intravenous regional anesthesia, a drug of low toxicity, such as prilocaine, would be the first choice, to obviate the hazard of accidental release of the tourniquet shortly after injection (Fig. 4-1; also see Table 4-1).

All local anesthetic drugs are toxic substances, with a margin between the safe and toxic doses of only two (see Table 3-4). However, they have two important advantages over most other drugs. First, they are applied at their site of action, which enables a very high local concentration around the nerves to be blocked with only a low systemic concentration. Second, they are administered by practitioners who will be in attendance at the time toxicity is likely to occur; that is, within the first minute if the drug is inadvertently injected into a blood vessel or up to 30 minutes after uneventful injection, at the time of peak blood concentration. Appropriate supervision and treatment of any untoward reaction are thus possible and require prompt and informed action to prevent serious sequelae.

Surface Activity. While most local anesthetics are absorbed from mucous membranes and may, therefore, produce anesthesia of those membranes, this is not universal. The most effective anesthetics for mucous membranes are cocaine, tetracaine, and lidocaine; the least effective are procaine and mepivacaine which do not possess significant local anesthetic activity when they are applied topically (Table 4-1).

(Text continues on p. 90.)

Table 4-1. Local Anesthetic Agents, Concentrations and Clinical Uses of

Agent	Concentration (%) and Clinical Use	Onset and Duration	Peak Blood Concentration C_{max} (mcg/ml) Epidural Block	Threshold Toxic Blood Concentration C_{tox} (mcg/ml)	$\frac{C_{max}}{C_{tox}}$	Maximum Single Dose (mg)	Comments
Amides							
Lidocaine	0.5–1; infiltration or IV 1–1.5; peripheral nerve 1–2; epidural/caudal 4; topical 5; spinal	Rapid onset; short to intermediate duration (60–120 min)	3.5 20 ml, 2% 2.4 20 ml, 2% + epinephrine	5–6	1.6 2.3	300* 500 epinephrine	Excellent spreading ability; wide range of applications
Prilocaine	0.5–1; infiltration or IV 1; peripheral nerve 2–3; epidural/caudal	Slow onset (faster with 3% for epidural); short to intermediate duration (60–120 min)	2.5 20 ml, 2% 1.8 20 ml, 2% + epinephrine	5–6	3.2 4.4	400* 600 epinephrine	0.5% is drug of choice for intravenous block; most rapidly metabolized and safest of all amide-type agents; doses in excess of 600 mg produce significant amounts of MetHb; therefore, avoid doses above 600 mg and repeated doses; probably also drug of choice in outpatient block
Mepivacaine	1; infiltration 1–1.5; peripheral nerve 1.5–2; epidural/caudal	Slow onset; intermediate to longer duration (90–180 min)	3.5 20 ml, 2% 2.8 20 ml, 2% + epinephrine	5–6	1.6 2	300* 500 epinephrine	Duration slightly longer than equal dose of lidocaine and blood levels not as sensitive to inclusion of epinephrine as lidocaine; thus may be useful if epinephrine not desirable
Etidocaine	0.5; infiltration 0.5–1; peripheral nerve 1–1.5; epidural/caudal	Rapid onset; long duration (4–8 h)	0.8 20 ml, 1% 0.6 20 ml, 1% + epinephrine	~2	2.5 3.3	300 400 epinephrine	Capable of producing profound motor block; excellent for intraoperative analgesia and muscle relaxation; useful for postoperative pain relief by peripheral nerve block
Bupivacaine	0.25–0.5; infiltration 0.25–0.5; peripheral nerve 0.5–0.75; epidural/caudal (surgical) 0.5; spinal 0.25; epidural (obstetrics)	Slow onset; long duration (4–8 h) Slow onset and reduced duration with low concentration for epidural	0.8 20 ml, 0.5% 0.6 20 ml, 0.5% + epinephrine	~1.6	2 2.7	175 250 epinephrine	Favored for obstetric nerve blocks because of minimal fetal effects; excellent for postoperative analgesia because of minimal motor block
Dibucaine	0.5; spinal	Rapid onset; long duration (3–4 h)		Unknown		50	Relatively toxic; for spinal block only; no information on blood levels

Esters				
Procaine	1; infiltration 2; epidural/caudal (only if amides not usable) 2; spinal	Slow onset; short duration (30–45 min)	500 without epinephrine 600 with	Indicated when history of malignant hyperpyrexia (MH) ideal for skin infiltration; very rapidly metabolized
Chloroprocaine	1–2 same as procaine	Rapid onset; medium duration	600 without epinephrine + 50 with	Drug of choice in USA and UK for obstetric and outpatient neural blockade; metabolized four times more rapidly than procaine
Tetracaine	0.5–1 topical 0.1–0.2 infiltration, peripheral nerve 0.4–0.5; epidural/caudal 0.25; epidural/caudal 1; spinal	Slow onset; long duration	100, approximately	May be useful alternative if amides contraindicated (*e.g.*, MH); metabolized four times more slowly than procaine
Cocaine	4–10; topical	Slow onset; medium duration	150, approximately (1.5 ml of 10% or 4 ml of 4%)	Topical use only; addictive; indirect adrenoceptor stimulation; no evidence that 10% solution more effective than 4%; patients sensitive to exogenous catecholamines should receive topical lidocaine rather than cocaine
Benzocaine	0.4–5; topical only (usually dispensed in admixture with other therapeutic ingredients, related to site of application)	Rapid onset; short duration	Unknown	Occasionally dispensed in urethane solution; urethane is a suspect carcinogen and should not be used

* When used by nonspecialists, should not exceed 200 mg.

Table 4-2. Effects of Dose and Epinephrine on Local Anesthetic Properties

	Increased Dose (Concentration or Volume)	*Addition of Epinephrine*
Onset time	↓	↓ (Minimal effect for etidocaine)
Degree of motor blockade	↑	↑
Degree of sensory blockade	↑	↑
Duration of blockade	↑	↑
Peak plasma Local anesthetic concentration	↑	↓ (See also Table 3-5)
Area of blockade	↑	↑

LOCAL ANESTHETIC DRUGS

The two major groups of local anesthetics are amides and esters. As discussed in the text and illustrated in Table 4-1 and Figures 3-1 and 3-5, these two chemical groups possess several distinguishing characteristics. The esters are rapidly hydrolyzed in the plasma, whereas the breakdown of amides depends on hepatic metabolism. In addition, some patients manifest immune responses to the esters but not to the amides. In the following discussion of local anesthetic agents, it should be kept in mind that safe adult doses are provided for healthy adults. Doses are not given on a mg per kg basis since no such relationship has been established in adults (see Fig. 4-13; also Chap. 3). For the dosage for children, Chapter 21 should be consulted.

AMIDES

The amide group of local anesthetics can be divided into anilides and quinolines.

ANILIDES

The anilide group contains most of the local anesthetic drugs in common use, most notably lidocaine.

Lidocaine (Xylocaine)

The molecular formula for lidocaine appears at the top of the next column.

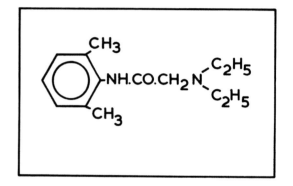

Physicochemical Properties. Lidocaine base has a partition coefficient of 2.9 and a pK_a of 7.9 (see also Table 3-1). The hydrochloride salt is water-soluble and has a pH of 6.5. It is 58 to 75 per cent protein-bound in plasma, and the blood plasma to erythrocyte concentration ratio of lidocaine is 1:0.8. There is a discrepancy between the U.S.P. and B.A.N. formulation (lignocaine), the former referring to lidocaine hydrochloride anhydrous and the latter to lidocaine hydrochloride salt. It should be remembered that 1 g of the hydrochloride salt is equivalent to 0.938 g of the hydrochloride anhydrous and 0.811 g of lidocaine base. Thus the B.A.N. form contains 6 per cent less local anesthetic than the U.S.P. form.

In addition to the hydrochloride salt, lidocaine can be prepared as a carbonated solution (see Chap. 2).

As a result of its slim molecular shape, a pK_a close to the physiologic pH, and a moderate lipid solubility, lidocaine has excellent spreading capabilities. Thus, it is generally preferred over procaine and mepivacaine, both of which are similar to lidocaine in other respects. Lidocaine is an ideal agent for most block procedures in which rapid onset is required (see Fig. 4-1; Table 4-1).

Effective Concentrations and Clinical Properties. Tables 4-1 to 4-5 and Figures 4-1 to 4-3 compare and contrast properties and forms of local anesthetics.

Topical Anesthesia. A 4-per-cent solution is available and provides effective topical anesthesia for oropharynx, tracheobronchial tree, and nose. A 2-per-cent solution also provides some degree of

Table 4-3. Topical Anesthesia

Agent	*Effective Concentration and Preparation Form*	*Clinical Application*	*Onset (min)*	*Duration (min)*
Benzocaine	20% ointment	Skin and mucous membrane	Slow	Prolonged
Cocaine	4% solution	Ear, nose, and throat	5–10	10–15
	10% solution	Ear, nose, and throat	2.5	30
Tetracaine	0.25–1% solution	Ear, nose, and throat	5–10	60
	0.5–1% cream	Skin, rectum, and mucous membrane		
Dibucaine	0.25–1% cream ointment	Skin		
	0.25% solution	Ear		
	2.5% suppositories	Rectum		
Lidocaine	2–4% solution	Oropharynx, tracheobronchial tree, and nose	5	15–30
	2% jelly	Urethra	5	15–30
	2.5–5% ointment	Skin, mucous membrane, rectum	5	15–30
	2% viscous	Oropharynx	5	15–30
	10% aerosol	Pharynx, larynx, possibly tracheobronchial tree, gingiva	5	15–30

topical anesthesia but is much less effective than the 4-per-cent solution. The 2-per-cent solution is useful in infants to avoid overdose. A 10-per-cent aerosol is available in some countries for anesthesia of the gingival mucosa, and some clinicians employ it for spraying the oropharynx and tracheobronchial tree; however, this must be done with extreme care because of the difficulty of determining the administered dose. A 2-per-cent viscous solution is also available and can be administered to patients in a small graduated medicine cup; the viscous solution is retained in the mouth for as long as possible and then discarded. A 2-per-cent jelly is available in a special tube with a nozzle to permit application into the urethra; a penile clamp is employed to allow retention in the male urethra until analgesia ensues. Ointments ranging in concentration from 2.5 to 5 per cent are also available for local anesthesia of skin, mucous membrane, and rectum, although they are only weakly effective; these ointments also contain ethylene and propylene glycols. Suppositories (10% lidocaine) are also available for local anesthesia of the rectum. Onset of anesthesia occurs within 5 to 10 minutes and is more rapid with the higher concentration, although precise objective data are lacking. Duration of anesthesia is approximately 30 minutes. An experimental solution of 30 to 40 per cent lidocaine has been reported to produce anesthesia of intact skin; however, this high concentration precludes clinical use. Comparative aspects of topical anesthetic solutions are shown in Table 4-3.

Infiltration Anesthesia. Effective blockade can be produced with 0.5 to 1-per-cent solutions either with or without epinephrine. Onset of anesthesia is almost immediate with all solutions. The 0.5-per-cent solution provides a duration of analgesia of approximately 75 minutes, or 240 minutes with 1:200,000 epinephrine. The 1-per-cent solution has a duration of approximately 120 minutes, or 420 minutes with epinephrine (Table 4-4). A special application is infiltration anesthesia for dentistry; here a 2-per-cent solution with 1:100,000 epinephrine is commonly employed, and this has been reported to provide a duration of soft-tissue analgesia for approximately 150 minutes (see Chap. 16).

Intravenous Regional Anesthesia. The popularity of 0.5-per-cent solution was revived in 1963 by Holmes and has probably been the most widely used drug and concentration for this technique (see Chap. 12). A 1-per-cent solution has also been used; however this increases peak blood concentrations by approximately 40 per cent and is less popular since 20 to 40 ml of solution are required even for upper limb anesthesia. A less toxic solution, 0.25

Table 4-4. Infiltration Anesthesia

Agent	Concentration (%)	Duration: Plain (min)	Duration: With Epinephrine 1:200,000 (min)
Procaine	0.5	20 (15–30)	60 (15–120)
Chloroprocaine	1	Possibly similar to procaine	(no data)
Lidocaine	0.5	75 (30–90)	200 (60–300)
	1	120 (90–140)	400 (360–420)
Mepivacaine	0.5	108 (30–120)	240 (140–310)
Prilocaine	1	100 (90–110)	280 (250–300)
Bupivacaine	0.25	190 (180–210)	430 (400–450)
Etidocaine	0.5	Possibly similar to bupivacaine	(no data)

per cent lidocaine, has been advocated for use in the lower limb since volumes of 75 to 100 mls may be required. Onset of anesthesia occurs in approximately 5 minutes and remains adequate for the duration of cuff inflation, which is commonly 60 minutes. A partial residual anesthesia may persist for approximately 1 hour following cuff deflation.

Peripheral Nerve Block. Minor nerve blocks such as ulnar and intercostal are adequately performed with concentrations of 0.5 per cent, and this concentration is preferred for larger volume blocks such as bilateral intercostal blocks. For major nerve blocks, such as brachial plexus block, 0.5- to 1-per-cent solutions are used, depending upon the degree of motor blockade desired. Epinephrine should be added to both the 0.5- and 1-per-cent solution if large volumes are required, for example, for bilateral intercostal or the larger volume axillary brachial plexus block.

Onset of anesthesia occurs in approximately 5 minutes for minor nerve blocks and 5 to 15 minutes with major nerve blocks. The carbon dioxide salt of lidocaine has a more rapid onset time than plain lidocaine and will produce brachial plexus block in approximately 8 minutes.[17]

Duration of anesthesia for minor nerve block is approximately 60 minutes without epinephrine and 120 minutes with epinephrine. Duration of anesthesia for major nerve block is approximately the same (Fig. 4-2).

Epidural and Caudal Block. Sympathetic blockade is produced by a 0.5-per-cent solution and leads to either minimal or no sensory blockade. Sensory blockade with minimal motor blockade is produced by a 1-per-cent solution. Motor blockade of minimal degree is produced by a 2-per-cent solution, with more profound motor blockade requiring a 2-per-cent solution with 1:200,000 epinephrine (Fig. 4-3).

Initial onset of blockade occurs in approximately 5 minutes, with complete onset requiring approximately 20 minutes.

Duration of anesthesia with untreated solutions is approximately 60 minutes, and this is extended to 100 minutes by the addition of epinephrine (see Table 4-2; also Chap. 8).

Spinal Anesthesia. A hyperbaric 5-per-cent solution of lidocaine in 7.5 per cent dextrose is available and has been widely used, despite criticism that its high specific gravity of 1.035 at 37°C causes very rapid spread in the subarachnoid space. Onset of anesthesia is almost immediate, and the duration is approximately 45 to 60 minutes with the unadulterated solution or 60 to 90 minutes if epinephrine is added (see Chap. 7).

Safe Dosage. Without epinephrine is 200 to 400 mg. With epinephrine, it is 500 mg, regardless of block technique or concentration, as long as the concentration is in the range of 0.5 to 2 per cent. For topical use, the safe dosage is (4%) 200 to 400 mg. As indicated in Table 3-4, lidocaine has a ratio of approximately 2 between the safe effective dose and the toxic dose. It is important to stress that for some blocks that require large doses, this ratio can be maintained only by the addition of epinephrine. The initial recommendation for a maximum safe dose of lidocaine was 200 mg if the drug was used without epinephrine. Recently, the availability of blood concentration measurements and a knowledge of the threshold blood concentration for toxicity has permitted a reappraisal of safe lidocaine dosages. Data from Table 3-4 indicate that 400 mg of lidocaine, administered as a single-dose epidural injection, resulted in blood concentrations of 2 to 4 μg per ml, which are below the threshold for toxic symptoms (5 μg/ml) and considerably below the level of 10 μg per ml associated with convul-

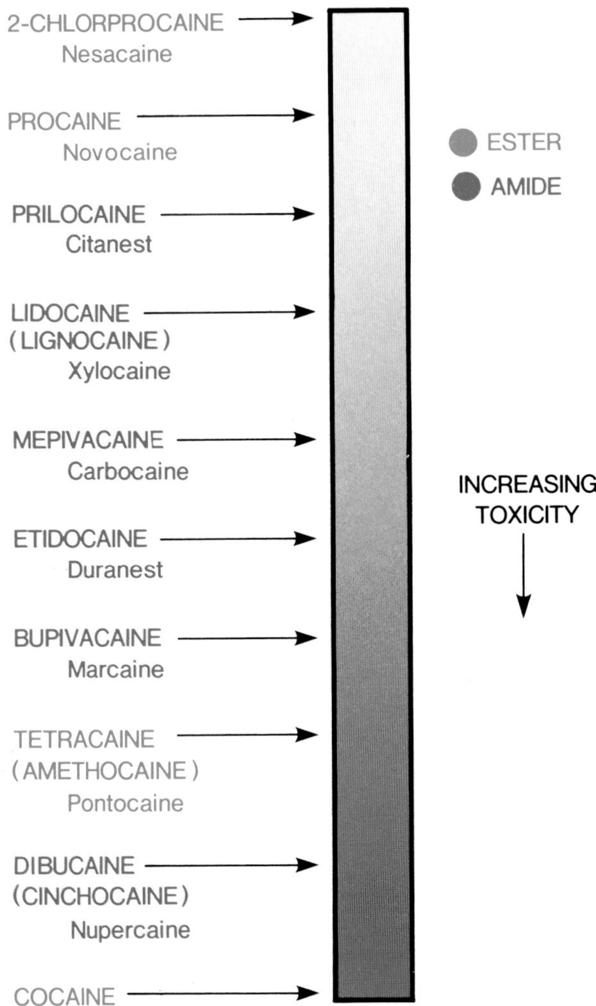

Fig. 4-1. Spectrum of local anesthetic agents. Agents are arranged in approximate order of increasing toxicity; it should be noted, however, that comparisons of all of the agents at "equi-effect" concentration, under the same conditions, have not yet been made in humans.

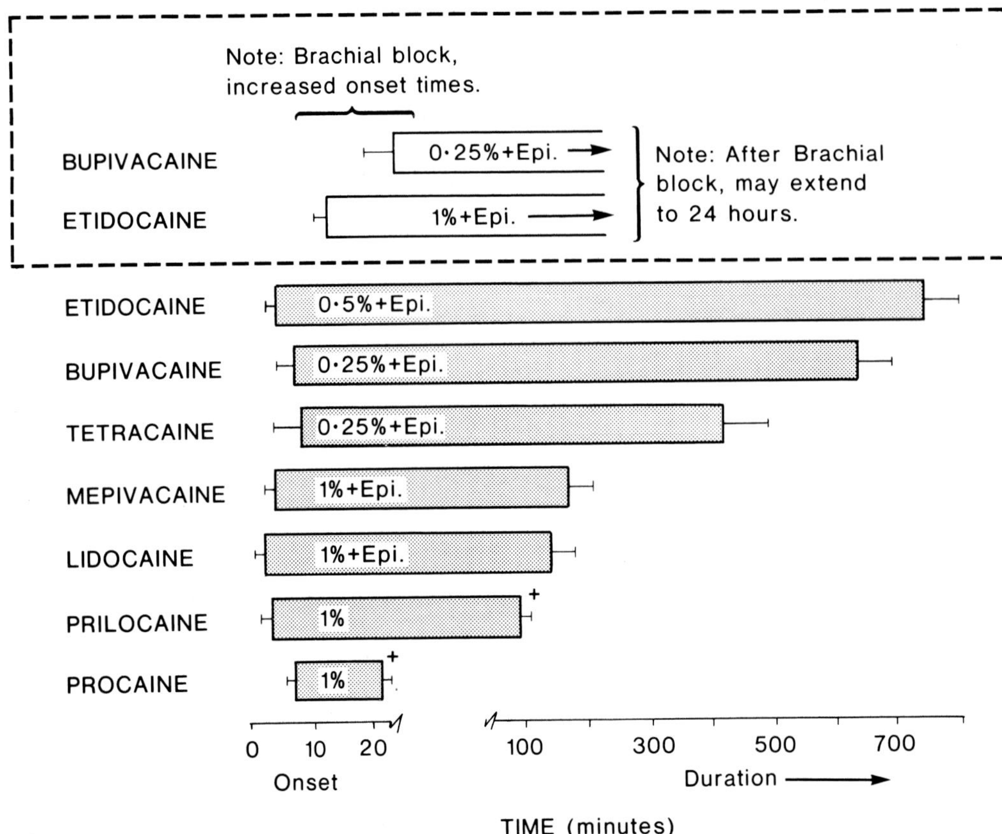

Fig. 4-2. Comparison of onset and duration of sensory block for peripheral nerve block. Onset times for peripheral nerve block are very similar for all of the agents; however, note the larger standard deviation for bupivacaine. For major plexus blocks, such as brachial, onset times are increased more than two times (*above dotted line*), and here the large standard deviation for bupivacaine becomes a significant clinical problem since it is difficult to predict onset time for each patient. (Data from Bromage, P.R., and Gertel, M.: An evaluation of two new local anesthetics for major conduction blockade. Can. Anaesth. Soc. J., *17*:557, 1970.) Duration of block may also be highly variable with bupivacaine and etidocaine, sometimes extending to 24 hours (*e.g.*, after brachial plexus block; *inset*). (Data for prilocaine and procaine are obtained from double-blind bilateral ulnar nerve block [Lofstrom, J.B.: Ulnar nerve blockade for the evaluation of local anaesthetic agents. Br. J. Anaesth., *47*:297, 1975]. Other data are from double-blind bilateral intercostal nerve block [Bridenbaugh, P.O.: Intercostal nerve blockade for the evaluation of local anaesthetic agents. Br. J. Anaesth., *47*:306, 1975])

sions. It also appears reasonable to increase the safe dose to 500 mg if epinephrine is added, since the resulting blood levels are similar to the 400-mg dose of lidocaine.

When repeated administration of lidocaine or the other agents is under consideration, the data in Tables 3-7 and 3-8 become of prime importance. Lidocaine is cleared quite rapidly from the body (total body clearance [CL] = 0.99 L/min), owing largely to rapid extraction by the liver (estimated hepatic extraction ratio [E] = 0.63); that is, 63 per cent of lidocaine in the blood is removed at each pass through the liver. It takes approximately 1.6 hours for the lidocaine blood concentration to be halved (half-life [T½] = 1.6 hr).

Thus, it should be remembered that a second dose of lidocaine 90 minutes after an initial maximum safe dose should be reduced by at least one-half if the cumulation of blood level is to be avoided (see Fig. 3-14*B*). A comparison of safe adult dosages of lidocaine with those for other agents is shown in Table 3-4.

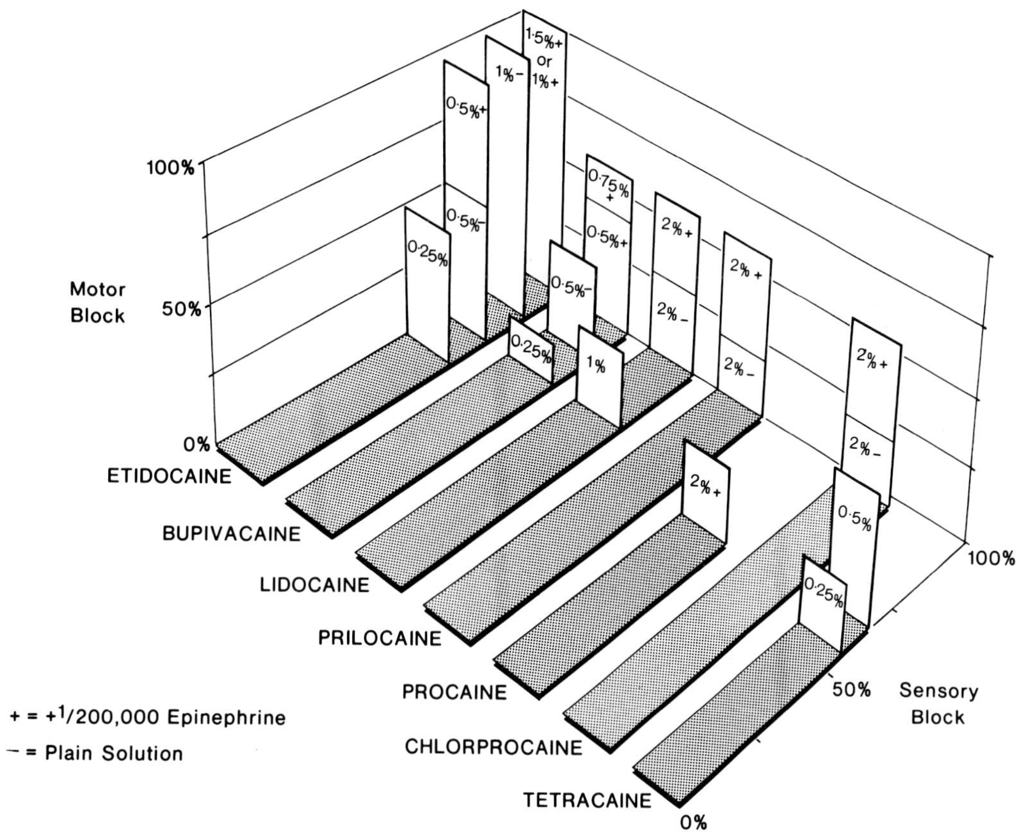

Fig. 4-3. Comparison of agents in epidural block. The percentage of motor blockade and the percentage of success of sensory blockade are illustrated for each agent. This illustration is based upon subjective clinical data and thus only approximate comparisons can be drawn.

It was originally claimed that, as the concentration of lidocaine was increased from 0.5 to 2 per cent for nerve block, the dosage should be reduced. However, within the clinical range of lidocaine concentrations, blood concentration is related to dosage, regardless of concentration of local anesthetic solution (see Fig. 4-6).[73] Also, it has now been shown that topical administration of 4 per cent or 10 per cent lidocaine results in blood levels similar to the level reached by the same dose given by injection.[78] Thus, safe dosages are the same, within the clinical range of 0.5 to 2 per cent for injection and 4 to 10 per cent for topical application.[36,78]

Degradation and Elimination. Lidocaine is primarily detoxified in the liver, less than 3 per cent being excreted unchanged in the urine (see also Fig. 3-24).

Because the liver is so important in the degradation of lidocaine, adequate hepatic function is critical to the normal elimination of the drug. Liver function will depend upon the integrity of the hepatic cells and the blood flow through the liver. The hepatic cells will be disturbed in liver disease, and blood flow can be considerably decreased in conditions of low cardiac output, such as shock.[43] These factors may be of great importance in block procedures that require the higher dosages of lidocaine (see also Table 3-8).

Mepivacaine

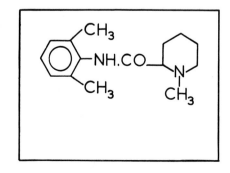

CH_3 — NH.CO — N — CH_3 — CH_3

The amine group is represented in mepivacaine by a piperidine ring.

Physicochemical Properties. Mepivacaine base has a partition coefficient of 0.8 and a pK_a of 7.6. The drug is 68 to 84 per cent bound to plasma protein. The hydrochloride salt is highly soluble in water, and the 2-per-cent solution has a pH of 4.5 (see also Table 3-1).

Effective Concentrations and Clinical Properties. Mepivacaine is approximately equipotent and equitoxic to lidocaine. It is not effective topically. Effective concentrations are the same as for lidocaine for infiltration, intravenous regional, nerve block, and epidural and caudal anesthesia. Although not commercially available for spinal block, the drug has been prepared as a 4-per-cent solution in 9.5 per cent dextrose, which has a specific gravity of 1.048 at 37°C. The addition of epinephrine to solutions of mepivacaine appears to have less effect on its clinical properties than on those of lidocaine. Thus, it is sometimes regarded as a useful alternative for medium duration blockade if epinephrine is to be avoided (Fig. 4-1; Table 4-1). Onset times and durations for the various block procedures are similar when mepivacaine is untreated or combined with 1:200,000 epinephrine and can be equated to those described previously for lidocaine with 1:200,000 epinephrine.

Safe dosage of mepivacaine is the same as for lidocaine, 400 mg or 500 mg with epinephrine. It should be noted that, particularly in association with epidural block, the addition of epinephrine has much less of an effect in lowering blood concentration (see Table 3-6). Although clinically mepivacaine appears to have a potency and toxicity very similar to lidocaine, studies in mice have shown that it is slightly more toxic than lidocaine. As described in Chapter 3, some data indicate that the transplacental transfer of mepivacaine may be greater than for lidocaine, and its neonatal metabolism may be slower. Thus, it may be a less satisfactory agent in obstetric practice (see Fig. 3-31).[63]

Degradation and Elimination. As with lidocaine, only a small fraction (1%) of mepivacaine is excreted unchanged (see Fig. 3-26).

Prilocaine (Citanest)

The molecular formula for prilocaine appears at the top of the next column.

CH3 / C3H7
NH.CO.CH.N
CH3 H

Physicochemical Properties. Prilocaine base has a partition coefficient of 0.4, and is 55 per cent protein-bound. In whole blood, the plasma to erythrocyte ratio is 1:1.2. The hydrochloride salt is very soluble, and the 2 per cent solution has a pH of 4.6 and a pK_a of 7.9 (see Table 3-1).

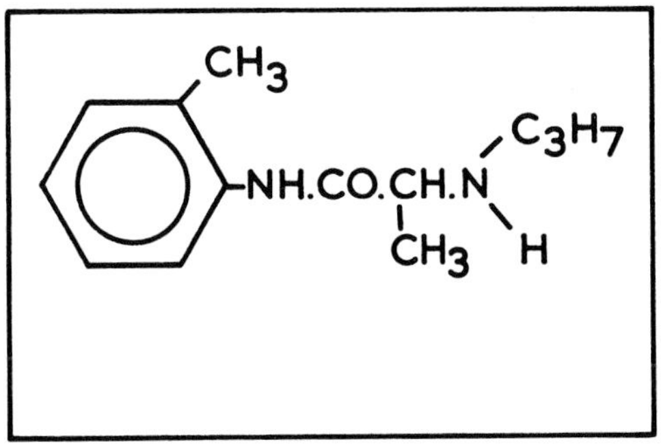

Effective Concentration and Clinical Properties. Prilocaine is equipotent to lidocaine but is less toxic, owing to a greater volume of distribution and more rapid metabolism (see Fig. 4-5).

Topical Anesthesia. Although this drug is effective topically, it is not presently available commercially for this purpose.

Infiltration Anesthesia. Satisfactory blockade is provided by 0.5 to 1 per cent solutions, both with and without epinephrine.

Onset of anesthesia is almost immediate and duration is approximately 75 to 90 minutes without epinephrine and 280 minutes with the epinephrine-containing solution (see Table 4-4).

Intravenous Regional Block. A 0.5-per-cent solution of prilocaine is now regarded as the solution of choice for intravenous regional block (see Table 4-1; also Fig. 4-1 and Chap. 12).

Peripheral Nerve Block. Solutions of 0.5 to 1 per cent prilocaine are available with and without epinephrine. Clinical properties are similar to those observed for lidocaine.

For medium-duration procedures, prilocaine may be a good choice if a large volume is to be injected, because of its rapid clearance and low toxicity.

Epidural and Caudal Block. Solutions of 2 per cent and 3 per cent are available with and without epinephrine. The 2-per-cent solution appears to have onset and duration characteristics similar to those of lidocaine. The 3-per-cent solution has been reported to have a more rapid onset but is not widely available; the use of this higher concentration is made possible by the toxicity of prilocaine being lower than that of lidocaine. For caudal block, the 2-per-cent solution is sometimes preferred over lidocaine for nonobstetrical uses, such as outpatient perineal surgery (Table 4-1). If the dosage is kept below 400 mg, the untreated solution can be used with no significant increase in blood concentration over the epinephrine-containing solution, but with a considerable reduction in the degree of motor blockade (Fig. 4-3; see also Table 3-6).

Onset and duration of anesthesia and degree of motor blockade are similar to those observed for the corresponding solutions of lidocaine.

Spinal Anesthesia. Prilocaine has been prepared as a 5-per-cent solution in either 6 per cent or 5 per cent dextrose, the former having a specific gravity of 1.023, and the latter, 1.022 at 37°C. It is not commercially available, however!

Safe dosage without epinephrine is 400 to 500 mg, with epinephrine, 600 mg. In animal studies, acute administration of prilocaine was 25 to 50 per cent less toxic than lidocaine. In humans, intravenous infusion of prilocaine is better tolerated than lidocaine, and the toxic effects are of shorter duration.[37] When prilocaine is used clinically in extradural and intercostal block, lower plasma concentrations are achieved with prilocaine than with lidocaine, the reduction being on the order of 25 to 30 per cent (Fig. 4-5).[73]

When prilocaine is used at a high dosage (usually above 600 mg)—for example, in a continuous extradural block—methemoglobinemia occurs, with the appearance of cyanosis.[75] The amount of methemoglobin formed is related to the dosage of prilocaine.[47] As prilocaine itself does not have any effect on hemoglobin *in vitro,* the formation of methemoglobin is most probably due to the action of one or more of its metabolites related to aniline (see Fig. 3-25).

Methemoglobinemia seldom produces symptoms in most patients, and comparatively little is required to cause cyanosis—1.5 g % as opposed to 5 g % of reduced hemoglobin. However, if methemoglobinemia is unsuspected, it can confuse the clinical picture. Once recognized, it may be rapidly treated, the intravenous administration of methylene blue, 1 mg per kg, causing return to normal hemoglobin levels in 15 to 20 minutes. However, it is advisable to limit the dose of prilocaine to 600 mg and not to administer additional doses. It is also advisable to avoid prilocaine in obstetric practice since cyanosis in mother and baby cause highly undesirable difficulties in the differential diagnosis of neonatal hypoxia. Like lidocaine, blood concentration depends on dosage rather than on concentration of local anesthetic solution within the usual clinical range (see Fig. 4-12).

Degradation and Elimination. Although in theory hydrolysis is more likely to occur with prilocaine than with lidocaine, the primary pathway of degradation appears to be found in the liver with the production of O-toluidine (see Fig. 3-25).[41]

Bupivacaine (Marcain)

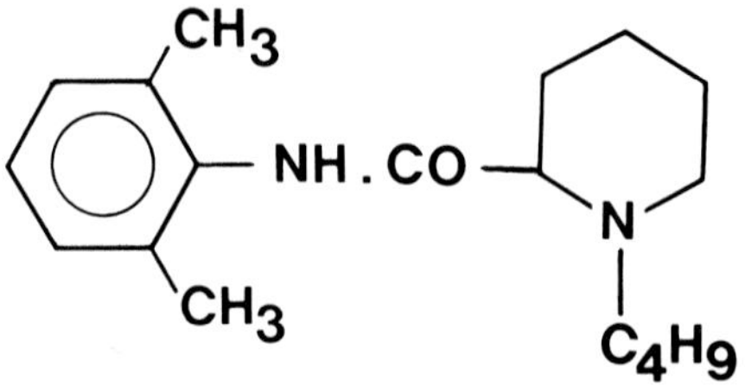

CH_3

NH . CO

N

CH_3

C_4H_9

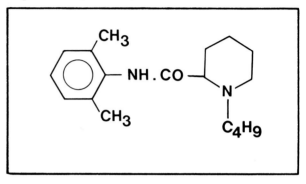

The structure of bupivacaine is essentially the same as mepivacaine, with a butyl group replacing the methyl group on the piperidine ring.

Physicochemical Properties. Bupivacaine base, which is an oil, is highly soluble in fat, the partition coefficient being 28. It has a pK_a of 8.01 and is 88 to 96 per cent bound in plasma protein. It is not taken up by erythrocytes to any extent, and, therefore, whole blood concentrations are considerably lower than the plasma concentrations. The hydrochloride salt is water-soluble, and at 1-per-cent concentration, the pH is between 4.5 and 6 (Table 3-1).

Effective Concentrations and Clinical Properties. Bupivacaine is approximately four times more potent than lidocaine, though this increase in potency is outweighed by a greater increase in toxicity.

Topical Anesthesia. Although bupivacaine is effective topically, such solutions are not currently available.

Infiltration Anesthesia. Effective concentrations are 0.125 per cent to 0.25 per cent with and without epinephrine. Onset is rapid, and duration of anesthesia is approximately 200 minutes to 400 minutes with epinephrine. In view of the very long duration of action it is, perhaps, not a good choice for dental anesthesia because of the risk of injury to the anesthetized area after the surgery. However, this solution has gained popularity for infiltration in hemorrhoidectomy and other procedures benefitting from a residuum of postoperative analgesia in a hospitalized patient.

Peripheral Nerve Block. Solutions of 0.25 to 0.5 per cent are effective with and without epinephrine. Onset is slow (approximately 10–20 min). However, there is a very wide variation, and the precise onset time is impossible to predict for a particular patient. The 0.25-per-cent solution is somewhat unreliable for major plexus blockade, and most clinicians prefer the 0.5-per-cent solution with epinephrine. Degree of motor blockade is quite satisfactory with the 0.5-per-cent solution but often only minimal with the 0.25-per-cent solution. Duration of anesthesia is approximately 400 minutes with both solutions, and the addition of epinephrine has only a minimal effect in increasing duration. There is a very wide range of duration of anesthesia, about which patients should be warned since it is not uncommon for anesthesia to continue for up to 24 hours (Fig. 4-2).

Epidural and Caudal Block. Autonomic blockade is provided by a 0.125-per-cent solution, and this has been reported to relieve the pain of labor.[82] Sensory blockade with very minimal motor blockade is provided by a 0.25-per-cent solution. Motor blockade is provided by a 0.5-per-cent solution, although this is still only moderate and is minimally enhanced by the addition of epinephrine. In the United States, a 0.75-per-cent solution is also available, this high concentration giving a more intense and longer-lasting sensory block and a more profound motor block than the 0.5-per-cent solution.[62] Bupivacaine has a much more pronounced effect upon sensory nerves than on motor nerves, and intense anesthesia may often be obtained without any motor blockade (Fig. 4-3). This is a special advantage in the treatment of pain, such as postoperative, and post-traumatic, and labor pain. Controlled data now indicate that the 0.25-per-cent solution provides adequate anesthesia for labor and produces significantly less motor blockade than the 0.5-per-cent solution.*

The duration of blockade is reduced if the 0.25-per-cent rather than the 0.5-per-cent solution is employed. Bupivacaine is currently preferred to lidocaine for obstetric analgesia because lidocaine is associated with a higher incidence of neurobehavioral defects in the newborn (see Chap. 3).

Spinal Anesthesia. Bupivacaine may become cloudy when it is mixed with cerebrospinal fluid, owing to bupivacaine base coming out of solution, and is currently not approved for spinal anesthesia. However, a series of 4000 cases in which the 0.5-per-cent solution was used without ill effect has been reported.[67]

Safe dosage without epinephrine is 150 mg; with epinephrine, 200 mg.

Toxicity. In toxicity tests on small animals, bupivacaine was four to six times more toxic than lidocaine.[64] Munson, Martucci, and Wagman found that seizures occurred in monkeys at plasma concentrations of 5.51 μg per ml with bupivacaine, and 26.1 μg per ml with lidocaine, which were achieved after doses of 4.3 and 22.7 mg per kg, respectively.[64] There are very little human data. Considerably more lidocaine than bupivacaine can be infused intravenously without toxic effects, and it appears that in humans bupivacaine is about four to five times more toxic than lidocaine (see Table 3-4).[70]

Degradation and Elimination. The metabolic pathway of bupivacaine in humans has not been fully established, and certainly wide species differences exist (see Fig. 3-27).

Etidocaine (Duranest)

The structure of etidocaine is similar to that of lidocaine.

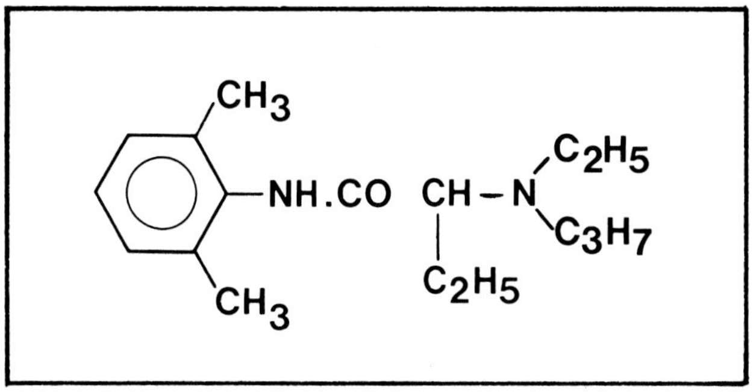

(2,6-dimethylphenyl ring, with CH_3 groups) —NH.CO CH—N(C_2H_5)(C_3H_7), with C_2H_5 on the CH

Physicochemical Properties. Etidocaine has a partition coefficient of 141, much higher than any other local anesthetic in clinical use. It is highly bound (94%) to plasma protein, and little is present in erythrocytes. Its pK_a is 7.74 (see Table 3-1).

Effective Concentrations and Clinical Procedures. Etidocaine is two to three times more potent than lidocaine and is, thus, a little less potent than bupivacaine; however, etidocaine is less toxic than bupivacaine.[70]

Topical Anesthesia. Etidocaine is very effective topically, and this may be of some clinical importance if prolonged topical anesthesia is desired. However, at present no topical preparation is commercially available.

Infiltration Anesthesia. Effective blockade is provided by a 0.5-per-cent solution without epinephrine. Onset is extremely rapid, and duration, similar to that of bupivacaine (Table 4-4).

Peripheral Nerve Block. Solutions of 0.5 per cent are available with and without epinephrine. Etidocaine appears to have advantages over bupivacaine since its onset is much more rapid (approximately 5 min), and the variability among patients is much less marked than that seen for bupivacaine (Fig. 4-2). In addition, if a prolonged duration of block is required for the larger-volume peripheral block pro-

* Lips, F.J., and Cousins, M.J.: Bupivacaine and motor blockade. Unpublished data.

cedures, such as bilateral intercostal and axillary brachial plexus block, the lower toxicity of etidocaine makes it more useful than bupivacaine (Table 3-4).

Duration of anesthesia appears to be similar to that of bupivacaine. Data available at present for some block procedures indicate that the addition of epinephrine has a significant effect in lowering the peak plasma concentration of etidocaine, but it does not greatly enhance block characteristics (see Table 3-6).

Epidural and Caudal Block. Sympathetic blockade is produced by 0.5-per-cent solutions with minimal sensory block but often significant motor block. Sensory blockade is produced by 1-per-cent solutions; however, these concentrations are associated with a very high degree of motor blockade. In this respect, etidocaine appears to differ from other local anesthetics in that even low concentrations produce considerable motor blockade, sometimes even without significant sensory blockade (Fig. 4-3). This feature appears to make etidocaine less suitable for obstetrical anesthesia or postoperative epidural anesthesia. The agent does have considerable advantages, however, when it is used for epidural blockade in surgery because there is a shorter time for obtaining complete sensory and motor blockade than with bupivacaine. In general, complete spread of sensory and motor blockade is achieved in approximately 20 minutes, in comparison to more than 30 minutes for bupivacaine (see Chap. 8). Etidocaine also appears to have a more reliable spread of anesthesia with excellent continuity of anesthesia in adjacent segments on both sides of the body.[25] Some clinicians prefer a 1.5-per-cent solution of etidocaine, which yields a more prolonged block. Epinephrine does not prolong the anesthesia but increases the degree of motor block.[19]

Spinal Anesthesia. Etidocaine is unsuitable for spinal anesthesia since it becomes opalescent when it is mixed with cerebrospinal fluid.

Safe dosage is 300 mg, 400 mg with epinephrine. Blood levels are moderately influenced by the addition of epinephrine (Table 3-6). The plasma clearance of etidocaine is second only to prilocaine in the amide group, with a hepatic extraction ratio 30 per cent greater than lidocaine and almost three times that of bupivacaine (see Table 3-7). Thus, if twice the dose of etidocaine (1%) is necessary for blockade equipotent with bupivacaine (0.5%), then an inadvertent intravenous injection of etidocaine would be less likely to induce undesirable effects. Furthermore, the extensive tissue-binding of etidocaine probably enhances its safety over that of bupivacaine when either drug is used for major conduction blockade. This rapid plasma clearance and the greater degree of tissue-binding appear to lessen the hazard of cumulative toxicity compared to that for bupivacaine (see Table 3-7).

Degradation and Elimination. Less than 1 per cent is excreted unchanged, but the metabolic products have not been fully elucidated. Although the structure of etidocaine is similar to that of lidocaine, the metabolites differ considerably from those of lidocaine (see Fig. 3-28).

QUINOLINES

Dibucaine (Nupercaine)

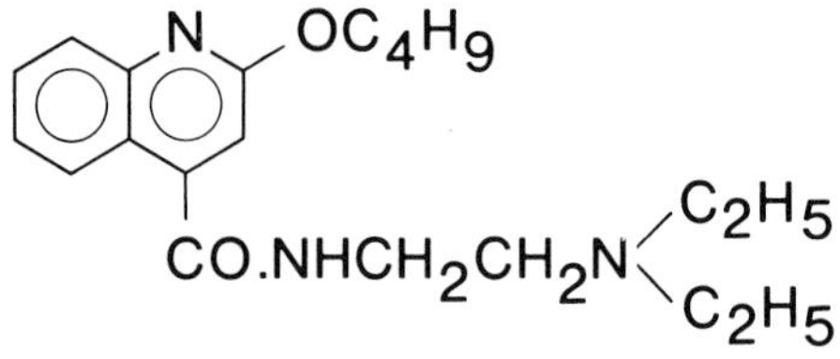

N, OC_4H_9

$CO.NHCH_2CH_2N(C_2H_5)_2$

Dibucaine is a quinoline derivative with an amide bond in the intermediate chain.

Physicochemical Properties. Dibucaine base is highly soluble in lipid but only slightly soluble in water. It is used in this water form in some preparations of creams and ointments for topical application. It has a pK_a of 8.5. Because of its stable amide bond, it may be autoclaved repeatedly.

Effective Concentrations and Clinical Properties. Dibucaine is available for spinal anesthesia as a hyperbaric 0.5-per-cent solution in 6 per cent dextrose, which has a specific gravity of 1.025 at 37°C. Hypobaric solutions of dibucaine, 1:1500, are also available. It has an onset of action of 5 to 10 minutes and a duration of action of 2.5 to 3 hours; the addition of epinephrine extends its action to 3 to 4 hours. It is also used in topical creams for surface anesthesia.

Safe Dosage. For subarachnoid block, dosages of 5 to 15 mg are required, which is well within the safe maximum dose of 50 mg (see Chap. 7).

Degradation and Elimination. Dibucaine is metabolized in the liver and is the most slowly eliminated of all the amides.

ESTERS

Cocaine and its first synthetic substitute procaine both have ester linkages (–COO–) in their intermediate chain. Other compounds with a similar linkage are tetracaine and chloroprocaine. The primary difference between esters and amides is their degradation in the body, the former being chiefly hydrolyzed by pseudocholinesterase in plasma. The rate of hydrolysis varies with each ester, being slow with tetracaine and rapid with chloroprocaine (see Fig. 3-23). More rapid hydrolysis occurs with the less toxic esters, procaine (4 times more rapid) and chloroprocaine (16 times more rapid) compared with slow hydrolysis of tetracaine; however, rapid hydrolysis is associated with a short duration of action. It should be remembered that cocaine is only minimally metabolized in the plasma and relies on relatively slow hepatic metabolism. Cocaine is derived from benzoic acid, but the remainder of the esters derive from para-aminobenzoic acid. This compound is formed during the process of hydrolysis and may induce, in a small minority of patients, an allergic-type reaction. The ester linkage being less stable than the amide renders these compounds less resistant to heat, especially in solution. This has important implications for their sterilization.

Cocaine

Cocaine is an alkaloid obtained from leaves of the coca tree which is indigenous to Peru and Bolivia. It has the formula:

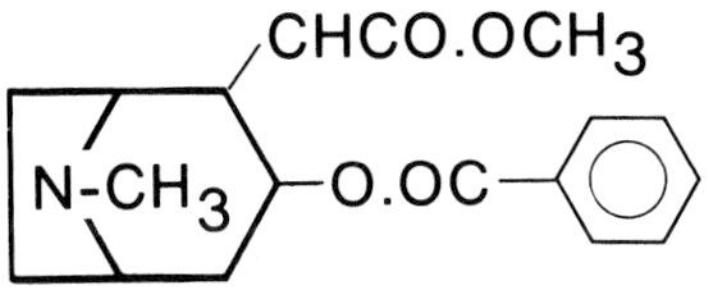

$CHCO.OCH_3$

$N\text{-}CH_3$ — O.OC —

It is related chemically to atropine and is an ester of benzoic acid.

Physicochemical Properties. Cocaine has a partition coefficient of 90. The hydrochloride is freely soluble in water and has a pK_a of 8.6. It does not withstand autoclaving.

Effective Concentration and Clinical Properties. Cocaine is only used for surface anesthesia, its high toxicity and addictive properties precluding it from parenteral use. It is presented in solutions of the hydrochloride varying in strength from 1 to 20 per cent or as a 25 per cent paste. Concentrations of 1 per cent are suitable for corneal anesthesia. Four- to 5-per-cent concentrations are adequate for anesthesia of the mucous membranes in the mouth, nose, and throat; increasing the concentration to 10 per cent decreases the onset time from 4 minutes to 2 minutes. Duration of anesthesia is approximately 60 minutes. Although epinephrine is often mixed with solutions, this is unnecessary as, unlike all other local anesthetics, cocaine is a vasoconstrictor in its own right. Recent studies have shown no difference in hemostasis during ear, nose, and throat surgery when 4 per cent cocaine alone is compared with 4-per-cent cocaine plus 1:80,000 epinephrine.[32] Since cocaine sensitizes the myocardium to catecholamines, it is wise to avoid its combination with epinephrine. Cocaine is thought to cause vasoconstriction by preventing the normal reuptake of catecholamine released at the sympathetic nerve endings.[46] The catecholamine is thus not removed as rapidly as normally, and a prolongation of sympathetic activity results. This effect also explains the mydriasis that occurs when cocaine is instilled into the eye.

Safe Dosage. Precise guidelines are not available since until recently blood levels had not been measured. Current practice is to regard 150 to 200 mg as a safe dose, depending on volume and concentration used.

Central Nervous System Effects. Cocaine differs from the other local anesthetics in its effects on the CNS because of its effect on sympathetic activity. Moderate blood levels initially result in mild euphoria and mental alertness and progressively become closer to the classic "fight and flight" reaction as cocaine blood level increases (Table 4-5).

At very high blood cocaine levels, extreme excitement is followed by convulsions and coma. Because of its euphoric effects, it is a powerful drug of addiction.

Cocaine also increases the capacity for both muscular and mental work, a feature observed for centuries by the natives of Peru and Bolivia where the drug occurs naturally. It also reduces the pangs of hunger and may stimulate the vomiting center.

Cardiovascular Effects. Again, because of the effect of cocaine on the sympathetic nervous system, circulatory effects are seen initially as tachycardia and elevation of arterial pressure, followed by myocardial depression, which, with a large dose, may be rapidly fatal.

Effects of Cocaine on Other Organs. Cocaine may result in an increase in body temperature, owing to interference with normal temperature control centers, combined with increased muscular activity and vasoconstriction in the skin.

Degradation and Elimination. When cocaine is used for anesthesia of mucous membranes in the mouth and throat, there is a tendency for the patient to swallow the drug, whereupon it is hydrolyzed in the intestines before absorption. However, considerable amounts may be absorbed from mucous membranes (or from lung alveoli if intratracheal insufflation is used). The liver is the primary site of degradation, only 10 per cent being excreted unchanged in the urine.

Table 4-5. Comparative Clinical Pharmacology of Cocaine and Lidocaine

Pharmacology	*Cocaine*	*Lidocaine*
Chemical class	Ester	Amide
Major use	Topical	All types of neural blockade
Metabolism	Liver and serum pseudo-cholinesterase	Liver
Plasma clearance	Probably slow (no data)	Rapid compared with other drugs but slower than procaine
CNS effects	"Fight and flight response" Extreme nervousness, talkative, dilated pupils, etc. (ultimately convulsions)	Initially mild sedation and anticonvulsive actions then increasing stimulation (ultimately convulsions)
Peripheral vascular effects	Vasoconstriction (prevents reuptake of noradrenaline into granules in sympathetic nerve endings); tissue slough (eye)	Vasodilation Tissue irritation not proven
Cardiac effects	Similar to sympathetic stimulation: ↑ HR, ↑ BP, ventricular arrhythmias, potentiation of adrenaline, arrhymogenicity	Some stimulation HR ↑ , CO ↑ , antiarrhythmic

The drug is slowly hydrolyzed in the plasma as a secondary method of elimination.

Procaine (Novocaine)

$$H_2N-C_6H_4-COOCH_2CH_2N(C_2H_5)_2$$

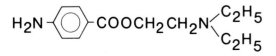

Procaine is a simple derivative of para-aminobenzoic acid.

Physicochemical Properties. Procaine has a partition coefficient of only 0.02 and a pK_a of 9. The hydrochloride is unstable at a pH above 5.5; and, as a 2-per-cent solution, has a pH of 5 to 6.5. It does not have a long shelf life. It must be protected from light and alkalies since its ester bond is unstable. Its high pK_a and very low partition coefficient provide an explanation for its very poor spreading qualities and the so-called missed segments in epidural block (see Table 3-1).

Effective Concentrations and Clinical Properties. Procaine is ineffective topically. For infiltration and nerve block, effective concentrations are similar to those of lidocaine, but its onset is longer and duration, shorter. Epidural block resulting from 2-per-cent solutions is barely satisfactory and often leads to so-called missed segments. Both procaine and chloroprocaine appear to be safe for regional block in patients with a family history of malignant hyperpyrexia (Table 4-1).

Spinal Anesthesia. Procaine, 5 per cent, is mixed with an equal volume of 5 per cent dextrose (see Chap. 7). Onset is rapid, and the block will last 30 to 45 minutes.

Safe Dosage. Procaine is four times less toxic than cocaine, is 25 to 50 per cent less toxic than lidocaine, and is one of the least toxic of the local anesthetics. Safe dose is 500 mg, 750 mg with epinephrine. Much higher doses have reportedly been tolerated but are not recommended.

Degradation and Elimination. The drug is hydrolyzed by plasma cholinesterase to para-aminobenzoic acid and diethylaminoethanol.[52] About 80 per cent of the former and 30 per cent of the latter are excreted unchanged. The remainder undergoes further degradation in the liver (see Fig. 3-22).

Chloroprocaine (Nesacaine)

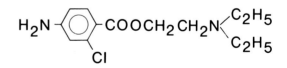

$$H_2N-C_6H_3(Cl)-COOCH_2CH_2N(C_2H_5)_2$$

Physicochemical Properties. Chloroprocaine has properties similar to procaine. The pH of the 2-per-cent solution untreated is 2.7 to 4; pK_a is 8.7. However, its partition coefficient in n-heptone is 0.14 compared to 0.02 for procaine. The difference in pK_a and partition coefficient provides at least a partial explanation for the improved spreading ability and more reliable blockade of chloroprocaine compared to procaine (see Table 3-1).

Effective Concentration and Clinical Properties. The essential difference between chloroprocaine and procaine is its more rapid hydrolysis (4 times more rapid) in the blood, leading to extremely low plasma concentrations after absorption (see Fig. 3-23).[39,69] Its primary disadvantage is its short duration of action, which, in extradural block, is in the region of 30 to 45 minutes. This may be prolonged to 60 to 75 minutes by adding 1:200,000 epinephrine. Its great advantage is that its toxicity is extremely low, only half that of procaine. It is available in 1-per-cent, 2-per-cent, and 3-per-cent solutions, ampules of which may be autoclaved although not repeatedly. It is by far the least toxic local anesthetic (Fig. 4-1).

Topical anesthesia is ineffective.

Infiltration Anesthesia. A 1-per-cent solution of chloroprocaine has a rapid onset and a duration of 45 to 60 minutes, which is prolonged to 70 to 80 minutes by adding epinephrine.

Intravenous Regional Anesthesia. A 1-per-cent solution has been employed; however, it appears to lead to a higher incidence of venous thrombosis than either lidocaine or prilocaine.

Peripheral Nerve Block. A 1-per-cent solution has a rapid onset similar to that of lidocaine, but the duration is only 45 minutes or 70 minutes with epinephrine.

Epidural and Caudal Block. A 2-per-cent solution provides excellent rapid analgesia similar to that of lidocaine but with a duration of only 45 minutes. Increasing the concentration to 3 per cent diminishes the onset time to some extent. Like procaine, chloroprocaine is a useful agent in patients with a family history of malignant hyperpyrexia; it is much more satisfactory than procaine for epidural and caudal blocks, with a lesser incidence of partial blockade (Table 4-1). It is also an attractive agent for outpatient perineal procedures because of its low toxicity and the early ambulation provided by its short duration and minimal motor block (Fig. 4-3). These same properties, together with low fetal levels of local anesthetic, make it a very attractive agent for obstetric analgesia.

Safe dosage is 600 mg, 800 mg with epinephrine.

Degradation and elimination are by rapid hydrolysis in serum except in the presence of low normal or abnormal pseudocholinesterase (see Fig. 3-23).

Tetracaine (Pontocaine)

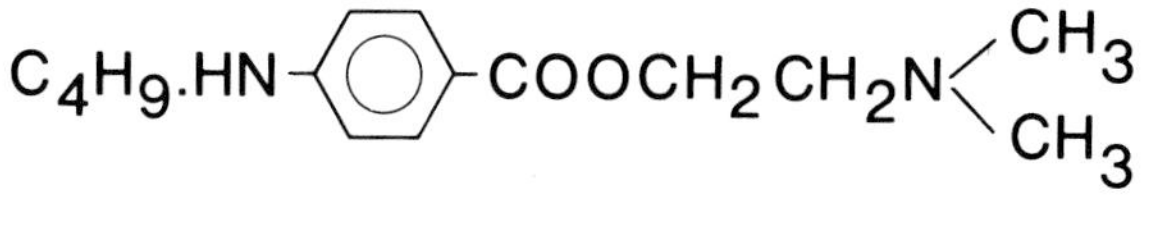

$$C_4H_9.HN-C_6H_4-COOCH_2CH_2N(CH_3)_2$$

Tetracaine is another ester derivative of para-aminobenzoic acid.

Physicochemical Properties. Tetracaine has a partition coefficient of 80 and is 70-per-cent bound to plasma proteins. It has a pK_a of 8.5. The hydrochloride is water-soluble with a pH of 4.5 to 6.5. The solution does not resist repeated autoclaving.[22] Tetracaine is also marketed in the crystalline form, which is more stable during both boiling and autoclaving.

Effective Concentrations and Clinical Properties. Tetracaine has been traditionally regarded as approximately four times more potent than lidocaine; however, it is effective for infiltration and nerve blocks at a concentration of 0.1 to 0.15 per cent so that it may be closer to six times more potent than lidocaine. Unfortunately, its increased potency is outweighed by an approximately tenfold increase in toxicity. Nevertheless, if it is used in the minimal effective concentrations, it has been shown to be a useful alternative for infiltration and nerve block anesthesia for the administration of many thousands of effective and safe block procedures.[60]

Topical Anesthesia. A 1-per-cent solution is said to be as effective as a 10-per-cent solution of cocaine but with a longer duration of action, approximately 50 to 90 minutes (Table 4-3).

Infiltration and Peripheral Nerve Block. Solutions of 0.1 to 0.2 per cent are used for infiltration and large-volume peripheral nerve blocks, such as bilateral intercostal block. Epinephrine should be added to all solutions of tetracaine because of the very slow plasma hydrolysis of tetracaine; however, to date it has not been possible to measure the anticipated effect of epinephrine in reducing blood levels of tetracaine. Onset of blockade is slow and may take as long as 30 minutes (Fig. 4-2).

Duration of anesthesia is very long and usually exceeds 4 to 6 hours when epinephrine-containing solutions are employed.

Epidural and Caudal Block. A 0.25-per-cent solution of tetracaine is required for epidural and caudal block; however, this usually produces relatively partial anesthesia, and it has been common in the past to add tetracaine—to achieve a concentration of 0.25 per cent—to a solution of lidocaine in order to prolong the action of lidocaine. At present, the availability of safer and more effective drugs for epidural block, such as bupivacaine and etidocaine, has greatly diminished the use of tetracaine for epidural block (Fig. 4-3).

Spinal Anesthesia. Solutions of 1 per cent are available for mixing either with distilled water for hypobaric anesthesia or with 10 per cent dextrose for hyperbaric anesthesia or with cerebrospinal fluid for isobaric anesthesia. Onset of blockade is achieved in approximately 5 to 10 minutes, and the duration of anesthesia is 60 to 90 minutes, lengthened to approximately 2 to 3 hours when epinephrine is added (see Chap. 7).

Safe Dosage. For spinal anesthesia, it is not necessary to exceed a dose of 15 to 20 mg, which is well below the maximum safe dose for infiltration and nerve block anesthesia of 100 mg, or 150 mg with epinephrine. Maximum safe dose of the topical solution (1%) is 100 mg.

Degradation and Elimination. Tetracaine is metabolized in the plasma at a much slower rate than either procaine or chloroprocaine (see Fig. 3-23).

OTHER DRUGS

Benzocaine

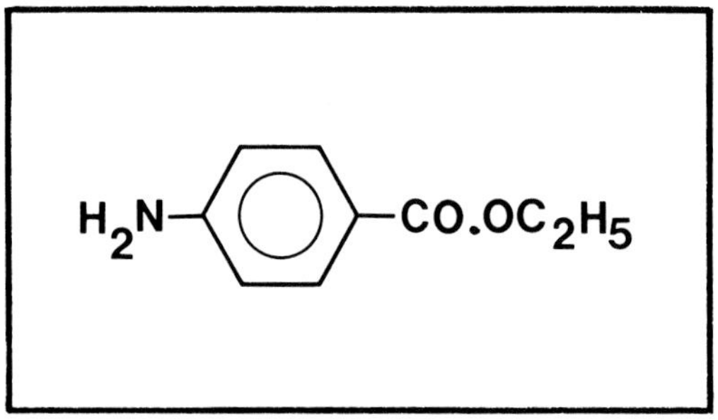

$$H_2N-C_6H_4-CO.OC_2H_5$$

Benzocaine, alone, is not marketed commercially; however, it is used clinically in Australia, Great Britain, and the United States in a variety of surface preparations for the relief of pain and pruritis (Table 4-3). A simple derivative of para-aminobenzoic acid, benzocaine is relatively insoluble in water (a partition coefficient of 50). More important, it can be dissolved in urethane and used as a 2-per-cent solution for injection. Because of its relative insolubility in water, benzocaine remains at the injection site for a long time and can cause nerve block that lasts many hours or even days.[56] It is a useful preparation for relieving the pain of fractured ribs by intercostal nerve block. Since urethane is now known to be carcinogenic, it is preferable to use benzocaine, for injection, suspended in dextran.

Toxicity. Benzocaine is hydrolyzed in the body to para-aminobenzoic acid and should not be used in patients being treated with sulfonamides. Methemoglobinemia has been reported in infants.[48]

Biotoxins

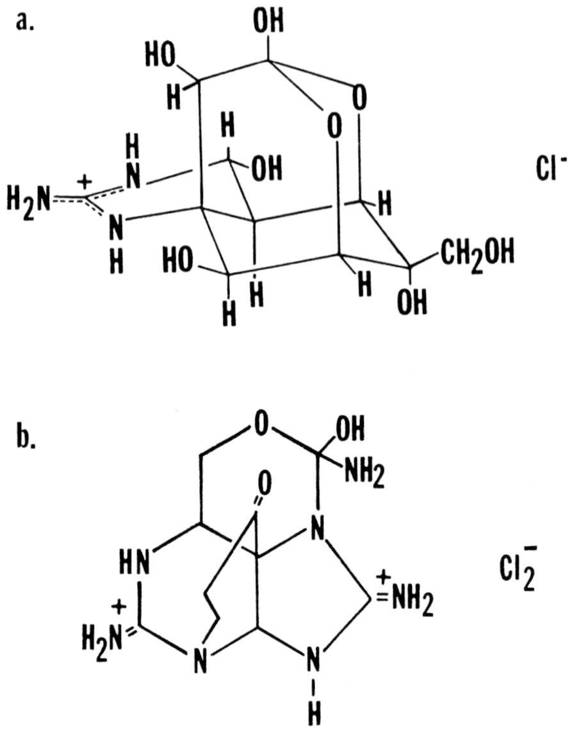

a.

b.

Biotoxins of Class A. **a.** Tetrodotoxin. **b.** Saxitoxin (as suggested by Wong, Oesterlin and Rapoport, 1971).

Another group of substances possessing local anesthetic activity includes those with a quinidine-type molecule. Certain animal species produce these nonprotein toxic substances. The puffer fish found mainly along the coast of Japan produces *tetrodotoxin,* and the marine dinoflagellates, which contaminate shellfish and are responsible for paralytic shell fish poisoning, produce *saxitoxin.*[27] These two substances are of interest in that they are by a wide margin the most powerful inhibitors of nerve conduction known, causing conduction block in nanomolar concentrations.[23,24] In animals they have poor penetrating qualities; thus while they are potent agents in the subarachnoid space, they are much less potent in the extradural space. However, if they are combined with a synthetic agent such as lidocaine, penetration can occur and a very prolonged but reversible block ensues, lasting up to several days.

Although not presently available for clinical use, such compounds may be of importance in the future.

DRUGS USED WITH LOCAL ANESTHETICS

Vasoconstrictors

In order to slow the absorption of local anesthetics from their site of injection—thus allowing a more prolonged application to the nerve fibers and to reduce systemic toxicity—vasoconstrictors may be added to local anesthetic solutions prior to injection (Table 4-2). The most commonly used agent is epinephrine, although others have been tried, such as norepinephrine. Nonsympathomimetic drugs, such as felypressin, have also been used.

Epinephrine is, of course, the active principle of the adrenal medulla. It is a powerful vasoconstrictor and has effects on both alpha- and beta-adrenergic receptors.

On exposure to air or light, epinephrine may rapidly lose potency as a result of degradation. For this reason, stabilizing agents, such as sodium metabisulphite, are used. They slow the breakdown of the drug to as little as 2 per cent per year. These agents also allow epinephrine-containing solutions to be autoclaved once without appreciable loss of activity. However, epinephrine-containing solutions cannot be re-autoclaved.[14] Epinephrine-containing solutions have a lower *p*H (3–4.5), owing to the added antioxidant, compared to untreated solutions (*p*H 6.5–6.8).

When epinephrine is used with local anesthetic solutions, it must be in a concentration and dose to produce the desired vasoconstriction without leading to epinephrine overdose. While the optimal concentration has been controversial, most authorities now agree on 1:200,000. More dilute solutions are of doubtful value; increasing the concentration does not achieve a correspondingly more effective vasoconstriction and increases the likelihood of toxicity. Even with 1:200,000, a total dose of 200 μg should not be exceeded.[53] The use of epinephrine-containing solutions may cause cardiac arrhythmias unless strict criteria for dosage, ventilation, and depth of supplemental anesthesia are observed.[53]

The principle side-effects of epinephrine are hypertension, bradycardia or tachycardia, and cardiac arrhythmias. Such reactions are likely to occur if the local anesthetic solution is accidentally injected intravenously. Animal experiments have shown that epinephrine increases the toxicity of local anesthetics when it is given directly into the circulation. The favorable cardiovascular effects of slowly absorbed 1:200,000 epinephrine are similar to those observed during recently developed "low-dose" constant infusion of epinephrine in intensive therapy; this differs markedly from the adverse effects of a relatively large bolus-dose rapidly injected directly into the circulation. It is wise to avoid the use of epinephrine in patients sensitive to catecholamines (*e.g.*, patients with hypertension, thyrotoxicosis; see Table 4-7).

Epinephrine also has local side-effects, the most important being vasoconstriction of terminal arteries leading to gangrene; for example, in the digits if the drug is used in a local anesthetic for ring blocks.

Norepinephrine. Because norepinephrine lacks much of the beta-sympathetic activity of epinephrine, it has been considered more suitable for adding to local anesthetics. In practice, however, it has not become popular for this purpose, probably because it is a tissue irritant.

Phenylephrine (Neosynephrine) is a sympathomimetic drug with predominately alpha-receptor activity. It has been extensively used in spinal anesthesia, in which it is reported to prolong nerve block by 100 per cent (as opposed to 50% by epinephrine).[61] In epidural and peripheral nerve block, it produces significant systemic sympathomimetic effects.

Felypressin (Octapressin) is a synthetic drug similar to the naturally occurring vasopressin, but without the antidiuretic and coronary vasoconstrictor effects of vasopressin. It has been shown to increase the intensity and duration of dental nerve blocks, and it is used in local anesthesia for this purpose in a concentration of 0.03 units per ml. It is a useful alternative in patients who are sensitive to catecholamines.

Ornipressin (POR-8) is another octapeptide related to vasopressin. It is supplied in ampules of 5 IU in 1 ml. A dose of 5 IU in 50 ml of 2 per cent lidocaine has been used for plastic surgery. It is claimed to have a direct effect on the peripheral vasculature with minimal or no direct cardiac effects. Animal studies have revealed teratogenicity in high, subcutaneous doses considerably in excess of the maximum clinical level.

Levonordefrin (Neo-cobefrin) is an alpha-receptor stimulator used with mepivacaine in dental blocks in a 1:20,000 concentration.

Hyaluronidase

Hyaluronidase is a mucolytic enzyme that renders tissues more permeable to injected fluids. It has been used to aid the spread of local anesthetic drugs, but as most modern local anesthetics have excellent spreading powers, its use is now limited.

Preservatives and Antibacterial Additives

Most of the commonly used local anesthetics, especially of the amide-type, are extremely stable compounds and will remain unchanged in solution indefinitely. Thus, solutions do not require additives if they are stored in ampules. If epinephrine is included in the preparation, however, then antioxidants must be added to prevent breakdown of the vasoconstrictor. The agent used for this purpose is sodium metabisulphite in a concentration of 0.1 per cent. Epinephrine-containing solutions will retain their potency for 2 years with this agent, and they will withstand single autoclaving.

Antimicrobial agents, such as methylparaben, are also added to local anesthetics if the solution is presented in multidose vials. In ampules such additives are unnecessary, but ampules have their own drawbacks, particularly the likelihood of small pieces of glass falling into the ampule when it is opened. Thus, rubber-capped vials are still popular. The ideal form of preparation is a preservative-free, rubber-capped single-dose vial; unfortunately, in some countries this form is not approved. The antimicrobial agents most commonly used are methylparaben and chlorocresol.

Methylparaben is effective against gram-positive organisms and fungi but less so against gram-negative bacteria. It is possible that it may be responsible for some of the allergic reactions that are attributed to local anesthetics—in theory, it should be considerably more antigenic than the local anesthetics.[4] Chlorocresol has been used as an antibacterial agent and is more effective than methylparaben, but, like phenol, it is neurotoxic and should not be used in spinal, IV, or plexus blocks or extradural injections.

LOCAL ANESTHETIC EFFECTS AND REACTIONS

Systemic Effects

Local anesthetics are absorbed from their site of injection into the bloodstream. Their ability to penetrate membranes and affect impulse conduction elsewhere is responsible for their systemic toxic effects, particularly on the CNS and the heart. In addition, they have effects upon the vasculature and also on myoneural junctions.

Central Nervous System Effects

CNS effects are by far the most common side-effects of local anesthetic drugs. They are common to most mammalian species and consist of muscular twitching progressing to epileptiform convulsions followed by coma and severe depression. In humans, the earliest symptoms are a characteristic feeling of light-headedness accompanied by numbness of the tongue and circumoral tissues (Fig. 4-14). The last effects are presumably due to the rich blood supply that allows the drug to cause blockade of nerve endings. Visual disturbances, such as the sensation that the surroundings move, are common, causing the eyes to oscillate in a way that resembles nystagmus. Tinnitus is experienced by some patients, and some become irrational. The exact features of these early premonitory symptoms vary from subject to subject but are highly reproducible in a patient, regardless of the local anesthetic used.

Some local anesthetics, particularly lidocaine, cause initial sleepiness in many patients, and, indeed, this agent has been used as an adjunct to general anesthesia. In contrast, cocaine causes excitement consistently (Table 4-5). The clinical picture, therefore, demonstrates increasing irritability of the brain, which reaches a climax in convulsions followed by depression. It now seems certain, however, that the primary effect of the drugs is depressive, the initial stimulation being the result of preferentially depressing higher cortical centers and allowing uncontrolled activity of the lower centers. This explains how the drugs can both cause epileptiform convulsions and be used to control status epilepticus where the latter is the result of a focus of abnormal activity in the cortex. Lidocaine is thus an anticonvulsant in certain circumstances.[10]

The depression of the brain, which reaches its maximum with coma after convulsions have occurred, causes respiratory arrest. Unless this is treated, death will result from the hypoxia. If respiration is artificially controlled, it is difficult to kill animals with these drugs, but extremely easy if respiration is unaided. In heavily sedated patients, muscular twitching and convulsions may not occur, and severe depression leads to coma, the true cause of which is not recognized.

Electroencephalography in cats being infused intravenously with various local anesthetic agents shows that the patterns of electrical activity produced are different with different drugs. Moreover, the brain toxicity is highly dependent upon the acid/

Table 4-6. Cardiovascular Effects of Increasing Doses of Local Anesthetic (Lidocaine)

Dose of Solution	*Plasma Concentration (μg/ml)*	*Hemodynamic Effects*			
		Heart Rate	*Cardiac Output*	*Blood Pressure*	*Peripheral Resistance*
400 mg (epidural)	3–4	↑ or ∅	↑ or ∅	↑ or ∅	∅ or ↓
500 mg (epidural)	5–6	↓	↓	↓	↓
>75 μg/kg/min (IV)	10–20	↓ or asystole	↓ ↓	Cardiovascular collapse	↓ ↓

∅ = No change

base status, being much more marked in acidotic states (see Chap. 2).[36]

Cardiovascular Effects

It has been generally accepted that local anesthetic drugs cause a depression of the myocardium and have a direct vasodilatory effect upon the peripheral vasculature, thus explaining the severe hypotension sometimes seen. However, recent evidence indicates that the situation is not quite this simple. As mentioned above, if hypoxia occurs as a result of untreated respiratory depression, then this may well be the major cause of myocardial failure and hypotension. If gas exchange is maintained, then severe depression of the myocardium will result only with massive overdose. At blood levels of approximately 3 μg per ml lidocaine, myocardial function is not greatly altered and may in fact be improved (Table 4-6).[50,51,55] Such data are not available for other local anesthetics except procaine, which causes dose-related depression of cardiac output less than that produced by procaine amide.[44]

Thus, in subconvulsive doses, a drug such as lidocaine has minimal effects on the circulation, and, if at all, the effect on the myocardium is positively inotropic.[51] For lidocaine this may be due to increased sympathetic activity counterbalancing any direct depressive effects on the myocardium. The use of lidocaine in the treatment of arrhythmias associated with myocardial infarction is testimony to the lack of deleterious effects upon the heart. Negative inotropic effects occur in the presence of drugs that themselves depress both myocardial function and sympathetic nervous system responses (*e.g.*, during general anesthesia with halothane), but such effects are transient and probably of little clinical importance.[72]

Local anesthetic solutions that contain epinephrine have been reported to result in significant beta-stimulating effects attributable to the epinephrine, particularly in large-volume blocks such as epidural blockade (Table 4-7).

Local anesthetic drugs also have effects upon the blood vessels. This effect is predominantly vasodilatory at the site of injection and occurs with almost all drugs (when used without epinephrine), with the exception of cocaine (see Table 4-5).

Table 4-7. Cardiovascular Effects of Epinephrine

Effect	*Low Dose**	*High Dose†*
Cardiac output	↑	↑ ↑ or ↓ (if high heart rate or arrhythmias)
Heart rate	∅ or ↑	↑ ↑ or ↓ (if massive increase in afterload)
Blood pressure		
Systolic	↓	↑ ↑
Mean	↑ or ∅	↑ ↑
Diastolic	↓	↑ ↑
Tissue blood flow		
e.g., urine output	↑ ↑	↓ ↓

∅ = No change
* 20 ml of 1:200,000 by epidural injection
† *e.g.*, approximately 500 μg rapidly IV

However, it should be remembered that, at the site of injection, the concentration of the drug is enormous compared to the concentration that acts on remote vessels following absorption. Evidence is now available that on certain vascular beds, these drugs cause an increase in myogenic tone, owing to a direct action on the muscular components within the vessel wall.[11]

Thus, the first discernible effects of local anesthetics on the circulation are increases in cardiac output, arterial pressure, heart rate, and peripheral resistance. With a high dosage, depressant effects predominate (see also Table 3-5).

Neuromuscular Junction. If procaine and lidocaine are given intravenously during general anesthesia, they have been observed to cause respiratory inadequacy in the presence of suxamethonium.[31,40] This led to speculation that pseudocholinesterase was depleted by the local anesthetics, lengthening the paralysis caused by suxamethonium. However, Katz and Gissen (1969) showed that the respiratory inadequacy seen was due to central depression and that the twitch response in the muscles was not affected by local anesthetics given in normal intravenous doses.[54] If, however, they were given intra-arterially into the brachial artery, depression of the twitch response in that arm did occur. Intra-arterial injection produces a much higher concentration of the drug in the arm than does an intravenous injection, and this can cause a short period of nerve block (similar to IV regional block), which would account for the depression of the twitch response.[79]

Reactions

All local anesthetics are relatively toxic substances with a therapeutic ratio that is not high. Thus, it is important to be able to recognize and treat adverse effects (see Table 4-8).

Accidental Intravascular Injection. Intravenous injection is probably the most common cause of overt toxicity from local anesthetics. Symptoms and signs, as described previously, appear very rapidly, often before the injection has been completed. Any complaint about numbness of the tongue and circumoral tissues should warn the anesthesiologist to stop the injection. Direct intra-arterial injection will result in toxic symptoms very rapidly if the artery leads directly to the brain, for example, injection of small doses into the vertebral artery during stellate ganglion or interscalene block.

Intravenous injection can often be avoided by simple aspiration prior to the injection, but this is not entirely foolproof because the flow of blood back into the syringe may not occur, especially if the vein is a small one or if the negative pressure of aspiration is excessive. Epidural veins are particularly easy to enter, especially with a catheter.

Effects Related to Additives. The effects of epinephrine may also be confused with local anesthetic effects, particularly in dentistry in which high concentrations of epinephrine (up to 1:50,000) are used. Thus, a history of sweating, tachycardia, and palpitations immediately after injection is more indicative of rapid absorption of epinephrine than local anesthetic effects. It would seem worth reconsidering the concentration and indications for the use of epinephrine in dentistry as discussed in Chapter 16.

Allergy is often blamed for reactions to local anesthetics, particularly in dentistry. Reported cases that are unquestionably due to allergy, however, are extremely rare and are usually associated with the ester-type drugs. Methylparaben used as a preservative is capable of causing allergic effects and may be responsible for some of the cases seen. A great majority of reactions labeled as "allergy" are probably due to vasovagal fainting in the dental chair, and are often paradoxically associated with the use of epinephrine-containing solutions. Some may also be due to intra-arterial injection, which might enable the local anesthetic to gain access to the carotid artery and thus access directly to the brain[5] (Table 4-8).

LOCAL ANESTHETIC TOXICITY

TOXICITY DUE TO IMBALANCE BETWEEN ABSORPTION AND DISPOSITION

Blood Concentration and Toxicity

The concentration of a drug in the blood depends on its absorption from the site of injection or application, its distribution throughout the tissues of the body, and its degradation. With the advent of methods of measuring accurately small quantities of drugs in whole blood or plasma, there are now considerable data that give a reasonably clear indication of these processes when local anesthetic drugs are injected into humans (see Figs. 3-12–3-20).

Because of the affinity of local anesthetics for nervous tissue and the ability of the nonionized drug to pass through membranes, there is a close relationship between the concentrations in arterial blood and the brain. Venous blood is a less reliable guide when the drug is given rapidly intravenously or if the limb from which blood is taken is vasocon-

Table 4-8. Differential Diagnosis of Local Anesthetic Reactions

Etiology	*Major Clinical Features*	*Comments*
Local anesthetic toxicity		
Intravascular injection	Immediate convulsion	Injection into vertebral or a carotid artery may cause convulsion after administration of small dose
Relative overdose	Onset in 5 to 15 min of irritability, progressing to convulsions	
Reaction to vasoconstrictor	Tachycardia, hypertension, headache, apprehension	May vary with vasopressor used
Vasovagal	Rapid onset Bradycardia Hypotension Pallor, faintness	Rapidly reversible with elevation of legs
Allergy		
Immediate	Anaphylaxis (↓ BP, bronchospasm, edema)	Allergy to amides extremely rare
Delayed	Urticaria	
High spinal or epidural block	Gradual onset Bradycardia* Hypotension Possible respiratory arrest	May lose consciousness with total spinal block

* Sympathetic block above T4 adds cardioaccelerator nerve blockade to the vasodilatation seen with blockade below T4; total spinal block may have rapid onset.

stricted (see Figs. 4-10; 4-11).[81] However, venous blood provides values close to those of arterial blood if the limb is not constricted and if the drug has not gained very rapid access to the blood. Thus, there is a relationship between the appearance of CNS toxicity and the venous blood level, factors that raise that level and increase toxicity or lower the level and decrease toxicity.

Basis of Local Anesthetic Toxicity

Toxicity affects mainly CNS as a result of high plasma concentration.

Plasma concentration is determined by a balance between absorption and disposition (distribution/metabolism-excretion).

- Absorption is influenced by choice of drug, dosage, vasopressor, site of injection, speed of injection, and pathophysiology (*e.g.*, cardiovascular disease).
- Disposition is influenced by distribution effects (see Chap. 3) and metabolism, that is, rate of plasma clearance (esters) and rate of hepatic clearance (amides).

Factors That Affect Blood Concentrations

For the practicing anesthesiologist several factors, which one can either control or take into account, determine the blood concentration and thus the toxicity of the injected local anesthetic drug. The most important are site of injection, choice of drug, dosage, addition of epinephrine, speed of injection, and pathophysiologic factors.

Site of Injection. Absorption from any site depends upon the blood supply to that site, richly supplied areas favoring rapid absorption.[13] Figure 4-4 shows mean plasma concentration curves following the injection of 400 mg of lidocaine at four different sites. The highest concentrations occurred after intercostal block and the lowest after subcutaneous abdominal infiltration. These results are in accord with the relative blood supplies of the four anatomical areas.

Choice of Drug. Figure 4-5 shows the plasma concentrations after epidural block, using the same doses of either lidocaine or prilocaine. As can be seen whether untreated solutions or those containing epinephrine are used, prilocaine yields lower plasma concentrations than does lidocaine. These differences may indicate a slower absorption for prilocaine, but it is more likely that they result from more rapid metabolism and a larger volume of distribution than for lidocaine. They explain the fact that intravenous prilocaine causes less toxicity and for a shorter time than the same doses of lidocaine.[37]

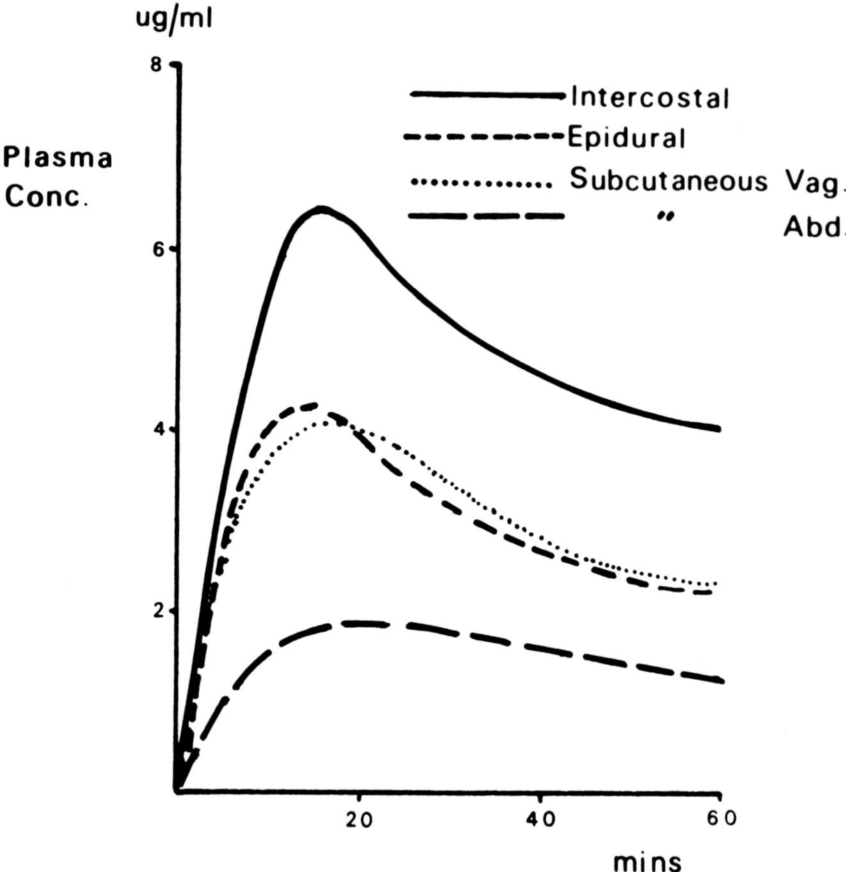

Fig. 4-4. Plasma concentrations of lidocaine following injection of 400 mg at four different sites.

It does not necessarily follow that a drug that is associated with lower plasma concentrations is less toxic. The concentrations that are associated with toxic effects must be established. With lidocaine and prilocaine, early toxicity is seen at concentrations of approximately 5 μg per ml.[39] From 5 μg per ml to 10 μg per ml, the likelihood of severe CNS toxicity progressively increases. In unmedicated subjects, the threshold is approximately 5 μg per ml; however, under light general anesthesia, the threshold increases to approximately 10 μg per ml.[18] The values for toxic concentrations for mepivacaine are somewhat lower, toxicity being experienced around a value of 4 μg per ml, while with bupivacaine and etidocaine, the threshold is in the range of 1 to 2 μg per ml. These figures should be treated with some caution as individual variations are considerable.[71]

Dosage. Within the clinical range of dosages for most local anesthetics, the relationship between dosage and maximum plasma concentration appears reasonably linear (Fig. 4-6).

Addition of Epinephrine. The efficacy of epinephrine in reducing the absorption of local anesthetics depends upon the sensitivity of the vasculature at the site of injection and the local anesthetic drug itself (Figs. 4-7, and 4-8; see also Table 3-6; Fig. 3-12).

Speed of injection has a small but definite effect on the absorption of local anesthetics from the epidural space, rapid bolus injections raising the plasma concentrations more quickly than slow injections, although this is probably of little clinical importance (Fig. 4-9). However, in the case of drugs injected intravenously, either purposely or accidentally, the effect of speed of injection is very critical. The concentration in arterial blood depends primarily on the speed of injection, the dose given, and the cardiac output (Fig. 4-10). Whether CNS toxicity develops also depends upon the proportion of the cardiac output that perfuses the brain. Quite small doses may give rise to toxicity if they are administered rapidly intravenously when cardiac output is reduced (Fig. 4-11). Under these conditions, not only is the plasma concentration high, but the proportion of the cardiac output going to the brain is also increased.

Insignificant Factors. *Concentration of solution* used was for many years considered to be of importance, increasing the concentration being thought to increase toxicity, even though dosage was unchanged. This has now been shown to be incorrect (Fig. 4-12). Three-per-cent and 2-per-cent solutions of prilocaine have been shown to yield the same plasma concentrations as would be expected for a 1-per-cent solution.[13] The use of 10 per cent lidocaine intramuscularly does not yield plasma concentrations greater than those achieved by the same dose of 2-per-cent lidocaine given intramuscularly.[49]

Body weight is commonly used to determine the dosage of drugs, but it is valid only if the distribu-

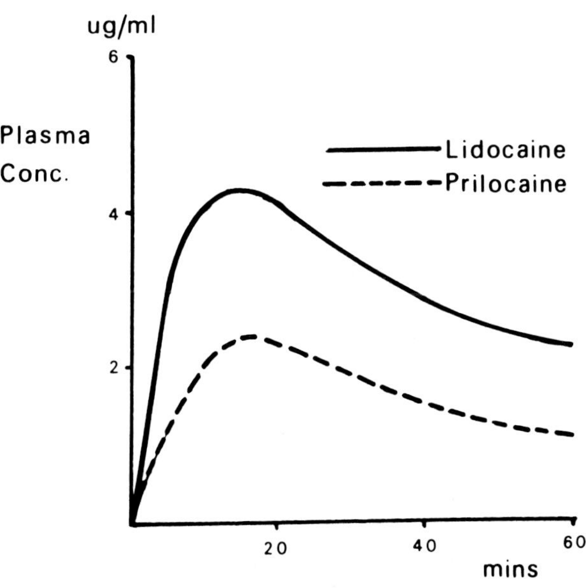

Fig. 4-5. Plasma concentrations of lidocaine and prilocaine following the epidural injection of 400 mg of each agent.

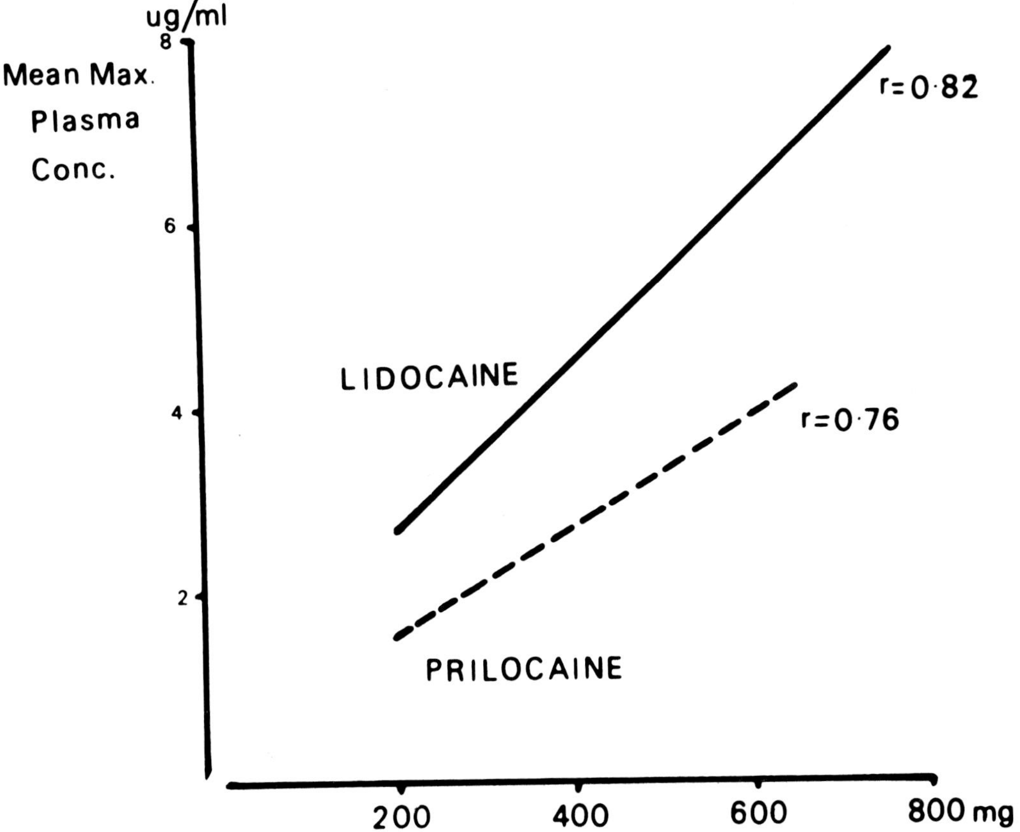

Fig. 4-6. Regression lines of mean maximum plasma concentration for lidocaine and prilocaine following epidural injection.

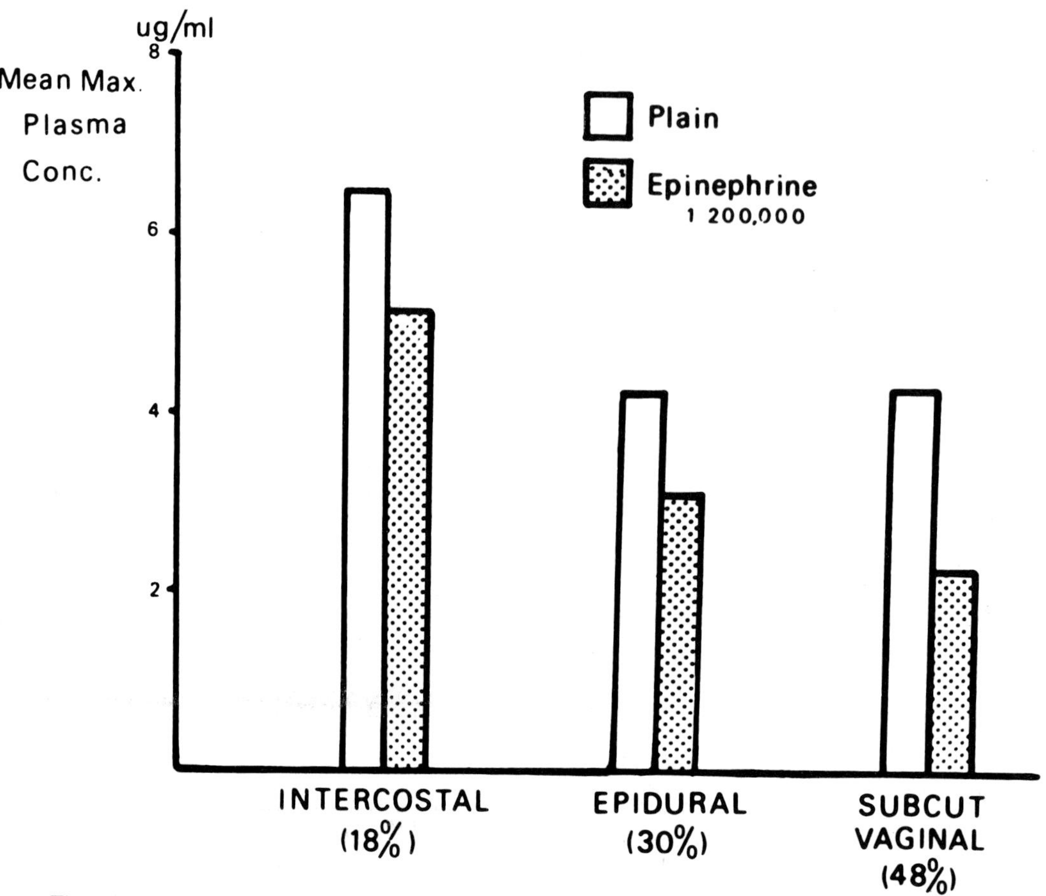

Fig. 4-7. Mean maximum concentrations of lidocaine with and without epinephrine, 1:200,000, given at three different sites. The most marked reduction caused by epinephrine occurs with the subcutaneous injection (48%), compared to 30 per cent for epidural and 18 per cent for intercostal (see also Fig. 3-13).

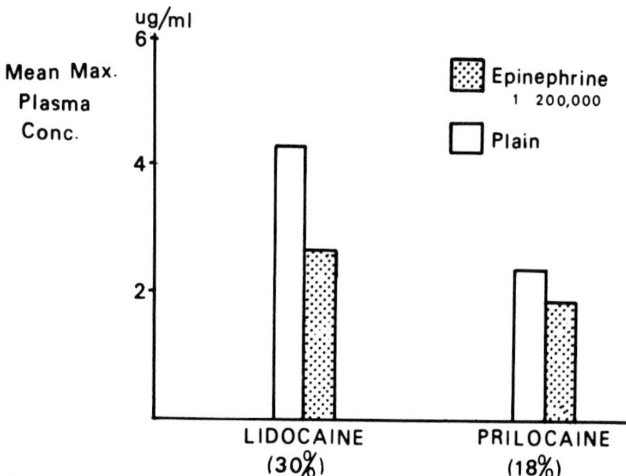

Fig. 4-8. Mean maximum concentration of lidocaine and prilocaine with and without epinephrine, 1:200,000, given epidurally. Epinephrine gives a larger reduction in plasma concentrations with lidocaine than with prilocaine (30% and 18%, respectively).

tion through the body is relatively uniform (Chap. 3). This is seldom the case, and with local anesthetics, much tissue (the fat and the muscle) equilibrates with the blood concentration very slowly and long after the peak plasma concentration has passed. Thus, it is not true that an obese patient either requires or can tolerate a higher dose than a thin patient. No correlation can be demonstrated between body weight of adults and peak plasma concentration of local anesthetics (Fig. 4-13).

Pathologic States. Cardiovascular disease may increase the hazard of toxicity due to local anesthetics given in normal safe dosage (see Table 3-8). Patients with a low cardiac output are particularly liable to this hazard (*e.g.*, a patient with a myocardial infarct who receives lidocaine antiarrhythmic therapy). In such cases, an intravenous bolus injection results in a much higher blood concentration (as the drug is being diluted in a smaller volume of blood) and the proportion of the drug reaching the

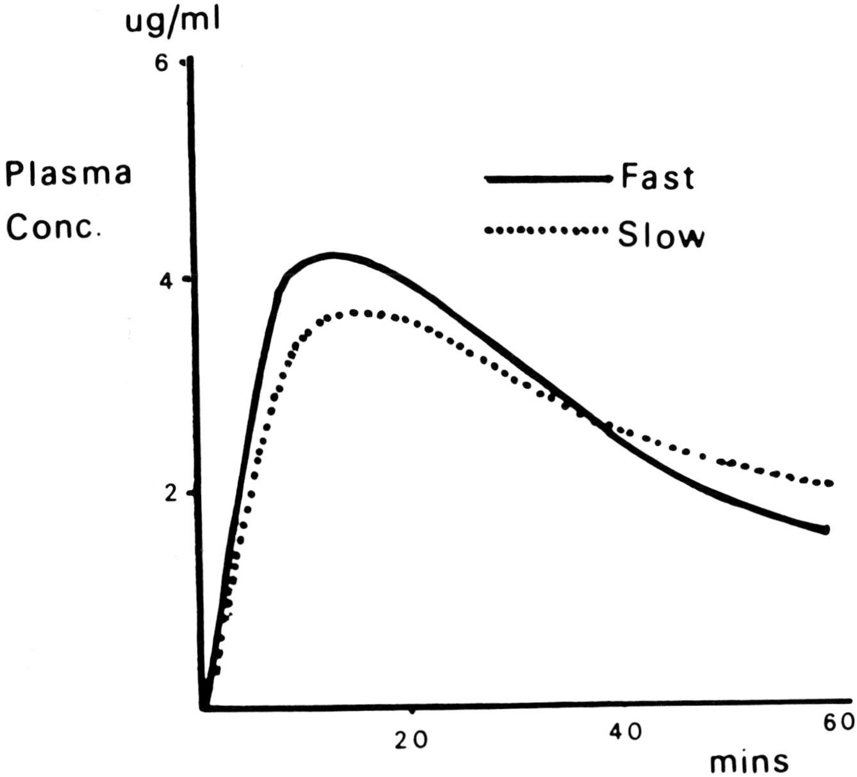

Fig. 4-9. Plasma concentrations of lidocaine following epidural injection given either fast or slow.

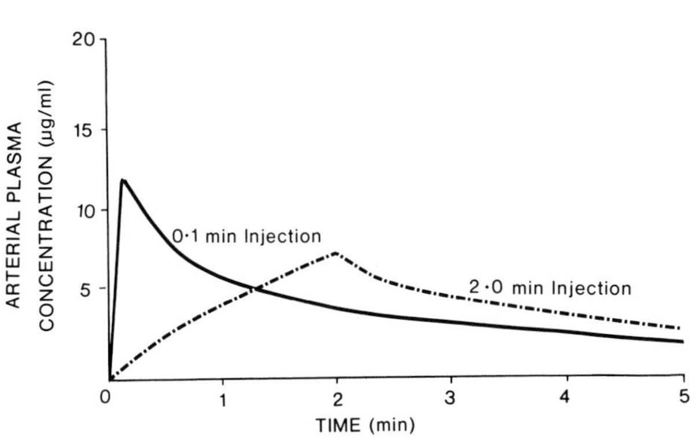

Fig. 4-10. Arterial plasma concentrations following intravenous injection of 100mg lidocaine hydrochloride over 0.1 and 2 minutes, to simulate concentrations of an inadvertent intravenous injection during a block procedure. Note the reduction in peak concentrations brought about by prolonging injection time. (Data from Tucker, G.T., and Boas, R.A.: Pharmacokinetic aspects of intravenous regional anesthesia. Anesthesiology, *34:*538, 1971)

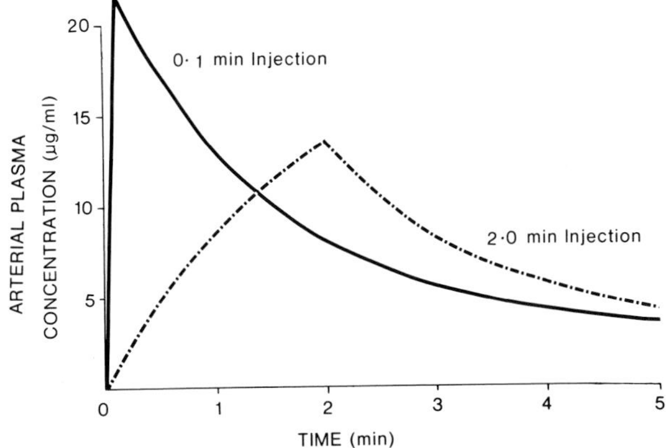

Fig. 4-11. Simulated arterial plasma concentrations of lidocaine, as described in Figure 4-10, show the likely outcome in patients with cardiac output reduced to around 50 per cent of normal. (Data from Thomson, S.P., *et al.:* Lidocaine pharmacokinetics in advanced heart failure, liver disease, and renal failure in humans. Ann. Intern. Med., *78*:499, 1973)

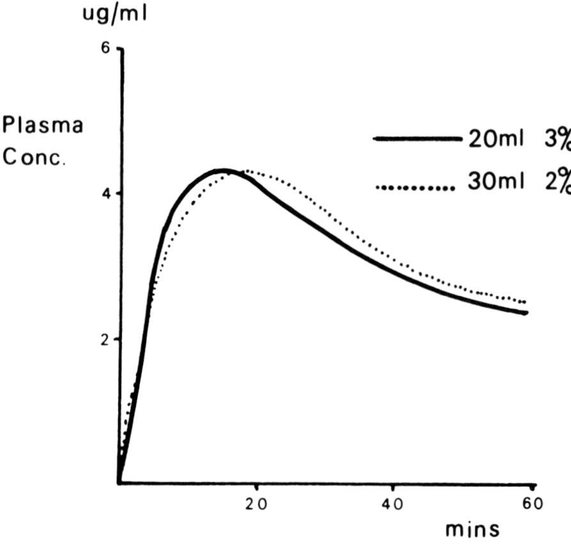

Fig. 4-12. Plasma concentrations of prilocaine following the epidural injection of 600mg, either as a 3-per-cent or a 2-per-cent solution.

brain and the myocardium in the first circulation will be higher (see Fig. 4-11). Normally, about 15 per cent of the cardiac output goes to the brain, and thus 15 per cent of the injected dose reaches the brain in the first circulation. In shock, this may increase up to 24 to 30 per cent (cerebral flow remaining constant as output decreases), thus increasing the amount of drug reaching the brain, and explaining why serious toxicity has occasionally been seen when quite small bolus injections of lidocaine have been given in myocardial infarction (see Fig. 4-11).

Low cardiac output states are, in addition, often associated with a considerable reduction in liver blood flow[43] (see Table 3-8).[43] Because the liver is responsible for detoxifying amide local anesthetics, reducing the liver blood flow will reduce the amount of drug available for degradation. This may produce very high blood concentrations during continuous intravenous infusion.[68] Hepatocellular disease could likewise reduce the speed of degradation and must be borne in mind if high or repeated doses of local anesthetic are contemplated (see Table 3-8).

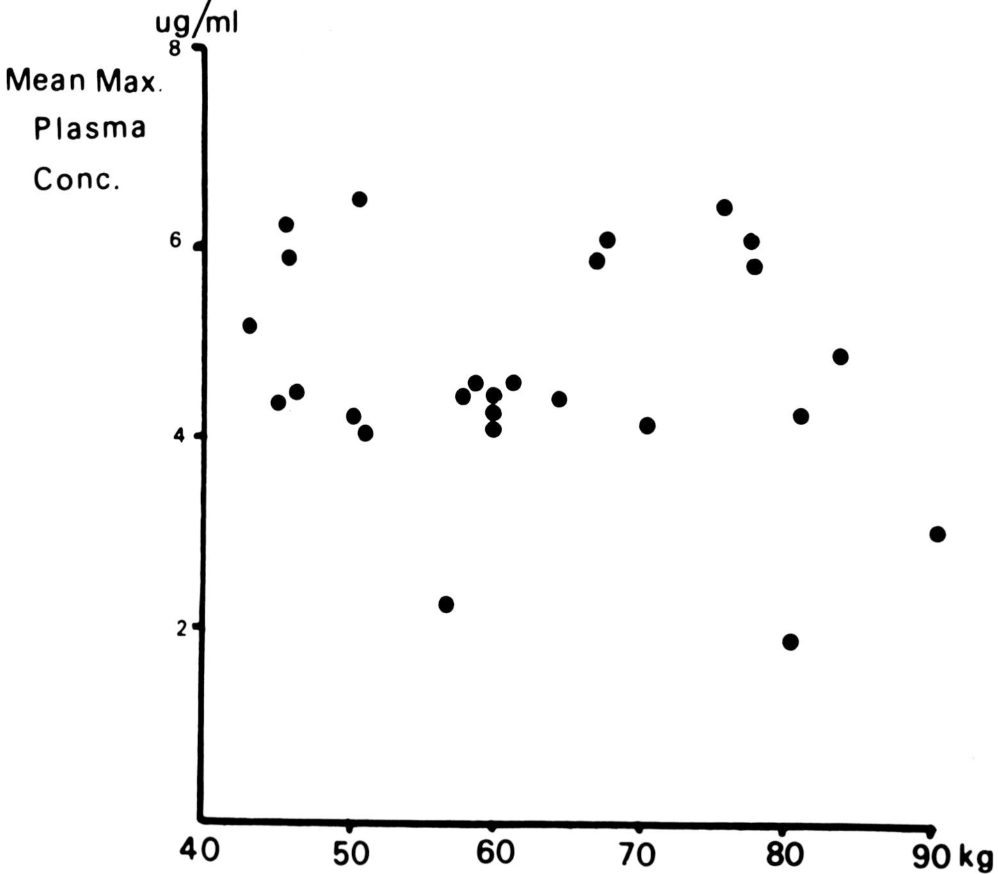

Fig. 4-13. Scatter diagram of the maximum plasma concentration of lidocaine following the epidural injection of 400mg, plotted against body weight. No correlation between the two variables could be discerned.

CLINICAL FEATURES AND DIAGNOSIS

The clinical features of toxicity are shown in Figure 4-14. They primarily affect the CNS while the cardiovascular system may be involved secondarily as a result of hypoxia or primarily as a result of gross overdose.

In diagnosing toxicity, the time course from the injection to the appearance of symptoms is important (Table 4-8). Thus, accidental intravenous injection will cause a rapid onset (*i.e.*, within 15–30 sec), while overdose will be associated with symptoms occurring 5 to 20 minutes later. Apparent evidence of toxicity appearing later than this should be viewed cautiously because it is unlikely that signs and symptoms would be delayed beyond 20 or 30 minutes. After treatment has been instituted, it is valuable to withdraw blood for the determination of the plasma concentration whenever toxicity is suspected.

Measures to Prevent Toxicity from Neural Blockade*

Patient evaluation
- Identification of significant systemic disease, age, and other factors, to permit individualization of local anesthetic dose

Premedication
- Diazepam or other appropriate CNS depressant in moderate dosage

Preparation
- Resucitative drugs
  - Diazepam or thiopentone, succinylcholine, atropine, vasopressor
- Equipment
  - Oxygen administration and suction
  - Airway (Oropharyngeal airway, laryngoscope, endotracheal suction tube)
- Ensure adequate IV available
- Discard any cloudy solutions or those containing crystals
- Physically separate neural blockade tray from any other drugs

Prevention
- Personally check dose of local anesthetic and vasoconstrictor
- Use test dose, 5–10% of total dose
- Aspirate frequently and discard solution colored by blood
- Monitor cardiovascular signs (rapid ↑ heart rate if epinephrine injected IV)
- Constant verbal contact with patient past time of peak plasma concentration

* Local anesthetic toxicity may result in convulsions; however, with rapid and appropriate treatment, these should never be fatal in themselves.

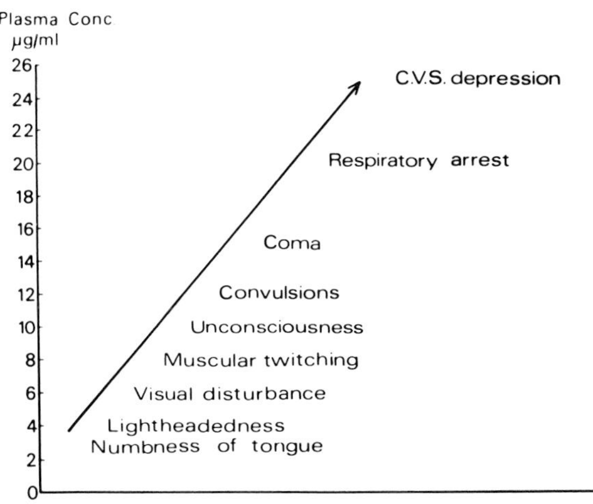

Fig. 4-14. Diagrammatic representation of the development of toxic effects with rising plasma concentrations of lidocaine.

Because the signs and symptoms of toxicity tend to be nonspecific (with the exception of numbness of the tongue and circumoral tissues, which is diagnostic) the diagnosis is prone to considerable error. Muscular twitching may be the result of shivering or nervousness rather than toxicity. Convulsions may be due to epilepsy or eclampsia, and there are many possible explanations of cardiovascular collapse. It is possible that hypotension is due to the local anesthetic procedure (*e.g.*, high extradural or spinal block) rather than the local anesthetic drug itself (see Table 4-8). The signs of toxicity may, on the other hand, be missed, especially if the patient is also taking anticonvulsive drugs, general anesthetics, or diazepam. Prolonged unconsciousness due to lidocaine given intravenously after cardiac surgery has been seen, muscular twitching having been abolished by sedative drugs.

Treatment of Acute Local Anesthetic Toxicity

Airway
- Establish clear airway, suction if required

Breathing
- Oxygen with face mask
- Encourage adequate ventilation (prevent cycle of acidosis, increased uptake of local anesthetic into CNS, and lowered seizure threshold)[30]
- Artificial ventilation, if required

Circulation
- Elevate legs
- Increase IV fluids if ↓ blood pressure
- CVS support drug if ↓ blood pressure persists (see below) or ↓ heart rate

Drugs
- CNS depressant

Diazepam 5–10 mg, IV
Thiopentone 50 mg, IV, incremental doses until seizures cease
Muscle relaxant
Succinylcholine, 1 mg/kg—if inadequate control of ventilation with above measures (Requires artificial ventilation and may necessitate intubation)
CVS support drugs
Atropine 0.6 mg, IV, if ↓ heart rate
Ephedrine, 12.5–25 mg, IV, to restore adequate blood pressure

---

TREATMENT

It is seldom necessary to treat the signs and symptoms of toxicity, excluding convulsions, provided adequate respiration and cardiovascular function are maintained.[30] Nevertheless, early signs of toxicity warrant constant verbal contact, cardiovascular monitoring, administration of oxygen, and encouragement to breathe at a normal minute volume.

If convulsions occur, then the aim of treatment is to stop them and treat any respiratory or cardiovascular depression before further cerebral hypoxia occurs.

Currently, three pharmacologic approaches to controlling convulsions are available. It should be stressed that the simple, nonpharmacologic measures on the list are carried out before any drug treatment is begun.

Pharmacologic Treatment

Intravenous barbiturates, such as thiopentone, can be used to treat local anesthetic toxicity. Even in small doses (50–100 mg), these drugs rapidly abort convulsions. They have been criticized because they may exaggerate both respiratory depression and cardiovascular depression, but in the small doses required, such effects would be minimal and short-lived. They have the great advantage of being extremely familiar (and generally readily available) to anesthesiologists.

Suxamethonium, (50 mg), given intravenously, will also stop convulsions rapidly, but administration is accompanied by paralysis and cessation of respiration. This would not be a disadvantage for a competent anesthesiologist who can intubate and ventilate the patient, but the drug should be avoided by the less experienced. Suxamethonium has less deleterious effect on the cardiovascular system than intravenous barbiturates. It is possible that suxamethonium would not affect the convulsive process in the brain and that this might increase the oxygen demand of the brain, which has been depressed by barbiturates. However, if respiration is assisted and cardiovascular function is adequate, this possibility is most unlikely to affect the outcome of treatment (see Chap. 2).

Diazepam, (5–10 mg), may be given intravenously. This drug is a powerful anticonvulsant and exerts its effect in little more time than does thipentone (although even 20–30 sec may seem a long time in these circumstances). It is virtually free from depressive effects on the circulation (see Chap. 2). Respiration must be carefully observed and a clear airway obtained, if necessary by endotracheal intubation. If depression or apnea supervene, artificial ventilation with oxygen is required. Provided oxygenation is maintained, it is very unlikely that serious consequences will ensue.

The prevention of hypoxia is the single most important feature of treatment (see Chap. 2).

Cardiovascular depression, as evidenced by a weak pulse and hypotension, should be treated by: correction of hypoxia, if present; elevation of legs and an increased rate of intravenous infusion; and intravenous injection of a vasopressor. Because the hypotension is due to a combination of myocardial depression and vasodilatation, it is preferable to use a vasopressor, which stimulates both alpha- and beta-adrenergic receptors, such as ephedrine (15–30 mg).

PREVENTION

The anesthesiologist has many courses of action to prevent overt toxicity due to local anesthetic drugs. Overdose can be avoided by a proper understanding of the pharmacology, especially the factors that affect absorption, distribution, and elimination.

Inadvertent intravenous injection can often be avoided by careful technique and by allowing sufficient time for reflux of blood down the needle or catheter used for injection. Very gentle syringe aspiration prior to injection is also useful, although a negative result may be due to collapse of the vessel wall against the needle orifice rather than correct placement extravascularly. The use of short bevel needles permits better recognition of vascular entry. The early discovery of toxicity before the entire planned dose is administered will prevent severe overdose. Although premedication of patients with anticonvulsant drugs such as diazepam will raise the threshold of toxicity, its use does not justify the administration of local anesthetics in excess of safe recommended dosages.

A knowledge of the blood concentration profile for the agent and technique employed will help to indicate the time when peak blood levels are likely to occur. Constant verbal contact and cardiorespiratory monitoring during this period are essential. As shown in Figure 3-14, after peridural block, peak concentrations may occur 20 to 30 minutes after drug administration and remain close enough to peak levels that a sudden change in cardiac output may cause a toxic plasma concentration to occur at least 30 minutes after the block. Also, if a second injection is required, then a knowledge of the drug clearance rate will determine safe timing and dosage.

LOCAL TOXICITY

New local anesthetics are carefully screened for tissue reactions at the site of injection before being released for clinical use. In normal drug concentrations, tissue reactions are very rare, if causes such as direct trauma (to nerves or blood vessels) and infection are eliminated.

The possible role of lidocaine intramuscularly as an antiarrhythmic agent has called for the use of concentrations higher than those generally used in anesthetic practice. This has led to an examination of the possible toxic effects upon muscle tissue. It has been found that changes can be produced in muscle especially with long-acting agents.

DRUG INTERACTION

Many drugs can affect the pharmacologic action of local anesthetics. At the site of injection, epinephrine and carbon dioxide (as a carbonated solution) can increase the effectiveness and duration of the block. General anesthetics and agents such as diazepam are powerful CNS anticonvulsants and will prevent or modify the toxicity of local anesthetics.[29] On the other hand, iproniazid, isoniazid, chloramphenicol, promethazine, and meperidine have been reported capable of enhancing or prolonging the convulsive effects of local anesthetics in animals; the clinical significance of this at doses used in clinical practice is unknown at present.[45,77] Procaine is metabolized to para-aminobenzoic acid, which inhibits the action of sulphonamide antimicrobial agents. Ester local anesthetics, which rely on metabolism by plasma pseudocholinesterase, potentiate the action of any other drug with a similar mode of biodegradation, such as suxamethonium, trimetaphan, and, to a lesser extent, propanidid.

Plasma levels of local anesthetics following neural blockade usually have clinically insignificant effects at the neuromuscular junction; however, at very high dosages, these effects significantly enhance the action of both depolarizing and nondepolarizing muscle relaxants.[54,79] Duration of apnea produced by succinylcholine or curare can be considerably increased by concomitant administration of lidocaine.[31,42] There is a synergistic depressant effect on the myocardium when drugs such as halothane,[73] ether, and pentobarbitone are used with lidocaine.[59,72]

Enzyme induction by phenobarbitone and barbital has been shown experimentally to cause an increase in the rate of elimination of lidocaine and mepivacaine.[33,45]

COMPARISON OF CLINICAL EFFECTS

Animal Studies

Animal studies *in vitro* have employed isolated nerve preparations to determine the relative potency of different local anesthetic agents. The minimum concentration required to produce a 50 to 60 per cent reduction in amplitude of the action potential of an A fiber within 5 minutes has been termed the *intrinsic potency*. If conditions of measurements are standardized (*e.g.*, *p*H 7.2–7.4, supramaximal stimulus at a frequency of 30 pulses/sec), then useful comparisons of intrinsic potency may be made between different local anesthetics.[27] Unfortunately, many early reports of effective concentrations of local anesthetics *in vitro* employed widely differing conditions of measurement, which introduce the added effects of stimulus intensity, stimulus frequency, *p*H effects,[21] and differences in fiber sensitivity (see Chap. 2). Under standardized conditions, it is possible to obtain useful comparative data that appear to correspond well with the small amount of controlled clinical data currently available.[27] Thus, procaine has the least intrinsic potency, with mepivacaine, prilocaine, chloroprocaine, and lidocaine having intermediate potency; and bupivacaine, etidocaine, and tetracaine, high potency (Table 4-9).

The data on Table 4-9 should not be used to predict values for clinical responses. Various animal models, *in vivo* have been used, which include the following: guinea pig intradermal wheals to assess infiltration anesthesia; rat sciatic nerve block and guinea pig brachial plexus block to assess peripheral nerve blockade; implanted epidural catheters in guinea pigs, cats, dogs, and sheep to assess epidural blockade; spinal anesthesia in various animals and application to rabbit cornea and trachea to assess topical anesthesia.[1,6,7,20,34,79] By means of a standard

***Table 4-9. Comparative Local Anesthetic Potency in Animals* in Vitro *and* in Vivo**

		C_m (in vivo)	
Agent	*Relative Intrinsic Potency** (in Vitro)	*Rat Sciatic Nerve†*	*Cat Epidural Block‡*
Procaine	1	1	4
Mepivacaine	2	0.5	2
Prilocaine	3	0.5	2
Chloroprocaine	4	1	2
Lidocaine	4	0.5	2
Bupivacaine	16	0.125	0.5
Etidocaine	16	0.125	0.5
Tetracaine	16	0.125	0.5

* Minimum concentration required to produce 50 percent reduction in A spike amplitude of sheathed frog sciatic nerve within 5 minutes at *p*H 7.2 to 7.4 and stimulus frequency 30 pulses per second.

† Minimum concentration (0.2 ml) required to produce 50 per cent frequency of sensory blockade

‡ Minimum concentration (1.5 ml) required to produce 50 per cent frequency of flexor reflex blockade

(Covino, B. G., and Vassallo, H. G.: Latency and duration of action of some local anesthetic mixtures. Anesth. Analg. (Cleve.), *45*:106, 1966)

preparation for comparison of agents, and sometimes an indwelling catheter, useful comparative data permit some degree of quantitative extrapolation to humans, but differences in degradation of agents between human and animal species remain (see Fig. 3-23).

Thus the maximum blocking concentration (C_m) of injected solution for peripheral nerve block is similar (0.5%) for mepivacaine, prilocaine, and lidocaine, and this bears a close relationship to clinical values for C_m. Procaine and chloroprocaine require the same C_m *in vivo,* whereas chloroprocaine has four times the intrinsic potency of procaine *in vitro;* chloroprocaine presumably loses its advantage *in vivo* because of its very rapid metabolism. Another discrepancy is seen between the potency *in vitro* of lidocaine (1.5–2 times greater than mepivacaine and prilocaine) and the potency *in vivo,* which is similar for the three agents. Once again, this similarity obtains in clinical findings, and it is possible that lidocaine's greater vasodilator action compared to mepivacaine and prilocaine may require a higher concentration *in vivo* to compensate for rapid vascular uptake.

The rat sciatic nerve data for bupivacaine, etidocaine, and tetracaine correlate quite well with clinical data when it is remembered that a concentration of 0.125 per cent prevents response to painful stimulus only 50 per cent of the time (median effective dose, or ED_{50}). It is in fact possible to achieve sympathetic block and mild sensory block clinically with 0.125 per cent of these drugs, although more satisfactory block requires 0.25 to 0.5 per cent.

The cat epidural data are even closer to clinical data and appear to correlate well for all of the amides, although some clinicians report that 1 per cent etidocaine is necessary for satisfactory sensory block, and 0.75 per cent bupivacaine is required for adequate motor block. Once again, the 50-per-cent block of flexor response achieved in the animal study is significant, but a similarly precise value is not yet available from clinical studies. Epidural studies in sheep indicate that 1 per cent etidocaine is required to produce blockade comparable to 0.75 per cent bupivacaine. These higher concentrations of the fat-soluble agents may be occasioned by the sequestration of very large amounts of agent in epidural fat (see Fig. 3-11).

Assessment of topical activity in rabbit cornea indicates that in decreasing order of potency, the drugs rank as follows: tetracaine, etidocaine, cocaine, bupivacaine, lidocaine, and prilocaine.[7,26] Procaine and mepivacaine require very high concentrations (10–20%) to produce even mild topical anesthesia. This is in keeping with clinical findings.

Animal models *in vivo* have also provided quite useful estimates of onset and duration of action of local anesthetics. Thus, spinal anesthesia in sheep, assessed by digital pain, has a duration of 36 to 42 minutes for lidocaine and 60 to 140 minutes for tetracaine, using solutions without epinephrine.[6] These figures are very similar to clinical data, although there has not been a randomized "blind" study. Controlled data on onset time for epidural block indicate that increasing the dose, either by increasing the concentration or volume, decreases the onset time of lidocaine by half.[34] In contrast, an alteration in *p*H of the solution and the addition of epinephrine produce inconsistent changes; the effect of the dosage is similar to that seen in humans.

Compounding of local anesthetic agents can be examined, for example, in the dog epidural preparation. This has provided initial information about an area that lacks clinical definition and shows that a combination of the short-acting agent lidocaine with the long-acting agent tetracaine results in a mixture that possesses the most favorable properties of the two agents, that is, an onset as rapid as lidocaine alone and a duration similar to tetracaine alone.[28] However, there are still no data on the relative proportions of agents required to produce the "best effects" of each component agent in humans.

It can no longer be argued that animal studies of local anesthetic neural blockade have no relevance for humans. As described above, careful control of conditions of measurement and a knowledge of the method of assessment of blockade provide data that are very useful in determining comparative efficacy of local anesthetics.

Relative toxicity of local anesthetics can also initially be assessed in animals. Local tissue toxicity, in particular, has been investigated in tissues from various animals. Local anesthetics have long been known to inhibit platelet and leukocyte aggregation at blood concentrations achieved during neural blockade.[27]

The clinical significance of these findings is unclear and is not thought to indicate clinically important toxicity. Studies in isolated frog nerves have shown that concentrations of local anesthetics required to produce irreversible conduction blockade are far in excess of those required for clinical nerve block.[76] Similarly, the inhibitory effect of local anesthetics on rapid axonal transport is achieved at concentrations in excess of those used clinically.[38] Studies of subarachnoid administration of the preservatives in local anesthetics have been useful in investigating claims that they may cause neurotoxicity; for example, methylparaben was shown not to be neurotoxic with or without lidocaine.[66] Studies of skeletal muscle structure have shown that high concentrations of local anesthetics may cause reversible changes if they are injected directly into skeletal muscle; regeneration is said to be complete within 2 weeks.[8,9] Such changes are not produced by the muscle concentration of local anesthetic associated with regional block procedures but relate to the current use of intramuscular solutions, such as 20 per cent lidocaine, for arrhythmia control.

Systemic toxicity is less satisfactorily evaluated in animals since the early clinical symptoms of toxicity are subjective and cannot be documented in animals. Nevertheless, an estimate can be obtained of the relative dosage of local anesthetic agent and blood level required to cause seizures (see Table 4-1).[30,65] As discussed in Chapter 2, this has allowed confirmation of data at subconvulsive doses in humans, which indicates that a direct relationship exists between the potency of the drug and the dose required to produce toxicity.[70] Thus, in order to test convulsions, procaine with low potency must be administered in the largest intravenous dose that will cause convulsions, whereas bupivacaine with a high potency requires very low doses. Unfortunately, blood levels associated with convulsions in animals are not the same as in humans. Thus the most meaningful comparison of toxic potential appears to require measurement of arterial blood concentrations and CNS response in humans during intravenous administration at a constant rate.

To evaluate the usefulness of animal data, the following ratio is important:

$$\frac{\text{Toxic dose}}{\text{Effective dose for nerve block}}$$

A high intrinsic potency will be of little value if it is outweighed by very high toxicity. Here, the following ratio is useful:

$$\frac{\text{Relative toxicity}}{\text{Intrinsic potency}}$$

Previous attempts to determine the following in animals have proved less useful:

$$\frac{\text{Effective dose}_{50}}{\text{Lethal dose}_{50}}\left(\frac{\text{ED}_{50}}{\text{LD}_{50}}\right)$$

Evaluation in Humans

Local anesthetics should be compared by considering their relative efficacy in the light of their relative toxicity. Until recently, precise data on relative toxicity in humans were lacking. However, because of the difficulty in measurement, data on the esters are still minimal. Table 3-4 illustrates the ratio of blood concentration associated with maximum effective doses (C_{Max}) and blood concentration associated with early signs of toxicity (C_{Tox}). This ratio, $\frac{C_{Tox}}{C_{Max}}$, is termed a *toxicity ratio* and is perhaps the most meaningful estimate of the clinical safety of a local anesthetic.

Having obtained data that indicate the maximum concentration (and dose) of a new drug that can be used to achieve a similar $\frac{C_{Tox}}{C_{Max}}$ ratio to a standard drug (*e.g.*, lidocaine), it is then necessary to determine if the new drug has any greater efficacy at this equitoxic dose.

Compounding of local anesthetics in clinical practice has recently gained popularity; however, definitive data on clinical benefits (if any) and toxicity are lacking. It is hoped that mixing a rapid-acting agent with one of long duration may combine the best effects of both; to date, this has not been conclusively established in humans. It seems likely, if animal data are confirmed in humans, that toxicity of mixtures of amides will be directly additive. Compounding an ester, cleared by plasma hydrolysis, with an amide, cleared by liver metabolism, would seem to offer advantages because of the alternative routes of metabolism. Initial clinical data tend to support this; however, confirmatory studies are required.[84]

The greatest possibilities for gathering controlled objective data on clinical aspects of local anesthetic action are in the field of clinical effects. Unfortunately, the use of controlled study design and objective criteria for assessment of neural blockade have not been frequently employed in clinical evaluation of local anesthetics.

The need for such objective data and suggestions for controlled study design were outlined at least 20 years ago by Bonica.[12] More recently, Covino and Bush have reviewed the difficulties encountered in clinical evaluation of local anesthetics.[26] In particular, attention was drawn to the unique problem of the effect of technical skill in administration of the local anesthetic agent; this can affect both safety and efficacy. This problem does not come into play in the comparative assessment of other classes of drugs. Important factors influencing comparative evaluation of local anesthetics are the following:

Procedural factors
- Type of regional block
- Skill of the clinician and the technique employed for that particular block (*e.g.*, for epidural block)
- Level of needle insertion, position of patient, speed of injection

Patient factors
- Age
- Height
- Weight
- Clinical status (*e.g.*, pregnancy, atherosclerosis)

Circumstances associated with local anesthetic administration and its subsequent assessment
- Presence or lack of premedication
- Use of adjunctive drugs such as sedatives and vasopressors
- Assessment in operated or nonoperated patients, etc.

Drug factors
- Dosage
- Concentration and volume
- Presence or absence of vasoconstrictor (see Table 4-2)
- *p*H of injected solution

Investigation factors
- Method of evaluation
  - Subjective, variable methods (*e.g.*, pinprick, Allis clamp, etc.) for sensory block testing in general use not recommended
  - More objective methods for sympathetic block testing (*e.g.*, skin temperature, skin resistance, limb blood flow) preferred

Timing of observations
- Adequate frequency of measurement
- Identical timing for each agent under evaluation

Study design
- Elimination of investigation bias
- Randomized prospective controlled design
- Standard and test drug in coded ampules and at equitoxic concentrations
- Drug administration "triple blind"

Single patient studies ideal (*e.g.*, bilateral ulnar nerve block, bilateral intercostal block, or crossover studies using two agents for epidural block or brachial plexus block in same patient[15,58,83]
- Alternatively, between patient studies with controlled design for nonbiased data[16,25,35]

It is clear that comparison of data from one study to another even within one institution is fraught with difficulties. It is still more difficult to make valid comparisons between studies in different institutions. These difficulties are much reduced if frequency and methods of testing are carefully defined and a randomized prospective controlled study design is employed. It is recommended that specific pharmacologic data, such as onset time, duration, and motor blockade in a limited number of patients with rigid control of design and without supplemental drugs, surgery, or other factors be obtained. Even before these measures are taken, of course, it will always be necessary to obtain additional data under the actual conditions of clinical use (*e.g.*, operative surgery, postoperative pain relief, obstetric analgesia, etc.). It must be remembered that the requirements of a local anesthetic may be quite different in each clinical application (*e.g.*, profound sensory and motor block for operative surgery, profound sensory but no motor block for obstetric analgesia and postoperative pain relief, and special characteristics of placental transfer for obstetric use).

Topical Anesthesia. Controlled clinical data on topical anesthesia are lacking, owing to difficulties in designing objective techniques for evaluation of topical efficacy, variability in method of application of topical agent, and lack of a method to determine the dose of agent taken up by the topical area. A great variety of topical anesthetic preparations also increases the likelihood of variations in effect, as does the site of topical application (*e.g.*, eye, trachea, bladder, etc.). Table 4-3 summarizes the common sites of topical application, the appropriate agent and one useful preparation, and its onset time and duration of action. Since only minimal comparative clinical data are available, it has been necessary to rely on data from certain standardized animal preparations.[7,20] By using the rabbit cornea, it has been determined that topical agents can be ranked for their relative potency in decreasing order: tetracaine, etidocaine, cocaine, bupivacaine, lidocaine, and prilocaine.[7] Procaine and mepivacaine do not have significant topical anesthetic activity. By means of intravesical application, the LD_{50} of tetracaine has been reported to be only five times the intravenous LD_{50}, whereas the intravesical LD_{50} values of cocaine, lidocaine, and prilocaine were 22 to 44 times their intravenous LD_{50} values.[7] Tetracaine has also been reported to be potentially hazardous when it is used topically for clinical purposes.[2]

At present, cocaine and lidocaine appear to be the best choices for topical anesthesia; lidocaine being preferred for tracheobronchial tree and eye; cocaine being reserved for nasopharynx and ear, particularly if vasoconstriction is desirable. As with injection techniques, data indicate that increasing the concentration decreases the onset time and increases the duration. Thus, 4 per cent cocaine has an onset time of 5 minutes and a duration of 10 minutes, while with 10 per cent the values are 2 minutes and over 30 minutes, respectively (Table 4-3). It should be remembered, however, that a manageable volume of agent is necessary, and the 10-per-cent solution permits the administration of only 2 ml as a maximum safe dose. As previously discussed, there is no longer any rationale for the addition of epinephrine to topical anesthetic solutions.[3,32]

In some countries, a 10-per-cent aerosol preparation of lidocaine is available and has been used for spraying oropharynx, larynx, and trachea. Each press of the release button delivers 0.1 ml (10 mg). Plasma concentration studies indicate that 15 to 20 presses (150–200 mg) would be the maximum safe dose.[74] Rapid absorption from the lower respiratory tract may occur, especially in paralyzed patients, when the ability to cough and swallow is lost. Conscious patients achieve much lower plasma concentrations than those who are anesthetized and paralyzed.[78]

Infiltration Anesthesia. The clinically effective concentrations of local anesthetics employed for infiltration anesthesia are similar to their relative intrinsic potencies determined *in vitro* (Tables 4-4; 4-9). Thus, 1 to 2 per cent procaine; 0.5 to 1 per cent lidocaine, mepivacaine, and prilocaine; 0.25 per cent bupivacaine; and 0.5 per cent etidocaine will produce equally adequate infiltration analgesia. At present, 1 per cent lidocaine has considerable advantage over most other agents because of its spreading capacities. In addition, its duration of action is increased from approximately 2 hours to at least 6 hours by the addition of epinephrine. Large-volume infiltration blocks are best accomplished with a weaker solution of 0.5 per cent lidocaine or the equivalent. Even with this solution, the duration of analgesia can be extended from 1 hour to almost 4 hours with epinephrine. Although the other amides are capable of highly satisfactory infiltration block, none appear to offer any significant advantage beyond prolonged duration without epinephrine, for instance, 0.25 per cent bupivacaine, which has a duration of action of approximately 3 hours (see Table 4-4).

Peripheral Nerve Block. Some of the best objective data available compare local anesthetics at the level of peripheral nerve blockade. Albert and Löfstrom performed single-patient comparisons using bilateral ulnar nerve blocks to obtain some of the block duration data reproduced in Figure 4-2. The data obtained from these controlled studies in humans correlates well with data from standardized animal studies *in vivo* and *in vitro*.[58] Because the ulnar nerve block evaluation employs direct intraneural injection, it is less suitable for assessment of onset time. Here the technique of bilateral intercostal block has been invaluable.[16] The data in Figure 4-2 indicate relative onset and duration for the long-acting agents etidocaine, bupivacaine, and tetracaine. It can be seen that all three agents provide blockade of quite long duration but that etidocaine has a more rapid onset of blockade. Another method of assessment, with similar results to ulnar nerve block, is bilateral axillary brachial plexus block, which also permits an estimate of the duration of sympathetic blockade.[83]

Intravenous regional block, caudal, epidural, and spinal anesthesia are described in detail in Chapters 7, 8, 9, and 12 and comparative data about the action of individual local anesthetics are illustrated.

Comparison of Systemic Effects of Regional Block. When there is no overt toxicity, local anesthetics have minimal but measurable effects on various body systems. Of much greater importance are the systemic effects of the regional block procedure, particularly for cardiovascular and respiratory function. The application of strict criteria for study design is equally important in this area of evaluation. The most important cardiorespiratory changes are seen following spinal and epidural anesthesia and are described in Chapters 7 and 8.

REFERENCES

1. Adams, H.J., Kronberg, G.H., and Takman, B.H.: Local anesthetic activity and acute toxicity of (±)-2-(N-ethypropylamino)-2′, 6′-butyrexylidide, a new long-acting agent. J. Pharm. Sci., *61*:1829, 1972.

2. Adriani, J., and Campbell, D.: Fatalities following topical application of local anesthetics to mucous membranes. J.A.M.A., *162*:1527, 1956.
3. Adriani, J., Zepernick, R., Arens, J., and Authement, E.: The comparative potency and effectiveness of topical anesthetics in man. Clin. Pharmacol. Ther., *5*:49, 1964.
4. Aldrete, J.A., and Johnson, D.A.: Evaluation of intracutaneous testing for investigation of allergy to local anesthetic agents. Anesth. Analg. (Cleve.), *49*:173, 1970.
5. Aldrete, J.A., *et al.:* Untoward reactions to local anesthetics via reverse intracarotid flow. J. Dent. Res., *54*:145, 1975.
6. Astrom, A., and Persson, N.H. Some pharmacological properties of o-methyl-N propylaminopropionanilide a new local anaesthetic. Br. J. Pharmacol., *16*:32, 1961.
7. ______: The toxicity of some local anaesthetics after application on different mucous membranes and its relation to anaesthetic action on the nasal mucosa of the rabbit. J. Pharmacol. Exp. Ther., *132*:87, 1961.
8. Benoit, P.W., and Belt, W.D.: Destruction and regeneration of skeletal muscle after treatment with a local anaesthetic bupivacaine (Marcaine). J. Anat., *107*:547, 1970.
9. ______: Some effects of local anaesthetic agents on skeletal muscle. Exp. Neurol., *34*:264, 1972.
10. Bernhard, C.G., and Bohm, E.: Local Anaesthetics as Anticonvulsants. Stockholm, Almqvist & Wiksel, 1965.
11. Blair, M.R.: Cardiovascular pharmacology of local anaesthetics. Br. J. Anaesth., *47*:247, 1975.
12. Bonica, J.J.: Clinical investigation of local anesthetics. Anesthesiology, *18*:110, 1957.
13. Braid, D.P., and Scott, D.B.: The systemic absorption of local analgesic drugs. Br. J. Anaesth., *37*:394, 1965.
14. Bridenbaugh, L.D., and Moore, D.C.: Does repeated heat sterilization of local anesthetic drugs affect potency? Anesthesiology, *25*:372, 1964.
15. Bridenbaugh, P.O.: Intercostal nerve blockade for the evaluation of local anaesthetic agents. Br. J. Anaesth., *47*:306, 1975.
16. Bridenbaugh, P.O., Tucker, G.T., Moore, D.C., Bridenbaugh, L.D., and Thompson, G.E.: Etidocaine: Clinical evaluation for intercostal nerve block and lumbar epidural block. Anesth. Analg. (Cleve.), *52*:407, 1973.
17. Bromage, P.R., and Gertel, M.: An evaluation of two new local anesthetics for major conduction blockade. Can. Anaesth. Soc. J., *17*:557, 1970.
18. Bromage, P.R., and Robson, J.G.: Concentrations of lignocaine in the blood after intravenous, intramuscular epidural and endotracheal administration. Anaesthesia, *16*:461, 1961.
19. Buckley, P.B., *et al.:* Effects of adrenaline and the concentration of solution on extradural block with etidocaine. Br. J. Anaesth., *50*:171–175, 1978.
20. Camougis, G., and Takman, B.H.: Nerve and nerve-muscle preparation (as applied to local anaesthetics). Methods in Pharmacology, *1*:1, 1971.
21. Catchlove, R.F.H.: The influence of CO_2 and *p*H on local anesthetic action. J. Pharmacol. Exp. Ther., *181*:298, 1972.
22. Chalaresunthernvatee, P., and Thomas, R.E.: The stability of solutions of amethocaine hydrochloride. Australas. J. Pharm., *42*:800, 1961.
23. Colquhoun, D., and Ritchie, J.M.: The interaction at equilibrium between tetrodotoxin and mammalian nonmyelinated nerve fibres. J. Physiol., *221*:533, 1972.
24. ______: The kinetics of the interaction between tetrodotoxin and mammalian nonmyelinated nerve fibres. Mol. Pharmacol., *8*:285, 1972.
25. Cousins, M.J., Augustus, J.A., Gleason, M., Morgan, D.J., and Thomas, J.: Epidural block for abdominal surgery: Aspects of clinical pharmacology of etidocaine. Anaesth. Intensive Care, *6*:105, 1978.
26. Covino, B.G., and Bush, D.F.: Clinical evaluation of local anaesthetic agents. Br. J. Anaesth., *47*:289, 1975.
27. Covino, B.G., and Vassallo, H.G.: Local Anesthetics: Mechanisms of Action and Clinical Use. New York, Grune & Stratton, 1976.
28. Defalque, R.J., and Stoelting, V.K.: Latency and duration of action of some local anaesthetic mixtures. Anesth. Analg. (Cleve.), *45*:106, 1966.
29. de Jong, R.H., Heavner, J.E., and Oliveira, L.F.: Effects of nitrous oxide on the lidocaine seizure threshold and diazepam protection. Anesthesiology, *37*:299, 1972.
30. de Jong, R.H., Wagman, I.H., and Prince, D.A.: Effect of carbon dioxide on the cortical seizure threshold of lidocaine. Exp. Neurol., *17*:221, 1967.
31. de Kornfeld, T.J., and Steinhaus, J.E.: The effect of intravenously administered lidocaine and succinylcholine on respiratory activity of dogs. Anesth. Analg. (Cleve.), *38*:173, 1959.
32. Delikan, A.E.: Topical cocaine/adrenaline combination in intranasal surgery—is it necessary? Anaesth. Intensive Care, *6*:328–332, 1978.
33. Difazio, C.A., and Brown, R.E.: Lidocaine metabolism in normal and phenobarbital-pretreated dogs. Anesthesiology, *36*:238, 1972.
34. Duce, B.R., Zelechowski, K., Camougis, G., and Smith, E.R.: Experimental epidural anaesthesia in the cat with lignocaine and amethocaine. Br. J. Anaesth., *41*:579, 1969.
35. Engberg, G., Holmdahl, M.H., and Edstrom, H.H.: A comparison of local anesthetic properties of bupivacaine and two new long-acting agents, HS 37 and etidocaine, in epidural analgesia. Acta Anaesth. Scand., *18*:277, 1974.
36. Englesson, S., and Matousek, M.: Central nervous system effects of local anaesthetic agents. Br. J. Anaesth., *47*:241, 1975.
37. Eriksson, E., Englesson, S., Wahlqvist, S., and Ortengren, B.: Study of the intravenous toxicity in man and some *in vitro* studies on the distribution and absorbability. Acta Chir. Scand., *358*[*Suppl.*]:25, 1966.
38. Fink, B.R., Kennedy, R.D., Hendrickson, A.E., and Middaugh, M.E.: Lidocaine inhibition of rapid axonal transport. Anesthesiology, *36*:422, 1972.
39. Foldes, F.F., Davidson, G.M., Duncalf, D., and Kuwabara, S.: The intravenous toxicity of local anesthetic agents in man. Clin. Pharmacol. Ther., *6*:328, 1965.
40. Foldes, F.F., *et al.:* Substrate competition between procaine and succinylcholine diiodide for plasma cholinesterase. Science, *117*:383, 1953.
41. Geddes, I.C.: Chemical structure of local anaesthetics. Br. J. Anaesth., *34*:229, 1962.
42. Hall, D.R., McGibbon, D.H., Evans, C.C., and Meadows, G.A.: Gentamicin, tubocurarine, lignocaine and neuromuscular blockade. Br. J. Anaesth., *44*:1329, 1972.
43. Harrison, D.C., and Alderman, E.L.: Relation of blood levels to clinical effectiveness of lidocaine. *In* Scott, D.B., and Julian, D.C. (eds.): Lidocaine in the Treatment of Ventricular Arrhythmias. Pp. 178–188. Edinburgh, E & S Livingstone, 1971.
44. Harrison, D.C., Sprouse, H., and Morrow, A.G.: The antiarrhythmic properties of lidocaine and procaine amide. Circulation, *28*:486, 1963.
45. Heinonen, J.: The effect of drugs on the duration of toxic symptoms caused by sublethal doses of local anaesthetics. An experimental study on mice. Acta Pharmacol. Toxicol. (Kbh.), *21*:155, 1964.

46. Hertting, G., Axelrod, J., and Whitby, L.G.: Effect of drugs on the uptake and metabolism of H_3-norepinephrine. J. Pharmacol. Exp. Ther., *134*:146, 1961.
47. Hjelm, M., and Holmdahl, M.H.: Clinical chemistry of prilocaine and clinical evaluation of methaemoglobinaemia induced by this agent. Acta Anaesthesiol. Scand., *16*[*Suppl*]:161, 1965.
48. Hughes, J.R.: Infantile methemoglobinemia due to benzocaine suppository. J. Pediatr., *66*:797, 1965.
49. Jebson, P.R.: Intramuscular lignocaine 2% and 10%. Br. Med. J., *3*:566, 1971.
50. Jewitt, D.: Comparison of the haemodynamic effects of antiarrhythmic drugs. *In* Scott, D.B., and Julian, D.C. (eds.): Lidocaine in the Treatment of Ventricular Arrhythmias. P. 208. Edinburgh, E & S Livingstone, 1971.
51. Jorfeldt, L., *et al.:* The effect of local anaesthetics on the central circulation and respiration in man and dog. Acta Anaesthesiol. Scand., *12*:153, 1968.
52. Kalow, W.: Hydrolysis of local anesthetics by human serum cholinesterase. J. Pharmacol. Exp. Ther., *104*:122, 1952.
53. Katz, R.L., and Epstein, R.A.: The interaction of anesthetic agents and adrenergic drugs to produce cardiac arrhythmias. Anesthesiology, *29*:763, 1968.
54. Katz, R.L., and Gissen, A.J.: Effects on intravenous and intra-arterial procaine and lidocaine on neuromuscular transmission in man. Acta Anaesthesiol. Scand., *36*[*Suppl.*]:103, 1969.
55. Klein, S., Sutherland, R.I.L., and Morch, J.: Haemodynamic effects on intravenous lignocaine in man. Can. Med. Assoc. J., *99*:472, 1968.
56. Kohn, J., Rutter, A.G., and Vitali, M.: Prolonged local analgesia with benzocaine-urethane solution. Br. Med. J., *1*:682, 1954.
57. Littlewood, D.G., *et al.:* Comparative anaesthetic properties of various local anaesthetic agents in extradural block for labour. Br. J. Anaesth., *49*:75, 1977.
58. Lofstrom, J.B.: Ulnar nerve blockade for the evaluation of local anaesthetic agents. Br. J. Anaesth., *47*:297, 1975.
59. McWhirter, W., Frederickson, E., and Steinhaus, J.: Interactions of lidocaine with general anaesthetics. South. Med. J., *65*:398, 1972.
60. Moore, D.C., and Bridenbaugh, L.D.: Intercostal nerve block in 4,333 patients: Indication, technique and complications. Anesth. Analg. (Cleve.), *41*:1, 1962.
61. Moore, D.C., Bridenbaugh, L.D., Bagdi, P.A., Bridenbaugh, P.O., and Stander, H.: The present status of spinal (subarachnoid) and epidural (peridural) block. Anesth. Analg. (Cleve.), *47*:40, 1968.
62. Moore, D.C., Bridenbaugh, L.D., Bridenbaugh, P.O., and Thompson, G.E.: Bupivacaine hydrochloride: A summary of investigational use in 3,274 cases. Anesth. Analg. (Cleve.), *50*:856, 1971.
63. Morishima, H.O., Daniel, S.S., Finster, M., Poppers, P.J., and James, L.S.: Transmission of mepivacaine hydrochloride (Carbocaine) across human placenta. Anesthesiology, *27*:147, 1966.
64. Munson, E.S., Martucci, R.W., and Wagman, I.H.: Bupivacaine and lignocaine induced seizures in rhesus monkeys. Br. J. Anaesth., *44*:1025, 1972.
65. Munson, E.S., Tucker, W.K., Ausinsch, B., and Malagodi, H.: Etidocaine, bupivacaine and lidocaine seizure threshold in monkeys. Anesthesiology, *42*:471, 1975.
66. Nathan, P.W., and Spears, T.A.: Action of methyl hydroxybenzoate on nervous conduction. Nature (Lond.), *192*:668, 1961.
67. Nolte, H., *et al.:* Zur frage der Spinalanaesthesie mit isobarem Bupivacain 0.5%. Anaesthesist, *26*:33, 1977.
68. Prescott, L.F., and Nimmo, J.: Plasma lidocaine concentrations during and after prolonged infusions in patients with myocardial infarction. *In* Scott, D.B., and Julian, D.C. (eds.): Lidocaine in the Treatment of Ventricular Arrhythmias. P. 168. Edinburgh, E & S Livingstone, 1971.
69. Raj, P.P., Rosenblatt, R., Miller, J., Katz, R.L., and Carden, E.: Dynamics of local anesthetic compounds in regional anesthesia. Anesth. Analg. (Cleve.), *56*:110, 1977.
70. Scott, D.B.: Evaluation of the toxicity of local anaesthetic agents in man. Br. J. Anaesth., *47*:56, 1975.
71. ———: Evaluation of clinical tolerance of local anaesthetic agents. Br. J. Anaesth., *47*:328, 1975.
72. Scott, D.B., Davie, I.T., and Stephen, G.W.: Cardiovascular effects of intravenous lignocaine during nitrous oxide/halothane anaesthesia. Br. J. Anaesth., *43*:595, 1971.
73. Scott, D.B., Jebson, P.J.R., Braid, D.P., Ortengren, B., and Frisch, P.: Factors affecting plasma levels of lignocaine and prilocaine. Br. J. Anaesth., *44*:1040, 1972.
74. Scott, D.B., Littlewood, D.G., Covino, B.G., and Drummond, G.B.: Plasma lignocaine concentrations following endotracheal spraying with an aerosol. Br. J. Anaesth., *48*:899, 1976.
75. Scott, D.B., Owen, J.A., and Richmond, J.: Methaemoglobinaemia due to prilocaine. Lancet, *2*:728, 1964.
76. Skou, J.C.: Local anaesthetics. Part II: The toxic potency of some local anaesthetics and of butyl alcohol determined on peripheral nerves. Acta Pharmacol. Toxicol. (Kbh.), *10*:292, 1954.
77. Smudski, J.W., Sprecher, R.L., and Elliott, H.W.: Convulsive interaction of promethazine, meperidine and lidocaine. Arch. Oral. Biol., *9*:595, 1964.
78. Telivuo, L.: An experimental study on the absorption of some local anaesthetics through the lower respiratory tract. Acta Anaesthesiol. Scand. *16*[*Suppl.*]:121, 1965.
79. ———: The effects of intra-arterial mepivacaine and bupivacaine on neuromuscular transmission in man. Acta Anaesthesiol. Scand., *11*:327, 1976.
80. Truant, A.P.: Studies on the pharmacology of meprylcaine (Oracaine), a local anesthetic. Arch. Int. Pharmacodyn. Ther., *115*:483, 1958.
81. Tucker, G.T., and Mather, L.E.: Pharmacokinetics of local anaesthetic agents. Br. J. Anaesth., *47*:213, 1975.
82. Vanderick, G., Geerinckx, K., Van Steenberge, A.L., and de Muylder, E.: Bupivacaine 0.125% in epidural block analgesia during childbirth: Clinical evaluation. Br. J. Anaesth., *46*:838, 1974.
83. Wencker, K.H., Nolte, H., and Fruhstorfer, H.: Brachial plexus blockade for evaluation of local anaesthetic agents. Br. J. Anaesth., *47*:301, 1975.
84. Winnie, A.P., Lavallee, D.A., Sosa, B.P., and Masud, K.Z.: Clinical pharmacokinetics of local anaesthetics. Can. Anaesth. Soc. J., *24*:252, 1977.

5 Neuropathology of Neurolytic and Semidestructive Agents

Jordan Katz and Jon W. Joseph

BASIC MORPHOLOGY

There are three kinds of nerve fibers described by neurophysiologists—A, B, and C (see Table 3-2). The A fibers are the typical myelinated fibers of spinal nerves and have been divided into A-alpha (motor and proprioception); A-beta (touch and kinesthesia); A-gamma (touch, excitation of muscle spindles, and pressure); and A-delta (pain, heat, cold, and pressure).[11]

The B fibers are preganglionic autonomic nerves that are myelinated, but to a lesser extent than A fibers. They vary from 1 to 3 μ in diameter.

C fibers are unmyelinated nerves that transmit smell, pain, heat, cold, pressure, and postganglionic autonomic impulses. C fibers seem to be responsible for delayed pain sensation following a stimulus and reflex sympathetic discharge accompanying painful stimuli.[12]

All peripheral nerves have certain common structures. Within each axon there are five basic organelles: mitochondria, endoplasmic reticula, neurofilaments, microtubules, and dense particles (Fig. 5-1).

The *mitochondria* are double membrane structures that vary in size from 0.1 to 0.5 μ in diameter and up to 20 μ in length. Each mitochondron is divided into an outer and inner compartment. The outer compartment contains monoamine oxidase, which is responsible for degradation of catecholamines. The inner compartment, bound by highly infolded membranes called *cristae,* contains the respiratory electron transport and energy transport enzymes and coenzymes involved in the Krebs cycle. Adenosine triphosphate (ATP) is stored here.[27,29]

The mitochondria are usually randomly located throughout the peripheral nerve and are constantly moving, changing size and shape. Their movement is dictated by the location of microtubules and neurofilaments.[29]

The *smooth endoplasmic reticulum* (SER) is generally an agranular, irregular structure in the peripheral axon. Under electron microscopy, it may appear as vesicles, tubules, or cisternae generally arranged in rows parallel to the length of the axon. The wall of the endoplasmic reticulum has a trilaminar appearance. It contains none of the ribosomes observed in the *granular* (*rough*) *endoplasmic reticulum* (RER). The SER probably does not take part in protein synthesis, as does the RER. The granular and agranular endoplasmic reticulum systems are anatomically continuous.[27]

The *neurofilament* is a tubular structure 100 Å in diameter with a single wall 30 Å thick. The wall seems to be a helically coiled thread composed of globular protein. The function of the neurofilament is thought to be the intracellular transport of ions and metabolites and skeletal support of the cell.

The *microtubules* are comprised of tubules that measure 200 to 260 Å in diameter with walls about 60 Å thick. The center may contain a thin central filament or row of granules. Microtubules seem to be most prevalent in unmyelinated axons where neurofilaments are rare. The function of the microtubules is still under study but is believed to be similar to the neurofilaments.

Dense particles are often aligned in the cytoplasm adjacent to the plasma membrane that abuts the axolemma. Sometimes, there are groups of dense particles in the cytoplasm near the node of Ranvier. The function of dense particles is not known.

Each axon is bound by a trilaminar plasma membrane, with each layer approximately 25 to 30 Å thick. The axon is either partially or totally enveloped by Schwann cells. Some unmyelinated axons, or C fibers, only indent Schwann cells to varying depths along their paths. If the cell is larger than 1 to 2 μ, myelinization will occur. In myelinization, the Schwann cell wraps around an axon in concentric layers of cell membrane and cytoplasm (Fig. 5-2*A* and *B*).

RESPONSE TO INJURY

There are a limited number of ways a nerve cell can respond to injury. If the central nerve cell body is injured, the neuron dies and no regeneration occurs. It is possible for a neuron to lose the myelin over a segment of injured axon with the actual underlying nerve cell remaining intact. This is known as *segmental demyelinization*.

Classically, injury to the axon has been described as an event that results from trauma.[36] However, the basic processes are probably applicable to neurolytic damage as well. There are three phases to this reaction.

First, the central nerve body triples in volume by absorbing water. There is increased RNA synthesis in the nucleus and increased rate of transportation of synthesized RNA into the cytoplasm. A subsequent increase in protein synthesis is evident.

Second, the peripheral portion of the nerve fiber proximal to the site of injury undergoes *primary degeneration*. Some breakdown of the myelin sheath and axon back to the nearest unaffected node of Ranvier occurs.

Third, the nerve fiber distal to the trauma undergoes secondary or Wallerian degeneration. This is usually evident within 1 to 12 hours after the injury with some loosening of the myelin sheath. At about 24 hours, SER dilates, mitochondria swell, and spaces between lamellae of myelin increase. Within 2 days, the swollen mitochondria tend to cling together. There is an increase in dense particles and some dilated vesicles of SER can be noted (Fig. 5-3*A* and *B*).

At 5 days, fragmentation of myelin sheaths and further vesiculation of the SER are seen, more so in the large rather than small myelinated fibers. By 1 to 2 weeks, the axoplasmic organelles of myelinated fibers gradually disappear, leaving empty fragmented myelin sheaths. The lamellar structure of the myelin sheath is still discernible. At this time, unmyelinated fibers begin showing degeneration with loss of mitochondrial cristae, confluence of dense granules of mitochondria, and dilatation of endoplasmic reticulum.

By 2 weeks after injury, degeneration of all axons is complete. The myelin sheaths of large and small fibers are collapsed and fragmented and evidence of cellular organelles can be found. Regeneration of the proximal portion of the axon has begun.

Regeneration Process

The regeneration of the proximal portion of the axon is usually marked by the formation of a spheroidal axo-plasmic mass at the free end of the severed axon. Inside this growth tip can be seen increased mitochondria, dense bodies, vesicular elements, and neurofilaments. Variation in mitochondrial shape and size may also be noted. Dense bodies are generally round or oval and occasionally continuous with mitochondria. One axon may actually send out many growth tips (Fig. 5-4).

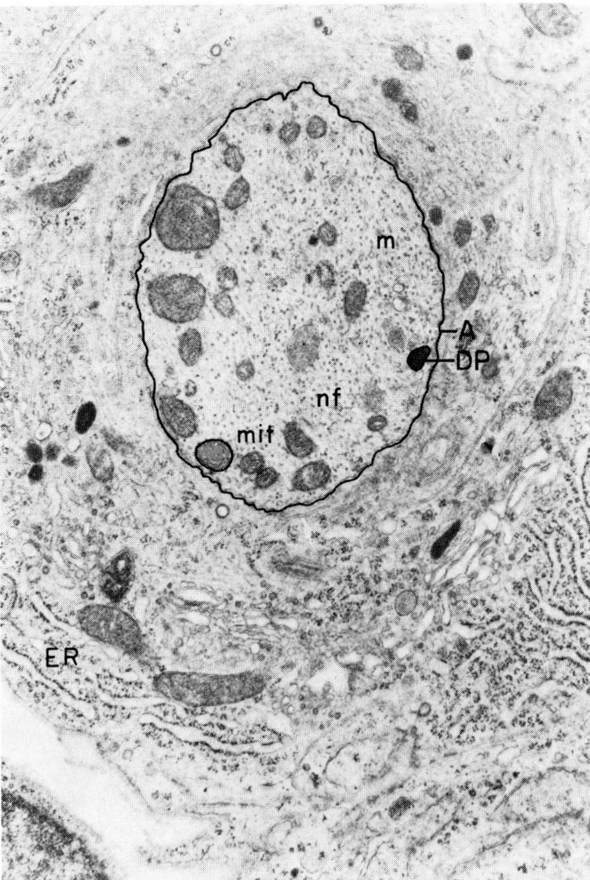

Fig. 5-1. Peripheral nerve, subcellular structure. This electron micrograph shows, within the axolemma (*A*): microtubules, the small rosette structure (*m*); neurofilaments, the smaller dense dots (*nf*); mitochondria, the large laminated structures (*mit*); and dense particles (*DP*). Rough endoplasmic reticulum (*ER*) is also depicted (×28,000). (Peters, A., Palay, S.L., and de F., Webster, H.: The Fine Structure of the Nervous System. Hagerstown, Hoeber Medical Division (Harper & Row), 1975)

Accompanying the development of the growth tip, the Schwann cells undergo mitotic activity and form tubes that guide the growth tips. If all regenerating growth tips reach the end organ, there may actually be more fibers distally than proximally.

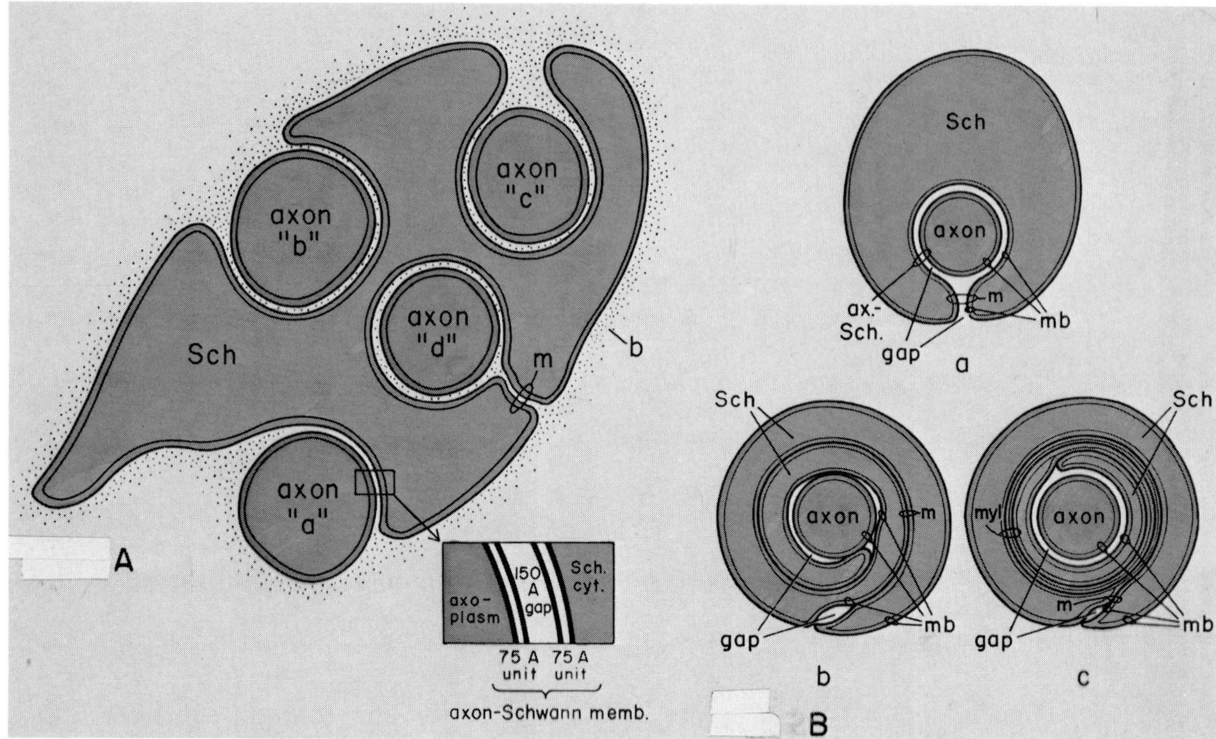

Fig. 5-2. (*A*) The natural structure of nonmyelinated nerve fiber. This drawing demonstrates the degree of embedding of axons in the Schwann cell by nonmyelinated nerve fibers. Also shown is a relative magnification of the axon and Schwann (*Sch*) cell interface. *m* designates the Schwann cell membrane. *b* is the matrix material that forms the "basement membrane." (*B*) The natural structure of myelinated nerve fiber. This drawing represents the development of a multilaminar myelin sheath (*myl*) as the Schwann cell (*Sch*) wraps itself around the axon. *a*, *b* and *c* denote progressive envelopment of the axon. *mb* designates the cell membrane of the Schwann cell. The gap is a space between layers of Schwann cell membrane. (Redrawn from Robertson, J.D.: Structural alterations in nerve fibers produced by hypotonic and hypertonic solutions. J. Biophysic. Biochem. Cytol., *4*:349, 1958)

Many of these additional fibers degenerate over the course of 1 year. The growth of the regenerating axon is occasionally blocked by glial scars and cystic spaces, which develop from lysis of neural debris. If a sensory fiber reaches a motor endplate or a motor fiber reaches a sensory terminal, the fiber will eventually degenerate.[22]

Regeneration occurs at the rate of 1 mm per day, so that reinnervation of a structure 5 cm away would take approximately 50 days. However, recovery of function may not always depend upon regeneration since alternative pathways may take over the impulse route. For example, after thoracic neurolytic subarachnoid block of posterior roots, pain conduction may "reroute" by way of the anterior roots, which are known to possess about 10 to 12 per cent of afferent C fibers. Alternatively, overlapping innervation from adjacent dermatomes may compensate for denervated axons (See Chap. 24).

Clinically, after simple injuries, the ulnar nerve requires approximately 8 weeks until the beginning of recovery. However, the healing after major wounds (*i.e.*, gunshot) requires a minimum of 4 months. Return of voluntary muscle action after brachial plexus injury may be as early as 3 months, or it may be delayed for 2 or more years, depending on the severity of injury.[36]

NEUROPATHOLOGIC CHANGES DUE TO NEUROLYTIC AGENTS

Hypertonic and Hypotonic Solutions

A simple method for achieving neurolysis is by the subarachnoid injection of either distilled water (hypotonic) or hypertonic salt solutions. It was believed from clinical observation that pain fibers were preferentially affected.[14]

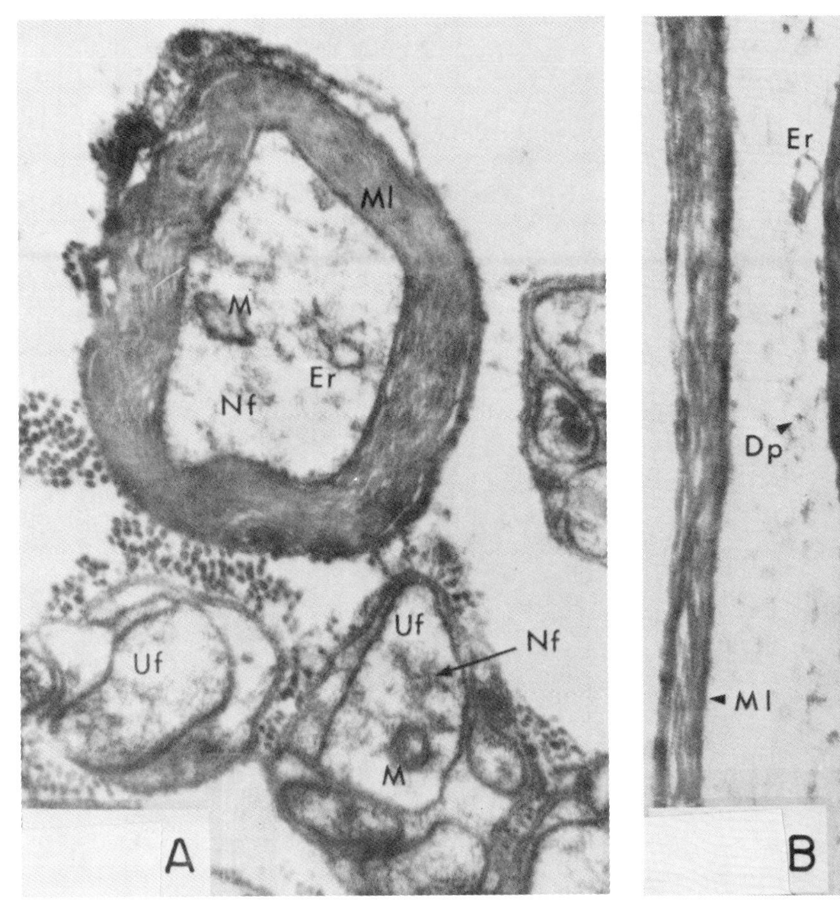

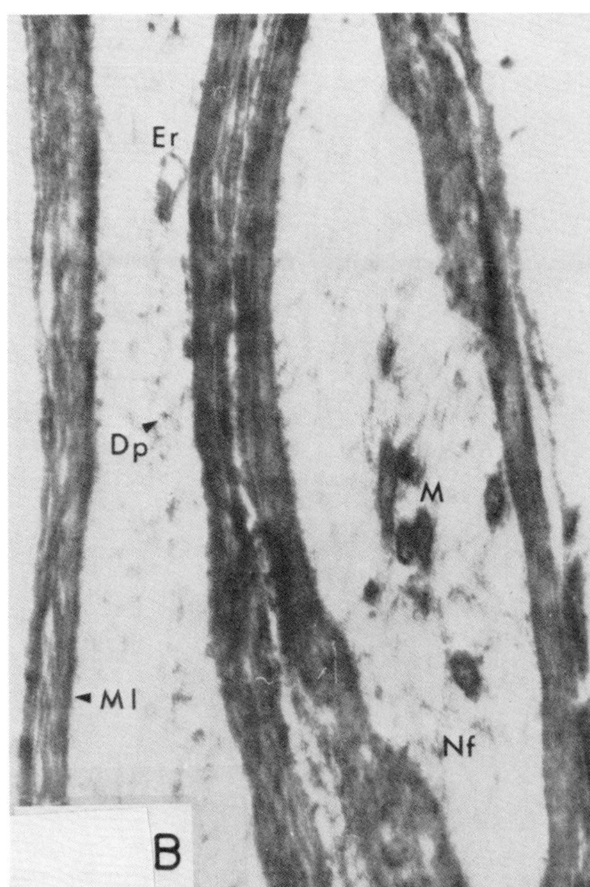

Fig. 5-3. Response to an injury distal to the neurotomy, 1 day later (rat sciatic nerve). Both cross-sectional (*A*) and longitudinal (*B*) views show loosening of myelin lamellae (*Ml*), dilatation of the endoplasmic reticulum (*Er*), mitochondrial swelling (*M*), and aggregation of neurofilaments (*Nf*). *Uf* is unmyelinated fiber, *Dp*, dense particles (×25,000). (Lee, J.C.: Comp. Neurol., *120*:65, 1963)

Pathologic changes due to hypertonic and hypotonic solutions have been studied extensively by both soaking peripheral nerves and intrathecal irrigation.[16,19,30]

Microscopic studies that demonstrate the effects of hyper- or hypotonic solutions on peripheral nerve fibers do not seem to correlate with clinical results. Demonstrable microscopic changes appear only after prolonged soaking for at least 1 hour and only after using distilled water or solutions of osmolality of greater than 1000 mmol per L. If a peripheral nerve is soaked for at least 1 hour in distilled water, the lamellae of the myelin sheath become separated, and each layer of myelin widens. Unmyelinated fibers occasionally show total destruction of all neuronal elements, but more commonly there is no significant pathology.

Myelinated nerves seem to be more resistant to hypertonic solutions. In order to see any microscopic change in animal tissue, a solution with osmolality of at least 1000 mOsm per L for 4 hours must be used. If these conditions are met, the myelin sheath appears irregularly swollen and fragmented, and the underlying axon becomes shrunken. Unmyelinated fibers in hypertonic solutions show a decrease in the distance between the inner and outer membranes of their mitochondria. The associated Schwann cell appears to be more closely bound to the axon.

The microscopic studies do not help to explain the differential C fiber blockade that is reported clinically and experimentally.[26,30] In the monkey dorsal root preparation, application of distilled water for 5 minutes produced a differential C fiber blockade similar to that noted with hypertonic solutions *in vitro*. Studies *in vitro* seem to indicate that

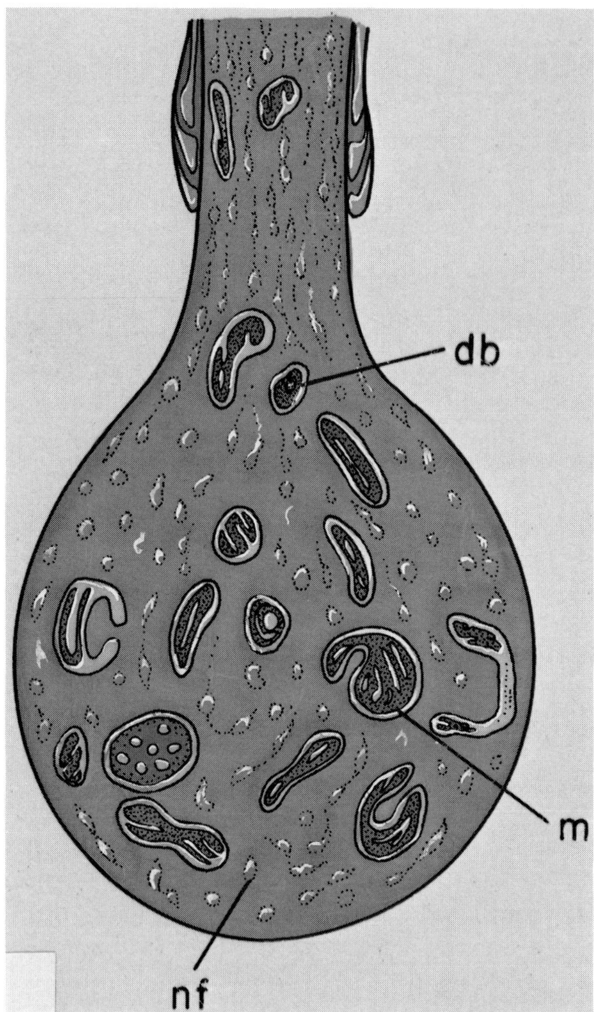

Fig. 5-4. Regeneration process in the proximal axon, 2 weeks after injury. This drawing represents regenerating axon tip, depicting dense body (*db*), multiple mitochondria (*m*), neurofilaments (*nf*), and other tubular and vesicular structures. (Redrawn from Lampert, P.W.: A comparative electron microscopic study of reactive degenerating, regenerating, and dystrophic axons. J. Neuropathol. Exp. Neurol., *26*:345, 1967)

hypotonic solutions* are more effective than hypertonic solutions in achieving a selective block.

Explanations for the production of differential block are based on the presence of myelin, which impedes the flux of water in larger unaffected fibers, and the relationship of volume to surface area, which makes smaller fibers more susceptible to intracellular water shifts when extracellular osmolarities are changed. As described in Chapter 27, hypertonic saline by subarachnoid injection has been reported to result in significant pain relief with no other sensory loss for periods of 2 days to 2 to 3 weeks, which would be in keeping with a minor neurolytic injury.

Hypothermia

In 1945, a report on the pathology of a segment of cat sciatic nerve after exposure to freezing by carbon dioxide spray noted that myelinated fibers seemed more susceptible to hypothermia. The temperature threshold for damage to A-delta and C sensory fibers was the lowest of all fibers.[6]

Stimulated by clinical evidence that spinal cord hypothermia might relieve chronic pain, studies have attempted to define the pathophysiologic changes of hypothermia.[1,9,28] In peripheral nerves, cooling to temperatures of 5°C for up to 2 hours decreases the velocity of conduction and amplitude of all fiber action potentials. Each type of fiber (A, B, and C) has a prolonged action potential, and, within each fiber group, individual neurons fire asynchronously.

There is conflicting evidence in the literature about the sequence of blockade of the different fibers in a mixed nerve. Most authors agree that C fibers are most resistant to blockade by hypothermia. The area of conflict is the sequence of blockade of the myelinated fibers. Although experimental results differ, the magnitude of change in the myelinated fibers is generally in proportion to decreased temperature, with clinically detectable signs.

Early cytopathology of the cooled peripheral nerve generally shows abnormalities of Schwann cells and endoneural capillaries. The Schwann cell develops electron-dense cytoplasm, increased numbers of filaments, vesicular structures, and ribosomes. It has been suggested that these changes may be due to accelerated enzyme production secondary to injury or disturbances in Schwann cell metabolism. The endoneural capillaries also show increased numbers of endothelial vesicles, which probably indicate cellular edema. Amorphous deposits can be seen in both the axon and the adjacent capillary.

If cooling is prolonged, axonal changes occur with swelling and separation of the perineurium. Neurofilaments and vesicular bodies begin congregating. In several days, demyelination takes place, with phagocytic activity of macrophage and

* Recent studies (Fink, B.R. personal communication) indicate that hypotonicity **per se** results in neural blockade, without neurolysis, and this blockade enhances local anesthetic blockade.

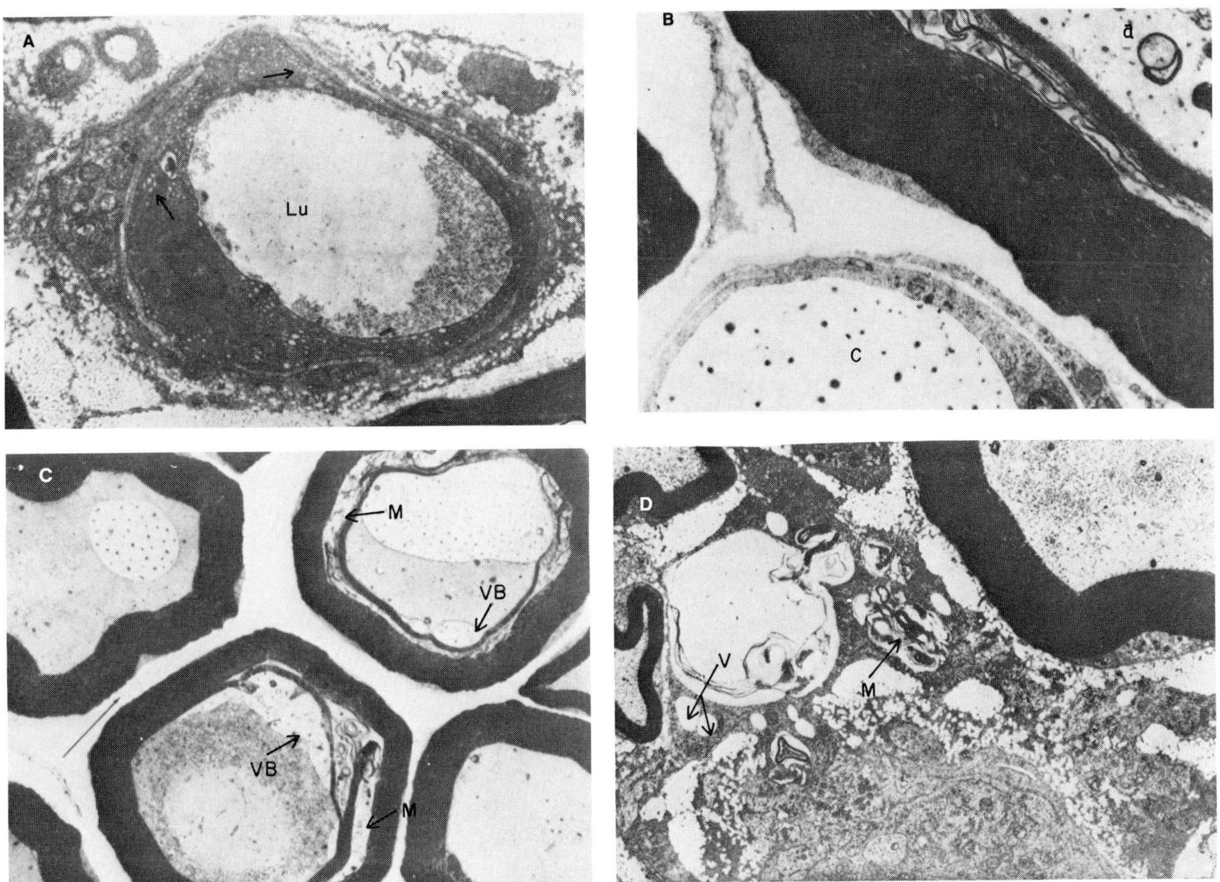

Fig. 5-5. (*A*) Effect of hypothermia on a peripheral nerve, 1 hour after application. This electron micrograph shows a transverse section through a capillary lumen after hypothermic injury. Note endothelial vesicles, indicating cellular edema, marked with arrows (×9,200). (*B*) Effect of hypothermia on a peripheral nerve, 7 hours after application. This electron micrograph shows the accumulation of amorphous material in both the axon (*a*) and capillary lumen (*c*) (×13,332). (*C*) Effect of hypothermia on peripheral nerve, 7 hours after application. This electron micrograph shows a transverse section of several axons. Note separation of the myelin (*M*) and numerous vesicular bodies (*VB*), indicating early injury to both the myelin sheath and the axon within (×3,200). (*D*) Effect of hypothermia on peripheral nerve, 3 days after application. This electron micrograph shows a phagocytic cell that contains vacuoles of amorphous material (*V*) and vacuoles in some laminated material that appears to be myelin (*M*; ×10,000). (Basbaum, C.B.: Electrophysiological observations. J. Neurocytol., *2*:171, 1973)

Schwann cells noted. Smaller myelinated and unmyelinated fibers seem more resistant to destruction by cold (Fig. 5-5*A*, *B*, *C*, and *D*).

Hypothermic techniques are currently administered by means of subarachnoid injection of iced saline, blockade of peripheral nerves using a cryoprobe, and, more rarely, refrigeration analgesia, produced by applying ice packs around a limb for amputation. A promising technique, cryoprobe blockade, produces its effects by repeated freeze-thaw cycles of the peripheral nerves. The resultant change in pain conduction persists for approximately 10 days (with a range of up to 224 days), but it is associated with sensory and motor loss.[23]

Ammonium Salts

The first reported use of salts for long-term relief of pain was in 1935, when Judovich used pitcher plant distillate (*Sarracenia purpnea*) for certain forms of neuralgia.[17] It was later reported that the ammonium ion in the form of ammonium chloride or ammonium hydroxide (depending on the PH of the distillate) was the active component.[35]

In 1942, a report on the use of ammonium salts for nerve pain stated the following:

> . . . In no instance has there been any motor weakness, following injection of peripheral nerves nor loss of touch, pressure, pinprick, and temperature sensibility. In some instances, one infiltration of the distillate is sufficient to provide permanent relief of pain even in cases of long duration . . .
>
> . . . In man, perineural infiltration of 0.5% to 1% solutions of ammonium chloride produces the same effects as does the filtration of pitcher plant extract. The immediate effect of the injection is an increased intensity of the pain which then subsides during the first 30 minutes after injection. The neuralgic pain is relieved, the zone of hyperesthesia contracts and disappears, and when injected around the sciatic nerve there results no weakness and the sensations of touch, pressure, pinprick, and temperature on the outer aspect of the leg are unimpaired . . .[2]

The action of ammonium salts on nerve impulses produces obliteration of C fiber potentials with only small effect on A fibers.[5,18] Subsequent clinical information has shown that with concentrations of 10 per cent of ammonium salts, motor function can be retained despite good analgesia. Limited pathologic studies suggest that injection of ammonium salts around a peripheral nerve causes an acute degenerative neuropathy affecting all fibers.

Anesthetic Oil Mixtures

In the late 30's and early 40's, it was quite popular to attempt long-term nerve blockade with mixtures of a short-acting local anesthetic and oil. It was thought that the oil suppressed absorption of the local anesthetic drug.

There were several preparations in use. In 1943, the ingredient most likely to cause the long-term neurolytic blockade was shown to be benzyl alcohol, which was common to all mixtures.[7] No further pathologic studies are noted in the literature.

Alcohol

Ethyl alcohol is an extremely potent neurolytic agent. It acts on the neuron by extraction of cholesterol, phospholipid, and cerebroside. It also causes precipitation of lipoproteins and mucoproteins.[31] The most common modes of administration are subarachnoid, celiac plexus, and lumbar sympathetic blockade or, more rarely, trigeminal nerve block (see Chaps. 15 and 27). The subarachnoid method allows protection of the motor nerve roots by the positioning of the patient so that only sensory roots come in contact with the alcohol (see Chap. 27). The concentration of alcohol in the spinal fluid is quickly reduced, presumably by uptake into neural tissue. Ninety per cent cannot be accounted for within the cerebrospinal fluid in 10 minutes.[24]

After *subarachnoid block* with absolute alcohol, the gross pathology of the spinal cord and meninges is unremarkable. Spotty areas of sclerosis of the posterior columns and mild focal inflammatory changes of the meninges are usually seen.[10]

Histologic sections usually show much more extensive changes. Occasionally, a superficial layer of necrosis around the total circumference of the spinal cord is noted. Usually, the injury is confined to the posterior portion of the cord, involving Lissauer's tract, but may be as deep as Clark's nucleus (Fig. 5-6*A* and *B*).

These localized areas of neurolysis of spinal cord cells are caused by direct contact with the alcohol. Myelin sheath disruption and beading of the axis cylinder are seen. Subsequently, an inflammatory response followed by proliferation of glial cells and formation of glial scars are noted.

There is a delayed and more remote degeneration of the spinal cord in areas that probably did not come in direct contact with the alcohol (most likely Wallerian degeneration). Contralateral degeneration of the lateral spinothalamic tract can be demonstrated. The gray matter of dorsal and lateral horns has been shown to be affected. Chromatolysis, nuclear eccentricity, and shrinkage of the nerve cell bodies are probably a function of both direct contact with alcohol and retrograde degeneration of injured nerve fibers.

When a *peripheral nerve* comes in contact with absolute alcohol (100% ethyl alcohol), both the Schwann cell and the axon show evidence of edema. The myelin sheath separates, while the actual Schwann cell cytoplasm has dilated endoplasmic reticulum and swollen mitochondria. Within the actual axon, dilated vesicles can be found. Intracellular edema progresses, and classical Wallerian degeneration begins (Fig. 5-7*A*,*B*,*C*,*D*, and *E*).[37]

The resistance of certain fibers to alcohol lysis is still unproven. Conduction studies with nerves treated with dilute alcohol solutions are equivocal and seem to indicate that differential blockade is difficult, if at all possible, to obtain.[8]

In summary, ethyl alcohol is a potent neurolytic

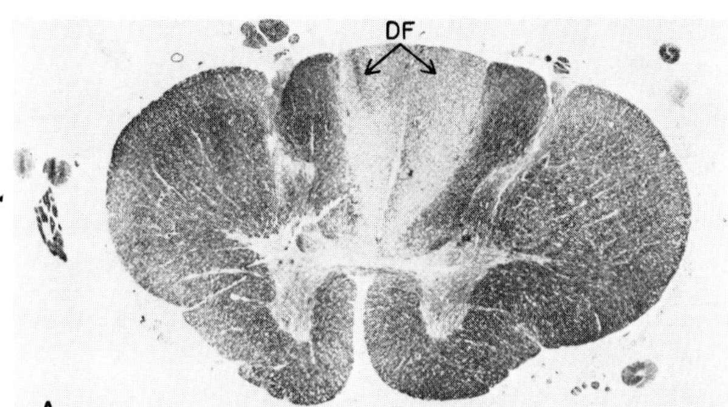

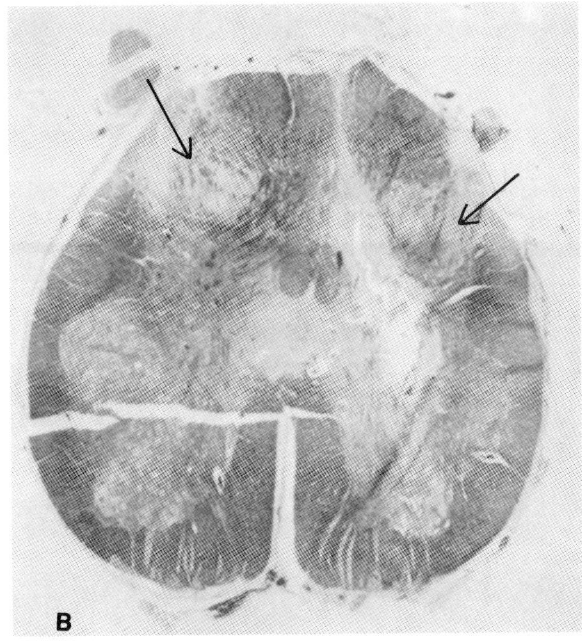

Fig. 5-6. (*A*) Effect of alcohol on spinal cord, 4 days after neurolytic block. Cross-section through spinal cord at T4 shows dorsal fasciculus (*DF*) degeneration after subarachnoid 100 per cent alcohol injection several interspaces lower. (*B*) Effect of alcohol on spinal cord, 50 days after direct cord injection. Necrosis and degeneration (*arrows*) following accidental injection of 100% alcohol into the spinal cord. (Gallager, H.S., Yonezawa, T., Hay, R.C., and Derrick, W.S.: Subarachnoid alcohol block II. Histologic changes in the central nervous system. Am. J. Pathol., *35*:679, 1961)

agent, commonly administered in the subarachnoid space. Even with positioning to control the concentration that bathes the cord, histologic evidence of early neurolysis of the posterior columns and Lissauer's tracts with late retrograde Wallerian degeneration of the lateral spinothalamic tract is seen. Peripherally, direct contact with alcohol leads to early edema of Schwann cells and neurons with subsequent degeneration. Differential resistance of certain fibers to alcohol is uncertain.

Phenol

Most studies on morphologic changes caused by neurolytic agents have been done with phenol.[3,4,13,15,25,33,34] It is commonly used for chronic pain relief and has its primary neurolytic effect as a result of protein denaturation. Similar to ethyl alcohol, it is extremely potent and essentially nonselective in its nerve destruction and in its electrophysiologic blockade.

The spinal cord and meninges of patients who receive subarachnoid blocks with 5 to 8-per cent phenol solutions have been studied. Grossly, the meningeal reaction can be very mild; however, thickening of the arachnoid has been reported. On primary inspection, the spinal cord usually appears unaffected by phenol injection of 5 to 8-per cent. Injection of 20 per cent phenol into the subarachnoid space causes much more extensive arachnoid thickening and fibrosis. Softening and flattening of the spinal cord have also been noted.

Histologically, after injection of 5 to 8-per cent phenol in iophendylate, the finding of degeneration of fibers in the posterior nerve roots and in the posterior columns is parallel to that noted previously with ethyl alcohol. The anterior horn cells are sometimes affected, showing chromatolysis, which may actually be secondary to lesions in the ventral nerve roots. The cause for this pattern in the posterior columns is most likely degeneration after peripheral damage, but direct contact with phenol may also play a part (Fig. 5-8).

Axons of all sizes are affected by therapeutic con-

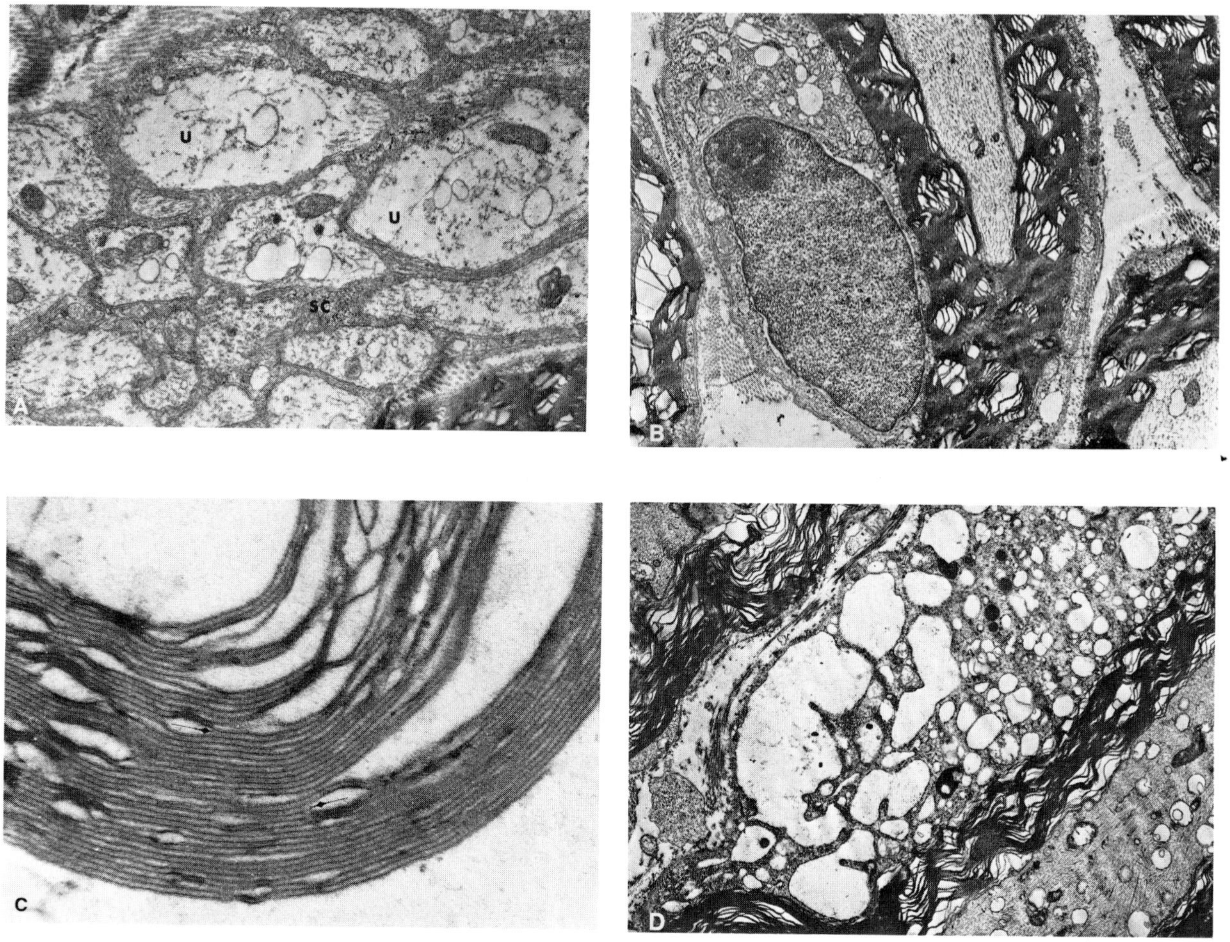

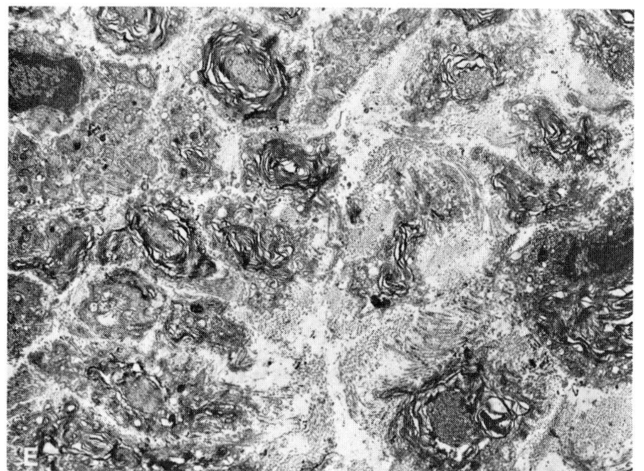

Fig. 5-7. (*A*) Effect of alcohol on peripheral nerve, 15 seconds after application. This electron micrograph shows the sciatic nerve of a mouse after topical 100 per cent alcohol application. The arrows denote swelling of unmyelinated nerve fibers; *S* denotes Schwann cell cytoplasm that is clumped and granular—Schwann cell destruction (×5,000). (*B*) Effect of alcohol on peripheral nerve, 15 seconds after application. This electron micrograph shows the Schwann cell after 100 per cent alcohol exposure. Note splitting of myelin sheath (*MS*) and dilated endoplasmic reticulum (*ER*), indicating acute injury to Schwann cell and myelin sheath (×4,300). (*C*) Effect of alcohol on peripheral nerve, 1 minute after application. This electron micrograph shows splitting of myelin sheath after exposure to topical 100 per cent alcohol (×9,600). (*D*) Effect of alcohol on peripheral nerve, 24 hours after a 15-second exposure to 100 per cent alcohol. Note degenerating axons (*A*), splitting myelin lamellae (*M*), and beginning of connective tissue reaction (*CR*; ×2,200). (*E*) Effect of alcohol on peripheral nerve, 4 hours after a 15-second exposure. This electron micrograph shows vacuolization in Schwann cell (*V*) after 100 per cent alcohol exposure. (Woolsey, R.M., Taylor, J.J., and Nagel, J.H.: Acute effects of topical ethyl alcohol on the sciatic nerve of the mouse. Arch. Phys. Med. Rehabil., *53*:410, 1972)

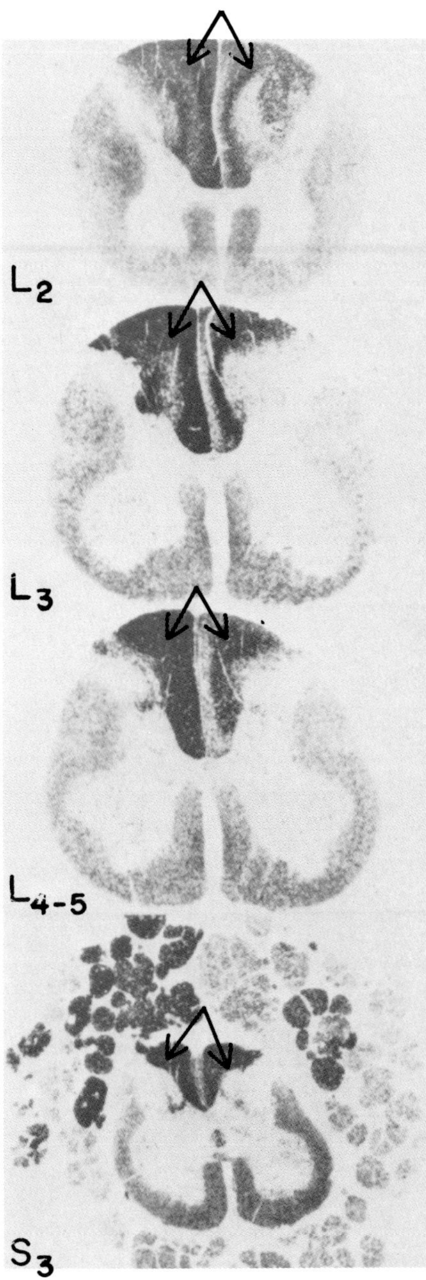

Fig. 5-8. Effect of phenol on spinal cord. These micrographs show transverse sections through a patient's spinal cord. Note posterior column degeneration (*arrows*), following injection of phenol subarachnoid. The sections were taken at levels (*top to bottom*) L2, L3, L4–5, and S3 of spinal cord. Injection was made at bony spine level L3–4. (Smith, M.C.: Histological findings following intrathecal injections of phenol solutions for relief of pain. Br. J. Anaesth., *36*:387, 1964)

centrations and usually appear swollen and edematous before they fragment. Phagocytosis by Schwann cells and tissue macrophages occurs. Characteristically, the posterior root ganglia are not affected by phenol. The histology of the peripheral nerve is similar to what is seen in the posterior nerve root.

There is debate over specific sensitivities of the peripheral nerves to very dilute solutions of phenol. In concentrations over 2 per cent phenol, most authors agree that phenol is nonselective in its fiber destruction. Adjuvants that have been tested to date neither significantly enhance the neurolytic effect of phenol nor make phenol more selective.[20,21,32] An extensive review of the neuropathology and clinical effects of phenol has recently been published.[38]

Clinical Correlation

As this review indicates, a spectrum of pathologic changes have been reported in both animal and human studies. Unfortunately, the pathologic changes do not necessarily correlate well with clinical observations. One author (J. Katz) has examined at postmortem the intraspinal contents of patients with cancer pain who had absolute alcohol injected into the subarachnoid space. In some cases, the pathology caused by the alcohol was extensive, but significant pain relief was not obtained. The reverse has also been seen—total pain relief with minimal pathology. The symptom of pain is a complex physiologic–psychologic event. Hence, the variances in correlation between the anatomic pathology and subjective (clinical) pain relief are not unexpected.

Many of the unwanted sequellae secondary to neurolytic injection are better understood in light of the known neuropathology. These complications are discussed in Chapter 23.

REFERENCES

1. Basbaum, C.B.: Electrophysiological observations. J. Neurocytol., *2*:171, 1973.
2. Bates, W., and Judovich, B.D.: Intractable pain. Anesthesiology, *3*:663, 1942.
3. Baxter, D.W., and Schacherl, U.: Experimental studies on the morphological changes produced by intrathecal phenol. Can. Med. Assoc. J., *86*:1200, 1962.
4. Berry, K., and Olszewski, J.: Pathology of intrathecal phenol injection in man. Neurology (Minneap.), *13*:152, 1963.
5. Davies, J.I., Steward, P.B., and Fink, P.: Prolonged sensory block using ammonium salts. Anesthesiology, *28*:244, 1967.
6. Denny-Brown, D., Adams, R., Brenner, C., and Doherty, M.M.: The pathology of injury to nerve induced by cold. J. Neuropathol. Exp. Neurol., *4*:305, 1945.
7. Duncan, D., and Jarvis, W.H.: A comparison of the actions

on nerve fibers of certain anesthetic mixtures and substances in oil. Anesthesiology, *4*:465, 1943.

8. Fischer, E., Cress, R.H., Haines, G., Panin, N., and Paul, B.J.: Evoked nerve conduction after nerve block by chemical means. Am. J. Phys. Med., *49*:333, 1970.
9. Franz, D.N., and Iggo, A.: Conduction failure in myelinated and non-myelinated axons at low temperatures. J. Physiol., *199*:319, 1968.
10. Gallager, H.S., Yonezawa, T., Hay, R.C., and Derrick, W.S.: Subarachnoid alcohol block II. Histologic changes in the central nervous system. Am. J. Pathol., *35*:679, 1961.
11. Guyton, A.C.: Textbook of Medical Physiology. pp. 563–564. Philadelphia, W.B. Saunders, 1971.
12. Hallin, R.G., and Torebjork, H.E.: Activity in unmyelinated nerve fibers in man. Adv. Neurol. Sci. (Tokyo), *4*:19, 1974.
13. Hansebout, R.R., and Cosgrove, J.B.R.: Effects of intrathecal phenol in man—A histological study. Neurology (Minneap.), *16*:277, 1966.
14. Hitchcock, E.: Osmolytic neurolysis for intractable facial pain. Lancet, *1*:434, 1969.
15. Iggo, A., and Walsh, E.G.: Selective block of small fibres in the spinal roots by phenol. Brain, *83*:701, 1960.
16. Jewett, D.L., and King, J.S.: Conduction block of monkey dorsal rootlets by water and hypertonic saline solutions. Exp. Neurol., *33*:225, 1971.
17. Judovich, B.D.: Relief of pain. M.J., & Rec., *141*:583, 1935.
18. Judovich, B.D., Bates, W., and Bishop, K.: Intraspinal ammonium salts for the intractable pain of malignancy. Anesthesiology, *5*:341, 1944.
19. King, J.S., Jewett, D.L., Phil, D., and Sundberg, H.R.: Differential blockade of cat dorsal root C fibers by various chloride solutions. J. Neurosurg., *36*:569, 1972.
20. Knott, L.W., Katz, J., and Rubinstein, L.J.: Separate and combined effects of phenol, hyaluronidase and dimethyl sulfoxide on the sciatic nerve of the rat—I. Acute studies. Arch. Phys. Med. Rehabil., *49*:100, 1968.
21. ———: Separate and combined effects of phenol, hyaluronidase, and dimethyl sulfoxide on the sciatic nerve of the rat—II. Chronic studies. Neurology (Minneap.), *19*:926, 1969.
22. Lampert, P.W.: A comparative electron microscopic study of reactive, degenerating, regenerating, and dystrophic axons. J. Neuropathol. Exp. Neurol., *26*:345, 1967.
23. Lloyd, J.W., Barnard, J.D.W., and Glynn, C.J.: Cryoanalgesia: A new approach to pain relief. Lancet, *2*:932, 1976.
24. Matsuki, M., Kato, Y., and Ichiyanagi, K.: Progressive changes in the concentration of ethyl alcohol in the human and canine subarachnoid spaces. Anesthesiology, *36*:617, 1972.
25. Nathan, P.W., Sears, T.A., and Smith, M.C.: Effects of phenol solutions on the nerve roots of the cat: An electrophysiological and histological study. J. Neurol., *2*:7, 1965.
26. Nicholson, M.F., and Roberts, F.W.: Refief of pain by intrathecal injection of hypothermic saline. Med. J. Aust., *1*:61, 1968.
27. Noback, C.R.: Human Nervous System. p. 45. New York, McGraw-Hill, 1975.
28. Paintal, A.S.: Block of conduction in mammalian myelinated nerve fibres by low temperatures. J. Physiol., *180*:1, 1965.
29. Peters, A., Palay, S.L., and de F. Webster, H.: The Fine Structure of the Nervous System. pp. 7–26. Hagerstown, Hoeber Medical Division (Harper & Row), 1975.
30. Robertson, J.D.: Structural alterations in nerve fibers produced by hypotonic and hypertonic solutions. J. Biophysic. Biochem. Cytol., *4*:349, 1958.
31. Rumsby, M.G., and Finean, J.B.: The action of organic solvents on the myelin sheath of peripheral nerve tissue—II (short-chain aliphatic alcohols). J. Neurochem., *13*:1509, 1966.
32. Schaumburg, H.H., Byck, R., and Weller, R.O.: The effect of phenol on peripheral nerve. A histological and electrophysiological study. J. Neuropathol. Exp. Neurol., *29*:615, 1970.
33. Smith, M.C.: Histological findings following intrathecal injections of phenol solutions for relief of pain. Br. J. Anaesth., *36*:387, 1964.
34. Stefanko, S., and Zebrowski, S.: Histological changes in the nerve roots and spinal cord after intrathecal administration of phenol for relief of spasticity. Pol. Med. J., *7*:1204, 1968.
35. Stewart, W.B., Judovich, B.D., Hughes, J., and Walti, A.: Ammonium chloride in the relief of pain. Am. J. Physiol., *129*:474, 1940.
36. Sunderland, S.: Nerve and Nerve Injuries. Churchill Livingstone, Edinburgh, London and New York, 1978.
37. Woolsey, R.M., Taylor, J.J., and Nagel, J.H.: Acute effects of topical ethyl alcohol on the sciatic nerve of the mouse. Arch. Phys. Med. Rehabil., *53*:410, 1972.
38. Wood, K.A.: The use of phenol as a neurolytic agent: A review. Pain, *5*:205, 1978.

PART TWO

Techniques of Neural Blockade

6 Preparation for Neural Blockade: The Patient, Block Equipment, Resuscitation, and Supplementation

William F. Kennedy, Jr.

There are several important requisites for optimal results in regional anesthesia. In order to have consistently good results, the anesthesiologist must have a genuine interest in and be convinced of the advantages of regional anesthesia. Initially, teaching and close supervision by someone expert in the field is required; subsequently, continued clinical application is necessary in order to maintain these skills. Thorough knowledge of the pertinent anatomy, obtained from review of anatomical dissections, textbooks, and atlases of anatomy, is essential. In addition, the physician should be intimately familiar with the pharmacology of the local anesthetic agent as well as the physiologic changes that accompany these anesthetics; he can thus anticipate any changes and be prepared to institute immediate treatment if necessary (*i.e.*, intravenous fluids, atropine, and possibly vasopressors). Equally important is the careful preparation and management of the individual patient and the availability of appropriate anesthesia equipment as well as equipment for resuscitation and the treatment of adverse reactions.

PREANESTHETIC MANAGEMENT

It is now generally accepted that an essential feature of the preparation of the surgical/obstetric patient is the active participation of the anesthesiologist. Thus, the importance of a visit prior to the administration of a regional anesthetic for a surgical/obstetric procedure, ideally by the anesthesiologist who will actually be performing the anesthetic, cannot be too greatly emphasized.

During the preanesthetic visit, the anesthesiologist should review the patient's history (including a review of use of previous anesthetics and examination of old anesthetic records), physical findings, and laboratory data. This interview should also focus on the presence or lack of coexisting medical/surgical problems and related drug therapy (*i.e.*, steroids for obstructive lung disease or arthritis, insulin for diabetes, etc.). A physical examination that includes measurements of blood pressure and pulse rates, auscultation of the heart and lungs, and any additional testing that is indicated should be performed. During the course of the preanesthetic interview and examination, it is important that the anesthesiologist establish sound rapport with the patient, a requisite for all preanesthetic visits, but most especially when regional anesthesia is to be performed. Further, it is essential that the anesthesiologist convey to the patient his own convictions about the advantages of the regional anesthetic and his ability to perform it in a completely satisfactory fashion. It is important to point out to the patient that with the blocks that do not require the patient's cooperation in reporting presence of paraesthesia, the patient can be so well sedated that he has little, if any, recall of the events during the anesthesia or surgical procedure.

The most appropriate anesthetic is selected based on these findings, and discussed in detail with the patient. It is essential that a preanesthetic note that summarizes the important history, physical findings, and laboratory data be included in the patient's clinical record along with a record that a specific kind of anesthesia has been selected and was discussed with and accepted by the patient. The note should also include a statement that the possible risks or complications of the anesthetic were described, as well as their incidence and severity. Finally, the anesthesiologist should order night and premedicant drugs appropriate to the individual physiologic and psychologic needs of the patient and, equally important, make certain that they are administered at the time when they will afford maximal benefit to the patient.

Although there is a variety of opinion on premedication prior to regional anesthesia, many prefer moderate-to-heavy premedication, including a nar-

Table 6-1. Therapeutic Procedure
Safe and Effective Use of Local Anesthetic Agents

1. *Correct Preparation*
   (a) Physiological and pathophysiological status.
   (b) Selection of correct agent and dose procedure.
   (c) Appropriate premedication
   (d) Assembly of resuscitative drugs and equipment.
   (e) Insertion of intravenous line.
   (f) Separation of neural blockade tray from other drugs.
2. *Correct Practice*
   (a) Personally check doses of local anesthetic and vasoconstrictor (if used).
   (b) Inject test dose.
   (c) Aspirate frequently to check for vascular penetration.
   (d) Monitor cardiovascular signs.
   (e) Maintain verbal contact with patient past time of peak blood concentration.
3. *Correction of Problems Arising*
   (a) Observe early warnings.
   (b) Maintain airway and oxygenation.
   (c) Maintain blood pressure.
   (d) Abort convulsions.

cotic analgesic. The narcotic is important for several reasons. First, it has been found that the vast majority of patients scheduled for regional anesthesia prefer being well sedated with little recall of either the induction of anesthesia or the intra-anesthetic part of the procedures. Second, with the use of narcotic analgesics together with other sedative drugs, both physical and psychological discomfort associated with the performance of the regional anesthetic, slight as it may be, can be avoided entirely or at least kept to a minimum. This is especially important when physicians in training are being taught these anesthetic techniques. Third, patients with preoperative pain obviously should receive an analgesic. And last, little cooperation is required on the part of the patient except to determine the resulting level when spinal, epidural, and caudal anesthesia is performed. Recommended premedication of the normal 70 kg adult man is as follows: pentobarbital, 100 mg; fentanyl 50–100 μg and droperidol 5–10 mg (or morphine, 10–15 mg, and hydroxyzine, 75–100 mg, or diazepam, 5–10 mg); atropine, 0.2–0.4 mg, may also be administered intramuscularly 1 hour before the anesthetic.

INDUCTION OF ANESTHESIA

In order to achieve optimal results, the anesthesiologist must plan carefully. This entails taking the patient to the location where the anesthetic will be administered well in advance of the time of the surgery; the duration of time required to perform various regional anesthetics is directly related to the skill of the anesthesiologist. The block tray should be prepared prior to the patient's arrival, together with the necessary resuscitative equipment as part of a therapeutic procedure (Table 6-1).

Upon arrival, the identification of the patient and the effects of the premedicant drugs are noted. Following this, an intravenous infusion of a balanced electrolyte solution or normal saline without dextrose is established with a large-bore catheter (radiopaque Teflon) needle. If the proposed regional anesthetic produces a significant amount of sympathetic blockade, 8 to 10 ml per kg of the intravenous solution should be administered prior to performing the block. In general, dextrose-containing solutions should be avoided because of the resulting osmotic diuresis, which may lead to full urinary bladder. If the urinary bladder becomes overdistended during spinal, epidural, or caudal anesthesia, the need for bladder catheterization postoperatively is significantly increased. Moreover, a full bladder in a patient with an extremity block may be most disruptive.

Appropriate monitoring equipment is set up, (*i.e.*, a blood pressure cuff, precordial stethoscope, and an electrocardiograph). Baseline measurements are recorded and compared with those from the preanesthetic visit. After the patient is placed in the proper position, the skin is prepared with either an organic or an inorganic iodine solution, care being taken to clean the skin physically as well as chemically.

The prescribed techniques should be performed with dispatch, careful attention being paid to the comfort and vital functions of the patient. If the desired effects of the premedication are not obtained, additional increments of the sedative/analgesic drugs should be administered intravenously, either by intermittent injection (50–100 μg fentanyl, and/or 5–10 μg droperidol), 5–10 mg of diazepam, 25–50 mg of thiopental or thiamylal, or 10–20 mg of methohexital) or by continuous infusion (0.1–0.2% methohexital). Although opinions vary widely on the optimal time to check the resultant analgesic level, 5 minutes for spinal anesthesia and 10 minutes for epidural and caudal anesthesia and peripheral nerve blocks is reasonable. A safety pin with a right-angle configuration is preferable to a disposable needle because needles not infrequently make holes in the skin, whereas a safety pin does not. An alcohol sponge can also be used to determine the temperature (analgesic) level of spinal, epidural, and caudal anesthesia. It should be noted that if the analgesic level is checked too early or too frequently, the anesthesiologist risks alarming the patient. It is imperative that the adequacy of the block be determined by the anesthesiologist and not by the surgeon or by surgical incision. Immediately after completing the block, the arterial pressure, pulse, electrocardiogram, respirations, and state of consciousness should be monitored continuously. With epidural, caudal, and peripheral blocks, the maximum cardiovascular effects and the peak blood levels of local anesthetics occur 15 to 30 minutes (during the first 30 minutes) after injection.[1,2,7,8,11]

INTRA-ANESTHETIC MANAGEMENT OF THE PATIENT

In many instances, the most difficult part of a regional anesthetic is the management of the patient once the desired analgesic effect has been achieved. Attention must be directed to the prevention of positional discomfort, apprehension, anxiety, and restlessness. At the same time, the anesthesiologist must guard against cardiovascular and respiratory depression as well as depression of other vital physiologic functions brought on by the use of excessive sedative drugs. Although a host of drugs and techniques have been used for sedation of the patient during these forms of regional anesthesia, many prefer the following technique: 2 to 4 L of 100 per cent oxygen administered either by nasal prongs or by a disposable oxygen mask. Incremental doses of sedative, analgesic drugs (fentanyl and/or droperidol, meperidine [Demerol], diazepam or an ultra-short-acting barbiturate—methohexital, thiopental, or thiamylal) are administered, depending on the patient's responsiveness and the duration of the surgical procedure. The barbiturates may be administered by a slow continuous infusion of a dilute solution (*e.g.*, 0.1–0.2% methohexital), or intermittently by using 25- to 50-mg increments of thiopental or thiamylal or 10- to 20-mg doses of methohexital. In this way, a patient's desire to be "asleep" is satisfied, and yet the patient may have the advantages of the regional anesthetic—profound motor and sensory blockade, postoperative analgesia, less nausea and vomiting, fewer adverse physiologic effects—and still not be aware of the events surrounding the anesthetic and operation.

In addition to monitoring and maintaining vital physiologic functions as well as providing for the physical and psychological comforts of the patient, the anesthesiologist must protect the tracheobronchial tree from aspiration of gastric contents when regional anesthesia is used for intra-abdominal procedures. When spinal and extradural anesthesia and intercostal, celiac plexus blocks are used for upper intra-abdominal procedures, a cuffed endotracheal tube should be inserted after topically anesthetizing the larynx and trachea. The administration of 50 to 70 per cent nitrous oxide usually provides adequate sedation as well as tolerance of the endotracheal tube. The adequacy of ventilation can be determined by the continuous use of a ventilation meter and periodic arterial blood gas determinations. Thus, the regional anesthetic becomes a component of a balanced anesthesia by providing anesthesia and relaxation in the operative area.

REGIONAL ANESTHETIC EQUIPMENT

The availability of appropriate equipment is another important component of regional anesthesia. Thus, Departments of Anesthesiology in which regional anesthesia is to be performed in a sophisticated fashion must have a significant inventory of regional anesthesia equipment.

Regional Anesthesia Carts

Although not absolutely essential, it is certainly both desirable and convenient to have carts designated exclusively for use in regional anesthesia (Fig. 6-1). The cart should be lightweight, mobile, and have at least three shelves with dimensions approximately 45 by 68 cm. The top shelf is reserved for the regional anesthesia tray being used, but the two lower shelves allow storage of other block trays, commonly employed local anesthetic agents, needles, epidural catheters, preparation solution, tape, and so forth. The advantages of this item are readily apparent.

Block Trays

Depending upon the preference of the anesthesiologist, disposable, commercially prepared, or reusable, department-prepared block trays may be used (Figs. 6-2 and 6-3). Department-prepared block trays must be meticulously assembled by con-

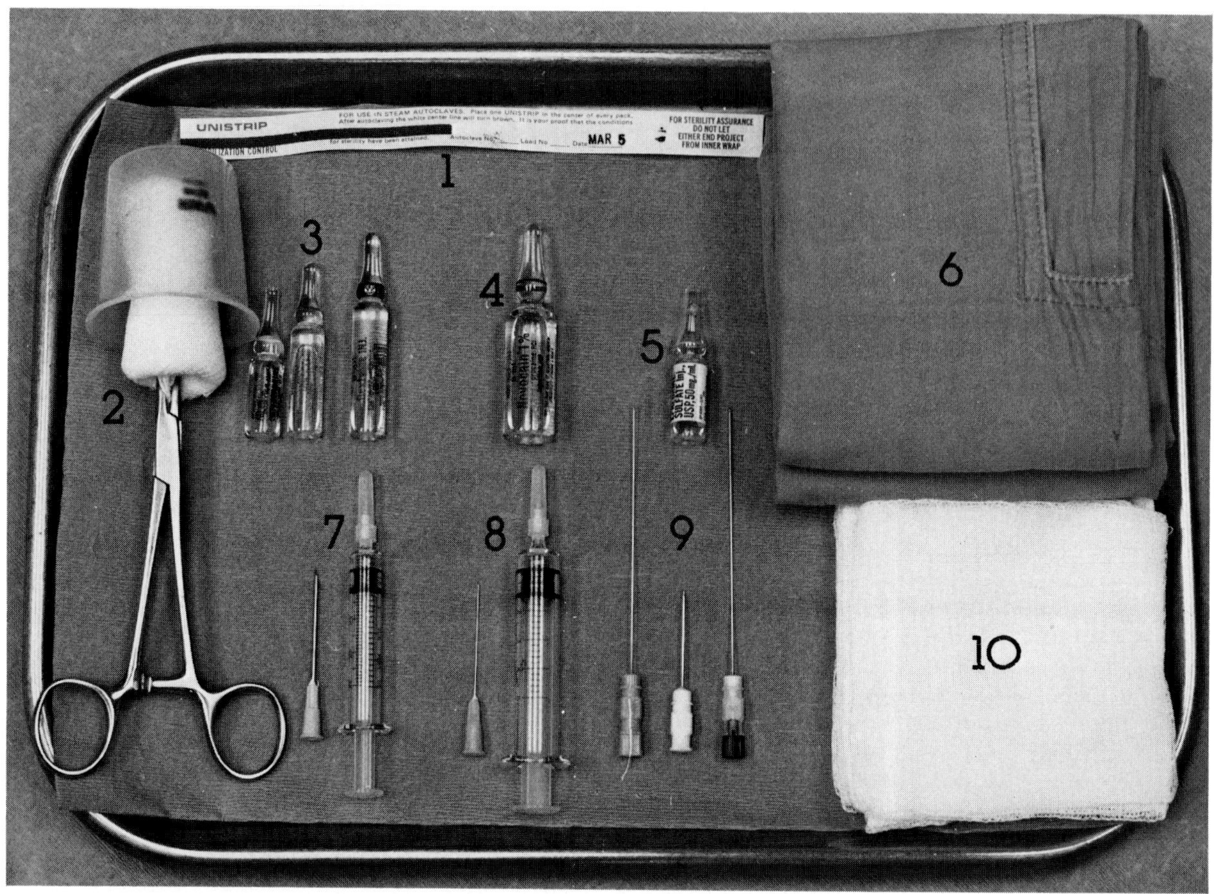

Fig. 6-1. Spinal tray, department-prepared with disposable components. (*1*) Sterility indicator; (*2*) preparation sponge and forceps for antiseptic solution (iodine tincture, 1% or povidone-iodine); (*3*) drugs for spinal anesthesia; (*4*) local anesthetic solution for infiltration; (*5*) vasopressor; (*6*) fenestrated drape; (*7*) mixing needle and disposable syringe for spinal anesthesia drugs; (*8*) disposable syringe and 25-gauge needle for local infiltration; (*9*) disposable needles for spinal anesthesia—22-gauge and 25-gauge with 20-gauge introducer; (*10*) sponges.

scientious, well-trained workers, with care being taken to prevent chemical and bacterial contamination.

Department-prepared trays are more versatile and have the added advantage of satisfying the personal preferences of the anesthesiologist. Regardless of the origin of the block tray, only high quality components are acceptable.

Local Anesthetic Agents

Although local anesthetics are discussed in detail in Chapters 3 and 4, it bears repeating that in order to achieve optimal results, the selection of the local anesthetic agents should be tailored to the anticipated duration of the surgical/obstetric procedure and in concentrations that will produce required sensory and motor blockade. For epidural and peripheral nerve blocks, local anesthetic agents that contain a 1:200,000 concentration of epinephrine should be used because the intensity of motor and sensory blockade is enhanced; the blood levels of the local anesthetic agent are lower; and the given dose of the local anesthetic lasts longer—as a consequence, with continuous blocks, the number of reinjections is reduced, thus retarding the development of tachyphylaxis or cumulative toxicity.

The recommended concentrations and doses of the frequently employed local anesthetics are listed in Table 6-2 (see also Chapter 4).

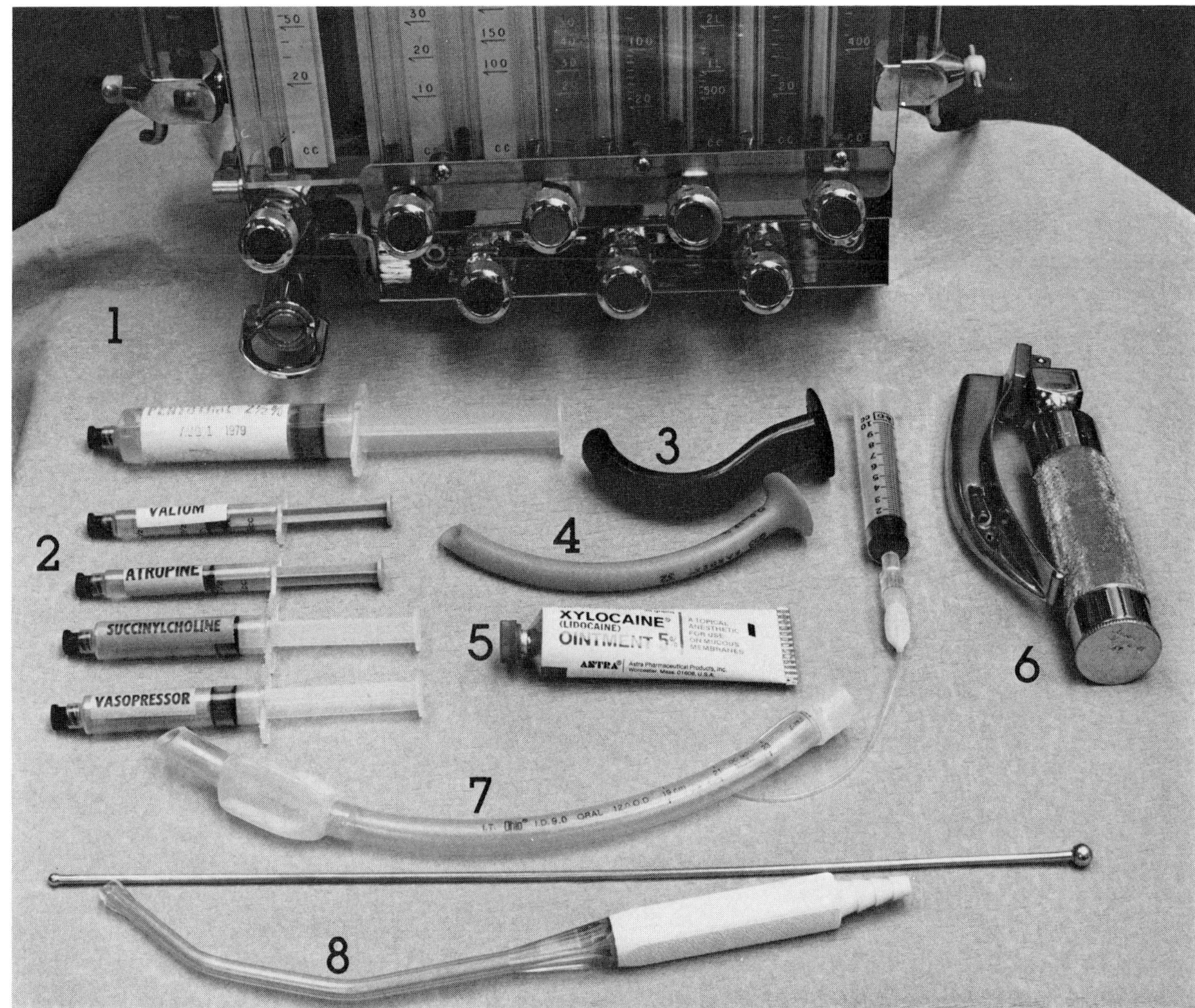

Fig. 6-2. Equipment for resuscitation and the treatment of adverse reactions. (*1*) Anesthesia machine as source of oxygen and ventilation; (*2*) labeled syringes containing succinylcholine, atropine, vasopressor (ephedrine, 5 mg/ml), diazepam, and thiopental; (*3*) oropharyngeal airway; (*4*) nasopharyngeal airway; (*5*) topical anesthetic; (*6*) laryngoscope and blade; (*7*) endotracheal tube with stylet and cuff syringe; (*8*) Yankauer suction.

Thus, in a normal 70-kg patient in whom bilateral intercostal nerve blocks of T5–T12 (16 nerves) are being performed, the injection of 5 ml per nerve of 0.5 per cent lidocaine with epinephrine, 1:200,000 (5 mg/ml, lidocaine and 5μg/mg epinephrine; total 400 mg, 400μg respectively) would not exceed the maximum safe amount of lidocaine (7–8 mg × 70 kg = 490–560 mg).

Needles

A wide selection of high quality needles of various lengths, gauges, and kinds of bevel for spinal, epidural, caudal, and peripheral nerve blocks should be available. Needles for spinal, epidural, and caudal anesthesia should not only be free of barbs but also have close-fitting stylets. Needles for peripheral nerve blocks should be sharp, free of barbs, and short-beveled.

Selander observed less nerve damage using short-beveled needles.[10] Thus, when available, short-beveled needles are preferred for peripheral nerve blocks.

Needles for Spinal Anesthesia. A needle with a close-fitting, removable stylet is essential (see

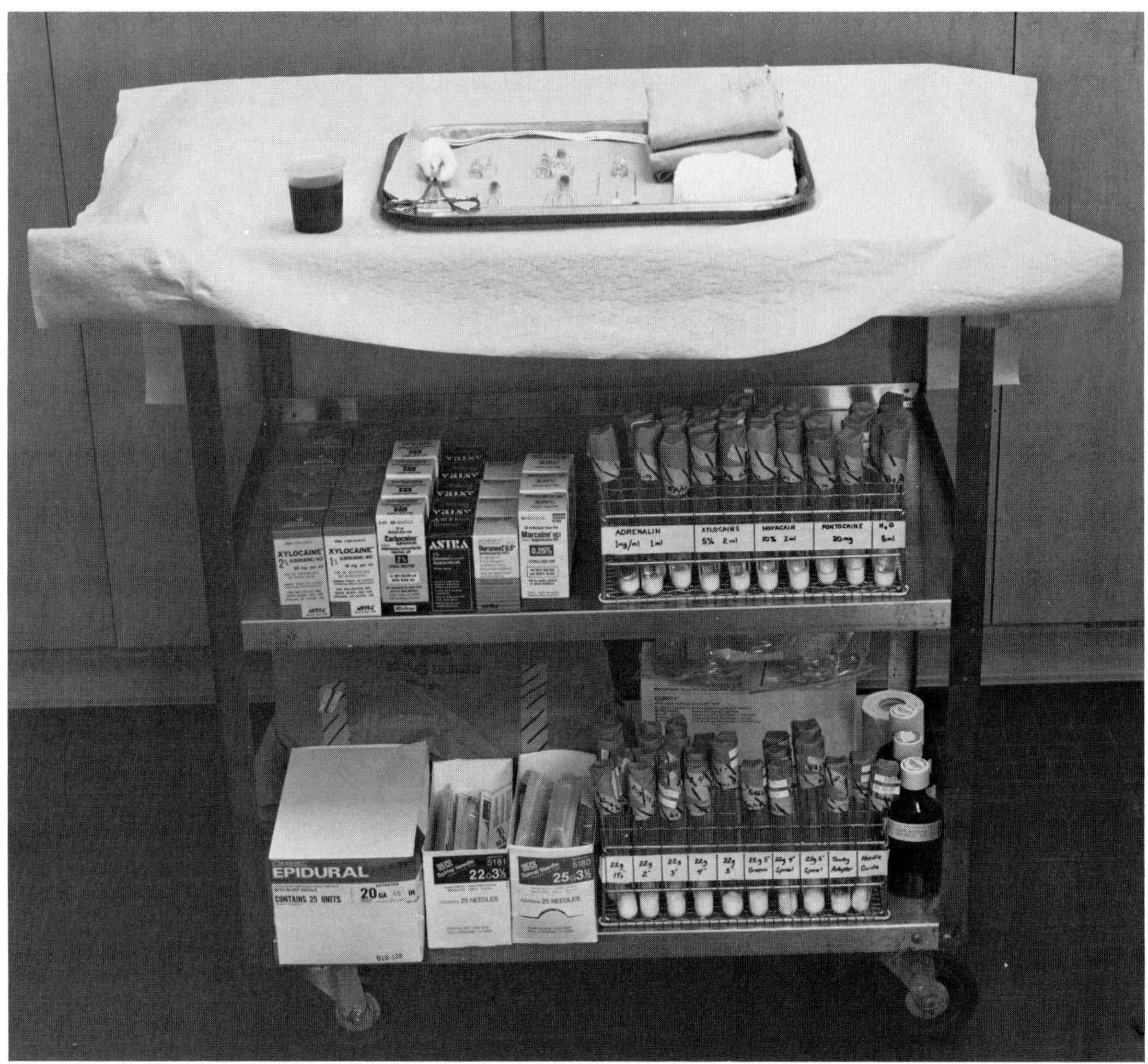

Fig. 6-3. Mobile regional anesthesia cart. Top shelf, work surface for block tray. Middle shelf, assortment of local anesthetic solutions for spinal, epidural, and caudal anesthesia and peripheral nerve blocks. Bottom shelf, disposable and reuseable needles for spinal, epidural, and caudal anesthesia and peripheral nerve blocks, epidural catheters, block trays, tape, preparation solution, and nasal oxygen cannulae.

Chap. 7). This will prevent coring of the skin and the rare, though possible occurrence of epidermoid spinal cord tumors from the introduction of bits of epidermis into the subarachnoid space. Over the years, a host of spinal needles of various diameters with numerous kinds of points have been developed. In general, in order to keep the incidence of post-puncture headache to a minimum, either needles of small-bore (25- or 26-gauge) or with a rounded, noncutting bevel (Greene or Whitacre) should be used. A few of the more popular spinal needles will be described.

The *Quincke-Babcock spinal needle,* the so-called standard spinal needle, has a sharp point with a medium-length cutting bevel. The *Pitkin spinal needle* has a sharp point but short-bevel with cutting edges and a rounded heel. Despite Pitkin's original claims, the incidence of post-puncture head-

Table 6-2. Recommended Concentrations and Doses of the Frequently Employed Local Anesthetics

Local Anesthetic Agents	*Maximum† Safe Amount (mg/kg)*	*Concentration (%)*					
		Local Infiltration	*Small Nerve Block*	*Epidural*	*Plexus, Large Nerves*	*Intravenous Regional*	*Spinal*
Lidocaine	7–8	0.5	0.5–1	1–2	1–1.5	0.5	2.5–5
Mepivacaine	7–8	0.5	0.5–1	1–2	1–1.5	0.5–0.6	
Tetracaine	2	0.05	0.1	0.2	0.15		0.5 Hyperbaric 0.5 Isobaric 0.1 Hypobaric
Procaine	10–12	0.5	1	2	2		5
Chloroprocaine	10–15	1	1	2–3	2		
Bupivacaine	3–4	0.25	0.25	0.5–0.75	0.5	0.25	0.5–0.75
Etidocaine	4–5	0.25–0.5	0.5	1–1.5	1		
Prilocaine	8	1	1–2	2–3	2–3	0.5	

† Maximum doses of epinephrine-containing solutions in healthy adults. See appropriate chapters for doses in individual block procedures.

ache with this needle is relatively high. *The Greene spinal needle* has a rounded point and a rounded noncutting bevel of medium length.[5] The *Whitacre spinal needle,* or the pencil-point needle, has a completely rounded, noncutting bevel with a solid tip; the opening of the needle being on the side, 2-mm proximal to the tip of the needle.[6] For the inexperienced, the use of either a 22-gauge Greene needle or 22-gauge Whitacre needle for younger patients will provide a characteristic "feel" of the various structures which may then be learned more readily than with the smaller-bore spinal needles, while simultaneously keeping the incidence of postpuncture headache low (2–7%).[9]

Several combination, or double-needle, sets are available but the 21- to 26-gauge is preferred. This needle set is composed of the standard 5 cm, 21-gauge Quincke-Babcock spinal needle with a stylet, and a 9 cm, 26-gauge Quincke-Babcock needle with a close-fitting stylet.[4] The 21-gauge introducer is inserted into the epidural space, and puncture of the dura-arachnoid is made with the fine 26-gauge needle.

Regardless of the size of the needle used, care must be taken that the dural fibers that run longitudinally are separated rather than transected. It should be borne in mind that, again, regardless of the type of needle used, the opening is always on the side of the notch on the hub of the needle.

Selection of the Spinal Needle. Headache is probably the most common and certainly the most annoying complication of spinal anesthesia and is directly related to the diameter of the needle and the age and sex of the patient. It is more common in patients under the age of 50, especially young women. In men over the age of 35 to 40 and in nonpregnant women over the age of 40 to 45, a 22-gauge Quincke-Babcock spinal needle is recommended. In men under the age of 35 to 40 and in nonpregnant women younger than 40 to 45 years of age, either a 22-gauge Greene or Whitacre needle, a 25-gauge needle, or a 21- to 26-gauge, double-needle technique is preferred; in pregnancy, 25- to 26-gauge is used.

Introducers. Various introducers have been developed both to facilitate the introduction of small-bore spinal needles, which are not easily directed, and to prevent contact of the spinal needle with the skin, hence reducing the incidence of coring and the introduction of bits of epidermis or bacteria into the subarachnoid space.

Epidural Needles. As with spinal anesthesia, a variety of epidural needles have been produced (see Chap. 8). A few of the more popular needles will be described.

The *Crawford point epidural needle,* a short-beveled (40°) needle with smooth edges, is one of the most popular needles used for epidural anesthesia today.[3]

The *Touhy needle,* originally designed for continuous spinal anesthesia, was also the original needle for continuous epidural anesthesia because its Huber point facilitated the insertion of an epidural catheter. Several modifications have been made in this needle since its introduction.

Hustead needle, is a modified Touhy needle,

10 cm in length, with a rounded tip and the bevel opening constant at 2.7 mm in the 18 gauge size. The heel of the bevel opening is smoother, thus reducing the incidence of shearing of epidural catheters.*

Caudal Needles. To facilitate insertion of the needle through the sacrococcygeal ligament, needles for caudal anesthesia should have a sharp point and a bevel of moderate length. A 6.5 cm, thin-wall, 8-gauge needle incorporating both of these features is most popular for performing caudal anesthesia. It can be used for either continuous or single-dose caudal anesthesia. Single-dose caudal anesthesia can also be performed with Quincke-Babcock or Pitkin spinal needles or with disposable 22- or 25-gauge 4 cm needles with a short bevel.

Needles for Peripheral Nerve Blocks. Traditionally, needles for peripheral nerve blocks have been predominantly 22- or 25-gauge in diameter, 2–15 cm in length, with a security bead and a regular bevel and have been reusable. In recent years, disposable needles with short bevels have been used with increasing frequency. These have the advantage of being extremely sharp. Because they are very inexpensive, they can be discarded whenever they become dull or when barbs develop, (*e.g.*, during supraclavicular brachial plexus blocks or intercostal nerve blocks after repeated contact with the bone).

Epidural and Caudal Catheters

There are several catheters available today for continuous epidural or caudal anesthesia. Preferred are the disposable, radiopaque teflon catheters, 20-gauge by 90–100 cm, fitted with a fine-wire stylet and a syringe adapter, marked at 5, 10, 15, and 20 cm from the distal end. This catheter will pass through an 18-gauge thin-wall needle.

Resuscitation

Prior to starting a regional anesthetic, an intravenous infusion of a balanced electrolyte solution or normal saline is established with a large-bore catheter/needle. Appropriate monitoring equipment is set up; that is, a blood pressure cuff, a precordial stethoscope, and an electrocardiograph; baseline measurements are recorded and compared with those from the preanesthetic visit.

Regional anesthesia should not be performed unless equipment and drugs for resuscitation and treatment of complications are immediately available. This should include: a means of administering oxygen by positive pressure, such as an anesthesia machine or an anesthetic bag and mask connected to a source of oxygen; airway equipment—laryngoscope, oropharyngeal airways of several sizes, a cuffed endotracheal tube, and a suction catheter connected to wall suction; and labeled syringes that contain an ultra-short-acting barbiturate, diazepam, succinylcholine, and a dilute solution of vasopressor (ephedrine, 5–10 mg/ml). [See also Chapter 4.]

Double Tourniquet for Regional Anesthesia

To minimize patient discomfort during intravenous regional anesthesia, the proximal cuff is inflated initially and maintained until the block is established. The distal cuff is then inflated and the proximal cuff deflated. Thus, the area under the tourniquet contains the local anesthetic (is analgesic) and allows longer toleration of the tourniquet.

Syringes

Glass-barrel syringes, with close-fitting metal (or glass) plungers and finger controls, are recommended for epidural, caudal, and peripheral nerve blocks. Disposable 2-ml and 5-ml glass syringes are preferred for spinal anesthesia.

Induction/Block Room

Because one of the most common complaints about regional anesthesia is that it is too time-consuming, the availability of an induction/block room will aid in reducing "turnover time." With adequate personnel, the patient to be followed can be brought to the block room and the regional anesthetic performed as the preceding surgical procedure is being completed. In addition, there is a need for adequate storage and work space within the anesthesia arena to store and process the equipment.

* Hustead, R. F.: Personal communication.

REFERENCES

1. Bonica, J.J., Kennedy, W.F., Jr., Ward, R.J., and Tolas, A.G.: A comparison of the effects of high subarachnoid and epidural anesthesia, Acta Anaesthesiol. Scand., [Suppl.] *23*, 429, 1966.
2. Braid, D.P., and Scott, D.B.: The systemic absorption of local analgesic drugs, Br. J. Anaesth., *37*:394, 1965.
3. Crawford, O.B.: Peridural anesthesia for thoracic surgery, N. Y. State J. Med., *52*:637, 1952.
4. Greene, B.A.: A 26-gauge lumbar puncture needle: its value in the prophylaxis of headache following spinal analgesia for vaginal delivery, Anesthesiology, *11*:464, 1950.

5. Green, H.M.: A technic to reduce the incidence of headache following lumbar puncture in ambulatory patients with a plea for more frequent examination of cerebrospinal fluid, Northwest Med., *22*:240, 1923.
6. Hart, J.R., and Whitacre, R.J.: Pencil-point needle in prevention of postspinal headache, J.A.M.A., *147*:657, 1951.
7. Kennedy, W.F., Jr., et al.: Cardiorespiratory effects of epinephrine when used in regional anesthesia, Acta Anaesthesiol. Scand., [Suppl.] *23*, 320, 1966.
8. Lund, P.C., and Covino, B.G.: Distribution of local anesthetics in man following peridural anesthesia. J. Clin. Pharmacol., *7*:324, 1967.
9. Moore, D.C.: Complications of Regional Anesthesia. Springfield, Charles C Thomas, 1955.
10. Selander, D., Dhuner, K.-G., and Lundborg, G.: Peripheral nerve injury due to injection needles used for regional anesthesia, Acta Anaesthesiol. Scand., *21*:182, 1977.
11. Thomas, J., *et al.*: The influence of adrenaline on the maternal plasma levels and placental transfer of lignocaine following lumbar epidural administration, Br. J. Anaesth., *41*:1029, 1969.

PART TWO

Techniques of Neural Blockade

Section A: Central Neural Blockade

7 Spinal, Subarachnoid Neural Blockade

Phillip O. Bridenbaugh and William F. Kennedy, Jr.

Spinal anesthesia—the temporary interruption of nerve transmission following injection of a local anesthetic solution into the subarachnoid space—is without any doubt a versatile and, in many institutions, a frequently employed method of regional anesthesia. It is used in surgical and obstetric anesthesia as well as in the management of certain pain problems. This regional anesthetic technique offers significant advantages over general anesthesia for surgical procedures of the lower extremities, pelvis, perineum, lower abdomen, and abdominal wall by producing specific sensory, motor, and sympathetic blockade.

In order to obtain optimal results, a thorough knowledge of the pertinent anatomy, obtained from a review of anatomic dissections, textbooks, and atlases of anatomy, is essential. In addition, the physician should be well versed in the pharmacology of the local anesthetic agent as well as in the physiologic changes that accompany this anesthetic; thus he can anticipate any untoward side-effects and be prepared to institute treatment. Initially, teaching and close supervision by someone expert in the field is required; subsequently, continued clinical application is necessary in order to maintain these skills.

HISTORY

Although J. L. Corning, the New York neurologist, first described the anesthetic effects following intervertebral (probably epidural) injection of cocaine in 1885, regional anesthesia, as such, had its actual beginning with the introduction of spinal anesthesia by the famous German surgeon August Bier in 1898.[6,14] The following year, the French physician Tuffier also reported successful surgical anesthesia by the subarachnoid injection of cocaine, the same year that the Americans, Tait and Caglieri, in San Francisco, and Matas, in New Orleans, reported its use in the United States (see Chap. 1).[44,57,62]

The toxicity of cocaine was recognized early, and, as a result, spinal anesthesia fell into relative disuse until 1904 with the synthesis of stovaine, a local anesthetic less toxic and more stable than cocaine. Tuffier and other French surgeons used stovaine extensively for spinal anesthesia, as did the Philadelphia surgeon W. Wayne Babcock, who had learned spinal anesthesia in France. (By 1938, Babcock had performed more than 40,000 spinal anesthetics and, perhaps more than anyone else, was responsible for perpetuating spinal anesthesia in the United States.[3]) In 1907, Arthur Barker, a London surgeon, reported the use of hyperbaric spinal anesthesia with a stovaine-dextrose solution.[4] Although procaine was synthesized by Einhorn in 1905, it did not displace stovaine as a spinal anesthetic agent until the 1920s, as a direct consequence of the studies of the French physician, Gaston Labat.[38] In 1927, George P. Pitkin devised spinocaine, a hypobaric procaine-containing solution.[52,53] Pitkin was an enthusiastic proponent of spinal and regional anesthesia and generated nationwide interest in this form of anesthesia. In 1938, Louis Maxson published his classic book on spinal anesthesia.[45]

Other milestones in the history of spinal anesthesia include the introduction of the tetracaine-dextrose technique by Sise in 1935 (although Sise's original technique has subsequently been modified, tetracaine-dextrose is the most common anesthetic solution in use in the United States today); Lemmon's continuous spinal anesthesia technique with a malleable needle in 1940; Touhy's continuous catheter (ureteral) technique in 1944; the continuous polyethylene and vinyl tubing method used by Davidson, Hingson, and Hellman in 1951; and, more recently, the continuous technique of Bizzari, and colleagues, using an ultra-fine vinyl catheter inserted through a special thin-wall 21-gauge needle.[7,15,39,55,61] The most recent contributions have been investigations of the physiologic consequences of spinal blockade.[2,8,20,32–34,59,64]

INDICATIONS

The selection of any anesthetic technique must be based on a perspective broader than just the surgical procedure. The decision must take into account the patient's physical and mental status, the surgeon performing the procedure, the postoperative care facility, and even the professional and legal climate of the community. Such considerations are especially applicable in the selection of spinal anesthesia. Anesthesiologists, like all medical practitioners, are being admonished to inform their patients fully of the risks and benefits of the selected as well as the alternate methods. This helps the anesthesiologist analyze what special benefits of spinal anesthesia might render it the anesthetic of choice for a particular patient.

Indications for spinal anesthesia, which follow, can be broadly categorized according to kinds of patients and kinds of procedures. There is a risk that listing "indications" may lead to rigid interpretation—that is, that omitted situations must be contraindications or that spinal anesthesia is always appropriate for the listed circumstances. Rather, the following is a discussion of patients and procedures for which spinal anesthesia should be given special consideration.

Patients

The major and most predictable of side-effects from spinal anesthesia is hypotension of a magnitude related to the level of the sympathetic block and the blood-volume status of the patient. It is, therefore, easy to state that high spinal anesthesia is not suited for hypovolemic patients.

Specifically, then, spinal anesthesia to almost any level is suitable for healthy patients (rated ASA Status 1). Patients with significant systemic diseases (rated ASA 2 or ASA 3) provide an important opportunity to exploit the specific advantages of spinal anesthesia.[43a] A very small quantity of drug placed into the subarachnoid space provides complete anesthesia to a given level, which avoids reliance on the respiratory system for administration of anesthesia and avoids the liver or kidneys for the metabolism of those or supplemental intravenous anesthetics. Therefore, patients with significant pulmonary disease can frequently be given a spinal anesthetic more safely than an endotracheal inhalation anesthetic. Similarly, patients with renal failure or diffuse liver disease, in which drug metabolism and excretion might be impaired, may also undergo spinal anesthesia with less risk. Although, of course, patients with nervous system disease, especially of the lower motor neuron or cord, are usually deemed unsuitable for spinal anesthesia, for patients with neuromuscular disease, muscular disease, or, particularly, malignant hyperpyrexia history, spinal anesthesia may be the preferred technique.

Special consideration is necessary in selecting spinal anesthesia for patients with cardiovascular disease. A careful preanesthetic evaluation of these patients is as essential as an understanding of the physiology of spinal anesthesia. It is important to recall that the higher the spinal anesthetic level, the higher the sympathetic block, and the greater the resulting vasodilatation. (A more thorough presentation of the physiology of spinal anesthesia appears later in this chapter.) Compensation for sympathetic vasodilatation occurs initially through alterations in cardiac output (*i.e.*, rate and stroke volume). The same endogenous catecholamines that stimulate cardiac activity have a mild effect on all vessels, but the vessels above the level of the spinal anesthesia will react to both neural and humoral elements and undergo marked vasoconstriction. Answers to the following questions are important when considering spinal anesthesia for patients with heart disease: "Will the level of anesthesia required be likely to produce significant hypotension?" and "Will this patient's heart and blood volume status adequately compensate for the degree of hypotension anticipated?" For example, a patient with mild congestive heart failure may be transiently improved with spinal vasodilatation until diuresis can reduce the total cardiac workload. In contrast, a patient with severe mitral stenosis may incur serious problems with spinal anesthesia if hypotension of any degree develops.

Finally, there are certain extremely poor-risk patients (ASA Status 4), for whom spinal anesthesia may be the anesthetic of choice. In general, this is true when the ability of spinal anesthesia to provide a very restricted area of blockade, with profound bilateral anesthesia of the lower extremities and pelvis and virtually no side-effects, can be exploited (Table 7-1). These are the same patients, of course, in whom general anesthesia may represent significant risk to an already compromised cardiorespiratory system.[43a]

Procedures

The selection of the appropriate anesthetic technique, whether it be inhalation, intravenous, or regional, must take into account the patient (as just

Table 7-1. Cardiovascular Effects of Spinal Anesthesia

	Saddle Block S2–5 Anesthesia	*T10 Spinal Anesthesia*	*T4 Spinal Anesthesia*
Example of use	Cystoscopy Perineal surgery	Lower limb Lower abdominal	Upper abdominal surgery
Major mechanism of CVS effects		Lower extremity vasodilatation (peripheral block of T11L2 sympathetic ganglia)	1) Lower limb vasodilatation (T11L2) 2) Mesenteric vasodilatation (celiac plexus) 3) Blockade of cardio accelerator fibers
Effect on blood pressure	Unchanged	↓*	↓↓
Effect on heart rate	Unchanged	Unchanged or slight ↑	↓
Effect on cardiac output	Unchanged	Unchanged or slight ↑	↓

* Can be reduced if "hemianalgesia" achieved with block of lumbar sympathetic outflow in only one lower extremity.

discussed) and also the special requirements of the procedure to be performed. These procedural requirements include location of the operation, time required to complete the procedure, anticipated blood loss, and muscle relaxation required.

Surgery

Spinal anesthesia is especially suited for surgical procedures below the level of the umbilicus (T10). This includes all orthopedic procedures of the lower extremities, most major urologic procedures on the genitourinary system distal to the ureters (*i.e.*, bladder and below), and general surgical or gynecologic procedures approached perineally. These kinds of procedures are especially suitable for spinal anesthesia in poor-risk patients, in patients with a full stomach, in patients with difficult airway management problems, and in patients in the prone position.

Spinal anesthesia at somatic levels as far as T6 permits the performance of many additional intra-abdominal surgical procedures. These include most intestinal surgery, especially in the rectosigmoid area, and gynecologic pelvic surgery of all kinds, as well as bladder, ureteral, and renal pelvic surgery. However, cardiorespiratory and airway management require special consideration.

There are significant numbers of anesthesiologists and surgeons who are advocates of "high" spinal anesthesia (T4 to C8) for all upper abdominal procedures such as cholecystectomy, gastrectomy, and splenic surgery. As previously mentioned, as the level of spinal anesthetic rises, the risk of hypotension increases and the patient's physical status, especially his cardiocirculatory status, becomes more important. Of equal concern in patients who undergo upper abdominal surgery with "high" spinal anesthesia is management of the airway. The visceral (vagal) responses elicited from traction on the esophagus, stomach, and diaphragm, in addition to the opportunity for surgically expressed gastric contents to be aspirated, make endotracheal intubation a requirement in the anesthetic management of most of these patients (Table 7-2).

Of equal concern with the location of the anticipated procedure are duration, anticipated blood loss, and required muscle relaxation. Extremely long or extremely short durations of action are important in the selection of spinal anesthesia. If no other factors were to be considered, it would seem inappropriate to select spinal anesthesia for a 10-minute outpatient procedure. Similarly, procedures expected to exceed 3 to 4 hours may not all be completed under pure spinal anesthesia, if it were to be administered as a single injection. Current drugs available for spinal anesthesia provide a minimum anesthetic duration of 30 to 45 minutes and a maximum predictable surgical anesthetic duration of 180 to 210 minutes (Table 7-3). This, too, depends on

Table 7-2. Level of Spinal Anesthesia Required for Common Surgical Procedures

Level	*Surgical Procedure*
T4–5 (Nipple)	Upper abdominal surgery
T6–8 (Xiphoid)	Intestinal surgery (including appendectomy),* gynecologic pelvic surgery, and ureter and renal pelvic surgery
T10 (Umbilicus)	Transurethral resection, obstetric vaginal delivery, and hip surgery
L1 (Inguinal ligament)	Transurethral resection, if no bladder distention; thigh surgery; lower limb amputations, and so forth
L2–3 (Knee and below)	Foot surgery
S2–5 (Perineal)	Perineal surgery, hemorrhoidectomy, anal dilation, and so forth

* Blockade to T10 is not adequate for appendectomy because of splanchnic supply to peritoneum (T6–L1).

the location of the procedure since sacral anesthesia is the last to subside in spinal anesthesia.

Spinal anesthesia may be indicated in certain patients in whom general anesthesia is relatively contraindicated. Inasmuch as muscle relaxation is a frequent requirement for adequate surgical conditions, it is accomplished in general anesthetic techniques through the use of depolarizing or nondepolarizing muscle relaxants. A small number of patients may pose potential problems with these drugs, for example, patients with myasthenia gravis, Eaton-Lambert syndrome, atypical pseudocholinesterase, or malignant hyperthermia; spinal anesthesia may be used in these patients to avoid possible problems from the relaxants.

Although spinal anesthesia is not empirically indicated in procedures in which significant hemorrhage has occurred or is anticipated, neither is it empirically contraindicated. For physiologic reasons, significant sympathetic blockade should be avoided in hypovolemic patients, and significant hypovolemia should be avoided in patients who undergo major sympathetic blockade. If, for other reasons then, spinal anesthesia is deemed the technique of choice, the anesthesiologist is obligated to achieve and maintain an adequate circulating blood volume.

Obstetrics

Several regional anesthetic techniques are increasingly being employed for elective obstetric procedures. There is little doubt that spinal anesthesia has traditionally been the most frequently employed of these techniques. However, current data are not readily available. The safety of the technique has been well documented in the literature with a variety of clinical series from a few hundred cases to the 18,559 and 34,000 case series reported by both Ebner and Macer.[17,42] Spinal anesthesia provides optimal operative conditions, including some degree of active maternal participation with the least risk of fetal depression. It is a safe, simple technique that can rapidly be administered and provides rapid and complete analgesia (see Chap. 18).

The indications for spinal anesthesia in obstetrics are relative to general anesthesia or other regional anesthesia techniques, and, therefore, the decision to use it is elective rather than absolute. In years past, sound data were not available on the physiologic changes of pregnancy and how these might be affected by the imposition of spinal anesthesia, in comparison to the effects of spinal anesthesia on the nonpregnant state. Lund discusses some of the early (generally 1928–1948) misconceptions about spinal anesthesia.[41]

In general, spinal anesthesia may be selected on the basis of fetal or maternal considerations. Fetal considerations include prematurity; fetal distress, which would benefit from administration of 100 per cent oxygen to the mother; and the delivery of a large fetus—especially that of a diabetic mother in whom maximum relaxation of perineal musculature

Table 7-3. Drugs for Spinal Anesthesia

Drug and Concentration	*Dose (in mg)*		*Onset (in min)*	*Duration (in min)*	
	To T10	*To T4*		*Plain*	*With 0.2 mg Epinephrine*
Procaine (5%)	100–150	150–200	5–10	30–45	60–75
Tetracaine (0.5%)	6–8	12–16	4–6	60–90	120–180
Dibucaine (0.5%)	6–8	10–15	5–7	150–180	180–240
Lidocaine (5%)	30–50	75–100	2–4	45–60	60–90

may be accomplished without the need for a deep general anesthetic.

Maternal indications are similar to those previously noted under Patients Suited for Spinal Anesthesia (see p. 147). These include patients with major organ disease, such as pulmonary problems; heart disease, especially if it is accompanied by congestive failure or pulmonary edema; diabetes; and toxemia of pregnancy. If the patient is allowed to remain awake during the delivery, many anesthesiologists believe spinal anesthesia is the anesthetic of choice for patients thought to have food in their stomach.

Special Techniques

Generally, anesthesiologists use the phrase *spinal anesthesia* to refer to a single-injection hyperbaric spinal anesthetic, which provides total anesthesia to a desired segmental level. There are, however, variations in technique that have limited but specific value. These include hypobaric spinal, isobaric spinal, continuous spinal, and unilateral spinal anesthesia.

Hypobaric Spinal Anesthesia. Authorities on spinal anesthesia agree that figures for the specific gravity of cerebrospinal fluid (CSF) are not in agreement and that density is a more appropriate measure.[25,41,44] Clinically, the position of the patient after injection of a spinal anesthetic is related to the relative specific gravities of the CSF and the injected solution. Thus, if the local anesthetic solution, containing dextrose, for example, has a specific gravity in excess of 1.020 and if the CSF has an average specific gravity of 1.001 to 1.005, then gravity should influence the flow of the heavier anesthetic solution within the CSF.

The reverse was applied to the use of hypobaric spinal solutions, that is that solutions lighter than CSF would "float up." Ernst measured densities and specific gravities of the various spinal anesthetic solutions and listed the specific gravity of dibucaine, 0.15 per cent, as 1.0036, distilled water as 1.000, and tetracaine, 1 per cent, as 1.0014.[19] Lund wrote, "It is generally stated that if a local anesthetic is to be considered hypobaric it must have a specific gravity less than 1.003."[41] Macintosh thought that the reporting of the specific gravity to the fourth decimal is clinically irrelevant.[43] He even doubted if minor variations in the third figure are of clinical significance and, therefore, believed that "light dibucaine" is probably isobaric. The foregoing should illustrate that the indications for hypobaric spinal anesthesia include isobaric solutions, which are to be managed by positioning the patient so that the injected anesthetic solution will migrate to the highest point in the vertebral column (see Fig. 27-4).

The indications for the hypobaric technique are primarily procedural or positional rather than patient-related. Procedures that require the patient to be prone, jackknifed, or lateral may be performed with hypobaric spinal anesthesia to avoid repositioning of the anesthetized patient. This is especially helpful, for example, in total hip arthroplasty in which the anesthetic is administered with the patient lateral and with the operative side obviously upward. As soon as analgesia ensues, the patient may undergo the elaborate orthopedic positioning and preparation without jeopardizing the level of anesthesia. Other procedures especially suited to hypobaric spinal anesthesia include anorectal surgery, surgery on the back and dorsal trunk, and some renal or ureteral procedures. Of course, there is no reason why the hypobaric technique could not be used in place of nearly all hyperbaric techniques as long as the anesthesiologist positions the patient appropriately after injection of the drug (see Chap. 27 for application of hypobaric technique to neurolytic blockades).

Isobaric Spinal Anesthesia. The purported advantage of a true isobaric technique is that patient position has no effect on the spread of anesthesia. This, however, limits its practical application to procedures on the perineum and lower extremities. Since position has no effect on level, thoracic analgesia may be achieved only through the use of large volumes of anesthetic solution or by performing the subarachnoid puncture at the thoracic level. Individual variation in the specific gravity of the CSF is sufficient to preclude predictable results from diluents other than the patients' own CSF. The usual mixture for perineal surgery is 4 to 6 mg of tetracaine diluted in 2 to 4 ml of CSF and injected slowly through the needle, which is placed in a lumbar interspace. This reportedly provides good sensory analgesia, lasting 100 to 150 minutes, to a level of L1. Little motor anesthesia results.[40] This procedure is seldom used, primarily because it has little to offer over either a hyperbaric or a hypobaric positional technique.

Continuous Spinal Anesthesia. The use of continuous spinal anesthesia illustrates especially that indications are the application of the maximum benefits provided with the fewest risks or side-effects. Underwood reported on his experiences with this technique in the poor-risk patient.[63] In his report, however, he identified three specific features of continuous spinal anesthesia that relate to its indications for use in specific patients or procedures. First, continuous spinal anesthesia has the ability to produce a precise level of sensory anesthesia, where it is administered, if necessary, as small serial doses of anesthetic solutions until the desired level is obtained. This helps avoid the unnecessarily high level of sympathetic blockade that may result from a single-dose injection and may be undesirable in the hypovolemic high-risk patient. Second, with continuous spinal anesthesia, the patient can be placed in the exact position to be used for surgery before injecting the anesthetic drugs. This avoids the problems associated with moving an anesthetized patient as well as the risk that the spinal level might be forced higher by a straining helpful patient during repositioning. Finally, the continuous technique allows the use of short-acting non-epinephrine-containing solutions. In this context, spinal anesthesia can be considered similar to general anesthesia in that it is induced at the start of surgery, continued as long as the surgery—whether it be 30 minutes or 6 hours and 30 minutes, and will subside very soon after the operation is completed. There are still anesthesiologists and institutions that view the addition of epinephrine to the spinal anesthetic solution with disfavor. However, since use of non-epinephrine-containing solutions severely limits the duration of single-injection techniques, the use of the continuous technique for certain situations would be of significant value.

Unilateral Spinal Anesthesia. There are some potentially valuable indications for unilateral spinal anesthesia, which are based on the principle that letting the patient lie on the side will produce anesthesia of the ventral and dorsal roots on the operative side. The technique has less practical value, however, than its theory would suggest. Because of the extreme care required to produce a neurolytic blockade of only dorsal roots, and the difficulty in doing so, the relative impracticality of attempting unilateral spinal analgesia for surgery becomes apparent. It would seem preferable to use small volumes of hyperbaric (rather than hypobaric) solutions. This would, however, necessitate putting the operative side down and delaying the procedure for an empiric time period (15–30 min). If unilateral anesthesia is absolutely necessary to avoid the hazards of bilateral sympathetic blockade, then segmental regional nerve block would be a better choice. Tanasichuk and co-workers reported on 42 patients who received what they termed *spinal hemianalgesia*.[58] Even with meticulous control of technique and the use of a directional needle, they were successful in only 67 per cent of their patients. The incidence of reduced hypotension was statistically significant, however, when the level of anesthesia was below T7 and in poor-risk patients (ASA Status 3). Surgical anesthesia was satisfactory in 80 per cent of their cases. These percentages should be kept in mind before undertaking use of this technique.

SPINAL ANESTHESIA VERSUS EPIDURAL ANESTHESIA

The dilemma for the anesthesiologist, who appreciates the physiologic differences between spinal and epidural anesthesia, is to establish the clinical relevance of that information (see Chaps. 8 and 9).[9]

Spinal anesthesia provides profound, predictable, controllable anesthesia with a very low dose of drug, yet frequently epidural anesthesia is preferred, perhaps because it avoids "spinal headache." Depending upon such variables as age of the patient, surgical procedure, and needle size, the incidence of headaches after spinal anesthesia has been reported to vary from 24 to 0.2 per cent.[23,24,27,59] Certainly, the dura may inadvertently be penetrated during the administration of epidural anesthesia, and if a large-bore needle has been used, headache is very likely.

The advent of long-acting local anesthetic agents (bupivacaine and etidocaine), which provide epidural analgesia of 4 to 6 hours' duration, was an improvement over single-injection spinal anesthesia, the duration of which is 3 to 4 hours. This latter duration is achieved, of course, with the addition of epinephrine or phenylephrine to the spinal mixture. As was mentioned previously under Continuous Spinal Anesthesia, many anesthetists, especially English and Australian, are reluctant to inject vasopressors into the subarachnoid space. Epidural anesthesia with a long-acting agent provides an alternative to the continuous spinal technique.

With the exceptions, then, of inducing headache and of an unwillingness to use epinephrine, spinal anesthesia may be chosen over epidural anesthesia primarily on the basis of the personal preference of the anesthesiologist, his patient, or the surgeon. Many believe, however, that spinal anesthesia is the technique of choice for profound visceral sensory and motor anesthesia to a predictable level.

ANATOMY

Vertebral column, composed of 33 vertebrae (7 cervical, 12 thoracic, 5 lumbar, 5 fused sacral, and 4 coccygeal) has four curves (Fig. 7-1). The cervical

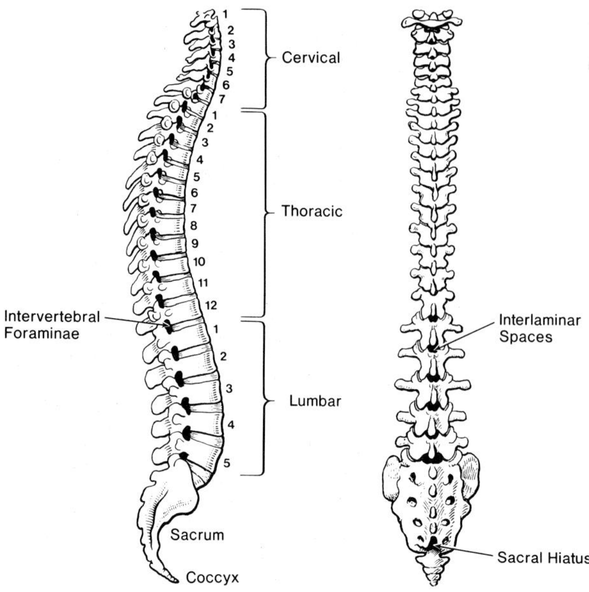

Fig. 7-1. Vertebral column, lateral (*left*) and posterior (*right*) views, illustrating curvatures and interlaminar spaces.

and lumbar curves are convex anteriorly while the thoracic and sacral curves are convex posteriorly. The curves of the vertebral column have a significant influence on the spread of local anesthetics in the subarachnoid space. In the supine position, the high points of the cervical and lumbar curves are at C5 and L5; the low points of the thoracic and sacral curves are at T5 and S2, respectively. The vertebral column is bound together by several ligaments, which give it stability and elasticity (Fig. 7-2).

Supraspinous ligament is a strong fibrous cord that connects the apices of the spinous processes from the sacrum to C7, where it is continued upward to the external occipital protuberance as the ligamentum nuchae. It is thickest and broadest in the lumbar region and varies with patient age, sex, and body build.

Interspinous ligament is a thin, membranous ligament that connects the spinous processes, blending anteriorly with the ligamentum flavum and posteriorly with the supraspinous ligaments. Like the supraspinous ligaments, the interspinous ligaments are broadest and thickest in the lumbar region.

Ligamentum flavum, or the "yellow ligament," consists of yellow elastic fibers and connects adjacent laminae that run from the caudal edge of the vertebra, above, to the cephalad edge of the lamina, below. Laterally, this ligament begins at the roots of the articular processes and extends posteriorly and medially to the point where the lamina join to form the spinous process. Here, the two components of the ligaments are united, thus covering the interlaminar space.

Longitudinal Ligaments. The anterior and posterior longitudinal ligaments bind the vertebral bodies together.

Epidural space surrounds the spinal meninges and extends from the foramen magnum, where the dura is fused to the base of the skull, to the sacral hiatus, which is covered by the sacrococcygeal ligament (see Chap. 8). It is bounded anteriorly by the posterior longitudinal ligament, laterally by the pedicles and the intervertebral foramina, and posteriorly by the ligamentum flavum and the anterior surface of the lamina. The anterior epidural space is very narrow because of the close proximity of the dura and the anterior surface of the vertebral canal. The epidural space is widest posteriorly and varies with the vertebral level, ranging from 1 to 1.5 mm at C5 to 2.5 to 3 mm at T6, to its widest point 5 to 6 mm at the level of L2. In addition to nerve roots that traverse the epidural space, the contents of the epidural space are fat, areolar tissue, lymphatics, arteries, and the extensive internal vertebral venous plexus of Batson.[5]

Although a negative pressure has been demonstrated in the epidural space, its exact cause is unknown. It has been attributed to transmission of the negative intrathoracic pressure, flexion of the vertebral column, or indentation of the dura by the epidural needle.

Spinal Meninges. The spinal cord is protected by both the bony vertebral column and three connective tissue coverings, the meninges (Fig. 7-3).

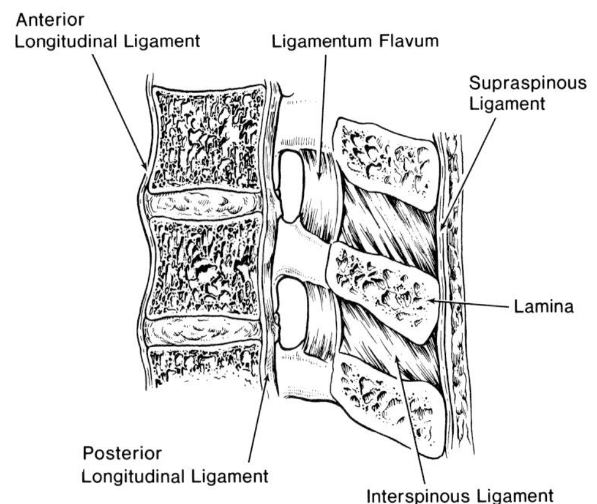

Fig. 7-2. Sagittal section of vertebral column, showing ligaments.

Dura mater, the outermost membrane, is a tough, fibroelastic tube whose fibers run longitudinally. Although continuous, it can be described in two parts, the *cranial* and the *spinal.* The cranial dura consists of an outer layer (endosteal), which lines the skull, and the inner layer (meningeal), which invests the brain and folds inward to form the falx cerebri. The two layers are closely united except where they enclose the great venous sinuses that drain the blood from the brain (Fig. 7-4).

At the spinal level, the outer (endosteal) layer continues down the vertebral canal as periosteal lining. The inner (meningeal) layer continues caudad as the spinal dura, or *theca.* Superiorly, it is firmly attached to the circumference of the foramen magnum of the occipital bone. Inferiorly, or caudally, the dural sac ends at the lower border of S2, where it is pierced by the filum terminale. The filum terminale is the terminal thread of the pia mater, which extends from the tip of the spinal cord to blend with the periosteum on the back of the coccyx. The filum terminale anchors the cord and spinal dura, the latter being further steadied in the lower end of the vertebral column by a few fibrous strips from the posterior longitudinal ligament. The spinal dura also provides a thin cover for the spinal nerve roots, becoming progressively thinner near the intervertebral foramina, where it continues as the epineural and perineural connective tissue of the peripheral nerves (Fig. 7-5).

Arachnoid mater is the middle of the three coverings of the brain and spinal cord. It is a delicate nonvascular membrane closely attached to the dura and, with it, ends at the lower border of S2. There is a capillary interval, called the *subdural space,* between the dura and the arachnoid. It contains a minute quantity of serous fluid, but it has no connection with the subarachnoid space that contains the CSF. The dura and arachnoid are in such close contact that in the process of lumbar puncture, it is not possible to pierce the dura without piercing the arachnoid as well. This does account, however, for the confusion that arises when spinal anesthesia is called, at times, a *subdural block* and, at other times, a *subarachnoid block.*

Pia mater is a delicate, highly vascular membrane closely investing the spinal cord and brain. It clings to the surface of both throughout their entire course. The space between the arachnoid and the pia is thus called the *subarachnoid space.* A large number of cobweblike trabeculae run between these two membranes, and, of course, the space contains the spinal nerves and the CSF as well. The many blood vessels that supply the spinal cord are also found in this space. Lateral projections of the pia, the denticulate ligaments, are attached to the dura and aid in supporting the spinal cord (Fig. 7-6).

Spinal cord, continuous above with the medulla oblongata, begins at the level of the foramen magnum and ends below as the conus medullaris. At birth, the cord ends at the level of L3, but rises to end in adult life at the lower border of L1 (Fig. 7-7).

Spinal Nerves. There are 31 pairs of symmetrically arranged spinal nerves, which are attached to the spinal cord by two roots. Both the anterior and posterior roots arise from the cord as several filaments, or rootlets. The lumbar and sacral roots are the longest and largest and extend over several vertebrae. This greater surface area, together with the fact that the rootlets and roots are covered by only a thin layer of pia, allows for a rapid onset of anesthesia when local anesthetics are injected into the subarachnoid space.

Subarachnoid space, bounded internally by the pia and externally by the arachnoid, is filled with cerebrospinal fluid and contains numerous arachnoid trabeculae, which form a delicate, spongelike mass. This space has three divisions: cranial (surrounding the brain), spinal (surrounding the spinal cord), and root (surrounding the dorsal and ventral spinal nerve roots). All of these components are in "free communication" with each other. Again, as the dorsal and ventral nerve roots leave the spinal cord, they are covered only by pia and bathed in CSF (see Fig. 7-3). As these spinal nerve roots pass beyond the spinal dura and traverse the epidural space, they carry with them all three meningeal layers and have distinct epidural, subdural, subarachnoid, and subpial spaces. As indicated above, as the dura extends further out toward the intervertebral foramen, it becomes much thinner. The subarachnoid space extends separately along both the dorsal and ventral roots to the level of the dorsal root ganglion where the arachnoid and the pia continue as the perineural epithelium of the peripheral nerve. The spinal nerve root arachnoid contains proliferations of arachnoid cells, or villi, which have been identified in humans and other animals, along with dorsal and ventral roots.[54] These proliferations are of many shapes and sizes and may protrude into adjacent subdural spaces (see Chap. 8).

Cerebrospinal fluid is an ultrafiltrate of the blood plasma with which it is in hydrostatic and osmotic equilibrium. It is a clear, colorless fluid found in the spinal and cranial subarachnoid spaces and in the ventricles of the brain. At 37°C, its specific gravity is 1003 to 1009, and its pH is physiologic at 7.4 to

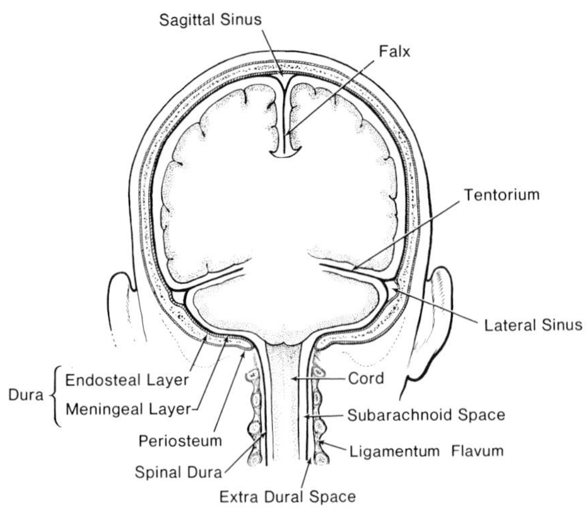

Fig. 7-4. Meningeal coverings of brain and proximal cord.

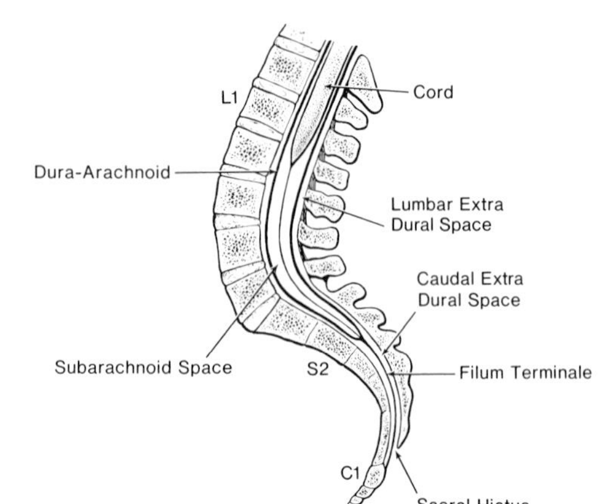

Fig. 7-5. Lumbosacral portion of vertebral column, showing terminal spinal cord and its coverings.

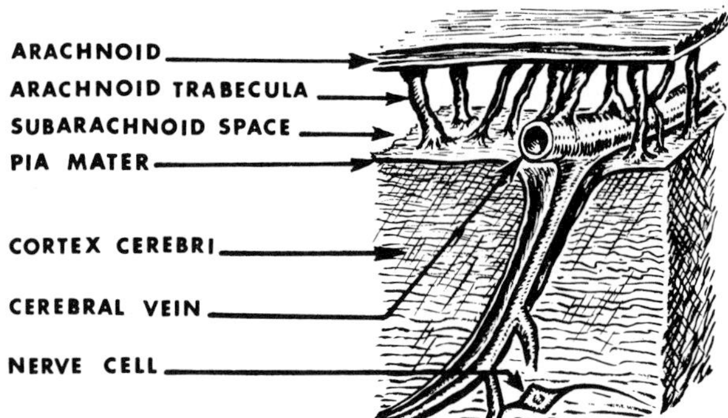

Fig. 7-6. Diagram of subarachnoid space showing blood vessels and arachnoid trabecula. (Redrawn after Strong, O.S., and Elwyn, A.: Human Neuroanatomy. Baltimore, Williams & Wilkins, 1959)

7.6 (see p. 156). The electrolyte concentration is similar to that of plasma but with a sodium and chloride ion content slightly higher and a protein content slightly lower. The total volume of CSF in the average adult ranges from 120 to 150 ml, of which 25 to 35 ml are in the spinal subarachnoid space. In the horizontal position, the pressure of CSF ranges from 60 to 80 mm of water.

Cerebrospinal fluid is formed by either secretion or ultrafiltration from the choroid arterial plexuses of the lateral, third, and fourth ventricles. The choroid plexus is composed of invaginations of capillaries from the subarachnoid space (Fig. 7-8). These capillaries are supported in a flimsy connective tissue framework of pia mater, which, in turn, is in intimate contact with the ependyma, a single layered epithelium lining the ventricle. It is presumed that these ependymal cells are primarily responsible for the secretion of CSF. The rate of formation of CSF is highly variable, related in part to change in osmotic and hydrostatic pressures of blood and CSF. Normal daily secretion is believed to be equal to the volume present (*i.e.*, 150 ml). It has been shown that after removal of small volumes of CSF, it is reformed at an increased rate of approximately 0.3 ml per minute (432 ml/day).

The circulation and elimination of CSF are important to the understanding and treatment of

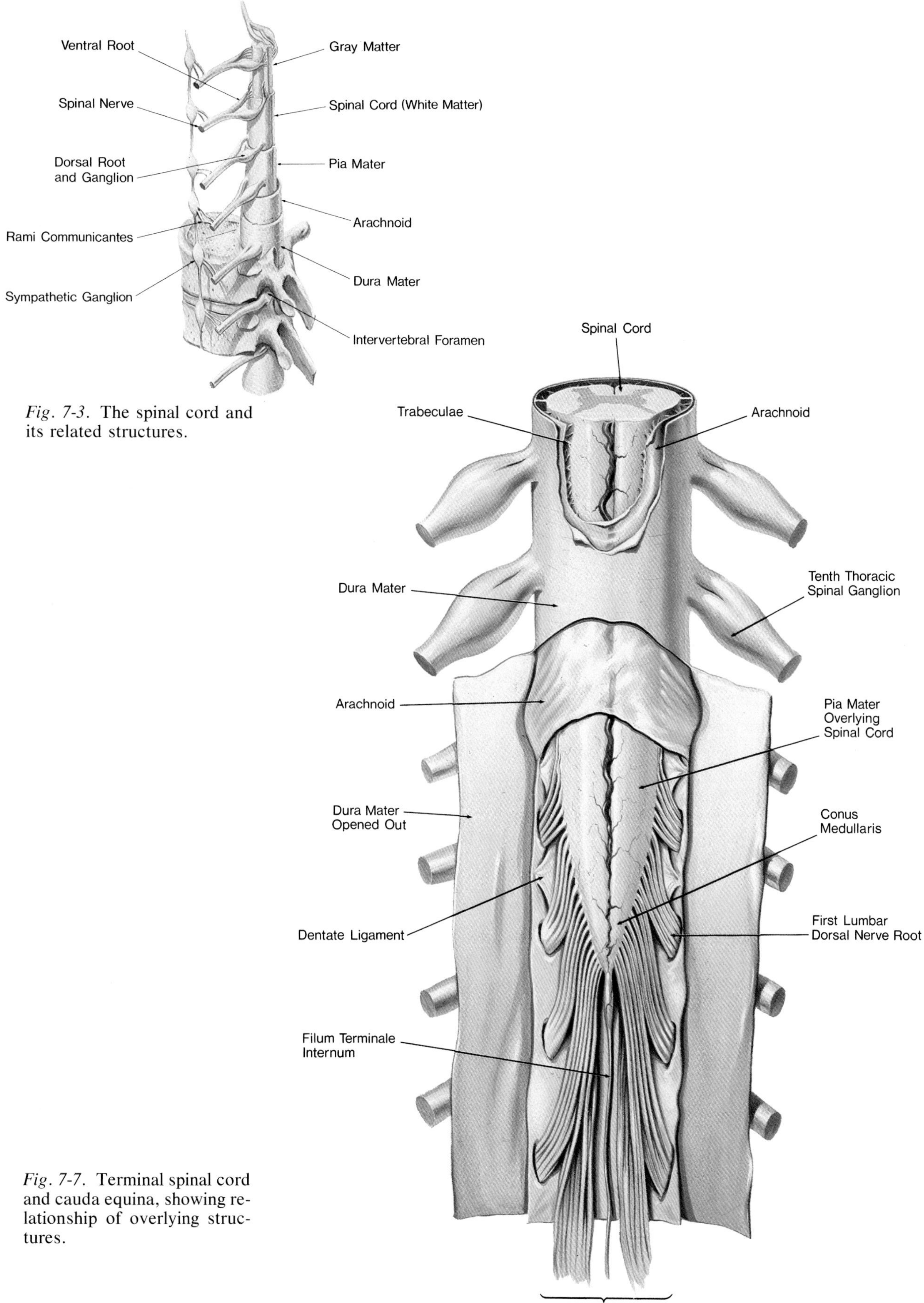

Fig. 7-3. The spinal cord and its related structures.

Fig. 7-7. Terminal spinal cord and cauda equina, showing relationship of overlying structures.

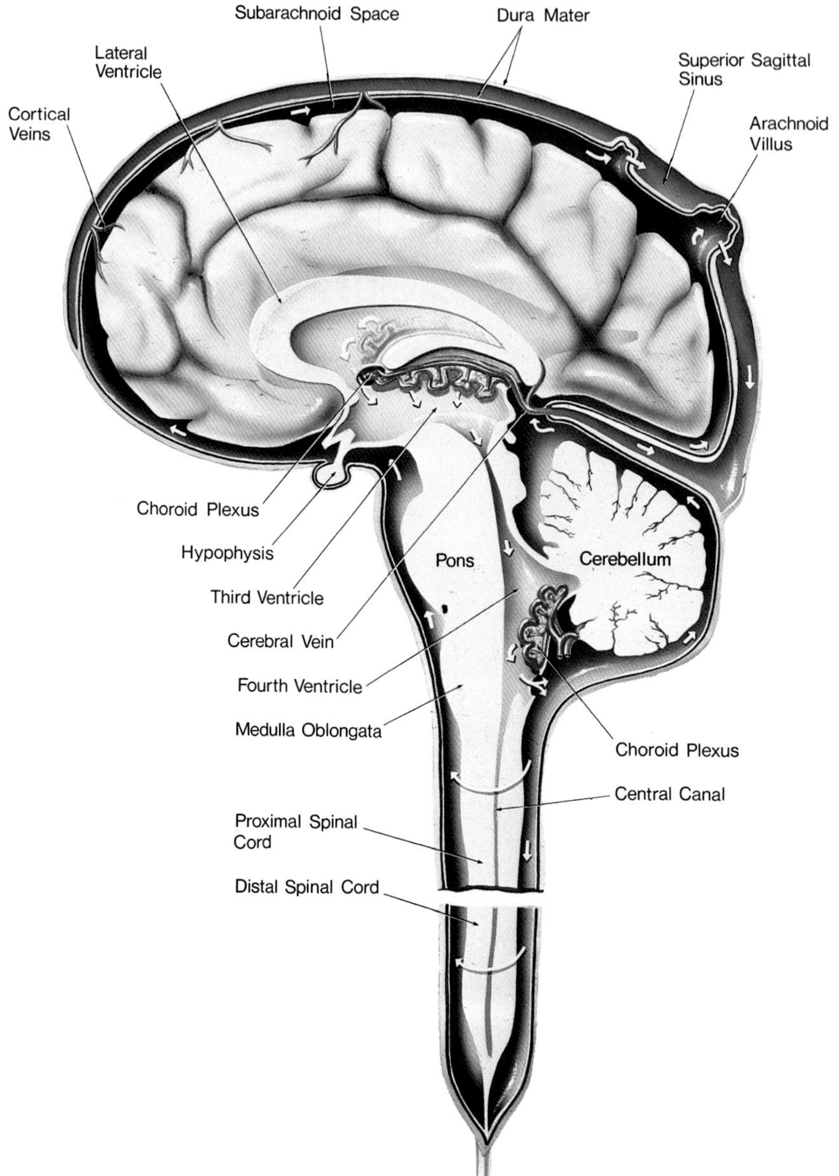

Fig. 7-8. Production, circulation, and resorption of cerebrospinal fluid.

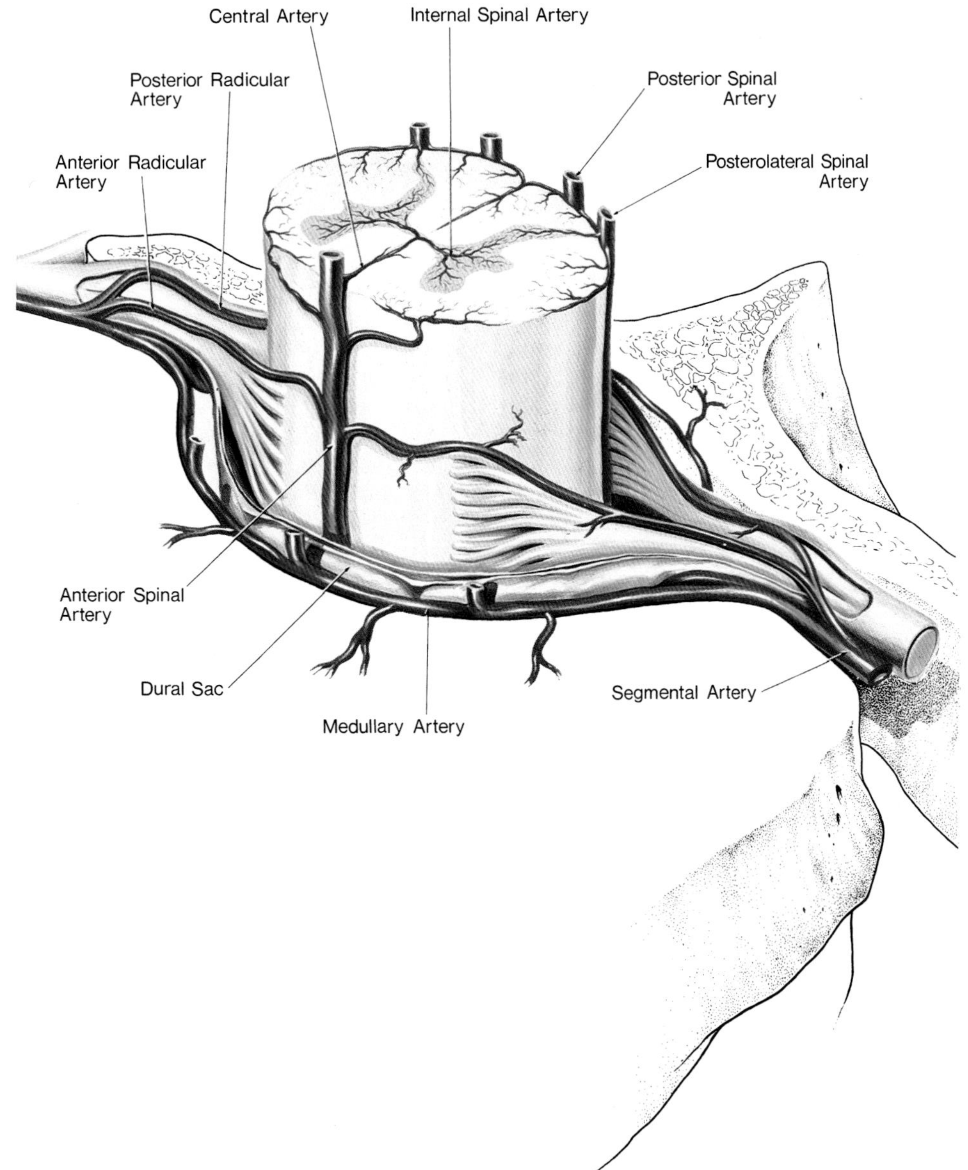

Fig. 7-9. Arterial supply of the spinal cord.

The Composition of Cerebrospinal Fluid

Protein, 15–45 mg%
Glucose, 50–80 mg%
Nonprotein nitrogen, 20–30 mg%
Chloride, 120–130 mEq/L
Sodium, 140–150 mEq/L
Bicarbonate, 25–30 mEq/L
*p*H, 7.4–7.6

(Lund, P. C.: Principles and Practice of Spinal Anesthesia. pp. 504–601. Springfield, Charles C Thomas, 1971)

postdural puncture headache. Although the choroid plexuses are in all four ventricles, the bulk of fluid is formed in the lateral ventricles and then passes into the third and fourth ventricles. In the fourth ventricle, it departs through the two foramen of Lushka and circulates upward over the surface of the brain. It also passes through the median foramen of Magendie to proceed downward into the medullary and spinal cord areas. It is generally accepted that there is no active circulation of the CSF in the spinal subarachnoid space but that osmosis, alterations in posture, and arterial pulsations keep the composition of the fluid constant.

The CSF passes back into the bloodstream by filtration and osmosis, transference taking place in the supratentorial region through the arachnoid villi and granulations. These villi are formed where the arachnoid penetrates the meningeal dura, which, in turn, comes in contact with the endothelium of the large venous sinuses.

The significance of the following kinds of arachnoid villi is discussed in Chapter 8 in conjunction with the spread of local anesthetic solutions in the epidural space.

Type II are arachnoid villi that partially protrude into the dural sheath without breaching the dural continuity, but at the same time, reduce the thickness of the dura at that site.

Type III are villi that completely breach the dura but do not protrude beyond it.

Type IV are villi that protrude out of the dura lying in the epidural space.

Type V are villi that protrude beyond the dura in proximity to epidural veins and partially protrude into the veins.

Blood Supply to the Spinal Cord. Because of the concern about direct trauma to, or the effects of vasoconstricting agents on, the vascular supply to the cord, it is important to understand its anatomy (Fig. 7-9).

The anterior spinal artery is formed between the pyramids of the medulla oblongata by the union of a root from the terminal part of each vertebral artery and descends in front of the anterior longitudinal sulcus of the spinal cord and the corresponding vein to the filum terminale. It gives off numerous circumferential vessels, which clasp the cord and supply its periphery, and sends some 200 branches into the sulcus toward the center of the cord. These turn either right or left, not necessarily alternately, sending radiating twigs into the anterior and lateral gray and white columns and into the anterior part of the posterior gray column.

The posterior spinal arteries (two on each side) arise from the posterior inferior cerebellar arteries and descend medial to the posterior nerve roots, sending penetrating twigs to the posterior white columns and the remainder of the posterior gray columns. These three longitudinal channels—anterior and posterior—are reinforced by the *spinal branches* of the vertebral arteries, deep cervical ascending cervical arteries, posterior intercostal arteries, lumbar arteries, and lateral sacral arteries. The spinal branches enter the intervertebral foramina and divide into twigs along the nerve roots, but the majority are insignificant, only some six or seven contributing materially to the anterior channel, and the same number, not at the same level, to the posterior channels (which are, moreover, rarely continuous). More often, they are broken into a series of short lengths freely anastamosing across the midline with the anterior spinal artery. The largest root vessels are in the upper lumbar region, and in parts of the cord, the blood may actually be flowing upward. Some authors have challenged the presence of anastamoses between these channels. The main communicating branches at T1 and T11 are larger than the others (called the *arteries of Adamkiewicz*). The artery of T11 supplies the cord both upward and downward; that at T1 only downward. Thus, there may be three vascular areas in the cord with no anastamoses between them (see also Chap. 8).

FUNDAMENTAL CONSIDERATIONS

The Spread of Local Anesthetic Solutions in the Subarachnoid Space

The spread of local anesthetic agents injected into the subarachnoid space is influenced by a multitude of factors, primarily, the physical principles of fluid dynamics related to spinal anesthesia.

Dispersion is the actual mixing of the injected material with the CSF, therefore, is primarily a function of the speed of injection of a given volume of solution. Barbotage—the technique of partial injection, aspiration of CSF, and reinjection of several amounts of solution—certainly has an effect on the dispersion of the drug in the CSF. Another physical factor that influences the spread of the local anesthetic solution in the CSF is that of *displacement*. The magnitude of that effect is directly related to the volume injected. Clearly, if 1 to 3 ml of solution is injected into the 30 ml reservoir of spinal fluid, the displacement would be minimal. However, with hypobaric spinal techniques, 8 to 12 ml of solution frequently is used. It is likely, therefore, that the spread of such solutions is as much a function of their volume as of their specific gravity.

Apart from these purely physical factors, there are a number of anatomic, physiologic, and technical factors with which the anesthesiologist must be familiar, if he is to have control over the level of spinal anesthesia. Some of these factors are beyond his control, but he can deal with and even exploit them by manipulation of the equally important factors that he can control. Examples of uncontrollable factors are the following: curvatures and calcification of the vertebral column; age of the patient; intra-abdominal pressure (affected by pregnancy, obesity, tumor, ascites); and *p*H of spinal fluid.

Briefly, the effects on spread attributable to either age of the patient or *p*H of the CSF can be discounted.[50] The curvature of the spine affects spread primarily at the lumbar area, whereby small doses placed caudally (below L5) will likely pool over the sacral area rather than spreading cephalad.

The effect of increased abdominal pressure is the same whether caused by obesity, pregnancy, or fluid. As inferior vena cava flow becomes reduced, progressively more venous blood is shunted through epidural venous plexuses. This, in turn, decreases the volume of CSF in the vertebral column and the greater spread of a dose of local anesthetic in the subarachnoid space. Obese people may have increased amounts of fatty tissue in the epidural space, which would further exaggerate this phenomenon.

However, knowing of these uncontrollable factors, the anesthesiologist may exploit factors under his control. These include the following: specific gravity of the solution, dose of drug injected, site of injection, and position of the patient both during and after injection.

Certainly, proper selection of the above factors is influenced by many other considerations. These include site and duration of surgical procedure, physical status of the patient, and the position of the patient during surgery. The intent here is to draw attention only to their role in the spread of local anesthetics in the subarachnoid space. Detailed discussion of those factors will be found elsewhere in the chapter.

The Fate of Local Anesthetic Solutions in the Subarachnoid Space

Koster and colleagues demonstrated that, immediately following the injection of a local anesthetic solution into the subarachnoid space, there is a rapid decrease in the concentration of the anesthetic agent in the CSF at the point of injection.[37] The greatest decrease occurs within the first 5 minutes, followed by a more gradual decline. The amounts present in solution are, however, so small that after 20 to 30 minutes, they are insufficient to produce spinal anesthesia. After this time, changes in patient position will not, likely, produce changes in the level of anesthesia. Further, the concentration decreases as the distance from the point of injection increases. This is because the local anesthetic agent is diluted by the CSF as well as its being taken up by the neural elements.[29] Kitahara, using a local anesthetic solution to which radioactive iodine (^{131}I) had been added, demonstrated that a hyperbaric solution such as dibucaine-dextrose (specific gravity, 1.039) injected at L2–3 or L3–4, spread predominantly in a cephalad direction when the patient was supine on a level table.[35] These investigators also demonstrated the spread of hyperbaric anesthetic solutions with other positions and compared these results with the spread of isobaric solutions (Fig. 7-10).

As the local anesthetic solution spreads, a differential block occurs; that is, there is a zone where the concentration of the local anesthetic solution is highest and motor and all sensory modalities are blocked; at the most cephalad extent, however, only the sympathetic nerves are involved in the blockade. Although the B fibers—preganglionic autonomic (sympathetic and parasympathetic) fibers—are larger than C fibers, Heavner and colleagues have demonstrated that they are more susceptible to local anesthetic solutions.[28] At present under clinical conditions, it is not possible to determine the exact extent of vasomotor blockade above the sensory (analgesic) level. Further, Freund and associates have demonstrated that a differential exists between motor and sensory levels, averaging two spinal segments.

Immediately after injection, the local anesthetic agent is taken up by neural elements, although like epidural anesthesia, the exact site of action is con-

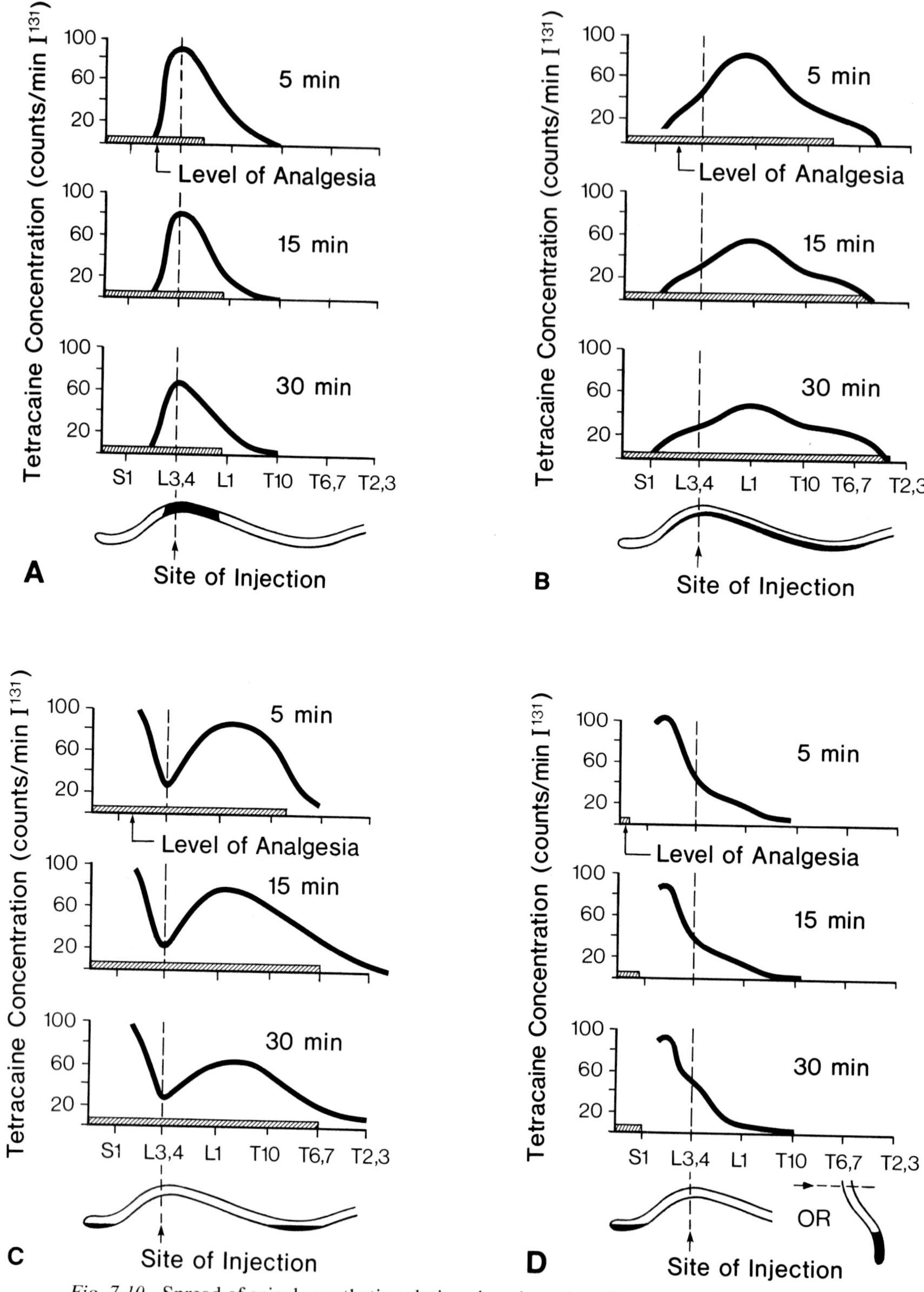

Fig. 7-10. Spread of spinal anesthetic solutions in subarachnoid space: (*A*) isobaric, (*B*) hyperbaric—head down, (*C*) hyperbaric—supine, and (*D*) saddle block.

troversial at present. Traditionally, it has been believed that the site of action of local anesthetic agents injected into the subarachnoid space is the spinal nerve roots.[44] However, Howarth, Bromage, and Cohen, using radioactive-isotope-labeled local anesthetic agents, have demonstrated in experimental animals that the local anesthetic accumulates along the posterior and lateral aspects of the spinal cord itself, as well as in the spinal nerve roots.[11,13,30]

The egress of local anesthetic agents following subarachnoid injection is primarily by vascular absorption with no hydrolysis or degradation taking place in the spinal fluid. Depending upon the type of local anesthetic, the drug is metabolized either in the plasma by pseudocholinesterase (*e.g.*, procaine and tetracaine), or in the liver (lidocaine and other amide-type local anesthetic agents; see Chap. 3). As the duration of anesthesia is, in part, a result of the rate of absorption from the subarachnoid space, the addition of a vasoconstrictor to the local anesthetic solution will retard absorption of the drug and, thus, increase the duration of anesthesia. Generally speaking, epinephrine will prolong the block about 50 per cent and phenylephrine, 100 per cent.[46,48]

PREOPERATIVE MANAGEMENT

The first step in the successful application of spinal anesthesia is proper patient selection. This is accomplished preanesthetically by evaluation of the patient through history, physical examination, laboratory data, and communication with the patient and surgical staff about details of the anticipated procedure.

Patient History

Every preanesthetic history is directed toward alternative techniques the anesthesiologist thinks might be used for the scheduled procedure. In this chapter, only spinal anesthesia, and its primary considerations, are discussed specifically. Some of these considerations are discussed earlier (Patients Suited for Spinal Anesthesia) in this chapter. It is certainly mandatory that the history of the organ systems elicit an accurate cardiorespiratory evaluation, related to the patient's blood volume and potential to develop or compensate for hypotension, and the implications of respiratory status for the level of spinal anesthesia. A careful neurologic history should be taken to elicit existing neurologic conditions that might complicate the evaluation of postspinal anesthesia recovery, immediate or latent, physically or psychologically. No reliable data show that the initiation of spinal anesthesia in itself will exacerbate preexisting neurologic disease such as multiple sclerosis, poliomyelitis, or even tertiary syphilis. However, there is, unfortunately, no proof that it will not. Spinal anesthesia is, therefore, usually avoided in patients with a history of such diseases.

Finally, an accurate drug history is important. Patients who receive drugs that affect the heart or circulation should be carefully considered for the possible interactions that may result after spinal anesthesia. For example, the effects of beta-blockade or peripheral sympathetic blockade may alter the usual response of the cardiovascular system to spinal anesthesia.

Physical Examination

Although physical findings of all systems are pertinent, careful documentation of preexisting neurologic findings is essential. This is extremely important in considering a spinal anesthetic for a patient following trauma. It might be extremely difficult, otherwise, to explain to consultants, the patient, or even the courts that the postanesthetic neurologic sequelae were a result of the patient's trauma and not the spinal anesthetic. Early recognition of neurologic deficits is essential to therapy (see pp. 172–173 for a discussion of complications from spinal anesthesia). If the presence or degree of preexisting neurologic signs and symptoms is not noted and recorded, it is impossible to determine what constitutes new findings. Finally, from a more technical standpoint, the examination of the skeletal system, especially the spine, will indicate potential difficulties that may be encountered in administering the spinal anesthetic. Patients with severe arthritis may be painfully or physically impossible to position appropriately. Conversely, intubation for general anesthesia is often difficult in patients with severe cervical arthritis. Such a finding may incline the anesthesiologist toward spinal rather than general anesthesia. Similarly, significant respiratory disease may also suggest the use of spinal anesthesia if there are no other contraindications.

Laboratory Data

The foregoing discussion of the history and physical examination reflects the special concerns that the cardiorespiratory and nervous systems pose for the anesthesiologist who plans spinal anesthesia. He must use the laboratory data then to provide additional documentation about these systems. Appropriate tests include the electrocardiogram (ECG), the hematocrit or blood volume, urine specific gravity, and coagulation deficits, such as abnormal prothrombin time or thrombocytopenia. Abnormal ventilatory studies would support the choice of spinal anesthesia and be an aid in subsequent management.

Communication With the Surgical Staff

Most surgical procedures are so routine as to require no advance discussion between the anesthesiologist and the surgeon. However, most anesthesiologists have had the perplexing experience of having a patient under spinal anesthesia because they assumed that the surgical requirements were clearly defined, only to have the surgeon enter the theater and alter the procedure sufficiently to compromise the anesthetic. The way to avoid this kind of unsatisfactory or inappropriate use of spinal anesthesia is to communicate with the surgeon before the operation so that the anesthesiologist will know the proper position of the patient and the extent and duration of the anticipated procedure. Examples of such problems are ureteral surgery, which may be undertaken through a pelvic approach in the supine position or from the high flank position to approach the renal pelvis. There are many other examples with which the anesthesiologist who uses spinal anesthesia is probably familiar.

Communication With the Patient

The final step in the selection of a spinal anesthetic should be the discussion of this and alternative anesthetic techniques with the patient. The two most common objections that patients raise to spinal anesthesia are their fear of being awake during the operation and their fear of having a "needle in their back." A few have also had or heard of the headache that sometimes may follow a spinal anesthetic. Usually, it is not at all difficult to reassure patients by outlining the sequence of events that lead to the operation. The patient should initially be told that he will have nothing to eat or drink after midnight of the day of surgery. Also, he should be informed that he will be given a sleeping pill at bedtime to ensure an adequate night's rest. He is told that the preanesthetic medication given 1 to 2 hours before surgery will make him relax and give him a dry mouth (narcotic + atropine). He should be told that when he arrives in the operating room, an intravenous line will be started and additional sedation given as necessary to keep him relaxed and comfortable during administration of the spinal anesthetic. He should know that next he will receive supplemental sedation up to and including complete general anesthesia, as needed, to keep him comfortable during the operation. Usually this narrative of events about supplemental sedation is sufficient to allay most of the patient's resistance to spinal anesthesia.

An extensive discourse on the advantages and disadvantages of premedication is inappropriate. Although it might be argued that prior to the administration of general anesthesia, patients need drugs that allay apprehension rather than provide analgesia, there is merit in combined sedation and analgesia for patients who undergo spinal anesthesia. Some barbiturates and tranquilizers produce states of tranquility in the quiet patient, but patients may become uncooperative and overreactive if they are painfully stimulated during and after the administration of the spinal anesthetic. However, with narcotics the patient will be cooperative. He will have analgesia for the mild discomfort of the needle and the awkward position on firm operating tables. In other words, preanesthetic narcotics not only add to the comfort and ease of administering the spinal anesthetic but supplement its effects during the operation, as well. The use of a belladonna drug before the spinal anesthetic, intravenously at the time of anesthesia, or not at all is a personal decision that takes into account such variables as patient dissatisfaction with a dry mouth, excess secretions, bradycardia, or hypotension. Ward and co-workers have shown that intravenous atropine was unusually effective in removing the nausea associated with high subarachnoid anesthesia.[65]

Contraindications

A disservice of medical writing, especially in textbooks and review articles, is the perpetuation of outdated, anecdotal, or undocumented statements. This seems to be especially pronounced in discussions of the risks and complications of a procedure or drug. Specifically, nearly every textbook of anesthesia has a section on the absolute and relative contraindications to spinal anesthesia. The proper function of lists of contraindications is to alert the anesthesiologist to the possibility that the frequency or magnitude of the potential complication may not justify the use of the technique. This hazard, of course, must be balanced with the perceived benefits that spinal anesthesia offers to a particular patient. The listing of "relative" contraindications implies, "Don't use spinal unless its benefits outweigh these potential risks or complications." Such an attitude is more in keeping with medical and surgical therapeutics. There, the risks and benefits of selected surgical procedures, even those with significant mortality and morbidity, are presented to the patient for his "informed consent." Such would be a more rational approach to the use of spinal anesthesia. The following list should be interpreted in this manner.

The "Contraindications" of Spinal Anesthesia

Absolute
- Localized infections of puncture site
- Generalized infections
  - septicemia, bacteremia
- Severe blood loss or shock
- Central nervous system diseases
- Abnormality of blood clotting mechanism (possibly)
- Specific cardiovascular diseases
- Miscellaneous conditions or disease states
  - Vasomotor instability
  - Various simulators of neurologic sequelae
- Patient refusal

Relative
- Diseases of the spinal column (deformities)
  - Arthritis, osteoporosis, metastases, extruded disc (possibly)
- Severe headache or backache
- Persistent bloody spinal taps
- The poor-risk patient (possibly, especially if there is specific pathology)
- Neurologic diseases or simulators
  - Poliomyelitis, PA, residual paralysis, vitamin deficiency (possibly)
- History of viral diseases
- Medicolegal considerations

(Lund, P.C.: Principles and Practice of Spinal Anesthesia. pp. 504–601. Springfield, Charles C Thomas, 1971)

The anesthesiologist wants to avoid infections or bleeding in the subarachnoid or peridural space. Any condition that might potentiate this risk should be fully assessed before instituting spinal anesthesia. Examples of these risks include localized or systemic infection and coagulopathies. Similarly, it is necessary to avoid cardiac arrest or irreversible hypoxic organ damage secondary to hypoperfusion (*i.e.*, hypotension). To that end, caution is warranted when patients with extremes of hypovolemia or cardiovascular disease are considered for spinal anesthesia, with the exception of saddle block. There are other conditions (neurologic and metabolic) that may contraindicate spinal anesthesia, but these should be evaluated on an individual basis. The empiric and generalized condemnation of spinal anesthesia for procedures or patients may deny some patients the opportunity to have the anesthetic of choice and subject the anesthesiologist to legal and professional censure if he acts against the advice of the textbooks.

TECHNIQUE

Equipment

The preference of the anesthesiologist can dictate whether disposable, commercially prepared, or reusable department-prepared spinal anesthesia trays are used. Reusable department-prepared trays must be meticulously prepared by conscientious, well-trained personnel, with care being taken to prevent chemical and bacterial contamination. Because the manufacturers of disposable trays have been able to duplicate almost completely the traditional reusable tray for spinal anesthesia, it appears that disposable spinal trays will eventually replace the traditional reusable tray.

Needles for Spinal Anesthesia. A needle with a close-fitting, removable stylet is essential. This will prevent coring of the skin and the rare, though possible, occurrence of epidermoid spinal cord tumors from the introduction of pieces of epidermis into the subarachnoid space. Over the years, a large number of spinal needles of various diameters with numerous types of points have been developed. In general, in order to keep the incidence of postpuncture headache to a minimum, needles either of small bore or with a rounded, noncutting bevel (Greene or Whitacre) should be used.

A description of a few of the more popular spinal needles follows (Fig. 7-11). The Quincke-Babcock spinal needle, the so-called standard spinal needle, has a sharp point with a medium-length cutting bevel. The Pitkin spinal needle has a sharp point, but short bevel with cutting edges and a rounded heel. Despite Pitkin's original claims, the incidence of postpuncture headache with this needle is relatively high. The Greene spinal needle has a rounded point and a rounded noncutting bevel of medium length. The Whitacre spinal needle, or the pencil-point needle, has a completely rounded, noncutting bevel with a solid tip, the opening of the needle being on the side, 2 mm proximal to the tip of the needle.[27] The Huber point needle has a curved tip for introducing catheters into the subarachnoid space. For the inexperienced, the use of either a 22-gauge Greene needle or a 22-gauge Whitacre needle is recommended because the characteristic "feel"

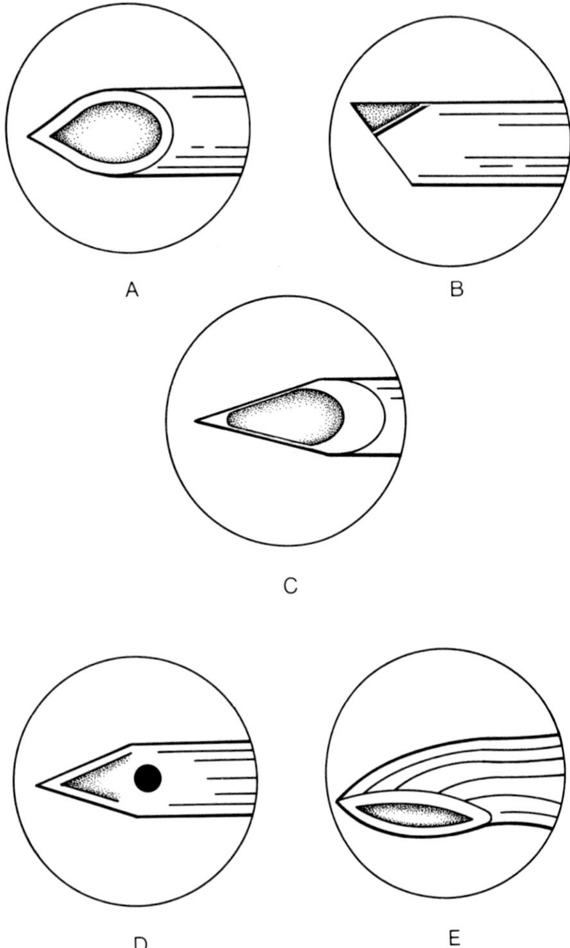

Fig. 7-11. Spinal needles: (*A*) Quincke-Babcock, (*B*) Pitkin, (*C*) Greene, (*D*) Whitacre, and (*E*) Touhy.

of the various structures can more readily be learned than with smaller-bore spinal needles, while simultaneously keeping the incidence of postpuncture headache low (2–7%).

Several combination, or double-needle, sets are available. One such set is composed of the standard 2-inch, 21-gauge Quincke-Babcock spinal needle with a stylet and a 3-½-inch, 26-gauge Quincke-Babcock needle with a close-fitting stylet. The 21-gauge introducer is inserted into either the ligamentum flavum or the epidural space, and puncture of the dura-arachnoid is made with the fine 26-gauge needle.

Regardless of the size of the needle used, care must be taken that the dural fibers that run longitudinally are separated rather than transected. With that in mind, regardless of the type of needle used, the opening bevel is always on the side of the notch on the hub of the needle, then the notch is arranged so that the needle bevel is parallel to the longitudinal dural fibers.

Introducers. Various introducers have been developed both to facilitate the introduction of small-bore spinal needles, which are not easily directed, and to prevent contact of the spinal needle with the skin, hence reducing the incidence of coring and the introduction of pieces of epidermis or bacteria into the subarachnoid space. As an alternative, a disposable 18-gauge needle may be used. The use of an introducer is particularly helpful with 25-gauge or 26-gauge needles (Fig. 7-12).

Drugs and Additives

The versatility of spinal anesthesia is afforded by a wide range of local anesthetic agents and additives that allow control over level and time of onset and duration of anesthesia. Discussion of some of the more common drugs used for spinal anesthesia follows (see Table 7-3; also Chap. 4 for a full description of each agent).

Procaine hydrochloride may be given subarachnoidally as a 2 per cent to 10 per cent aqueous solution or as a 5 per cent to 10 per cent solution in cerebrospinal fluid. A 5-per-cent solution in water is isosmotic with serum; to increase its specific gravity, 5 per cent dextrose may be added (hyperbaric technique). Procaine is marketed in ampules of dry crystals in amounts that vary from 50 mg to 300 mg

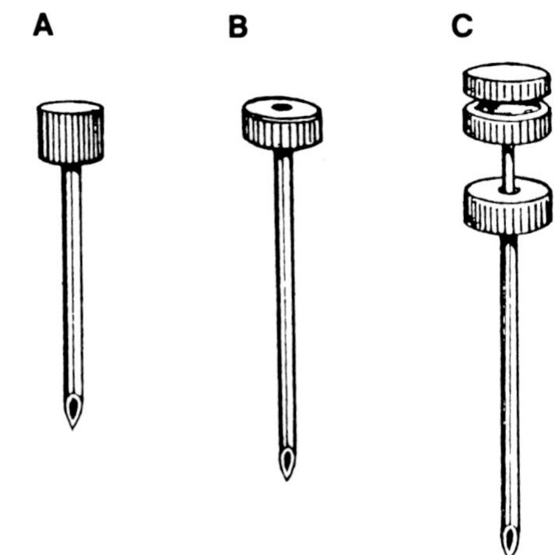

Fig. 7-12. Spinal needle guides and introducers: (*A*) Pitkin guide, (*B*) Sise introducer for 20-gauge or smaller spinal needles, and (*C*) Lundy modification of Sise with locking stylet. (Lund, P.C.: Principles and Practice of Spinal Anesthesia. Springfield, Charles C Thomas, 1971)

and in solutions of 5 per cent to 10 per cent. It can be autoclaved and is compatible with epinephrine. Procaine is preferably administered in strengths not to exceed 5 per cent, with the crystals being diluted in CSF, 1 ml per 50 mg of procaine. The 10-per-cent solution is often diluted with an equal volume of CSF before injection (isobaric technique). The duration of action of procaine is rarely more than 45 minutes. The suggested dosage ranges from 50 to 100 mg for perineal and lower extremity surgery to 150 to 200 mg for upper abdominal surgery.

Tetracaine may be administered subarachnoidally in strengths of 0.1 per cent to 0.5 per cent. It is marketed in ampules that contain 20 mg of crystals, which may be mixed with CSF prior to injection for the isobaric technique, and in a 1-per-cent solution that usually contains 10 to 20 mg. It may be autoclaved and is compatible with dextrose and epinephrine. Tetracaine, 0.1 per cent, in sterile water (1 mg/ml) is suitable for hypobaric techniques. The 1-per-cent solution with equal volumes of 10 per cent dextrose (0.5% tetracaine in 5% dextrose) is the usual mixture for hyperbaric techniques. The suggested dosage ranges from 5 mg for lower extremity and perineal surgery to 15 mg for upper abdominal surgery. It should be noted that although the volumes of solution vary with hypo- and hyperbaric spinal anesthesia, the dosage is nearly the same. The onset of analgesia with tetracaine occurs in 3 to 5 minutes. The duration of action for plain solutions is 60 to 90 minutes, that for solutions that contain epinephrine, 120 to 180 minutes.

Dibucaine hydrochloride is used for spinal anesthesia in concentrations of 0.1 per cent to 0.5 per cent dissolved in 6 per cent dextrose. The usual mixture is 0.5 per cent (5 mg/ml) in dextrose (1:200). A hypobaric solution that contains 0.067 per cent in 0.5 per cent sodium chloride is also available (1:1500). It may be autoclaved and is compatible with epinephrine. It darkens on exposure to light and should be protected. The recommended dosage is 3 to 5 mg for lower extremity and perineal surgery and 12 to 15 mg for upper abdominal surgery. Onset of analgesia is slightly slower for hypobaric solutions, being 3 to 5 minutes for hyperbaric and 5 to 16 minutes for hypobaric. The duration of anesthesia is 150 to 180 minutes for plain solutions and 180 to 240 minutes for solutions that contain epinephrine.

Lidocaine for spinal anesthesia is, almost universally, employed in the 5 per cent form (50 mg/ml) in a solution of 7.5 per cent dextrose. It is stable to autoclaving and is compatible with epinephrine. The recommended dosage varies from 30 to 50 mg for lower extremity and perineal surgery to 75 to 100 mg for upper abdominal surgery. The onset of analgesia is rapid, 3 to 5 minutes, but its duration is extremely short, 45 to 60 minutes with the plain solution and 75 to 90 minutes with solutions that contain epinephrine.

Other Drugs. It should be mentioned for the sake of completeness that mepivacaine, prilocaine, and bupivacaine have been used for spinal anesthesia.[51] None are currently in use, however. It was hoped that bupivacaine, with its extreme length of action for peripheral nerve and extradural blocks, would produce an equally lengthy duration of action for the subarachnoid block. Results of studies thus far have failed to demonstrate a duration of action greater than tetracaine or dibucaine.

Additives. *Vasoconstrictors.* There is still considerable difference of opinion, geographic and personal, about the role of adding vasoconstrictors to prolong the duration of anesthetic action of the various spinal anesthetic agents. At one extreme are case reports and articles that appeared 20 to 50 years ago reporting neurologic sequelae subsequent to spinal anesthesia when vasoconstrictors were used. At the other extreme are clinical papers that report a total in excess of 500,000 cases with no report of serious neurologic sequelae from spinal anesthesia, with or without vasoconstrictors (Table 7-4). One prospective study of 222 patients compared solutions that contained tetracaine with dextrose and tetracaine with epinephrine, 0.2 mg, or phenyl-

Table 7-4. Summary of Large Series of Spinal Anesthesia*

Authors	*Year of Publication*	*Number of Cases*
Dripps and Vandam	1954	10,098
Sadove and Levin	1961	20,000
Bonica	1953	12,000
Moore and Bridenbaugh	1966	11,574
Macer	1956	34,936
Ebner	1959	21,545
El-Sherbiny, et al.	1966	20,000
Jackson and Petch	1955	10,350
Romberger and Ratcliff	1948	10,000
Lund and Cwik	1967	25,000
Various series over 5000	1935–1965	31,098
Various series over 2000	1947–1965	16,589
Bridenbaugh, et al., survey	1967	359,000
Total		582,190

* No incidence of permanent motor paralysis reported
(Lund, P.C.: Principles and Practice of Spinal Anesthesia. pp. 504–601. Springfield, Charles C Thomas, 1971)

Table 7-5. Prolongation of Spinal Anesthesia by Vasopressors

		Prolongation by Vasopressors (%)		
Investigators	*Year*	*Epinephrine (mg)*	*Phenylephrine (mg)*	*Ephedrine (mg)*
Bray	1949	60 (1)	8 (5)	7 (50)
Sergent	1949	51 (0.5)	45 (1)	14 (50)
Bonica	1951	51 (0.2–0.5)	50 (2–5)	30 (20–50)
Brockmyer	1949		100 (3)	
Egbert	1960	12 (0.2) 27 (0.5)		
Moore	1966	50 (0.2)	100 (5)	Not significant (50)
Park	1974	53 (0.2)	72 (2)	

(Park, W. Y., Balingit, P. E., and Macnamara, T. E.: Effects of patient age, *p*H of cerebrospinal fluid and vasopressors on onset and duration of spinal anesthesia. Anesth. Analg., *54*:455, 1975)

ephrine, 2 mg. The results of this study showed 53 per cent prolongation with epinephrine and 72 per cent prolongation with phenylephrine. Their results have also been compared with previous authors (Table 7-5).[50]

EPINEPHRINE. The dose of epinephrine added to spinal solutions has, to date, been a standard 0.2 mg (0.2 ml of 1:1000) without regard to the volume or dose being injected; however, the minimum effective concentration is not known. Epinephrine has been shown to prolong the duration of tetracaine and lidocaine by 12 to 60 per cent.[50] Clearly, it is unnecessary to use vasoconstriction if the duration of action of the selected drug is adequate for the expected duration of surgery.

PHENYLEPHRINE. The recommended dose of phenylephrine is a standard 5 mg (0.5 ml of a 1% solution). It has been used primarily with tetracaine. Reports of prolongation vary from 8 to 100%.[46,50]

EPHEDRINE has been used and its results reported, but the results vary from no significant change to 30 per cent prolongation. It is seldom used.

Dextrose. The use of dextrose with all local anesthetic agents for spinal anesthesia is widespread. Since its role is to increase the specific gravity of the injectate for hyperbaric techniques, the concentration varies from 3 per cent to 5 per cent.

Steroids. Recently, the addition of steroids to the solutions injected subarachnoidally have been advocated for the treatment of low back pain (This is discussed in detail in Chap. 26).

Radiopaque dyes are commonly used by neuroradiologists in the diagnosis of spinal cord tumors and herniated intervertebral discs. Their reactivity in the subarachnoid space has been suggested as an explanation of the higher incidence of postdural puncture headache after myelography.

Position of the Patient

Inasmuch as all conduction anesthetics may potentially become general anesthetics, the preparation for spinal anesthesia should be the same as the preparation for general anesthesia. This includes a functional intravenous line, blood pressure monitor, and appropriate equipment for airway management. In the management of any technique, the spinal anesthesia should be administered to a cooperative patient who is lying on a table that can be tipped upward or downward. The primary advantage of spinal over epidural anesthesia is the ability to control the spread of the anesthetic by manipulation of the specific gravity of the solution and the position of the patient. Failure to utilize a movable table will lead to a higher incidence of both unsatisfactory anesthetics and of complications. Similarly, the anesthesiologist must be able to assess the spread if it is to be controlled. The spread in overly sedated or anesthetized patients is virtually impossible to assess, and, again, this will lead to a greater degree of failure or complications.

Lateral decubitus position is undoubtedly the most popular position for the performance of spinal anesthesia because of the comparative comfort it affords the patient (Fig. 7-13). The patient should be placed on the very edge of the table closest to the anesthesiologist. The vertebral column is then flexed to widen the interlaminal spaces, which is accomplished by drawing the knees up to the chest and putting the chin down on the chest, the head supported by a pillow. (Care must be taken that the vertebral column remains parallel with the edge of the table and the iliac crest and shoulders perpendicular to the table.) An assistant must stand in front of the patient to help the patient maintain the correct position. If the anesthesiologist is right-handed, the left lateral decubitus position should be used with the spinal anesthesia tray at the right of the anesthesiologist. If the patient is to be positioned prone or supine at the conclusion of administering the spinal anesthetic, the location of the operative site is immaterial. If, on the other hand, unilateral or hypobaric techniques are being employed, then position of the operative site appropriate to the relative baricity of solution is essential.

Sitting position is used less frequently than lateral decubitus, with the exceptions of low spinal anesthesia in obstetrics, certain gynecologic and uro-

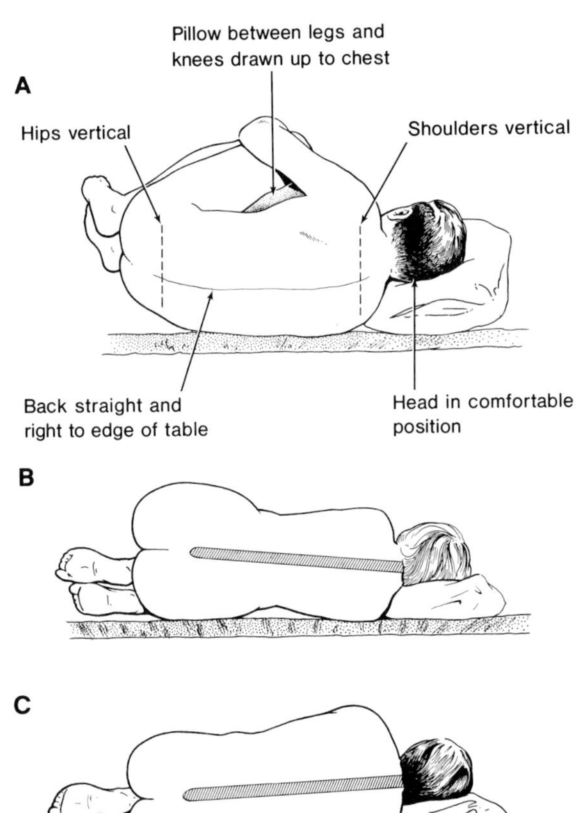

Fig. 7-13. Lateral decubitous position for spinal anesthesia. Note skeletal differences of (*B*) female and (*C*) male on level of subarachnoid space.

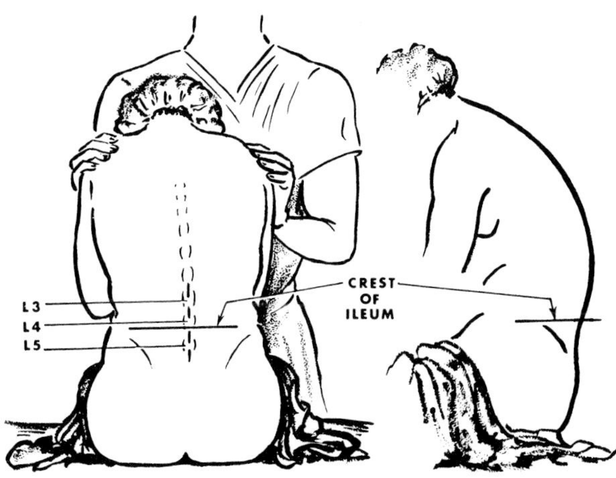

Fig. 7-14. Sitting position correctly demonstrated for spinal anesthesia. (Lund, P.C.: Principles and Practice of Spinal Anesthesia. Springfield, Charles C Thomas, 1971)

logic procedures, and certain hypobaric (and hyperbaric) techniques (Fig. 7-14). Precautions must be taken against hypotension when patients who have received moderate to heavy premedication or are prone to fainting are in the sitting position. As in the lateral decubitus position, the patient sits on the table as close to the anesthesiologist as possible, the feet supported by a stool. The patient's neck and back are flexed again to provide maximum opening of the interlaminal spaces. An assistant must stand in front of the patient at all times both to support and also to maintain the correct position of the patient.

Prone position is used primarily for the hypobaric technique for procedures on rectum, sacrum, and lower vertebral column. Preferably, the patient is placed on his abdomen on the operating table to avoid repositioning after induction of spinal anesthesia. The technique is most easily accomplished if the lumbar curve is extended by flexion of the table or by placing a pillow under the patient's abdomen. The spinal fluid pressure is low in this position, and, therefore, aspiration may be necessary to obtain a free flow of spinal fluid. Flow of spinal fluid may be facilitated by elevating the head of the table. If this is to be done and the technique is hypobaric, it is critical that the table be repositioned before injection of the anesthetic so that the highest portion of the vertebral column is at the desired level of anesthesia.

Preparation

Prior to the induction of any major anesthetic technique, there are fundamental preparations to be

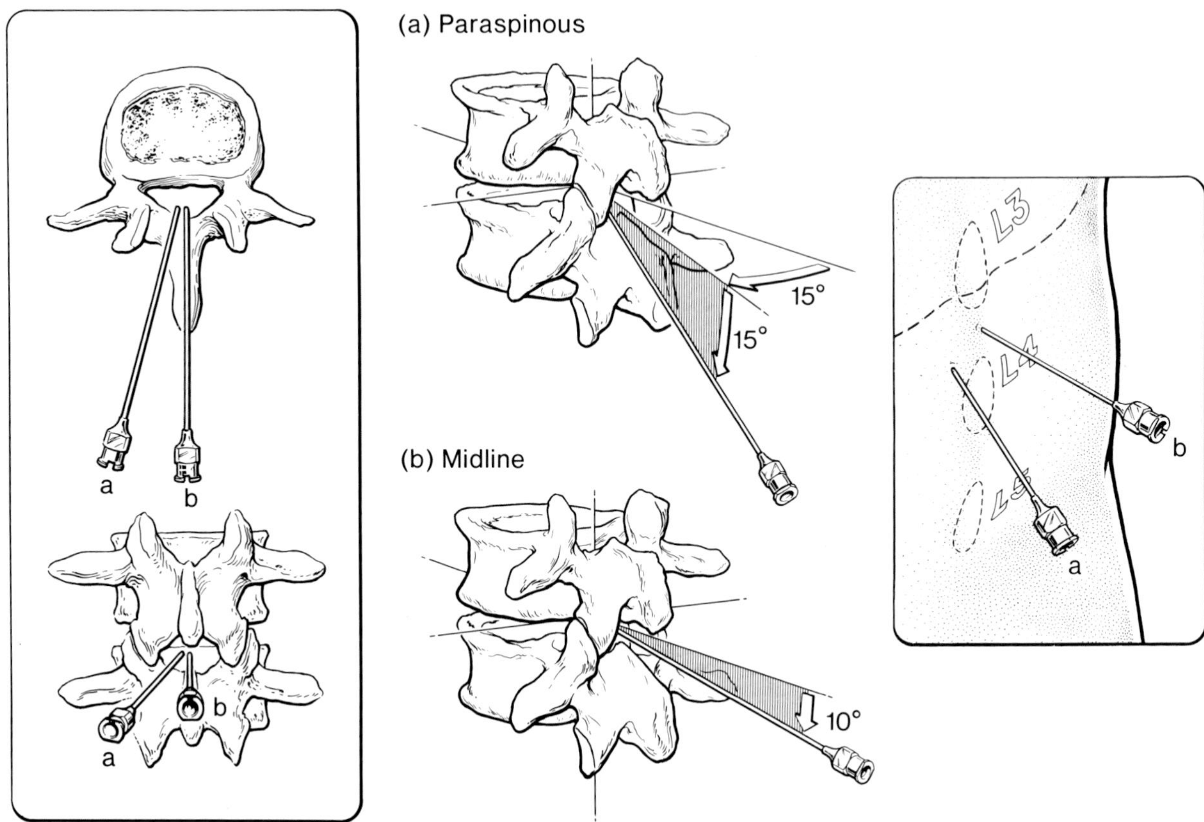

Fig. 7-15. Illustration of two common techniques of lumbar puncture for spinal anesthesia. (*top*) Paraspinous, paramedian, or lateral approach. (*bottom*) Midline.

accomplished. With rare exception, all patients who undergo a spinal anesthetic technique should initially have an intravenous cannula in place. Blood pressure and heart rate must be measured before anesthesia. The patient is then placed in the appropriate position, and the puncture area (usually lumbar), exposed.

Preparation of Equipment and Puncture Site. A previously prepared tray (hospital or commercial) should then be opened, and its sterility noted by checking the sterilization indicator. All subsequent activity should be performed using careful aseptic technique. The patient's back is then widely prepared with an antiseptic solution, and sterile drapes applied. After discarding the preparation solution, the anesthetic drugs may be prepared, being careful at all times to ensure no contamination of drugs or equipment with the preparation solution.

A line between the upper border of the iliac crest passes through either the spinous process of L4 or the interspace between L4 and L5. The anesthesiologist should position himself with the tray on his right (if right-handed) and the patient as nearly at eye level as possible. He may sit or stand as he prefers. Prior to any injection, he should inspect the spinal needle to make certain the stylet fits properly and that there are no barbs or foreign material on the tip of the needle. Care is taken not to handle the plunger of the syringe, which contains the spinal anesthetic solution, nor to touch the shaft of the spinal needle, which will subsequently be introduced into the subarachnoid space.

Depending upon the interspace and approach selected, an intracutaneous skin wheal is made at the puncture site with a 25- to 27-gauge, 1-cm needle attached to a 2- to 5-ml syringe. One to 2 ml of procaine, 1 per cent, or lidocaine, 1 per cent, are the usual drugs for skin wheals. Following this, subcutaneous infiltration may be accomplished with a 2- to 3-cm, 22-gauge needle. The patient is then ready for the introduction of the spinal needle.

Technique of Lumbar Puncture

Midline. Traditionally, midline with the patient lateral is the most popular approach (Fig. 7-15). If an introducer is being used, it is inserted through the skin wheal firmly into the interspinous ligament. Then the spinal needle is held like a dart (*i.e.*, the hub is held between the thumb and index finger with the third finger along the proximal part of the shaft of the needle). If no introducer is used, the skin and soft tissues are fixed against the bony landmarks by the second and third fingers of the left hand, which straddle the interspace.

The spinal needle is inserted through the same hole in the skin that was used to perform the intracutaneous wheal and subcutaneous infiltration. The bevel of the spinal needle should be directed laterally (notch facing upward), so that the dural fibers that run longitudinally are spread rather than transected. After traversing the skin and subcutaneous tissues, the needle is advanced in a slightly cephalad direction (100°–105° on the cephalad side) with the long axis of the vertebral column, care again being taken to stay absolutely in the midline. (Even in the lumbar area where the spinous processes of the lumbar vertebrae are relatively straight, the interlaminal space is slightly cephalad to the interspinous space.) There is a characteristic change in resistance as the needle traverses the ligamentum flavum and the dura-arachnoid, which becomes quite recognizable as experience is gained with this technique. The stylet is removed and CSF allowed to appear at the hub of the needle. If proper flow of spinal fluid does not occur, the needle is rotated in 90° increments until good flow is achieved. Occasionally, with patients in the prone position or if a small-bore spinal needle is being used, free flow of CSF will not be apparent. Gentle aspiration with a small, sterile syringe may then be used to obtain fluid.

With the hub of the spinal needle held firmly between the thumb and index finger of the left hand, the back of the left hand against the patient's back to prevent either withdrawal or advance of the spinal needle, the syringe containing the local anesthetic solution is firmly attached to the needle. Aspiration of spinal fluid is then performed, and if there is free flow, the local anesthetic solution is injected. Prior to removal of the spinal needle, aspiration and reinjection of a small amount of fluid are again performed to reconfirm that the tip of the needle is still in the subarachnoid space. The patient is then placed in the desired position; cardiovascular and respiratory functions are monitored frequently; and the analgesic level to pinprick or temperature level with alcohol is checked at 5-minute intervals until the desired level is achieved. The patient should be repositioned as necessary, according to the baricity of the injected solution to achieve this desired level. However, this must be accomplished within the "fixing time" of approximately 20 minutes for the local anesthetic.

Paramedian (Lateral) Approach. There are many variations of the paramedian (lateral) approach that avoid traversing the sometimes narrowed or calcified interspinous space. This approach is especially useful when degenerative changes are encountered in the interspinous structures (*e.g.*, in elderly patients) and when ideal positioning of the patient cannot be achieved, owing to pain (*e.g.*, fractures and dislocations involving the hips and lower extremities).

The patient is placed in the flexed lateral decubitus position, and a skin wheal raised 1.5 cm lateral to the midline directly opposite the cephalad tip of the spinous process below the selected interspace. The direction of the spinal needle is at an angle of approximately 15° to 20° with the midline and slightly cephalad, 100° to 105° on the cephalad side. As with the midline approach, there is a characteristic "feel" encountered as the needle passes through the ligamentum flavum and dura-arachnoid. At this point, the advance is stopped and the stylet withdrawn to allow spinal fluid to appear in the hub of the needle. If periosteum rather than the subarachnoid space is encountered, the needle should be redirected slightly cephalad, thus walked off the laminae into the interspace. Anesthesiologists should remember that the interlaminal space is created by the failure of the laminae to unite in the midline. If the needle is walked off the laminae, it must enter the interlaminal space and on into the subarachnoid space. Once the tip of the needle lies within the subarachnoid space, the remainder of the technique for administering spinal anesthesia is identical to that described previously for the midline approach.

The Taylor approach is a special paramedian approach to enter the L5 interspace (the largest interlaminal space). It was originally described for urologic procedures but was subsequently used for other operations in the pelvis and perineum.[60] The patient is placed in the flexed lateral decubitus position, and a 12-cm spinal needle is inserted through a skin wheal made 1 cm medial and 1 cm caudad to the lowest part of the posterior–superior iliac spine. The needle is directed medially and cephalad at an angle of 55° into the subarachnoid space. Again, if periosteum is encountered, the needle is withdrawn and redirected slightly cephalad or walked into the correct location. Once the needle has been placed in the subarachnoid space, the remaining steps are identical to those described for the midline approach (Fig. 7-16).

The continuous catheter approach is a standard

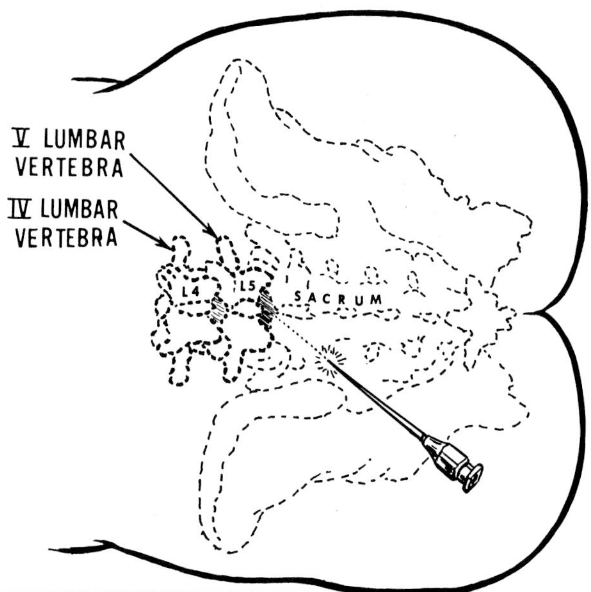

Fig. 7-16. Taylor approach to spinal anesthesia. (Lund, P.C.: Principles and Practice of Spinal Anesthesia. Springfield, Charles C Thomas, 1971)

midline approach but with a Huber-tip needle that will allow passage of a plastic catheter through its lumen. The bevel of the needle is most advantageously directed cephalad during the advancement of the needle through the interspinous ligament. The tip acts like a ski directing the needle between the spines along their natural slant, whereas if it were turned longitudinally, the tendency would be to direct the needle laterally out of the interspinous ligament. Once the needle is on, or just through the ligamentum flavum, then the bevel is rotated 90° to be parallel to the dural fibers prior to entry into the subarachnoid space. Once free flow of CSF is observed, the needle should be advanced another 1 to 2 mm to ensure that the entire tip of the needle is within the subarachnoid space; otherwise, the catheter will impinge on the dura as it emerges from the tip of the needle. The threading and fixation of the catheter are identical to the technique used for epidural anesthesia. Because stimulation of the nerve roots by the catheter tip is painful and because the catheter could conceivably enter a subarachnoid vessel, it is preferable to thread it only 2 to 4 cm beyond the top of the needle. Once free flow of CSF through the catheter has been demonstrated, local anesthetic may be injected. The use of a millipore filter at the injection end of the catheter is recommended for all doses not administered at the time of initiation of the catheter.

There is obviously no advantage to adding epinephrine to agents being injected through the catheter since the duration is limitless anyway. Subsequent doses through the catheter may be reduced by 30 per cent to 50 per cent from the original dose.

PHYSIOLOGIC EFFECTS

In the past 10 to 15 years, there have been extensive, carefully controlled studies in humans that have defined the systemic cardiovascular and respiratory effects of spinal anesthesia, as well as the effects of this anesthetic on renal, hepatic, coronary, and cerebral circulations.

Systemic Cardiovascular Effects. During high spinal anesthesia, there is a reduction in coronary blood flow and myocardial oxygen consumption that parallels the decrease in mean arterial pressure.[26]

The degree of arterial hypotension that accompanies spinal anesthesia is directly related to the degree of sympathetic blockade; that is, the more spinal segments that are blocked, the greater the decrease in arterial pressure. In studies of healthy, young, unmedicated male volunteers in whom no surgical procedures were performed, a 15 to 20 per cent decrease in mean arterial pressure, central venous pressure, and total peripheral resistance with high, T5, spinal anesthesia was observed (Fig. 7-17).[32,33] Although only minimal reductions in cardiac output, cardiac rate, and stroke volume were observed, two subjects developed transient asystole accompanied by a marked drop in blood pressure when the analgesic level rose to T2–3.[22] Although these patients were readily resuscitated, it is recommended that, prior to the induction of a high spinal anesthetic, atropine be administered intravenously (see Fig. 8-21).

It should be emphasized that older patients and those with poor physical status do not tolerate high spinal anesthesia as well as younger patients, and more profound hypotension should be anticipated. Depending upon the circumstances, often the administration of 500 to 1000 ml of normal saline or a balanced electrolyte solution immediately before administering the block will reduce the magnitude of cardiovascular changes. Unlike epidural anesthesia, the addition of epinephrine to the local anesthetic solution injected into the subarachnoid space does not have any effect on the systemic circulation (see Table 8-7).[10] Low spinal (saddle block) anesthesia produces no change in cardiovascular function, provided the upper lumbar segments are not blocked (Table 7-1).

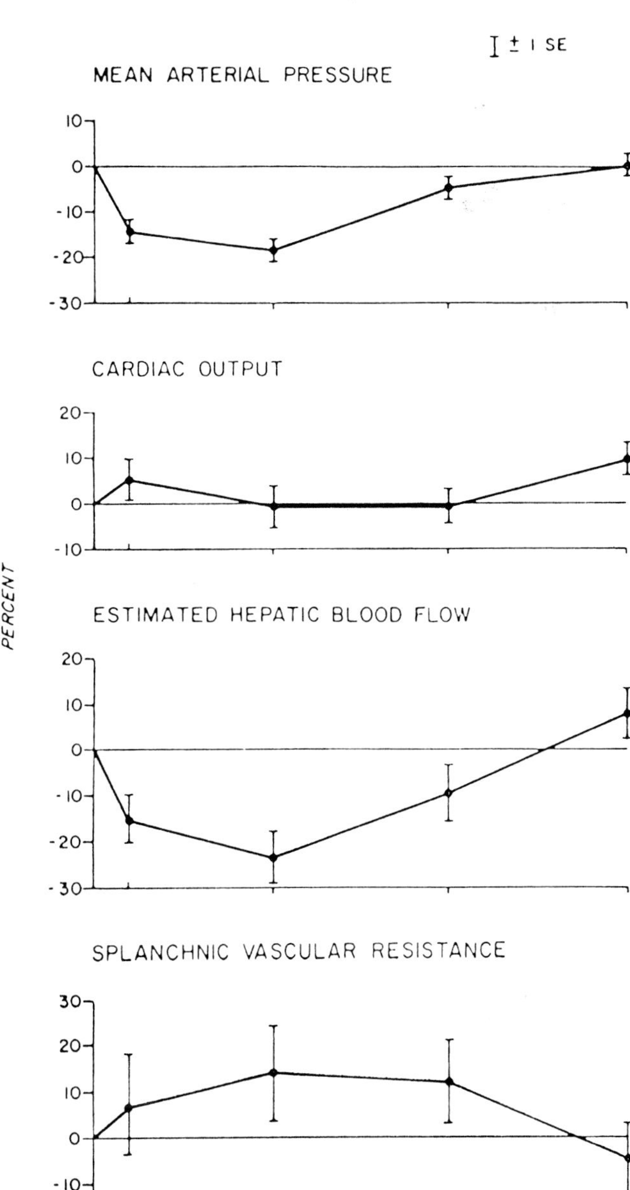

Fig. 7-17. Effect of high (T5) spinal anesthesia on circulation. (*A*) mean arterial pressure, (*B*) cardiac output, (*C*) estimated hepatic blood flow, and (*D*) splanchnic vascular resistance. (Kennedy, W.F., Jr.: Effects of spinal and peridural blocks on renal and hepatic functions. *In* Bonica, J.J. [ed.]: Regional Anesthesia: Recent Advances and Current Status. Clinical Anesthesia Series. vol. 2. p. 117. Philadelphia, F.A. Davis, 1969)

Respiratory Effects. Although it has traditionally been maintained that high spinal anesthesia impairs respiration, recent evidence indicates that resting ventilation is not impaired. As mentioned above, during spinal anesthesia the motor level is two to three segments below the sensory level. The degree of motor blockade is usually more profound at each blocked segment than that produced by epidural block; thus, for a given sensory level, spinal anesthesia produces a more profound effect on respiration than does epidural. Freund and colleagues and Egbert and associates observed only a 20 per cent decrease in the inspiratory capacity with motor block of all the thoracic spinal nerve roots.[18,21,22] In contrast, the expiratory reserve volume decreased sharply and was eventually reduced to zero when motor block of all the thoracic spinal nerve roots was achieved. Again, resting ventilation was not impaired, nor were there significant alterations in blood gas measurements. However, it is likely that

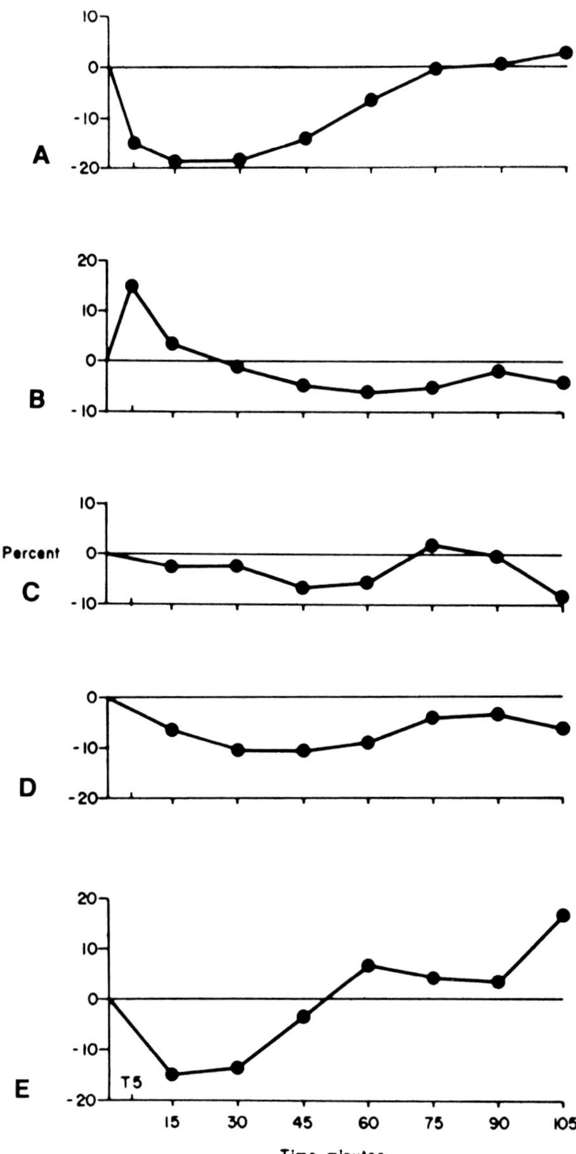

Fig. 7-18. Effect of high (T5) spinal anesthesia on renal function. (*A*) mean arterial pressure, (*B*) cardiac output, (*C*) effective renal plasma flow, (*D*) glomerular filtration rate, and (*E*) renal vascular resistance. (Kennedy, W.F., Jr.: Effects of spinal and peridural blocks on renal and hepatic function. *In* Bonica, J.J. [ed.]: Regional Anesthesia: Recent Advances and Current Status. Clinical Anesthesia Series. vol. 2. p. 112. Philadelphia, F.A. Davis, 1969)

ability to cough was effectively reduced. Low spinal (saddle block) anesthesia has no effect on respiratory function.

Renal Circulation and the Genitourinary System. Both Smith and associates and Kennedy and associates demonstrated that, in normal men who did not undergo surgical procedures, high spinal anesthesia had only a slight effect (5–10% reduction) on renal function, glomerular filtration rate (GFR), and effective renal plasma flow (ERPF) (Fig. 7-18).[32,56*] These changes, though statistically significant, are probably of little clinical significance in the normotensive, normovolemic patient. Sphincters of the bladder are not relaxed, in contrast to the anal sphincter, which is. Although the GFR may be reduced with blood pressure, the bladder (S2 and S3) is innervated by small autonomic fibers, which are the last to regain function, and, therefore, postoperative urinary retention is not uncommon. The penis is flaccid and engorged, owing to paralysis of the nervi erigentes (S2 and S3). This is a useful sign of successful block and is also the basis for the use of spinal anesthesia to relieve the pain of priapism.

Hepatic Circulation. In humans in whom no surgical procedures were performed, Mueller and associates and Kennedy and associates studied the effects of high spinal anesthesia on hepatic blood flow by the hepatic clearances of Bromsulphalein (BSP) and indocyanine green, respectively.[32,49] Both groups of investigators demonstrated that the decrease in estimated hepatic blood flow paralleled the decrease in arterial pressure; blood flow to this vital organ returned to normal with the recovery of the arterial pressure as the spinal anesthetic level receded (Fig. 7-17).

Cerebral Circulation. Kleinerman and associates observed only minimal alterations in cerebral blood flow during high spinal anesthesia; a decrease in cerebrovascular resistance maintained cerebral blood flow at the preblock level.[36]

Gastrointestinal System. Preganglionic sympathetic fibers from T5 to L1 are inhibitory to the gut. The small intestine, under spinal anesthesia, is contracted, owing to the relatively unopposed activity of the vagus nerve. Sphincters are relaxed, and peristalsis in normally active. The spleen may enlarge two- to threefold if its efferent fibers (splanchnic nerves) are blocked. Stimuli from surgical activity in the upper abdomen may be perceived as "visceral pain" by the lightly sedated patient as these impulses ascend by way of the unblocked vagal fibers. Paraesophageal infiltration of local anesthetic solution to block the vagus nerve will eliminate this response.

Endocrine System. Spinal anesthesia may delay adrenal response to trauma. Whereas operations under general anesthesia may increase blood

* Kennedy, W.F., Jr.: Unpublished data.

steroid levels and cause eosinopenia, this does not occur with spinal anesthesia. Increases in 17 hydroxycorticosteroids also do not occur with spinal anesthesia, compared to marked increases with general anesthesia (see Fig. 8-22).

POSTOPERATIVE MORTALITY

A randomized prospective controlled study of mortality following surgery for fractured neck of the femur compared mortality rates of spinal and general anesthesia.[43a] Two weeks postoperatively, no patients who had had spinal anesthesia had died, but the mortality rate with general anesthesia was 25 per cent. At 4 weeks following surgery, the mortality rate was 31 per cent in the general anesthesia group and 3.6 per cent in the spinal group. The only weakness of this study was the small number of patients studied (55); however, the differences between spinal and general anesthesia were significant even after applying the Yate's correction factor to allow for the small sample size. It is of interest that unilateral spinal blockade was performed in this study with hyperbaric tetracaine without epinephrine. However, patients were kept on the blocked side for only 3 minutes after the injection so that bilateral sympathetic blockade almost certainly resulted in most patients.

INTRAOPERATIVE MANAGEMENT

The first 5 to 10 minutes after administration of the spinal anesthetic are probably the most critical, especially in assessing the pure effect of the spinal on the circulation and adjusting the level of anesthesia (see Table 7-2). Frequent checks of blood pressure and pulse will allow diagnosis and treatment of any degree of hypotension. Once that baseline is established, superimposed effects of sedation and surgery can be better appreciated and treated accordingly. Treatment of spinal hypotension must be individualized to the status of the patient's cardiovascular and renal function. If he is healthy but relatively volume-depleted from enemas, vomiting, reduced fluid intake, fever, and so forth, then volume expansion with crystalloid solutions is indicated. However, if the patient has significant renal or cardiac disease, then colloids, blood, or vasopressors, alone or in combination, may be indicated. In brief, the volume most likely lacking can usually be added to the dilated vascular bed.

Having achieved cardiocirculatory stability of the administered spinal anesthetic, the anesthesiologist may then proceed with the assessment and management of ventilation. This may vary from administration of supplemental insufflated oxygen to the lightly sedated patient under low spinal anesthesia to intubated inhalation anesthesia to protect the airway and assist ventilation in the unconscious patient under high spinal anesthesia or the patient with severe respiratory disease. Loss of the intercostal musculature *per se* with high spinal anesthesia has virtually no detrimental effect on resting ventilation (see pp. 169–170).

The remaining organ system to be considered in the intraoperative management of spinal analgesia is the nervous system. The diversity of opinion on kinds and degrees of supplemental CNS depression (sedation) is great and probably reflects the lack of objective data to document superior efficacy of any single approach or agent. Primary consideration should be given to the patient's physical and psychological status. Very poor-risk patients are often given spinal anesthesia to avoid the use of systemic depressants. In contrast, an agitated healthy, young patient who undergoes major prolonged surgery with spinal anesthesia may receive inhalation anesthesia. All degrees of supplementation between these extremes may be used to meet the needs of the particular patient and surgeon for a given procedure.

POSTOPERATIVE MANAGEMENT

The anesthesiologist's role postoperatively can be divided into two periods. The first is actually a continued monitoring of the anesthetized patient in the recovery unit until complete cessation of the spinal anesthesia has occurred. Concerns during this period commence with the careful movement and transport of the patient from the operating room to the unit. It is not uncommon for such activities to precipitate some degree of hypotension owing to redistribution of blood volume with movement, so careful monitoring of the blood pressure is essential. If the patient does not have an indwelling urinary catheter, then recovery-room personnel should be watchful for a distended bladder. The voiding mechanism is mediated through sacral autonomic fibers, which are the last to regain function after spinal anesthesia. Even after patients are able to move their extremities and respond to sensory stimuli, they may have some residual autonomic blockade that not only would prevent voiding but would also cause postural hypotension if they were to be prematurely placed in a sitting or standing position.

The second phase of the postoperative period is the postanesthetic period. The role of the anesthesiologist becomes surveillance with special attention to the possible development of postanesthetic complications. Equally as important as the detection of bona fide complications is good rapport with the patient, which will permit the explanation of postsurgical aches and pains and the dismissal of them as not being caused by spinal anesthesia.

Complications and treatment

Backache. One of the most frequent complaints in the postanesthetic period is backache. Lund, in reviewing the literature, found an incidence of backache varying from 2 to 25 per cent.[41] Although it is remotely possible that needle puncture of an intervertebral disc might result in postanesthetic backache, the more likely and understandable cause is the flattening of the normal lordotic lumbar curve secondary to relaxation of the muscles and ligaments of the back. This, presumably, results in stretching of joint capsules, ligaments, and muscles beyond their normal "self-protective" range and results in pain. To this extent, it seems just as likely that a patient who receives paralyzing doses of muscle relaxants would suffer the same problem and that the lithotomy position might even exaggerate the condition. A study by Brown evaluated patients who received both general and spinal anesthesia.[12] The incidence of backache in this study showed no significant differences between the two techniques.

Headache. The next most common complication of spinal anesthesia postoperatively is headache. This is more appropriately called *post-dural-puncture headache* rather than *spinal headache*. Although it can be a post-spinal-anesthetic problem, it is more likely to occur after diagnostic lumbar puncture and myelography. Just as many patients have backache in the postoperative period; they also have headache. Not *all postspinal anesthesia* headaches are due to the dural puncture. It is important, therefore, to be conversant with the diagnostic features that are unique to this complication.

Features of Post-lumbar-puncture Headache

Onset, 24–48 hr after puncture
Postural headache, exacerbated by standing
Location, occipital and cervical and may also be frontal
Accompanying symptoms, blurred vision, tinnitus, etc., if headache severe

They include some or most of the following: onset—usually not until 24 to 48 hours postoperatively; postural headache—headache is first noted when patient sits or stands for a brief period and subsides or disappears upon resumption of the horizontal position; location—the most common complaint is occipital with radiation down the posterior cervical region (however, it may also be described as frontal and posterior orbital); auditory and visual disturbances—very infrequently (<1%). The severe spinal headache will be accompanied by visual disturbances such as diplopia, dizziness, or blurred vision, or auditory complaints of tinnitus or decreased hearing acuity.

Once the diagnosis of post-dural-puncture headache is established, prompt treatment is essential. Until the past few years, treatment was conservative and serially progressive to the point that therapeutic efficacy could not be separated from the self-limiting nature of the process itself. The earliest measure was prophylactic in the form of enforced flat bedrest for 24 to 48 hours. This, of course, became therapeutic once the headache had occurred. Symptomatic treatment with analgesics or sedatives is just that and probably has no beneficial effect in reversing the process. The most popular current concept of the pathophysiology is loss of CSF through the puncture site with resultant intracranial tension on meningeal vessels and nerves. Therapeutic modalities have, therefore, been directed at restoring the pressure relationships in the peridural and subarachnoid spaces. This has included such measures as the following: abdominal binders forcing more venous blood through epidural plexuses, injection of saline in large volumes into the epidural space, overhydration of the patient—orally or intravenously—to stimulate production of CSF, and antidiuresis. In practical terms, many mild headaches may be resolved with forced fluid intake of 3 or more liters per day, plus the use of a tight abdominal binder when the patient is sitting or standing.

In 1970, DiGiovanni reported on 50 patients who received epidural injections of autologous blood as treatment for post-lumbar-puncture headache.[16] Subsequently, and despite fears of infection and neurologic sequelae, the procedure has become an important therapy, employed progressively earlier. Abouleish summarized 524 cases reported by 11 centers.[1] He also reported a prospective study of an additional 118 patients. The technique of autologous blood patch is simply the establishment of a needle in the epidural space by the usual methods, followed by the injection of 5 to 10 ml of blood drawn aseptically from the patient's own antecubital vein. If patients are at all volume-depleted, it is desirable simultaneously to infuse 1000 ml of intravenous fluid. Subsequent to the injection, the patient remains supine for 30 to 60 minutes. The success rate after the first injection varies from 89 to 95 per cent. The procedure may be repeated 24 hours later and will provide equivalent success. Reported complications are few and mild. They include backache (35%), neck ache (0.9%), and transient temperature elevation (5%) of 24 to 48 hours' duration. It appears, then, that this is a worthwhile procedure with minor known risk, which should be considered if early conservative measures fail.

Neurologic Sequelae. The remaining complications of postspinal anesthesia fall in the category of neurologic sequelae. Although these are the most feared and most serious of all complications, they are extremely rare.[16a,47] Lund tabulated the major series of spinal anesthesia reported between 1948 and 1958.[41] Of these 582,190 cases of spinal anesthesia, he stated that "no incidence of permanent motor paralysis reported" (Table 7-4). Nonetheless, cases have been reported. It is obviously important to both patient and anesthetist alike that every postanesthetic complication be examined critically with reference to prevention of similar complications. This is especially important with neurologic sequelae after spinal anesthesia.

Nowhere in the foregoing have any of these neurologic complications been identified as being caused by spinal anesthesia. This is not to say that that is not possible but rather that not all post-spinal-anesthetic neurologic complications are directly related to the anesthetic; perhaps, they are not even indirectly related to the anesthetic and, even more perplexing, may never have a proven etiology. Much of the negative image of spinal anesthesia had been a result of "speculative etiology by association."

It is important to keep the perspective that determination of etiology should not be fault-motivated but rather therapy-oriented. To that end, the important first step in any neurologic complication is early detection, diagnosis, and treatment. The degree of irreversibility of many of these complications is time-related. Since most anesthesiologists are not trained neurologists, an early neurologic consultation is mandatory. There are two potential categories of neurologic complications, which may aid in the diagnosis and treatment. Etiologically, the injury to the nervous structures may be toxic (*e.g.*, chemicals and drugs) viral or bacterial, traumatic, or ischemic (*e.g.*, subdural or peridural hemorrhage or vascular occlusion). Anatomically, injuries may be categorized as peripheral nerve, cauda equina, spinal cord, and intracranial. Of these two classifications, the anatomic is more helpful in diagnosis. Peripheral nerves usually have multiple nerve root origins. A complication in a unilateral peripheral nerve distribution (*e.g.*, hypoesthesia or weakness), is more likely secondary to trauma to the nerve, secondary to positioning, or secondary to operative trauma than to spinal anesthesia. The precise location, by a neurologist, of the neural distribution of the lesion is essential in arriving at an appropriate differential diagnosis and treatment. In contrast, bilateral involvement, whether cauda equina or higher up the spinal cord, would be more indicative or a peridural or subarachnoid injury with totally different therapeutic and prognostic implications. Anesthesiologists and surgeons alike should realize that patients who have complications are not interested in fault if they are assured that everyone is working together for an early diagnosis and treatment.

From the prophylactic viewpoint, there is merit in the anesthesiologist's reviewing the etiologic categorization. Strict attention must be paid to the cleansing of the patient, particularly the locally or systemically infected patient. Care should be exercised to eliminate introduction of detergents or chemicals into the subarachnoid space and extreme caution to ensure use of the correct drugs and vasopressors in the correct concentrations. Traumatic complications can usually be avoided by careful and cooperative positioning of the patient by the surgeon and the anesthesiologist with awareness of the vulnerability of peripheral nerves for the particular surgical procedure. Certainly, the anesthesiologist always endeavors to use an atraumatic spinal technique but should be sensitive to early abandonment rather than perseverance in extremely difficult cases. The risks of hemorrhage can be lessened with knowledge of (and perhaps avoidance of) patients with coagulopathies. The safe use of spinal anesthesia in patients with low-dose heparin is yet to be resolved. Bloody taps should be watched carefully in the postanesthetic period. Most perplexing of all is the question of vascular occlusion (*i.e.*, anterior spinal artery thrombosis). If, why, and how often this occurs is also not established. In most of the reported cases thus far, it seems to be a diagnosis of presumption or exclusion. Therapeutically and prognostically, it is probably not important to know the etiology, but prophylactically that may be an important factor.

NEUROLYTIC SUBARACHNOID BLOCK

Subarachnoid block with alcohol, phenol, and hypertonic saline (warm or cold) are useful techniques in the treatment of chronic pain problems. The techniques, agents, indications, and complications of this utilization of spinal anesthesia are discussed in Chapter 27.

REFERENCES

1. Abouleish, E., Vega, S., Blendinger, I., and Tio, T.: Long term follow-up of epidural blood patch. Anesth. Analg., *54*:459, 1975.
2. Akamatsu, T.J.: Cardiovascular response to spinal anesthesia. *In* Bonica, J.J. (ed.): Regional Anesthesia. Recent Advances and Current Status. Clinical Anesthesia Series. vol. 2. Pp. 84–96. Philadelphia, F. A. Davis, 1969.
3. Babcock, W.W.: Foreward. *In* Maxson, L.H.: Spinal Anesthesia. Philadelphia, J.B. Lippincott, 1938.
4. Barker, A.E.: A report in clinical experiences with spinal anesthesia in 100 cases and some reflections on the procedure. Br. Med. J., *1*:665, 1907.
5. Batson, O.V.: The function of the vertebral veins and their role in the spread of metastases. Ann. Surg., *112*:138, 1940.
6. Bier, A.: Versuche Uber Cocainisirung des Ruckenmarkes. Deutsch. Z. Chir., *51*:361, 1899.
7. Bizarri, D., Giuffrida, J.G., Bandoc, L., and Fierro, F.E.: Continuous spinal anesthesia using a special needle and catheter. Anesth. Analg. (Cleve.), *43*:393, 1964.
8. Bonica, J.J., Kennedy, W.F., Jr., Ward, R.J., and Tolas, A.G.: A comparison of the effects of high subarachnoid and epidural anesthesia. Acta Anaesth. Scand. *23* [*Suppl.*]:429, 1966.
9. Bonica, P.R.: Cardiovascular effects of peridural block. *In* Bonica, J.J. (ed.): Regional Anesthesia: Recent Advances and Current Status. Clinical Anesthesia Series. vol. 2. Pp. 64–81. Philadelphia, F.A. Davis, 1969.
10. Bromage, R.P.: The physiology and pharmacology of epidural blockade. *In* Bonica, J.J. (ed.): Regional Anesthesia: Recent Advances and Current Status. Clinical Anesthesia Series. vol. 2. Philadelphia, F.A. Davis, 1969.
11. Bromage, P.R., Joyal, A.D., and Binney, J.C.: Local anesthetic drugs: Penetration from the spinal extradural space into the neuraxis. Science, *140*:392, 1963.
12. Brown, E.M., and Elman, D.S.: Postoperative backache. Anesth. Analg. (Cleve.), *40*:683, 1961.
13. Cohen, E.N.: Distribution of local anesthetic agents in the neuraxis of the dog. Anesthesiology, *29*:1002, 1968.
14. Corning, J.L.: Spinal anesthesia and local medication of the cord. N. Y. State J. Med., *42*:483, 1885.
15. Davidson, H.H., Hingson, R.A., and Helman, L.M.: Use of various plastic catheters in the subarachnoid and peridural spaces. Arch. Surg., *62*:540, 1951.
16. DiGiovanni, A.J., and Dunbar, B.S.: Epidural injections of autologous blood for postlumbar puncture headache. Anesth. Analg. (Cleve.), *49*:268, 1970.

16a. Dripps, R.D., and Vandam, L.D.: Long term follow-up of patients who received 10,098 spinal anesthetics. I. Failure to discover major neurological sequelae. J.A.M.A., *156*:1486, 1954.

17. Ebner, H.: An evaluation of spinal anesthesia in obstetrics. Anesth. Analg. (Cleve.), *38*:378, 1959.
18. Egbert, L.D., Tamersoy, K., and Deas, T.C.: Pulmonary function during spinal anesthesia: The mechanism of cough depression. Anesthesiology, *22*:882, 1961.
19. Ernst, E.A.: In-vitro changes of osmolality and density of spinal anesthetic solutions. Anesthesiology, *29*:104, 1968.
20. Freund, F.G.: Respiratory effects of subarachnoid and epidural block. *In* Bonica, J.J. (ed.): Regional Anesthesia: Recent Advances and Current Status. Clinical Anesthesia Series. vol. 2. Pp. 98–107. Philadelphia, F.A. Davis, 1969.
21. Freund, F.G., Bonica, J.J., Ward, R.J., Akamatsu, T.J., and Kennedy, W.F., Jr.: Ventilatory reserve and level of motor block during high spinal and epidural anesthesia. Anesthesiology, *28*:834, 1967.
22. Gerbershagen, H.U., and Kennedy, W.F., Jr.: Hertzstillstand nach hoher spinalanaesthesia. Anaesthetist, *20*:192, 1971.
23. Greene, B.A.: A 26-gauge lumbar puncture needle: Its value in the prophylaxis of headache following spinal analgesia for vaginal delivery. Anesthesiology, *11*:464, 1950.
24. Greene, H.M.: A technic to reduce the incidence of headache following lumbar puncture in ambulatory patients with a plea for more frequent examination of cerebrospinal fluids. Northwest Med., *22*:240, 1923.
25. Greene, N.M.: Physiology of Spinal Anesthesia. pp. 1–3. Baltimore, Williams & Wilkins, 1958.
26. Hackel, D.B., Sancetta, S.M., and Kleinerman, J.: Effect of hypotension due to spinal anesthesia on coronary blood flow and myocardial metabolism. Circulation, *13*:92, 1956.
27. Hart, J.R., and Whitacre, J.J.: Pencil-point needle in prevention of postspinal headache. J.A.M.A., *147*:657, 1951.
28. Heavner, J.E., and deJong, R.J.: Lidocaine blocking concentrations for B- and C-nerve fibers. Anesthesiology, *40*:228, 1974.
29. Helrich, M., Papper, E.M., Brodie, B.B., Fink, M., and Rovenstine, E.A.: The fate of intrathecal procaine and the spinal fluid level required for surgical anesthesia. J. Pharmacol. Exp. Ther., *100*:78, 1950.
30. Howarth, F.: Studied with a radioactive spinal anesthetic. Br. J. Pharmacol., *4*:333, 1949.
31. Kennedy, W.F., Jr.: Effects of spinal and peridural blocks on renal and hepatic functions. *In* Bonica, J.J. (ed.): Regional Anesthesia: Recent Advances and Current Status. Clinical Anesthesia Series. vol. 2. Pp. 110–121. Philadelphia, F.A. Davis, 1969.
32. Kennedy, W.F., Jr., *et al.*: Cardiorespiratory effects of epinephrine when used in regional anesthesia. Acta Anaesth. Scand., *23* [*Suppl.*]:320, 1966.
33. Kennedy, W.F., Jr., Everett, G.B., Cobb, L.A., and Allen, G.D.: Simultaneous systemic and hepatic hemodynamic measurements during high spinal anesthesia in normal man. Anesth. Analg. (Cleve.), *49*:1016, 1970.
34. Kennedy, W.F., Jr., *et al.*: Simultaneous systemic cardiovascular and renal hemodynamic measurements during high spinal anesthesia in normal man. Acta Anaesth. Scand., *37*:163, 1970.
35. Kitahara, T., Juri, S., and Yoshida, J.: The spread of drugs used for spinal anesthesia. Anesthesiology, *17*:205, 1959.
36. Kleinerman, J., Sancetta, S.M., and Hackel, D.B.: Effects of high spinal anesthesia on cerebral circulation and metabolism in man. J. Clin. Invest., *37*:285, 1958.
37. Koster, H., Shapiro, A., and Leikensohn, A.: Procaine concentration changes at the site of injection in subarachnoid anesthesia. Am. J. Surg., *33*:245, 1936.

38. Labat, G.: Regional Anesthesia: Its Technique and Clinical Application. Philadelphia, W.B. Saunders, 1922.
39. Lemmon, W.T.: A method for continuous spinal anesthesia. A preliminary report. Ann. Surg., *111*:141, 1940.
40. Louthan, B.W., Jones, J.R., Henschel, E.O., and Jacoby, J.J.: Isobaric spinal anesthesia for anorectal surgery. Anesth. Analg. (Cleve.), *44*:6, 1965.
41. Lund, P.C.: Principles and Practice of Spinal Anesthesia. pp. 504–601. Springfield, Charles C Thomas, 1971.
42. Macer, G.A.: Spinal anesthesia in more than 34,000 vaginal deliveries. West. J. Surg., *64*:625, 1956.
43. MacIntosh, R.R.: Lumbar Puncture and Spinal Analgesia. P. 125. E & S Livingstone, Edinburgh, 1951.
43a. McLaren, A.D., Stockwell, M.C., and Reid, V.T.: Anesthetic techniques for surgical correction of fractured neck of femur. Anaesthesia, *33*:10, 1978.
44. Matas, R.: Report of successful spinal anesthesia. Medical News. J.A.M.A., *33*:1659, 1899.
45. Maxson, L.H.: Spinal Anesthesia. Philadelphia, J.B. Lippincott, 1938.
46. Meagher, R.P., Moore, D.C., and DeVries, J.C.: Phenylephrine: The most effective potentiator of tetracaine spinal anesthesia. Anesth. Analg. (Cleve.), 45:34, 1966.
47. Moore, D.C.: Complications of Regional Anesthesia. Springfield, Charles C Thomas, 1955.
48. Moore, D.C., and Bridenbaugh, L.D.: Spinal (subarachnoid) block. A review of 11,574 cases. J.A.M.A., *195*:907, 1966.
49. Mueller, R.P., Lynn, R.B., and Sancetta, S.M.: Studies of hemodynamic changes in humans following induction of low and high spinal anesthesia. II. The changes in splanchnic blood flow, oxygen extraction and consumption and splanchnic vascular resistance in humans not undergoing surgery. Circulation, *6*:894, 1952.
50. Park, W.Y., Balingit, P.E., and Macnamara, T.E.: Effects of patient age, *p*H of cerebrospinal fluid, and vasopressors on onset and duration of spinal anesthesia. Anesth. & Analg. (Cleve.), *54*:455, 1975.
51. Pflug, A.E., Aasheim, G.M., and Beck, H.A.: Spinal Anesthesia: Bupivacaine versus tetracaine. Anesth. Analg. (Cleve.), *55*:489, 1976.
52. Pitkin, G.P.: Controllable spinal anesthesia. J. Med. Soc. N. J., *24*:425, 1927.
53. ———: Controllable spinal anesthesia. Am. J. Surg., *5*:537, 1928.
54. Shantha, T.R., and Evans, J.A.: The relationship of epidural anesthesia to neural membranes and arachnoid villi. Anesthesiology, *37*:543, 1972.
55. Sise, L.F.: Pontocaine-glucose solution for spinal anesthesia. Surg. Clin. North Am., *14*:1501, 1935.
56. Smith, H.W., Rovenstine, E.A., Goldring, W., Chasis, H., and Ranges, H.A.: The effects of spinal anesthesia on the circulation in normal unoperated man with reference to the autonomy of the arterioles and especially those of the renal circulation. J. Clin. Invest., *18*:319, 1939.
57. Tait, D., and Caglieri, G.: Experimental and clinical notes on the subarachnoid space. Trans. Med. Soc. Calif. [Abstr.] J.A.M.A., *35*:6, 1900.
58. Tanasichuk, M.A., Schultz, E.A., Matthews, J.H., and Van Bergen, F.H.: Spinal hemianalgesia: An evaluation of a method, its applicability and influence on the incidence of hypotension. Anesthesiology, *22*:74, 1961.
59. Tarrow, A.B.: Solution to spinal headaches. Int. Anesthesiol. Clin., *1*:877, 1963.
60. Taylor, J.A.: Lumbosacral subarachnoid tap. J. Urol., *43*:561, 1940.
61. Touhy, E.B.: Continuous spinal anesthesia: Its usefulness and technic involved. Anesthesiology, *5*:142, 1944.
62. Tuffier, T.: Analgesie chirurgicale per l'injection sous-arachnoidienne lombaire de cocaine. C. R. Soc. Bull. (Paris), *51*:882, 1899.
63. Underwood, R.J.: Experiences with continuous spinal anesthesia in physical status group IV patients. Anesth. Analg. (Cleve.), *47*:18, 1968.
64. Ward, R.J., *et al.*: Epidural and subarachnoid anesthesia; cardiovascular and respiratory effects. J.A.M.A., *191*:275, 1965.
65. Ward, R.J., *et al.*: Experimental evaluation of atropine and vasopressors for the treatment of hypotension of high subarachnoid anesthesia. Anesth. Analg. (Cleve.), *45*:621, 1966.

8 Epidural Neural Blockade

Michael J. Cousins

Although techniques of epidural anesthesia do not offer the economy of drug dosage or degrees of blockade of spinal anesthesia, they are currently more versatile and better studied. No other neural blockade techniques are used as extensively in each of the fields of surgical anesthesia, obstetric anesthesia, and diagnosis and management of acute and chronic pain. Epidural blockade is also unique because of special features of the anatomical site of injection and the resultant diverse sites of action of the local anesthetic solution (see below).

The most practical and widely used continuous method of neural blockade is spinal epidural blockade; continuous caudal blockade has useful but limited applications, and continuous spinal anesthesia has not been accepted in some countries. As indicated in Chapters 24 and 31, new developments in the understanding of pain conduction seem likely to extend the use of continuous epidural blockade to the administration of drugs that selectively block pain conduction, while leaving sensation, motor power, and sympathetic function essentially unchanged. The safety and reliability of spinal epidural catheter techniques, with the addition of bacterial filters, raises the possibility of long-duration relief of acute pain, even in ambulatory patients. This may herald an even more vigorous and fruitful era of investigation and clinical application of epidural blockade than the unprecedented development of the past 20 years.

HISTORY AND RECENT DEVELOPMENT

The study of epidural blockade sustained interest in neural blockade techniques in the 1940s and 1950s, when they seemed doomed to obscurity, and it played an important part in a recent resurgence of interest. By a coincidence, the introduction of curare in 1946 and its meteoric rise of popularity in the 1950s occurred at a similar time to the rise in popularity of obstetrical caudal analgesia.[101,219] However, for many years, caudal rather than lumbar epidural blockade was the preferred method of obstetrical and postoperative pain relief.[169,219] The adaptation of Tuohy's subarachnoid needle[421] for use with epidural blockade in 1949,[133] and the use of continuous catheter techniques, both caudal[220] and lumbar epidural,[100] played a major part in enabling improvements to be made in epidural neural blockade: its efficacy, safety, and duration of action for surgical analgesia, postoperative pain management, and obstetrical pain relief. Although lumbar epidural anesthesia, by continuous catheter techniques, was first used extensively in surgical operations and for postoperative pain,[100] it was the obstetrical application of this technique that most sustained its use in the 1950s. A gradual recognition of the greater anatomical difficulty of caudal block in adults,[76,418] the higher dose required, and the "nonselective" nature of this block in obstetrical applications[53] increased the popularity of lumbar epidural block over caudal block. In the early 1950s, the availability of a new drug, lidocaine,[278] with rapid onset and superior neural penetration, greatly increased enthusiasm for use of epidural block. More important, studies by Bromage of the spread of analgesia and site of action of epidural blockade supported and rationalized the use of the technique.[55,56,62] During the 1960s, epidural blockade became the most widely used technique of neural blockade for pain relief in obstetrics in Canada,[53] in the U.S.A.,[214] and in other countries such as Australia[339] and New Zealand[235]; it was used in Britain initially in surgery and postoperative pain relief by Dawkins.[137,138]

By the early 1970s, there was an increased understanding of the advantages of segmental blockade, with minimal local anesthetic dosage and, thus, reduced toxicity. Controlled clinical studies had clearly demonstrated the long duration of action of the new drug bupivacaine, originally introduced in the early 1960s (see Chap. 4). This now made prolonged segmental blockade a practical re-

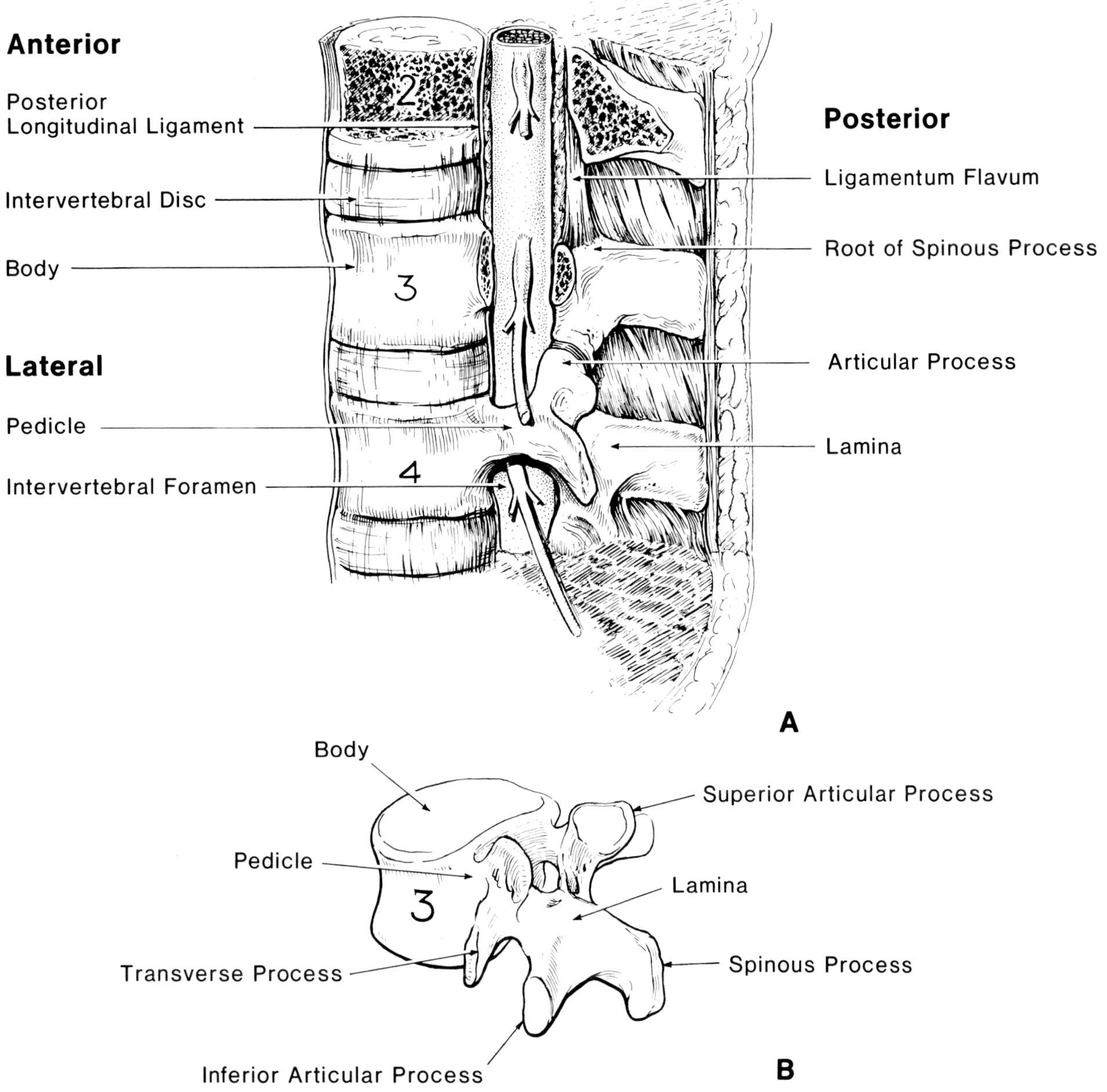

Fig. 8-1. (*A*) Boundaries of the epidural space. Note the superior portion of ligamentum flavum, hidden from posterior view because of attachment to the anterior aspect of the lamina, and the inferior attachment of the ligamentum flavum to the posterior aspect of the lamina (see also Fig. 8-9). (*B*) Lumbar vertebra. (Macintosh, R.R.: Lumbar Puncture and Spinal Analgesia. Edinburgh, E. & S. Livingstone, 1957)

ality. Previous attempts to provide long-duration epidural analgesia with lidocaine alone often led to tachyphylaxis and sometimes caused toxicity (see below). The addition of small doses of long-acting agents, such as tetracaine, to solutions of lidocaine was said to be successful in some institutions,[309] but tetracaine is not available throughout the world. Prolonged pain relief with bupivacaine by continuous catheter epidural blockade became very attractive when it was demonstrated that excellent analgesia after surgery, or in obstetrics, could be obtained with minimal motor blockade.[60,148] De-

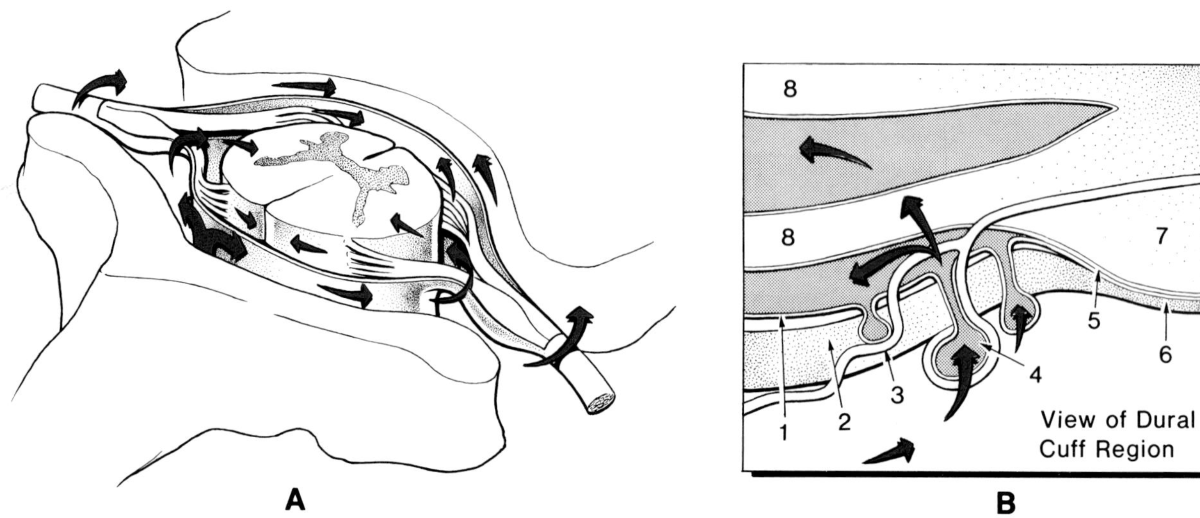

Fig. 8-2. (*A*) Horizontal spread of local anesthetic in epidural space. Major spread posteriorly to the region of "dural cuff" (root sleeve) region is shown, with subsequent entry to cerebrospinal fluid (CSF) and spinal cord. Minor spread into anterior epidural space is also shown. (*B*) Enlarged view of dural cuff region shows rapid entry of local anesthetic into CSF by way of arachnoid granulations: *1*, arachnoid membrane; *2*, dura; *3*, epidural vein; *4*, arachnoid "granulation" protruding through dura and contacting epidural vein; *5*, perineural epithelium of spinal nerve in continuity with arachnoid; *6*, epineurium of spinal nerve in continuity with dura; *7*, dorsal root ganglion; *8*, intradural spinal nerve roots.

tailed pharmacokinetic studies of local anesthetic drugs administered by epidural injection[420] and comparative studies of toxic blood concentrations of local anesthetics in humans[35,376] permitted meaningful estimations of toxicity ratios for the various local anesthetics in the clinical application of epidural blockade (see also Chaps. 3 and 4).[420] Concurrently, detailed studies of the cardiorespiratory effects of epidural blockade[24,26,27,28,438,439] provided important information to increase the safety of the technique by careful attention to level of blockade, maintenance of blood volume, and other factors.

APPLIED ANATOMY OF EPIDURAL BLOCKADE

The reader should review the description of the anatomy of bony spine, ligaments, meninges, and cerebrospinal fluid in Chapter 7, since this is directly applicable to epidural blockade.

The epidural space is not as voluminous as the subarachnoid space. Nevertheless, it extends from the base of the skull to the sacrococcygeal membrane and has complicated direct communications with the paravertebral space and indirect communications with the cerebrospinal fluid. It also leads directly to the vascular system by way of its large epidural veins, which have no valves and connect with intracranial veins; this is a potential direct route to the brain for drugs, air, or other material inadvertently injected into an epidural vein. Within the cranium, there is no epidural space, as the meningeal dura and endosteal dura are closely adherent, except where they separate to form the venous sinuses. At the foramen magnum, these two layers separate: the former becomes the spinal dura, and the latter becomes the periosteum of the spinal canal (Figs. 8-1,2,3). Thus, although local anesthetics cannot enter between the endosteal and meningeal layer of the cerebral dura, they can diffuse across the spinal dura at the base of the brain into the cerebrospinal fluid (CSF) and, thence, to the brain (Figs. 8-2,3). Between the spinal dura and

Fig. 8-3. Longitudinal spread in the epidural space. (*A*) Spread superiorly to *base of skull,* with rapid diffusion by way of cervical arachnoid granulations into CSF or with slow diffusion across dura. (*B*) Spread inferiorly to caudal canal with seepage by way of anterior sacral foramina. There is also seepage through the intervertebral foramen into the paravertebral space.

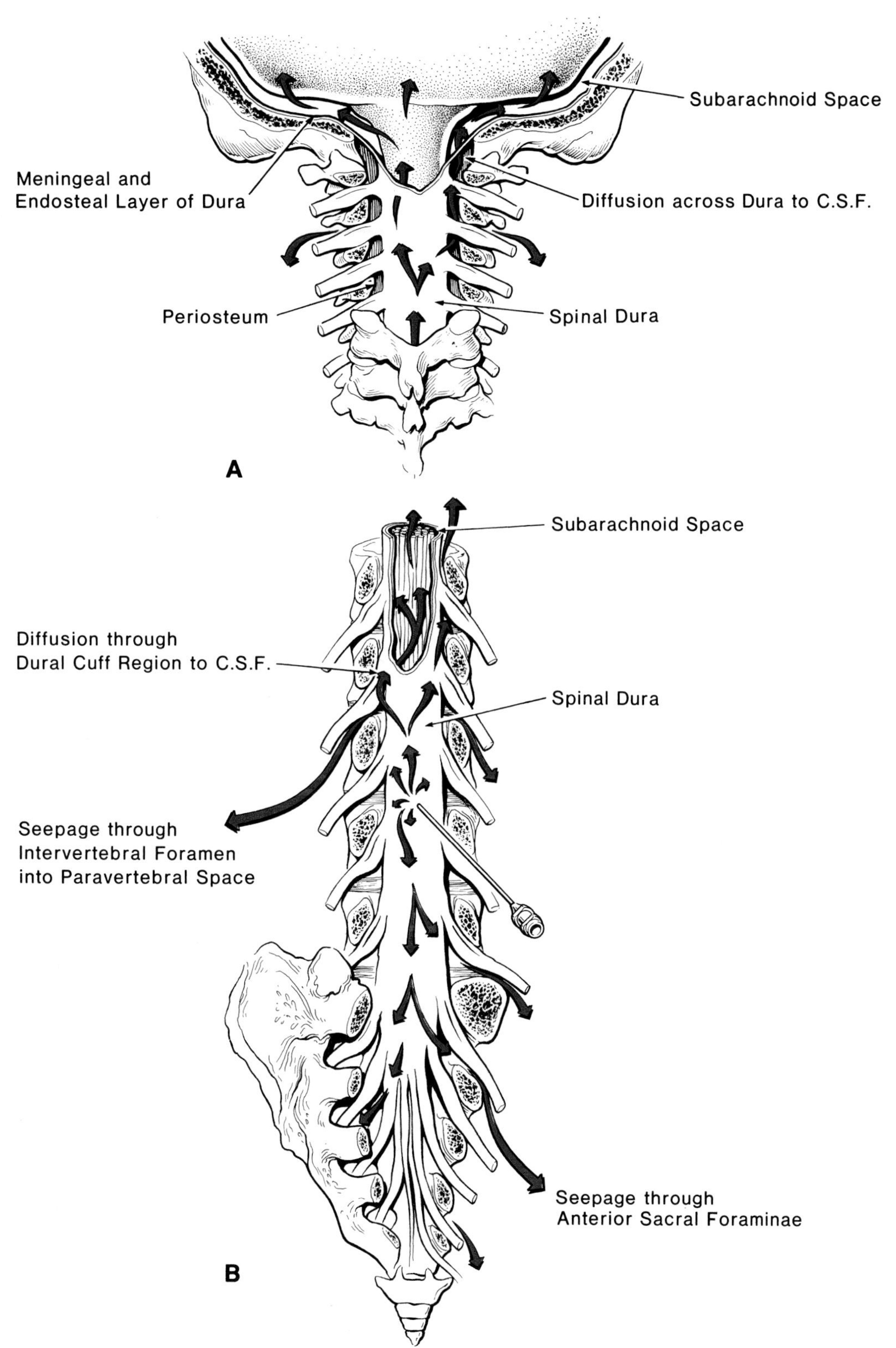
Subarachnoid Space
Meningeal and
Endosteal Layer of Dura
Diffusion across Dura to C.S.F.
Periosteum
Spinal Dura
A
Subarachnoid Space
Diffusion through
Dural Cuff Region to C.S.F.
Spinal Dura
Seepage through
Intervertebral Foramen
into Paravertebral Space
Seepage through
Anterior Sacral Foraminae
B

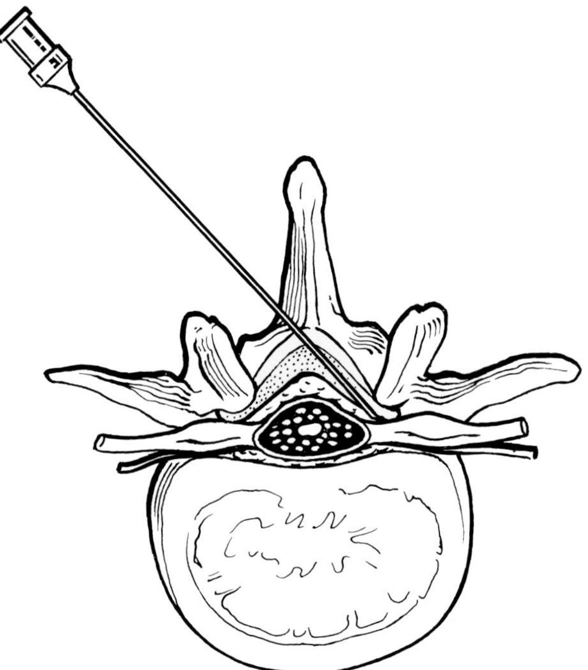

Fig. 8-4. Ligamentum flavum, cross sectional view. The triangular shape of each half of the ligament is apparent. They narrow toward the articular processes, as does the underlying epidural space. Also, incorrect extreme lateral angulation of a needle is shown. Oblique penetration of the ligamentum flavum results, with continued resistance for several millimeters and eventual loss of resistance in the dural cuff region, where there are two main hazards: the epidural space is very narrow and the dura is thin (see also Fig. 8-2); the needle is close to spinal nerve and vessels. (Macintosh, R.R.: Lumbar Puncture and Spinal Analgesia. Edinburgh, E. & S. Livingstone, 1957)

the spinal periosteum lies the epidural space. The ligamentum flavum completes the posterior wall in direct continuity with the periosteum of the spinal canal (Fig. 8-1). Since the spinal canal is approximately triangular in cross-section and the articular processes indent the triangle (Fig. 8-4), the epidural space narrows posterolaterally and then widens again laterally towards the intervertebral foramina (Fig. 8-5). Thus, the safest point of entry into the epidural space is in the midline.

Surface Anatomy

The key anatomy for safe placement of a needle in the epidural space is summarized in Tables 8-1 to 8-3. However, before considering deep structures, the anesthesiologist should be certain of the level and direction of insertion of the needle; thus, sur-

Summary of Boundaries of the Epidural Space

Superior
- The foramen magnum where the periosteum of the spinal canal and the spinal dura fuse together to form the endosteal and meningeal layer of the cerebral dura (Fig. 8-3)

Inferior
- The sacral hiatus and sacrococcygeal membrane (Fig. 8-3)

Lateral
- The periosteum of the pedicles of the vertebrae and the intervertebral foramina (Fig. 1)

Anterior
- The posterior longitudinal ligament covering the vertebral bodies and intervertebral discs (Fig. 1)

Posterior
- The periosteum of the anterior surfaces of the laminae, the articular processes, and their connecting ligaments, the roots of the vertebral spines, and the interlaminar spaces filled by the ligamenta flava (Figs. 8-1 and 8-5,6).

Summary of Spread of Injected Solutions in Epidural Space

Contrast medium, local anesthetic, or other agent injected into the spinal (or caudal) epidural space may potentially spread as follows:
- Superior and Inferior spread is mainly in posterior portion of epidural space between dura and ligamentum flavum (Fig. 8-3).
- Superiorly to foramen magnum. Note the possibility of diffusion across dura at base of brain to cerebral CSF, with possibility of blockade of cranial nerves, vasomotor and respiratory centers, and other vital centers.
- Inferiorly to sacral hiatus, caudal canal, and through anterior sacral foramina (Fig. 8-3).
- Laterally through intervertebral foramina to paravertebral space, to produce paravertebral neural blockade. Note rapid access to CSF at "dural cuff" region (Figs. 8-1,2) to produce spinal nerve root blockade and also subsequent access to spinal cord (see below).
- Anteriorly in thin epidural space between dura and anterior longitudinal ligament (Fig. 8-2).

Note also:
- Access to CSF by slow diffusion across spinal dura, subdural space, and subarachnoid membrane into subarachnoid space
- Vascular absorption by way of epidural veins may convey drug directly to brain (see below).
- Profuse epidural fat may take up drug (see below).

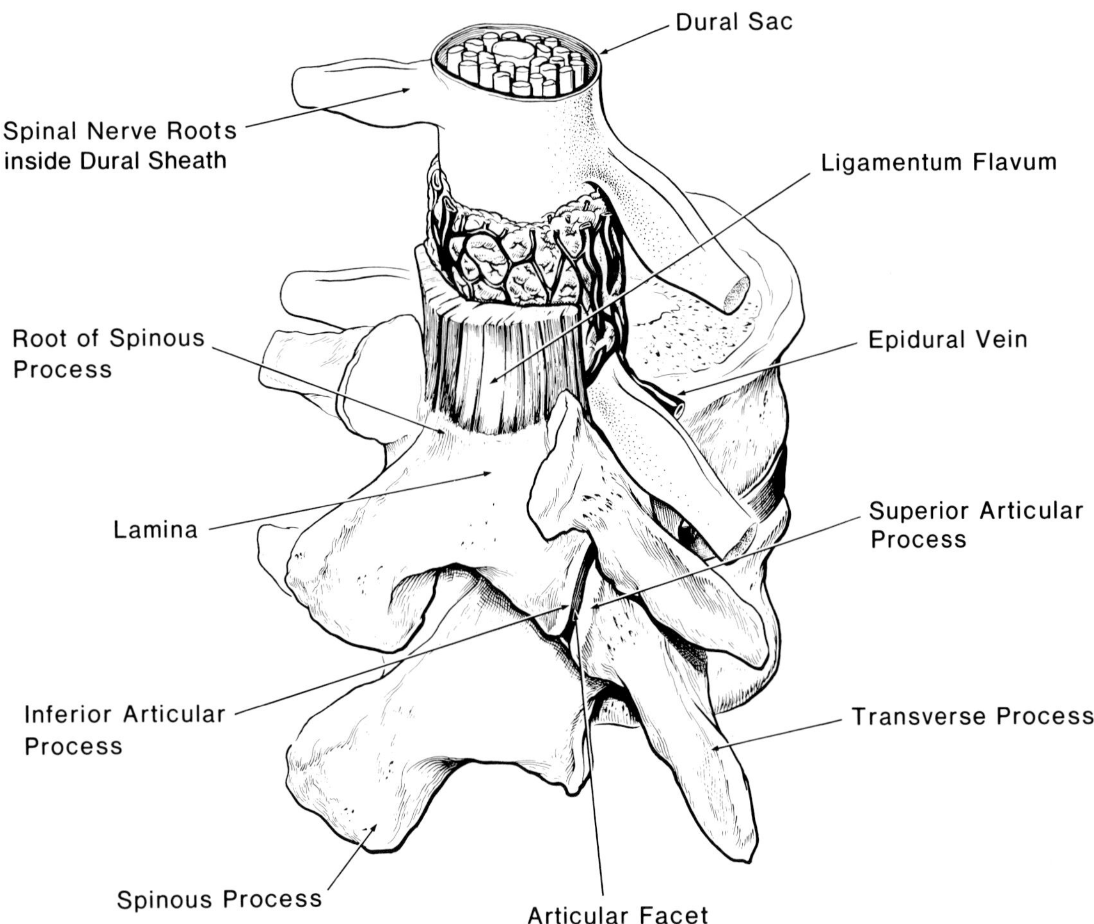

Fig. 8-5. Epidural space, relationships from the posterior view. Note the increased prevalence of epidural veins lateral to the midline; narrowing of the ligamentum flavum and epidural space laterally; slight downward slope of spinous processes; proximity of articular facets at lateral aspect of lamina (see also Fig. 8-12B). (Macintosh, R.R.: Lumbar Puncture and Spinal Analgesia. Edinburgh, E. & S. Livingstone, 1957)

face anatomy is important. Since the easiest and safest point of entry into the epidural space is in the midlumbar region, a reliable surface marking for this level is of great importance: The line drawn between the highest points of the two iliac crests passes through the spinous process of the fourth lumbar vertebra (Fig. 8-7A). The interspinous space immediately above this spinous process (L3–4) or one higher (L2–3) is the standard site of needle insertion for epidural block in adults, since the spinal cord usually ends at the lower border of vertebra L1. As noted in Chapter 21, this is not the case in children and is one reason the caudal route of entry is preferred to the spinal route in young children. Also, the dural sac terminates at the level of S2 in adults (S3 in small children): A line through the posterior superior iliac spines crosses this level. As noted in Table 8-1, puncture below L4 increases the difficulty of "midline" epidural block because of the ill-defined interspinous ligament; also, puncture above L2 increases the risk of damage to conus medullaris, so that the interspaces of L2–3 and L3–4 are both the safest and easiest; identification of L4 reassures that an easy entry may be achieved. Identification of L1 acts as a "double check" and confirms that the point of entry is safely below the conus medullaris. There is no difference in the potential danger of damaging the cord if one chooses the T12–L1 interspace or the C8–T1 interspace, both of which can often be technically easy; however, the spinal cord lies directly beneath the epidural space in both instances. Thus, only anes-

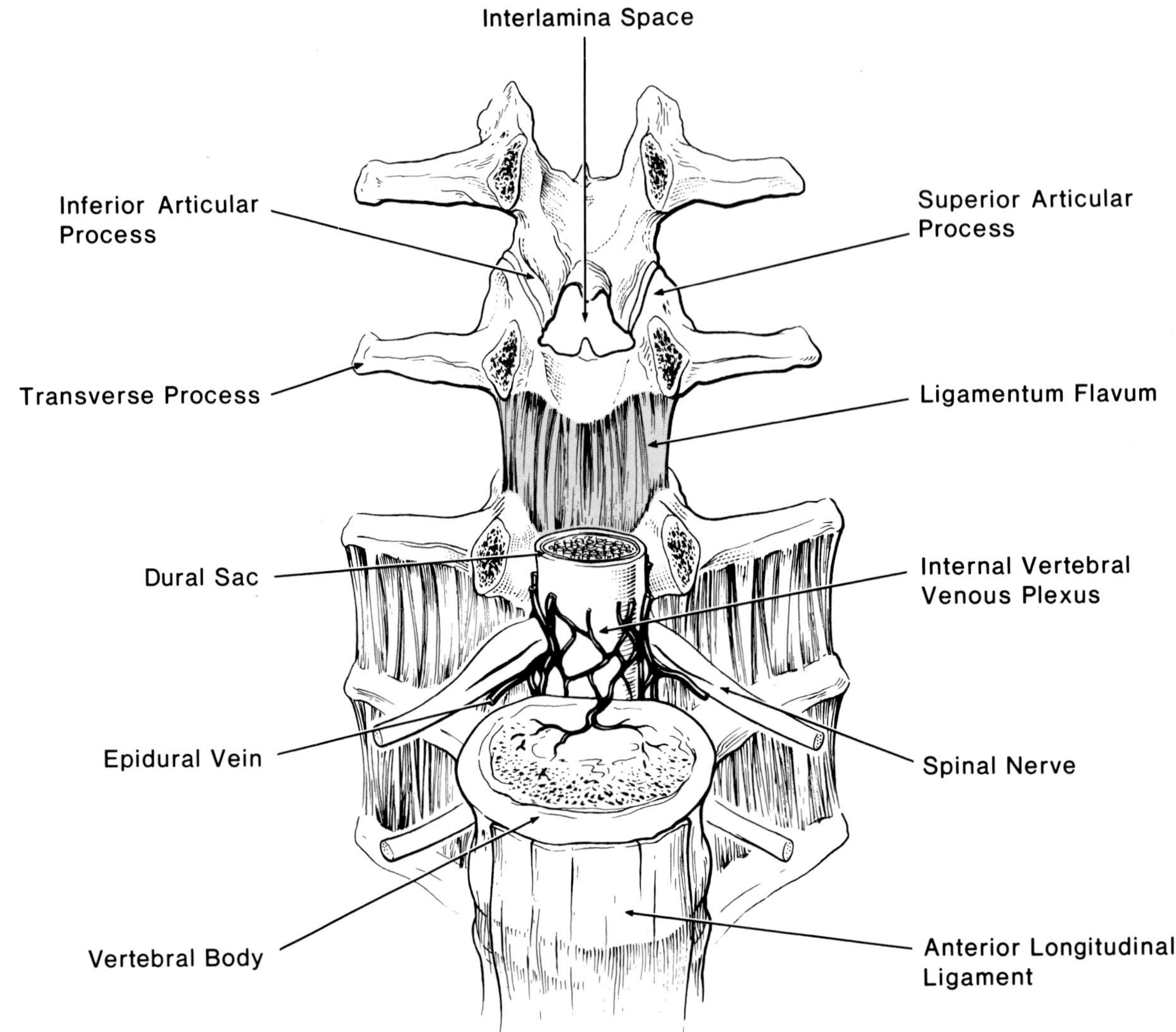

Fig. 8-6. Epidural space, relationships from anterior view. Note "interlaminar space" at one level and covered by ligamentum flavum at the level below. Epidural veins are in continuity with veins draining vertebral body ("internal vertebral venous plexus"). (Macintosh, R.R.: Lumbar Puncture and Spinal Analgesia. Edinburgh, E. & S. Livingstone, 1957)

thesiologists experienced with epidural techniques require the anatomical landmarks above L1: the inferior angle of scapula (T7), the root of the spine of the scapula (T3), and the vertebra prominens (C7).

Because of the extreme angulation of the spinous processes in the midthoracic region, midline puncture is very difficult, and the paraspinous (paramedian) approach is preferable. In contrast, there is excellent access to the interlaminar space in the midline at C7–T1 and T1–2, and the same applies in the low thoracic region. However, it should be noted that anatomical differences, such as a narrower epidural space (Tables 8-2,3), require greater technical skill at these levels and require a technique different from that usually employed for lumbar epidural block.

In the lumbar region, correct needle insertion takes full advantage of the fact that it is both easier and safer to insert the needle at the L2–3 or L3–4 interspace, with the needle entering the epidural space in the midline. The latter does not necessarily imply that the needle must start in the midline, although in most cases this is an easy approach. As shown in Figures 8-1 and 8-12B, the inferior aspects

Table 8-1. Key Anatomical Features for Administration of Lumbar Epidural Anesthesia

Spine and Ligaments

- Spinous process
  - Widest in midlumbar region
  - Only slight downward angulation (see Fig. 8-1)
  - Inferior border opposite widest point of interlaminar space (see Fig. 8-12B)
  - Superior border over upward sloping lamina (see Fig. 8-12B)
  - Narrower superiorly. Needle inserted beside spinous process guided into midline by lateral aspect of spinous process (see Fig. 8-30A)
- Interspinous ligament
  - Well defined above L4. Below L4 narrower and loose—may offer less resistance
- Lamina
  - Posterior surface slopes down and back
  - Needle may strike lamina superficially at inferior aspect of slope or deep at superior aspect of slope (see Fig. 8-5)
- Interlaminar space
  - Increased by flexing lumbar spine
  - Larger "target" area in midline, and in midlumbar region
  - Smaller target laterally (see Fig. 8-12B)
- Articular facets
  - Needle directed past lateral aspect of interlaminar space may impinge on articular facets causing severe radiating pain and muscle spasm (see Fig. 8-12B)
- Ligamentum flavum
  - Thickest in mid lumbar region, in midline (see Fig. 8-8)
  - Attached to anteroinferior aspects of lamina above and posterosuperior aspects of lamina below; thus, needle entering at inferior aspect may be held up by lamina (see Fig. 8-9).

Relationships of Epidural Space

- Epidural space
  - Widest in midlumbar region in midline (5–6 mm), narrower next to articular processes where ligamentum flavum and dura almost touch (see Fig. 8-4)
  - Widens laterally where spinal nerve surrounded by dural cuff (see Fig. 8-2A)
  - Communicates with paravertebral space via intervertebral foramen (see Fig. 8-1); therefore, epidural catheter may stimulate spinal nerve—unisegmental paresthesia.
- Spinal nerve
  - Needle inserted past depth of lamina with lateral angulation on *same* side may penetrate past spinous process to spinal nerve (Fig. 8-5).
  - Needle angled across midline to *opposite* side may run in substance of ligamentum flavum laterally to reach spinal nerve and/or dural cuff (see Fig. 8-4).
- Arterial supply of spinal cord (see Figs. 8-10, 11).
  - Only one anterior spinal artery
  - In thoracolumbar region fed mainly by "Radicularis Magna," which usually enters by way of an intervertebral foramen on left side at T11–12 (T8–L3).
  - Supply to thoracolumbar cord is discontinuous with higher levels.
  - Sharp demarcation between anterior and posterior spinal artery territory
- Epidural veins
  - Prominent in lateral portion of epidural space (see Fig. 8-5)
  - Drain to azygos vein and connect to pelvic veins providing an alternative route from pelvis to right heart. Therefore, they become distended when IVC is obstructed (see Fig. 8-13).
  - Also connect to cerebral venous sinuses

Table 8-2. Key Anatomical Features for Administration of Midthoracic Epidural Anesthesia

Spinous process
- Extreme downward slope, inferior border opposite mid point of *lamina* below.
- Small posterior surface, processes very close together and difficult to identify
- Therefore, the paraspinous (paramedian) technique is easier (see Fig. 8-30B)

Interspinous ligament
- Difficult to identify because spinous processes close to each other

Lamina
- Broader but shorter in vertical dimension
- Large area available for location of depth of ligamentum flavum with less fear of accidental puncture of dura

Ligamentum flavum
- Thick but less so than midlumbar

Epidural space
- In midline 3–5 mm, very narrow laterally

of the spinous processes, in the midlumbar region, lie opposite the line across the widest lateral extent of the interlaminar space. Thus, needle insertion should be close to the superior spinous process, since the upper border of the inferior spine lies over the lamina of its underlying vertebral body. A needle inserted with due regard to this requires very slight upward angulation to give an unobstructed approach to the interlaminar space. A surface anatomical aid that is often neglected involves checking that the needle is inserted in the center of a line running through the middle of the superior and inferior aspects of the spinous processes: that is, in the center of the supraspinous ligament. This is best achieved by grasping the spinous processes adjacent to the site of puncture between thumb and forefinger, while needle is inserted through skin and subcutaneous tissue into the supraspinous ligament (Fig. 8-7B). If this is done, the needle should sit firmly in the supraspinous ligament without angulation to one side.

Table 8-3. Key Anatomical Features for Administration of Cervicothoracic Epidural Anesthesia

Spinous process
- At C7 (vertebra prominens) and T1, direction is almost horizontal
- Inferior border C7 opposite widest point of C7–T1 interlaminar space

Lamina
- Shaped like narrow rectangle

Interlaminar space
- Accessible with midline puncture if neck flexed

Ligamentum flavum
- Thinner than at any other level

Epidural space
- Width at first thoracic interspace is 3 to 4 mm (note width at C3–6 is 2 mm)
- Increased width if neck flexed
- Usually marked negative pressure (increased if sitting)

Segmental Levels

In assessing the level of epidural blockade, it is important for the anesthesiologist to have a method of using simple surface landmarks to indicate level of dermatomal blockade and, thus, segmental spinal nerve and sympathetic blockade. Table 8-4 lists the key levels (Fig. 8-35).

There is no point in testing for blockade of T1–2 by testing above the nipple line, since this area has double innervation from T1–2 and C3–4, so that normal sensation remains even when T1–T2 are blocked. Thus, residual activity in the important cardiac sympathetics T1 and T2 is checked by testing skin sensation on the inside of the arm above the elbow (T2) and below the elbow (T1). Residual motor activity in T1 can also be checked by testing the ability of the patient to hold a sheet of paper between the outstretched fingers (interossei C8, T1). In an anesthetized patient, spinal reflexes are useful for testing level of blockade: epigastric (T7–8), abdominal (T9,12), cremasteric (L1,2), plantar (S1,2), knee-jerk (L2–4), ankle-jerk (S1,2).

Structures Encountered During Midline Insertion of Epidural Needle

If *correct* use of surface anatomy described above is observed and prior skin puncture is made with a larger needle (introducer), an epidural needle should encounter no resistance in the skin and subcutaneous tissue, but should then penetrate the tough supraspinous ligament, which will support it at right angles to the skin in all directions (Fig. 8-8); the *interspinous* ligament then offers continued resistance to advancing the needle; an increase in resistance to advancement of the needle signals that the needle tip has entered the thick, elastic ligamentum flavum; after only a few millimeters of advancement, a sudden loss of all resistance occurs as the needle tip enters the epidural space.

The distance of the epidural space from the skin

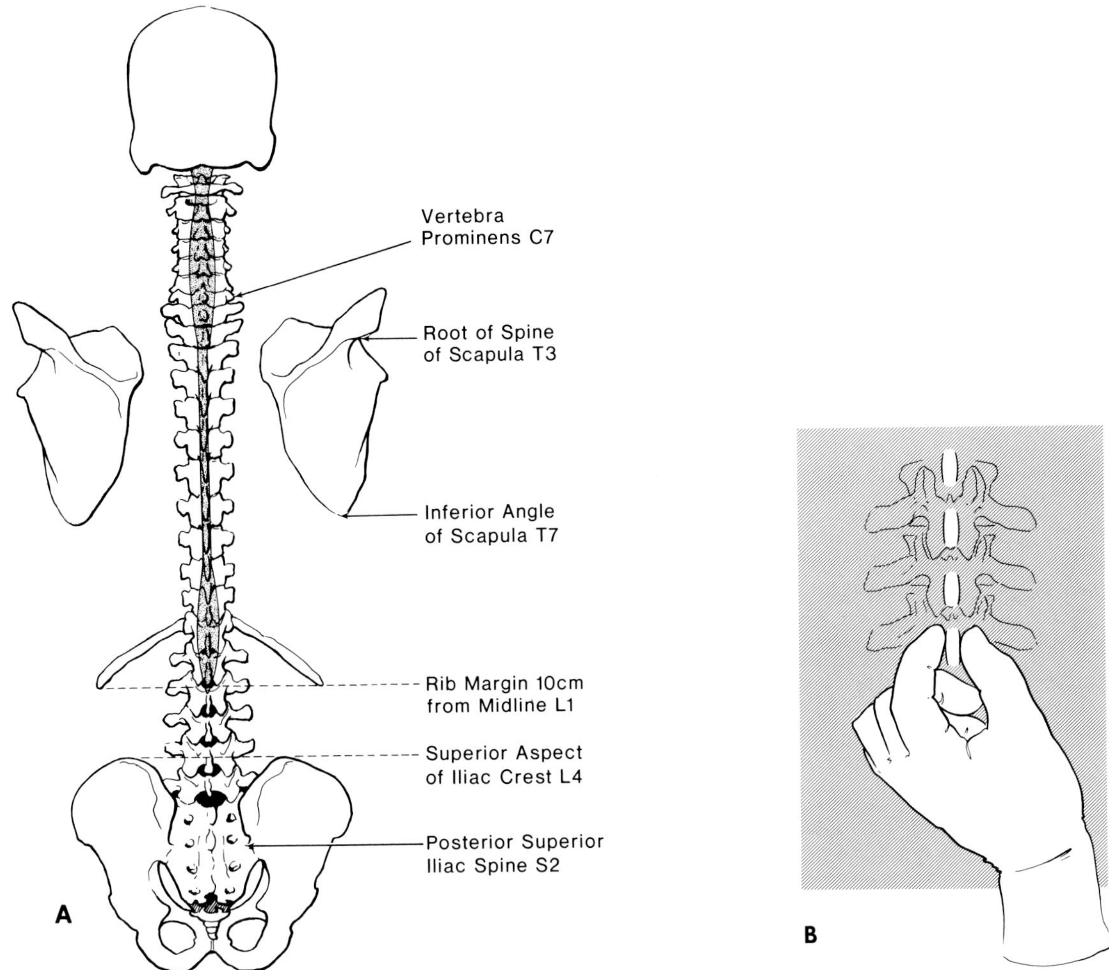

Fig. 8-7. (*A*) Surface anatomy and landmarks for epidural blockade. The spinous process (vertebra prominens) at C7 is the most prominent spinous process when the neck is flexed. The spinous process at T3 lies opposite the root of the spine of the scapula (arm by side). The spinous process at T7 lies opposite the inferior angle of the scapula (arm by side). For puncture between C7 and T1, there is direct access to the interlaminal space but there are other hazards (see text). Puncture below T3 and above T7 is difficult due to angled spinous processes. Puncture below T7 becomes progressively similar to L2–3. Other hazards are the same as those for high puncture (see text). The spinous process at L1 (lower border) is noted by a line meeting the costal margin 10 cm from midline. The spinous process at L4 (center) lies at the top of the iliac crests. S2 is noted by the posterior superior iliac spines. Puncture at C7, at T7, and at L1 to L4 is *safest* and *easiest* in lumbar region. L2–3 and L3–4 are the preferred levels. (*B*) Method of checking midline. Labat's method of checking center of spinous processes uses the thumb and forefinger to grasp the spinous processes above and below the site of the needle puncture.

is most commonly 4 cm (50%) and is 4 to 6 cm in 80 per cent of the population according to detailed records of 3,200 cases.[206] However, in obese patients, this distance may be greater than 8 cm.

Incorrect procedure (Tables 8-5,6) or sometimes inadvertent aberrant needle placement owing to anatomical difficulties may result in quite a different sequence of events than that described above and contact with different anatomical structures. Failure to clearly define the midline results in needle entry beside the supraspinous ligament. If the anesthesiologist persists with this unsatisfactory start, it

Table 8-4. Key Levels of Dermatomal Blockade

Cutaneous Landmark	*Segmental Level*	*Significance*
Little finger	C_8	All cardio-accelerator fibers (T1–T4) blocked
Nipple line (midway sternal notch and xiphisternum)	T4–5	Beginning of cardio-accelerator blockade
Tip of xiphoid	T7	Splanchnics (T5–L1) may become blocked
Umbilicus	T10	Sympathetic blockade limited to lower limbs
Inguinal ligament	T12	
Outer side of foot	S1	No lumbar sympathetic blockade Most difficult nerve root to block

is likely that the needle will next enter the interspinous ligament obliquely, resulting in only a very transient resistance, followed by loss of resistance; or, it may miss the ligament completely, resulting immediately in a feeling of no resistance, in the paravertebral muscles. Both of these situations may be interpreted as rapid entry into the epidural space. However, injection of local anesthetic is followed by marked "drip back" and subsequent attempts to thread an epidural catheter will be met with considerable resistance. If the needle is inserted too close to the spinous process (or during any attempt at midline puncture in the midthoracic region), it is not uncommon for the needle to contact the spinous process. Perhaps the commonest obstruction to the needle is the lamina of the vertebral body. Since the posterior surface of the lamina slopes from its anterior end gently down and back to its posterior end (Fig. 8-5), an epidural needle inserted too far laterally may encounter lamina either at a superficial depth or deeper, close to its junction with the ligamentum flavum (see Fig. 8-9). Even more extreme lateral insertion or lateral angulation of the needle may result in the needle point contacting the superior or inferior articular processes or the joint space (Fig. 8-12B), where their articular facets meet. The latter can be particularly painful, since the articular facets have a rich nerve supply, and needle trauma may result in sudden severe localized pain on one side of the back with accompanying paravertebral muscle spasm on that side. This pain is not dissimilar to that caused by direct contact with a nerve root: "radicular pain." Both may result in pain which radiates into the leg. Radicular pain is usually more discreet with only one area involved (*e.g.*, the inside of the knee for L3 or inside of the leg for L4). Facet pain may radiate but is somewhat more diffuse and usually does not radiate below the knee.

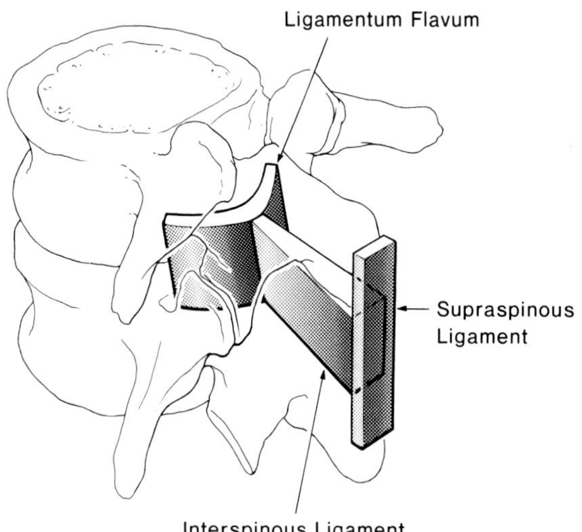

Fig. 8-8. Ligaments encountered during a midline puncture.

The ligamentum flavum should be entered in the center of the interlaminar gap, regardless of where the needle enters the skin (midline or paraspinous). Even with midline puncture, failure to control the penetration of the ligament results in a second loss of resistance signalling dural puncture. Entry at the lateral aspect of the interlaminar gap may also result in dural puncture, since the epidural space is narrow at this point (Fig. 8-4); there is also an increased risk of puncturing an epidural vein with return of blood from the epidural needle.

The epidural space should permit easy injection of solution and easy threading of an epidural catheter, if it is entered in the midline in a controlled manner. Uncontrolled entry or failure to fix the needle securely during subsequent injections or insertion of catheter may result in pushing the needle tip forward until it touches the dura. This results in some resistance to injected local anesthetic and may cause the epidural catheter to puncture the dura if

Table 8-5. Structures Encountered During Epidural Block

Structure	Comment
With Correct Procedure (Midline Technique)	
Skin	Prior puncture with 19-gauge needle should ensure no "drag" on epidural needle
Supraspinous ligament	Needle sits *firmly* in midline
Interspinous ligament	Clear-cut resistance to syringe plunger (above L4) ? Poorly defined resistance (below L4) ? choose another interspace
Ligamentum flavum	Increase in resistance to syringe plunger, with marked "elastic" quality Increased resistance to advancing needle
Epidural space	*Controlled* and well-defined loss of resistance No resistance to injected solution No, or minimal, "drip back" of injected solution Catheter passes easily
Incorrect Procedure or Inadvertant Misplacement of Needle	
Skin	No prior puncture causes marked "drag" on epidural needle
Supraspinous ligament	Entered to one side, causes needle to angle laterally Missed completely, causes needle to flop to one side and appear to have no support
Interspinous ligament	Entered obliquely, results in transient resistance, then loss of resistance, which is interpreted as entrance to epidural space; however, there is marked run back of injected solution, and catheter will not thread Missed completely, results in low resistance—needle in paravertebral muscles
Spinous process	Very superficial contact: interspace not marked ?; spine flexed? (see Fig. 8-12B) Deep contact: needle angled much too acutely?
Lamina	Posterior end of slope: superficial obstruction to needle advancement Anterior end of slope: Deep obstruction (see Fig. 8-9)
Articular processes	Sudden pain in back Muscle spasm on one side of back
Ligamentum flavum	
Pierced midline but with poor control of entry	Needle "overshoots" through epidural space and punctures dura (see Table 8-6)
Pierced to side of midline where dura close and veins prominent	Dural puncture ± CSF flow; or cannulation of epidural vein, +/− bleeding
1 or 2 above with entry into SUBDURAL SPACE	No CSF aspirated some resistance to injected solution and "drip back" which is local anesthetic catheter passes with difficulty small dose of local anesthetic results in widespread block with bizarre distribution
Needle enters lateral aspect from opposite side and continues within ligament to region of spinal nerve (see Fig. 4).	Continued "elastic resistance" for several millimeters then sudden unisegmental paresthesia May be followed by CSF flow if dural cuff entered

(*Continued*)

Table 8-5. (Continued)

Structure	*Comment*
Epidural space	
Entry uncontrolled, needle against dura, no solution injected to expand epidural space	Catheter threads with difficulty or sudden loss of resistance—CSF in catheter
Entry to side of midline into epidural vein or CSF	Blood or CSF via needle or bleeding as catheter threaded—clot in catheter unless flushed with saline
Entry at extreme inferior aspect of ligamentum flavum at attachment to lamina of lower vertebra	Loss of resistance to syringe plunger but needle progress halted by upper edge of lamina and catheter will not thread Danger of dural puncture if needle forced above lamina since epidural space narrower at this point (see Fig. 8-1)
Entry at extreme superior aspect with only tip of needle piercing ligament	Loss of resistance to syringe plunger but some resistance to injected solution and catheter will not thread Further progress of needle easy
Entry at lateral aspect	Catheter may impinge on spinal nerve

Table 8-6. Suspected Dural Puncture

Sign	*Cause*	*Management*
Second loss of resistance and fluid flows from needle	Dural puncture	Convert to spinal anesthetic or move to another interspace for epidural
Second loss of resistance after identifying ligamentum flavum with No CSF from needle Injected solution → some "drip back"	?Entry into subdural space ?Dural puncture	*Test* "drip back" on arm: Cold = LA; warm = CSF With glucose test tape: CSF → color change Drip into thiopentone syringe; CSF → precipitate If drip back only LA, withdraw needle and re-identify epidural space If drip back = CSF ± LA, move to another interspace or convert to spinal anesthetic
One loss of resistance only, however "drip back" at: A shallow level	Interspinous ligament pierced and needle in paravertebral muscle	Reinsert needle in midline
A deeper level	Low compliance of epidural fat	Test as above, if drip back only LA: Attempt to pass catheter → easy passage
	Needle only partially through ligamentum flavum	Attempt to pass catheter → does not pass: Superiorly needle can be advanced and then catheter threaded Inferiorly needle will not advance
	Needle in CSF	Test for CSF, if positive move to another interspace or convert to spinal

LA = Local Anesthetic CSF = Cerebrospinal Fluid.

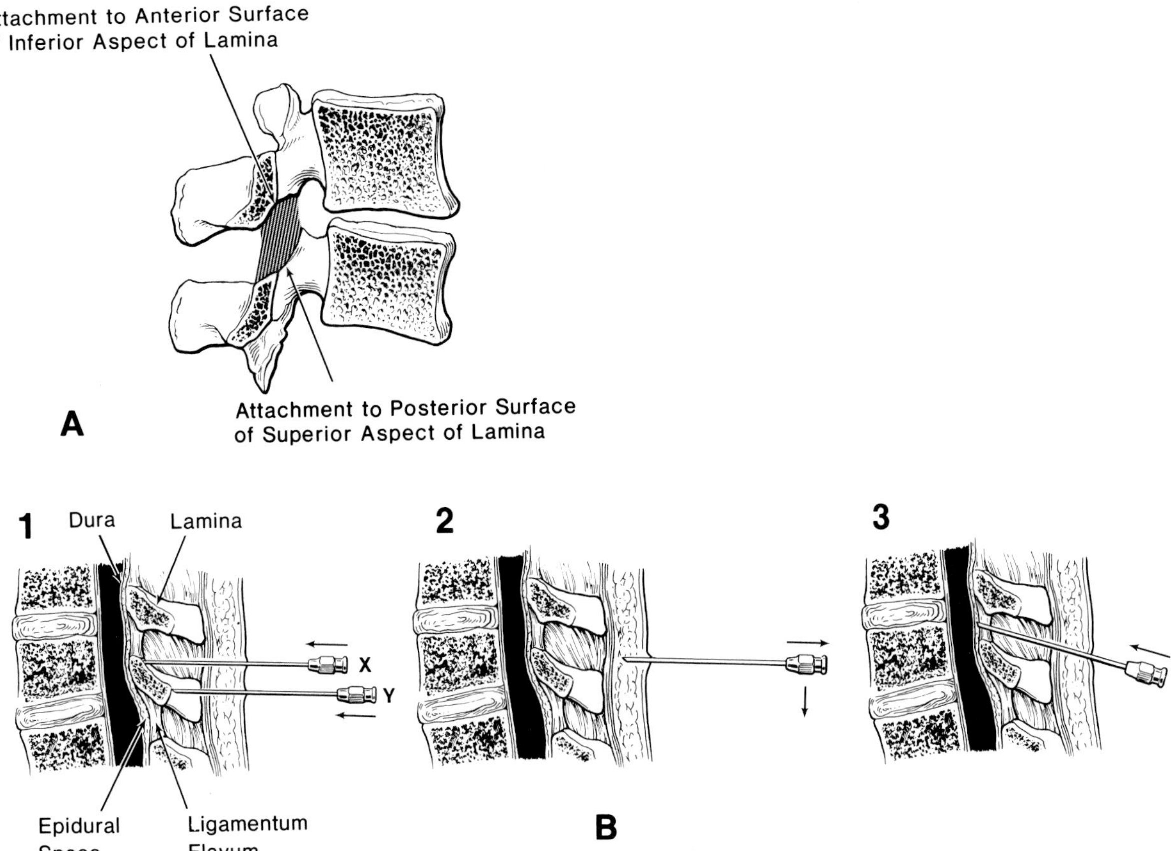

Fig. 8-9. (*A*) Attachment of ligamentum flavum, superiorly and inferiorly. (*B*) *1.* Insertion of epidural needle too close to inferior spinous process may result in contact with lamina superficially (*Y*) or at the superior end of its posterior surface (*X*) where the ligamentum flavum attaches. *2.* Needle is withdrawn to the level of subcutaneous tissues and angled superiorly. *3.* Successful penetration of the ligamentum flavum occurs in the interlaminar space. (From Macintosh, R.R.: Lumbar Puncture and Spinal Analgesia. Edinburgh, E. & S. Livingstone, 1957)

undue force is used when catheter insertion becomes difficult. Many textbooks fail to explain why catheter insertion is impossible, and why further progress of the needle is obstructed immediately after an otherwise impeccably correct loss of resistance through the ligamentum flavum. The explanation lies in the anatomy of the lamina and ligamentum flavum; the latter attaches to the anteroinferior aspects of the lamina below (Figs. 8-1,6). Thus, a needle piercing the ligamentum flavum at its extreme inferior aspect may be held up by the upper edge of the sloping lamina (see also Fig. 8-9). Usually reinsertion of the needle, more to the center of the interlaminar space, is then necessary. Less commonly, a needle angled sharply upwards may undergo a clear-cut loss of resistance as its tip penetrates the ligamentum flavum, but attempts to pass a catheter meet with bony resistance. In this case, the recurved tip of an epidural needle still lies partially in the ligamentum flavum immediately adjacent to its attachment to the lamina above. If the epidural needle can be advanced without further resistance, and the catheter then threads easily without aspiration of CSF, this confirms a high entry through the interlaminar gap. More rarely, but of great importance, a needle angled acutely laterally may penetrate the ligamentum flavum very close to a spinal nerve. Subsequent attempts to pass a catheter may lead to resistance and the immediate report of a unisegmental paresthesia. This calls for repositioning of the needle, since persistance may lead to spinal nerve trauma.

It is very unusual not to obtain a jet of CSF back through an 18-gauge (or larger) needle if it enters the

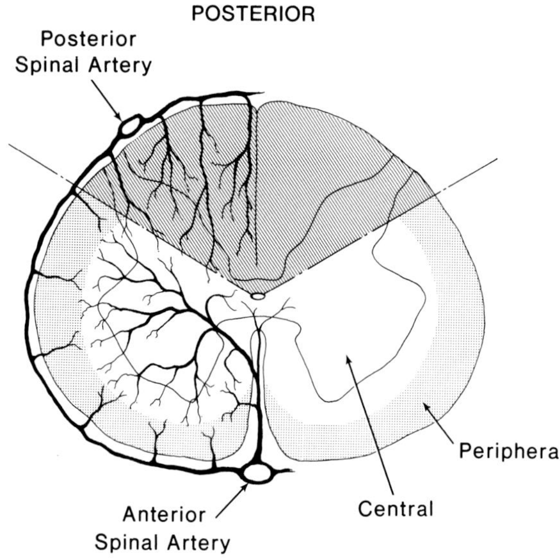

Fig. 8-10. Blood supply of spinal cord, horizontal distribution. The "central" area, supplied only by anterior spinal artery, is predominantly a motor area (see text).

subarachnoid space. Thus, the syringe should always be disconnected as soon as the loss of resistance through the ligamentum flavum is obtained, or if a subsequent second loss of resistance is noted. The width of the epidural space, accessible by means of ligamentum flavum, varies considerably, depending upon the level of the bony spine at which it is approached and the horizontal point of needle entry (Tables 8-1,2,3). It is widest in the midline in the midlumbar region (5–6 mm) but narrows next to the articular processes (Fig. 8-4). In the midthoracic region, it is 3 to 5 mm in the midline and very narrow laterally. In the lower cervical region, the distance between ligamentum flavum and dura is only 1.5 to 2 mm in the midline; however, this increases below C7 to 3 to 4 mm, particularly if the neck is flexed.

The epidural veins are most prominent along the lateral walls of the spinal canal in the lateral portion of the epidural space.

The spinal arteries reach the spinal cord by way of the intervertebral foraminae and enter the epidural space to reach spinal nerve roots in the region of the dural cuffs (Figs. 8-2,4). It is thus possible to cause spinal cord ischemia if a spinal artery is traumatized by a needle inserted toward a spinal nerve root. The spinal cord territory supplied by the anterior spinal artery is most vulnerable, since there is only one anterior artery, and since the major feeder to this artery usually enters unilaterally (on the left in 78%) by way of a single intervertebral foramen, between T8 and L3 (Figs. 8-10,11). This further supports the practice of ensuring that the needle enters the epidural space in the midline and suggests that the L3–4 interspace is the best choice for beginners.

Aspects of Individual Anatomic Structures With Relevance to Epidural Block

The above description of applied anatomy of epidural puncture highlights relevant aspects of the anatomy of the bony spine, ligaments, meninges, spinal nerves, and blood vessels. Anesthesiologists are strongly advised to study the detailed anatomy of the individual lumbar vertebrae, as well as the articulated skeleton, with the aid of an atlas of anatomy.

Only by direct handling of the bony spine and its articulations will the reader fully appreciate the important relationships discussed (Tables 8-1,2,3).

The vertebrae and vertebral column hold the key to both spinal subarachnoid and epidural blockade (Figs. 8-1, 12, and 30). These are discussed also in Chapter 7. However, the following are of particular importance to epidural blockade. The spinous processes are widest in the midlumbar region and have only very slight angulation, making insertion of the 16- to 18-gauge Tuohy needle into the center of the supraspinous ligament relatively easy compared to elsewhere in the spine. The inferior border of the spinous process lies over the widest part of the interlaminar space (Fig. 8-12). The process becomes somewhat narrower superiorly, so that a needle can be guided by the lateral aspect of the spinous process to enter the midpoint of the ligamentum flavum. In the midthoracic region, the spinous processes are much narrower and closer together and are angulated sharply downward, thus obscuring the interlaminar space completely (see Fig. 7-1). The inferior border of spinous processes in this region lies opposite the lamina of the vertebral body below. Insertion of an epidural needle may require a paraspinous (paramedian) approach. If the needle is inserted beside the lower border of the spinous process and angled upwards at 130 degrees, the lateral aspect of the process can once again be used to guide the needle inwards 15 degrees toward the center of the ligamentum flavum (Fig. 8-30). In the cervical region, the spinous processes become widened and bifid with a wide supraspinous ligament. They are almost horizontal in the

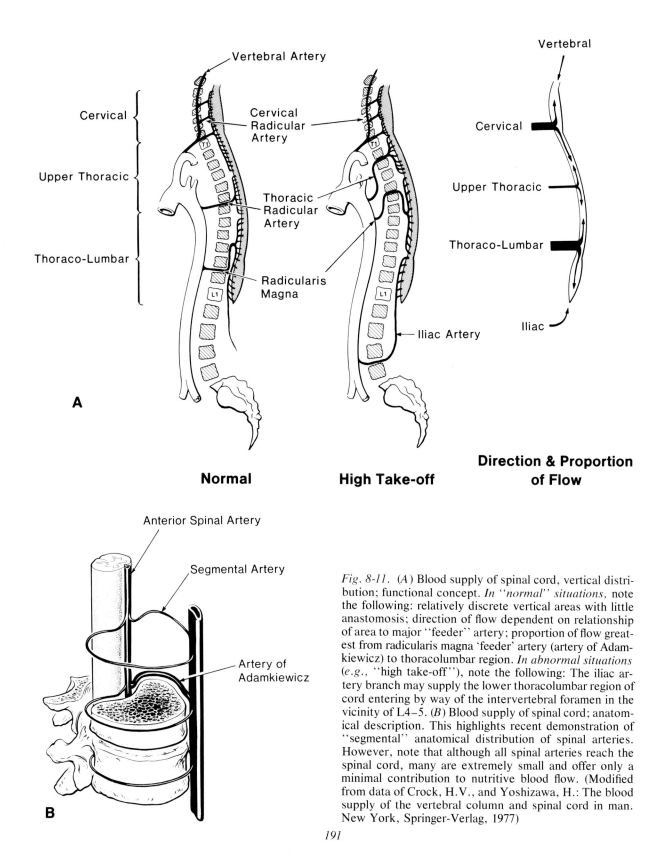

Vertebral Artery

Cervical

Upper Thoracic

Thoraco-Lumbar

Cervical Radicular Artery

Thoracic Radicular Artery

Radicularis Magna

Iliac Artery

A

Vertebral

Cervical

Upper Thoracic

Thoraco-Lumbar

Iliac

Normal **High Take-off** **Direction & Proportion of Flow**

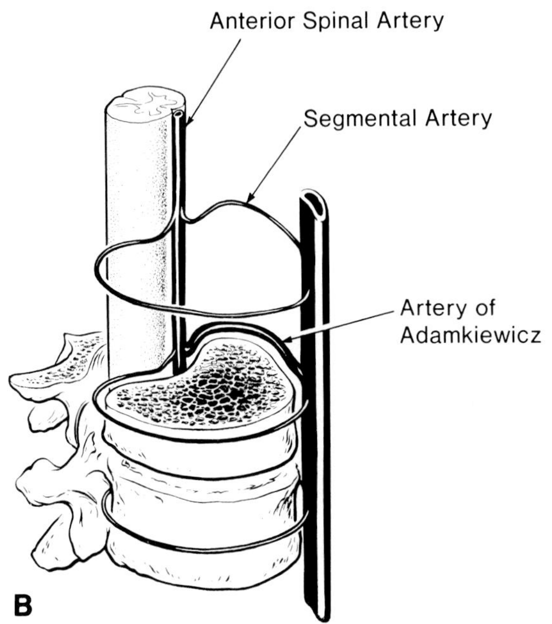

Fig. 8-11. (*A*) Blood supply of spinal cord, vertical distribution; functional concept. *In "normal" situations,* note the following: relatively discrete vertical areas with little anastomosis; direction of flow dependent on relationship of area to major "feeder" artery; proportion of flow greatest from radicularis magna 'feeder' artery (artery of Adamkiewicz) to thoracolumbar region. *In abnormal situations* (*e.g.*, "high take-off"), note the following: The iliac artery branch may supply the lower thoracolumbar region of cord entering by way of the intervertebral foramen in the vicinity of L4–5. (*B*) Blood supply of spinal cord; anatomical description. This highlights recent demonstration of "segmental" anatomical distribution of spinal arteries. However, note that although all spinal arteries reach the spinal cord, many are extremely small and offer only a minimal contribution to nutritive blood flow. (Modified from data of Crock, H.V., and Yoshizawa, H.: The blood supply of the vertebral column and spinal cord in man. New York, Springer-Verlag, 1977)

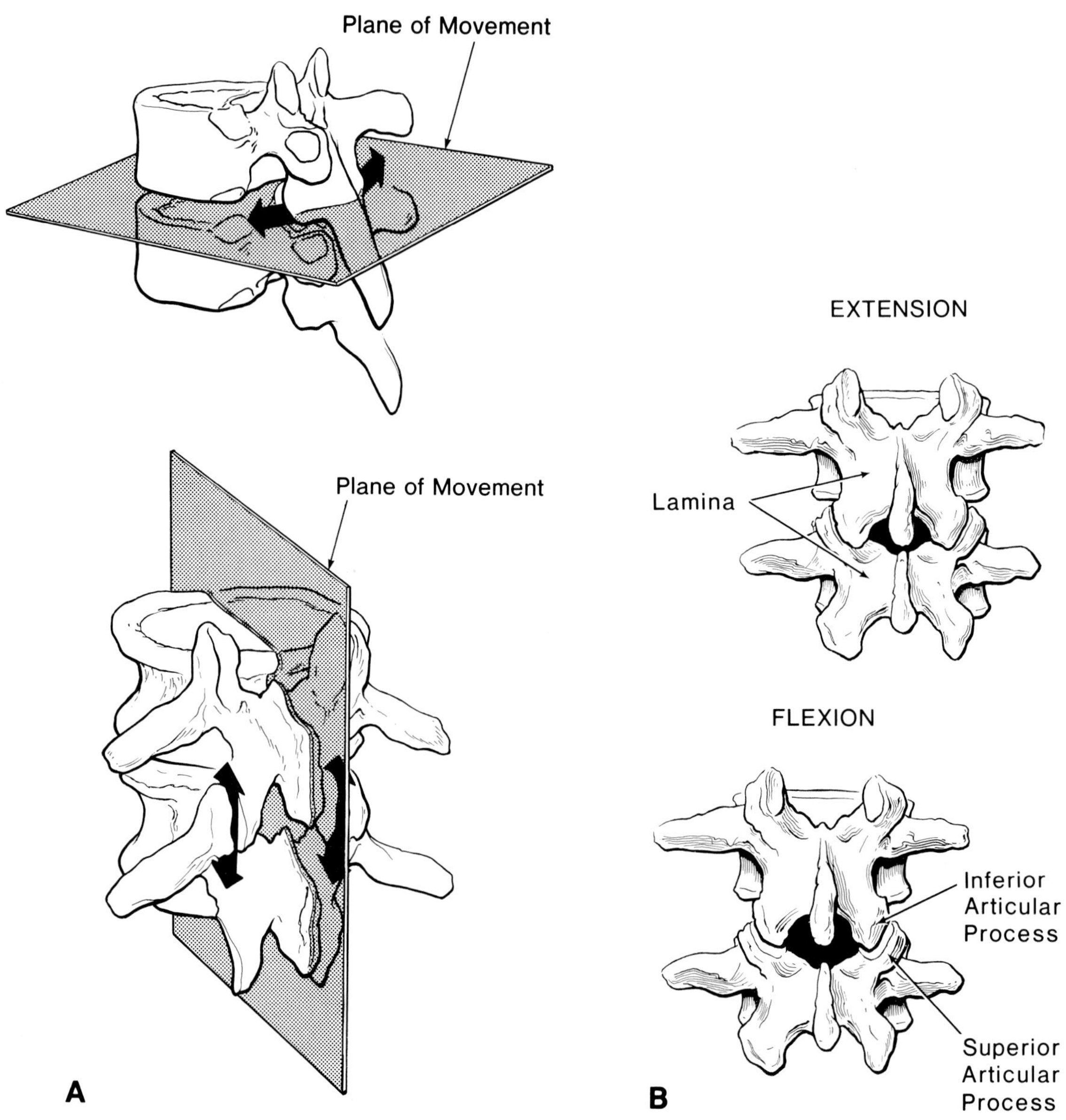

Fig. 8-12. (*A*) Articular facets, plane of rotation. In the thoracic region, the plane through the facets is a horizontal circle, so that lateral rotation can occur. In the lumbar region, the plane through the facets is a vertical circle, so that lateral rotation cannot occur and the only possible movement is flexion and extension. (Arrows indicate direction of movement.) (*B*) Interlaminar space, lumbar region, in extension and flexion. In extension, the boundaries are roots of spinous processes and laminae. With flexion, articular processes form the lateral boundary, and articular facets are exposed at the lateral extremity of the interlaminar space. (Part B modified from Macintosh, R.R.: Lumbar Puncture and Spinal Analgesia. Edinburgh, E. & S. Livingstone, 1957)

lower cervical region and permit easy access to the interlaminar space.

The supraspinous ligament runs vertically between the apices of the spinous processes of lumbar and thoracic vertebrae and continues above as ligamentum nuchae. It varies in width directly with the width of the spinous process; in the lumbar region, it may be as much as 1 cm wide (Fig. 8-8). In persons who engage in heavy physical activity and in laborers and the aged, the ligament may become ossified, making midline puncture impossible.

The interspinous ligament runs obliquely between the spinous processes and is continuous anteriorly with the ligamentum flavum and posteriorly with the supraspinous ligament. As indicated in Tables 8-1,2, and 3 its thickness is greatest above L4 in the lumbar region. Although it is a thin ligament, its fibers are attached along the entire superior and inferior surfaces of the spinous processes; thus, in the lumbar region the ligament is rectangular in shape and provides an identifiable resistance to injected air or solution (Fig. 8-8).

The laminae and articular processes form the boundaries of the interlaminar foramen: In the lumbar region the foramen is triangular in shape when the lumbar spine is extended, with the base being formed by the upper borders of the laminae of the lower vertebra and the sides by the medial aspects of the inferior articular processes of the vertebra above. However, if the lumbar spine is flexed, the inferior articular processes glide upward by means of the synovial joints between facets of articular processes, thus enlarging the interlaminar foramen to a diamond shape (Fig. 8-12B); borders of the superior articular process of the vertebra below now form the lower part of the lateral boundaries of the foramen. It is worth noting that, in the lumbar region, the facets of the articular processes articulate at right angles to a circle with its center in the middle of the vertebral body, so that rotation cannot take place; in contrast, in the thoracic region, the facets articulate in the same plane as such a circle, so that rotation of one vertebra on another readily occurs.[285] This further indicates the potential increase in difficulty in puncture in the thoracic compared to the lumbar region (Fig. 8-12A).

The lamina itself slopes down and back on its posterior surface, so that it may be contacted by a needle either superficially or deep (Figs. 8-5 and 8-9B). Indicated above, the lamina forms only the wide base of the interlaminar space. The remaining boundaries are formed laterally and superiorly by the articular processes (Fig. 8-6).

The ligamentum flavum is composed almost entirely of elastic fibers and is aptly named, since it is indeed yellow in color. Because of its tough elasticity and its thickness of several millimeters in the lumbar region, the ligament imparts a characteristic "springy" resistance, particularly to a large-bore needle with an upturned end (Tuohy needle). The ligament runs from the anterior and inferior aspects of the lamina above to the posterior and superior aspects of the lamina below. Laterally, the ligament narrows as it blends with the capsule of the joint between the articular processes (Figs. 8-4,5,6). Since developmentally two laminae fuse at each level to form the root of the spinous process, two ligamenta flava meet in the median plane and here become continuous with the deep fibers of the interspinous ligament (Fig. 8-8). Thus, an epidural needle advancing in the midline encounters continuing resistance that increases immediately as the needle passes into the ligamentum flavum.

The pedicles that join the laminae to the vertebral bodies complete the bony spinal canal that protects the dural sac. Each pedicle is notched, so that pedicles of adjacent vertebral bodies form the intervertebral foramen. The inferior pedicle of each foramen is notched more deeply. The intervertebral foramina are completed posteriorly by the capsule surrounding the articular processes of adjoining vertebrae and anteriorly by an intervertebral disc and the lower part of the body above it (Fig. 8-1). Since the epidural space is continuous with the paravertebral space, it is possible to produce an epidural block by injection close to an intervertebral foramen (see Chap. 10), or to penetrate the dura at the dural cuff region if a needle is inserted into an intervertebral foramen. The degree of patency of intervertebral foramina is thought to influence the spread of local anesthetics and contrast media injected into the epidural space[386]; it has been shown that extensive "leakage" of local anesthetic occurs through intervertebral foramina.[171,286,392] There are a total of 58 foramina, so the potential for "leakage" is considerable. However, the density of areolar tissue around the foramina varies considerably, and with advancing age it forms a recognizable "operculum" that effectively blocks off foramina.[171] This appears to play a part in the declining dose requirements with advancing age[59,386] although a declining neural population probably also contributes.[110] Similar mechanisms probably result in reduction in dose requirements in atherosclerosis.[56]

The contents of the epidural space are also discussed in Chapter 7. However, several aspects de-

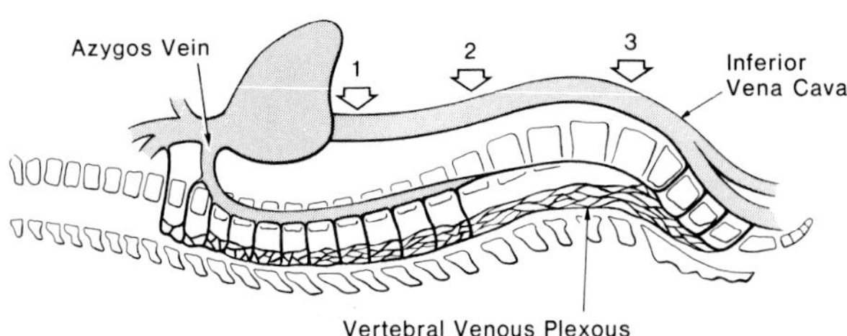

Fig. 8-13. Epidural veins (vertebral venous plexus) and their connections with inferior vena cava (IVC) and azygos vein. Epidural veins are protected from compression by the vertebral canal; thus, obstruction to IVC results in rerouting of venous return by way of epidural veins and, thence, to the azygos vein above the level of obstruction. Some common sites of IVC obstruction are shown: (*1*) below the liver (*e.g.*, severe ascites); (*2*) thoracolumbar junction (*e.g.*, abdominal pressure) in prone position; (*3*) pelvic brim (*e.g.*, lordotic posture, pregnancy). (Modified from Bromage, P.R.: Epidural Analgesia. Philadelphia, W.B. Saunders, 1978)

serve further comment with relation to epidural block.

The epidural fat is semifluid lobulated areolar tissue that extends throughout the spinal and caudal epidural space. It is most abundant posteriorly, diminishes adjacent to the articular processes, and then increases laterally round the spinal nerve roots, where it is continuous with the fat surrounding the spinal nerves in the intervertebral foramina and thence with the fat in the paravertebral space. Anteriorly, it is very sparse, and thus, the dura may lie very close to the posterior longitudinal ligament. Overall, the amount of fat in the epidural space tends to vary in direct relation to that present elsewhere in the body, so that obese patients may have epidural spaces that are occupied by generous amounts of fat. Mostly, the epidural fat lies free in the epidural space except near the nerve roots, where connective tissue tends to tether the fat in the intervertebral foramina. The epidural fat is surprisingly vascular, with small capillaries that form a rich network in its substance.[350,415] The fat itself has a great affinity for drugs with high-lipid solubility, such as bupivacaine and etidocaine, which may remain in epidural fat for very long periods of time (see Chap. 3); uptake of local anesthetic into epidural fat competes with vascular and neural uptake. The compliance of the epidural fat varies considerably between persons and with increasing age.[431,432] In children and young adults, it offers very little resistance to injection, but in some adults a low compliance may result in considerable "drip back" of injected local anesthetic.

Epidural Veins. The large valveless epidural veins form the internal vertebral venous plexus,[8,9] draining the neural tissue of spinal cord, the cerebrospinal fluid (CSF), and the bony spinal canal. The major portion of this plexus lies in the anterolateral part of the epidural space,[31] out of reach of a correctly placed epidural needle (Figs. 8-5,6). The plexus has rich segmental connections at all levels within intervertebral foramina and epidural space, and within the body of the vertebrae. Superiorly, the plexus communicates with the occipital, sigmoid, and basilar venous sinuses within the cranium. Inferiorly, anastomoses by way of the sacral venous plexus link the vertebral plexus to uterine and iliac veins. By way of the intervertebral foramina at each level, the vertebral plexus communicates with thoracic and abdominal veins,[453] so that pressure changes in these cavities are transmitted to the epidural veins but not to the supporting bony elements of the neural arch and the vertebral bodies. Thus, marked increases in intra-abdominal pressure may compress the inferior vena cava while distending the epidural veins and increasing flow up the vertebrobasilar plexus. This increased flow is accommodated mostly by means of the azygos vein, which ascends in the right chest over the root of the right lung into the superior vena cava (Fig. 8-13). However, it is also possible for a small dose of local anesthetic injected into an epidural vein to be channeled directly up the basivertebral system to a cerebral venous sinus; this is most likely to occur in a pregnant woman in the supine position when the inferior vena cava is obstructed, and intrathoracic pressure rises during active bearing down, so that the azygos flow is temporarily increased. Clearly, local anesthetic should not be injected into the epidural space under such conditions. Distention of epidural veins, owing to direct inferior vena caval obstruction (*e.g.*, by the uterus) or owing to increased thoracoabdominal pressure, will also diminish the effective volume of the epidural space, with the result that injected local anesthetics spread more widely up and down the epidural space. In addition, the potential absorptive area of venules and capillaries is increased. The impressive size of the epidural veins on the lateral wall of the spinal canal (Figs. 8-5,6) can be confirmed by epidural phlebography during a valsalva maneuver.[187,369] Three important aspects of safety emerge:

The epidural needle should pierce the ligamentum flavum in the midline to avoid the large laterally placed epidural veins.

Insertion of epidural needles or catheters or injection of local anesthetic should be avoided during episodes of marked increase in size of epidural veins, such as that which occurs with increased thoracoabdominal pressure during straining.

The presence of vena caval obstruction calls for a reduction in dosage, a decrease of rate of injection, and an increase in care in aspirating for blood (see below) prior to epidural injection.

An intriguing feature of the epidural veins is of importance in draining CSF and also in the transfer of local anesthetic to the CSF. In the region of the dural cuffs, bulbs of arachnoid mater protrude through the dura into the epidural space, where they often invaginate the walls of epidural veins that drain spinal cord and nerve root area.[386,446] Although the primary purpose of these arachnoid granulations is to drain CSF[136] and to remove debris from the CSF into the vascular system,[232] they also provide a favorable site for transfer of local anesthetic into the spinal fluid (Fig. 8-2).

Spinal Arteries. The spinal cord receives its blood supply from arteries on the surface of the brain above or from arteries that enter the intervertebral foramina and then gain access to the spinal cord by way of the spinal nerve roots (Fig. 7-9).

It is of significance to epidural block that the spinal branches of the subclavian, aortic, and iliac arteries cross the epidural space and enter the subarachnoid space in the region of the dural cuffs (Fig. 8-2). The purpose of many of these branches is to provide a blood supply only as far as the spinal nerve roots. Only a few actually act as "feeder arteries" to the anterior spinal artery and, thence, to the spinal cord.[422] However, it has recently been shown that, although "nonfeeder" arteries may be very small, they do actually reach the spinal cord, and thus, the arterial supply of the cord is potentially segmental.[132] The paired *posterior spinal arteries* fare quite well, receiving 25 to 40 well developed radicular tributaries. In contrast, the single midline *anterior spinal artery* is really a composite vessel, fed by only a small number of "feeder" arteries, which appear to be critical in maintaining adequate blood flow over three large and relatively discreet segments of the spinal cord (Figs. 8-10,11).[268,269] The largest feeder is the radicularis magna (artery of Adamkiewicz), which supplies the anterior spinal artery in the area of the lumbar enlargement of the cord.[3] It enters by way of a single intervertebral foramen, usually (in 78%) on the left side between T8 and L3 foramina. Damage to this artery by needle trauma or by other means[351] can result in ischemia to the entire lumbar enlargement of the cord. This is possible because there is poor vertical anastomosis between cervical, thoracic, and lumbar segments of the anterior spinal artery (Fig. 8-11) and only minimal horizontal anastomosis between anterior spinal artery territory and that of the posterior spinal artery. Anterior spinal artery ischemia results in a predominantly motor lesion,[191] since the anterior two-thirds of the spinal cord, including the anterior horn cells, are supplied almost exclusively by anterior spinal artery. In a small percentage of cases (15%), the artery of Adamkiewicz takes off high (T5), and the usually slender contribution of iliac tributaries to the conus medullaris and lumbar cord enlarges; under these circumstances, iliac tributaries may feed the anterior spinal artery by means of low lumbar intervertebral foramina. Ligation of these iliac tributaries during pelvic surgery or trauma during epidural block may result in a lesion in the region of the conus medullaris. In the midthoracic region, relatively small feeder arteries reach the anterior spinal artery by way of intervertebral foramina between T4 and T9. In the cervical and upper thoracic region, the anterior spinal artery commences with a contribution descending from both vertebral arteries and then receives feeder branches, through intervertebral foramina, from the subclavian artery to help maintain anterior spinal artery blood flow in the upper thoracic region; but, this is reduced near T4. The T4 region appears to be the most tenuously supplied, since blood flow from the midthoracic region also becomes sluggish near T4.[453]

Apart from the cervical region, the entire blood supply of the spinal cord passes through the epidural space. The anterior spinal artery is more susceptible, because it is nonpaired, has three distinct levels of supply with little anastomosis between them, and has only minimal horizontal anastomosis with the posterior spinal arteries. Thus, although epidural puncture below the level of L2 avoids direct trauma to the cord, the dangers of trauma to anterior spinal artery may be minimized by puncture at L3–4.

Epidural Lymphatics. The dural cuff region is supplied with a rich lymphatic network that rapidly conveys debris from arachnoid villi out through intervertebral foramina to reach lymph channels in front of the vertebral bodies.[41,452] It is reassuring that foreign material can be carried away rapidly by an efficient system that runs in a direction away from spinal fluid and spinal cord.

Dural sac, containing dura, arachnoid, spinal fluid, pia, spinal nerves, and spinal cord, is, strictly speaking, contained within the annular epidural space. A detailed description of the meninges and CSF is given in Chapter 7. For the purposes of this chapter, it is important to examine some aspects of the anatomy of the dura, arachnoid, and spinal nerves in the region adjacent to the intervertebral foramina, the so-called dural cuff region.

The dura can be considered as a protective tube that is pierced by and gives a short "cuff" to each pair of spinal nerves; at this point, the dura becomes markedly thinner and is closely adherent to the dorsal surfaces of the dorsal root ganglia as far as the point where anterior and posterior roots fuse to form the spinal nerve. Within these dural cuffs, there is a small blind pocket of CSF, which is separated from the epidural space only by the greatly thinned dura (Fig. 8-2). Here, the dura is pierced by veins, arteries, and lymphatics, running to and from the underlying subarachnoid space. Also, the arachnoid membrane pushes small "granulations"[386] through the dura; these may either indent epidural veins or come into contact with epidural lymphatics, to facilitate drainage of CSF and elimination of foreign material.[41,452] This region also provides a ready route for passage of local anesthetics into the spinal fluid. Although the dura and arachnoid are usually in close apposition, they are easily separated, and it is possible to inadvertently insert an epidural catheter into the subdural space.[32]

Arachnoid Membrane. It is now known that the arachnoid membrane is metabolically active[436] and is capable of forming giant vacuoles, which may temporarily communicate with the subdural space or, in the dural cuff region, directly with the epidural space. This probably provides a system for rapid drainage of CSF and clearance of debris from the CSF.[416,417]

Spinal Nerves. Some recent advances in neuroanatomy have helped to explain the segmental onset of epidural blockade. Studies of the size of dorsal roots indicate a large variation in size with very large roots at C8 and S1 and a "valley" between these two peak sizes in the thoracic region.[184,237] Studies of the number of myelinated and nonmyelinated fibers in ventral roots also revealed a peak at S1 and in the lower cervical region at C5–8.[102] This is in keeping with the relative resistance of the lower cervical region and S1 to neural blockade. It has recently been suggested that the pia of the spinal cord and spinal nerve roots is continuous with the perineurium of the spinal nerves. Since the epineurium of spinal nerves is continuous with the dura, this raises the possibility of continuity between the subarachnoid space and a subepineurial space.[387] This would explain reports of transverse myelitis after injection of neurolytic agents directly beneath spinal nerve epineurium.[310] All that is required for rapid spread of injected solution from spinal nerve to CSF is accurate needle placement beneath the spinal nerve epineurium (Fig. 8-2).

Spinal Cord. It is known that local anesthetics, injected into the epidural space, can subsequently be detected in spinal nerve roots and the peripheral areas of the spinal cord[68] in concentrations sufficient to block nerve conduction.[177] The peripheral part of the spinal cord in the dorsolateral funiculus contains descending excitatory sympathetic fibers, the descending pyramidal tracts, and medullary reticulospinal fibers. The pyramidal tract synapses in Rexed's layers IV, V and VI, which are involved in the modulation of sensory input (see Chap. 24). It has been hypothesized that local anesthetics with a high propensity to penetrate the spinal cord may produce a rapid and long-lasting sympathetic blockade, followed closely by motor blockade owing to the superficial placement of the appropriate tracts. At the same time, the modulating influences on lamina V and VI may be blocked with a resultant expansion of segmental receptive fields[440] and a relative "antianalgesic" state.[434] This anatomical basis may emerge as an explanation for the "sensory motor dissociation" exhibited by drugs such as bupivacaine and etidocaine (see below). However, at present there are no data to support differential penetration of the spinal cord for the various local anesthetics (see also Chap. 3). Recent support for rapid transport of drugs from epidural space to spinal fluid is provided by studies of epidural narcotics[121]: High concentrations of pethidine are measured in the CSF within 5 minutes of epidural administration, and this coincides with onset of pain relief (see Fig. 31-1), without signs of blockade of other modalities.

Epidural Pressures

In the **lumbar region,** the major cause of generation of a negative pressure lies in "coning" of the dura by the advancing needle point. Since Janzen's original observation of negative pressure in the lumbar epidural space, a number of studies have substantially agreed with his conclusions regarding the etiology of this negative pressure.[30,47,75,151,216,431,432]

The negative pressure increases as the needle advances across the epidural space towards the dura.

Blunt needles with side openings produce the greatest negative pressure: They produce a good "coning" effect on the dura without puncturing it and also transmit the negative pressure well because of their side opening.

Slow introduction of the needle produces the greatest negative pressure. Even if the needle is halted and the pressure equalized, further advances of the needle will continue to produce a negative pressure until the dura is eventually punctured.

Greater negative pressure can be obtained if the dura is not distended (*e.g.*, by gravity in the sitting position or by high abdominal or thoracic pressure).

Eaton[151] provided key data when he showed that tenting the dura with a blunt stylet in the interspace above an epidural needle caused negative pressures of up to -14 cm H_2O, which were recorded by means of the epidural needle. The pressure could be returned to zero by withdrawing the stylet from the dura, and then the same level of negative pressure could be obtained by advancing the stylet again. Despite the convincing nature of the above data, Bryce-Smith[75] was able to record an increase in negative pressure in the epidural space during deep inspiration with no associated change in CSF pressure. In all four patients studied, the epidural pressure was zero at rest and varied from -2 to -8 cm H_2O with deep inspiration. It is noted that the contribution of negativity from deep inspiration was quite small compared to the potential effect of tenting the dura. Of further interest, it was shown that coughing caused a small positive swing in epidural pressure. Thus, although under resting conditions any negativity in the lumbar epidural space is produced by tenting of the dura, it appears that large changes of intrathoracic pressure are transmitted to the lumbar epidural space. Care was taken in the studies of Bryce-Smith[75] and in many hundreds of measurements by Usubiaga and colleagues,[431,432] to ensure that pressure was measured as soon as the needle entered the epidural space. These results then should apply to a carefully performed epidural block, in which the needle is halted immediately when it enters the epidural space. Bromage[47] measured pressure immediately on entering the lumbar epidural space with the patient sitting and during expiration. His results agreed with those of Usubiaga.[431,432] There was still a recordable negative pressure in ten out of 16 cases, pointing to a tenting effect on the dura in 60 per cent of cases, even with very careful entry into the epidural space. The present author's view is that the absence of initial negative pressure in Bryce-Smith's studies, and in at least 12 per cent of Usubiaga's patients in the lying position, means that negative pressure is an unreliable sign of *initial entry* into the lumbar epidural space. Obviously further advancement of the needle in the epidural space may be able to demonstrate negativity where it is initially absent, as reported in the studies of Janzen[239] and Eaton.[151] This appears to conflict with the optimal clinical technique of halting the epidural needle as soon as it enters the epidural space. Techniques of lumbar epidural puncture that are based on a "loss of resistance" tests through ligamentum flavum with air-filled or fluid-filled syringes offer a more reliable means of achieving this optimal technique in the lumbar area (see below). If the anesthesiologist finds it easier to employ the two-handed grip employed in the "hanging-drop" negative pressure test, then it is important to ensure that pressure in the lumbar epidural space is as low as possible by arranging for the patient to be in the lateral position, with a slight head-down tilt, to lower intra-abdominal pressure as the diaphragm moves upwards.[30]

In the **thoracic region** the major determinant of negative pressure is the transmission of negative respiratory pressures from the thorax by way of the paravertebral space and intervertebral foramina to the epidural space. The direct communication between adjacent and contralateral paravertebral spaces by way of the epidural space was strikingly demonstrated by injecting dye from one paravertebral space and showing its distribution by way of the epidural space to other paravertebral spaces on the same and opposite sides.[285] Since the mean intrapleural pressure is -7 cm H_2O (-5 to -10 cm H_2O), it is not surprising that Usubiaga found thoracic epidural pressures of -1 to -9 cm H_2O at the point of needle entry into the epidural space.[431,432] In contrast to the lumbar region, Usubiaga found negative pressure in the thoracic epidural space in 100 per cent of patients, regardless of whether they were sitting or lying; there was a slight increase in negative pressure on moving from a lying to sitting position. The same results were obtained in the cervical region, except that a larger increase in negative pressure was obtained in the sitting position. Since the needle is inserted obliquely in the midthoracic region, it is less likely that the dura will be tented, and negative pressure effects are predominantly due to transmitted intrathoracic negative pressure. The reliability of a "hanging-drop" negative pressure sign has led to the recommendation that this technique be used at least in the midthoracic region.[63] The narrowness of the epidural space in this region and the excellent control afforded by the two-handed grip of the winged "hanging-drop" needle give strong support to this recommendation, although this author prefers loss of resistance.

If one routinely employs a *negative pressure test* for epidural puncture, it is important to be aware of factors that result in marked changes in epidural pressure:

In severe lung diseases such as emphysema, epidural negative pressure may sometimes be abolished, particularly if the patient is lying down.[174,343]

Any factor that causes increased abdominal pressure and/or occlusion of the inferior vena cava may cause distention of epidural veins (see above) and increased pressure in the lumbar epidural space. This, however, results in only slight changes in the thoracic epidural space, particularly if the patient is sitting.[431]

During labor, baseline lumbar epidural pressures are higher in women in the supine position compared to those in the lateral position. As labor progresses, baseline pressures increase to as high as +10 cm H_2O at full dilatation.[183] Also, there are peaks of epidural pressure during each uterine contraction, with increases of 8 to 15 cm H_2O.[53]

Coughing or a valsalva maneuver increases both intrathoracic and intra-abdominal pressure, so that pressure in thoracic and lumbar epidural space is increased,[431,432] with the result that high positive pressures are recorded throughout the epidural space.

Changes in pressure in the epidural space also have implications for the ease of injection into the epidural space and the spread of local anesthetic solutions. Studies by Usubiaga[431,432] have helped to explain why successful entry into the epidural space is sometimes followed by "drip back" when local anesthetic is subsequently injected; classic pressure-volume compliance studies showed that compliance decreased with increasing age and that residual pressure after injection of 10 ml of solution at a standard rate had a positive correlation with age. Thus, some patients with a low compliance in the epidural space will be unable to accommodate a large volume of solution if it is injected rapidly; "drip back" will be less common in young patients and if injection is made slowly, because although there was an increase in epidural pressure in young patients, Usubiaga found that pressure was essentially back to baseline in 30 seconds.

As expected from the above data, Usubiaga found that spread of analgesia was positively correlated with residual epidural pressure, and, in turn, with age. These studies tend to support radiologic studies, in which peridurograms with contrast media showed a reduced longitudinal spread of injected solutions in young patients because of widely patent intervertebral foramina.[64,386,393] In contrast, in old patients with relatively obstructed foramina, longitudinal spread was increased.

PHYSIOLOGIC EFFECTS OF EPIDURAL BLOCKADE

With currently available local anesthetic agents, spinal epidural neural blockade implies sympathetic blockade accompanied by somatic blockade, which may involve sensory and motor blockade alone or in combination. Although it is possible to avoid blockade of "peripheral" lumbar sympathetic fibers if only sacral segments are blocked by a caudal approach to the epidural space, spinal epidural blockade almost invariably results in some degree of sympathetic blockade (Fig. 8-14A). Some of the most important (but not all) of the physiologic effects of epidural blockade can be discussed in relation to either sympathetic blockade of vasoconstrictor fibers (below T4) and/or of cardiac sympathetic fibers (T1–4; Fig. 8-14B; see also Chap. 13). Many clinicians prefer to have a wide margin of safety if they are intent on avoiding major sympathetic blockade. Thus they aim to restrict the level of analgesia to T10. This division of sympathetic blockade is a very practical approach in considering the physiologic effects of epidural blockade, because lower abdominal, inguinal, perineal, urological, and lower limb surgical procedures can be carried out satisfactorily and will only produce a "peripheral" sympathetic blockade. In examining the data that follow, it is useful to think in terms of the use of epidural blockade essentially either above or below the umbilicus and to consider the effects of the resulting sympathetic blockade as one important aspect of epidural blockade. More subtle and somewhat indirect is the reduced input to the central nervous system (CNS), which accompanies various levels of sensory blockade. This "deafferentation" has long been thought capable of exerting a "protective" effect that reduces the efferent neurohumoral response to surgical stimulation or trauma; although very little objective data have been available to support this hypothesis, quite convincing recent evidence is available (Figs. 8-22 and 8-32).

Finally, it is important to remember that extensive epidural blockade often requires quite large doses of local anesthetic (with or without epinephrine). Large doses themselves may cause physiologic changes as a result of the direct pharmacological effects of circulating blood concentrations. These are an inevitable outcome of vascular absorption from the epidural space. Because of the unique epidural venous system (see above), direct intravascular injection may result in the rapid attainment of very high concentrations of local anesthetic in the brain and/or heart with the potential for convulsions and/or sudden depression of cardiac output (see Chaps. 2–4). Also, important changes in vagal tone accompany sympathetic block (Fig. 8-21). The various mechanisms for physiologic effects of epidural block are summarized in Table 8-7.

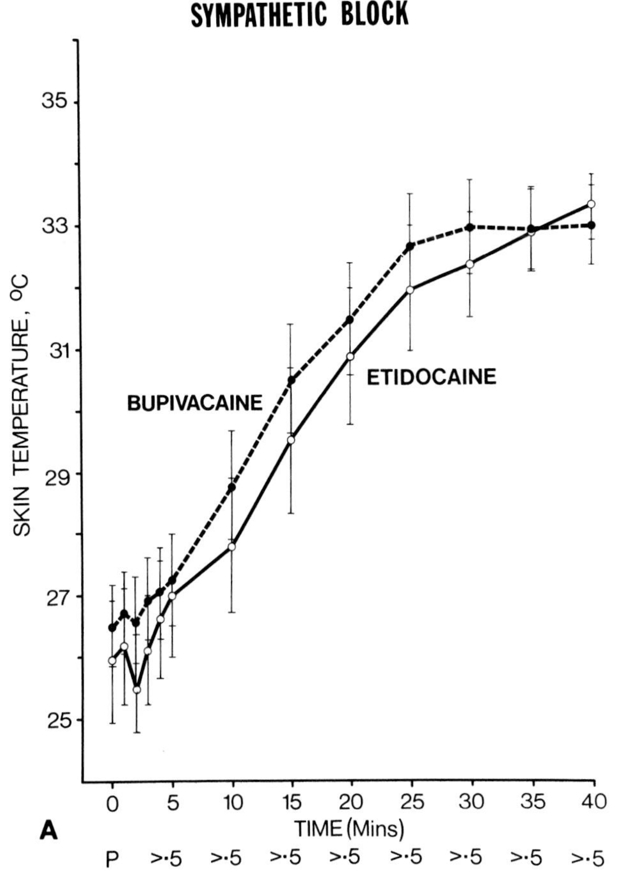

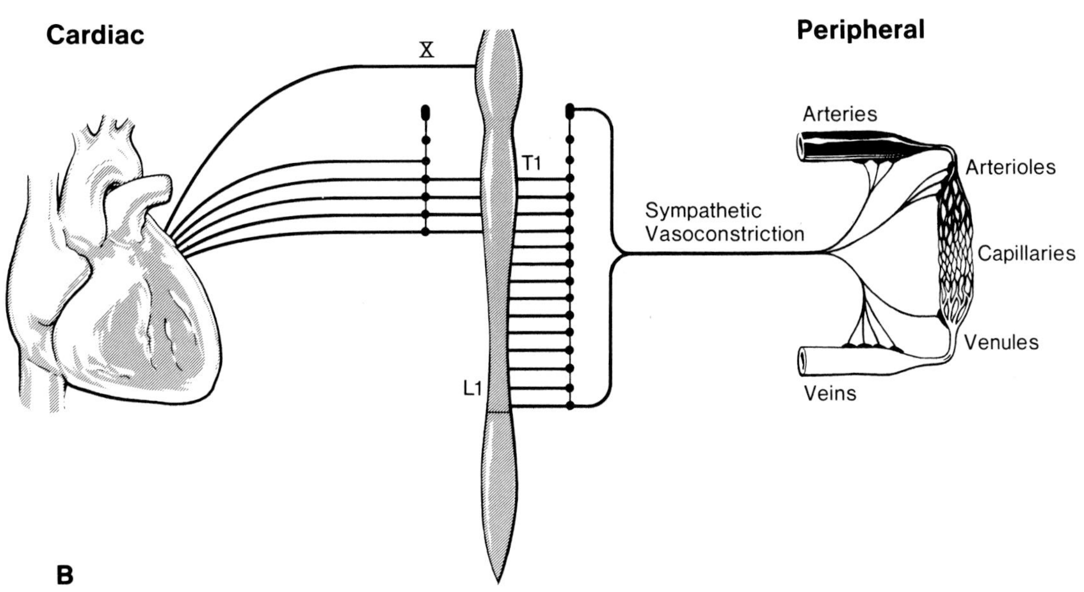

Fig. 8-14. (*A*) Sympathetic blockade: graph. Onset profile of "peripheral" sympathetic blockade is indicated by skin temperature measurements in the lower limbs. (*B*) Sympathetic blockade: "Central" (cardiac) and "peripheral" components. These consist of T1–4 cardiac sympathetic fibers; T1–L2, "peripheral" sympathetic fibers. Note important innervation of veins and venules. *Vagal* cardiac fibers are also shown. (Part A from Cousins, M.J., et al.: Anaesthesia and Intensive Care, *21*:108, 1978)

Table 8-7. Mechanisms for Physiologic Effects of Epidural Analgesia

By Way of Vascular Absorption of Local Anesthetic (LA) or Epinephrine (EPI)	*By Way of Direct Neural Blocking Effects or Indirect Results of Blockade*
Receptor	Spinal nerves (roots and trunks) by axonal blockade
β-stimulation by EPI	*Sympathetic*
α-stimulation by EPI	Efferent blockade
or phenylephrine	Peripheral (T1–L2) vasoconstrictor
Smooth muscle	"Central" T1–T4 cardiac sympathetic
Blood vessels, LA or EPI	Afferent blockade of visceral pain fibres
Heart, LA or EPI	*Sensory*
Other organs, LA or EPI	Afferent blockade
Cardiac muscle	Reduced peripheral sensation
By LA or EPI	Reduced efferent neurohumoral response to surgical or other stimulus within the blocked area
Neural Tissue	
CNS, by LA	*Motor*
Conducting system of	Efferent blockade
heart, by LA	Varying degrees of motor paralysis
Miscellaneous	Reflex muscle relaxation without paralysis (Deafferentation)
Neuromuscular	Spinal cord
junction by LA	*Axons*
	Superficial (*e.g.*, bupivacaine)
	Sensory tracts blocked
	Deep (*e.g.*, etidocaine)
	Sensory tracts blocked
	Motor paths blocked
	Dorsal horn modulation of pain transmission (?axons, ?cells)
	Possibility of "antianalgesic" effect
	Cell Bodies: "selective" narcotic blockade
	Secondary changes in parasympathetic activity
	Sympathetic block to T5 + $\downarrow$ venous return may $\rightarrow$ $\uparrow\uparrow$ vagus
	Sympathetic block to T1 $\rightarrow$ unopposed vagus (see Fig. 8-21)

CARDIOVASCULAR EFFECTS OF EPIDURAL BLOCKADE

In order to understand the cardiovascular effects of epidural blockade, a sound knowledge of the autonomic control of circulation is required (see Chap. 13).[274,295] Although it has been claimed that epidural block results in a lesser degree of sympathetic block and much greater cardiovascular stability than subarachnoid block,[137,145] there are no controlled data to support this. In general, cardiovascular depression may occur with both epidural and subarachnoid blockade (Fig. 8-15) and is at least partly related to the level of sympathetic blockade (Figs. 8-17,18; see also Chap. 7).[26,28,255,256] While the potential for cardiovascular changes owing to sympathetic block to the same level* is similar for epidural and subarachnoid blockade, vascular absorption of local anesthetic and vasoconstrictor may result in significant hemodynamic changes after epidural but not after subarachnoid blockade; the reason for this lies predominantly in the much larger doses of drugs employed in epidural blockade and also in the proximity of the large epidural veins, which, owing to their anatomy, have considerable potential for rapid transport of drug to heart (Table

* Level of sympathetic block is the same as sensory with epidural blockade. In comparison, sympathetic block is 2 to 3 segments higher than sensory level with subarachnoid block.

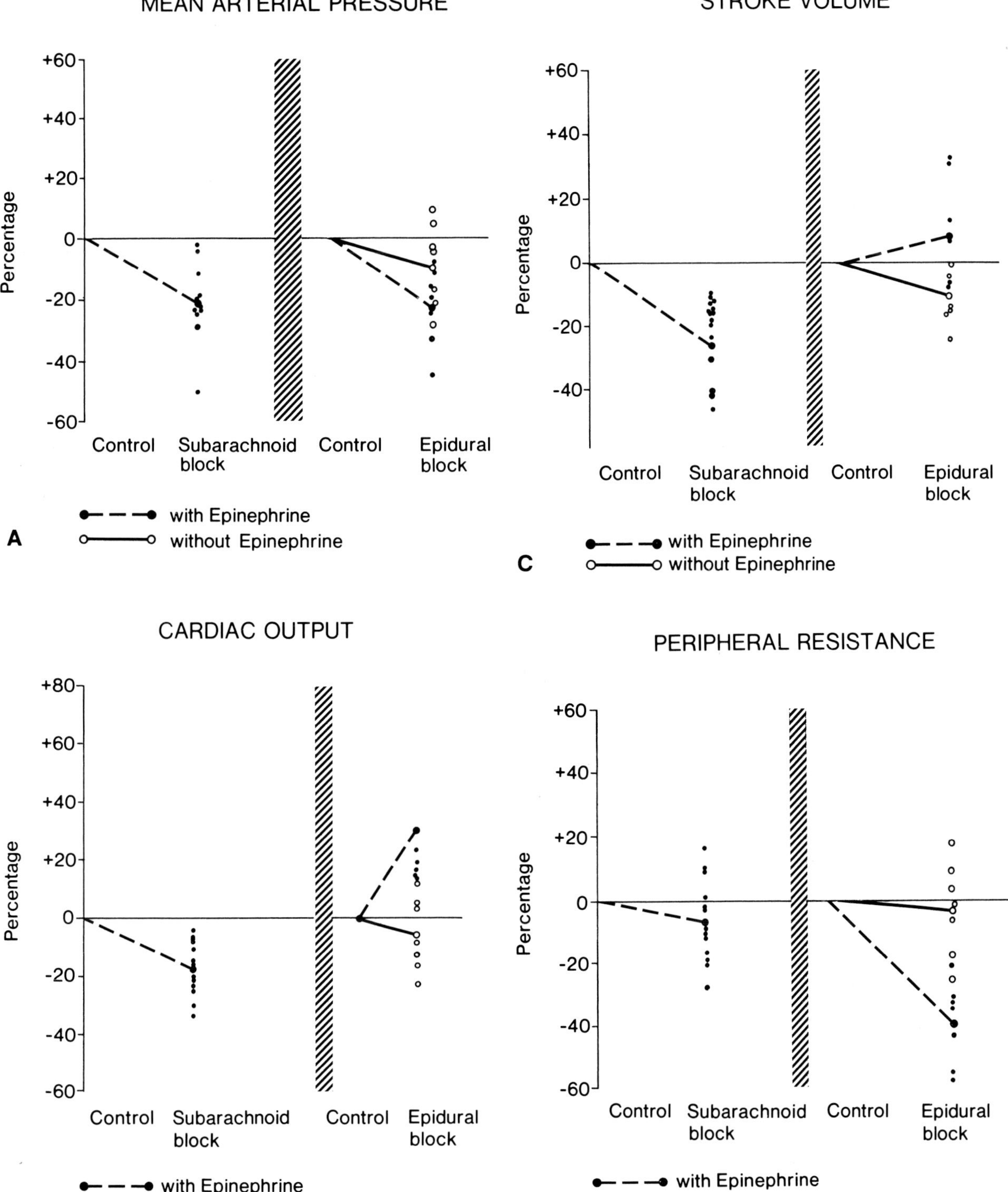

Fig. 8-15. Cardiovascular effects of epidural block, with and without epinephrine. (*A*) Mean arterial pressure. (*B*) Cardiac output. (*C*) Stroke volume. (*D*) Peripheral resistance. Percentage changes for each variable are shown after epidural block, with a comparison given for a similar level of subarachnoid block. (Ward, R.J., et al.: Epidural and subarachnoid anesthesia. Cardiovascular and respiratory effects. J.A.M.A., *25*:275, 1965. Copyright 1965, American Medical Association)

Table 8-8. Cardiovascular Effects of Epidural Blockade

Neural Effects	
Mechanism	*Effect*
"Peripheral" sympathetic block (T10–L2)	
Blockade of vasoconstrictor fibers to lower limbs	Arteriolar dilatation. Increased venous capacitance and pooling of blood in lower limbs → decreased venous return → ↓ CO
Reflex increase in vasoconstrictor fiber activity in upper limbs via baroreceptors	Increased vasomotor tone in upper limbs → ↑ venous return → ↑ CO
Reflex increase in cardioaccelerator nerve activity	↑ HR ↑ CO
Reduced right atrial pressure, due to ↓ venous return	↑ HR (Note ↓↓ RA pressure may → ↓↓ HR; see Fig. 8-21)
Adrenal medullary sympathetic block (T5–L2)	
(Blockade of splanchnic nerves)	
Vasoconstrictor fibers to abdominal viscera	Pooling of blood in gut → decreased venous return
Adrenal medullary catecholamine secretion	Decreased levels of circulating catecholamines → ↓ HR ↓ CO
"Central" sympathetic block (T1–T4)	
Blockade of	
Cardiac sympathetic outflow from vasomotor center Cardiac sympathetic reflexes at segmental level	↓ HR ↓ CO
Vasoconstrictor fibers to head, neck, and arms	Vasodilatation in upper limbs. Blockade of compensatory vasoconstriction resulting from T5–L1 blockade
Vagal predominance	"Inappropriate bradycardia"; "Sudden Bradycardia"; vagal arrest (see Fig. 8-21 and Table 8-11)
Effects of Drug Absorption	
Absorbed local anesthetic	Usually no measurable effects on HR, CO, MAP, or TPR even in patients with vascular disease
Moderate blood levels	Lidocaine may→ ↑ CO which is balanced by ↓ TPR so that MAP is unchanged
Antiarrhythmic	
Maintenance of normal CO	
Minimal reduction in vascular tone	
High blood levels (*toxic*)	↓ CO↓ HR
Decreased contractility	↓ MAP
If convulsions occur hypoxia results in further reduction in C.O.	
Vascular dilatation	↓ TPR
Absorbed epinephrine	↑ CO↑ HR↓ TPR
β-stimulation	MAP may be unchanged or slightly reduced Antagonism of Reflex Vasoconstriction above level of blockade because of β effects on muscle vasculature (→ ↓ TPR)

CO = Cardiac output
HR = Heart rate
MAP = Mean arterial pressure
TPR = Total peripheral resistance

8-8) and CNS. The more gradual onset of sympathetic blockade following epidural analgesia (Fig. 8-14A) of approximately 25 minutes compared to approximately 12 minutes for subarachnoid block may provide a mechanism for initial responses that are less severe for epidural block.[391] Animal studies have shown that autoregulation at the level of the precapillary sphincters develops within 30 minutes of complete ablation of neural activity.[196]

Although controlled studies are not available, experience with large series of thoracic epidural blocks administered in intensive care units by continuous catheter techniques further supports the allowance of adequate time for autoregulation. A common management protocol for "topping up" thoracic epidural blockade for chest trauma involves keeping the patient supine during and for 20 to 30 minutes after "top-up." Using this procedure, serious hypotension is very rare, whereas topping up in the semirecumbent position or allowing inadequate time in the supine position after blockade may result in large reductions in blood pressure (see Chap. 25).

Blockade Below T4

Epidural blockade which is restricted to the level of the low thoracic and lumbar region (T5–L4) results in a "peripheral" sympathetic blockade with vascular dilatation in the pelvis and lower limbs; if all splanchnic fibers are blocked (T5–L1), then pooling of blood in the gut and abdominal viscera also may occur. This "peripheral" blockade has been demonstrated by measurements of large increases in lower limb blood flow owing to arteriolar vasodilation[26,125,397] and "pooling" of blood in the venous capacitance vessels.[391] Since the latter contain 80 per cent of blood volume, venodilatation has a potential for dramatic changes in venous return, reduction in right atrial pressure, and reduced cardiac output. In healthy unmedicated subjects, there is a potential for at least an eight-fold increase in skin blood flow in the lower limbs[299] and the possibility of pooling up to 1 L of blood in the venous capacitance vessels. The magnitude of this change can be appreciated by observing the increase of great toe skin temperature of more than 8°C that often accompanies onset of lumbar epidural sympathetic blockade (Fig. 8-14A). A precise quantitative measurement of increased venous capacitance requires venous occlusion plethysmography of the calf.

Compensatory Mechanisms. *Peripheral Sympathetic Activity*. Even without intravenous "rehydration," healthy subjects in the supine position compensate for a decrease in mean arterial pressure with a reflex increase in efferent sympathetic vasoconstriction above the level of the block. Thus, blood flow and venous capacitance are reduced in the head, neck, and upper limbs.[26,391,397] This increased efferent sympathetic activity is mediated predominantly (by means of the baroreceptors) by those sympathetic vasocontrictor nerves (T1–5) that remain unblocked and also by circulating catecholamines released from the adrenal medulla owing to increased activity in any unblocked fibers in the splanchnic nerves (T5–L1). Although blood vessels in some viscera, such as the kidney, appear to be more responsive to direct neural stimuli,[1] in other vascular beds both neural and hormonal influences have major effects, though at different levels of the vasculature: Major arterioles respond mostly to neural stimuli, while small arterioles and venules near the capillary bed respond predominantly to circulating catecholamines. Thus, while any splanchnic fibers remain unblocked, there is a potential for vasoconstrictor activity below (as well as above) the level of blockade, by release of catecholamines from adrenal medulla. Finally, the ability of precapillary sphincters to achieve autoregulation within a short time of cessation of neural activity[196] provides a further mechanism for regaining vascular tone and minimizing vascular pooling below the level of blockade.

Increased activity in cardiac sympathetic fibers (T1–4) may result in increased cardiac contractility and increased heart rate; similar effects are produced by increased levels of circulating catecholamines. Evidence that the latter are important in maintaining homeostasis in some clinical situations is provided by the surprisingly small changes in heart rate and cardiac output (−16%) with blockade of C5–T4, but with splanchnic fibers to the adrenal medulla (T5–L1) intact (Fig. 8-16).[334] Although quite large compensatory cardiac effects may be observed in unmedicated volunteers (*e.g.*, a 20% increase in heart rate and cardiac output[26]), these changes are not seen in premedicated patients (Table 8-9).[190] In premedicated patients, despite decreased peripheral resistance, an unchanged heart rate, and cardiac output, mean arterial pressure was reduced by only 10 per cent, since changes in total vascular resistances were held to only a 25-per-cent reduction by increased sympathetic activity in unblocked areas (Fig. 8-20).

The studies by Germann and colleagues[190] and Sjögren and Wright[397] report changes that are close to those the anesthesiologist may anticipate in clinical practice, although patients in the latter study

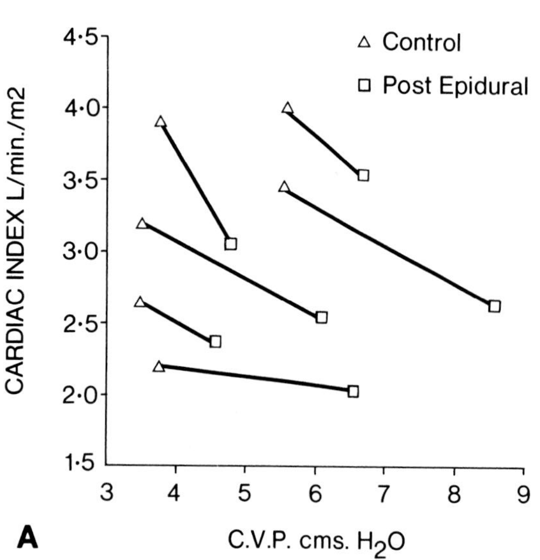

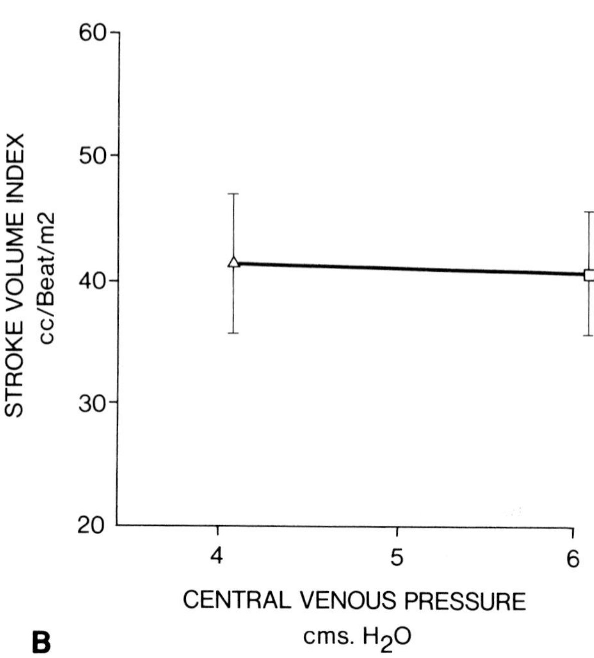

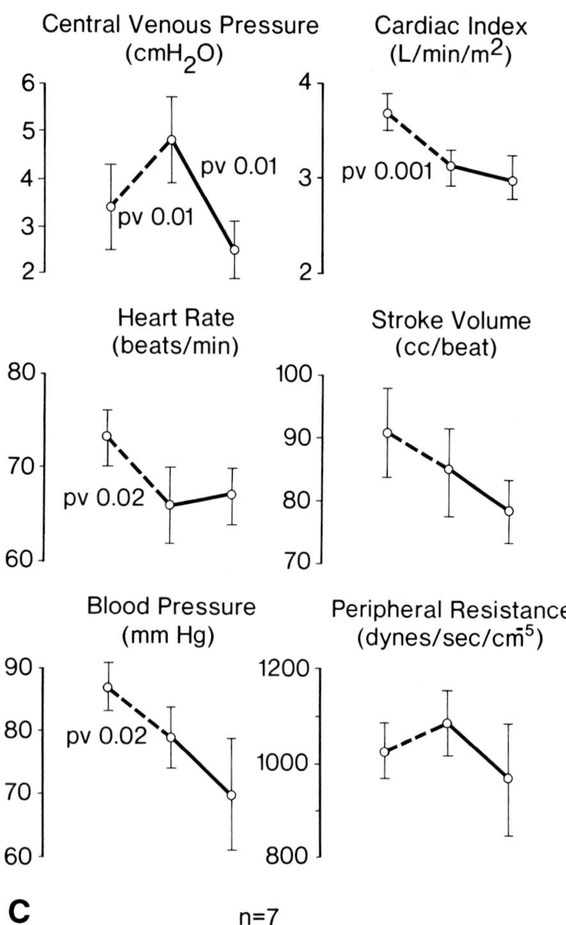

Fig. 8-16. Cardiovascular effects of epidural block. (*A*, *B*) *"Central" blockade of T1–4 alone.* (*A*) Central venous pressure (CVP) is plotted against cardiac index. (*B*) CVP is plotted against stroke volume index. Cardiovascular changes in A and B are compared to controls. (*C*) *"Central" blockade of T1–4 alone compared to "total" epidural blockade* of T1–S5. Block of T1–4 alone results in reductions in blood pressure and heart rate, cardiac index, and a rise in central venous pressure. Extension of block to total blockade is associated with a further fall in CVP and cardiac index. (Part A and B from Otton, P.E., and Wilson, E.J.: The cardiocirculatory effects of upper thoracic epidural analgesia. Can. Anaesth. Soc. J., *13*:541, 1966; Part C from McLean, A.P.H., Mulligan, G.W., Otton, P., and MacLean, L.D.: Hemodynamic alterations associated with epidural anesthesia. Surgery, *62*:79, 1967)

were not rehydrated. The practice of preblock "rehydration" with intravenous balanced salt solution is capable of maintaining mean arterial blood pressure close to preblock levels in healthy patients, including parturients, provided the level of blockade is below T4 and inferior vena caval obstruction is avoided.[26,451]

Is there any reason to believe that blockade to T10 is any safer than that extending up to T5? Data available from studies in healthy volunteers[26] and healthy patients[190,397] indicate that changes are minimal, provided bradycardia is avoided. However, there are several inescapable differences if blockade is extended right up to T5: (1) A larger number of vasoconstrictor fibers are blocked; (2) the level of blockade is very close to the cardiac sympathetics, so that any "overshoot" with initial or "top up" doses will produce changes similar to those shown for blockade to T1 in Figure 8-16; and (3) the splanchnic nerves T5–L1 are blocked—thus varying degrees of blockade of visceral pain are provided, but also blockade of adrenal medullary activity and splanchnic vasoconstrictor fibers is produced.

The combination of (1) and (3) may become important if a patient's state of hydration has been wrongly assessed, if blood volume is reduced,[27] owing to occult blood loss or disease states, or if compensatory mechanisms are for any other reason impaired. It is to be expected that the cardiovascular effects of other sedative and narcotic drugs will be additive. Such effects are mild if anesthesia is light and patients are healthy (Fig. 8-20). However, the additional cardiovascular depression can be clearly documented even in healthy patients[190,408] and may be much greater in ill patients (Table 8-9). It seems wise, then, to be most cautious about the level of blockade and the dose of sedative/narcotic in patients with any compromise of compensatory mechanisms.

While the benefits of retaining activity in vasoconstrictor fibers are fairly clear, what evidence is there that splanchnic neural activity may produce significant cardiovascular effects? The potential for circulating catecholamines to provide cardiovascular activity and overshoot hypertension is seen most dramatically in patients with pheochromocytoma (Fig. 8-32). Although in routine surgery there is recent support for the modification of the stress response in suitable patients,[72] the removal of this emergency response in a patient whose compensatory mechanisms are impaired may be undesirable. Direct stimulation of the splanchnic nerve in cats results in a 20-fold increase in catecholamine secretion,[94] and in humans, catecholamine secretion is thought to increase by at least this amount during emergency situations.[97] Thus, while volunteers and healthy patients appear to be able to maintain cardiovascular stability after blockade to T5, which is similar to that seen with more limited blockade to T10, it should not be assumed that this can be extrapolated to patients with varying degrees of pathology.

The role of the splanchnic blood vessels in hypotension after epidural blockade has not been clearly defined. It is well known that blockade of the celiac plexus may produce marked pooling of blood in the splanchnic region, which receives 25 per cent of cardiac output ("splanchnicectomy faint"), although this pooling is no greater than in the limbs; the potential for hypotension owing to both these mechanisms is markedly accentuated in patients with hypovolemia.

Blockade Above T4 (High Thoracic Block)

"Total Sympathetic Blockade" (T1–L4). It has been thought that control of cardiac rate (chronotropy) and force of contraction (inotropy) resided in the vasomotor center and was mediated by means of the cardiac sympathetic fibers (T1–T4). While this is substantially true, it now appears that changes of cardiac sympathetic activity of approximately 20 per cent[291] can be accomplished at a spinal cord level by reflex activity in the upper four or five thoracic segments, without vasomotor center control[108,109,400]; this can still be overridden by changes in parasympathetic activity.[274] Thus, epidural blockade of T1–5 segments has the following effects on cardiac sympathetic activity: blockade of segmental cardiac reflexes in segments T1–4; blockade of outflow from vasomotor center to cardiac sympathetic fibers (T1–4); vasoconstrictor nerve blockade in head, neck, and upper limbs.

If, as is often the case, blockade extends from T1 to L4, the following effects will be added to the above: splanchnic nerve blockade (T5–L1) with resultant blockade of adrenal medullary secretion of catecholamines and blockade of splanchnic vasoconstrictor fibers; blockade of vasoconstrictor fibers in the lower part of the body, most importantly the capacitance vessels of the lower limbs (Table 8-8).

The magnitude of cardiovascular changes has been documented in unmedicated volunteers[24,26] and in unmedicated patients[287,397] (Fig. 8-16). In general, the mean arterial blood pressure was reduced approximately 20 per cent, with a similar re-

Table 8-9. Cardiovascular Effects of Epidural Blockade by Level of Blockade with Plain Solutions

		Percent Change from Control Value										
Extent of Block	*Dose of Local Anesthetic*	*Venous Capacitance*	*Cardiac Output*	*HR*	*MAP*	*SV*	*CVP*	*TPR*	*dp/dt*	*Arm Flow*	*Leg Flow*	*Reference*
	Lower abdominal block											
T10–S5	20–25 ml 1.5% lidocaine				−6*							142
T10–S5	10 ml 2% lidocaine		0	+5	0	0	0	0	−25	+300	+300	26
	Upper abdominal block											
T4/5–S5	20–25 ml 1.5% lidocaine				−21*							142
T4/7–S5	30 ml 1.5% lidocaine	+20	0	0	−16	0		0		0	+64	391
T5–S5	25–40 ml 2% lidocaine		−5	+7	−9		−10	−3				442
T3–S5	20–35 ml 2% lidocaine⁺		+21	+22	+5	+1	+13	−17	+23	−51	+287	26
T4–L4	15 ml 2% lidocaine		+7	+3	−1	+6	+6	−13		−35	+510	397
T7–S5	15–20 ml 1.5% lidocaine		0	0	−20	0		−24				190
	High thoracic block											
C5–T4	6–8 ml 1% mepivacaine		−17	−17	−8	0	+45	+8				334
C8–S5	30–40 ml 2% lidocaine⁺		+2	+6	−17	−3	+26	−21	−12	+91	+177	26
C5–S5	24–32 ml 1% mepivacaine		−19	−8	−20	−13	−27	−6				287
T2–12	8 ml 2% lidocaine		−1	−7	−12	+10	−3	−3		+47	+21	397
T3–	20–25 ml 1.5% lidocaine				−23*							142

⁺ Incremental doses
* Systolic pressure

duction in total peripheral resistance. Although Bonica and colleagues found that cardiac output was increased slightly or unchanged, McLean and colleagues found a 15 to 20 per cent reduction.[287] Bonica and colleagues found that central venous pressure was markedly raised (26%).[24,26] Since only the studies of McLean and Bonica achieved blockade above T1, their results are more indicative of the effects of complete cardiac sympathetic block. Most surprising was the minimal change in heart rate observed despite blockade of C5–S5: complete blockade of cardio-accelerator fibers and also adrenal medullary catecholamine secretion. Since changes in cardiac rate are known to be controlled chiefly by the balance of sympathetic and parasympathetic tone at any moment, it must be assumed that parasympathetic tone was reduced to almost the same degree as sympathetic tone to maintain heart rate at a normal or near normal level (see Table 8-11). This small change in heart rate gives a deceptive picture of cardiac sympathetic activity, since Otton and Wilson have shown that blockade of T1–4 alone produced an increase in central venous pressure (CVP) without an increase in stroke volume output of the heart (Fig. 8-16).[334] That is, the heart did not empty as well as prior to blockade —a reduced response of the Frank-Starling mechanism. Since the other major determinant of stroke volume is catecholamine stimulation determining the level of Frank-Starling response, the patient with blockade extending from T1 to L2 potentially has both mechanisms obtunded. Thus, one may view the rise in CVP in Bonica's study[26] as a warning sign that the myocardium has exhausted its compensatory mechanisms. Although the associated changes in mean arterial pressure (MAP) and cardiac output were surprisingly small in the studies of T1 blockade (see Table 8-9), the cardiovascular system has essentially no further mechanisms to respond if called upon to do so. In this situation, the anesthesiologist has "assumed control of the circulation" and must be prepared to make rapid adjustments in body position, blood volume, vascular tone, cardiac rate, and cardiac contractile state; this may require administration of various combinations of crystalloids, colloids, atropine, ephedrine, catecholamines. Although such control can (see Table 8-21) and has been accomplished, it is by no means easy to mimic the subtle interbalance achieved by the vasomotor center.

Absorbed Local Anesthetics

Pharmacokinetic studies (see Chap. 3) have provided a very precise picture of the blood concentration profile resulting from absorption of local anesthetics from the epidural space.[420] This formed the basis for determining systemic effects after intravenous infusion of local anesthetics to achieve blood concentrations similar to those occurring with epidural block. Early observations came from intravenous use of lidocaine in the treatment of cardiac arrhythmias.[212] At blood concentrations of lidocaine very similar to those resulting from epidural blockade (3–5 μg/ml), Harrison reported excellent cardiovascular stability, even in patients with severe myocardial disease. Subsequent studies in healthy patients reported minimal changes in cardiovascular function with blood concentrations of lidocaine of 4 to 8 μg per ml.[244] Indeed, there was even some evidence of cardiovascular stimulation. The latter was postulated as the cause of surprising increases in cardiac output, cardiac rate, and mean arterial pressure associated with thoracic epidural block accomplished with large incremental doses of lidocaine (1500 mg). Since these changes were not reported by other studies of thoracic blockade, Bonica and colleagues postulated that the high blood concentrations of lidocaine (4–7 μg/ml) resulted in stimulatory effects on the circulation.[26] Such stimulation was thought to be due to a central effect of lidocaine enhancing sympathetic activity by means of remaining cardiac sympathetic fibers. An alternative peripheral mechanism would have to invoke potentiation of peripheral sympathetic activity. Although local anesthetics can exert a biphasic effect on vascular smooth muscle (see Chap. 3), it seems unlikely that a peripheral mechanism is responsible for the changes observed by Bonica and colleagues.[26]

More recent studies of bupivacaine and etidocaine administered intravenously to volunteers failed to show significant cardiovascular changes when blood concentration profiles were carefully matched to those expected for epidural block.[298]

Epinephrine-Containing Solutions. The preceding discussion has focussed on studies employing plain solutions of local anesthetic. Vascular absorption of added epinephrine does result in systemic actions on β-adrenergic receptors. It is now well established that the cardiovascular effects of low-dosage epinephrine are quite different from its traditional picture of tachycardia, hypertension, and peripheral ischemia. Systemic effects of doses of epinephrine in the range of 80 to 130 μg, as used in epidural block, are a moderate increase in heart rate; increased cardiac output; decreased peripheral resistance; and decreased mean arterial pressure (Fig. 8-17). These effects are attributed solely to β-adrenergic stimulation by Bonica and colleagues.[24] In

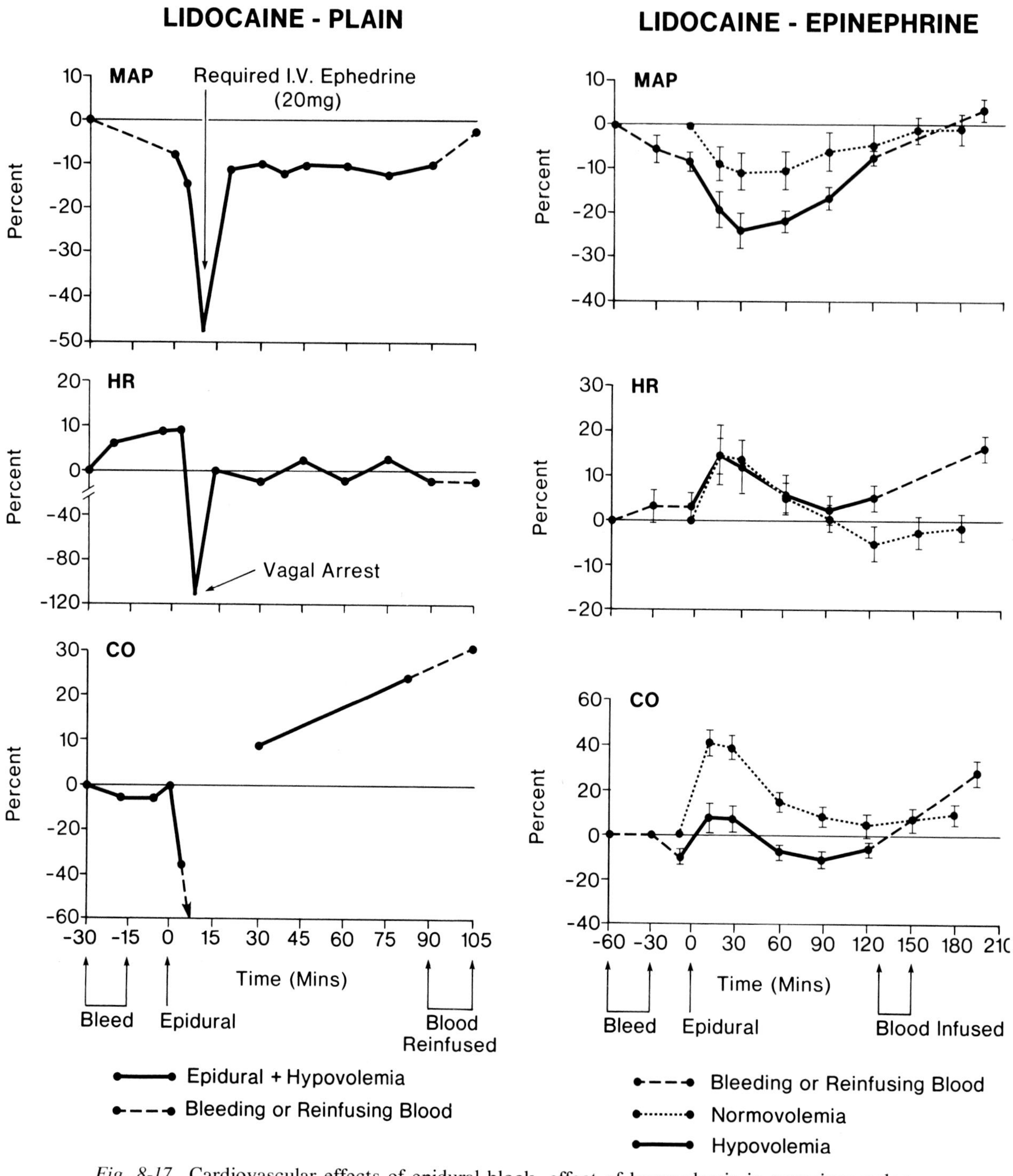

Fig. 8-17. Cardiovascular effects of epidural block, effect of hypovolemia in conscious volunteers; epidural block to T5 with plain and epinephrine-containing solutions. The mean percent changes are shown for each variable. Lidocaine-epinephrine (*right*). The cardiovascular changes after lidocaine-epinephrine in the presence of normovolemia are compared with hypovolemia (−13%). During normovolemia, note the marked increase in heart rate and cardiac output, lasting approximately 60 minutes. During hypovolemia, mean arterial pressure is significantly lower

order to investigate this hypothesis, they administered epinephrine epidurally without local anesthetic, in doses similar to those usually incorporated in local anesthetic solutions (80–130 μg). The epinephrine per se produced changes similar to those seen with epinephrine-containing local anesthetics, except that the changes were of lesser magnitude and shorter lived. Also Bromage[63] has postulated that the epinephrine-containing solutions result in more profound sympathetic neural blockade, in a manner similar to the increase in intensity of motor blockade that results from epinephrine-containing solutions.[66] At present, however, there is no direct evidence to confirm that sympathetic block is sometimes incomplete with plain local anesthetic solutions but not with epinephrine-containing solutions. Indirect support is provided by Bonica's observation, that two out of ten of his subjects failed to develop evidence of sympathetic blockade despite sensory analgesia to T1.[26] Also Cousins and Wright[125] observed that, in patients with postoperative pain, abolition of vasoconstrictor responses sometimes did not occur with 1-per-cent plain lidocaine but appeared more satisfactory with 2-per-cent plain lidocaine. They attributed this effect to more profound sensory blockade with better "deafferentation" of the operative site and prevention of adrenal medullary release of catecholamines; level of blockade was only T7–10 in these studies (i.e., incomplete denervation of adrenal medulla). However, it is entirely possible that the stronger solution produced more effective sympathetic nerve penetration over the same number of segments or over a more extensive area. The latter may be important, since there is ample evidence of large individual variations in extent of sympathetic innervation of upper and lower limbs.[170]

The most likely explanations for the more pronounced cardiovascular effects of epinephrine-containing local anesthetic solutions appear to be as follows:

1. Systemic absorption of epinephrine: β-adrenergic effects on the heart, resulting in increased heart rate and cardiac output; peripheral vascular β-adrenergic effects, resulting in further vasodilatation within the area of sympathetic block and antagonism of compensatory vasoconstrictor responses outside the area of blockade. Thus, total peripheral resistance falls and mean arterial blood pressure is reduced to a comparable degree to that seen with equivalent levels of subarachnoid blockade (Fig. 8-13).

2. More intense neural penetration or more extensive spread of neural blockade, resulting in more reliable sympathetic block.

Hypovolemia and Epidural Block

It has long been said that subarachnoid or epidural neural blockade may result in dangerously accentuated cardiovascular depression in the presence of uncorrected hypovolemia. However, this was largely anecdotal until the studies of Bonica and colleagues: Healthy volunteers received epidural block to T5 with and without epinephrine. Subjects were normovolemic or had undergone withdrawal of 13 per cent of blood volume.[24,26,27] In comparison to the mild cardiovascular changes at normovolemia, major reductions in heart rate, cardiac output, and mean arterial pressure occurred in the presence of hypovolemia; in five out of seven patients who had received plain solutions of lidocaine, vigorous resuscitation, including ephedrine administration, was required. Cardiovascular homeostasis was better maintained with epinephrine-lidocaine blockade. However, marked reductions in mean arterial blood pressure still occurred (Fig. 8-17). Since cardiac sympathetic fibers were thought not to be blocked in these patients, an explanation was sought for the large reductions in heart rate and cardiac output. Morikawa and colleagues repeated the above studies of plain lidocaine in anesthetized dogs.[312] Although they recorded large reductions in mean arterial pressure and cardiac output, heart rate was not reduced and cardiovascular collapse did not occur in the presence of withdrawal of 13 per cent of blood volume. It thus seemed likely that the sudden bradycardia resulting in cardiovascular

(−23%), but cardiac output remains close to control levels as a result of an elevated heart rate. Lidocaine plain (*left*). A representation of a typical response is shown. Severe bradycardia is associated with extreme hypotension, and in two subjects, vagal arrest occurred which required rapid resuscitation with ephedrine and oxygen. In only one subject studied, hypotension was associated with increased heart rate, and this prevented the extreme hypotension seen in the other five subjects. (Modified from data of Bonica, J.J., Berges, P.U., and Morikawa, K.: Circulatory effects of epidural block: I. Effects of levels of analgesia and dose of lidocaine. Anesthesiology, *33*:1619, 1970; Bonica, J.J., Akamatsu, T.J., Berges, P.U., Morikawa, K., and Kennedy, W.F.: Circulatory effects of epidural block. II: Effects of epinephrine. Anesthesiology, *34*:514, 1971 and Bonica, J.J., et al.: Anesthesiology, *36*:219, 1972)

Table 8-10. Danger Signals: Cardiovascular Effects of Epidural Block

Signal	*Mechanisms and Potential Sequelae*	*Treatment*
↑HR ↓BP in Supine Parturient with sensory level T11–L4 or ↓HR ↓BP—a more dangerous sign	Inferior Vena Cava Occlusion + venodilatation in lower limbs →↓Venous return, ↓CO, ↓organ perfusion (incl. fetus) →Epidural vein engorgement → ↓spinal cord perfusion → "spinal stroke" →↑Sympathetic activity (above level of block) → ↑HR + vasoconstriction in upper limbs →↓RA pressure → ↑HR (also ↓BP → ↑HR via baroreceptors (Note ⇊RV pressure may → ⇊HR; see Table 8-11 & LV Fig. 21)	Lateral Position IV fluids, oxygen until MAP normal
Gradual ↓HR ↓BP with sensory level above T4	Venodilation (as above) + ↓ cardiac sympathetic activity → ↓CO ↓HR ↓MAP → ↓Cardiac Sympathetic Activity initially accompanied by ↓ Parasympathetic (see also Fig. 8-21). → However ⇊ venous return → ↑ vagal activity. Therefore, ⇊HR may occur before blockade of all T1–T4	IV fluids. Elevate legs. Atropine. Oxygen until MAP normal. Rarely, Vasopressor (ephedrine)
"Sudden bradycardia" in either condition above	⇊Venous return may result in sudden ↑parasympathetic tone ("faint response"); see table 8-11; Fig. 8-21) ⇊HR → cardiac arrest	As above, but emphasis on sequence: elevate legs, oxygen, IV atropine, IV fluids—ephedrine rapidly if no response to above
"Inappropriate" bradycardia (i.e., "normal" HR in face of ↓MAP with sensory level T3–4)	Peripheral vasodilatation should evoke an ↑HR. Blockade above T4 may impair this response, so HR remains at pre-block rate but is "inappropriately" slow	IV atropine if MAP does not respond to fluids and elevation of legs, and relief of venous obstruction
Reduced blood volume or known obstruction of inferior vena	Hemorrhage Increased intra-abdominal pressure	Restore blood volume Relieve vena caval obstruction } Prior to epidural block
↓HR with visceral traction, in presence of blockade to T1	Total sympathetic block Unopposed vagus Changes in vagal tone → profound changes in HR; may → transient asystole (see Table 8-11; Fig. 8-21)	IV atropine(?) Local infiltration to block vagal stimulus Ensure venous return adequate + arterial P_{O_2} adequate since ↑HR → ↑myocardial oxygen demand

Table 8-11. Vagal and Sympathetic Activity: Effects on Heart Rate

	Venous Return "Sensors" in Great Veins, Atria, Ventricles	*Arterial Pressure "Sensors" in Carotid Sinus and Aortic Arch*
Afferent path	Vagus	Vagus, glossopharyngeal
Efferent path	Vagus	Sympathetic
Effect of increased venous return + ↑ BP	↑ Venous return ↘ ↓ Vagal activity → ↑ HR	↑ BP ↘ ↓ sympathetic activity → ↓ HR
Effect of decreased venous return + ↓ BP	↓ Venous return ↘	
Mild (↓ atrial *volume*)	↓ Vagal activity → ↑ HR	↓ BP → ↑ sympathetic activity → ↑ HR
Severe (↓ ventricular *pressure*)	↑ Vagal activity → ↓↓ HR	?↓↓ BP† → ↑↑ Sympathetic activity ↓ ? Accentuates activation of vagal receptors in ventricle

† ↓↓ BP also → ↓ carotid body oxygen supply. This initiates a "hypoxic" response and further increases vagal efferent activity.

collapse in human subjects may have been due to parasympathetic activity similar to that seen in the "faint" response to decreased venous return.[42] This sudden increase in parasympathetic activity is a vagal response to marked reductions in venous return (Tables 8-10,11; Fig. 8-21). Usually this response only occurs in conscious humans (and in no other species) and is abolished by general anesthesia.[388] It is worth emphasizing that severe reductions in venous return, such as those observed in Bonica's study,[27] result in a very sudden large increase in vagal activity[201,328–331] (Fig. 8-21). Thus, a patient's condition may suddenly deteriorate to the point of loss of consciousness and, perhaps, asystole.

What factors were responsible for the somewhat less pronounced cardiovascular depression in hypovolemic subjects receiving epidural block with lidocaine-epinephrine? It has already been noted that absorbed lidocaine-epinephrine results in increased heart rate and cardiac output, but a lower mean arterial pressure owing to decreased peripheral resistance, compared to plain lidocaine. However, the higher cardiac rate may protect the heart from increases in vagal activity, although it has been noted that a high level of sympathetic activity may accentuate cholinergic effects in patients with poor venous return.[331] It is also possible that peak arterial blood concentrations of lidocaine were higher after plain lidocaine in patients with hypovolemia owing to decreased cardiac output and, thus, a smaller volume of distribution (see Fig. 4-10). In this situation, the myocardium receives a larger percentage of cardiac output and, thus, is potentially exposed to higher concentrations of local anesthetics. Any coexistent hypercapnia or acidosis would tend to accentuate the transfer of local anesthetic into the myocardium by the "ion trapping" mechanism (see Chap. 3). The moral of Bonica's study is clear:[27] Epidural block should be avoided or used with great care in patients with uncorrected hypovolemia or in any other patient in whom venous return is markedly impaired (*e.g.*, patients with large intra-abdominal masses, in whom the pressure of the mass on the vena cava cannot be relieved prior to blockade; Fig. 8-13).

Epidural Block and General Anesthesia

It has been a standard practice in many institutions to employ a combination of light general anesthesia and epidural block for lower abdominal and pelvic surgery.[375] Despite anecdotes suggesting that the combination has dangerous hemodynamic consequences, until recently there were few objective data available. Stephen and colleagues studied the combination of epidural block administered approx-

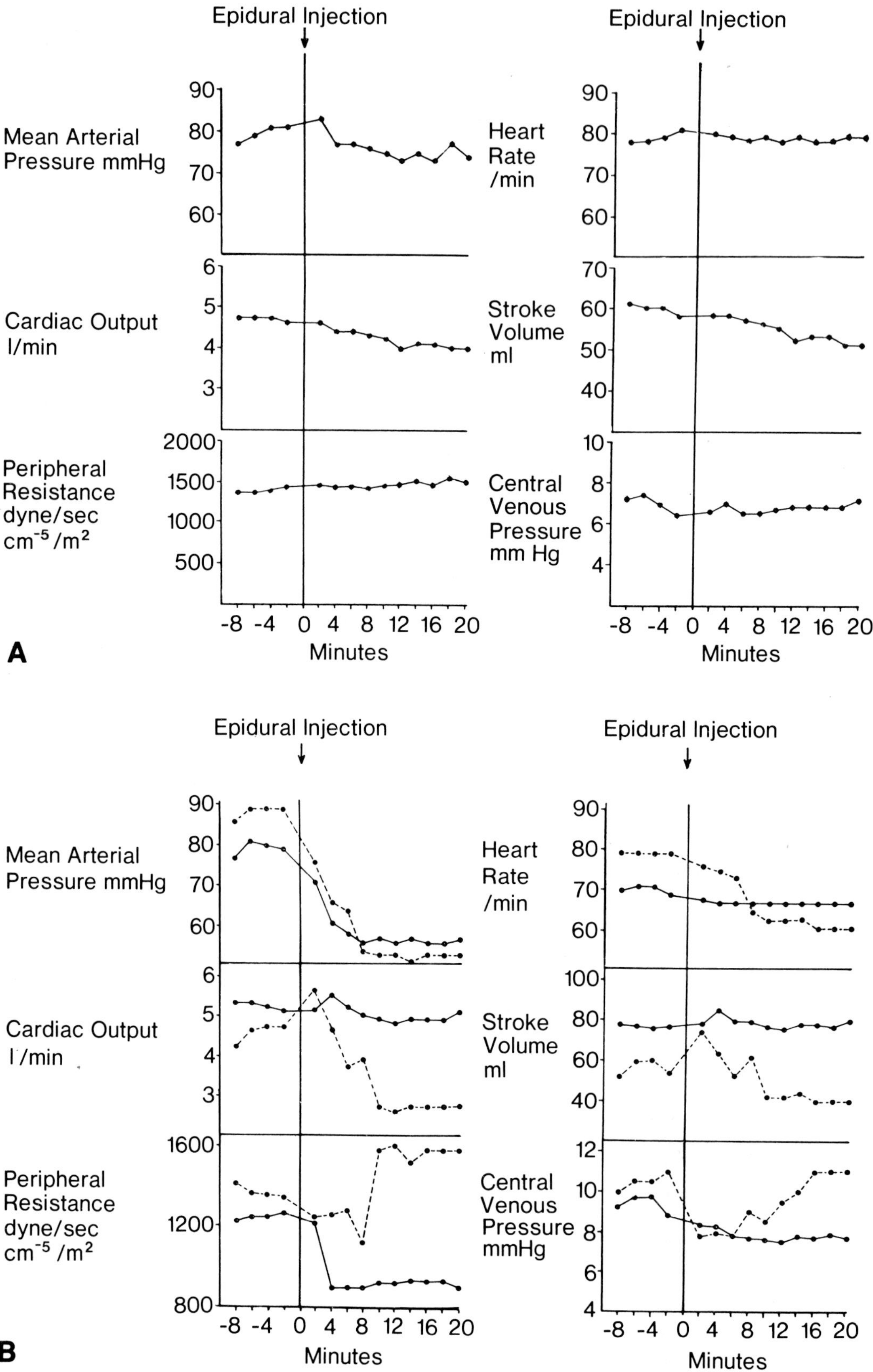
Epidural Injection
Mean Arterial Pressure mmHg
90
80
70
60
Heart Rate /min
Cardiac Output l/min
6
5
4
3
Stroke Volume ml
Peripheral Resistance dyne/sec cm^{-5}/m^2
2000
1500
1000
500
Central Venous Pressure mm Hg
10
8
6
4
-8 -4 0 4 8 12 16 20
Minutes
A
Epidural Injection
Mean Arterial Pressure mmHg
Heart Rate /min
Cardiac Output l/min
Stroke Volume ml
100
Peripheral Resistance dyne/sec cm^{-5}/m^2
1600
1200
800
Central Venous Pressure mmHg
12
-8 -4 0 4 8 12 16 20
Minutes
B

imately 20 minutes after the induction of light general anesthesia, consisting of thiopentone-nitrous-oxide-oxygen.[408] In six of the 11 patients studied, there were no significant hemodynamic changes resulting from the epidural injection of 30 ml of 2-per-cent plain lidocaine at the L3 interspace. The remaining five patients had significant reductions of mean arterial blood pressure (−30%). However, only one of these five also had a reduced cardiac output (−40%) which was associated with bradycardia (−25%). Unfortunately, level of blockade could not be recorded in this study, although it was likely to be in the region of T5, considering the dose of local anesthetic employed (Fig. 8-18). Interesting additional observations were made by Stephen and colleagues in patients given epidural block and general anesthesia:[408] Elevation of the legs resulted in increased mean arterial pressure, central venous pressure, and peripheral resistance, but no change in cardiac output; intravenous ephedrine (10 mg) was more effective in producing the above changes and also increased cardiac output (Fig. 8-19). Scott's group extended this study to epidural block with lidocaine and epinephrine (1:200,000).[381] Although hemodynamic changes were quite variable, their findings were similar to those of Bonica and colleagues in conscious subjects.[24] In particular, total peripheral resistance was much lower than when plain solutions were used. More recently, Germann and colleagues addressed themselves to important gaps in knowledge of the cardiovascular effects of epidural block combined with general anesthesia (thiopentone-nitrous-oxide-oxygen-succinylcholine):[190] precise documentation of level of epidural block and hemodynamic effects of superimposed general anesthesia; the effect of order of performance of epidural block either before or after general anesthesia; the comparative effects of 10-degree, head-down tilt and intravenous atropine during established epidural block and general anesthesia.

Epidural block was carried out in healthy patients by using an indwelling epidural catheter (L3–4), with a dose of 15 to 20 ml of 1.5-per-cent plain lidocaine. Level of analgesia extended to T6 (± 2 segments) in patients who received epidural block prior to general anesthesia, and it was assumed that similar levels were achieved in those who had general anesthesia induced first. Since the protocol for this study was complicated, a summary of the sequence of events is given in Table 8-12. In patients receiving general anesthesia first (group A), epidural block resulted in reductions of mean arterial pressure (− 22%) which were the only significant changes (Fig. 8-20; Table 8-13). In those receiving epidural block first (group B), mean arterial pressure was reduced by 20 per cent from awake control values after epidural block, and there was a further reduction to 35 per cent below control values when general anesthesia was induced (Table 8-13). Heart rate and cardiac output were not significantly changed. However, it seems reasonable to postulate that a heart rate of approximately 60 beats per minute is *inappropriately slow* in the face of reduced mean arterial pressure and reduced peripheral vascular resistance. Subsequent administration of 0.6 mg intravenous atropine returned mean arterial blood pressure to control values in both groups and was associated with a heart rate of approximately 110 beats per minute; as indicated in Table 8-24, smaller doses of atropine seem to be preferable. Head-down tilt (10 degrees) resulted in a small increase in stroke volume but no other significant hemodynamic changes in either group. Right atrial pressure was not significantly altered at any stage of the studies. Blood gases were not significantly altered, except that Pa_{O_2} was reduced when epidural block was added to established general anesthesia; however, there was no change in oxygen consumption (Table 8-13). When the sequence of performance of epidural block and general anesthesia was examined, no significant differences in hemodynamics or blood gases were found; these findings indicated that order of performance of epidural block did not affect hemodynamic variables. However, technical and anatomical considerations also influence the decision, since the awake patient can signal contact of needle with nerve root, facet, and other important structures (Table 8-21). Also, the ability to determine level of blockade prior to induc-

←

Fig. 8-18. Cardiovascular effects of epidural block and general anesthesia. (*A*) Patients (n = 6) who did not become markedly hypotensive maintained normal heart rate and cardiac output. (*B*) Patients (n = 5) who developed marked hypotension. Four of the patients (*continuous line*) had cardiac output and heart rate that were essentially unchanged so that hypotension was due to the marked reduction in peripheral resistance. In one patient (*dotted line*) cardiac output fell coincident with reduced heart rate. (Stephen, G.W., Lees, M.M., and Scott, D.B.: Cardiovascular effects of epidural block combined with general anaesthesia. Br. J. Anaesth., *41*:933, 1969)

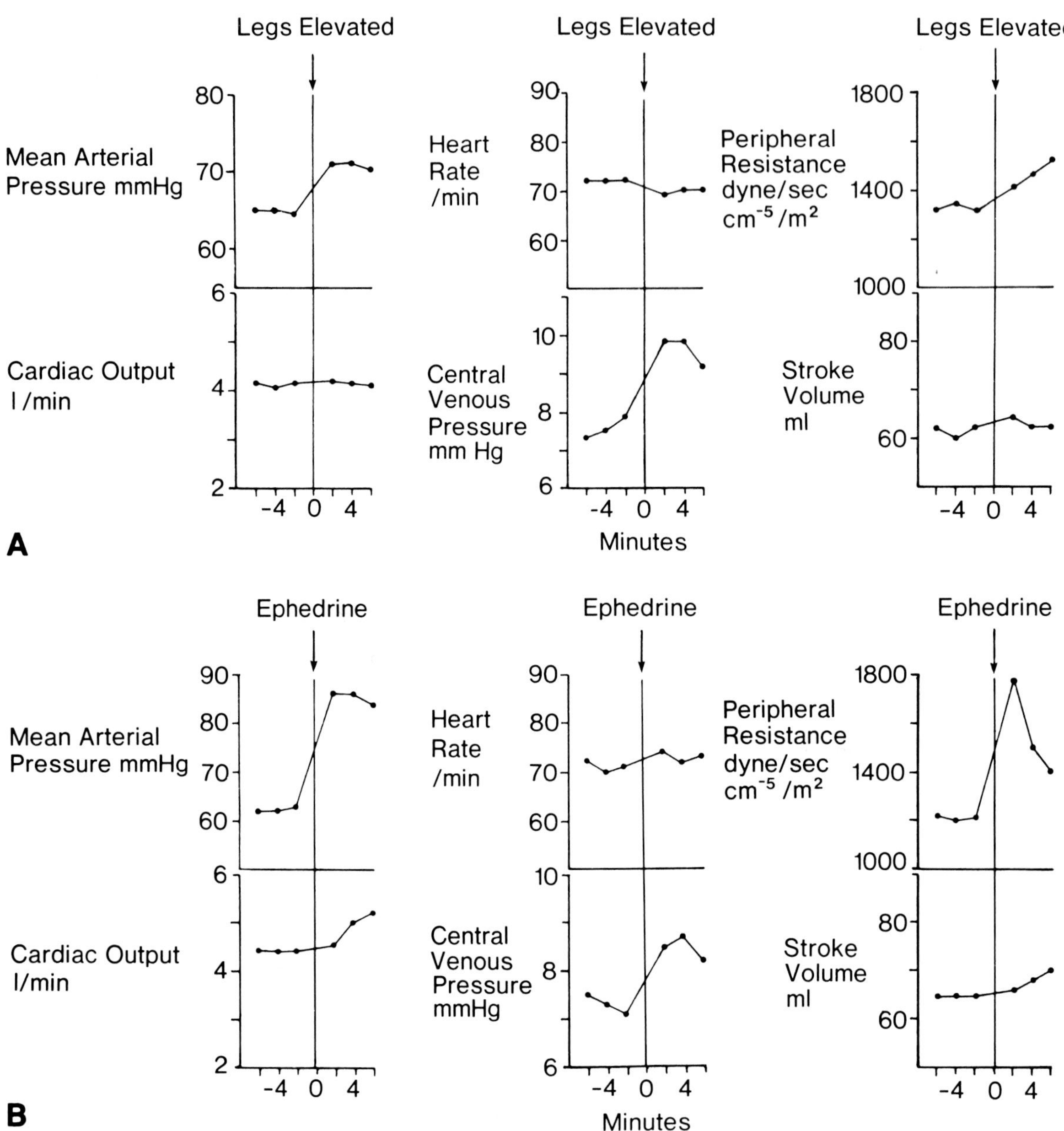

Fig. 8-19. CVS changes with epidural block and general anesthesia; effect of ephedrine and leg elevation. (*A*) Leg elevation results in increased mean arterial blood pressure and central venous pressure, but no change in cardiac output. (*B*) Ephedrine (10 mg IV) results in increased mean arterial blood pressure initially due to increased peripheral resistance and subsequently due to increased cardiac output. (Stephen, G.W., Lees, M.M., and Scott, D.B.: Cardiovascular effects of epidural block combined with general anaesthesia. Br. J. Anaesth., *41*:933, 1969)

tion of anesthesia permits more informed decisions about cardiovascular support and also confirms adequacy of blockade of operative field.

In summary it appears that light general anesthesia can be safely combined with epidural block to the level of T5 in healthy patients. The studies of both Stephen and colleagues[408] and Germann and colleagues[190] recommend the use of small incremental doses of atropine in this situation to maintain heart rates of approximately 90 to 100 beats per

Table 8-12. Summary of Protocol for Study of Epidural Block and General Anesthesia

Stage	*Time (min)*	*Procedure*
	0	Insertion of epidural and vascular catheters
		20 minutes rest period
1	20	Hemodynamic and blood gas measurements
	30	Group A receives general anesthesia
		Group B receives epidural block
		20 minutes stabilization
2	60	Hemodynamic and blood gas measurements
	65	10-degree head-down tilt
3	70	Hemodynamic and blood gas measurements (Patient returned to horizontal position)
	75	Group A epidural block
		Group B general anesthesia
		20 minutes stabilization
4	100	Hemodynamic and blood gas measurements
	105	10-degree head-down tilt
5	110	Hemodynamic and blood gas measurements
		Groups A and B
	115	Return to horizontal position
	125	Atropine (0.6 mg IV)
6	130	Hemodynamic and blood gas measurements

(Germann, P. A. S., Roberts, J. G., and Prys-Roberts, C.: The combination of general anaesthesia and epidural block. I: The effects of sequence of induction on haemodynamic variables and blood gas measurements in healthy patients. Anaes. Intens. Care, 7:229, 1979)

Table 8-13. Epidural Block and General Anesthesia, Hemodynamics

		Stage 1 (*Control*)	*Stage 2* (*GA or Epidural*)	*Stage 4* (*GA + Epidural*)
Heart rate (beats/min)	A (GA 1st)	67 ± 18	63 ± 11	63 ± 8
	B (epidural 1st)	60 ± 4	64 ± 8	57 ± 13
Mean arterial pressure (torr)	A	82 ± 10	75 ± 6	*64 ± 5
	B	89 ± 10	*71 ± 18	*58 ± 16
Cardiac output (L/min/70 kg)	A	4.95 ± 0.70	4.35 ± 0.90	4.25 ± 0.75
	B	4.35 ± 0.90	4.50 ± 1.00	3.60 ± 1.00
Stroke volume (ml)	A	79 ± 19	70 ± 10	68 ± 11
	B	73 ± 14	70 ± 9	64 ± 11
Systemic vascular resistance	A	1487 ± 277	1528 ± 305	1344 ± 206
(dyn. sec. cm − 5)	B	1889 ± 239	*1428 ± 177	*1447 ± 233

* Significant change ($p < 0.05$) Vs control
\+ Significant change ($p < 0.05$) Vs stage 2
(Germann, P. A. S., Roberts, J. G., and Prys-Roberts, C.: The combination of general anaesthesia and epidural block. I: The effects of sequence of induction on haemodynamic variables and blood gas measurements in healthy patients. Anaes. Intens. Care, 7:229, 1979)

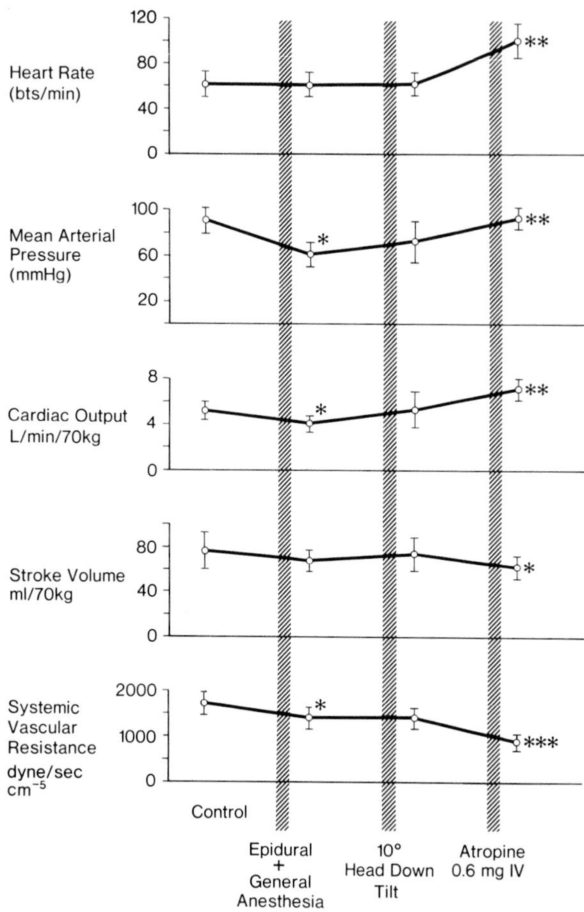

Fig. 8-20. CVS effects of epidural block and general anesthesia; effect of sequence of block, atropine, and 10-degree head down tilt. Epidural block (to T6) plus general anesthesia result in a similar degree of reduction in mean arterial blood pressure (MAP) whether epidural block is induced before or after general anesthesia. Administration of atropine (0.6 mg IV) returned MAP to control values in both groups. Head-down tilt (10 degrees) was not effective in reversing hemodynamic changes. (Germann, P.A.S., Roberts, J.G., and Prys-Roberts, C.: The combination of general anaesthesia and epidural block. I: The effects of sequence of induction on haemodynamic variables and blood gas measurements in healthy patients. Anaesth. Intens. Care, *7*:229, 1979)

minute. If additional cardiovascular support is required, elevation of the legs, increased intravenous fluid administration, or ephedrine should be employed, depending upon each patient's cardiovascular status and likely response to such maneuvers. Although significant changes in Pa_{O_2} were only observed by Germann and colleagues with the sequence of general anesthesia followed by epidural block, it seems wise to administer at least 30-percent inspired oxygen whenever epidural block is combined with general anesthesia or with intravenous sedation.

IMPORTANT ASPECTS OF VENOUS RETURN AND EPIDURAL BLOCKADE

As indicated in Tables 8-10,11 and Figure 8-21, reduced venous return may play a dominant role in initiating sudden reductions in cardiac rate, which should be viewed as a danger signal that oxygenation of the myocardium is at risk. There is little doubt that obstruction to venous return, by whatever means, must be avoided in patients being given epidural block. If postural changes are added to obstruction in the presence of the increased venous capacitance of epidural block, then serious impairment of venous return will follow. In addition, pressure in epidural veins will rise due to channeling of blood from the pelvis by way of the alternative route of the vertebral venous plexus and azygos vein to the right atrium; this has important consequences for increased spread of segmental analgesia and also may impair arterial blood flow to the spinal cord.[395] Situations in which venous return may be compromised may be summarized (Fig. 8-13):

Supine hypotensive syndrome in pregnancy owing to uterine compression of the vena cava is accentuated by increased venous capacitance due to sympathetic block of epidural analgesia and postural changes favoring pooling of blood in the lower limbs.[228,373,374,379]

Uterine contraction during labor in supine position. Mean brachial arterial pressure may be maintained at deceptively normal levels because of simultaneous compression of vena cava and aorta (Poseiro effect). However, mean femoral arterial pressure drops precipitously, as does uterine blood flow.[19] These effects are accentuated by epidural block if the patient is allowed to remain supine.

Intestinal obstruction, ascites, and large intra-abdominal tumors may compress the vena cava at three main sites: *below the liver,* due to abdominal distention, by intestinal obstruction[11] or by ascites.[352] (This site is also commonly occluded by overenthusiastic retraction or by abdominal packs during upper abdominal surgery); *in the upper lumbar region,* by large intraabdominal tumors, (including the uterus); *at the pelvic brim,* by stretching of the iliac vessels due to extreme backward tilting of the pelvis. This is sometimes an accompaniment of later pregnancy and may also occur due to extreme lordotic posturing on the operating table. The "extended lordotic posture" may also occlude the vena cava below the liver—with potential for venous congestion in the kidney and resultant proteinuria.[80]

The most common causes of vena caval obstruction in surgical applications of epidural block are poor posturing, heavy-handed retraction, and incorrect use of abdominal packs. Extreme postures, such as the jack knife prone, lateral "kidney," and hyperflexed lithotomy should be avoided in association with any anesthetic and with epidural block in particular.[289,373] Whenever possible, caval obstruction should be relieved prior to epidural block or carefully avoided after epidural block. If it occurs and can not be corrected for a period of time, then venous return may be assisted by restoring venous capacitance to normal levels by using carefully titrated doses of ephedrine (5–10 mg), intravenously. In some patients with large abdominal tumors, the aorta and vena cava may both be partially obstructed, but with maintenance of sufficient venous return to keep mean arterial pressure normal, with a partly occluded aorta. Sudden relief of the aortic obstruction as the tumor is removed may cause a precipitous fall in blood pressure owing to the reactive hyperemia below the level of obstruction. This situation may be avoided by ensuring adequate hydration and, perhaps, by using appropriate amounts of colloid prior to tumor removal. Also, one should be prepared to use small doses of ephedrine until reactive hyperemia subsides.

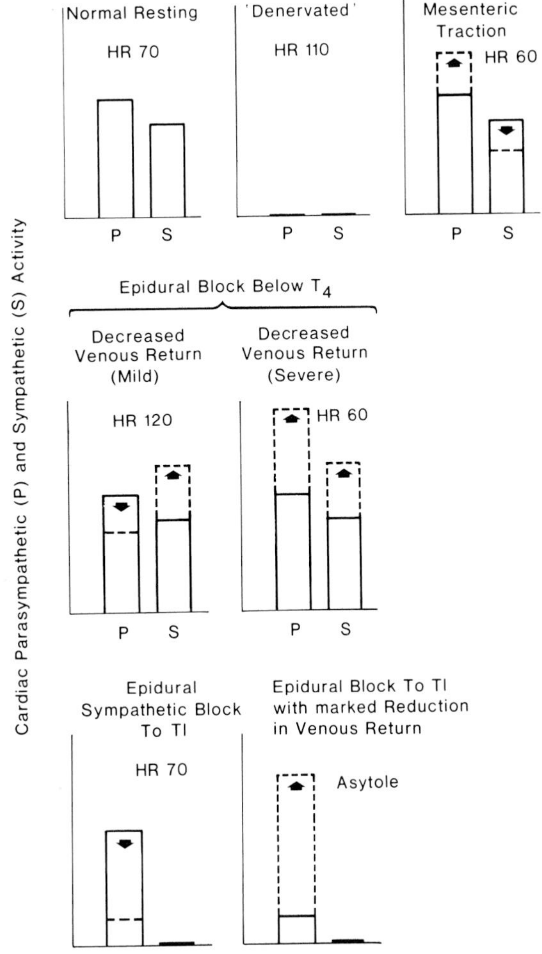

Fig. 8-21. Vagal effects of epidural block. (*Top, left*). The balance of cardiac parasympathetic (P) activity and sympathetic (S) activity is shown with a normal resting heart rate of 70. (*Top, middle*) The presence of a heart rate of 110 following complete "denervation" of the heart emphasizes the dominant action of the vagus. (*Top, right*) Autonomic reflexes such as mesentric traction usually result in bradycardia by an opposite change in P and S. (*Center*) With epidural block to T4. (*Center, left*) A mild reduction in venous return results in tachycardia by an opposite change in P and S. (*Center, right*) Marked reduction in venous return stimulates an increase in P, and S increases in an attempt to minimise the bradycardia. (*Bottom*) Epidural block to T1. (*Bottom, left*) Usual situation, in which P has diminished to compensate for a blocked S. A heart rate of 70 is the result of the same dominance of P over S that exists at rest. However, P is now completely unopposed. (*Bottom, right*) Marked reduction in venous return (or other stimulus to P) results in unopposed increase in P, which may lead to asystole. Such responses are much more likely in the conscious patient.

Epidural Blockade and Reduction of Blood Loss

Although initial emphasis on methods to reduce operative blood loss focussed on reduction of arterial blood pressure,[155,200] it was also well known that posture played an important part.[155]

More recently, there has been a gradual recognition of the importance of avoidance of venous obstruction and the use of posture in combination with sympathetic blockade to aid venous pooling away from the operative site. Thus, although epidural blockade has been used to produce hypotension and, in turn, control operative blood loss,[426,427] others have found that blood loss can be reduced *without* the levels of hypotension commonly required if general anesthesia and ganglion blockade are employed.[166,253,280,304,414,459] Keith deliberately avoided arterial hypotension in a randomized prospective study of blood loss using epidural or general anesthesia for surgery for total hip replacement.[253] Blood loss intraoperatively was determined by a colorimetric technique and postoperatively, by closed suction drains. Patients receiving epidural block had operative blood losses that were half those associated with general anesthesia. In contrast, there was no difference in postoperative blood losses between the two groups. Stanton-Hicks also reported a reduction of blood loss by half if epidural block is used for hip surgery.[404] Thus, it appears that epidural block may reduce operative blood loss by factors other than a mild reduction in arterial blood pressure, increased venous capacitance,[391] and the use of appropriate posture. Additional factors may include the prevention of high venous pressure in response to sympathetic activity resulting from pain:[63] avoidance of "reactive arterial hypertension"[221] and avoidance of increased airway pressure with resultant effects on venous pressure.[303]

FUNCTION OF HOLLOW VISCERA AFTER EPIDURAL BLOCKADE

The Bladder

One of the most commonly observed sequela of lumbar epidural block is temporary atonia of the bladder owing to blockade of sacral segments S2–4. This is similar to lower motor neuron lesions in which bladder sensation is lost. Fortunately, this type of effect after epidural blockade is usually short-lived and causes no or minimal increases in post-block bladder dysfunction.[128,305]

However, when continuous epidural techniques are employed, catheterization of the bladder may be necessary.[227] On the other hand, segmental thoracic epidural block (*e.g.*, T5-L1) may spare the sacral segments and thus leave bladder sensation intact. In addition, relief of severe abdominal pain by epidural block from T5 to L1 may prevent reflex sympathetic activity (via T12–L1 spinal segments), which increases bladder sphincter tone and may predispose to acute retention.

The Gut

Epidural block extending from T5 to L1 effectively denervates the splanchnic sympathetic supply to the abdominal viscera (see Figs. 13-1,2). The sympathetic blockade results in a small contracted gut due to parasympathetic dominance. This may greatly enhance access during surgery. However, the question has been raised whether this predisposes to postoperative ileus. In 1977 electroenterographic studies were carried out in patients after cholecystectomy under general anaesthesia, with or without thoracic epidural blockade.[189] The electrical activity of the stomach and intestine decreased after surgery in all patients and did not return to normal until the third or fourth postoperative day. However, a marked increase in amplitude and frequency of electrical oscillations was recorded in 80 per cent of patients who received epidural block. Also, eating resulted in markedly increased electrical activity in patients whose postoperative pain was treated by epidural block, whereas eating in association with nicomorphine injection resulted in no change in electrical activity. These interesting results suggest that intra- and postoperative epidural block may be useful in preventing and treating postoperative adynamic ileus. However, a note of caution is necessary: The use of epidural block should not distract attention from the treatment of important causes of ileus, such as obstruction and peritonitis. Further work to elucidate the effects of epidural block on gut motility is warranted.

Gastric emptying, as assessed by paracetamol absorption, was much closer to normal following epidural block compared to the use of morphine for postoperative pain.[324]

THERMOREGULATION, SHIVERING, AND MALIGNANT HYPERPYREXIA

The vasodilatation of extensive epidural block may predispose to hypothermia if vasodilated areas of the patient are left exposed in a cold environment. However, this reduction in body temperature occurs slowly and does not explain the rapid onset of shivering that sometimes immediately follows the injection of local anaesthetic solutions into the epidural space.[148] The mechanism of this shivering is not known. However, the following factors may be involved: vasodilatation of skin blood vessels and heat loss; stimulation of epidural temperature sensors by cold fluid, with resultant shivering (this response occurs in animals,[260] but these sensors have not been found in humans); a short period of differential loss of warm sensation, which sometimes occurs prior to loss of cold sensation.[319] It appears that shivering is more common after bupivacaine, and the slow onset of blockade would certainly permit a longer period of differential loss of warm sensation with associated shivering. A controlled study comparing incidence of shivering with saline, lidocaine, and bupivacaine, all at a similar temperature, is not available.

Malignant hyperthermia until recently was thought to be due to genetic abnormalities in skeletal muscle.[313] However, Kerr and colleagues recently reported that porcine malignant hyperthermia could be prevented by epidural block: Surprisingly, if epidural block only involved the hind limbs, these remained flaccid while the rest of the body became rigid and the temperature rise was prevented.[256a]

In contrast, spinal cord transection in the cervical region delayed the rise in temperature but did not prevent it. Thus, it appears that maintenance of some spinal cord activity is necessary, but modification of sensory, sympathetic, and, perhaps, efferent motor activity is somehow involved in preventing the explosive temperature rise of malignant hyperpyrexia. Further investigations are required to determine the implications of these observations for human malignant hyperpyrexia.

NEUROENDOCRINE EFFECTS OF EPIDURAL BLOCKADE

Does "deafferentation" of the surgical field by epidural block favorably modify the "stress" response to surgery? The difficulty in answering this question has been two-fold: methodological problems in measuring neuroendocrine responses and uncertainty about the clinical significance of changes that have been observed. In interpreting the results of such studies, it should be remembered that epidural block to T5 level abolishes efferent splanchnic outflow to adrenal medulla as well as noxious afferent somatic and sympathetic impulses, provided blockade extends outside the upper and lower limits of the operative field. However, epidural block does not block vagal afferent fibers from the upper abdominal viscera, and this may be responsible for afferent stimulation of release from the hypothalamus of hormones (*e.g.*, ADH) or of humoral "trophic" hormones (*e.g.*, ACTH), which in turn may result in humoral release from target organs (*e.g.*, cortisol from adrenal cortex). The relative importance of the various components of the neurohumoral "stress" response in the surgical patient has not been elucidated, so that it is not possible to say if the failure of epidural block to obtund vagal afferents negates its favorable effect on adrenal medullary function[70,124] and hepatic release of blood glucose.[72] However, a gross indication that the net effect may be favorable is a markedly diminished hospital stay of patients who received continuous epidural block for perioperative management of upper abdominal surgery compared to those who received general anesthesia and narcotic medication.[341] Further evidence is provided by a favorable influence of epidural block on incidence of deep vein thrombosis after major surgery.[264]

Adrenal Medulla

Although it is known that surgery and pain increase sympathetic activity with resultant rises in circulating catecholamine levels,[323] precise quantitation has had to await the development of assay techniques capable of measuring basal levels of catecholamines in humans.[87] These techniques are currently being applied to investigate the perioperative changes in catecholamine output associated with general and/or regional anesthesia.

Early animal studies indicate that during surgery, general anesthesia alone may be sufficient to dampen catecholamine release.[149,358] More recent studies in humans report that insignificant changes in serum catecholamine levels occur during surgery under general anesthesia.[83] However, it is possible that the assay technique employed was not of sufficient sensitivity to detect clinically important changes or that measurements were not made at the most appropriate times. Evidence now accumulating indicates that catecholamine levels may be high preoperatively, "breakthrough" may occur under light general anesthesia, and levels may again be very high in the postoperative period as a result of postoperative pain.* Epidural block modifies the pentazocine stimulated increase in catecholamines.[412] Since epidural block prevents catecholamine release due to surgical stimulus in patients with pheochromocytoma,[70,124] it is likely that it is capable of preventing intraoperative catechol release in normal patients. Recent studies of the antihypertensive effects of epidural block after cardiac surgery[221] indicate that postoperative catecholamine release and associated reduction in myocardial oxygen delivery may also be prevented by the "deafferentation" of epidural block. Obstetrical studies indicate that epidural block prevents increased catecholamine secretion and resultant reductions in uterine blood flow that are associated with severe pain.[454] Further circumstantial evidence of reduced catecholamine secretion by epidural block is the maintenance of normal blood sugar

* Hamilton, W.: Personal communication, 1979.

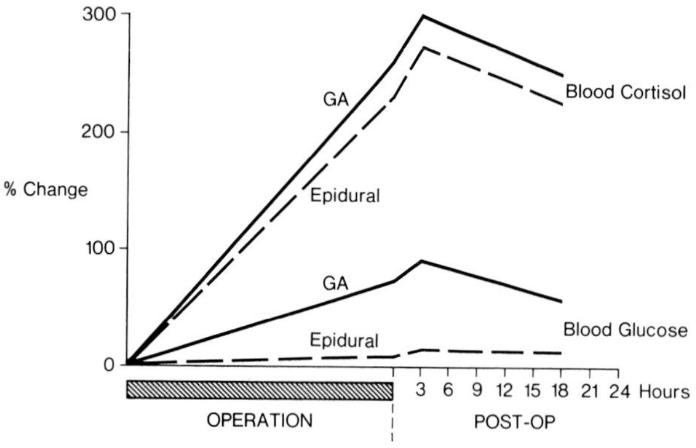

Fig. 8-22. Neuroendocrine effects of epidural block. The blood sugar response to surgery is completely abolished by epidural block which "deafferents" the operative site. The increase in plasma cortisol is little affected by epidural block in upper abdominal and thoracic surgery, presumably because afferent vagal impulses to the hypothalamus release cortisol by means of blood-borne ACTH.

response and glucose tolerance during surgery under epidural block.[72,230]

Adrenal Cortex

It is well known that adrenal cortical output of cortisol may be increased up to ten times by surgical trauma[234] to result in five-fold rises in plasma cortisol levels.[70] Epidural or subarachnoid blockade may delay the normal increase in cortisol secretion[208,433]; however, even in lower abdominal surgery, epidural block provides only a temporary effect, and cortisol levels may eventually reach the same concentration as with general anesthesia, even if postoperative analgesia is managed with epidural block.[38,115,158,194,283] Gordon and colleagues interpreted their results,[194] in gynecological surgery, as an indication that cortisol response could be prevented if complete deafferentation of the lower abdomen was obtained and continued into the postoperative period. They reported that patients with satisfactory "continuous" blockade did not manifest an increase in plasma cortisol in the perioperative period. Only patients with unsatisfactory or discontinuous block developed a delayed increase in plasma cortisol.

Upper abdominal and thoracic surgery show a more consistent picture. There is little difference in plasma cortisol levels between general anesthesia alone and/or epidural block.[36,72] In the study by Bromage and colleagues, epidural block was maintained above T4 during and for 19 hours after abdominal surgery and above T1 in association with thoracic surgery.[72] Despite meticulous attention to adequate blockade, plasma cortisol levels increased as much as with general anesthesia, presumably because vagal afferents were unblocked (Fig. 8-22). It was suggested that vagal impulses to the hypothalamus initiated ACTH release, which then produced a humoral release of cortisol from the adrenal cortex. No studies of the effect on cortisol secretion of celiac plexus or splanchnic nerve blockade combined with epidural or intercostal block are available.

Blood Sugar Level

Epidural block in animals capable of abolishing reflex efferent stimuli to the adrenal medulla and liver usually results in increased blood glucose during surgical stress under general anesthesia, provided the entire splanchnic outflow is blocked.[242] Bromage and colleagues[72] and Brandt and colleagues[36] were able to show complete abolition of blood glucose response if effective blockade was maintained during and after upper abdominal and thoracic surgery (Fig. 8-22). More recently, Houghton and colleagues[230] reported that epidural block maintained normal glucose tolerance and insulin release during surgery, whereas general anesthesia resulted in decreased insulin release and glucose tolerance. Since sympathetic stimulation may occur under general anesthesia, the finding of decreased insulin release by Houghton and colleagues[230] is supportive of animal studies, in which sympathetic stimulation reduced insulin secretion[345] and resulted in increased glucagon secretion. However, other studies in humans have failed to measure a decrease in insulin secretion during surgery under general anesthesia.[36,37] On the contrary, Brandt and colleagues reported that insulin secretion remained low and unchanged during both general and epidural anesthesia.[37] Thus, the "inappropriately" low insulin secretion in the face of hyperglycemia during general anesthesia and surgery indicates that the secretion of insulin in response to hyperglycemia is blocked during general anesthesia. The abolition of the hyperglycemic response by epidural analgesia is not caused by an increased insulin secretion. It is still possible that glucagon secretion is increased by general anesthesia, thus raising blood sugar, and that this increase is prevented by epidural block. However, it is more likely that abolition of reflex sympathetic activity during surgery by epidural block prevents sympathetic neural and humoral effects on the liver, which would otherwise result in glycogenolysis and increased blood glucose.

Important clinical implications of the effect of epidural block on blood sugar are as follows:

Diabetic patients may be managed very satisfactorily by this method, provided that insulin is not given to such patients unless added glucose is administered intravenously; otherwise, blood sugar levels may become dangerously low. The combination of hypotension of epidural block with reduced oxygen delivery to the brain and the added insult of hypoglycemia may have disastrous effects on cerebral function.

If insulin is administered on the basis of a high blood glucose measurement, it should be remembered that the subsequent reduction in blood glucose may be much greater than that without epidural block, since additional factors, such as increased catecholamine levels, that usually elevate blood glucose are probably not present.

Other Hormonal Effects

Some hormonal effects of epidural block are listed below.

A suppression of the rise in plasma renin which occurs during surgery under general anesthesia*
A suppression of the increase in plasma cortisol response during late stages of labor under epidural block[78]
Slightly lower concentrations of renin and angiotensin II during labor in patients with epidural block compared to controls[281]
Thyroid hormone concentration during surgery is unchanged in the presence of epidural block[335]
Cyclic-AMP rises after epidural block during the first stage of labor, and this may coincide with a decrease in uterine contraction[245]

The clinical implications of these observations are not yet known. However, it has been reported that epidural block prevents the increase in plasma cyclic-AMP and modifies the increase in glucose and cortisol that occurs during lower abdominal surgery and general anesthesia. This indicates a protective effect of epidural block in preventing the catabolic response to surgery provided that the operative area is "deafferented."[288]

* Bevan, D.R., Lightman, S., and Peart, W.S.: Plasma Renin Activity, Extradural Analgesia and Surgery. Anesthesiology *51*: 35, 5228.

EFFECTS OF EPIDURAL BLOCKADE ON RESPIRATION

Two important questions concerning respiration and epidural blockade require an answer: Does epidural block interfere with respiration? Is the ability to cough impaired?

The following aspects of epidural blockade may influence respiration:

Aspects of Epidural Blockade That May Influence Respiration

Sensory ("afferent") neural blockade
Motor ("efferent") neural blockade of intercostal muscles, abdominal muscles, and diaphram (rarely)
Sympathetic neural blockade with resultant changes in cardiac output and pulmonary blood flow
Vagal dominance in the presence of complete sympathetic blockade
Effects of systemically absorbed epinephrine and local anesthetic on:
  Respiratory control centre in mid-brain and on chemoreceptors in medulla and carotid bodies
  Myoneural junction
  Metabolism of succinylcholine in serum

The potential for phrenic (C3–5) palsy is extremely low with epidural block, since even blockade to T1 produces motor blockade to only the T4–5 level. The only exception may be intentional epidural block at the cervical level or inadvertant epidural block during interscalene brachial plexus block (see Chap. 10).

Respiratory arrest during high epidural blockade is usually not the result of the effects of sensory or motor blockade, nor is it due to depressant effects of local anaesthetic in the cerebrospinal fluid; the concentrations attained in the brain by means of this route are known not to depress neuronal activity unless gross overdosage is administered.[68] The most common cause of the rare instances of respiratory arrest associated with epidural block is extensive sympathetic blockade, reduced cardiac output, and reduced oxygen delivery to the CNS. It cannot be overemphasized that meticulous attention to maintenance of organ perfusion, by means of the clinical measures described above, should ensure that respiratory arrest in association with epidural block occurs extremely rarely; and, such an occurrence should be rapidly reversible.

It has been claimed that extensive sensory blockade may result in loss of consciousness owing to lack of input to the reticular activating system. However, epidural block to T1 does not cause loss of consciousness.[124] This requires complete efferent blockade, including blockade of the cranial nerves.[63] Although it is likely that such loss of consciousness would interfere with respiratory drive, cardiovascular depression associated with this level of blockade poses an even greater potential for respiratory depression unless appropriate supportive measures are applied; this classically occurs in patients with hypovolemia and with attempts to limit the spread of analgesia by use of the "head-up" position.

However, even patients with sensory loss extending to the level of the chin may have normal respiration and may be fully conscious provided that cardiovascular homeostasis is maintained.[124]

Many factors may contribute to the respiratory effects of epidural block. At present, our knowledge in this area is meager. However, the documented changes produced by epidural block per se appear to be mild. For example, a sensory level of T3, associated with a motor level of T8, may be expected to result in essentially no change in vital capacity (VC) and functional residual capacity (FRC) in normal patients, so that respiration and the ability to cough are not impaired.[176,284,438] In patients with severe pain, epidural block probably improves VC and FRC as well as Pa_{O_2}, at least in the early postoperative period (see also Chap. 25); this may result in improved respiratory exchange and more effective coughing.[49,63,227,301,396,397,401,439]

NEURAL EFFECTS OF EPIDURAL BLOCKADE

The differential neural effects of epidural block on motor, sensory, and sympathetic function are discussed in the context of the pharmacology of the local anesthetics employed for epidural block. Although epidural blockade aims to produce a reversible blockade of axonal activity, it has sometimes been questioned whether more permanent interference with the integrity of the nervous system may result. As discussed in Chapter 4, depressed rapid axonal transport[163,164] does result from profound neural blockade, such as that associated with epidural analgesia. This indicates reduced oxidative metabolism in the axoplasm of nerves. However, this is a reversible process, and the margin of safety appears to be large for local anesthetics compared to drugs producing an irreversible block (*e.g.*, batrachotoxin). It is not known whether some people have genetic abnormalities in neural structure that make them more susceptible to irreversible blockade or whether regenerating neurons are at greater risk. There is some evidence that the developing nervous system may be quite susceptible to some local anesthetics, since neurobehavioral changes in the newborn have been observed following obstetrical epidural block with lidocaine.[368] However, such changes are not seen with bupivacaine[111] or chloroprocaine.[222]

Spinal cord effects of epidural blockade have been proposed by Bromage[61] following his observations of changes in lower limb reflexes in association with thoracic epidural blockade. This is supported by autoradiographic studies: Quite high concentrations of radioactively labeled local anesthetic were found in or close to the peripheral areas of the spinal cord.[68] Thus, it appears likely that epidural block results in blockade of long tracts in the spinal cord and possibly in cell bodies. Further evidence for blockade of cell bodies is given in Chapter 31.

The brain is not immune from local anesthetic penetration, since local anesthetics reach the CSF by way of dural cuffs and are then conveyed to the brain (Figs. 8-2,3).[61] High-dosage epidural block thus exposes the brain to local anesthetic in significant amounts by means of vascular absorption and also by diffusion up the CSF. Although concentrations in the brain are usually below C_m,* it is possible for neural blocking concentrations to be reached if very large doses are employed epidurally or accidentally injected into the subarachnoid space.

Another neural effect of epidural analgesia relates to the deprivation of afferent input which results. Bromage and Melzack reported that patients often experienced "phantom" limb phenomena during epidural blockade, presumably owing to the loss of normal afferent input from body surface, joints, and other structures.[69]

Electromyographic (EMG) recording in animals after application of high concentrations of local anesthetic to the muscle's nerve supply shows temporary abolition of EMG activity. However, ischemic and toxic effects on nerves may result in permanent or semipermanent abolition of normal EMG activity. Denervation results in the development of a low-voltage "fibrillation" pattern in the muscle(s) supplied by the damaged nerve. Recording from appropriate muscle groups can be helpful

* C_m minimum concentration resulting in blockade (see Chapter 2).

in determining if only a single spinal nerve is involved distal to the intervertebral foramen. In such a situation, it is very unlikely that epidural injection of local anesthetic results in nerve damage.[292,293] At the present time, there is no evidence that permanent changes in EMG occur following the use of appropriate clinical concentrations of local anesthetics for epidural blockade. A more detailed examination of the potential for complications in association with epidural blockade reveals, however, that other factors, such as direct trauma by the needle, may result in neural damage.

Studies in humans, employing intra-arterial injection of lidocaine, indicate a significant reduction in response as assessed by evoked electromyography.[411] The pattern of response indicated that the results may be attributable to an effect of lidocaine on the motor nerve terminal. Thus, high blood concentrations of lidocaine might be expected to produce additive effects with both depolarizing and nondepolarizing muscle relaxants.

EPIDURAL BLOCKADE AND PREGNANCY

The known and potential physiologic effects of epidural block on mother, placenta, and fetus must be viewed in the light of contemporary knowledge of the physiology and pathophysiology of pregnancy,[22] and fetal physiology,[165] and pharmacology.[302,349,367] The detailed implications for regional anesthesia are discussed further in Chapter 18.

In brief, the following aspects of the physiologic effects of pregnancy have either proven or potential roles in the management of epidural block:

Pulmonary Changes in Pregnancy

A 50-per-cent increase in minute volume occurs at term, and a further increase occurs during labor. It may peak at 90 L per minute in the second stage of severe pain. Pa_{CO_2} decreases to 30 torr by the onset of labor, but pH remains normal owing to renal compensation; thus, buffer base decreases, and base excess is − 3 to − 5 mEq/L. Oxygen consumption is increased 20 per cent above nonpregnant levels; airway conductance is increased by unknown mechanisms; lung compliance is normal. However, chest wall compliance is reduced. Upward displacement of the diaphragm reduces function residual capacity (FRC) by 20-per-cent, and this is accentuated in the supine position and during contractions as pulmonary blood volume increases. Thus, one-third of parturients develop airway closure during tidal breathing in the supine position[17]; the anteroposterior diameter of the chest wall increases to maintain a normal total lung capacity (TLC), while vital capacity (VC), forced expiratory volume (FEV_1), maximal breathing capacity (MBC), and peak flow rates remain normal; administration of oxygen increases fetal PaO_2 and does not result in placental vasoconstriction.[349]

Clinical Significance. Hypoxia and hypocapnia ensue rapidly if hypoventilation is permitted to occur. During apnea in association with total spinal or epidural blockade or convulsions due to local anesthetic toxicity, Pa_{O_2} drops precipitously, so that administration of 100-per-cent oxygen by mask, or if the airway is obstructed, by rapid intubation, is urgent.

High respiratory minute volumes (MVs) use excess amounts of energy and further increase maternal oxygen consumption without improving fetal oxygenation. This may combine with reduced myocardial oxygen delivery in the supine position to seriously compromise myocardial oxygenation, if epidural block is permitted to reduce venous return.

Recent evidence indicates that high MVs and severe pain are a sign that uterine blood flow may be reduced by excess catecholamine output (see below).

If ventilation has to be controlled for any reason, the preexisting deficiency of base should be borne in mind. Together with the other changes noted above, a higher minute volume than the nonpregnant state is required.

If supplemental inhalation analgesia is required, uptake of soluble agents such as methoxyflurane is very rapid, and as minimum anesthetic concentration (MAC) requirements are reduced, the patient can lose consciousness rapidly.[337]

Maternal Cardiovascular Changes

A 30- to 50-per-cent increase in cardiac output is present by the eighth month of pregnancy. This increase persists if the supine position is avoided. Increasing fetal demands for oxygen occur during labor, with a superimposed 10- to 15-per-cent increase during each contraction. A final large increase in cardiac output to 80 percent above prelabor values occurs immediately after delivery of the placenta. There is also compensatory vasodilation to counteract the latter and maintain normal blood pressure. Compression of vena cava occurs in all parturients; significant hypotension occurs in a small percentage, but in all parturients there is some degree of redirection of venous return by epidural, basivertebral, and azygos veins, as well as a compensatory increase in sympathetic nervous system tone; aortoiliac artery compression occurs during each contraction in the supine position, with reduced femoral artery and uterine artery blood flow. There is a 40-per-cent increase in plasma volume, and a 20-per-cent increase in red cell volume.

Clinical Significance. Under epidural block, changes in cardiac output during labor are greatly reduced compared to "normal" labor. This reduction in cardiac work may be very beneficial to patients with poor myocardial reserves (*e.g.*, patients with valve disease, cardiomyopathy, hypertension, and congestive cardiac failure). However, careful monitoring of the fetus is indicated, particularly if the fetus is "at risk," since small reductions in cardiac output may critically reduce fetal oxygen delivery. Maternal hypotension, regardless of anesthetic technique, correlates directly with infant neurologic activity.[225]

The supine position must be avoided, in labor or during cesarean section.[129]

Hypovolemia should be carefully avoided, particularly in the preeclamptic patient who may require blood volume expansion prior to epidural block.

Epidural block abolishes the normal compensatory vasoconstriction noted above.

Epidural venous engorgement reduces dose requirements for local anesthetics to two-thirds of normal, and injections should not be made during a contraction, since spread may be even greater and potential for rapid vascular absorption may be increased.

Rapid offset of action of epidural block in the early postpartum period may result in large increases in blood pressure because of postpartum increase in cardiac output. This is particularly likely if severe pain and catecholamine release overcome the normal compensatory vasodilation. Overzealous infusion of fluid or colloid during the epidural block accentuate this problem. The administration of ergot derivatives or oxytoxin, subsequent to a dose of ephedrine employed with epidural block during labor, may result in precipitous increases in blood pressure.

Fetal Oxygen Delivery

Oxygen delivery to the fetus depends upon uteroplacental blood flow (UBF) and oxygen content difference across the placenta ($Cao_2 - Cvo_2$)

$$\text{Fetal } O_2 \text{ delivery} = \text{UBF} \times (Cao_2 - Cvo_2)$$

$$\text{UBF} = \frac{\text{Uterine arterial} - \text{venous pressure}}{\text{Uterine vascular resistance}}$$

(i.e., "Perfusion Pressure")

Uterine perfusion pressure may be reduced by the supine position[85]: uterine venous pressure rises, and if venous return is reduced under epidural block in the supine position, uterine arterial pressure may also fall. This may not be apparent by brachial artery blood pressure measurements but may be better reflected in femoral artery blood pressure. Uterine blood flow is increased at least 30-fold at term, and uterine blood vessels are less responsive to sympathetic stimulation or vasopressor agents. However, it is now known that high levels of sympathetic activity (*e.g.*, those associated with severe pain), may result in large increases in uterine vascular resistance and reduced oxygen delivery to the fetus, with fetal acidosis and bradycardia.[7,198,294] Further recent studies in both sheep and baboons have confirmed the adverse effects of severe unrelieved pain on uterine blood flow and oxygen delivery to the fetus.[454] Amounts of epinephrine contained in local anesthetic solutions of 1:200,000 concentration decrease uterine blood flow minimally (– 14%) and for a short period of time (15 min), with no change in fetal acid-base status.[441] On the other hand, large doses of exogenous epinephrine (0.5 μg/kg/min) and vasopressors with α-adrenergic stimulating properties result in large decreases in uterine blood flow. The only exception is ephedrine.[349]

Indirect changes in uterine vascular resistance (extrinsic vascular resistance) occur during uterine contraction and also with increased basal uterine tone during oxytoxic infusion in patients in the supine position.[86] However, fetal acid-base does not suffer if basal tone increase is limited to 20 torr, provided that the lateral position is maintained.[444] Uterine blood flow may be reduced, with fetal oxygenation marginal, in the presence of maternal essential hypertension or preeclampsia. However, uterine blood flow changes during epidural block do not appear to jeopardize oxygen delivery to fetal liver or to contribute to neonatal hyperbilirubinemia.[84] Increased maternal Pao_2 leads to a small gradual reduction in uterine blood flow over a period of 1 hour. However, the net result is an improvement in fetal oxygenation, with a peak increase of 30 per cent after 45 minutes of maternal hyperoxia.[257] Recent studies show maintenance of normal placental blood flow during epidural block in normal human labor.[246]

Clinical Significance. Uterine perfusion pressure must be maintained during epidural block by careful attention to cardiovascular management (see above), by avoidance of the supine position, by consideration of increased needs for volume expansion in patients with abruptio placenta and preeclampsia (after blood pressure control).

It is necessary to avoid increases in uterine vascular resistance that may be due to: excessive doses of epinephrine in local anesthetic solutions; α-adrenergic stimulating vasopressors; any vasopressor following ergot derivatives or oxytoxin; severe unrelieved pain due to inadequate epidural block; severe anxiety due to inadequate explanation of management of labor and epidural block.

Maternal pathophysiology such as preeclampsia requires special consideration of effects of epidural block and added epinephrine on fetal oxygen delivery.

The only vasopressor capable of increasing uterine blood flow is ephedrine.

Oxygen administration to the mother increases fetal oxygen delivery.

Maternal Gastrointestinal Changes

In women in labor, there is an increased danger of acid aspiration syndrome because of: upward displacement of pylorus; increased intragastric pressure, especially in the lithotomy position or when the abdomen is compressed; decreased tone of the cardioesophageal junction; decreased gastric motility and decreased gastric emptying time; decreased *p*H of gastric juice; further decreases in gastric *p*H and gastric emptying time as a result of severe pain and narcotics administration; and increased incidence of vomiting owing to emotional stress, prior administration of narcotics, hypotension and/or hypoxia due to supine hypotension, and local anesthetic toxicity.

Clinical Significance. The anesthesiologist must be aware that epidural block does not avoid most of the factors referred to above. Thus, the hazard of acid aspiration remains, particularly in the presence of supine hypotension, high epidural block with poor cardiovascular management, and local anesthetic toxicity.

Administration of atropine may increase smooth muscle tone at the cardioesophageal junction, in addition to its cardiovascular effects.

Oral antacid administration may be advisable in all pregnant patients receiving epidural block.

Maternal Liver Function Changes

At term bromsulphalein (BSP) excretion tests are abnormal in 80 per cent of parturients. Serum pseudocholinesterase is low in 10 per cent of patients during labor.

Clinical Significance. The small change in pseudocolinestrase makes very little difference to the metabolism of chlorprocaine, whereas the change in liver function could be significant for the amide local anesthetics used for epidural block.

Maternal Renal Function Changes

Renal blood flow and glomerular filtration rate are increased, provided that supine hypotension is avoided. Blood urea nitrogen (BUN; 8–9 mg%) and creatinine (Cr; 0.46 mg%) are normally low at term.

Clinical Significance. Significant preexisting renal disease should be suspected if BUN is elevated above "normal" pregnant levels. For example, a BUN of 20 mg% may indicate extensive renal disease. Such patients may be very sensitive to changes in cardiac output and oxygen delivery to the kidney, so that bladder catheterization and monitoring of urine flow rate may be advisable during epidural block.

Fetal Physiology and Epidural Blockade

Several aspects of fetal physiology are important in the management of epidural block. As far as the anesthesiologist is concerned, most of these considerations are exemplified by changes detectable by modern methods of fetal monitoring.[165] Important aspects include the following:

Antepartum Changes. *Urinary estriol* (E_3) that is low or rapidly declining indicates that the fetus is "at risk"; this implies the need for rapid delivery and careful maintenance of uterine perfusion (see above).

Serum "human placental lactogen" (*HPL*) that is low and accompanied by maternal hypertension indicates a very high risk of fetal death; considerations for epidural block are the same as for low urinary estriol.

Amniocentesis may reveal high levels of bilirubin (Rh disease), a low lecithin–sphingomyelin ratio (immature fetal lungs), or low creatinine (immaturity and low weight).

Ultrasound scanning may reveal a small fetus, and reduced fetal chest wall movements may indicate fetal hypoxia.

Intrapartum Changes. *Fetal scalp pH,* P_{O_2}, *and* P_{CO_2}, *and base excess* may reveal adverse effects of labor, oxytoxins, and/or epidural block on fetal oxygen delivery. A *p*H below 7.2 requires immediate investigation of the cause of reduced fetal oxygenation, and if a cause cannot be found and corrected, as evidenced by improved fetal *p*H, then urgent delivery should be carried out.

Fetal Heart Rate (*FHR*). Loss of beat-to-beat variability indicates possible fetal hypoxia, as does "late deceleration" (Type II dips; i.e., persistence of reduced FHR after a contraction ceases). Variable deceleration (Type III dips; i.e., reduced FHR variably related to contractions) indicates cord compression, and if FHR decreases to less than 60 beats per minute for more than 1 minute, immediate knee chest position, administration of oxygen, and preparations for delivery are required.

Clinical Significance. Continuous fetal monitoring is now almost routine and adds greatly to the safety of use of epidural block, since there is no other way to determine if oxygen delivery to the fetus is adequate. Older methods of intermittent auscultation of fetal heart sounds are very insensitive.

Certainly any parturient whose baby is classified as "at risk" by antepartum criteria should be continuously monitored for uterine contractions, FHR, and intermittent fetal scalp blood gases, whether epidural block is used or not.

Atropine administration to the mother may result in persistent increases in FHR, which may obscure important changes in FHR. Thus, it should only be given if specifically indicated by cardiovascular changes in the mother.

The anesthesiologist employing epidural block should be fully aware of prepartum signs of fetal distress and their implications. A full communication with the obstetrician should take place, and both should continue this dialogue as intrapartum monitoring is carried out.

Perinatal Pharmacology and Epidural Blockade

Special aspects of perinatal pharmacology raise important considerations that have a major bearing on the physiologic response to epidural block and its management:[302,349]

All drugs (local anesthetics, epinephrine) administered by epidural injection and as adjuncts to the management of epidural block cross the placenta. Thus, only essential drugs should be administered.

Local anesthetics, atropine, and sedatives may abolish fetal heart beat to beat variability; unfortunately, this may also be a sign of severe fetal distress. Thus, dosage should be the smallest possible.

Diazepam has a very long half-life in the neonate and may result in loss of muscle tone, hypothermia, and, rarely, icterus owing to displacement of bilirubin from albumin by sodium benzoate preservative in diazepam (large doses only). It should not be used in doses greater than 5 mg intravenously.

Supplemental analgesic doses of inhalation agents do not depress the fetus and are therefore safe to use if concentration is below 1/2 MAC.

Local anesthetics absorbed from the epidural space may have fetal effects as assessed by the Brazelton Neonatal Assessment Scale or Scanlon's modified scale.[367] Bupivacaine and chloroprocaine have such minimal effects in usual clinical doses that they are not detectable by the above tests and are therefore the drugs of choice. It appears that fetal stresses such as maternal hypotension are more important than the choice of local anesthetic.[225] Thus, using lidocaine for elective cesarean section, Hollmen found no neurologic differences between epidural block and general anesthesia, but in both groups maternal hypotension was significantly correlated with fetal neurologic changes, such as weak rooting and sucking reflexes.[225]

High concentrations of local anesthetics may cause uterine artery constriction. Thus, minimal doses of local anesthetic and slow injection with frequent aspiration is mandatory.

Large doses of salicylates may cause increased bleeding, so that epidural block may be unwise in a parturient who has a history of such a drug intake.

If magnesium is used in large doses to treat preeclampsia, it should be noted that it may cause maternal hypotonia and respiratory depression, and cardiovascular depression in the newborn. These effects may be additive with those of local anesthetics, which have crossed the placenta.

Fetal acidosis increases placental transfer of local anesthetics.[18]

Safe management of epidural block in parturients requires that the anesthesiologist be part of the obstetric team and be fully informed of the preexisting physiologic status of mother and fetus. He should fully understand the significance of changes in maternal and fetal physiology. With careful attention to such considerations, epidural block with bupivacaine and/or chloroprocaine has minimal effects on the fetus. In some patients it may *improve* oxygen delivery to the fetus, reduce maternal cardiac work, and permit an otherwise distressed mother to remember her delivery as a satisfying and fulfilling experience. This may enable her to look forward to a further delivery with confidence rather than dread.

PHARMACOLOGY OF EPIDURAL BLOCKADE

The essence of the clinical pharmacology of epidural block is the provision of safe and effective neural blockade. To institute an epidural block safely, a knowledge of the physiology of epidural block is necessary, as well as a revision of the pharmacokinetics of local anesthetics as related to their administration by means of the epidural route. The efficacy of epidural block depends upon this and upon the clinical effects of the local anesthetics employed.

Factors in "Safety" of Epidural Blockade. The majority of studies of absorption and disposition of local anesthetics have been carried out in patients receiving epidural blockade. Thus, this aspect of the pharmacology of epidural analgesia is discussed in detail in Chapter 3. Also, much of the work on local anesthetic toxicity has been obtained with reference to the epidural route of administration of local anesthetics; this is presented in Chapter 2 and in Chapter 4. It is worth emphasizing that epidural blockade often entails the use of maximum clinical doses of local anesthetic, with resultant blood levels that are nearly toxic.[420] Thus, a thorough knowledge of the pharmacokinetics and toxicity of local anesthetics is a prerequisite to the safe use of epidural analgesia.

The discussion below summarizes some important aspects that are covered in detail in Chapters 2, 3, and 4.

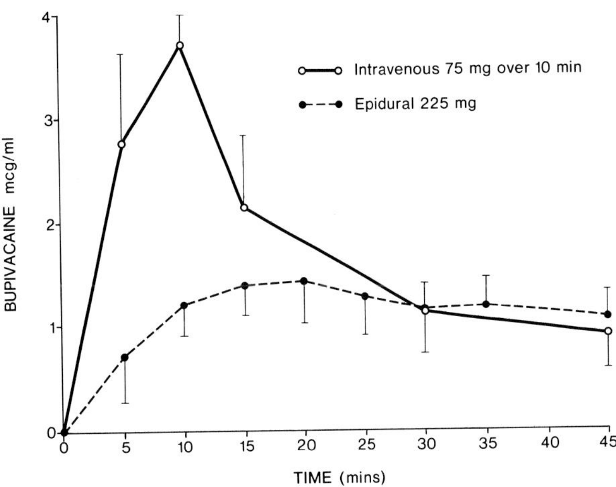

Fig. 8-23. Simulation of epidural blood concentration profile by intravenous infusion (IVI) to examine cardiovascular (CVS) and central nervous system (CNS) effects of absorbed local anesthetic. Although blood concentrations after IVI were slightly higher than computer simulation of absorption from epidural space, CVS and CNS effects were minimal (see text). (Mather, L.E., et al.: Anaesth. Intens. Care, *7*:215, 1979)

ABSORPTION

Epidural injection deposits local anesthetic some distance from the neural target, so that diffusion across tissue barriers is of great importance. Thus, local anesthetics with excellent qualities of penetration of lipid are desirable for rapid and effective epidural analgesia. Since a major site of action is within the dural sac, water solubility is of equal importance. Thus, agents with a *p*Ka close to physiologic *p*H (*e.g.*, lidocaine, *p*Ka = 7.87) are most effective, in that they are able to readily exhibit both lipid and water solubility. Procaine and tetracaine, with a high *p*Ka (8.92 and 8.50), suffer in this respect and perform poorly in epidural blockade.

Epidural fat provides a potential "reservoir" for deposition of fat-soluble local anesthetics. Thus, accumulation of long-acting fat-soluble agents, such as bupivacaine, occurs in epidural fat. This is not so for less fat-soluble agents, such as lidocaine. Thus, with repeated injections of bupivacaine, epidural fat concentrations rise, but blood concentrations tend to remain the same provided that dosage is appropriate. Repeated injections of lidocaine result in little accumulation in epidural fat, but progressive accumulation in the blood, with a potential for gradually increasing blood concentration (see Figs. 3-11, 14,15).

The epidural venous system provides a rich network for rapid absorption of local anesthetic (Fig. 8-13). Rapid injection into an epidural vein may dispatch local anesthetic directly to the brain by way of the basivertebral venous system.

The inclusion of epinephrine in local anesthetic solutions may greatly reduce vascular absorption (see Figs. 3-13,17), and thus enhance neural blocking properties and reduce the likelihood of systemic toxicity after epidural injection.[297]

The time profile of local anesthetic absorption, indicates a peak blood level at 10 to 20 minutes after injection, so that surveillance is necessary for at least 30 minutes after injection (Fig. 8-23).

Acidic solutions, containing antioxidants to stabilize epinephrine, may release local anesthetic base with difficulty and thus spread poorly across lipid barriers. Carbonated solutions release base very readily and have superior penetrating ability.[92]

Plasma protein binding greatly influences the amount of free local anesthetic available for action on the CNS after systemic absorption from the epidural space (see Figs. 3-6,21).

Hyaluronidase does not improve onset time of epidural block and reduces efficacy of motor and sensory block.[65]

Potassium additives to local anesthetics reduce sensory onset time but are not clinically acceptable for epidural block because of depolarizing phenomena that cause distressing muscle spasms.[65]

DISPOSITION

Disposition is influenced by distribution, metabolism, and renal excretion.

Distribution

Distribution of local anesthetics after epidural injection depends initially on the "initial dilution volume" (V), which reflects dilution of the dose in blood, and the "buffering" action of uptake of local anesthetic by the lung and transit time through the lung. Bupivacaine and etidocaine have higher values for V than mepivacaine and lidocaine.[420] Subsequent distribution of "unbound" drug is by the "volume of distribution" at steady state (V_{DSSF}), which reflects total distribution through the body tissues. This provides an approximate indication of tissue affinities, including epidural fat, plasma protein binding, and red cell uptake. Etidocaine has a very large V_{DSSF} (1478), followed by bupivacaine (1028), mepivacaine (382), and lidocaine (253). Surprisingly, a value is not yet available for prilocaine.

Metabolism and Excretion

Metabolism of ester agents procaine and chloroprocaine takes place at rapid rates in the serum. Chloroprocaine is effective in producing satisfactory epidural block, while procaine is not. Thus, the rapid plasma clearance of chloroprocaine combines with its efficacy to give it a high therapeutic index.

Metabolism of the amide agents in the liver is much slower. Hepatic extraction ratios are as follows: etidocaine, 0.74; bupivacaine, 0.39; mepivacaine, 0.52; and lidocaine, 0.63. Decreased hepatic blood flow in association with epidural block may reduce the clearance of amide agents[346,413]; the greatest effect is on slowly cleared agents, such as bupivacaine. Enhanced liver blood flow, after ephedrine administration, increases hepatic clearance (see Chapter 3).

Clearance is determined by the sum of values for distribution, metabolism, and renal excretion. Thus total clearance values are highest for etidocaine (1.11 L/min), followed by lidocaine (0.95 L/min), mepivacaine (0.78 L/min), and bupivacaine (0.58 L/min). However, since V values are similar for all four drugs, initial half-lives are quite similar (etidocaine = 2 min, bupivacaine = 3 min, mepivacaine = 1 min, lidocaine = 1 min), and maximum arterial concentrations following equipotent doses are similar. The larger V_{DSSF} and higher clearance of etidocaine contribute to a shorter intermediate half-life compared to bupivacaine (etidocaine = 18 min, bupivacaine = 29 min), so that duration of a toxic reaction should be shorter for etidocaine compared to bupivacaine following slow absorption from the epidural space. It would be expected that duration of toxicity for mepivacaine and lidocaine will be similar and much shorter than for the long-acting amides, because of shorter intermediate half-lives (lidocaine = 7 min, mepivacaine = 10 min). However, since etidocaine must be used in twice the dose of bupivacaine for effective epidural block, direct injection intravascularly is more likely to produce toxicity with etidocaine; under these circumstances, the rapid clearance and large V_{DSSF} of etidocaine are insufficient to compensate for the two-fold increase in blood concentration compared to bupivacaine.

Clearance of mepivacaine in neonates appears to be halved, and there is a prolonged half-life compared to adults, whereas lidocaine clearance is the same as in adults (see Fig. 3-31). Thus, mepivacaine appears less attractive for obstetric patients. In aged patients, the volume of distribution of lidocaine is reduced, and half-life is increased,[320] so that epidural dosage should be reduced if toxicity is to be avoided.

Biotransformation of lidocaine results in at least one active metabolite: monoethylglycylxylidine (MEGX). The half-life of MEGX may be greater than lidocaine, and its CNS toxicity is additive to that of lidocaine. Thus, prolonged administration of lidocaine into the epidural space may result in accumulation of MEGX, particularly in patients with cardiac disease where clearance of MEGX may be reduced.[346] MEGX is broken down to glycylxylidine (GX), which has a much longer half-life than lidocaine. Thus, GX has a high potential for accumulation and is also capable of CNS toxicity after prolonged administration of lidocaine. These two compounds may be responsible for a delayed onset of convulsions during the course of continuous epidural block with lidocaine.

Prilocaine biotransformation results in formation of *o*-toluidine and subsequent formation of an N-hydroxy metabolite. The latter causes methemoglobinemia, if the dose of prilocaine exceeds 600 mg. Single-dose epidural block can almost always be accomplished with a dose of prilocaine of less than 400 mg. Since blood concentrations of prilocaine following equipotent doses are 50 per cent of those of lidocaine, prilocaine is an attractive alternative for single-shot epidural blockade, except in obstetrical patients. The drug is not suitable for continuous epidural block.

ALTERATIONS IN ABSORPTION AND DISPOSITION

Age and Weight of Patient

As discussed in Chapter 3, plasma concentrations of local anesthetic after epidural block do not correlate well with age or weight. However, since dose requirements for epidural block diminish at the extremes of age, it is necessary to reduce dosage for this reason and because clearance of local anesthetics may be reduced in very young or in aged people.

Pathophysiologic Changes

Tissue acidosis results in increased uptake of local anesthetic into the brain. In addition, acidemia results in higher concentrations of unbound local anesthetic in the blood. Thus, local anesthetic toxicity is enhanced in the presence of acidosis (see Chap. 2), so that hypercapnia and other causes of acidosis must be avoided during epidural block.

Hypothermia may result in tissue acidosis, as well as reduced hepatic biotransformation of local anesthetics, so that amide-type local anesthetics may be more toxic in patients with hypothermia. The vasodilatation accompanying epidural block may predispose to hypothermia in surgical or obstetric patients; with regard to the latter, neonates are also susceptible to hypothermia unless they are rapidly dried and warmed.

Heart Disease. Clearance of amide agents may be greatly reduced owing to low hepatic blood flow. In addition, reduced cardiac output may result in higher peak arterial blood concentrations of local anesthetic (Figs. 4-10,11). This is particularly important for use of amide local anesthetics, such as lidocaine, during continuous epidural block, in which the cumulative dosage may be large.

Liver Disease. Reduced hepatic clearance of the amide agents suggests that long-acting amide agents should be used for continuous epidural block, so that cumulation of blood concentration does not occur; the large V_{DSSF} of etidocaine and bupivacaine may act as a buffer if hepatic metabolism is reduced, provided that injection is not made directly intravascularly.

Kidney Disease. Likelihood of local anesthetic toxicity is increased due to several contributing factors, such as acidosis and reduced plasma protein binding. Also, duration of action of local anesthetics is reduced, so that there is an increased risk of cumulative toxicity during continuous epidural block with short-acting agents such as lidocaine. Long-acting agents, such as bupivacaine, may be a better choice in these patients if continuous epidural block is employed.

Lung Disease. Despite the frequent use of epidural block in patients with pulmonary disease, very little is known about potential changes in drug kinetics and toxicity. Since the lung acts as an important "buffer" during absorption of local anesthetics, it is possible that pulmonary disease may increase the risk of acute toxicity.

FACTORS ASSOCIATED WITH ADMINISTRATION OF EPIDURAL BLOCKADE

Dosage

If dosage is kept constant, blood concentrations of local anesthetic are similar within the range of concentrations used for epidural block (*e.g.,* 40 ml of 1% lidocaine compared to 20 ml of 2% lidocaine). However, at high concentrations, the same dose (*e.g.,* 10 ml of 4% lidocaine) results in disproportionately higher blood concentrations.[34,35]

Thus, the use of very high concentrations of local anesthetic for epidural block should be avoided; previously, viscous "plombes" of concentrated agent were used in the mistaken belief that they would increase effectiveness of block without increasing toxicity (see Chapter 3).

Epinephrine

In general, epinephrine lowers peak plasma concentrations following epidural block. However, the effect is most pronounced with lidocaine. For other drugs, rather complicated effects are produced by the local anesthetic concentration and the agent employed (see Table 3-7). No benefit results from use of epinephrine concentrations in excess of 1:200,000.

Speed of Injection

Braid and Scott showed that peak plasma concentration of lidocaine was slightly higher after epidural injection over 15 seconds compared to 60 seconds (see Fig. 4-9).[34] If injection is made directly into a blood vessel, this difference is markedly accentuated (Figs. 4-10,11). The other advantage of a slow injection is the detection of impending toxicity, before all of the dose has been injected. Furthermore, rapid injection may be painful for the patient and may cause serious increases in CSF pressure.

Tachyphylaxis

Increasing dose requirements for maintenance of the same segmental spread of blockade may result in a high potential for cumulative toxicity. This is most likely to occur with short-acting agents; they are more likely to be associated with tachyphylaxis, as accumulation in epidural fat does not occur to sufficient degree to buffer the effects of repeated injection (see Figs. 3-14,15).

"EFFICACY" OF EPIDURAL BLOCK

Site of Action

Before discussing factors that influence the clinical efficacy of epidural blockade, it is helpful to summarize current data concerning the site(s) at which local anesthetics act following their injection into the epidural space. The anatomical spread of local anesthetic is summarized in Figures 8-2 and 8-3. It can be seen that local anesthetic comes into contact with the following structures; which are potential candidates for a site of action.

Spinal Nerves in Paravertebral Spaces. Local anesthetic readily seeps out through the intervertebral foramina (Fig. 8-3).[160,285]

Dorsal Root Ganglia Immediately Adjacent to The "Dural Cuff" Region. The dura is very thin in this region (Fig. 8-2B).

Individual Anterior and Posterior Spinal Nerve Roots within their Dural Root "Sleeves" or "Cuffs." Local anesthetic diffuses very rapidly into adjacent CSF in this region by way of "arachnoid granulations" (Fig. 8-2A,B).

Spinal nerve "rootlets" are very fine nerve filaments and have a large surface area, exposed to local anesthetic reaching the CSF by way of the adjacent dural cuff region (Fig. 8-2A).

Peripheral regions of the spinal cord are bathed by CSF with local anesthetic crossing from nearby dural cuffs (Fig. 8-2A).

The Brain. By way of spread of local anesthetic upward in the CSF or, indirectly, up the epidural space and then across dural cuffs in the upper cervical region (Fig. 8-3), the brain is exposed to local anesthetic.

Studies to Determine Sites of Action

Bromage et al provided the key data by injecting[14] C-labeled lidocaine into the epidural space of dogs and then carrying out autoradiography.[68] Their data suggested that rapid diffusion of local anesthetic into the CSF at the dural cuff region is the most important determinant of onset of epidural block: Peak local anesthetic concentrations in the CSF are reached within 10 to 20 minutes of epidural injection and concentrations are high enough to produce blockade in the spinal nerve roots and "rootlets."[68,181] This coincides with clinical onset of epidural block. Bromage and colleagues also showed that by 30 minutes after injection the C_m for lidocaine (0.28 μg/mg) had been exceeded in the peripheral spinal cord (1.38 μg/mg) and also in spinal nerves in the paravertebral space (1 μg/mg). Data from other studies in which local anesthetic was injected directly into the CSF indicate that C_m is not exceeded in the dorsal root ganglion or in the more central parts of the spinal cord.[104,231]

Bromage's studies also demonstrated local anesthetic in the brain but in insufficient concentrations to produce neural blockade. However, it seems likely that large overdoses of local anesthetic may be capable of achieving C_m in brain tissue.[68]

It is most likely that diffusion into intradural spinal nerve roots plays a major role during the early stages of epidural block, particularly when moderately small volumes of local anesthetic are employed. Subsequently, local anesthetic seepage through intervertebral foramina contributes by producing "multiple paravertebral block." Following lumbar epidural block, diffusion through the CSF to the spinal cord is probably a secondary phenomenon, although it may occur more rapidly when local anesthetic is injected closer to the spinal cord in thoracic blockade. Urban has reported that regression of analgesia after epidural block follows a circumferential pattern in the saggital plane, rather than the classic segmental pattern seen during onset of epidural block.[423] This is consistent with a persisting action of local anesthetic on the peripheral spinal cord after the initial effects on spinal nerve roots have abated. Also, Bromage has shown reflex changes in lower limbs during thoracic epidural blockade that spares the lumbar segments.[61] Changes typical of an upper motor neuron (long tract) lesion were seen: increased deep tendon reflexes, and an upgoing toe on Babinski's reflex.

Since epinephrine speeds the onset of epidural block, it is unlikely that local anesthetic is conducted from the epidural space to the spinal cord by way of spinal arteries; however, this remains a possibility, since spinal arteries pierce the dura in the region of the dural cuffs and then pass directly to the spinal cord. Nevertheless, the most likely mechanism for rapid appearance of local anesthetic in the CSF relates to the unique anatomy of the "arachnoid granulations" in the dural cuff region. This is extensively reviewed by Shantha and Evans,[386] who point out that arachnoid proliferations and villi are plentiful along both dorsal and ventral roots in humans. They are most plentiful in the region of the dural root sleeves ("cuffs"), immediately proximal to the dorsal root ganglion, where the dura becomes thin and is continuous with the epineurium of spinal nerves (Fig. 8-2B). Shantha and Evans described at least five different types of villi; three are shown in Figure 8-2B. The important point is that they provide a mechanism by which arachnoid protrudes either partially or completely through the dura into adjacent subdural and epidural spaces. This implies that local anesthetics may only have to diffuse across a layer of arachnoid epithelial cells to reach CSF. These anatomical and pharmacological data provide strong evidence that the major sites of action of local anesthetics after epidural block are the spinal nerve roots and spinal cord. It seems likely that future research in the epidural administration of drugs will indeed support the results of Corning's original experiment of 1885 (see Chap. 1).[112] He inadvertently injected anesthetic into the epidural space and claimed that he had produced "spinal anesthesia and local medication of the cord" (see also Chap. 31).

Longitudinal Spread of Solutions in the Epidural Space

Studies employing radiological contrast media and radioactively labeled solutions have mostly shown that these solutions tend to spread more in a cranial than a caudal direction.[82,96,180,325,393,432] However, radiologic contrast media cannot be expected to accurately reflect the spread of a local anesthetic drug; mixtures of local anesthetics and radioactive substances, such as ^{131}I, may result in different rates of diffusion of the local anesthetic and the radioactive substance. To date, no studies in humans have been possible with radiolabeled local anesthetics; in the meantime, it seems that clinical neural blockade extends beyond the spread of marker solutions in the epidural space.

CLINICAL CONSIDERATIONS FOR THE EFFICACY OF EPIDURAL BLOCKADE

There is no question now that epidural block can be effective in nearly all cases if attention is paid to the anatomy, physiology, and pharmacology of the technique. Yet there are still many major medical centers throughout the world that hold the belief that epidural blockade has a high failure rate compared to subarachnoid blockade. This merely serves to underline the relatively recent acquisition of relevant data on which to base the effective use of epidural block.

Assessment of Epidural Blockade

In defining important factors in effective epidural block, the development of standardized methods of assessment of epidural block has been essential:

Sensory block is graphed by testing for loss and return of pinprick sensation in each dermatome on both sides of the body (Fig. 8-34). An alternative method of testing initial onset is to use an alcohol swab to assess loss of temperature sensation, which is the most sensitive indicator of sensory block (see Table 3-2). *Complete* loss of touch sensation may also be charted (Fig. 8-24).[119]

From a "time-segment" graph, the following can be obtained: time to initial onset and complete spread of analgesia; time to regression of two segments and complete regression of analgesia; total number of segments blocked on both sides of the body; milliliters of local anesthetic per mean segmental spread (total segments R + L divided by two); and area of the segment-time diagram (segment minutes), which can be related to the dose of local anesthetic, in segment minutes per dose. The latter expression is used to assess the development of tachyphylaxis (see below).

Sympathetic block is assessed by measuring skin temperature with a telethermometer (Fig. 8-14) or temperature-sensitive papers. Alternatively, a digital plethysmogram may be employed (see Fig. 13-3). Skin resistance can be measured in the clinical setting by use of the psychogalvanic response; reliable measurements are much more difficult than usually acknowledged. More precise, but of research application only, are the use of various sweat tests such as cobalt blue and starch iodine or the response of skin plethysmography to ice during venous occulsion plethysmography (Figs. 13-3 and 13-13). A full discussion of the clinical and laboratory tests of sympathetic block is given in Chapter 13.

Motor block is usually assessed by use of the Bromage scale for motor blockade in the lower limbs.[58]

Bromage Scale

No Block (0%)	Full flexion of knees and feet possible
Partial (33%)	Just able to flex knees, still full flexion of feet possible
Almost complete (66%)	Unable to flex knees. Still flexion of feet
Complete (100%)	Unable to move legs or feet

Another alternative is to score the number of joints completely blocked in both lower limbs (Fig.

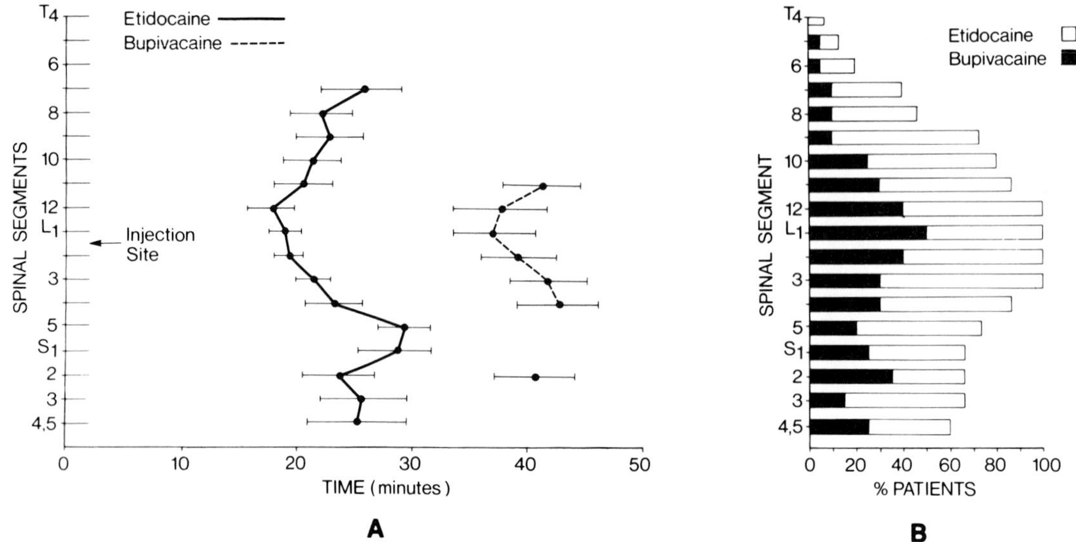

Fig. 8-24. Sensory blockade, onset profile. (*A*) Onset of *complete* blockade in each segment *bilaterally* is plotted against time; etidocaine (1%) is compared to bupivacaine (0.5%). (*B*) Percentage of patients with *complete bilateral* block in each segment is shown for etidocaine compared to bupivacaine. (Both solutions contain epinephrine, 1:200,000, injection at L1–2 average dose of 12 ml; Cousins, M.J., et al.: Epidural block for abdominal surgery: aspects of clinical pharmacology of etidocaine. Anaesth. Intens. Care, *6*:105, 1978)

8-25A).[119] Only an all or none decision need then be made at each joint. Thus, if a score of 0 is assigned for no block and 1 for complete block, the maximum score is 6:

	Right	Left	
Hip	1	1	
Knee	1	1	
Ankle	1	1	
Total	6		= complete block in both lower limbs

EMG. Few studies have employed the more quantitative method of electromyography (EMG), although this would provide more sensitive assessment.

Reflex Response. Under general anesthesia without muscle relaxation, sensation can still be crudely assessed by use of reflex response to pinch by a forceps at appropriate segmental levels. Alternatively, the tendon reflexes in the lower limbs give a gross index of both motor and sensory block, while reflexes such as those of the cremaster, anal, and abdominal may also be useful as a very gross guide to adequacy of blockade.

Site of Injection and Nerve Root Size

It can readily be seen from the time-segment diagram and "percentage of blockade" graph in Figure 8-24 that blockade tends to be most intense and has the most rapid onset close to the site of injection. The subsequent spread of analgesia depends to some extent on whether the injection is made in thoracic or lumbar regions. Following *lumbar epidural* injection, analgesia spreads in the manner shown in Figure 8-24. There is a somewhat greater cranial than caudal spread and a long delay in the L5 and S1 segments. The delay in onset at these segments appears to be due to the large size of these nerve roots.[184]

Following *midthoracic epidural* injection, analgesia spreads quite evenly from the site of injection. However, the upper thoracic and lower cervical segments are resistant to blockade, because of the large size of the nerve roots and the large number of nerve fibers within them. Repeated doses by the midthoracic route eventually may cause analgesia to spread into lumbar and sacral segments, with the expected lag in onset at L5–S1. Careful control of dose in the thoracic region permits sparing of the lumbar segments and, thus, avoidance of sympa-

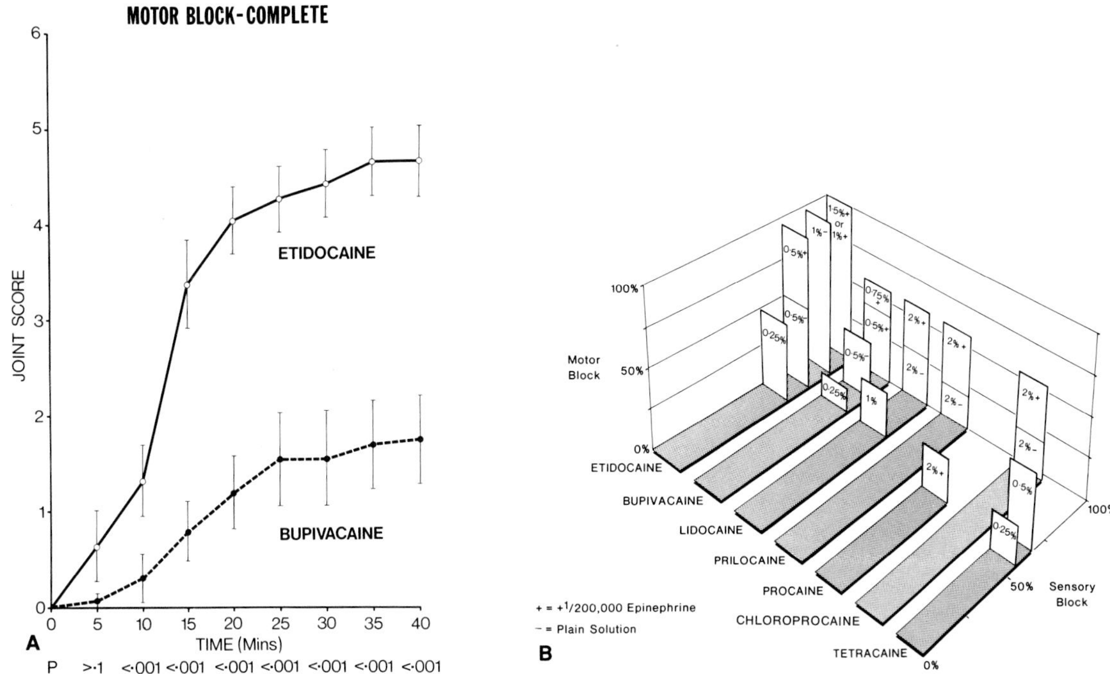

Fig. 8-25. (*A*) Motor blockade. Method of charting onset for comparison of agents. Complete blockade is charted following epidural block with 1-per-cent etidocaine or 0.5-per-cent bupivacaine, both solutions with 1:200,000 epinephrine. Each of the six major joints in the lower limbs received a score of 1 for complete blockade (see text). (*B*) Motor and sensory block, percentage success rate. Comparison of agents, concentrations, and addition of epinephrine are based on subjective data, so only approximate comparisons can be made. (Part A from Cousins, M.J., et al.: Epidural block for abdominal surgery: aspects of clinical pharmacology of etidocaine. Anaesth. Intens. Care, *6*:105, 1978)

thetic block in the lower limbs and maintenance of normal bladder function—that is, a true segmental block. Similarly, a very small dose injected at L2–3 for labor pain may block only T11 and L3–4 segments, while it spares the sacral segments.

The profile of onset of *caudal* epidural block spreads upward from S5, and the S1 segment is the last to be blocked, as expected (see Fig. 9-9).

Weight, Age, and Height

There appears to be no correlation between spread of analgesia and weight in adults. However, Bromage found a correlation between age and dose requirements when over 2,000 patients between ages 4 and 102 years were assessed by a standard technique:[55,62] An increase in dose requirements was found from age 4 to 18, and a gradual decrease in dose requirements from age 19 to 104. The increasing dose requirements from childhood to adulthood has been confirmed by Schulte-Steinberg and Rahlfs.[370,371] However, if one examines the data for dose requirements between age 20 and 40, there is a variation of 1 to 1.6 ml of 2-per-cent lidocaine per segment. This variation shows little difference in this age-group. At the extremes of age, it does seem necessary to reduce dosage. However, this is more predictable in children (see Chap. 21) on the basis of age; in adults, other factors, such as the presence of pregnancy[53,67,204] and arteriosclerosis,[56,202] also require consideration. Interestingly, a recent study showed high levels of blockade in patients 60 to 80 years of age regardless of dose.[389]

In practical terms, a range of 1 to 1.6 ml of 2-per-cent lidocaine per segment can be used in adults between age 20 to 40 years, and further adjustments are then made on the basis of height, site of injection (Table 8-14), and pathophysiological state.

Bromage reported a trend to increasing dose requirements with increased height, although the cor-

Table 8-14. Dose Calculation for Epidural Block with 2-per-cent Lidocaine in Normal Adults

Site of Injection	*Height*	*Volume*	*Maximum Dose**
Lumbar region	5 feet (150 cm)	1 ml/segment	(Lidocaine) or equipotent dose of other agent
	+2 inches (5 cm)	Add 0.1 ml/ segment for each 2 inches (5 cm) above 5 feet	500 mg at 20 yrs 200 mg at 80 yrs
Mid-thoracic region	70% of above		

* Caution should be taken with dosage in obstetrics. A 30% reduction may be required.[53,67] In patients with arteriosclerosis, a 50% reduction may be needed.[56] In both of these situations, *incremental* doses are advised. A further "rule of thumb" for 2-per-cent lidocaine solution (+ epi) or equivalent: 20–40 years—1 to 1.5 ml/segment, adjusted for height; 40–60 years—0.5 to 1 ml/segment, adjusted for height; 60–80 years—0.3 to 0.6 ml/segment, adjusted for height.

relation is weak when injections are made in the lumbar region.[55] A dose of 1 ml per segment is adequate for the majority of patients of height 5 feet (150 cm), while a dose of 1.6 ml per segment is sufficient for the majority of patients of height 6 feet (180 cm; see Table 8-14). A simple rule of thumb is to use 1 ml per segment for 5 feet of height, and then to add 0.1 ml per segment for each 2 inches (each 5 cm) over 5 feet.

It is wise to check that the dosage to be delivered is safe (see Table 3-5), and one should reduce dosage to about 50 per cent for aged patients. Thus, 500 mg plain lidocaine or 600 mg with epinephrine is acceptable in a healthy adult, while 200 to 250 mg of plain lidocaine is a reasonable dose in an 80-year-old. As noted below, 30-per-cent reductions are recommended for pregnancy, and 50-per-cent reductions for severe arteriosclerosis.

Posture

Despite continuing controversy, most data indicate that posture has a mild but significant effect on spread of epidural analgesia. Bromage reported that caudad spread of analgesia was favored by the sitting position, and dose requirements were slightly increased in comparison to the horizontal position.[55]

Cousins and Mazze, in a randomized prospective study of 164 patients in the age-group of 25 to 75 years, found that the sitting position greatly facilitated the onset of analgesia in sacral segments compared to injection in the horizontal position (Tables 8-15,16).[123] Further support for an effect of posture is given by recording the onset of sympathetic block following injection in a patient lying on one side. A large percentage of patients have more rapid onset of sympathetic block on the dependent side (Fig. 8-26). If the patient is maintained on this side, it is common to "miss" sensory block in some segments on the "up" side. Other studies agree with these findings.[203]

Table 8-15. Epidural Injection by Needle Compared to Catheter

	Injection by Needle	*Injection by Catheter*	
Number	84	80	
Total failures	2 (2.4%)*	12 (15%)*	
Cause of failure	Inadequate dose, 1	Catheter unable to thread 4†	
	Incorrect needle placement, 1	Catheter threaded, but no analgesia	3
		Patchy block	1
		Blood in catheter, unable to clear	2
		Unisegmental block	1
		Dural tap in effort to pass catheter	1
Irretrievable failure	1 (1.2%)	8 (10%)†	

* $P < 0.001$: Mann Whitney U test for nonparametric data (Cousins, M. J., and Mazze, R. I.: Anaesthesia and Intensive Care, 1980).
† It is possible that a catheter stilette may improve on the success rate for threading catheters, but may increase other complications, such as vascular cannulation. The group of catheter threading failures were potentially retrievable by injecting the whole dose via the needle or by moving to another interspace, thus necessitating a further needle insertion with its potential complications.

Speed of Injection

A slow rate of injection of 0.3 to 0.75 ml per sec results in the most reliable spread of analgesia, whereas rapid rates of injection may produce less satisfactory results.[159] This implies that attempting to force the solution up and down the epidural space has little effect on resultant blockade.

Volume, Concentration, and Dose of Local Anesthetic

Early concepts of epidural block as a "multiple paravertebral block" led to a firmly held view that the local anesthetic solution had to diffuse widely up and down the epidural space if extensive blockade was required. Thus, the early proponents of high epidural block used large volumes (60–100 ml) of dilute local anesthetic (1.0–1.5% procaine).[145,206]

Extensive studies by Bromage indicated that the dose of drug (concentration × volume) determined the spread of analgesia,[62] at least between the concentrations of 2- and 5-per-cent lidocaine and 0.2- and 0.5-per-cent tetracaine. However, data were not obtained to compare 0.5-per-cent lidocaine with a range of 1 to 2 per cent, which is a typical clinical range of concentrations. It did appear from Bromage's data that dose requirements diminished from about 30 mg per segment to 20 mg per segment when concentration was reduced from 2 to 1-per-cent lidocaine. Erdmeir and colleagues have shown that 30 ml of 1-per-cent lidocaine produced a higher sensory level than 10 ml of a 3-per-cent solution.[159] Burn and colleagues showed that large volumes of contrast media (40 ml) were more likely to spread into cervical regions compared to higher concentrations and smaller volumes (20 ml).[82]

With regard to motor blockade, dosage becomes less important when dilute solutions are employed. Below concentrations of 1-per-cent lidocaine, motor block is very minimal regardless of dose.

Increasing dosage results in a linear increase in degree of *sensory block* and duration of epidural

Table 8-16. The Effect of Gravity on Epidural Injection

	*Position After Injection**	
	Supine	*Sitting for 8–10 Minutes*
Number	53	31
% patients without S1 block at 10 minutes	30	6

* Injection of whole dose by needle

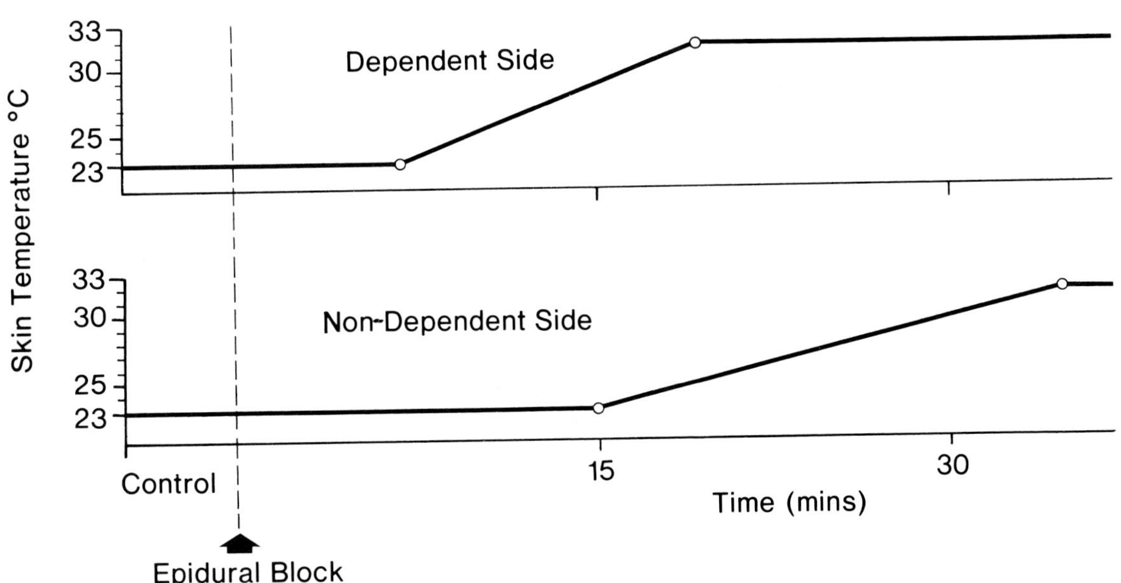

Fig. 8-26. Effect of posture. Onset of sympathetic block is much slower in non-dependent leg following injection of local anesthetic in lateral posture. A typical case is shown with continuous bilateral recording of skin temperature by telethermometry. (Courtesy of Lips, F.J., Seow, L.T., and Cousins, M.J.)

Table 8-17. Choice of Agent for Epidural Block

Application and Requirements	Agent(s)	Comment
Surgical analgesia	2% Lidocaine (HCl or CO_2) +	Rapid onset, excellent analgesia and motor block, medium duration
Sensory +++	3% Chloroprocaine	For very brief procedures only
Motor +++	1% Etidocaine ±	Rapid onset, profound analgesia and motor block, long duration
	0.75% Bupivacaine	Slow onset, good analgesia, moderate motor block, long duration
Medium to long duration	2% Mepivacaine −	Similar to Lidocaine. Can be used for medium duration if epinephrine is undesirable.
	3% Prilocaine −	Single shot techniques. Dose of <600 mg, low toxicity
Postop or Post-trauma pain	0.25–0.5% Bupivacaine −	Slow onset, long duration
Sensory +++		Sensory analgesia with very little motor blockade
Motor O Long Duration Obstetric analgesia	0.125%–0.5% Bupivacaine −	As above
Sensory ++ Motor O Long Duration Obstetric Surgery or Instrumental Delivery	1% Lidocaine-CO_2 + 3% Chloroprocaine +	Very useful for resistant "missed segments" Rapid onset, medium duration Considerations similar to surgical analgesia
Sensory +++	2% Lidocaine +	(Note: 0.25% bupivacaine is not potent enough and 0.5% bupivacaine provides inadequate analgesia in 5–10% of patients)
Motor ++ Medium to long duration Diagnostic & Therapeutic Neural Blockade	0.75% Bupivacaine + 0.5%–2% Lidocaine	0.5%− sympathetic, 1%− sensory, 2%+ motor blockade for diagnostic blockade
Range of blockade from sympathetic to motor	0.25% Bupivacaine	May be useful for diagnostic blockade requiring long duration sensory block with no motor block, also used for "therapeutic block" (see Chap. 26)

+ = with Epinephrine; − = without epinephrine

block, while increasing concentration results in a reduction in onset time and intensity of motor blockade (see Fig. 3-9). A general summary of the effects of local anesthetic dose and added epinephrine is given in Table 4-2. However, it should be recognized that choice of drug influences these effects.

Choice of Local Anesthetic

The concept of a "spectrum" of local anesthetics depicted in Figure 4-1 relates significantly to epidural block. The great flexibility of sensory and motor block that can be obtained by careful choice of drug is seen in Figure 8-25B. For example, 0.25-per-cent bupivacaine provides satisfactory analgesia for labor pain with close to zero motor block, while 0.25-per-cent etidocaine results in close to 50-per-cent motor block.

If more potent analgesia with minimal motor block is required, then 0.5-per-cent bupivacaine or 2-per-cent lidocaine may be chosen, although the former is the best choice for continuous techniques. The requirements of profound sensory block and excellent muscle relaxation (*e.g.*, for surgery or operative obstetrics) are best met by 2-per-cent lidocaine with epinephrine or by 1-per-cent etidocaine.[279]

Procaine, dibucaine, and tetracaine are usually not chosen for epidural block because of their rather inferior sensory and motor blocking properties. An exception may be the use of tetracaine if chloroprocaine is unavailable and amides are thought to be contraindicated.

Chloroprocaine has become an attractive alternative for short procedures and also for obstetric analgesia; it is a safe drug because of its high rate of metabolism.

Use of prilocaine for epidural block is worthy of consideration. It is still the safest amide agent when used in a dose of less than 600 mg and should be considered for single-shot epidural block, except in obstetrics. Of practical use, the 2-per-cent plain solution provides intense sensory block and minimal motor block which is associated with plasma levels similar to the 2-per-cent epinephrine-containing solution, provided dose is below 400 mg. This solution has appeal for outpatient caudal blocks or for single-shot epidural block for brief procedures. Alternatively, the 3-per-cent solution may be employed if very rapid onset is required, although a 20-ml dose produces some degree of motor block even with the plain solution (Table 8-17).

The differential capabilities of local anesthetics to block sensory and motor fibers has been referred to as "sensory-motor dissociation" (Fig. 8-25B). The basis for this phenomenon is unknown: Differential affinities for motor and sensory nerves based on lipid solubility seem unlikely; bupivacaine and etidocaine are both highly lipid-soluble, yet they have widely divergent potencies for motor blockade. Differential penetration of the spinal cord, as proposed by Bromage,[61] is also unlikely; sensory-motor dissociation can be seen with peripheral nerve block.[279]

Perhaps the best documented explanation lies in the phenomenon of "frequency dependent conduction block" (see Fig. 2-8).

Exciting new possibilities for providing selective blockade of pain conduction[121] while sensory, motor and sympathetic function remain intact are presented in Chapter 31.

Local Anesthetic Mixtures. Randomized controlled studies of local anesthetic mixtures have not been available to permit a rational decision concerning the safety and efficacy of such mixtures. Initial data indicate that toxicity of amide-amide mixtures is additive (see Chap. 4).[314] Mixtures of an ester and an amide may be less toxic than an equivalent mixture of amide-amide; however, definitive data are not available. A mixture of 0.2-per-cent tetracaine and 1.5-per-cent lidocaine has been popular with some groups of anesthesiologists to obtain rapid onset and long duration[309]; controlled studies of this time-honored mixture are unavailable to document if duration of blockade greatly exceeds that obtainable with lidocaine alone. In the obstetric setting, chloroprocaine-bupivacaine mixtures have been popular. The most promising mixture of modern amides appears to be lidocaine-bupivacaine for surgical blockade with residual postoperative analgesia. Initial results of a randomized prospective controlled study of various mixtures of lidocaine and bupivacaine are summarized in Figure 8-27. Only some of the characteristics of onset of action of the short-acting agent are retained by the 50-per-cent mixture. However, the most predictable effect is prolongation of action compared to the short-acting agent alone. It seems likely that it is preferable to inject lidocaine first for surgical analgesia and then switch to bupivacaine for postoperative analgesia, unless a single-shot technique is to be used. For this, the 50-per-cent mixture offers the best combination of onset and duration of action.

Epinephrine

There is general agreement that addition of epinephrine reduces vascular absorption to a variable extent (Table 7, Chapter 3) and enhances the effi-

1
2
3
4
DERMATOMES
THORACIC
LUMBAR
SACRAL
0
1
2
3
4
5
HOURS

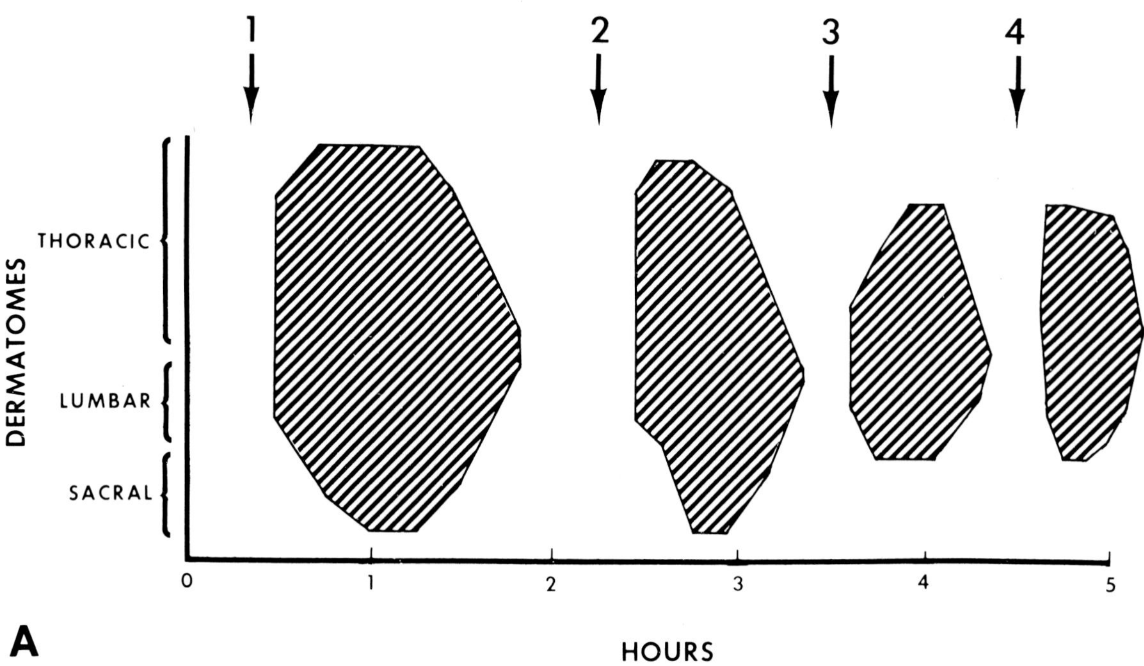

A

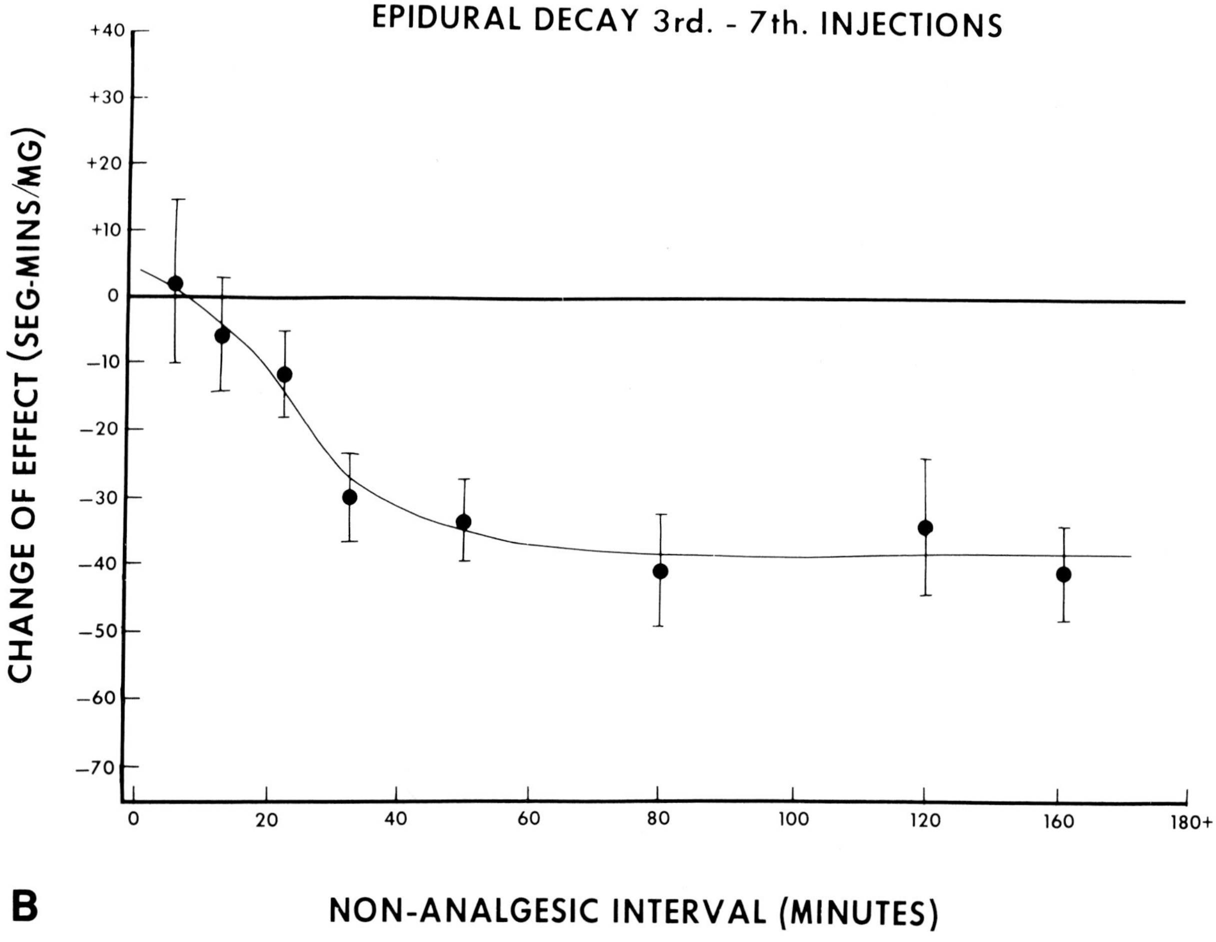

EPIDURAL DECAY 3rd. - 7th. INJECTIONS
CHANGE OF EFFECT (SEG-MINS/MG)
+40
+30
+20
+10
0
−10
−20
−30
−40
−50
−60
−70
0
20
40
60
80
100
120
160
180+
NON-ANALGESIC INTERVAL (MINUTES)

B

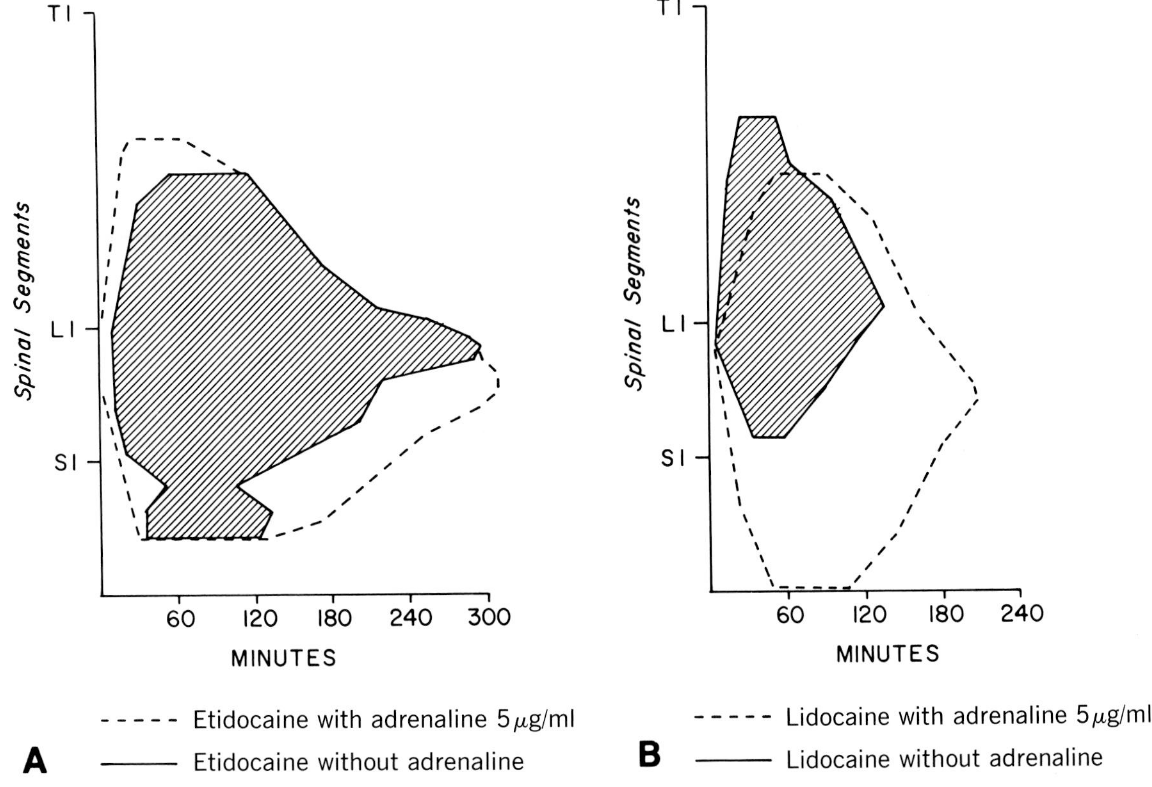

Fig. 8-28. Effect of epinephrine; segmental spread and duration of sensory blockade, comparison of lidocaine and etidocaine. Segmental spread and duration of analgesia are enhanced by addition of epinephrine. Caudad spread of analgesia is also markedly improved with epinephrine-containing solutions. *Broken line,* +epinephrine (5 μg/ml); *solid line,* plain solution. (Murphy, T.M., Mather, L.E., Stanton-Hicks, M.D.A., Bonica, J.J., and Tucker, G.T.: Effects of adding adrenaline to etidocaine and lignocaine in extradural anaesthesia. I: Block characteristics and cardiovascular effects. Br. J. Anaesth., *48*:893, 1976)

cacy of epidural blockade. However, with respect to efficacy, the following distinctions must be drawn: Enhancement of blockade is much less marked with the longer-acting agents bupivacaine and etidocaine; addition of fresh epinephrine in a concentration of 1:200,000 may enhance the intensity of motor block, quality of sensory blockade, and duration of blockade at least for lidocaine and prilocaine.[58,66]

As indicated in Table 3-3, the combination of local vasoconstriction owing to epinephrine and acidity due to anti-oxidants in premixed epinephrine-containing solutions may lower tissue *p*H below 7 for 150 to 250 minutes. This theoretically would result in reduced release of local anesthetic base and reduced penetration of neural tissue. It has been proposed that this may be responsible for increased latency to onset of sensory blockade, although data to support this view are not available. Bromage has reported that onset of sensory blockade is slightly longer when freshly prepared epinephrine is added to lidocaine for epidural

Fig. 8-27. Tachyphylaxis. (*A*) Diminished segmental spread and duration of action of repeated epidural injections of the same dose of local anesthetic, injected at each arrow. Note reinjection has been made at least 30 minutes after analgesia has regressed two segments. (*B*) "Nonanalgesic interval." As the time lag from loss of analgesia to reinjection exceeds 10 to 15 minutes, there is a progressive reduction in analgesic effect that reaches a maximum reduction of about 35 to 40 per cent at 60 minutes. (Bromage, P.R., Pettigrew, R.T., and Crowell, D.E.: Tachyphylaxis in epidural analgesia. I: Augmentation and decay of local anesthesia. J. Clin. Pharmacol., *9*:30, 1969) block.[57,66] However, recent double-blind studies of etidocaine and lidocaine reported statistically significant reductions in onset time with epinephrine-containing solutions[40,315] (Fig. 8-28).

Carbon Dioxide Salts

In *vitro* data indicate a ten-fold increase in uptake of lidocaine base into neural tissue when the same dose of lidocaine-carbon dioxide base is compared to lidocaine-hydrochloric acid base.[92] Clinical comparisons using lumbar epidural block and caudal block show a shortened latency to onset and a more extensive spread of analgesia when lidocaine-carbon dioxide is compared to lidocaine-hydrochloric acid.[58,120] The mechanism of this enhancement of blockade is discussed in detail in Chapters 2 and 3. Although peak blood lidocaine concentrations are slightly higher when lidocaine-carbon dioxide is employed for epidural block (Fig. 3-17), the enhanced neural blockade far outweighs this disadvantage. Unfortunately, the cost of manufacturing carbon dioxide salts of local anesthetics has so far precluded their release except in Canada.

Number and Frequency of Local Anesthetic Injections

Whether augmentation or diminution of neural blockade occurs following repeated epidural injection of local anesthetics depends on the local anesthetic agent, the number of injections, and the timing between injections.

A single "repeat" dose (20% of total dose) given approximately 20 minutes after the main dose of local anesthetic has been said to consolidate blockade, within the level of blockade already established. Thus, "missed segments" may be "filled in," but the level of blockade may not be extended.

A second dose of approximately 50 per cent of initial dosage will maintain the initial segmental level of analgesia if given when the upper level of segmental analgesia has receded one to two dermatomes. On the other hand, administration of the same dose as given for induction of block will result in augmentation of level of blockade at this time. Clinical practice relies on either mean duration times (Table 8-18) or careful monitoring for signs of regression of blockade, to determine the need for a second or refill dose.

A "refill" dose given more than 10 minutes outside regression of analgesia (the "interanalgesic interval") may result in tachyphylaxis. That is, an *increase* in dosage is required to maintain a constant level of blockade. Tachyphylaxis increases with the length of interanalgesic interval up to 60 minutes, but then it remains constant; at 60 minutes there is a 30- to 40-per-cent decrease in effect of a repeated dose (Fig. 8-29).[71]

Tachyphylaxis has been most clearly demonstrated in association with "continuous" epidural block in patients in whom repeated injections of the short-acting amides, lidocaine, prilocaine, or mepivacaine, are employed. Since the interanalgesic interval seems so important, it is not surprising that tachyphylaxis has been much less of a problem with the longer-acting agents, such as bupivacaine.

Bromage found that tachyphylaxis increased with the number of injections administered. This again indicates the desirability of using long-acting agents. Finally, it should be recalled that bupivacaine and etidocaine have a lesser tendency to accumulate in the blood, whereas the short-acting agents are associated with gradually increasing blood concentrations with increased risks of toxicity.

Table 8-18. Clinical Effects of Local Anesthetic Solutions Commonly used for Epidural Blockade

Drug	*Time spread to ± 4 Segments ±1 S.D. (min)*	*Approximate time to 2 Segment Regression ± 2 S.D.* (min)*	*Recommended "Top-Up" Time from Initial Dose* (min)*
Lidocaine, 2%	10 ± 3	100 ± 40	60
Prilocaine, 2–3%	12 ± 4	100 ± 40	60
Chloroprocaine, 2–3%	12 ± 5	60 ± 15	45
Mepivacaine, 2%	15 ± 5	120 ± 50	60
Bupivacaine, 0.5–0.75%	18 ± 10	200 ± 80	120
Etidocaine, 1–1.5%	10 ± 5	200 ± 80	120

* Note TOP UP time is based on duration −2 S.D. which encompasses the likely duration in 95% of the population. In a conscious, co-operative patient an alternative is to use frequent checks of segmental level to indicate need to "top up". All solutions contain 1:200,000 epinephrine.

(Data from studies of Bromage,[63] Cousins et al.,[121] Murphy et al.,[315] and Cousins [unpublished data])

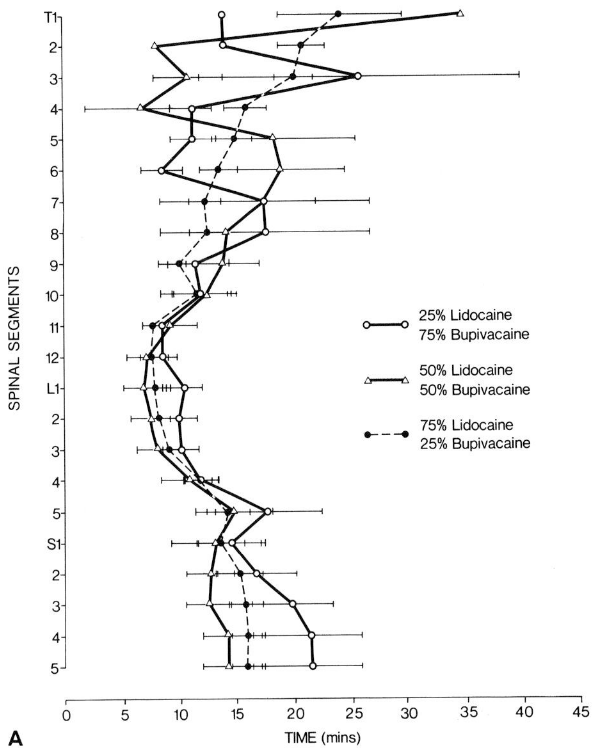

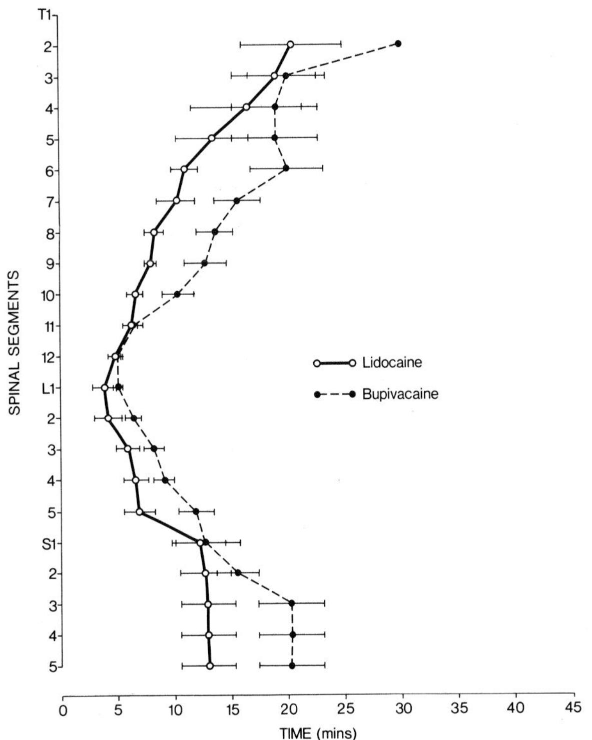

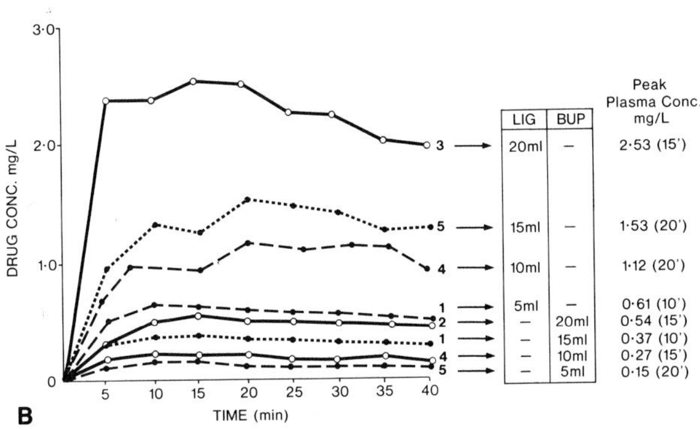

Fig. 8-29. Epidural block and local anesthetic mixtures. (*A*) Onset of analgesia. Solutions all contain 1:200,000 epinephrine. There were no significant differences among the solutions. (*B*) Epidural block and local anesthetic mixtures: pharmacokinetics. The solutions are the same as in *A*. Peak blood concentrations from components of mixtures are almost identical to those anticipated from injection of the same dose of the component by itself. However, the time to achievement of peak blood concentration is altered by mixtures of short- and long-acting agents. (Based on unpublished data from Lips, F.J., Seow, L.T., Mather, L.E., and Cousins, M.J.)

Injection by Needle or Catheter

Is there any difference in the spread of analgesia when injection is made with an epidural needle or catheter? Before answering this question, it should be noted that there is undoubtedly an increased incidence of outright failure with epidural catheter techniques and a higher incidence of complications. For example, Cousins and Mazze found an irretrievable failure rate of 10 per cent,[123] using catheters without stilletes in 80 patients. This compares to a rate of failure of 1.2 per cent in 84 cases when injection was made by needle. The major causes of "catheter failures" were complete inability to thread the catheter (5%); inability to clear the catheter of blood (2.5%); and threading the catheter through an intervertebral foramen (1.3%; see Table 8-15). The use of stilletes to introduce catheters may reduce the incidence of failure to thread the catheter but may increase vascular cannulation. Other studies report a similar failure rate for the use of a catheter.[39,215,366,385,429]

TECHNIQUE OF EPIDURAL BLOCKADE

Equipment

There are now a large number of commercially prepared disposable epidural trays that contain a variable number of the ideal components for epidural blockade. Individual preference plays a considerable part in choice of a tray. However, there are several desirable features:

Separation of a preparation section from the equipment section of the tray is preferable.

Glass syringes for testing loss of resistance should be of highest quality, with freely moving snug fitting plungers.

Disposable epidural needles should not have the "chisel" tip of the original Tuohy needle, since this increases the risk of dural puncture. Some current disposable epidural needles are dangerously sharp.

Epidural needle stylets should fit the needle precisely, particularly at the needle tip.

Epidural catheters should be of clear material so that aspirated blood can be clearly seen in the catheter. Also, catheters should be strong and flexible, should be inert, and should not have sharp tips capable of tearing blood vessels or puncturing dura. They should also be marked for roentgenographic detection.

Local anesthetics to be used in disposable trays should be packed in sterile protective covering on the tray or in individual sterile containers.

Mixing cups should be free of any particulate matter.

Unfortunately, many disposable trays fall short of these ideals. However, sterility is guaranteed by the manufacturer, and needles and syringes should be free of imperfections.

Many anesthesiologists still prefer department prepared trays, which contain all items decided upon by that particular group. This works well in a practice in which all can agree on a "standard" tray and a dedicated and skilled staff prepare the trays to ensure sterility and exclusion of chemical materials that may be neurolytic. In smaller hospitals that use epidural trays infrequently, commercial trays may be a valuable insurance against chemical and bacterial contamination. Larger units may prefer to design their own trays and to employ carefully maintained, reusable, high-quality needles and syringes. The following "traps" should be avoided:

Syringe barrels and plungers should be kept together, since "odds" may not fit with the precision required for loss of resistance testing. Powder or other material on syringe plungers may result in sticking, which can be very dangerous if entry into the epidural space is missed, particularly above the level of L1.

Epidural needles should be skilfully machined and maintained, so that rough and sharp edges are avoided. Stylets must fit perfectly to avoid tissue damage or plugs in the end of the needle.

Epidural local anesthetics must be sterilized very carefully, using a technique approved by a trained pharmacist, so that sterility, potency, and freedom from chemical contamination are ensured.

Epidural Needles

As for spinal analgesia, a close-fitting removable stylet is essential for epidural anesthesia, to prevent plugging of the needle tip with skin and failure to recognize loss of resistance. The possibility of a large epidermal plug being carried into the epidural or subarachnoid space must also be avoided. The epidural space can also be identified by compression of a 10- to 20-ml air-filled syringe attached to a 22-gauge Greene or Whitacre spinal needle; this is a useful teaching aid while performing lumbar puncture and may also be an alternative technique for single-shot epidural block. For the novice, the 18-gauge Tuohy needle[421] is probably the best choice because it has the lowest incidence of dural puncture. However, with the Tuohy needle, catheter threading is difficult if the needle is angled upward in the paraspinous (lateral) approach at any level or if a midline approach is used in the midthoracic region. Calibrated needles with centimeter markings also are available.[147,270]

The 18-gauge Crawford, thin-walled needle is preferred for the "paraspinous" (lateral) approach, since a catheter threads directly up the epidural space if the needle is angled at 45 to 60 degrees upward. Other needles, such as the large Cheng[95] and Crawley needles[131] and the fine 22-gauge Wagner needle[437] are less commonly used, since they have little advantage over standard needles.

"Winged needles" are ideal for "hanging-drop" techniques, since the grip on the needle should be well away from the fluid drop on the hub of the needle. Many variants of the original Labat winged needle are available, and detachable wings made of plastic have also been designed[450] for use with standard Tuohy needles. Some anesthesiologists prefer more versatile and more solid "spool" type needles with a Barker style of hub, (*e.g.*, the Bromage needle).[54]

Epidural equipment should be simple. A steady pair of hands with a highly trained feel for loss of resistance, a freely running glass syringe, and a high-quality epidural needle are far superior to the multitude of mechanical devices offered as aids to identify the epidural space.[139]

Required Equipment for Epidural Blockade

A satisfactory preparation tray or (section of tray)
1 × 2.5 cm, 25-gauge needle for skin analgesia
1 × 4 cm, 22-gauge needle for deep infiltration
1 × 18 gauge needle for drawing up epidural solutions and then for piercing skin prior to inserting the epidural needle
Epidural needle (Tuohy, Crawford)
Epidural catheter
1 × 2 ml, glass syringe for infiltration
2 × 10 ml, all glass syringes for loss of resistance tests and drawing up local anesthetic (preferable to "mixing" containers)
Normal saline
Local anesthetic
Filters and caps for epidural catheter (if desired)

Some practitioners prefer to have sterilized vials of local anesthetic on the tray and to drawn them up into 10-ml glass syringes, rather than using a "mixing" container and exposing the solution to possible contamination. Although millipore filters have not been conclusively shown to reduce the incidence of epidural infection, they may have other advantages. Particulate matter has been reported from mixing containers and "snap-neck" glass ampules.[252] The millipore filter offers some protection against this material reaching the epidural space. (Chapter 6 should be consulted for general information regarding equipment for neural blockade and preparation of the patient.)

Patient Evaluation and Preparation

As in any preanesthetic evaluation, certain essential information should be obtained. Its implications must be considered prior to selecting epidural blockade as part of the anesthetic regimen. If epidural block seems appropriate, then the necessary preoperative steps should be taken: The minimum entails adequate psychological preparation, adequate baseline data (*e.g.*, blood sugar levels in a diabetic), and correction of reversible abnormalities such as dehydration (Table 8-19).

Preoperative Discussion With Medical Staff

A discussion with the medical staff should not be omitted because the choice of anesthesia is considered the province of the anesthesiologist. Consultation with the surgeon is necessary to help determine the precise nature of operative approach and, therefore, the level of blockade required, the need for supplementation, and the necessity for intubation if exploration will markedly impinge on upper abdominal areas. Preoperative communication with nursing staff can be accomplished by a telephone call, to inform them beforehand of requirements for special equipment, timing of transportation of the patient to the operating room, and the need for assistance during positioning of the patient for a block (Table 8-19).

Planning for Technique of Block and Drug Dosage

Choice of patient posture for puncture follows the same principles outlined in Figures 7-13,14. Although the effect of gravity may be debatable, reliability of blockade of S1 is increased in the sitting position. Also, it is easier to enter the epidural space in obese patients if the sitting position is used. On the other hand, patients who have a history of fainting or who are heavily premedicated should have their block induced in the lateral position. Site of puncture is usually at L3–4 (Fig. 8-7A), unless the anesthesiologist is an experienced epiduralist; puncture at L5–S1 aids in ensuring blockade of the difficult S1 segment for ankle or knee surgery. At higher levels, experienced epiduralists may choose an interspace close to the center of the dermatomal segments required.[227] However, the degree of difficulty of needle insertion should also be considered. Thus, one may choose T9–10 for a thoracic operation, even though the more difficult T5–6 level may be closer to the center of the required dermatomes. Similarly, C7–T1 level may be chosen for an upper thoracic procedure rather than the more difficult T3–4 level. The author believes that the midline approach should be learned thoroughly prior to using the paraspinous (lateral) approach, since the chance of needle entry into the lateral aspects of ligamentum flavum (Fig. 8-4) may be greater if inexperienced attempts are made to "angle" the needle toward the midline. However, careful use of the spinous process to guide the needle for a paraspinous approach to a midline entry through the ligamentum flavum can be extremely reliable and easy in the hands of an experienced epiduralist (see Table 8-1), and this feature is very helpful in the midthoracic region (see Table 8-2). In the cervical region, midline puncture becomes more reliable again, and it is best to choose the C7–T1 level,

Table 8-19. Check List: A Safety Procedure Prior to Spinal Epidural Blockade

Patient Evaluation
Psychological suitability
Physical suitability with emphasis on the following:
Obesity and/or bony spine abnormalities
Preexisting neurological disease
Cardiorespiratory function (*e.g.*, ability to withstand sympathetic blockade)
Blood volume
Drug factors:
Anticoagulants, sensitivity to LA's, antihypertensive agents, monoamine oxidase inhibitors (and other drugs interferring with sympathetic function)
History of previous anesthetic and other drug administration
Family history of adverse drug effects
Patient Preparation
Explanation of blockade procedure and its benefits (intra- and postoperative)
Inquiry as to patient's desire for sedation or full unconsciousness
Baseline information
Spine radiograph for undefined pathology, blood sugar level for diabetics
Correction of reversible abnormalities (*e.g.*, dehydration)
Record history and management plan in notes
Order
Changes (if any) in current medication
Premedication
Preoperative Discussion
Operative details with surgeon to determine the following:
Level of blockade required
Appropriate supplementation
Necessity for intubation
Management plan with surgical staff: equipment and drug requirements
Timing for patient transport to operating room
Assistance from nursing staff

since the epidural space is wider than at higher cervical levels, and access between the spinous processes is easy if the neck is flexed (see Table 8-3).

The technique chosen for identification of epidural space depends largely on personal preference and familiarity with technique.[282,308] The author prefers the technique of loss of resistance, using an air-filled syringe at all levels, provided that the firm "Bromage" grip is used.[63] Certainly, the two-handed grip of the "hanging-drop" technique ensures excellent control; however, the slight risk that there is a plug in the needle tip and the occurrence of low or no negative pressure tends to outweigh the benefits of the "hanging-drop" or "Gutierriez" technique. The author prefers to employ the midline approach (Fig. 8-30), with an air-filled syringe (Fig. 8-31,32) at lumbar, low-thoracic, and C7–T1 levels, unless midline entry proves difficult; then a paraspinous approach is used. In the midthoracic region, the paraspinous (lateral) approach (Fig. 8-30) is routinely used with an air-filled syringe.

It is very desirable when puncture is made above the L2 level to routinely infiltrate down beside the spinous process and to check the depth of the lamina as a guide to the depth of the interlaminar space. This avoids the danger of continuing to advance a needle with a plug in the end. Experience with the use of the Bromage grip develops a keen sense of resistance in the hand advancing the needle and the hand compressing the syringe plunger. Unfortu-

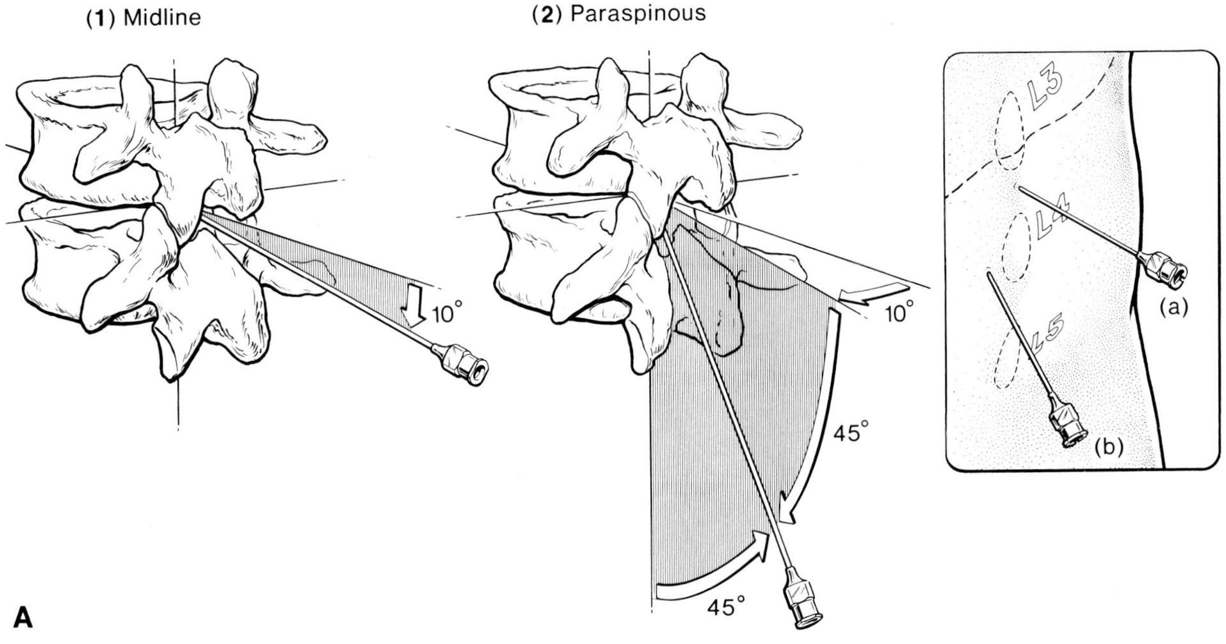

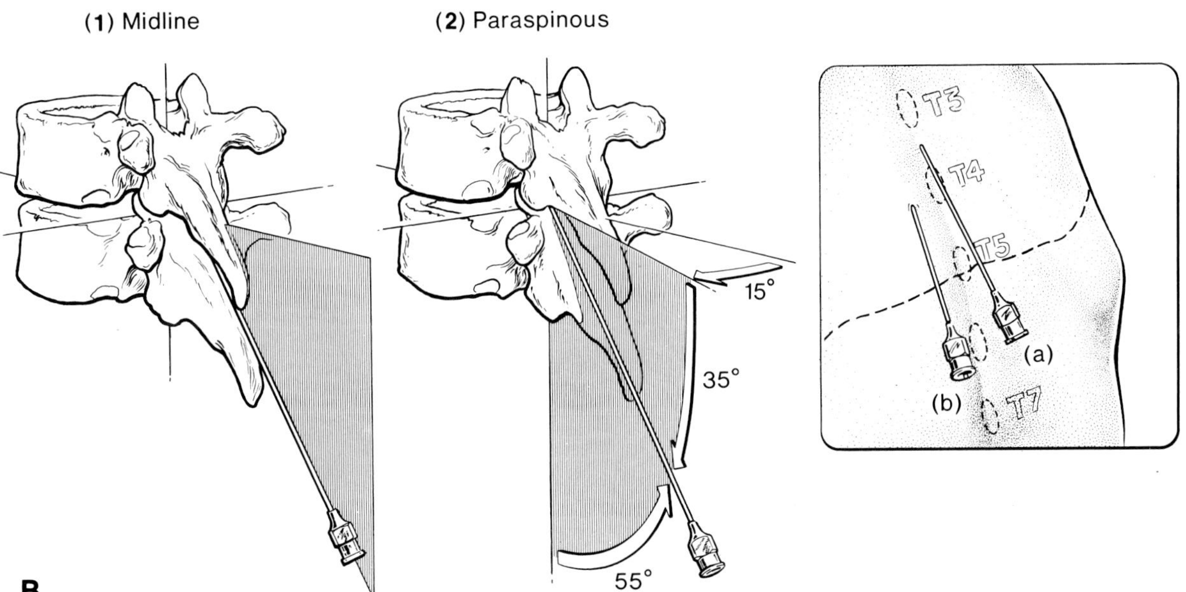

Fig. 8-30. Sites of needle insertion. (*A*) Lumbar epidural. (*1*) Midline. Note insertion closer to the superior spinous process and with a slight upward angulation. (*2*) Paraspinous (paramedian). Note insertion beside caudad edge of "inferior" spinous process, with 45-degree angulation to long axis of spine below. (*B*) Thoracic epidural. (*1*) Midline. Note extreme upward angulation required in midthoracic region. Therefore, a paraspinous approach may be easier. (*2*) Paraspinous. Note needle insertion next to caudad tip of the *same* spinous process as intended level of entry through ligamentum flavum. Upward angulation is 55 degrees to long axis of spine below and inward angulation is 10 to 15 degrees.

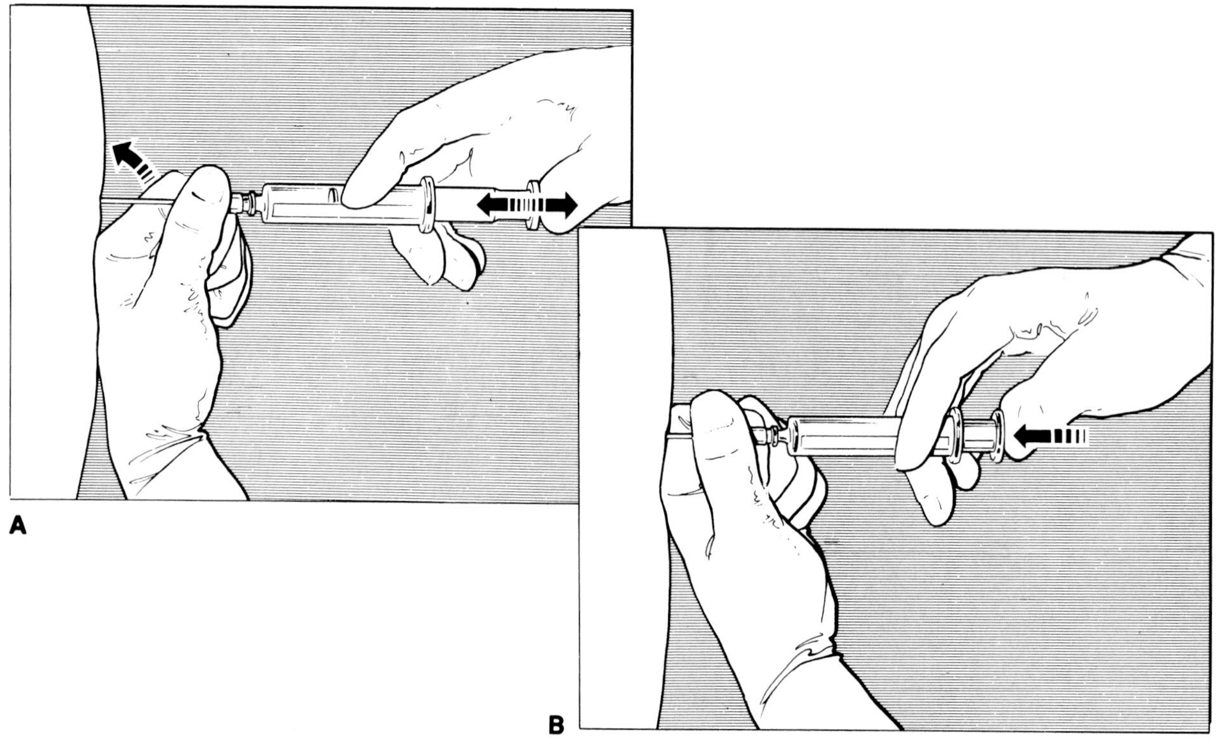

Fig. 8-31. "Bromage" grip for loss of resistance technique. (*A*) Note the vice-like grip of needle between thumb and *entire fist*. Metacarpal heads are braced against the back. The needle is advanced by rotation of the entire hand around the metacarpal heads; only a small, highly controlled movement is possible without repositioning the hand on the needle. There is continual compression of syringe plunger, with a "bouncing" movement. (*B*) As soon as the ligamentum flavum is pierced, resistance to syringe plunger is lost, and the needle is immediately halted. (Seen from above.)

nately, the "hanging-drop" is not under the anesthesiologists control; it may impart a visual sign only upon entry into the epidural space without premonitory sign of increased plunger resistance, which becomes highly developed during routine use of lumbar epidural block. Nevertheless, many anesthesiologists find that the two-handed grip of the "hanging-drop" technique gives them greater control. If this technique is used, the stylet must not be withdrawn until the needle is close to the ligamentum flavum. It should be reinserted if the needle contacts periosteum and requires repositioning. Also, it is preferable to advance the needle only during inspiration, so that negative pressure in the epidural space is maximal.[63]

The choice of single-shot or catheter technique depends on the patient and the type of operation. Catheter techniques are useful in debilitated and aged patients, since level of blockade can be gradually extended to the required level; this is also a wise approach in operative obstetrics. Prolonged surgery requires catheter techniques. Healthy patients undergoing brief procedures can be adequately managed with a single shot by the needle; even if it is planned to thread a catheter for "insurance," this author prefers to inject the dose via the needle, since up to 10 per cent of catheters malfunction owing to transforaminal escape or superficial placement,[39,215] "curling up,"[366] or, sometimes, passage into the anterior epidural space.[429] Threading catheters only 3 to 4 cm into the epidural space reduces but does not eliminate malfunction.[385]

Dosage calculation and choice of agent depend upon factors discussed on page 233. Single-shot techniques depend upon a generous calculation of dose requirements (Table 8-14), so that catheter techniques are prefereable if it is essential to restrict level of blockade. Considerations of the most appropriate drug and concentration and addition of epinephrine are also discussed on page 237 and are outlined in Table 8-17.

Needle insertion under general anesthesia is cer-

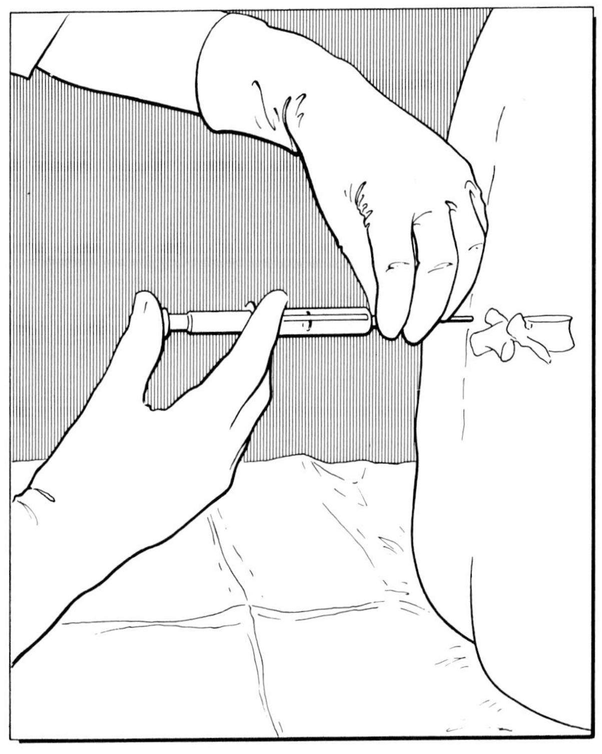

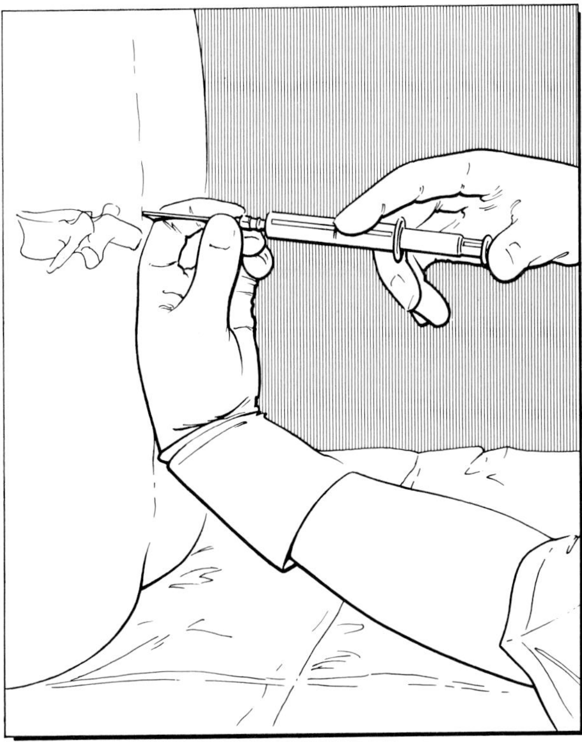

Fig. 8-32. Alternative, less controlled grips. (*A*) Hand gripping needle from above. (*B*) Hand gripping needle from below. Note that in both A and B the hand holding the needle is braced against the patient's back at all times, and the needle is advanced by forward movement of the forefinger and thumb.

tainly more comfortable for the patient. However, valuable signs of contact with neural tissue during intravascular or subarachnoid injection may be lost, so that considerable experience or supervision by an experienced epiduralist is required.

CONDUCT OF EPIDURAL BLOCKADE

Epidural neural blockade should be viewed as part of a complete anesthetic procedure (Table 8-20), which includes preparative steps, continuous surveillance, and appropriate responses (*e.g.*, supplementation if indicated); it should be stressed that insertion of the epidural needle is only part of the total anesthetic procedure.

Initial steps in the operating room must always include preparation of drugs and equipment for life support, the means of supplementation, and provision of a contingency plan for general anesthesia, to provide complete coverage for the operative procedure if the epidural block is inadequate. There should be no delay in deciding whether epidural block can be counted upon to provide analgesia and muscle relaxation (if required). Inadequate or patchy blockade should be swiftly covered by appropriate supplementation, and this should be done in a manner that is not discernable to the patient or the surgeon. This is extremely important in maintaining acceptibility of the technique to patient, surgeon, and other medical staff. Also, emphasis is placed on erecting a screen as soon as the patient is placed on the operating table.

Supplementation agents are discussed in Chapter 6. Some practitioners have a preference for supplementation with low-dose narcotic infusion (*e.g.*, pethidine[405]) or with low-dose infusion of rapidly cleared drugs, such as methohexitone, hexobarbital, or hemineurin.[296,372]

An exciting new approach uses infusion of hemineurin, since light sedation results in "natural"

(*Text continues on p. 250.*)

Table 8-20. Therapeutic Procedures for Epidural Block

Initial steps in the Operating Room

- Preparation
  - Support: drugs and equipment
    - Resuscitative drugs and equipment (Table 4-10)
    - Plastic oxygen mask and appropriate connection to anesthetic machine
  - Supplementation: drugs and equipment
    - Narcotic-sedative requests from drug "safe"
    - Stereo-headphones
    - Screen (to be erected *as soon as* patient in operating room)
    - Contingency plan for GA if needed, equipment and drugs prepared
- The patient
  - Inquire about adequacy of sedation and other problems
  - Insert IV line and rehydrate
  - Position correctly but *comfortably*
  - Reiterate steps of procedure
  - Mark landmarks with skin marker or other means
  - Check BP, HR

Skin Preparation and Preparation of Neural Block Tray

- Equipment physically separated from all other drugs
  - Sterile tray
  - Sterile wrapped drugs
- Check sterility control indicator
- Skin preparation
  - Keep equipment and drugs covered and separated from cleansing solutions, during skin preparation
  - Discard cleansing solution and equipment prior to uncovering block equipment
  - Discard entire block tray if cleansing solution splashed onto drugs/needles
  - Allow at least 3 minutes for solution to act (draw up drugs during this time)
- Preparation of drugs and equipment
  - Discard drug solutions that are cloudy or have crystals
  - Double check identity of drugs
  - Check dose of local anesthetic (and vasoconstrictor)
  - Draw up solution for epidural block in 10-ml syringes (to facilitate aspiration)
  - Draw up infiltration solution
  - Check fit of stillete, tip of epidural needle, fit of catheter through needle, patency of catheter
  - Check that "loss of resistance" syringe operates without sticking

Insertion of Needle (Midline Technique)

- Infiltrate skin and interspinous region (then recheck epidural equipment)
- Puncture skin with 19-gauge needle
- Check that epidural needle insertion is midline by "Labat" palpation of spinous process
- Maintain constant pressure on "testing" syringe
- Control needle advancement in vice-like grip with hand braced against patient at all times (Fig. 31)
- Halt needle immediately if resistance is lost or if there is any doubt about position (see Table 5)
- Aspirate gently and then immediately inject "test dose," 4 ml of prepared solution, again with hand holding needle braced against back
- Disconnect syringe and check temperature of any back-flow solution on arm (? cold = LA; ? warm = CSF)
- Question patient about warmth or numbness in lower limbs
- Maintain constant verbal contact, check heart rate, blood pressure

(*Continued*)

Table 8-20. (Continued)

Single shot
  Inject (<0.3 ml/sec) one-half the full dose, aspirate; then disconnect syringe, check as above, and inject remainder of dose if no adverse sequelae
Catheter technique
  Insert catheter and inject 4-ml dose through catheter; wait 5 minutes; check level, BP, HR, aspirate; then inject remainder of dose
Caution; reposition needle/catheter if the following occur:
  Paresthesia during insertion in a conscious patient
  Muscle twitching in segmental nerve distribution
  Excessive force appears necessary
  CSF or blood are aspirated
  Onset of analgesia appears excessivley prolonged
  No resistance is felt in interspinous ligament (? below L4)
Choose another interspace or use paraspinous approach to check depth of lamina and ligamentum flavum

Insertion of Needle (Paraspinous)

Infiltrate skin, ½–1 cm lateral to caudad edge of spinous process
Using 22-gauge "spinal needle," infiltrate at 90 degrees to skin down to lamina; note depth
Insert epidural needle **beside** spinous process (see Fig. 8-30) and angle toward midline 10–15 degrees
Lumbar epidural
  Epidural needle angled at 45 degrees to long axis of spine, caudad to point of insertion
  Needle beside spinous process, caudad to intended level of entry
Thoracic epidural
  Epidural needle angled at 55 degrees to long axis of spine, caudad to point of insertion
  Needle beside spinous same process as intended level of entry
Further steps in techniques are same as those for midline, except that little resistance is encountered until ligamentum flavum is engaged
Epidural needle should enter epidural space in midline

Continuing Management

Monitor
  By constant verbal contact (if patient conscious)
  Cardiorespiratory systems for "danger signals" (see Table 8-10)
  Level of blockade
Respond to altered physiology
  (See Tables 8-7 to 11 and Figs. 8-14 to 22)
Diagnose and treat local anesthetic "reactions"
  (See Table 4-8 and 4-10)
Supplement as needed
  With additional narcotic or sedative agents
  By superimposed GA if operative or patient requirements warrant it
Maintain adequate epidural block
  Check for "missed" segments
  Top-up at mean duration minus 2 S.D. (see Table 8-18) or when measured segmental level regresses 2 segments
  Diagnose and treat problems such as tachyphylaxis, vascular cannulation, delayed dural puncture
Follow-up
  Early
    Arrange continuing postoperative epidural analgesia if needed
    Prevent infection
  Late
    Check for any sequelae and, if present, participate in diagnosis and management

sleep with maintenance of an unobstructed airway, even in the prone position. This technique permits patients to tolerate uncomfortable positions without the long-standing problems associated with induction of general anesthesia and an obstructed airway. Since the drug is very rapidly cleared from the body, cessation of infusion results in a rapid recovery from sedation within a few minutes.[296]

Once the patient arrives in the operating room, all of the above should be ready, and activity should then concentrate on aspects relating directly to the patient (Table 8-20). For example, adequacy of sedation prior to needle insertion should be assessed. Any recent untoward events such as severe angina during the night should be elicited. The medical record should be checked. In particular, drug therapy should be scrutinized to determine if prescribed drugs (*e.g.*, insulin) have been given and undesired drugs (*e.g.*, heparin) have been discontinued. The steps of the procedure should be reassuringly outlined for the patient, and any changes in patient requirements determined (*e.g.*, a desire to be completely asleep rather than lightly sedated).

Although there are many approaches to *locating the desired interspace*, the author prefers to make an indentation with the thumb nail in the chosen interspace, to leave a mark at the level of the anterior superior iliac crest with the skin preparation solution, and then finally to palpate the rib margin as a guide to location of L1 (Fig. 8-7A). With this approach, the landmarks can be identified immediately prior to needle insertion. In contrast, marking with a skin "pen" is carried out prior to skin preparation, and the patient may move in the interim. Baseline blood pressure and heart rate should always be recorded on the anesthetic record prior to blockade.

Skin preparation and preparation of the neural block tray should require two separate steps. Also, it should be stressed that the neural block tray must be kept separate from all other drugs, since human error may result in injection of inappropriate agents into the epidural space with potentially disastrous sequelae.[428] It is preferable to complete the skin preparation before uncovering the epidural needles and drugs. In any event, splashing of preparatory solutions on neural block equipment must be avoided (Table 8-20).

Except for skin infiltration, complete preparation of neural block equipment should take place prior to commencing the block. The remaining steps are completed while skin analgesia ensues. It should be noted that the local anesthetic to be employed for epidural block is drawn up ready to inject, and the catheter (if used) has been checked and is ready to thread. Care should be taken that glove powder or other material does not soil the barrel of the "loss of resistance" syringe, since this may result in dangerous sticking of the barrel.

Midline Technique (see Fig. 8-30,31)

The essential anatomy of needle insertion in the midline is described in detail in the text accompanying Tables 8-1,2,3,5,6, and 7. The anesthesiologist should constantly think of the structures the needle encounters. The practical steps are outlined in Table 8-20, and the following aspects should be emphasized: Needle insertion should be in the center of the interspace; deep infiltration with a 22-gauge needle is important to "explore" the anatomy and to make subsequent insertion of the epidural needle comfortable; the skin should be punctured with a large-bore (18–19 gauge) needle to avoid "drag" on the epidural needle or carriage of an epidermal "plug" into the epidural space; if the midline approach is used, the spinous processes should be gripped as shown in Figure 8-7B, to assist in identification of the midline; constant pressure on the testing syringe should be maintained (Fig. 8-31A), and the epidural needle should be held in a vice-like grip that permits only a small forward movement at a time; the hand holding the needle must be braced firmly against the patient at all times; even in the lumbar region, a slight upward angulation is required to reach the interlaminar space (Fig. 8-8,9). If the "Bromage" grip illustrated in Figure 8-31 is employed, it is possible to readily identify changes in resistance, transmitted by the hand holding the needle and the syringe plunger, as the needle enters supraspinous, interspinous, and ligamentum flavum (Fig. 8-8). Constant pressure on the syringe plunger permits immediate recognition of loss of resistance as the needle tip enters the epidural space, and the vice-like grip on the needle permits immediate halting of needle progress (Table 8-20). Very gentle aspiration or, preferably, mere disconnection of syringe is carried out to check for flow of CSF or blood. If neither is present, 4 ml of solution is immediately injected to push the dura away from the needle tip. Two points require emphasis: The injected solution should meet no resistance at all, and the hand holding the needle must remain braced against the patient's back; otherwise, the needle may be advanced as the solution is injected. The syringe is disconnected again and any drip back is tested as in Table 8-6; while the patient is questioned about warmth and numbness in lower limbs;

a subarachnoid injection results in almost immediate onset of blockade of β-fibers (Table 8-2, Ch 3). If no evidence of onset of a subarachnoid block is present, one may proceed to inject the calculated epidural dose as follows:

Single-Shot Techniques. One-half the full dose is injected at 0.5 ml per second, with frequent aspiration; then the syringe is disconnected to check for reflux of CSF, and if negative, the remainder of the dose is injected.[159]

Catheter Techniques. The catheter is inserted 3 to 4 cm while the hand holding the needle is braced against the patient's back to ensure that the needle does not move. After removal of the needle and careful aspiration, a 5-ml test dose is then injected through the catheter. After 5 to 10 minutes, the level of blockade, heart rate, and blood pressure are checked; if satisfactory, a careful aspiration test is carried out, and then the remainder of the dose is injected. As noted in Table 8-20, needle or catheter insertion should be halted if undue force is required or if paresthesias or muscle twitches are elicited. If blood flows freely from an epidural needle, it may be necessary to move to an adjacent interspace and ensure that the subsequent entry through the ligamentum flavum is in the midline (see Figs. 8-5,6). If clear solution drips back or is aspirated from needle or catheter, then the steps outlined in Table 8-6 must be taken to determine if the fluid is local anesthetic or CSF.[93,188] Aspiration of blood from the epidural catheter may be overcome by withdrawing the catheter (*provided that the catheter is not still in the epidural needle*) or by injecting some saline. The catheter must not be left with blood in it, since it may rapidly become occluded. If blood aspiration does not cease, then the catheter should be reinserted at another level. Two further signs to reposition needles or catheters are important: If resistance is poorly defined at any level, then it is often helpful to either try another interspace or to choose the paraspinous (lateral) approach, which permits checking of the depth of the lamina by an exploring needle; if onset of analgesia is excessively prolonged, it is likely that injection has not been made into the epidural space.

Paraspinous Techniques ("Paramedian")

Paraspinous, paramedian (lateral) insertion is a useful alternative technique. The term *paraspinous* is favored for the following reasons:

The needle should be inserted precisely beside the spinous process, because in both lumbar and thoracic regions, the spinous process narrows superiorly and thus guides the needle to a midline entry through the ligamentum flavum.

Lateral angulation of the needle should be avoided, since it may result in oblique penetration of the ligamentum flavum (Fig. 8-4) and vascular or neural damage. In most instances, the needle need not be angulated at all and merely follows the spinous process; thus, "paraspinous" describes the essence of the technique.

Older techniques with more extreme angulation of the needle were referred to as "lateral" techniques; these techniques should be disgarded in favor of the safer paraspinous approach (Fig. 8-30).

In the lumbar region infiltration is made 1 to 1.5 cm lateral to the caudad tip of the inferior spinous process of the chosen interspace.[21] A 9- to 10-cm, 22-gauge spinal needle is then used to infiltrate perpendicular to the skin beside the spinous process; this enables the depth of the lamina to be determined prior to inserting the epidural needle. It is worth noting that the epidural space can be identified, for single shot techniques, if an air-filled syringe is attached to the 22-gauge needle, and constant pressure is applied to the plunger. However, in most patients an 18-gauge epidural needle is next inserted beside the spinous process and angled upward at 45 degrees to the skin (Fig. 8-30A); often the spinous process carries the needle slightly inward, 10 to 15 degrees to the saggital plane. However, this may not always be so, and the needle may pass directly to the ligamentum flavum without any necessity for inward angulation. With this technique, resistance to the advancing needle and syringe plunger is only encountered when the needle tip enters the ligamentum flavum. Thus, careful location of the depth of ligamentum flavum is essential; from this point the technique is identical to that at the midline.

In the thoracic region, skin infiltration is made 1 to 1.5 cm lateral to the caudad tip of the spinous process, corresponding to the intended level of needle insertion (Fig. 8-30B). Infiltration down to the level of the lamina is carried out as described above. The epidural needle is inserted beside the spinous process and 55 to 60 degrees to the skin (saggital plane); that is, a *steeper* angle is required to reach ligamentum flavum at the *same* level as the chosen spinous process (Fig. 8-30B). For both thoracic and lumbar paraspinous approaches, the Crawford 18-gauge thin-wall needle is preferred for single-shot and catheter techniques. The angulation of the needle permits easier threading of a catheter if a straight-tip Crawford needle is used rather than the Huber tip of the Tuohy needle.

Table 8-21. Cardiovascular Support—Epidural Block: Cardioactive Drugs (70 kg adult)

Drugs of Choice	
Atropine	0.3 mg I.V. increments[190]
Ephedrine	5–10 mg I.V. increments[27,46,156,157,408,443]
Epinephrine	1 mg in 250 ml solution (4 μg/ml) Infuse at rate 2–4 μg/min* (0.5–1 ml/min) *titrate* against heart rate, improved tissue perfusion, and mean arterial pressure. If mini drip is used, 60 mini drips = 1 ml ∴ Rate 30–60 drips/min

Other Drugs

Dopamine and *Dobutamine*[5] are alternatives to epinephrine, however dopaminergic receptors blocked by butyrophenones and phenothiazines. *Isuprel* (β) or *Norepinephrine* (α) are usually inadequate alone since both α and β effects are needed.[299] *Methoxamine, Metaraminol* and *Phenylephrine* produce mainly α effects with reflex slowing of the heart and decreased cardiac output.[276]

* Resting catechol output of 70-kg man is 3–4 μg/min.[106] This can be replaced exogenously by 3–10 μg/min epinephrine.[406] Note, however that these requirements need verification by modern catecholamine assay techniques.[87]

Continuing Management

As indicated in Table 8-20, monitoring and response to altered physiology are very important aspects of the conduct of epidural block. The management of sudden reactions to injection of local anesthetic requires a sound knowledge of the differential diagnosis of local anesthetic reactions[376] (Table 4-8) and their treatment as well as detailed knowledge of the cardiovascular effects of epidural block (Tables 8-7 to 8-13). Only with constant monitoring can the appropriate responses to physiologic changes be made (Table 8-21). Such surveillance also permits appropriate supplementation with sedative-narcotic or anesthetic agents and also appropriately timed "top-up" doses for the epidural block.

Maintenance of effective epidural block may entail overcoming common deficiencies in blockade and problems in the management of epidural catheters.

Blockade Too Low at Upper Level or Inadequate Blockade at Lower Level. Approximately one-half the initial dose is administered 30 minutes after the first dose. However, if the initial dose was small (*e.g.*, 4–8 ml), it may be necessary to repeat the initial dose. This is particularly so in the region of L5–S1, which are difficult to block.

"Missed Segments." Manage missed segments as above, depending on the size of initial dose and size of nerve root of "missed segment(s)." If a segment is missed on one side, it is worthwhile turning the patient on to that side prior to injection. Epinephrine-containing solutions are the most effective, particularly 2-per-cent lidocaine with 1:200,000 epinephrine, in dealing with missed segments or inadequate block. This is a useful practice even if another agent has been used for the initial injection. If available, 2-per-cent lidocaine-carbon dioxide is the best choice for such problems.

Inadequate motor block within the segmental area blocked requires further injection, 30 minutes after the initial dose, of approximately half this dose, preferably as 2-per-cent lidocaine with epinephrine.

Level Too High but Inadequate Sacral Analgesia. Careful monitoring of the physiologic effects of the high block and appropriate treatment are essential. Approximately 30 to 60 minutes after the initial dose, a small dose of 8 to 10 ml may be injected by a separate single-shot caudal needle. Such a dose will reliably block sacral segments without extending the upper level of lumbar epidural block. If access to the sacral hiatus is impossible, then it is preferable to wait as long as possible (approximately 60 min) and inject a small increment (*e.g.*, 5–8 ml by the epidural catheter), since blockade tends to spread progressively into the sacral segments with each repeat injection. However, careful monitoring is required for signs of total epidural block.

"Visceral" Pain During Lower Abdominal Surgery. It is not commonly recognized that peritoneal stimulation during appendectomy and sometimes during a difficult herniorrhaphy may require blockade to the level of T5–6. Thus, adequate provision should be made to block to this level or, alternatively, to "top-up" to this level if required. If there is a delay in onset of T5 block, then intravenous narcotic or light general anesthesia may be required.

Inability to Thread Epidural Catheter. If the planned operation could be accomplished with a single-shot of long-acting local anesthetic, then a generous dose of bupivacaine (0.5–0.75%) or etidocaine (1.0–1.5%) should be injected by the needle. If it is certain that a very long duration is required and the catheter is held up at the needle tip, then the epidural needle and catheter should be withdrawn together, the needle reinserted at the same or different level, and a further attempt made to thread the catheter. Flexible epidural catheter stylets are sometimes helpful.

Dural Puncture. Very often it is feasible to convert to a subarachnoid block merely by injecting the appropriate dose of tetracaine or dibucaine. If the anesthesiologist wants to persevere with epidural block, then another interspace should be chosen (preferably above), and a catheter should be threaded upward. Injection should be made entirely by the catheter and should be very slow.

Subarachnoid cannulation may occur at the time of initial insertion of needle or epidural catheter.[207,250,306] It has an incidence of 0.2 to 0.7 per cent.[250,306] Failure to recognize malplacement of needle or of catheter and injection of the usual epidural dose would result in a total spinal anesthesia (see Table 4-8). Epidural catheters have also been found to penetrate the dura at the time of a "top-up" dose, having initially functioned as if normally placed in the epidural space.[342] Thus, a small test dose administered by an epidural catheter is always advisable.

Subdural cannulation results from performation of the dura without penetration of the underlying arachnoid membrane. This is a rare result of intended epidural cannulation.[32] It occurs quite frequently during myelography[103] and in spinal anesthesia, with an incidence of up to 1 in 100. Spread of analgesia is patchy, markedly asymmetrical, and sometimes quite extensive.[32] Replacement of the epidural catheter at another level is required.

Cannulation of an epidural vein is a greater hazard, especially in pregnant women because of epidural venous distention during labor, particularly if the needle or catheter enters the epidural space other than in the midline (see Fig. 8-5). Usually the risk of epidural venous cannulation is small.[150,236,457] The best treatment is *prevention*, which depends on gentle insertion of catheters that do not have sharp ends, and avoidance of use of stylets; insertion of only 3 to 4 cm of the catheter length; aspiration before injection via an epidural catheter; use of a test dose, preferably with epinephrine (injected into an epidural vein results in a rapid increase in heart rate and blood pressure) (see also Table 8-15).

Injection of a small amount of saline and withdrawal of the catheter by 1 to 2 cm usually permits retrieval of the catheter from the vein; if not, then the catheter should be reinserted at another level. Delayed entry of a catheter into a vein may occur at the time of a "top-up" dose, with resulting CNS toxicity.[364] Once again, the catheter must be withdrawn, or if it is inaccessible, then epidural block must be discontinued.

Epidural Hematoma

Needle or catheter trauma to epidural veins may result in bleeding, but this is usually minimal and stops rapidly; it is extremely rare for an epidural hematoma and neurological symptoms to arise if coagulation is normal. Only one case is currently recorded.[272] However, patients on anticoagulant therapy may develop large epidural hematomas and, possibly, paraplegia if either an epidural needle or catheter is inserted.[141,179,193]

It should be remembered that more than 100 cases of spontaneous epidural hematoma have occurred in patients on anticoagulant therapy unassociated with epidural block.[210,402] Thus, spontaneous epidural hematoma may sometimes be erroneously attributed to epidural block. It is not known whether the tendency toward epidural hematoma in patients on anticoagulants is accentuated by the use of epidural block. Because there is still doubt, it is best to very carefully weigh the benefits of epidural block against the risks of epidural hematoma.[118] In the majority of cases, alternative means of providing most of the beneficial effects of epidural block are now available if anticoagulation is felt to be essential. For example, epidural block increases graft blood flow in association with vascular procedures on the lower limb.[125] However, limb blood flow may also be increased by prior sympathetic blockade using long-acting local anesthetics or intravascular reserpine injected into the affected limb, or even surgical sympathectomy (see Chap. 13). It is also important to note that surgical procedures involving the abdominal aorta may cause paraplegia. This may be the result of prolonged clamping of the aorta[116] or sectioning of nutrient arteries to nerve plexuses and the spinal cord.[430] Thus, while in lower limb vascular surgery, anticoagulation or epidural block, or both, may lead to epidural hematoma and paraplegia, in aortic surgery, direct cord ischemia must be added to the differential diagnosis of postoperative paraplegia.

The risk–benefit ratios of epidural block in both of these categories of patients need to better defined. In the meantime, the indication for epidural block in each patient should be carefully assessed. If epidural block is used, postoperative neurologic deficits should be viewed in the light of the differential diagnosis discussed above, and when it is necessary, surgical intervention should be early.

In particular, it is important to allow a continuous epidural block to wear off for long enough to assess motor and sensory function at some time during the first 24 postoperative hours. Failure to recover function fully and, in some cases, severe lumbar pain indicate the possibility of epidural hematoma. Anticoagulants should then be stopped and myelography carried out immediately, because most patients who have recovered from epidural hematoma have been decompressed within 12 hours of the onset of symptoms.[20] The variability in individual response to "low-dose" heparin therapy means that some patients may still develop epidural hematomas, and this risk will not be obviated until rapid methods are available to measure plasma levels of heparin and to assess the effect of heparin therapy on coagulation.[456]

Tachyphylaxis

Decreasing duration and segmental spread with successive doses of local anesthetic is called *tachyphylaxis*. The mechanism is discussed in Chap. 3, and the most important methods of avoiding the problem are as follows:use of long-acting local anesthetic for continuous catheter techniques; "topping-up" before analgesia wears off—usually at a time for mean duration—"2 S.D." for the agent employed or at the first sign of two segment regression (see Table 8-18); sometimes, changing to an alternative agent is said to help, but this is not supported by data (see also Fig. 8-29).

MANAGEMENT OF EPIDURAL CATHETERS

Accurate placement of a minimal length of catheter is described in the foregoing discussion as an essential aid to successful "continuous" catheter epidural blockade. The problems of patchy blockade, missed segments, intravascular cannulation, and subarachnoid and subdural cannulation can usually be effectively managed if the "correct procedure" is carefully followed and close monitoring is carried out (Table 8-20). The long-term complications of catheter placement, due to damage to neural tissue, should be avoidable if catheters are withdrawn at the first sign of pain or paraesthesias on insertion. The complications of epidural hematoma are mostly (but not always) avoidable.

Prevention of Infection

Perhaps the most important aspect of management of epidural catheters is the avoidance of infection:

A strict antiseptic routine should always be carried out during catheter insertion. Adequate time should be allowed for the skin preparation to exert its antibacterial effect, and great care should be taken not to contaminate the epidural catheter prior to insertion.

Multidose local anesthetic vials should not be used: Preservative-free, single-use, local anesthetic solutions should be used, and any residuum should be discarded after injection.

Local anesthetics should not be aspirated via "rubber bungs" in tops of local anesthetic vials; the top should be removed and the vial discarded after single use.

Glass syringes should be used only once and then resterilized, since the outside of the plunger may be contaminated during use. Many hospitals now use plastic single-use syringes.

During "top-up," the syringe nozzle and epidural catheter connection must not be contaminated, and if they are touched directly, then the appropriate components should be changed. Wiping with alcohol swabs is not advised, since it is possible that neurolytic alcohol solution may then be carried into the epidural space.

The use of micropore (millipore) filters has been shown in one study to reduce catheter contamination.[238] Although other studies have not substantiated this finding,[2] it seems reasonable to recommend the use of such filters. They provide at least some protection against infection and also reduce the chance of contamination with particulate matter.[252]

If reasonable precautions are taken, the risk of infection due to contamination of epidural catheters or local anesthetic solution should be very small (*e.g.*, 30,000 epidurals without a single infection[63]). However, endogenous infection owing to bloodborne spread from a preexisting focus on infection may be a hazard.[6] Also, patients with septicemia clearly pose a considerable risk of metastatic epidural infection, and insertion of an epidural catheter is best avoided in these patients. Infection in the pelvic region could possibly spread to the epidural space by way of the venous connections to epidural veins (Fig. 8-13); thus, the use of epidural catheters should be avoided unless the pelvic infection has been treated adequately with antibiotics.

More complex measures to combat contamination include the enclosure of large-volume syringes in sterile bags,[63] and the use of continuous drips and syringe pumps.[81,381] However, these techniques all potentially infringe on some or all of the important principles: aspiration for blood and CSF prior to injection; injection only after careful checking of segmental level of blockade; injection only by trained personnel (patients have been known to adjust drips and pumps themselves!); "continuous" drip or pump techniques are only safe if dilute solutions are used, and this results in a very high cumulative doses.[199,227,397]

In practice, intermittent injection is safer and

may be more effective if careful precautions are carried out and injection is made prior to two-segment regression.

PROCEDURE FOR "TOP-UP"

In conscious and cooperative patients, careful monitoring for signs of segmental regression will indicate the need for "top-up." In other situations, it is most convenient to top-up at the approximate time of regression of analgesia (minus 2 standard deviations) as determined in clinical studies (Table 8-18), provided that this timing coincides with safe blood concentrations of local anesthetic (see Fig. 3-14). The mean −2 S.D. predicts the duration in 95 per cent of patients. In practice, injection of one-half the initial dose of lidocaine approximately every hour results in maintenance of blockade associated with a small but significant gradual increase in blood lidocaine concentration (Fig. 3-14). This is usually not of importance during surgery, when one to two tops are usually sufficient. In contrast, with the long-acting agents bupivacaine and etidocaine, topping up with half the initial dose every 2 hours maintains level of blockade without appreciable increase in blood concentration over many successive top-ups. Thus, for long-term catheter techniques, bupivacaine is preferable with respect to toxicity and because the generous margin between top-up and two-segment regression lessens the chance that tachyphylaxis may occur. It should be clearly understood that we are interested in duration of blockade from time of complete spread to regression of two-segments, provided an appropriate level of blockade is achieved with the initial dose; duration to two-segment regression is considerably shorter than complete duration. If initial level of blockade is much too high, then initial top-up should be appropriately delayed, and size of top-up dose should be reduced in proportion to the level of "overshoot." A routine for topping-up is important.

Topping-Up Routine

Check level if possible: pin prick in conscious patients, reflexes and presence or absence of bradycardia (? level above T2) in anesthetised patients. Do not top-up if a high level is suspected.

Aspirate for CSF or blood.

Inject a small test dose (3–4 ml) of epinephrine-containing solution and check heart rate and blood pressure: Intravascular injection results in rapid increase in heart rate and blood pressure; subarachnoid injection results in extensive blockade with hypotension and sometimes bradycardia.

Inject remainder of top-up dose *slowly* with frequent aspiration, only if no complications ensue after the step above.

Monitor closely for one-half hour after top-up. If the patient is conscious and mobile, he should lie flat during top-up and for one-half hour afterward. In any patient, be prepared to increase rate of intravenous infusion or to manage local anesthetic reactions or extensive sympathetic blockade (Table 4-8).

Durations of maintenance of epidural catheters for over 2 weeks have been reported. Bromage advocates replacement of catheters at a different site every 72 hours.[63] However, if a catheter is functioning satisfactorily with no sequela, it is reasonable for it to remain in situ for approximately 1 week. Catheters should be removed gently, and the end of the catheter should be carefully checked for completeness. If difficulty is experienced in withdrawing the catheter, the spine should be flexed, and very gentle continuous traction exerted. There is a remote possibility that a knot may form in the catheter if excessively long lengths have been inserted; this is impossible if only 3 to 4 cm of catheter is inserted into the epidural space. There is an even more remote possibility that a catheter may loop around a spinal nerve if excess lengths are inserted; pain on removal of catheter should alert the anesthesiologist to this possibility. If subsequent radiographs, after injection of 0.3 ml of contrast media into the catheter, show that it is located in the region of a spinal nerve, removal by laminectomy may have to be considered. Sequestration of a small amount of catheter in the epidural space should be noted, and the patient must be carefully assessed over the ensuing weeks. However, it is usually not necessary to remove this foreign body, nor is it technically easy to locate it at laminectomy. Thus, in general, laminectomy is reserved for situations associated with symptoms or signs.

LOW-DOSE HEPARIN THERAPY AND IMPLICATIONS FOR EPIDURAL BLOCKADE

A major international multicenter study of low-dose heparin prophylaxis for postoperative deep venous thrombosis (DVT) recently reported the following impressive results: Only two patients receiving heparin (n = 2,045) developed fatal pulmonary embolus (0.09% of all patients), and there was a 7.7-per-cent incidence of DVT detected by ^{125}I fibrinogen scanning; 16 control patients (n = 2,076) developed fatal pulmonary embolus (0.7% of all patients), and there was a 24.0-per-cent incidence of DVT.[248] The incidence of deaths from hemorrhage was the same in both groups, but a breakdown of morbidity owing to hematoma formation was not given. Despite these impressive results, too little attention was paid to the variability in plasma heparin concentration, with the risk of either ineffective prophylaxis or overdose with hematoma formation; also there was insufficient emphasis on the increased risks of heparin therapy in some surgical procedures.

Nevertheless, an initial wave of enthusiasm for low-dose heparin therapy led to its almost routine use in some hospitals. Their aim was to lower a rather alarming recent rise in postoperative pulmonary embolism.[223,354] More objective assessment of benefits and risks of this treatment for surgical patients has gradually confirmed an approach directed at "at risk" groups,[249] in which the heparin treatment per se does not result in significant problems.[322] For example, the risk of hematoma and hemarthrosis in major orthopedic surgery far outweighs the benefits of low-dose heparin. Risks of excessive bleeding in pulmonary and prostatic surgery have resulted in a similar reluctance to use heparin. On the other hand, patients with cancer requiring major surgery are at considerable risk of postoperative thrombosis.[356] This risk has to be usefully weighed against the potential problems of heparin therapy for the proposed surgery. Unfortunately, even the responses to the low-dose regimen proposed by Kakkar and colleagues[248] vary considerably and unpredictably; this indicates the possibility of hematoma formation in susceptible patients. This may occur in major joints, behind the peritoneum and in other concealed sites, causing occult blood loss and acting as a site for infection. They may also result in neurological deficits (*e.g.*, from an epidural hematoma).

The author, in consultation with a hematologist experienced in heparin prophylaxis,[186] has developed the following approach to the conflict of interest of use of epidural block and heparin prophylaxis: The risks and benefits of epidural block are compared to low-dose heparin for the patient under consideration and the proposed operation; If the benefits of heparin are minimal and epidural block is the anesthetic technique of choice, then heparin therapy is omitted; on the other hand, if heparin prophylaxis is strongly indicated and is practicable for the proposed surgery, then a single-shot epidural technique with long-acting local anesthetic may be employed prior to starting heparin—in this situation, epidural catheters are not used, since there is a small chance that they may cause subsequent trauma or dislodge a previously formed clot on an epidural vein with resultant fresh bleeding. In some patients, heparin therapy should be started before the patient is brought to the operating room. In such a patient, epidural block is not used in any form.

If the patient is at a high risk for venous thrombosis, but heparin therapy is incompatible with the proposed surgery (*e.g.*, total hip replacement, prostatic surgery), then epidural block may be chosen in an attempt to modify the stress response and reduce coagulation changes. Also, the analgesia and freedom from sedation associated with epidural block are used to facilitate early and vigorous postoperative mobilization.

APPLICATIONS OF EPIDURAL BLOCKADE

A discussion of the "indications" and "contraindications" of epidural block is not the scope of this section. The preceding material in this chapter has provided a broad anatomical, technical, pharmacological, and physiological basis upon which to answer two important questions: Does epidural blockade offer significant benefits to the *individual* patient under consideration for the proposed operative or other application? Do the benefits outweigh the risks due to factors peculiar to the patient and/or procedure?

When viewed in this context, lists of "indications" and "contraindications" can be misleading and dangerous, since they cannot take into consideration factors that vary in individual patients. The only absolute contraindications to epidural blockade are patient refusal, major coagulation defects, uncorrected hypovolemia, infection in the area of proposed needle insertion, or severe systemic infection. As with spinal anesthesia, the benefits of epidural blockade in patients with neurologic disease should be carefully weighed; it appears wise, although there is no clear evidence, to avoid blockade in the patients with unstable neurologic disease, particularly if the spinal cord is involved. However, if epidural block offers significant benefits in patients with stable "peripheral" neurologic disease, such as diabetic neuropathy, then its use may be considered in light of individual patients and procedures. The use of epidural block in many thousands of patients with back pain and neurologic deficit following back surgery (see Chap. 26) attests to its safety in carefully selected patients with stable

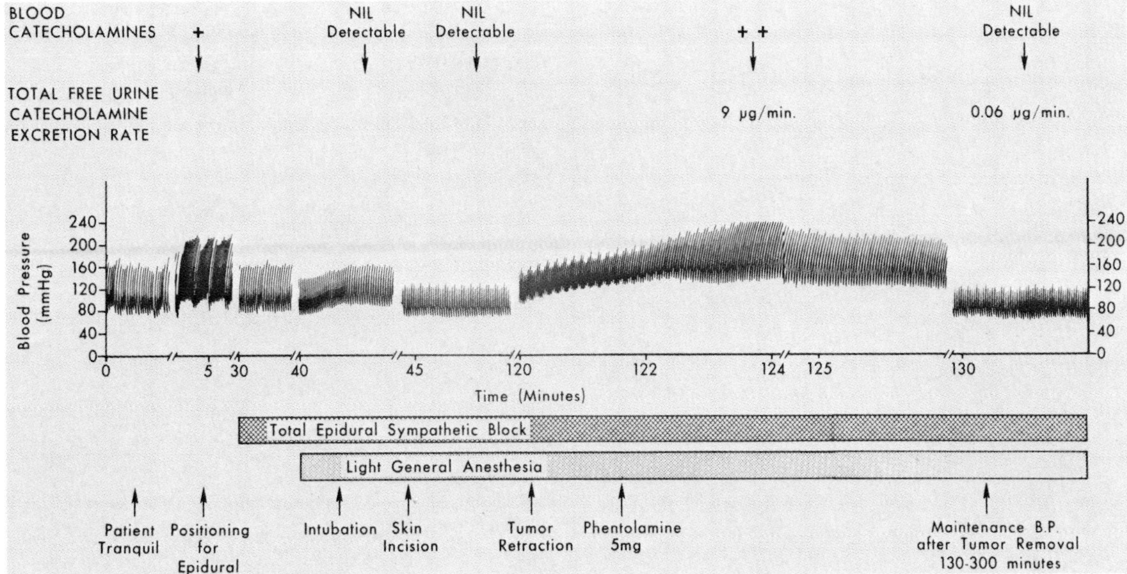

Fig. 8-33. Pheochromocytoma and total epidural blockade. Radial artery blood pressure, and urine and serum catecholamine levels were determined during surgery. Total epidural blockade was gradually accomplished by incremental doses of 1.5-per-cent mepivacaine administered by an epidural catheter, with essentially no change in blood pressure. Only a small change in blood pressure resulted from intubation, and there was no response to skin incision. Direct manipulation of the tumor required phentolamine to control the blood pressure rise. (Cousins, M.J., and Rubin, R.B.: The intraoperative management of phaeochromocytoma with total epidural sympathetic blockade. Br. J. Anaesth. *46*:78, 1974)

neurologic signs. Abnormalities of the bony spine may increase the difficulty of epidural block, although by no means do they make it impossible; this difficulty must be weighed against the skill of the anesthesiologist and the risk–benefit ratio for the patient and procedure; both anteroposterior and lateral radiographs of the lumbar spine should be available to assist in making such a decision.

Other anatomical, pharmacological, and physiological factors in individual patients may lead to a decision not to use epidural block. However, they cannot be merely "listed" here, since the balance of risk to benefit must be decided for each patient. For example, a patient with a low fixed cardiac output owing to constrictive pericarditis may be better managed during a perineal procedure by a saddle-block spinal anesthetic rather than an epidural anesthetic. A patient with severe congestive cardiac failure may be safely managed by epidural block for lower abdominal surgery, provided that incremental doses are used by a catheter and the "internal phlebotomy" due to sympathetic block has a slow onset and is confined to the lower limbs.

The above considerations enable the anesthesiologist to determine which benefits epidural blockade offers to each patient in each clinical setting. The potential applications may include: operative surgery; postoperative pain management; post-trauma pain management (see also Chap. 25); obstetric analgesia and operative obstetrics (see also Chap. 18); chronic pain diagnosis and management (see also Chaps. 24–27); and special applications in the management of particular medical and surgical conditions (*e.g.*, Fig. 8-33) [see Table 8-22].

COMPLICATIONS OF EPIDURAL BLOCKADE

The problems discussed on pp. 252–254 may be considered as minor complications. Any complication should be viewed in the light of a sound knowledge of the anatomy, pharmacology, and physiology of epidural block.

Complications Relating to Anatomical or Technical Problems

Several problems are discussed elsewhere: inadvertant dural puncture and total spinal blockade;

Table 8-22. Some Applications of Epidural Blockade

1. Surgery
   Upper and lower abdominal surgery,[63,233,375] urologic surgery,[161,459] pelvic surgery,[304] hip surgery,[253,303,404] vascular surgery,[125] surgery in the obese patient,[173] thoracic surgery,[130,182] (uncommon), surgery of neck and upper limb (uncommon)
   Surgery in patients with medical conditions (see Chap. 7), *e.g.*, buccal pemphigus [241] malignant hyperthermia[256]
   Specialized surgical procedures
   Pheochromocytoma[63,70,124]
   Surgery of spine[382]
   Bladder distention for bladder cancer
2. Postoperative and Post-Trauma Pain Relief
   See Chapter 25.
3. Obstetrics (see also Chap. 18)
   e.g., for patient comfort, to avoid incoordinate uterine action,[306] to minimize fetal acidosis,[326,360] to reduce use of "urgent" instrumental delivery or "painful delivery" under general anesthesia,[23,143,277] to relieve pain during labor for *medical*[152] indications, preeclampsia,[306] for cesarian section.[74,128,129]
4. Diagnosis and Management of Chronic Pain
   "Differential" epidural block (see Chap. 26)
   "Selective" epidural block (see Chap. 31)
   Epidurography with metrizamide[63,218]
   Neurolytic epidural block[63]
   Pain due to: vasospasm due to ergot poisoning,[4,383] cold injuries of extremities,[31,263] Raynaud's disease or phenomenon and other vasospastic problems,[271] phantom limb pain and causalgia,[300] post-herpetic neuralgia,[107,340] pancreatitis,[332] renal colic,[276,359] acute priapism.[307]
5. New Epidural Techniques
   Epidural electrical stimulation[390,424]
   Epidural narcotics[121]

massive subdural spread; total epidural blockade; epidural venous injection; epidural hematoma; epidural abscess; anterior spinal artery syndrome; ligation of spinal cord blood supply during major vascular surgery; injection of local anesthetics contaminated with neurolytic agents; injection of the "wrong drug" (*e.g.,* thiopentone); broken epidural catheters; and local anesthetic toxicity.

Rigid adherence to a "therapeutic procedure," as outlined in Table 8-20, greatly reduces the risks of major complications.

The occurrence and management of postdural puncture headache are discussed in Chapter 7. Unfortunately, the incidence of headache is high (70–80%) if the dura is punctured with a 16- to 18-gauge epidural needle.[126,127] Thus, routine prophylaxis is advisable if the dura is punctured with an epidural needle; this includes use of the supine posture, increased oral and intravenous fluid intake, the use of abdominal binders, and systemic analgesics. If an epidural catheter has been inserted at another level it should be left in situ and 1500 ml of saline should be infused over 24 hours.[126,127] The use of epidural blood patch is discussed in Chapter 7.

Backache is supposed to be more severe when large epidural needles (compared to spinal needles) are used. However, there are no data to support this. In obstetrics, the incidence of backache appears to be the same following delivery with or without epidural block.[128,195,247,305]

Bladder dysfunction is a distinct possibility if blockade of the sacral segments continues into the postoperative period. As discussed in more detail in Chapter 25, it is important to attempt to restrict epidural block to the required segments, which often do not include S2–5. Also, it is vital to ensure that the bladder does not become overdistended if epidural block extends into the sacral segments during surgery; this is particularly important in aged men with incipient prostatic obstruction. Careful management of level of blockade in obstetric patients results in a similar incidence of catheterization, whether or not epidural block is used.[127,305]

Major neurologic sequelae of epidural block are potentially the same as for spinal anesthesia (see Chap. 7). It was initially thought that these sequelae followed spinal anesthesia and not epidural block, but this has been disproved. In a major world review of the use of epidural blockade, Usubiaga uncovered a number of cases of neurological sequelae that were purportedly due to epidural block.[428] However, the retrospective nature of the documentation in many of these cases often make it impossible to determine the relative contribution of preexisting medical factors, the surgical procedure itself, and the epidural block. As with spinal anesthesia, several large epidural case series report no neurologic sequelae in major hospitals where a standard procedure is followed: Bromage reports over 40,000 epidural blocks without major neurological sequelae.[63] The majority of cases of serious neurologic sequelae occur in small hospitals or occur following epidural block by an inexperienced operator who violates some aspect of a reasonable therapeutic regimen. Even so, there is a *potential* for neurologic sequelae owing to anatomical or technical aspects of epidural block. These are summarized in Figure 8-34.

Direct trauma to the spinal cord can be eliminated if puncture is below L2. In all reported cases in which the patient was conscious, insertion of needle or catheter was followed by *severe lancinating pain* in dermatomes adjacent to or below the site of puncture.[63,229]

Epidural hematoma is discussed on page 253.[118,179,193] This complication can be prevented if the combination of coagulation defects or complete heparinization and epidural block is avoided. It is remotely possible for epidural hematoma to occur in patients without coagulation defects. Constant surveillance and early investigation are most important. In all reported cases, there is a rapid onset of signs of neurologic deficit and/or severe back pain. These signs should always be rapidly investigated by myelography, and if necessary, laminectomy should be performed within a maximum of 12 hours, since recovery is unlikely if decompression is delayed beyond this time.[20]

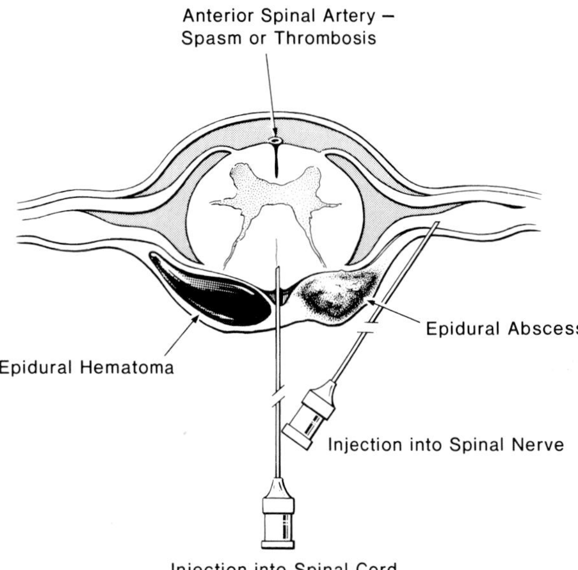

Fig. 8-34. Complications of epidural block (see text).

Epidural Abscess

In a series of 39 cases of epidural abscess, Baker and colleagues found that 38 cases were associated with endogenous infection.[6] In this series, an epidural abscess occurred in association with epidural block in only one case. Important diagnostic features present in all cases were severe back pain, local back tenderness, fever, leukocytosis, and abnormal myelogram with obstruction to flow of contrast medium. As for epidural hematoma, rapid investigation and laminectomy are essential for complete recovery. Since *Staphylococcus aureus* is the most common infecting organism,[209] antibiotic administration should include treatment for a staphylococcus infection if positive cultures are not available. The majority of reported cases of epidural abscess have followed continuous caudal blockade prior to the emphasis on sterile technique.[73,153,394] However, a disturbing case of extensive epidural empyema has been reported following midthoracic epidural blockade.[162] It should be noted that epidural abscess may occur in association with general systemic infection,[290] which reinforces the view that epidural block should be avoided in this situation.

Subarachnoid infection has also been reported following epidural block, and contamination of equipment or drugs appears to be responsible.[33,240]

Trauma to Spinal Nerves or Blood Vessels in Dural Cuff Region

Oblique lateral entry into the ligamentum flavum may direct the needle into the dural cuff region (Fig. 8-4. This may result in direct trauma to a nerve root, with resultant unisegmental paresthesia; such a sign should warn the anesthesiologist not to persist with needle insertion in this position and not to attempt to thread a catheter. It is also possible that a major "feeder" artery to the anterior spinal artery may be damaged as it enters by way of an intervertebral foramen (Fig. 8-11), resulting in the so-called anterior spinal artery syndrome, or possibly in a large epidural hematoma (even in a patient with normal coagulation).

Unexplained Causes of Anterior Spinal Artery Syndrome

The most likely explanations for unexplained cases of anterior spinal artery syndrome are direct trauma and reduced perfusion pressure and/or venous congestion. The contribution of the small doses of epinephrine (1:200,000) in modern epidural local anesthetic solutions is doubtful, except perhaps in patients with severe arteriosclerosis if epidural block has been used in association with hypotension (see also Chap. 7). Spinal cord ischemia and anterior spinal artery syndrome may result from low spinal cord perfusion unassociated with epidural block.[172] It is not known if epidural block increases the risk of low spinal cord perfusion. However, it is certain that the same percautions should be taken, whether or not epidural block is used.

It should be noted that angiomas of vertebrae or the spinal cord are relatively common and may compress the spinal cord, particularly if intraspinal pressure is increased (*e.g.*, during labor).[321] Once again, investigation by myelography and rapid exploration, if indicated, must be carried out if permanent sequelae are to be avoided.

Unexplained Arachnoiditis and Transverse Myelitis

Arachnoiditis and transverse myelitis are discussed in Chapter 7. Meticulous precautions must be taken to ensure that chemical agents capable of causing these lesions[258] are excluded from epidural block equipment and drugs (see Table 8-20). Only preservative-free local anesthetics from sterile single-use containers should be used for epidural block. The lack of neurotoxicity of any agent should be established before it is injected epidurally. Previous tragedies have occurred with the neurolytic carriers present in the so-called long-acting local anesthetic "efocaine."[99] As is the case with paraplegia following spinal anesthesia, it seems likely that reported cases of adhesive arachnoiditis following epidural blockade are due to chemical contamination.[63] However, the features of adhesive arachnoiditis may be produced by infection, trauma, and hemorrhage in the region of the arachnoid. Perhaps the best example of the latter is adhesive arachnoiditis following laminectomy or spinal fusion for "back pain." The author has seen a number of these patients, who were neurologically normal prior to laminectomy, apart from symptoms of back pain; they developed classic signs of adhesive arachnoiditis following operation. Subsequent reexploration revealed no infective process, but signs of extensive tissue trauma and classic features of adhesive arachnoiditis were present.

Partial or complete lesions of the cauda equina resulting in loss of bladder function, incontinence of feces, and sacral analgesia are sometimes attributed to epidural block. While these lesions are possible, owing to abscess, hematoma, or chemical contamination, a more widespread neurological deficit would be expected, considering the usual level of needle insertion. More likely causes are ligation of nutrient iliac vessels supplying the distal spinal cord in some patients or, alternatively, compression of sacral nerve roots or the pudendal nerve during pelvic surgery.

Complications Relating to Altered Physiology

The potential for complications owing to alteration in oxygen delivery to vital organs is outlined in detail in Tables 8-10, 11. Thus, like general anesthesia, it is possible for epidural block to result in compromise of oxygen delivery to heart, brain, liver, or kidney, with sequelae that depend on the degree and duration of compromise. Full knowledge of preexisting physical status and careful monitoring throughout the use of epidural block are essential to avoid such complications.

Complications of epidural block are given further consideration in Chapters 22 and 23.

DIFFERENTIAL DIAGNOSIS OF POSTOPERATIVE NEUROLOGICAL SEQUELAE

It is all too easy to attribute a serious neurologic deficit following anesthesia and surgery to epidural block if the latter has been employed as part of the anesthetic regimen. This is comforting for the surgical team, but it has no greater validity than does labeling all cases of postoperative jaundice as "halothane hepatitis." Factual evidence that links epidural blockade with neurological sequelae is scarce: Local anesthetics in clinical concentrations do not cause neural damage or meningeal irritation; a properly placed epidural needle or catheter with no evidence of contact with nerve root during insertion does not damage spinal nerves or spinal cord, unless gross infection or epidural hematoma results, usually from associated medical or surgical problems; epinephrine used in a concentration of 1:200,000 almost certainly does not result in anterior spinal artery spasm.

There are a large number of common causes of neurologic deficit following anesthesia and surgery, just as there are common causes of postoperative jaundice. The medical team must consider a differential diagnosis with these common causes at the top of the list and must ensure that a readily treatable condition is not overlooked.

The effective management of postoperative neurologic sequelae requires the collaboration of the anesthesiologist, surgeon, and a neurologist. The assistance of a radiologist and neurosurgeon may well also be required. A frank discussion aimed at defining etiology rather than fault should take place after each physician has had an opportunity to examine the patient and history. The investigative steps are as listed on the next page.

Anesthesiologists should have a thorough knowledge of the causes of postoperative **neurologic sequelae that have been reported in patient's who did**

Investigative Steps in the Management of Postoperative Neurologic Sequelae

1. Thorough review of preexisting medical problems and drug therapy (preexisting signs and symptoms of a spinal cord tumor may be elicited or a family history of neurologic problems, or drug therapy capable of causing neurologic side effects)
2. Review of anesthetic management and surgical procedure (*e.g.*, evidence of poor spinal cord perfusion see physiology section); dangerous posturing during surgery?; surgical section of nutrient vessels to spinal cord?; surgical section or retraction of spinal nerves or peripheral nerves?
3. An attempt to anatomically localize the lesion (see Fig. 8-35)
4. Consideration of most likely causes of a lesion located at such a level
5. Appropriate further investigations, such as blood culture, coagulation studies, myelography, electromyography
6. Careful surveillance for signs of progression of the lesion or associated medical problems
7. Rapid response to significant abnormalities (*e.g.*, progressive neurologic deficit, back pain, pyrexia, and leucocytosis require myelogram to identify possible epidural abscess and urgent laminectomy)
8. Follow-up documentation of outcome with appropriate investigation of progress of lesion (*e.g.*, repeated EMG, serial cystometric measurements to document return or otherwise of bladder function)
9. Careful postmortem examination of nervous system by a skilled neuropathologist, if possible in conjunction with the anesthesiologist and surgeon involved. The pertinence of the pathologist's examination is greatly enhanced by first-hand information, and the education of medical staff is best served by direct participation in examining the morbid anatomy of such major complications
10. Precise reporting in the medical literature, avoiding misleading titles. For example, an excellent report by Usubiaga[430] provided clear evidence that paraplegia following vascular surgery under epidural block was due to ligation of nutrient vessels to the spinal cord during the surgery; unfortunately, the title of this article was "Neurological Complications of Prevertebral Surgery Under Regional Anesthesia." This implies that the regional anesthesia was to blame.

not receive epidural block: (1) *Spinal cord lesions* resulting from: ligation of nutrient spinal cord vessels during abdominal surgery[430] or during pelvic surgery (iliac vessels, see anatomy section and Fig. 8-11); prolonged clamping of the aorta[116]; extreme posture and severe retraction causing epidural venous congestion, combined with low cardiac output and leading to "spinal stroke." (2) *Lesions of the cauda equina or spinal nerve roots:* "Adhesive arachnoiditis" has been found at reexploration following major back surgery, and damage to spinal nerve roots has also resulted from surgery in the paravertebral region. Epidural hematoma associated with coagulation defects and systemic heparinization are discussed on page 255. Bladder dysfunction or complete loss of bladder and bowel control is a difficult diagnostic problem. Careful neurologic examination, including cystometry, EMG, and, sometimes, myelography are required to determine etiology. Ligation of nutrient "iliac" supply to sacral segments of spinal cord may result in a clinical picture that mimics a cauda equina lesion. Severe retraction of sacral nerve roots during pelvic surgery may result in such a lesion. (3) *Peripheral nerve lesions* are the most common neurologic sequelae[43] and should be carefully distinguished from more "central" causes on the basis of distribution of sensory, motor, and autonomic deficit; and electromyography to determine pattern of "muscle denervation" (if present) and timing of onset of denervation. This assists in determining if spinal root(s) or peripheral nerves are involved and whether the lesion predates or postdates the operation or is consistent with an intraoperative episode.[292] However, this data alone is not definitive and provides only a guide.[63] Knowledge of potential sites of peripheral nerve injury during surgery, and a tendency for such lesions to be unilateral also serve as a basis for differentiation.

Examples of sites of peripheral lesions are: *lumbosacral trunk* (L4–5): compression on the ala of the sacrum during pregnancy with resultant foot drop and weakness or analgesia[316] at L4–5; *sacral nerves:* during delivery or pelvic surgery; *femoral nerve* (L2–4): during pelvic surgery; *lateral femoral cutaneous nerve* (L2–3): commonly damaged in the lithotomy position or because of direct pressure or retraction close to the inguinal ligament; *lateral popliteal nerve* (L4–S2): pressure over the head of the fibula. It should be noted that patients with preexisting neurologic disease, such as diabetic neuropathy, are at greater risk.[89]

CONCLUSION

Epidural neural blockade is capable of great diversity in terms of its range of neural blocking ef-

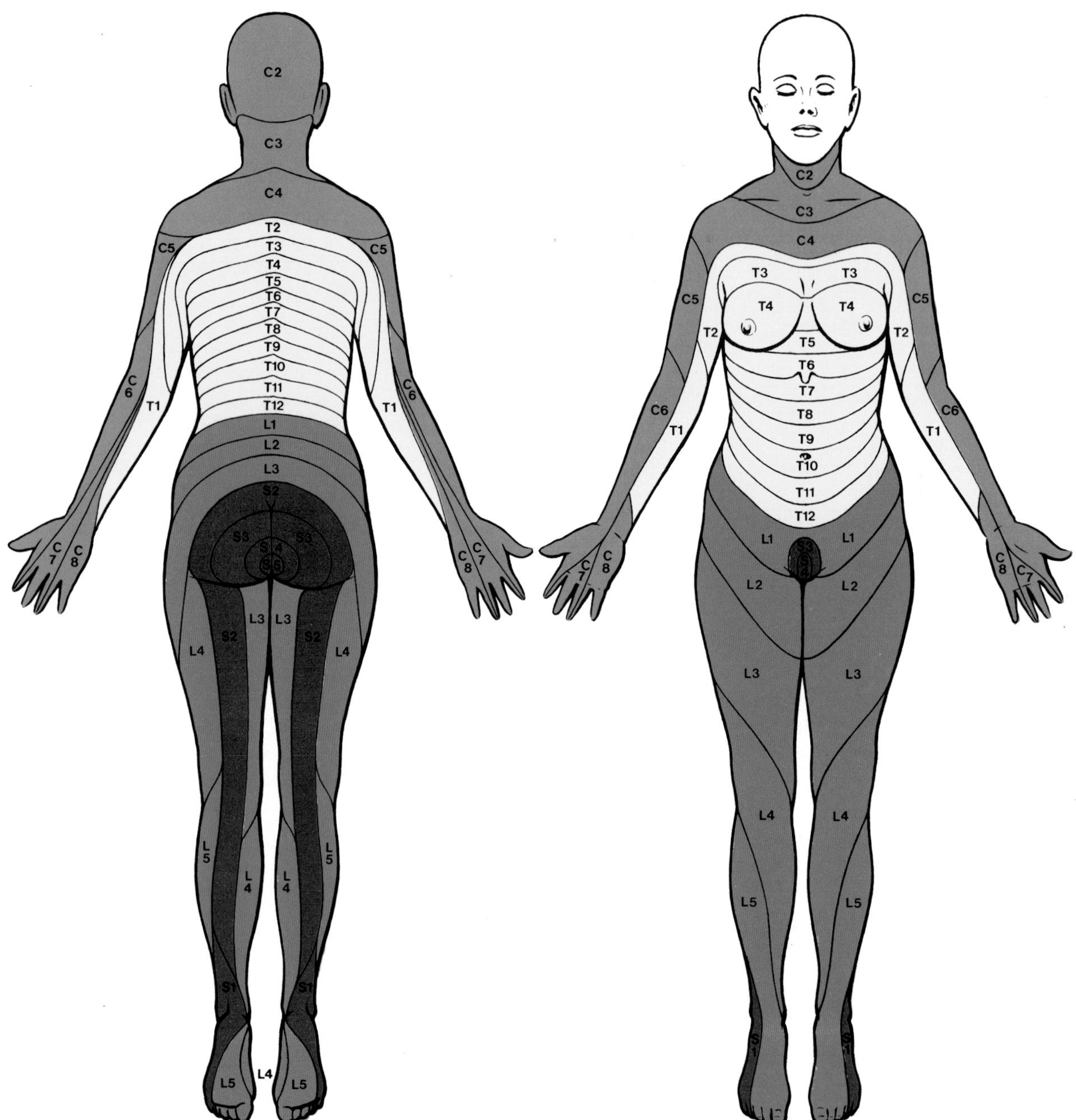

Fig. 8-35. Dermatomal chart. The segmental areas are illustrated to emphasize the most reliable cutaneous area to test for blockade of individual spinal cord segments.

fects and the clinical applications of these effects. It is undoubtedly the most complex technique in terms of its anatomy, site of action, physiology, and pharmacology. Because of this, it is a technique for the specialist—the anesthesiologist. However, if used with due attention to the data presented in this chapter, it can be done with a high degree of safety and efficacy.

APPENDIX

EPIDURAL BLOCK—FUTURE DEVELOPMENTS

Review of the physiology of epidural block points to a number of areas where basic information or further development of current data is indicated. A brief summary with some appropriate references is given in this appendix. References refer to studies of epidural block and also relevant source information where no studies of epidural block have yet been reported.

CARDIOVASCULAR PHYSIOLOGY

Cardic Output

??Effects of absorbed local anesthetics in presence of light anesthesia,[407] hypovolemia and acidosis.[27,377]

Left Atrial (LA) Pressure

LA pressure in patients with post thoracotomy pain is reduced by epidural block[221] ??Effects of epidural block or LA pressure[353] and myocardial oxygen supply[79] in surgical patients.

Oxygen Supply to Myocardium

??Use of systolic pressure × heart rate index to indicate critical changes in myocardial oxygenation[79] in patients with ischemic heart disease[363] or hypertension[225] receiving epidural block.

??Effects of α stimulation during epidural block on coronary vascular resistance[363] and coronary blood flow.[362] ??Usefulness of ECG monitoring during epidural block for myocardial ischemia.[251,261,348]

Cardiac Irritability and High Epidural Block

??Effects of total epidural block on cardiac irritability at normothermia[27,377,407] and hypothermia.[185]

Vagal Activity

??Does sudden reduction in venous return activate vagal reflexes in man in response to reduced ventricular filling[328,329] as a protective mechanism to prevent the ventricle contracting on an empty chamber?[330,331] Is this accentuated by norepinephrine?[201]

??Does reduced oxygen delivery to carotid and aortic bodies (in low blood flow states) activate increased vagal activity in man as it does in animals?[134,135,265,448]

Liver Blood Flow (LBF) and Liver Function

??LBF reduced by epidural block only if perfusion pressure reduced[255,256] or increase catecholamine secretion.[266]

??Is sympathetic block by epidural techniques capable of protecting the liver from toxic injury[44] or shock.[338]

Renal Blood Flow (RBF) and Renal Function

??RBF reduced by epidural block if perfusion pressure reduced or catecholamine secretion increased.[15,122,266,419]

??Sympathetic denervation by epidural block prevents renal changes associated with anesthesia.[15,435]

??When total RBF maintained under normotensive epidural block,[254] is the "key" inner cortical area normally perfused.[29,344]

??Epidural block prevents renal failure following trauma[113] or medical conditions such as pancreatitis.[447]

??Epidural block prevents BOTH sodium[16] and water retention following surgery.

Central Nervous System

Brain

??Safe reductions in cerebral blood flow in normal patients and those with diseased vessels.[409,627]

??Do rapid reductions in cerebral perfusion pressure with epidural block initiate neurogenic cerebral vasoconstriction which initially overcomes local vasodilatory mechanisms?[211]

??Usefulness of supplementation with moderate doses of thiopentone to reduce cerebral metabolic rate of oxygen consumption.[399]

Spinal Cord

??Is autoregulation present in man to maintain normal flow when epidural block reduces perfusion pressure?[259,398]

??Are clinical doses of epinephrine in local anesthetics responsible for spinal cord ischemia?[425]

Hematologic Effects

??Is reduced platelet aggregation[318] clinically significant after epidural block?

??Is increased lower limb blood flow after epidural block a significant factor in reducing venous thrombosis?[125,264,317,391]

??In major surgery of long duration is adjunctive epidural block useful in preventing the initiation of venous thrombosis?[168,217,403]

??In reducing venous thrombosis as judged by ^{125}I fibrinogen scanning,[355] which treatment(s) are most effective or in combination: ?epidural block,[264,404] ?electrical calf stimulation,[361] calf compression with a pump,[88,217,357] ?dextran, ?heparin.[13,243]

Respiratory Effects

?Changes in central and peripheral control of respiration after epidural block.[50–52,327,365,384]

?Compliance changes.[50–52,130,182]

?Precise pathways of afferents for noxious stimuli.[130,182,262]

?Changes in functional residual capacity and airway closure.[10,146,178]

?Reduced ability to cough due to motor block.[154,175,176]

?Blood gas changes and oxygen flux with epidural and general anesthesia.[63,233,311]

?Respiratory effects of relief of severe pain such as acute pancreatitis.[213]

?Does epidural block relieve asthma[12,14,63,90,97,167,273,458] or does it cause exacerbation?[449]

REFERENCES

1. Abboud, F.M.: Control of the various components of the peripheral vasculature. Fed. Proc., *31*:1226, 1972.
2. Abouleish, E., Amortegui, A.J., and Taylor, F.H.: Are bacterial filters needed in continuous epidural analgesia for obstetrics? Anesthesiology, *46*:351, 1977.
3. Adamkiewicz, A.: Die Blutgefasse des Menschlichen Ruckenmarkes. II. Die Gefasse der Ruckenmarksoberflache. S.B. Heidelberg Akad. Wiss., *85*:101, 1882.
4. Andersen, P.K., *et al.*: Sodium nitroprusside and epidural blockade in the treatment of ergotism. N. Engl. J. Med., *296*:1271, 1977.
5. Andy, J.J., *et al.*: Cardiovascular effects of dobutamine in severe congestive heart failure. Am. Heart J., *94*:175, 1977.
6. Baker, A.S., Ojemann, R.G., Swartz, M.N., and Richardson, E.P.: Spinal epidural abscess. N. Engl. J. Med., *293*:463, 1975.
7. Barton, M.D., Killam, A.P., and Meschia, G.: Response of ovine uterine blood flow to epinephrine and norepinephrine. Proc. Soc. Exp. Biol. Med., *145*:996, 1974.
8. Batson, O.V.: The function of the vertebral veins and their role in the spread of metastases. Ann. Surg., *112*:138, 1940.
9. ______: The vertebral vein system. A. J. R., *128*:195, 1957.
10. Beecher, H.K.: The measured effect of laparotomy on the respiration. J. Clin. Invest., *12*:639, 1933.
11. Bellis, C.J., and Wangensteen, O.H.: Venous circulatory changes in the abdomen and lower extremities attending intestinal distention. Proc. Soc. Exp. Biol. Med., *41*:490, 1939.
12. Benumof, J.L., and Wahrenbrock, E.A.: Blunted hypoxic pulmonary vasoconstriction by increased lung vascular pressures. J. Appl. Physiol., *38*:846, 1975.
13. Berquist, E., Bergqvist, D., Bronge, A., Dahlgren, S., and Lindquist, B.: An evaluation of early thrombosis prophylaxis following fracture of the femoral neck. Acta Chir. Scand., *138*:689, 1972.
14. Bergren, D.R., and Beckman, D.L.: Pulmonary surface tension and head injury. J. Trauma., *15*:336, 1975.
15. Berne, R.M.: Haemodynamics and sodium excretion of denervated kidney in anaesthetized and unanaesthetized dog. Am. J. Physiol., *171*:148, 1952.
16. Bevan, D.R.: The sodium story: Effects of anaesthesia and surgery on intrarenal mechanisms concerned with sodium homeostasis. Proc. R. Soc. Med., *66*:1215, 1973.
17. Bevan, D.R., *et al.*: Closing volume and pregnancy. Br. Med. J., *1*:13, 1974.
18. Biehl, D.B., Shnider, S.M., Levinson, G., and Callender, K.: Placental transfer of lidocaine: Effects of fetal acidosis. Anesthesiology, *48*:409, 1978.
19. Bieniarz, J., *et al.*: Aortocaval compression by the uterus in late human pregnancy. II: An arteriographic study. Am. J. Obstet. Gynecol., *100*:203, 1968.
20. Binnert, D., Thierry, A., Michiels, R., Soichot, P., and Perrin, M.: Presentation d'un nouveau cas d'hematome extradural rachidien spontane observe au cours d'un accouchement. J. Med. Lyon, *52*:1307, 1971.
21. Bonica, J.J.: Continuous peridural block. Anesthesiology, *17*:626, 1956.
22. ______: Maternal physiologic changes during pregnancy and anesthesia. In Shnider, S.M., and Moya, F. (eds.): The Anesthesiologist, Mother and Newborn. pp. 3–19. Baltimore, Williams & Wilkins, 1974.
23. ______: Principles and Practice of Obstetric Analgesia and Anesthesia. pp. 725, 745. Philadelphia, F.A. Davis, 1967.
24. Bonica, J.J., Akamatsu, T.J., Berges, P.U., Morikawa, K., and Kennedy, W.F.: Circulatory effects of peridural block. II. Effects of epinephrine. Anesthesiology, *34*:514, 1971.
25. Bonica, J.J., *et al.*: Peridural block: Analysis of 3637 cases and a review. Anesthesiology, *18*:723, 1957.
26. Bonica, J.J., Berges, P.U., and Morikawa, K.: Circulatory effects of peridural block: I. Effects of levels of analgesia and dose of lidocaine. Anesthesiology, *33*:619, 1970.
27. Bonica, J.J., Kennedy, W.F., Akamatsu, T.J., and Gerbershagen, H.U.: Circulatory effects of peridural block. III: Effects of acute blood loss. Anesthesiology, *36*:219, 1972.
28. Bonica, J.J., Kennedy, W.F., Ward, R.J., and Tolas, A.G.: A comparison of the effects of high subarachnoid and epidural anesthesia. Acta Anaesthesiol. Scand., *23* [*Suppl.*]:429, 1966.
29. Bonjour, J.P., Churchill, P.C., and Malvin, R.L.: Change of tubular reabsorption of sodium and water after renal denervation in the dog. J. Physiol. (Lond.), *204*:571, 1969.

30. Bonniot, A.: Note sur la pression epidurale negative. Bull. Soc. Nat. Chir., *60*:124, 1934.
31. Bowsher, D.: A comparative study of the azygos venous system in man, monkey, dog cat, rat and rabbit. J. Anat., *88*:400, 1954.
32. Boys, J.E., and Norman, P.F.: Accidental subdural analgesia. Br. J. Anaesth., *47*:1111, 1975.
33. Braham, J., and Saia, A.: Neurological complications of epidural anaesthesia. Br. Med. J., *2*:657, 1958.
34. Braid, D.P., and Scott, D.B.: The systemic absorption of local analgesic drugs. Br. J. Anaesth., *37*:394, 1965.
35. ______: Dosage of lignocaine in epidural block in relation to toxicity. Br. J. Anaesth., *38*:596, 1966.
36. Brandt, M.R., Kehlet, H., Binder, C., Hagen, C., and McNeilly, A.S.: Effect of epidural analgesia on the glycoregulatory endocrine response to surgery. Clin. Endocrinol. (Oxf.), *5*:107, 1976.
37. Brandt, M.R., *et al.*: C-Peptide and insulin during blockade of the hyperglycaemic response to surgery by epidural analgesia. Clin. Endocrinol. (Oxf)., *6*:167, 1977.
38. Brandt, M.R., Kehlet, H., Skovsted, L., and Hansen, J.M.: Rapid decrease in plasma-triiodothyronine during surgery and epidural analgesia independent of afferent neurogenic stimuli and of cortisol. Lancet, *2*:1333, 1976.
39. Bridenbaugh, L.D., Moore, D.C., Bagdi, P., and Bridenbaugh, P.O.: The position of plastic tubing in continuous-block techniques: An X-ray study of 552 patients. Anesthesiology, *29*:1047, 1968.
40. Bridenbaugh, P.O., *et al.*: Role of epinephrine in regional block anesthesia with etidocaine: A double-blind study. Anesth. Analg. (Cleve.), *53*:430, 1974.
41. Brierley, J.B., and Field, E.J.: The connexions of the spinal sub-arachnoid space with the lymphatic system. J. Anat., *82*:153, 1948.
42. Brigden, W., Howarth, S., and Sharpey–Schafer, E.P.: Postural changes in the peripheral blood-flow of normal subjects with observations on vasovagal fainting reactions as a result of tilting, the lordotic posture, pregnancy and spinal anaesthesia. Clin. Sci. Mol. Med., *9*:79, 1950.
43. Britt, B.A., and Gordon, R.A.: Peripheral nerve injuries associated with anaesthesia. Can. Anaesth. Soc. J., *11*:514, 1964.
44. Brody, T.M., Calvert, D.N., and Schneider, A.F.: Alteration of carbon tetrachloride induced pathologic changes in the rat by spinal transection, adrenalectomy and adrenergic blocking agents. J. Pharmacol. Exp. Ther., *131*:341, 1961.
45. Bromage, P.R.: Vascular hypotension in 150 cases of epidural analgesia. Anaesthesia, *6*:26, 1951.
46. ______: Comparison of vasoactive drugs in man. Br. Med. J., *2*:72, 1952.
47. ______: The 'hanging-drop' sign. Anaesthesia, *8*:237, 1953.
48. ______: Spinal epidural analgesia. Edinburgh, E. & S. Livingstone, 1954.
49. ______: Spirometry in assessment of analgesia after abdominal surgery. A method of comparing analgesic drugs. Br. Med. J., *2*:589, 1955.
50. ______: Hypotension and vital capacity. Anaesthesia, *11*:139, 1956.
51. ______: The phrenic reflex in epidural analgesia. Can. Anaesth. Soc. J., *5*:29, 1958.
52. ______: Total respiratory compliance in anaesthetized subjects and modifications produced by noxious stimuli. Clin. Sci. Mol. Med., *17*:217, 1958.
53. ______: Continuous lumbar epidural analgesia for obstetrics. Can. Med. Assoc. J., *85*:1136, 1961.
54. ______: Epidural needle. Anesthesiology, *22*:1018, 1961.
55. ______: Spread of analgesic solutions in the epidural space and their site of action: A statistical study. Br. J. Anaesth., *34*:161, 1962.
56. ______: Exaggerated spread of epidural analgesia in arteriosclerotic patients. Dosage in relation to biological and chronological ageing. Br. Med. J., *2*:1634, 1962.
57. ______: A comparison of the hydrochloride salts of lignocaine and prilocaine for epidural analgesia. Br. J. Anaesth., *37*:753, 1965.
58. ______: A comparison of the hydrochloride and carbon dioxide salts of lidocaine and prilocaine in epidural analgesia. Acta Anaesthesiol. Scand., *16* [*Suppl.*]:55, 1965.
59. ______: Ageing and epidural dose requirements. Segmental spread and predictability of epidural analgesia in youth and extreme age. Br. J. Anaesth., *41*:1016, 1969.
60. ______: An evaluation of bupivacaine in epidural analgesia for obstetrics. Can. Anaesth. Soc. J., *16*:46, 1969.
61. ______: Lower limb reflex changes in segmental epidural analgesia. Br. J. Anaesth., *46*:504, 1974.
62. ______: Mechanism of action of extradural analgesia. Br. J. Anaesth., *47*:199, 1975.
63. ______: Epidural Analgesia. Philadelphia, W.B. Saunders, 1978.
64. Bromage, P.R., Bramwell, R.S.B., Catchlove, R.F.H., Belanger, G. and Pearce, C.G.A.: Peridurography with metrizamide: Animal and human studies. Radiology, *128*:123, 1978.
65. Bromage, P.R., and Burfoot, M.F.: Quality of epidural blockade. II: Influence of physico-chemical factors: Hyaluronidase and potassium. Br. J. Anaesth., *38*:857, 1966.
66. Bromage, P.R., Burfoot, M.F., Crowell, D.F., and Pettigrew, R.T.: Quality of epidural blockade. I: Influence of physical factors. Br. J. Anaesth., *36*:342, 1964.
67. Bromage, P.R., Datta, S., and Dunford, L.A.: Etidocaine: An evaluation in epidural analgesia for obstetrics. Can. Anaesth. Soc. J., *21*:535, 1974.
68. Bromage, P.R., Joyal, A.C., and Binney, J.C.: Local anesthetic drugs: Penetration from the spinal extradural space into the neuraxis. Science, *140*:392, 1963.
69. Bromage, P.R., and Melzack, R.: Phantom limbs and the body schema. Can. Anaesth. Soc. J., *21*:267, 1974.
70. Bromage, P.R., and Millar, R.A.: Epidural blockade and circulating catecholamine levels in a child with phaeochromocytoma. Can. Anaesth. Soc. J., *5*:282, 1958.
71. Bromage, P.R., Pettigrew, R.T., and Crowell, D.E.: Tachyphylaxis in epidural analgesia. I: Augmentation and decay of local anesthesia. J. Clin. Pharmacol., *9*:30, 1969.
72. Bromage, P.R., Shibata, H.R., and Willoughby, H.W.: Influence of prolonged epidural blockade of blood sugar and cortisol responses to operations upon the upper part of abdomen and the thorax. Surg. Gynecol. Obstet., *132*:1051, 1971.
73. Brown, W.W.: Meningitis following continuous caudal anesthesia. Am. J. Obstet. Gynecol., *53*:682, 1947.
74. Brownridge, P.: Central neural blockade and caesarian section. Part I: Review and case series. Anaesth. Intens. Care, *7*:33, 1979.
75. Bryce-Smith, R.: Pressures in the extradural space. Anaesthesia, *5*:213, 1950.
76. ______: The spread of solutions in the extradural space. Anaesthesia, *9*:201, 1954.
77. Bryce–Smith, R., and Williams, E.O.: The treatment of eclampsia (imminent or actual) by continuous conduction analgesia. Lancet, *1*:1241, 1955.

78. Buchan, P.C., Milne, M.K., and Browning, M.C.K.: The effect of continuous epidural blockade of plasma 11-hydroxycorti-costeroid concentrations in labour. Br. J. Obstet. Gynaecol., *80*:974, 1973.
79. Buckberg, G.D., Fixler, D.E., Archie, J.P., and Hoffman, J.I.E.: Experimental subendocardial ischemia in dogs with normal coronary arteries. Circ. Res., *30*:67, 1972.
80. Bull, G.M.: Postural proteinuria. Clin. Sci. Mol. Med., *7*:77, 1948.
81. Burn, J.M.B.: A method of continuous epidural analgesia. Anaesthesia, *18*:78, 1963.
82. Burn, J.M., Guyer, P.B., and Langdon, L.: The spread of solutions injected into the epidural space: A study using epidurograms in patients with the lumbosciatic syndrome. Br. J. Anaesth., *45*:338, 1973.
83. Butler, M.J., *et al.*: Plasma catecholamine concentrations during operation. Br. J. Surg., *64*:786, 1977.
84. Calder, A.A., Moar, V.A., Qunsted, M.K., and Turnbull, A.C.: Increased bilirubin levels in neonates after induction of labour by intravenous prostaglandin E_2 or Oxytocin. Lancet, *2*:1339, 1974.
85. Caldeyro–Barcia, R., *et al.*: Effects of position changes on the intensity and frequency of uterine contractions during labor. Am. J. Obstet. Gynecol., *80*:284, 1960.
86. Caldeyro–Barcia, R., and Poseiro, J.J.: Physiology of the uterine contraction. Clin. Obstet. Gynecol., *3*:386, 1960.
87. Callingham, B.A., and Barrand, M.A.: Catecholamines in blood. J. Pharm. Pharmacol., *28*:356, 1976.
88. Calnan, J.S., and Allenby, F.: The prevention of deep vein thrombosis after surgery. Br. J. Anaesth., *47*:151, 1975.
89. Calverley, J.R., and Mulder, D.W.: Femoral neuropathy. Neurology, *10*:963, 1960.
90. Campbell, E.J.M.: The relationship of the sensation of breathlessness to the act of breathing. *In* Howell, J.B.L., and Campbell, E.J.M.: Breathlessness. pp. 55–64. Oxford, Blackwell Scientific Publications, 1966.
91. Campbell, H.H., and Walker, F.G.: Continuous epidural analgesia in the treatment of frostbite. A report of three cases. Can. Med. Assoc. J., *84*:87, 1961.
92. Catchlove, R.F.H.: The influence of CO_2 and *p*H on local anesthetic action. J. Pharmacol. Exp. Ther., *181*:298, 1972.
93. Catterberg, J.: Local anesthetic vs. spinal fluid. Anesthesiology, *46*:309, 1977.
94. Celander, O.: The range of control exercised by the sympathico-adrenal system. A quantitative study on blood vessels and other smooth muscle effectors in the cat. Acta Physiol. Scand., *32* [*Suppl. 116*]:1, 1954.
95. Cheng, P.A.: Blunt-tip needle for epidural anesthesia. Anesthesiology, *19*:556, 1958.
96. ———: The anatomical and clinical aspects of epidural anesthesia. Anesth. Analg. (Cleve.), *42*:398, 1963.
97. Christensen, N.J., and Brandsborg, O.: The relationship between plasma catecholamine concentration and pulse rate during exercise and standing. Eur. J. Clin. Invest., *3*:299, 1973.
98. Christensen, V., Ladengaard-Pedersen, H.J., and Skovsted, P.: Intravenous lidocaine as a suppressant of persistent cough caused by bronchoscopy. Acta Anaesthesiol. Scand., *67* [*Suppl.*]:84, 1978.
99. Clarke, E., Morrison, R., and Roberts, H.: Spinal cord damage by Efocaine. Lancet, *1*:896, 1955.
100. Cleland, J.G.P.: Continuous peridural and caudal analgesia in surgery and early ambulation. Northwest. Med. J., *48*:26, 1949.
101. ———: Continuous peridural and caudal analgesia in obstetrics. Anesth. Analg. (Cleve.), *28*:61, 1949.
102. Coggeshall, R.E., Coulter, J.D., and Willis, W.D.: Unmyelinated axons in the ventral roots of the cat lumbosacral enlargement. J. Comp. Neurol., *153*:39, 1974.
103. Cohen, C.A., and Kallos, T.: Failure of spinal anesthesia due to subdural catheter placement. Anesthesiology, *37*:352, 1972.
104. Cohen, E.N.: Distribution of local anesthetic agents in the neuraxis of the dog. Anesthesiology, *29*:1002, 1968.
105. Cohen, E.N., Levine, D.A., Colliss, J.E., and Gunther, R.E.: The role of pH in the development of tachyphylaxis to local anesthetic agents. Anesthesiology, *29*:994, 1968.
106. Cohen, G., Holland, B., Sha, J., and Goldenberg, M.: Plasma concentrations of epinephrine and norepinephrine during intravenous infusions in man. J. Clin. Invest., *38*:1935, 1959.
107. Colding, A.: The effect of regional sympathetic blocks in the treatment of herpes zoster. A survey of 300 cases. Acta Anaesthiol. Scand., *13*:133, 1969.
108. Corbett, J.L., Frankel, H.L., and Harris, P.J.: Cardiovascular reflex responses to cutaneous and visceral stimuli in spinal man. J. Physiol. (Lond.), *215*:395, 1971.
109. ———: Cardiovascular responses to tilting in tetraplegic man. J. Physiol. (Lond.), *215*:411, 1971.
110. Corbin, K.B., and Gardner, E.D.: Decrease in number of myelinated fibers in human spinal roots with age. Anat. Rec., *68*:63, 1937.
111. Corke, B.C.: Neurobehavioural responses of the newborn. The effect of different anaesthesia, *32*:539, 1977.
112. Corning, J.L.: Spinal anaesthesia and local medication of the cord. N.Y. Med. J., *42*:483, 1885.
113. Cort, J.H.: Relief of post-traumatic anuria. Am. J. Physiol., *164*:686, 1951.
114. ———: Effect of nervous stimulation on the arterio-venous oxygen and carbon dioxide differences across the kidney. Nature, *171*:784, 1953.
115. Cosgrove, D.O., and Jenkins, J.S.: The effects of epidural anaesthesia on the pituitary-adrenal response to surgery. Clin. Sci. Mol. Med., *46*:403, 1974.
116. Coupland, G.A.E., and Reeve, T.S.: Paraplegia: A complication of excision of abdominal aortic aneurysm. Surgery, *64*:878, 1968.
117. Cousins, M.J.: Vascular responses in arteriosclerotic patients. Anesthesiology, *35*:99, 1971.
118. ———: Hematoma following epidural block. Anesthesiology, *37*:263, 1972.
119. Cousins, M.J., *et al.*: Epidural block for abdominal surgery: Aspects of clinical pharmacology of etidocaine. Anaesth. Intens. Care, *6*:105, 1978.
120. Cousins, M.J., and Bromage, P.R.: A comparison of the hydrochloride and carbonated salts of lignocaine for caudal analgesia in out-patients. Br. J. Anaesth., *43*:1149, 1971.
121. Cousins, M.J., Mather, L.E., Glynn, C.J., Wilson, P.R., and Graham, J.R.: Selective spinal analgesia. Lancet, *1*:1141, 1979.
122. Cousins, M.J., and Mazze, R.I.: Anaesthesia, surgery and renal function. Immediate and delayed effects. Anaesth. Intens. Care, *1*:355, 1973.
123. ———: Epidural blockade by needle or catheter? Anaesth. Intens. Care. [In press]
124. Cousins, M.J., and Rubin, R.B.: The intraoperative management of phaeochromocytoma with total epidural sympathetic blockade. Br. J. Anaesth., *46*:78, 1974.
125. Cousins, M.J., and Wright, C.J.: Graft, muscle, skin blood flow after epidural block in vascular surgical procedures. Surg. Gynecol. Obstet., *133*:59, 1971.
126. Craft, J.B., Epstein, B.S., and Coakley, C.S.: Prophylaxis

of dural-puncture headache with epidural saline. Anesth. Analg. (Cleve.), *52*:228, 1973.

127. Crawford, J.S.: The prevention of headache consequent upon dural puncture. Br. J. Anaesth., *44*:598, 1972.
128. ______: Principles and Practice of Obstetric Anaesthesia. ed. 4. Oxford, Blackwell Scientific Publications, 1978.
129. Crawford, J.S., Burton, M., and Davies, P.: Time and lateral tilt at caesarean section. Br. J. Anaesth., *44*:477, 1972.
130. Crawford, O.B.: The technic of continuous peridural anesthesia for thoracic surgery. Anesthesiology, *14*:316, 1953.
131. Crawley, B.E.: Catheter sequestration. A complication of epidural analgesia. Anaesthesia, *23*:270, 1968.
132. Crock, H.V., and Yoshizawa, H.: The blood supply of the Vertebral Column and Spinal Cord in Man. New York, Springer-Verlag, 1977.
133. Curbelo, M.M.: Continuous peridural segmental anesthesia by means of a ureteral catheter. Anesth. Analg. (Cleve.), *28*:13, 1949.
134. Daly, M de B., and Scott, M.J.: An analysis of the primary cardiovascular reflex effects of stimulation of carotid body chemoreceptors in the dog. J. Physiol., (Lond.), *162*:555, 1962.
135. Daly, M. de B., *et al.*: Cardiovascular-respiratory reflex interactions between carotid bodies and upper-airways receptors in the monkey. Am. J. Physiol., *234*:H293, 1978.
136. Davson, H., Domer, F.R., and Hollingsworth, J.R.: The mechanism of drainage of the cerebrospinal fluid. Brain, *96*:329, 1973.
137. Dawkins, C.J.M.: Discussion on extradural spinal block. Proc. R. Soc. Med., *38*:299, 1945.
138. ______: Discussion of anaesthesia for caesarean section. Proc. R. Soc. Med., *40*:564, 1947.
139. ______: The identification of the epidural space. A critical analysis of the various methods employed. Anaesthesia, *18*:66, 1963.
140. ______: The relief of pain in labour by mean of continuous-drip epidural block. Acta Anaesthesiol. Scand., *37* [*Suppl.*]:248, 1970.
141. de Angelis, J.: Hazards of subdural and epidural anesthesia during anticoagulant therapy: A case report and review. Anesth. Analg. (Cleve.), *51*:676, 1972.
142. Defalque, R.J.: Compared effects of spinal and extradural anesthesia upon the blood pressure. Anesthesiology, *23*:627, 1962.
143. Dinnick, O.P.: Discussion on general anaesthesia for obstetrics: An evaluation of general and regional methods. Some aspects of general anaesthesia. Proc. R. Soc. Med., *50*:547, 1957.
144. Dogliotti, A.M.: Segmental peridural anesthesia. Am. J. Surg., *20*:107, 1933.
145. ______: Anesthesia. p. 537. Chicago, S.B. Debour, 1939.
146. Don, H.F., Wahba, M., Cuadrado, L., and Kelkar, K.: The effects of anesthesia and 100 per cent oxygen on the functional residual capacity of the lungs. Anesthesiology, *32*:521, 1970.
147. Doughty, A.: A precise method of cannulating the lumbar epidural space. Anaesthesia, *29*:63, 1974.
148. Downing, J.W.: Bupivacaine: A clinical assessment in lumbar extradural block. Br. J. Anaesth., *41*:427, 1969.
149. Dreyer, C., Bischoff, D., and Gothert, M.: Effects of methoxyflurane anesthesia on adrenal medullary catecholamine secretion: Inhibition of spontaneous secretion and secretion evoked by splanchnic-nerve stimulation. Anesthesiology, *41*:18, 1974.
150. Duncalf, D., and Foldes, F.F.: The use of radioiodinated serum albumin to confirm accidental intravascular insertion of epidural catheters. Anesthesiology, *25*:564, 1964.
151. Eaton, L.M.: Observations on the negative pressure in the epidural space. Mayo Clin. Proc., *14*:566, 1939.
152. Editorial: A time to be born. Lancet, *2*:1183, 1974.
153. Edwards, W.B., and Hingson, R.A.: The present status of continuous caudal analgesia in obstetrics. Bull. N.Y. Acad. Med., *19*:507, 1943.
154. Egbert, L.D., Tamersoy, K., and Deas, T.C.: Pulmonary function during spinal anesthesia: The mechanism of cough depression. Anesthesiology, *22*:882, 1961.
155. Enderby, G.E.H.: Controlled circulation with hypotensive drugs and posture to reduce bleeding in surgery. Preliminary results with pentamethonium iodide. Lancet, *1*:1145, 1950.
156. Engberg, G., and Wiklund, L.: The use of ephedrine for prevention of arterial hypotension during epidural blockade. A study of the central circulation after subcutaneous premedication. Acta Anaesthesiol. Scand., *66* [*Suppl.*]:1, 1978.
157. ______: The circulatory effects of intravenously administered ephedrine during epidural blockade. Acta Anaesthesiol. Scand. *66* [*Suppl.*]:27, 1978.
158. Engquist, A., Askgaard, B., and Funding, J.: Impairment of blood fibrinolytic activity during major surgical stress under combined extradural blockade and general anaesthesia. Br. J. Anaesth., *48*:903, 1976.
159. Erdemir, H.A., Soper, L.E., and Sweet, R.B.: Studies of factors affecting peridural anesthesia. Anesth. Analg. (Cleve.), *44*:400, 1965.
160. Evans, J.A., Dobben, G.D., and Gay, G.R.: Peridural effusion of drugs following sympathetic blockade. J.A.M.A., *200*:573, 1967.
161. Evans, T.I.: Regional anaesthesia for trans-urethral resection of the prostate—which method and which segments. Anaesth. Intens. Care, *2*:240, 1974.
162. Ferguson, J.F., and Kirsch, W.M.: Epidural empyema following thoracic extradural block. J. Neurosurg., *41*:762, 1974.
163. Fink, B.R., Aasheim, G., Kish, S.J., and Croley, T.S.: Neurokinetics of lidocaine in the infraorbital nerve of the rat in vivo: Relation to sensory block. Anesthesiology, *42*:731, 1975.
164. Fink, B.R., and Kish, S.J.: Reversible inhibition of rapid axonal transport in vivo by lidocaine hydrochloride. Anesthesiology, *44*:139, 1976.
165. Finster, M., and Petrie, R.H.: Monitoring of the fetus. Anesthesiology, *45*:198, 1976.
166. Fisher, A., and James, M.L.: Blood loss during major vaginal surgery. Br. J. Anaesth., *40*:710, 1968.
167. Fishman, A.P.: Pulmonary edema: The water-exchanging function of the lung. Circulation, *46*:390, 1972.
168. Flanc, C., Kakkar, V.V., and Clarke, M.B.: The detection of venous thrombosis of the legs using 125 I-labelled fibrinogen. Br. J. Surg., *55*:742, 1968.
169. Flowers, C.F.: Continuous peridural analgesia in obstetrics. Anaesthesia, *9*:146, 1954.
170. Folkow, B.: Nervous control of blood vessels. Physiol. Rev., *35*:629, 1955.
171. Forestier, J.: Le trou de conjugaison vertebral et l'espace epidural. p. 105. Paris, Jouve et Cie, 1922.
172. Forrester, A.C.: Mishaps in anaesthesia. Anaesthesia, *14*:388, 1959.
173. Fox, G.S.: Anaesthesia for intestinal short circuiting in the morbidly obese with reference to the pathophysiology of gross obesity. Can. Anaesth. Soc. J., *22*:307, 1975.

174. Frank, N.R., Mead, J., and Ferris, B.G.: The mechanical behaviour of the lungs in healthy elderly persons. J. Clin. Invest., *36*:1680, 1957.
175. Freund, F., Roos, A., and Dodd, R.B.: Expiratory activity of the abdominal muscles in man during general anesthesia. J. Appl. Physiol., *19*:693, 1964.
176. Freund, F.G., *et al.*: Ventilatory reserve and level of motor block during high spinal and epidural anesthesia. Anesthesiology, *28*:834, 1967.
177. Frey, H.H., and Soehring, K.: Untersuchungen uber die Durchlassigkeit der Dura Mater des Hundes fur Procain. Arch. Exp. Veterinaermed., *8*:804, 1954.
178. Froese, A.B., and Bryan, A.C.: Effects of anesthesia and paralysis on diaphragmatic mechanics in man. Anesthesiology, *41*:242, 1974.
179. Frumin, M.J., and Schwartz, H.: Continuous segmental peridural anesthesia. Anesthesiology, *13*:488, 1952.
180. Frumin, M.J., Schwartz, H., Burns, J.J., Brodie, B.B., and Papper, E.M.: Sites of sensory blockade during segmental spinal and segmental peridural anesthesia in man. Anesthesiology, *14*:576, 1953.
181. ——: The appearance of procaine in the spinal fluid during peridural block in man. J. Pharmacol. Exp. Ther., *109*:102, 1953.
182. Fujikawa, Y.F., Neves, A., Brasher, C.A., and Buckingham, W.W.: Epidural anesthesia in thoracic surgery: A preliminary report. J. Thorac. Surg., *17*:12W, 1948.
183. Galbert, M.W., and Marx, G.F.: Extradural pressures in the parturient patient. Anesthesiology, *40*:499, 1974.
184. Galindo, A., Hernandez, J., Benavides, O., Ortegon de Munoz, S., and Bonica, J.J.: Quality of spinal extradural anaesthesia: The influence of spinal nerve root diameter. Br. J. Anaesth., *47*:41, 1975.
185. Galindo, A., and Sprouse, J.H.: The influence of epidural anaesthesia on cardiac excitability in profound hypothermia. Can. Anaesth. Soc. J., *11*:614, 1964.
186. Gallus, A.S., *et al.*: Small subcutaneous doses of heparin in prevention of venous thrombosis. N. Engl. J. Med., *288*:545, 1973.
187. Gargano, F.P., Meyer, J.D., and Sheldon, J.J.: Transfemoral ascending lumbar catheterization of the epidural veins in lumbar disk disease. Radiology, *111*:329, 1974.
188. Gavin, R.: Continuous epidural analgesia, an unusual case of dural perforation during catheterisation of the epidural space. N.Z. Med. J., *64*:280, 1965.
189. Gelman, S., Feigenberg, Z., Dintzman, M., and Levy, E.: Electroenterography after cholecystectomy. The role of high epidural analgesia. Arch. Surg., *112*:580, 1977.
190. Germann, P.A.S., Roberts, J.G., and Prys-Roberts, C.: The combination of general anaesthesia and epidural block. I: The effects of sequence of induction of haemodynamic variables and blood gas measurements in healthy patients. Anaesth. Intens. Care, *7*:229, 1979.
191. Gilles, F.H., and Nag, D.: Vulnerability of human spinal cord in transient cardiac arrest. Neurology, *21*:833, 1971.
192. Gillies, I.D.S., and Morgan, M.: Accidental total spinal analgesia with bupivacaine. Anaesthesia, *28*:441, 1973.
193. Gingrich, T.F.: Spinal epidural hematoma following continuous epidural anesthesia. Anesthesiology, *29*:162, 1968.
194. Gordon, N.H., Scott, D.B., and Robb, I.W.P.: Modification of plasma corticosteroid concentrations during and after surgery by epidural blockade. Br. Med. J., *1*:581, 1973.
195. Gove, L.H.: Backache, headache and bladder dysfunction after delivery. Br. J. Anaesth., *45*:1147, 1973.
196. Granger, H.J., and Guyton, A.C.: Autoregulation of the total systemic circulation following destruction of the central nervous system in the dog. Circ. Res., *25*:379, 1969.
197. Greene, N.M.: Area of differential block in spinal anesthesia with hyperbaric tetracaine. Anesthesiology, *19*:45, 1958.
198. Greiss, F.C., and Gobble, F.L.: Effect of sympathetic nerve stimulation on the uterine vascular bed. Am. J. Obstet. Gynecol., *97*:962, 1967.
199. Griffiths, D.P.G., Diamond, A.W., and Cameron, J.D.: Postoperative extradural analgesia following thoracic surgery: A feasibility study. Br. J. Anaesth., *47*:48, 1975.
200. Griffiths, H.W.C., and Gillies, J.: Thoraco-lumbar splanchnicectomy and sympathectomy: Anaesthetic procedure. Anaesthesia, *3*:134, 1948.
201. Grodner, A.S., *et al.*: Neurotransmitter control of sinoatrial pacemaker frequency in isolated rat atria and in intact rabbits. Circ. Res., *27*:867, 1970.
202. Grundy, E.M., *et al.*: Extradural analgesia revisited. A statistical study. Br. J. Anaesth., *50*:805, 1978.
203. Grundy, E.M., Rao., L.N., and Winnie, A.P.: Epidural anesthesia and the lateral position. Anesth. Analg. (Cleve.), *57*:95, 1978.
204. Grundy, E.M., Zamora, A.M., and Winnie, A.P.: Comparison of spread of epidural anesthesia in pregnant and nonpregnant women. Anesth. Analg. (Cleve.), *57*:544, 1978.
205. Gutierrez, A.: Valor de la aspiracion liquida en el espacio peridural en la anestesia peridural. Review Circulation Buenos Aires, *12*:225, 1933.
206. ——: Anestesia Extradural. Review Cirugie Buenos Aires, p. 34, 1939.
207. Hamelberg, W., Siddall, J., and Claassen, L.: Perforation of dura by a plastic catheter during continuous caudal anesthesia. Arch. Surg., *78*:357, 1959.
208. Hammond, W.G., *et al.*: Studies in surgical endocrinology. IV. Anesthetic agents as stimuli to change in corticosteroids and metabolism. Ann. Surg., *148*:199, 1958.
209. Hancock, D.O.: A study of 49 patients with acute spinal extradural abscess. Paraplegia, *10*:285, 1973.
210. Harik, S.I., Raichle, M.E., and Reis, D.J.: Spontaneously remitting spinal epidural hematoma in a patient on anticoagulants. N. Engl. J. Med., *284*:1355, 1971.
211. Harper, A.M., Deshmukh, D., Rowan, J.O., and Jennett, W.B.: The influence of sympathetic nervous activity on cerebral blood flow. Arch. Neurol., *27*:1, 1972.
212. Harrison, D.C., Sprouse, J.H., and Morrow, A.G.: The antiarrhythmic properties of lidocaine and procaine amide. Clinical and physiologic studies of their cardiovascular effects in man. Circulation, *28*:486, 1963.
213. Hayes, M.F., Rosenbaum, R.W., Zibelman, M., and Matsumoto, T.: Adult respiratory distress syndrome in association with acute pancreatitis. Evaluation of positive end expiratory pressure ventilation and pharmacologic doses of steroids. Am. J. Surg., *127*:314, 1974.
214. Hehre, F.W., and Sayig, J.M.: Continuous lumbar peridural anesthesia in obstetrics. Am. J. Obstet. Gynecol., *80*:1173, 1960.
215. Hehre, F.W., Sayig, J.M., and Lowman, R.M.: Etiologic aspects of failure of continuous lumbar peridural anesthesia. Anesth. Analg. (Cleve.), *39*:511, 1960.
216. Heldt, J.H., and Moloney, J.C.: Negative pressure in the epidural space. Am. J. Med. Sci., *175*:371, 1928.
217. Hills, N.H., Pflug, J.J., Jeyasingh, K., Boardman, L., and Calnan, J.S.: Prevention of deep vein thrombosis by intermittent pneumatic compression of calf. Br. Med. J., *1*:131, 1972.

218. Hindmarsh, T.: Methiodal sodium and metrizamide in lumbar myelography. Acta Radiol. (Stockh.), *335* [*Suppl.*]:359, 1973.
219. Hingson, R.A., and Edwards, W.B.: An analysis of the first ten thousand confinements managed with continuous caudal analgesia with a report of the authors' first one thousand cases. J.A.M.A., *123*:538, 1943.
220. Hingson, R.A., and Southworth, J.L.: Continuous caudal anesthesia. Am. J. Surg., *58*:93, 1942.
221. Hoar, P.F., Hickey, R.F., and Ullyot, D.J.: Systemic hypertension following myocardial revascularization. A method of treatment using epidural anesthesia. J. Thorac. Cardiovasc. Surg., *71*:859, 1976.
222. Hodgkinson, R., *et al.*: Neonatal neurobehavioural tests following vaginal delivery under ketamine thiopental and extradural anesthesia. Anesth. Analg. (Cleve.), *56*:548, 1977.
223. Hodgson, D.C.: Venous stasis during surgery. Anaesthesia, *19*:96, 1964.
224. Hoffman, J.I.E., and Buckberg, G.D.: Transmural variations in myocardial perfusion. *In* Yu, P., and Goodwin, J. (eds.): Progress in Cardiology. Vol. V. pp. 37-89. Philadelphia, Lea & Febiger, 1976.
225. Hollmen, A.I., *et al.*: Neurologic activity of infants following anesthesia for cesarean section. Anesthesiology, *48*:350, 1978.
226. Hollmen, A., and Saukkonen, J.: The effects of postoperative epidural analgesia versus centrally acting opiate on physiological shunt after upper abdominal operation. Acta Anaesthesiol. Scand., *16*:147, 1972.
227. Holmdahl, M.H., Sjorgren, S., Strom, G., and Wright, B.: Clinical aspects of continuous epidural blockade for postoperative pain relief. Ups. J. Med. Sci., *77*:47, 1972.
228. Holmes, F.: Spinal analgesia and caesarean section. Maternal mortality. Br. J. Obstet. Gynaecol., *64*:229, 1957.
229. Honkomp, J.: Zur Begutachtung Bleibender Neurologischer Schaden nach Periduralanaesthesie. Der Anaesthesist, *15*:246, 1966.
230. Houghton, A., Hickey, J.B., Ross, S.A., and Dupre, J.: Glucose tolerance during anaesthesia and surgery. Comparison of general and extradural anaesthesia. Br. J. Anaesth., *50*:495, 1978.
231. Howarth, F.: Studies with a radioactive spinal anaesthetic. Br. J. Pharmacol., *4*:333, 1949.
232. ______: Observations on the passage of a colloid from cerebrospinal fluid to blood and tissues. Br. J. Pharmacol., *7*:573, 1952.
233. Howat, D.D.C.: President's address. Anaesthesia for biliary and pancreatic surgery. Proc. R. Soc. Med., *70*:152, 1977.
234. Hume, D.M., Bell, C.C., and Bartter, F.M.: Direct measurement of adrenal secretion during operative trauma and convalescence. Surgery, *52*:174, 1962.
235. Hutchinson, B.R.: Caudal analgesia in obstetrics. N.Z. Med. J., *65*:224, 1966.
236. Hylton, R.R., Eger, E.I., and Rovno, S.H.: Intravascular placement of epidural catheters. Anesth. Analg. (Cleve.), *43*:379, 1964.
237. Ingbert, C.: An enumeration of the medullated nerve fibers in the dorsal roots of the spinal nerves of man. J. Comp. Neurol., *13*:53, 1903.
238. James, F.M., George, R.H., Haiem, H., and White, G.J.: Bacteriologic aspects of epidural analgesia. Anesth. Analg. (Cleve.), *55*:187, 1976.
239. Janzen, E.: Der Negative Vorschlag bei Lumbalpunktion. Dtsch. Z. Nervenheilk., *94*:280, 1926.
240. Jenicek, J.A.: Aseptic meningitis following lumbar epidural block: Case report. Anesthesiology, *16*:464, 1955.
241. Jeyaram, C., and Torda, T.A.: Anesthetic management of cholecystectomy in a patient with buccal pemphigus. Anesthesiology, *40*:600, 1974.
242. Johnson, S.R.: The mechanism of hyperglycemia during anesthesia: An experimental study. Anesthesiology, *10*:379, 1949.
243. Johnsson, S.R., Bygdeman, S., and Eliasson, R.: Effect of dextran on postoperative thrombosis. Acta Chir. Scand., *387* [*Suppl.*]:80, 1968.
244. Jorfeldt, L., *et al.*: The effect of local anaesthetics on the central circulation and respiration in man and dog. Acta Anaesthesiol. Scand., *12*:153, 1968.
245. Jouppila, R., *et al.*: Cyclic amp and segmental epidural analgesia during labour. Acta Anaesthesiol. Scand., *21*:95, 1977.
246. Jouppila, R., *et al.*: Effect of segmental extradural analgesia on placental blood flow during normal labour. Br. J. Anaesth., *50*:563, 1978.
247. Jouppila, R., *et al.*: Segmental epidural analgesia and postpartum sequelae. Ann. Chir. Gynaecol., *67*:85, 1978.
248. Kakkar, V.V., *et al.*: Prevention of fatal postoperative pulmonary embolism by low doses of heparin. An international multicentre trial. Lancet, *2*:45, 1975.
249. Kakkar, V.V., Howe, C.T., Nicolaides, A.N., Renney, J.T.G., and Clarke, M.B.: Deep vein thrombosis of the leg. Is there a "high risk" group? Am. J. Surg., *120*:527, 1970.
250. Kalas, D.B., and Hehre, E.W.: Continuous lumbar peridural anesthesia in obstetrics VIII: Further observations on inadvertent lumbar puncture. Anesth. Analg. (Cleve.), *51*:192, 1972.
251. Kaplan, J.A., and King, S.B.: The precordial electrocardiographic lead (V5) in patients who have coronary-artery disease. Anesthesiology, *45*:570, 1976.
252. Katz, H., Borden, H., and Hirscher, D.: Glass-particle contamination of color-break ampules. Anesthesiology, *39*:354, 1973.
253. Keith, I.: Anaesthesia and blood loss in total hip replacement. Anaesthesia, *32*:444, 1977.
254. Kennedy, W.F., Jr.: Effects of spinal and peridural blocks on renal and hepatic functions. *In* Clinical Anesthesia Series. pp. 110–121. F.A. Davis, Philadelphia, 1969.
255. Kennedy, W.F., Everett, G.B., Cobb, L.A., and Allen, G.D.: Simultaneous systemic and hepatic hemodynamic measurements during high spinal anesthesia in normal man. Anesth. Analg. (Cleve.), *49*:1016, 1970.
256. ______: Simultaneous systemic and hepatic hemodynamic measurements during high peridural anesthesia in normal man. Anesth. Analg. (Cleve.), *50*:1069, 1971.
256a. Kerr, D.D., Wingard, D.W., and Gatz, E.E.: Prevention of porcine malignant hyperthermia by epidural block. Anesthesiology, *42*:307,1975.
257. Khazin, A.F., Hon, E.H., and Hehre, F.W.: Effects of maternal hyperoxia on the fetus. I. Oxygen tension. Am. J. Obstet. Gynecol., *109*:628, 1971.
258. Kliemann, F.A.D.: Paraplegia and intercranial hypertension following epidural anesthesia. Report of four cases. Arq. Neuropsiquiatr., *33*:217, 1975.
259. Kobrine, A.I., Doyle, T.F., and Rizzoli, H.V.: Spinal cord blood flow as affected by changes in systemic arterial blood pressure. J. Neurosurg., *44*:12, 1976.
260. Kosaka, M., Simon, E., and Thauer, R.: Shivering in intact and spinal rabbits during spinal cord cooling. Experientia, *23*:385, 1966.
261. Kossmann, C.E., *et al.*: Recommendations for standardisa-

tion of leads and of specifications for instruments in electrocardiography and vectorcardiography. Circulation, *35*:583, 1967.

262. Kostreva, D.R., Zuperku, E.J., Hess, G.L., Coon, R.L., and Kampine, J.P.: Pulmonary afferent activity recorded from sympathetic nerves. J. Appl. Physiol., *39*:37, 1975.
263. Kyosola, K.: Clinical experiences in the management of cold injuries: A study of 110 cases. J. Trauma., *14*:32, 1974.
264. Lahnborg, G., and Bergstrom, K.: Clinical and haemostatic parameters related to thromboembolism and low-dose heparin prophylaxis in major surgery. Acta Chir. Scand., *141*:590, 1975.
265. Landgren, S., and Neil, E.: The contribution of carotid chemoceptor mechanisms to the rise of blood pressure caused by carotid occlusion. Acta Physiol. Scand., *23*:152, 1951.
266. Larson, C.P., Mazze, R.I., Cooperman, L.H., and Wollman, H.: Effects of anesthetics on cerebral, renal and splanchnic circulations. Anesthesiology, *41*:169, 1974.
267. Lassen, N.A.: Control of cerebral circulation in health and disease. Circ. Res., *34*:749, 1974.
268. Lazorthes, G., *et al.*: La vascularisation arterielle du renflement lombaire. Etude des variations et des suppleances. Rev. Neurol. (Paris), *114*:109, 1966.
269. Lazorthes, G., Poulhes, J., Bastide, G., Chancolle, A.R., and Zadeh, O.: Le vascularisation de la moelle epiniere (etude anatomique et physiologique). Rev. Neurol. (Paris), *106*:535, 1962.
270. Lee, J.A.: Specially marked needle to facilitate extradural block. Anaesthesia, *15*:186, 1960.
271. Leriche, R.: Resultat eloigne de la ganglionectomie lombaire dans les troubles trophiques et vasomoteurs de la poliomyelite infantile. Lyon Chir., *44*:399, 1949.
272. Lerner, S.M., Gutterman, P., and Jenkins, F.: Epidural hematoma and paraplegia after numerous lumbar punctures. Anesthesiology, *39*:550, 1973.
273. Levin, G.L.L.: Treatment of bronchial asthma by dorsal perisympathetic injection of absolute alcohol. Lancet, *2*:249, 1934.
274. Levy, M.N.: Sympathetic-parasympathetic interactions in the heart. Circ. Res., *29*:437, 1971.
275. Li, T.-H., Shimosato, S., and Etsten, B.E.: Methoxamine and cardiac output in nonanesthetised man and during spinal anesthesia. Anesthesiology, *26*:21, 1965.
276. Lloyd, J.W., and Carrie, L.E.S.: A method of treating renal colic. Proc. R. Soc. Med., *58*:634, 1965.
277. Lock, R.F., Greiss, F.C., and Winston-Salem, N.C.: The anesthetic hazards in obstetrics. Am. J. Obstet. Gynecol., *70*:861, 1955.
278. Löfgren, N.: Studies on Local Anaesthetics. Xylocaine. A New Synthetic Drug. Stockholm. Haegggstroms, 1948.
279. Löfström, B.: Blocking characteristics of etidocaine (Duranest). Acta Anaesthesiol. Scand., *60* [*Suppl.*]:21, 1975.
280. Loudon, J.D.O., and Scott, D.B.: Blood loss in gynaecological operations. Br. J. Obstet. Gynaecol., *67*:561, 1960.
281. Lumbers, E.R., and Reid, G.C.: Effects of vaginal delivery and caesarian section on plasma renin activity and angiotension II levels in human umilical cord blood. Biol. Neonate, *31*:127, 1977.
282. Lund, P.C.: Peridural analgesia and anesthesia. pp. 71, 93. Springfield, Charles C Thomas, 1966.
283. Lush, D., Thorpe, J.N., Richardson, D.J., and Bowen, D.J.: The effect of epidural analgesia on the adrenocortical response to surgery. Br. J. Anaesth., *44*:1169, 1972.
284. McCarthy, G.S.: The effect of thoracic extradural analgesia on pulmonary gas distribution. Functional residual capacity and airway closure. Br. J. Anaesth., *48*:243, 1976.
285. Macintosh, R.R.: Lumbar Puncture and Spinal Analgesia. Edinburgh, E. & S. Livingstone, 1957.
286. Macintosh, R.R., and Mushin, W.W.: Observations on the epidural space. Anaesthesia, *2*:100, 1947.
287. McLean, A.P.H., Mulligan, G.W., Otton, P., and MacLean, L.D.: Hemodynamic alterations associated with epidural anesthesia. Surgery, *62*:79, 1967.
288. Madsen, S.N., Brandt, M.R., Endquist, A., Badawi, I., and Kehlet, H.: Inhibition of plasma cyclic amp, glucose and cortisol response to surgery by epidural analgesia. Br. J. Surg., *64*:669, 1977.
289. Malatinsky, J., and Kadlic, T.: Inferior vena caval occlusion in the left lateral position. Br. J. Anaesth., *46*:165, 1974.
290. Male, C.G., and Martin, R.: Puerperal spinal epidural abscess. Lancet, *1*:608, 1973.
291. Malliani, A., Peterson, D.F., Bishop, V.S., and Brown, A.M.: Spinal sympathetic cardiocardiac reflexes Circ. Res., *30*:158, 1972.
292. Marinacci, A.A.: Applied electromyography. pp. 163–180. Philadelphia, Lea & Febiger, 1968.
293. Marinacci, A.A., and Courville, C.B.: Electromyogram in evaluation of neurological complications of spinal anesthesia. J.A.M.A., *168*:1337, 1958.
294. Marx, G.F., and Greene, N.M.: Lactate-pyruvate ratio of umbilical vein blood. Am. J. Obstet. Gynecol., *92*:548, 1965.
295. Mason, D.T.: The autonomic nervous system and regulation of cardiovascular performance. Anesthesiology, *29*:670, 1968.
296. Mather, L.E., and Cousins, M.J.: Low-dose hemineurin infusion as a supplement to epidural blockade. I: Pharmacokinetics. Anaesth. Intens. Care. [In press]
297. Mather, L.E., Tucker, G.T., Murphy, T.M., Stanton-Hicks, M.D'A., and Bonica, J.J.: The effects of adding adrenaline to etidocaine and lignocaine in extradural anaesthesia. II: Pharmacokinetics. Br. J. Anaesth., *48*:989, 1976.
298. Mather, L.E., *et al.*: Cardiovascular and subjective central nervous system effects of long-acting local anaesthetics in man. Anaesth. Intens. Care, *7*:215, 1979.
299. Mellander, S., and Johansson, B.: Control of resistance, exchange and capacitance functions in the peripheral circulation. Pharmacol. Rev., *20*:117, 1968.
300. Melzack, R.: Phantom limb pain: Implications for treatment of pathalogic pain. Anesthesiology, *35*:409, 1971.
301. Miller, L., Gertel, M., Fox, G.S., and MacLean, L.D.: Comparison of effect of narcotic and epidural analgesia on postoperative respiratory function. Am. J. Surg., *131*:291, 1976.
302. Mirkin, B.L.: Perinatal Pharmacology and Therapeutics. New York, Academic Press, 1976.
303. Modig, J., and Malmberg, P.: Pulmonary and circulatory reactions during total hip replacement surgery. Acta Anaesthesiol. Scand., *19*:219, 1975.
304. Moir, D.D.: Blood loss during major vaginal surgery. A statistical study of the influence of general anaesthesia and epidural analgesia. Br. J. Anaesth., *40*:233, 1968.
305. Moir, D.D., and Davidson, S.: Postpartum complications of forceps delivery performed under epidural and pudendal nerve block. Br. J. Anaesth., *44*:1197, 1972.
306. Moir, D.D., and Willocks, J.: Epidural analgesia in British obstetrics. Br. J. Anaesth., *40*:129, 1968.
307. Moloney, P.J., Elliott, G.B., and Johnson, H.W.: Experience with priapism. J. Urol., *114*:72, 1975.
308. Moore, D.C.: Regional Block. ed. 4. Springfield, Charles C Thomas, 1976.
309. Moore, D.C., Bridenbaugh, L.D., Bridenbaugh, P.O.,

Thompson, G.E., and Tucker, G.T.: Does compounding of local anesthetic agents increase their toxicity in humans? Anesth. Analg. (Cleve.), *51*:579, 1972.

310. Moore, D.C., Hain, R.F., Ward, A., and Bridenbaugh, L.D.: Importance of the perineural spaces in nerve blocking. J.A.M.A., *156*:1050, 1954.

311. Morgan, M., and Norman, J.: The effect of extradural analgesia combined with light general anaesthesia and spontaneous ventilation on arterial blood-gases and physiological deadspace. Br. J. Anaesth., *47*:955, 1975.

312. Morikawa, K. -I., Bonica, J.J., Tucker, G.T., and Murphy, T.M.: Effect of acute hypovolaemia on lignocaine absorption and cardiovascular response following epidural block in dogs. Br. J. Anaesth., *46*:631, 1974.

313. Moulds, R.F.W., and Denborough, M.A.: Biochemical basis of malignant hyperpyrexia. Br. Med. J., *2*:241, 1974.

314. Munson, E.S., Paul, W.L., and Embro, W.J.,: Central-nervous-system toxicity of local anesthetic mixtures in monkeys. Anesthesiology, *46*:179, 1977.

315. Murphy, T.M., Mather, L.E., Stanton-Hicks, M.D'A., Bonica, J.J., and Tucker, G.T.: Effects of adding adrenaline to etidocaine and lignocaine in extradural anaesthesia. I: Block characteristics and cardiovascular effects. Br. J. Anaesth., *48*:893, 1976.

316. Murray, R.R.: Maternal obstetrical paralysis. Am. J. Obstet. Gynecol., *88*:399, 1964.

317. Mustard, J.F., Murphy, E.A., Rowsell, H.C., and Downie, H.G.: Factors influencing thrombus formation in vivo. Am. J. Med., *33*:621, 1962.

318. Nachmias, V.T., Sullender, J.S., and Fallon, J.R.: Effects of local anesthetics and human platelets. Filopodial suppression and endogenous proteolysis. Blood, *53*:63, 1979.

319. Nathan, P.W.: Observations on sensory and sympathetic function during intrathecal analgesia. J. Neurol. Neurosurg. Psychiatry, *39*:114, 1976.

320. Nation, R.L., Triggs, E.J., and Selig, M.: Lignocaine kinetics in cardiac patients and aged subjects. Br. J. Clin. Pharmacol., *4*:439, 1977.

321. Nelson, D.A.: Spinal cord compression due to vertebral angiomas during pregnancy. Arch. Surg., *11*:408, 1964.

322. Nicolaides, A.N., *et al.*: Small doses of subcutaneous sodium heparin in the prevention of deep vein thrombosis after elective hip operations. Br. J. Surg., *62*:348, 1975.

323. Nikki, P., Takki, S., Tammisto, T., and Jaattela, A.: Effect of operative stress on plasma catecholamine levels. Ann. Clin. Res., *4*:146, 1972.

324. Nimmo, W.S., *et al.*: Gastric emptying following hysterectomy with extradural analgesia. Br. J. Anaesth., *50*:559, 1978.

325. Nishimura, N., Kitahara, T., and Kusakabe, T.: The spread of lidocaine and 1-131 solution in the epidural space. Anesthesiology, *20*:785, 1959.

326. Noble, A.D., *et al.*: Continuous lumbar epidural analgesia using bupivacaine: A study of the fetus and newborn child. Br. J. Obstet. Gynaecol., *78*:559, 1971.

327. Nunn, J.F.: Applied respiratory physiology with special reference to anesthesia. *In* Control of Breathing. London, Butterworth, 1969.

328. Oberg, B., and Thoren, P.: Studies on left ventricular receptors signalling in non-medullated vagal afferents. Acta Physiol. Scand., *85*:145, 1972.

329. ______: Increased activity in left ventricular receptors during hemorrhage or occlusion of caval veins in the cat. A possible cause of vaso-vagal reaction. Acta Physiol. Scand., *85*:164, 1972.

330. Oberg, B., and White, S.: Circulatory effects of interruption and stimulation of cardiac vagal afferents. Acta Physiol. Scand., *80*:383, 1970.

331. ______: The role of vagal cardiac nerves and arterial baroreceptors in the circulatory adjustments to hemorrhage in the cat. Acta Physiol. Scand., *80*:395, 1970.

332. Orr, R.B., and Warren, K.W.: Continuous epidural analgesia in acute pancreatitis. Lahey Clin. Bull., *6*:204, 1950.

333. Ottesen, S., Renck, H., and Jynge, P.: Cardiovascular effects of epidural analgesia. An experimental study in sheep of the effects on central circulation, regional perfusion and myocardial performance during normoxia, hypoxia and isoproterenol administration. Nunt. Radiol., *69*:2, 1978.

334. Otton, P.E., and Wilson, E.J.: The cardiocirculatory effects of upper thoracic epidural analgesia. Can. Anaesth. Soc. J., *13*:541, 1966.

335. Oyama, T., and Matsuki, A.: Serum levels of thyroxine in man during epidural anesthesia and surgery. Der Anaesthetist, *19*:298, 1970.

356. Pages, F.: Anestesia metamerica. Rev. Sanid. Mil. (Madr.), *11*:351, 1921.

337. Palahniuk, R.J., Shnider, S.M., and Eger, E.I., II: Pregnancy decreases the requirement for inhaled anesthetic agents. Anesthesiology, *41*:82, 1974.

338. Palmeiro, C., *et al.*: Denervation of the abdominal viscera for the treatment of shock. N. Engl. J. Med., *269*:709, 1963.

339. Paton, A.S.: Lumbar epidural analgesia in obstetrics. Med. J. Aust., *2*:449, 1966.

340. Perkins, H.M., and Hanlon, P.R.: Epidural injection of local anesthetic and steroids for relief of pain secondary to herpes zoster. Arch. Surg., *113*:253, 1978.

341. Pflug, A.E., Murphy, T.M., Butler, S.H., and Tucker, G.T.: The effects of postoperative peridural analgesia on pulmonary therapy and pulmonary complications. Anesthesiology, *41*:8, 1974.

342. Philip, J.H., and Brown, W.U.: Total spinal anesthesia late in the course of obstetric bupivacaine epidural block. Anesthesiology, *44*:340, 1976.

343. Pierce, J.A., and Ebert, R.V.: The elastic properties of the lungs of the aged. J. Lab. Clin. Med., *51*:63, 1958.

344. Pomeranz, B.H., Birtch, A.G., and Barger, A.C.: Neural control of intrarenal blood flow. Am. J. Physiol., *215*:1067, 1968.

345. Porte, D., Girardier, L., Seydoux, J., Kanazawa, Y., and Posternak, J.: Neural regulation of insulin secretion in the dog. J. Clin. Invest., *52*:210, 1973.

346. Prescott, L.F., Adjepon-Yamoah, K.K., and Talbot, R.G.: Impaired lignocaine metabolism in patients with myocardial infarction and cardiac failure. Br. Med. J., *1*:939, 1976.

347. Price, H.L., *et al.*: Can general anesthetics produce splanchnic visceral hypoxia by reducing regional blood flow? Anesthesiology, *27*:24, 1966.

348. Prys-Roberts, C.: Monitoring of the cardiovascular system. *In* Saidman, L.J., and Smith, N.T. (eds.): Monitoring in Anesthesia. pp. 53–83. New York, John Wiley and Sons, 1978.

349. Ralston, D.H., and Shnider, S.M.: The fetal and neonatal effects of regional anesthesia in obstetrics. Anesthesiology, *48*:34, 1978.

350. Ramsey, H.J.: Fat in the epidural space of young and adult cats. Am. J. Anat., *104*:345, 1959.

351. Ramsey, R., and Doppman, J.L.: The effects of epidural masses on spinal cord blood flow. An experimental study in monkeys. Radiology, *107*:99, 1973.

352. Ranniger, K., and Switz, D.M.: Local obstruction of the inferior vena cava by massive ascites. A. J. R., *93*:935, 1965.

353. Risk, C., Rudo, N., and Falltrick, R.: Comparison of right

atrial and pulmonary capillary wedge pressures. Crit. Care Med., *6*:172, 1978.

354. Roberts, V.C.: Thrombosis and how to prevent it. New Scientist and Science Journal, September 16, p. 620, 1971.
355. ———: Fibrinogen uptake scanning for diagnosis of deep vein thrombosis: A plea for standardization. Br. Med. J., *3*:455, 1975.
356. Roberts, V.C., and Cotton, L.T.: Prevention of postoperative deep vein thrombosis in patients with malignant disease. Br. Med. J., *1*:358, 1974.
357. ———: Failure of low-dose heparin to improve efficacy of peroperative intermittent calf compression in preventing postoperative deep vein thrombosis. Br. Med. J., *3*:458, 1975.
358. Roizen, M.F., Moss, J., Henry, D.P., and Kopin, I.J.: Effects of halothane on plasma catecholamines. Anesthesiology, *41*:432, 1974.
359. Romagnoli, A., and Batra, M.S.: Continuous epidural block in the treatment of impacted ureteric stones. Can. Med. Assoc. J., *109*:968, 1973.
360. Rooth, G., McBride, R., and Ivy, B.J.: Fetal and maternal *p*H measurements—a basis for common normal values. Acta Obstet. Gynecol. Scand., *52*:47, 1973.
361. Rosenberg, I.L., Evans, M., and Pollock, A.V.: Prophylaxis of postoperative leg vein thrombosis by low dose subcutaneous heparin or peroperative calf muscle stimulation: A controlled clinical trial. Br. Med. J., *1*:649, 1975.
362. Ross, G.: Adrenergic responses of coronary vessels. Circ. Res., *39*:461, 1976.
363. Rowe, G.G.: Responses of the coronary circulation to physiologic changes and pharmacologic agents. Anesthesiology, *41*:182, 1974.
364. Ryan, D.W.: Accidental intravenous injection of bupivacaine: A complication of obstetrical epidural anaesthesia. Br. J. Anaesth., *45*:907, 1973.
365. Salmoiraghi, G.C.: Functional organization of brain stem respiratory neurones. Ann. N.Y. Acad. Sci., *109*:5771, 1963.
366. Sanchez, R., Acuna, L., and Rocha, F.: An analysis of the radiological visualization of the catheters placed in the epidural space. Br. J. Anaesth., *39*:485, 1967.
367. Scanlon, J.W.: Effects of local anesthetics administered to parturient women on the neurobehavioural and behavioural performance of newborn children. Bull. N.Y. Acad. Med., *52*:231, 1976.
368. Scanlon, J.W., Brown, W.U., Weiss, J.B., and Alper, M.H.: Neurobehavioral responses of newborn infants after maternal epidural anesthesia. Anesthesiology, *40*:121, 1974.
369. Schobinger, R.A., Krueger, E.G., and Sobel, G.L.: Comparison of intraosseous vertebral venography and pantopaque myelography in the diagnosis of surgical conditions of the lumbar spine and nerve roots. Radiology, *77*:376, 1961.
370. Schulte-Steinberg, O., and Rahlfs, V.W.: Caudal anaesthesia in children and spread of 1 per cent lignocaine. A statistical study. Br. J. Anaesth., *42*:1093, 1970.
371. ———: Spread of extradural analgesia following caudal injection in children. A statistical study. Br. J. Anaesth., *49*:1027, 1977.
372. Schweitzer, S.A.: Chloremethiazole (Hemineurin) infusion as supplemental sedation during epidural block. Anaesth. Intens. Care, *6*:248, 1978.
373. Scott, D.B.: Inferior vena caval pressure. Changes occurring during anaesthesia. Anaesthesia, *18*:135, 1963.
374. ———: Inferior vena caval occlusion in late pregnancy. Clinical Anesthesia. F.A. Davis & Co., Philadelphia, *10*:37, 1973.
375. ———: Management of extradural block during surgery. Br. J. Anaesth., *47*:271, 1975.
376. ———: Evaluation of the toxicity of local anaesthetic agents in man. Br. J. Anaesth., *47*:56, 1975.
377. Scott, D.B., Davie, I.T., and Stephen, G.W.: Cardiovascular effects of intravenous lignocaine during nitrous oxide/halothane anaesthesia. Br. J. Anaesth., *43*:595, 1971.
378. Scott, D.B., Jebson, P.J.R., and Boyes, R.N.: Pharmacokinetic study of the local anaesthetics bupivacaine (Marcaine) and etidocaine (Duranest) in man. Br. J. Anaesth., *45*:1010, 1973.
379. Scott, D.B., and Kerr, M.G.: Inferior vena caval pressure in late pregnancy. Br. J. Obstet. Gynaecol., *70*:1044, 1963.
380. Scott, D.B., Littlewood, D.G., Drummond, G.B., Buckley, P.F., and Covino, B.G.: Modification of the circulatory effects of extradural block combined with general anaesthesia by the addition of adrenaline to lignocaine solutions. Br. J. Anaesth., *49*:917, 1977.
381. Scott, D.B., and Walker, L.R.: Administration of continuous epidural analgesia. Anaesthesia, *18*:82, 1963.
382. Scoville, W.B.: Epidural anesthesia and lateral position for lumbar disc operations. Surg. Neurol., *7*:163, 1977.
383. Semb, B.K., *et al.*: Ergot-induced vasospasm of the lower extremities treated with epidural anaesthesia. Scand. J. Thorac. Cardiovasc. Surg., *9*:254, 1975.
384. Severinghaus, J.W., *et al.*: Respiratory control at high altitude suggesting active transport regulation of CSF *p*H. J. Appl. Physiol., *18*:1155, 1963.
385. Shanks, C.A.: Four cases of unilateral analgesia. Br. J. Anaesth., *40*:999, 1968.
386. Shantha, T.R., and Evans, J.A.: The relationship of epidural anesthesia to neural membranes and arachnoid villi. Anesthesiology, *37*:543, 1972.
387. Shanthaveerappa, T.R., and Bourne, G.H.: Perineural epithelium: A new concept of its role in the integrity of the peripheral nervous system. Science, *154*:1464, 1966.
388. Sharpey-Schafer, E.P.: Syncope. Br. Med. J., *1*:506, 1956.
389. Sharrock, N.E.: Epidural anesthetic dose responses in patients 20 to 80 years old. Anesthesiology, *49*:425, 1978.
390. Shimoji, K., *et al.*: Spinal hypalgesia and analgesia by low-frequency electric stimulation in the epidural space. Anesthesiology, *41*:91, 1974.
391. Shimosato, S., and Etsten, B.E.: The role of the venous system in cardiocirculatory dynamics during spinal and epidural anesthesia in man. Anesthesiology, *30*:619, 1969.
392. Sicard, J.A., and Forestier, J.: Radiographic method for exploration of the extradural space using lipiodol. Rev. Neurol. (Paris), *28*:1264, 1921.
393. ———: The use of lipiodol in diagnosis and treatment. p. 178. London, Oxford University Press, 1932.
394. Siever, J.M., and Mousel, L.H.: Continuous caudal anesthesia in three hundred unselected obstetric cases. J.A.M.A., *122*:424, 1943.
395. Silver, J.R., and Buxton, P.H.: Spinal stroke. Brain, *97*:539, 1974.
396. Simpson, B.R., Parkhouse, J., Marshall, R., and Lambrechts, W.: Extradural analgesia and the prevention of postoperative respiratory complications. Br. J. Anaesth., *33*:628, 1961.
397. Sjögren, S., and Wright, B.: Circulation, respiration and lidocaine concentration during continuous epidural blockade. Acta Anaesthiol. Scand., *16* [*Suppl. 46*]:5, 1972.
398. Smith, A.L., Pender, J.W., and Alexander, S.C.: Effects of

PCO_2 on spinal cord blood flow. Am. J. Physiol., *216*:1158, 1969.

399. Smith, A.L., and Wollman, H.: Cerebral blood flow and metabolism: Effects of anesthetic drugs and techniques. Anesthesiology, *36*:378, 1972.
400. Smith, O.A.: Reflex and central mechanisms involved in the control of the heart and circulation. Annu. Rev. Physiol., *36*:93, 1974.
401. Spence, A.A., and Smith, G.: Postoperative analgesia and lung function: A comparison of morphine with extradural block. Br. J. Anaesth., *43*:144, 1971.
402. Sreerama, V., Ivan, L.P., Dennery, J.M., and Richard, M.T.: Neurosurgical complications of anticoagulant therapy. Can. Med. Assoc. J., *108*:305, 1973.
403. Sripad, S., Antcliff, A.C., and Martin, P.: Deep-vein thrombosis in two district hospitals in Essex. Br. J. Surg., *58*:563, 1971.
404. Stanton-Hicks, M.D'A.: A study using bupivacaine for continuous pedridural analgesia in patients undergoing surgery of the hip. Acta Anaesthesiol. Scand., *15*:97, 1971.
405. Stapleton, J.V., Austin, K.L., and Mather, L.E.: A pharmacokinetic approach to postoperative pain: Continuous infusion of pethidine. Anaesth. Intens. Care, *7*:25, 1979.
406. Steen, P.A., *et al.*: Efficacy of dopamine, dobutamine and epinephrine during emergence from cardiopulmonary bypass in man. Circulation, *57*:378, 1978.
407. Steinhaus, J.E., and Howland, D.E.: Intravenously administered lidocaine as a supplement to nitrous oxide-thiobarbiturate anesthesia. Anesth. Analg. (Cleve.), *37*:40, 1958.
408. Stephen, G.W., Lees, M.M., and Scott, D.B.: Cardiovascullar effects of epidural block combined with general anaesthesia. Br. J. Anaesth., *41*:933, 1969.
409. Sundt, T.M., *et al.*: Cerebral blood flow measurements and electroencephalograms during carotid endarterectomy. J. Neurosurg., *41*:310, 1974.
410. Sutton, J.R., Cole, A., Gunning, J., Hickie, J.B., and Seldon, W.A.: Control of heart-rate in healthy young men. Lancet, *2*:1398, 1967.
411. Suzuki, H., *et al.*: Neuromuscular effects of i.a. infusion of lignocaine in man. Br. J. Anaesth., *49*:1117, 1977.
412. Takki, S., Nikki, P., Tammisto, T., and Jaattela, A.: Effect of epidural blockade on the pentazocine-induced increase in plasma catecholamines and blood pressure. Br. J. Anaesth., *45*:376, 1973.
413. Thomson, P.D., *et al.*: Lidocaine pharmacokinetics in advanced heart failure, liver disease, and renal failure in humans. Ann. Intern. Med., *78*:499, 1973.
414. Thorud, T., Lund, I., and Holme, I.: The effect of anesthesia on intraoperative and postoperative bleeding during abdominal prostatectomies: A comparison of neurolept anesthesia, halothane anesthesia and epidural anesthesia. Acta Anaesthesiol. Scand., *57* [*Suppl.*]:83, 1975.
415. Tretjakoff, D.: Das Epidurale Fettgewebe. Z. Anat., *79*:100, 1926.
416. Tripathi, R.C.: Ultrastructure of the arachnoid mater in relation to outflow of cerebrospinal fluid. Lancet, *2*:8, 1973.
417. Tripathi, B.J., and Tripathi, R.C.: Vacuolar transcellular channels as a drainage pathway for cerebrospinal fluid. J. Physiol., *239*:195, 1974.
418. Trotter, M.: Variations of the sacral canal: Their significance in the administration of caudal analgesia. Anesth. Analg. (Cleve.), *26*:192, 1947.
419. Trueta, J., Barclay, A.E., Daniel, P.M., Franklin, K.J., and Prichard, M.M.L.: Studies of the renal circulation. Oxford, Blackwell Scientific Publications, 1948.
420. Tucker, G.T., and Mather, L.E.: Pharmacokinetics of local anaesthetic agents. Br. J. Anaesth., *47*:213, 1975.
421. Tuohy, E.B.: Continuous spinal anesthesia: A new method of utilising a ureteral catheter. Surg. Clin. North. Am., *25*:834, 1945.
422. Turnbull, I.M.: Blood supply of the spinal cord: Normal and pathological considerations. Clin. Neurosurg., *20*:56, 1973.
423. Urban, B.J.: Clinical observations suggesting a changing site of action during induction and recession of spinal and epidural anesthesia. Anesthesiology, *39*:496, 1973.
424. Urban, B.J., and Nashold, B.S.: Percutaneous epidural stimulation of the spinal cord for relief of pain: Long term results. J. Neurosurg., *48*:323, 1978.
425. Urquhart-Hay, D.: Paraplegia following epidural analgesia. Anaesthesia, *24*:461, 1969.
426. Urquhart-Hay, D., Marshall, N.G., and Marsland, J.M.: Comparison of epidural and hypotensive anaesthesia in open prostatectomy. Series 1. N.Z. Med. J., *69*:280, 1969.
427. ———: Comparison of epidural and hypotensive anaesthesia in open prostatectomy. Series 2. N.Z. Med. J., *70*:223, 1969.
428. Usubiaga, J.E.: Neurological complications following epidural anesthesia. Int. Anaesthesiol. Clin., *13*:2, 1975.
429. Usubiaga, J.E., Dos Reis, A., and Usubiaga, L.E.: Epidural misplacement of catheters and mechanisms of unilateral blockade. Anesthesiology, *32*:158, 1970.
430. Usubiaga, J.E., Kolodny, J., and Usubiaga, L.E.: Neurological complications of prevertebral surgery under regional anesthesia. Surgery, *68*:304, 1970.
431. Usubiaga, J.E., Moya, F., and Usubiaga, L.E.: Effect of thoracic and abdominal pressure changes on the epidural space pressure. Br. J. Anaesth., *39*:612, 1967.
432. Usubiaga, J.E., Wikinski, J.A., and Usubiaga, L.E.: Epidural pressure and its relation to spread of anesthetic solutions in epidural space. Anesth. Analg. (Cleve.), *46*:440, 1967.
433. Virtue, R.W., Helmreich, M.L., and Gainza, E.: The adrenal cortical response to surgery. I. The effect of anesthesia on plasma 17-hydroxycorticosteroid levels. Surgery, *41*:549, 1975.
434. Vogt, M.: The effect of lowering the 5-hydroxytryptamine content of the rat spinal cord on analgesia produced by morphine. J. Physiol., *236*:483, 1974.
435. Wagenknecht, L.V., Zamora, M., and Madsen, P.O.: Continuous recording of renal clearance by external monitoring during epidural anesthesia. Invest. Urol., *8*:540, 1971.
436. Waggener, J.D., and Beggs, J.: The membranous coverings of neural tissues: An electron microscopy study. J. Neuropathol. Exp. Neurol., *26*:412, 1967.
437. Wagner, R.S.: A needle for single-dose peridural anesthesia. Anesth. Analg. (Cleve.), *36*:31, 1957.
438. Wahba, W.M., Craig, D.B., Don, H.F., and Becklake, M.R.: The cardio-respiratory effects of thoracic epidural anaesthesia. Can. Anaesth. Soc. J., *19*:8, 1972.
439. Wahba, W.M., Don, H.F., and Craig, D.B.: Post-operative epidural analgesia: Effects on lung volumes. Can. Anaesth. Soc. J., *22*:519, 1975.
440. Wall, P.D.: The laminar organization of the dorsal horn and effects of descending impulses. J. Physiol., *188*:403, 1967.
441. Wallis, K.L., Shnider, S.M., Hicks, J.S., and Spivey, H.T.: Epidural anesthesia in the normotensive pregnant ewe: Effects on uterine blood flow and fetal acid-base status. Anesthesiology, *44*:481, 1976.
442. Ward, R.J., *et al.*: Epidural and subarachnoid anesthesia.

Cardiovascular and respiratory effects. J.A.M.A., *191*:275, 1965.

443. Ward, R.J., *et al.*: Experimental evaluation of atropine and vasopressors for the treatment of hypotension of high subarachnoid anesthesia. Anesth. Analg. (Cleve.), *45*:621, 1966.
444. Weaver, J.B., Pearson, J.F., and Turnbull, A.C.: The effect upon the fetus of an oxytocin infusion in the absence of uterine hypertonus. Br. J. Obstet. Gynaecol., *81*:297, 1974.
445. Weil, J.V., McCullough, R.E., Kline, J.S., and Sodal, I.E.: Diminished ventilatory response to hypoxia and hypercapnia after morphine in normal man. N. Engl. J. Med., *292*:1103, 1975.
446. Welch, K., and Pollay, M.: The spinal arachnoid villi of the monkeys *Cercopitheus aethiops sabaeus* and *Macaca irus*. Anat. Rec., *145*:43, 1963.
447. Werner, M.H., Hayes, D.F., Lucas, C.E., and Rosenberg, I.K.: Renal vasoconstriction in association with acute pancreatitis. Am. J. Surg., *127*:185, 1974.
448. White, S.W., Traugott, F.M., and Quail, A.W.: Arterial chemoreflex in unanesthetized man, monkey and rabbit: Circulatory-respiratory interactions during severe arterial hypoxia. Proc. Aust. Phys. Pharmacol. Soc., *10*, 1979.
449. Willis, R.J., Germann, P.A.S., and Cousins, M.J.: Exacerbation of asthma by reflex vagal activity during central neural blockade. Anaesth. Intens. Care, [In press]
450. Winnie, A.P.: A grip to facilitate the insertion of epidural needles. Anesth. Analg. (Cleve.), *50*:23, 1971.
451. Wollman, S.B., and Marx, G.F.: Acute hydration for prevention of hypotension of spinal anesthesia in parturients. Anesthesiology, *29*:374, 1968.
452. Woollam, D.H.M., and Millen, J.W.: An anatomical approach to poliomyelitis. Lancet, *1*:364, 1953.
453. ———: The anatomical background to vascular disease of the spinal cord. Proc. R. Soc. Med., *51*:540, 1958.
454. Wright, R.G., *et al.*: The effect of maternal stress on plasma catecholamines and uterine blood flow in the pregnant ewe. Abstracts of Scientific Papers. p. 17. Memphis. Society of Obstetric Anesthesia and Perinatology. 1978.
455. Wugmeister, M., and Hehre, F.W.: The absence of differential blockade in peridural anaesthesia. Br. J. Anaesth., *39*:953, 1967.
456. Yin, E.I., Wessler, S., and Butler, J.V.: Plasma heparin: A unique, practical, submicrogramsensitive assay. J. Lab. Clin. Med., *81*:298, 1973.
457. Youngman, H.R.: Toxic reactions in epidural anesthesia. Anesthesiology, *17*:632, 1956.
458. Zapol, W.M., and Snider, M.T.: Pulmonary hypertension in severe acute respiratory failure. N. Engl. J. Med., *296*:476, 1977.
459. Zorgniotti, A.W., Narins, D.J., and Dell'Aria, S.L.: Anesthesia, Hemorrhage and prostatectomy. J. Urol., *103*:774, 1970.

9 Caudal Blockade

Kevin McCaul

GENERAL CONSIDERATIONS

Definitions

The term *caudal blockade* has been used to indicate several combinations of sacral, lumbar, and thoracic epidural analgesia following transhiatal injection of local anesthetic solution. However, despite the care taken by many authors to avoid confusion, much of the literature on the subject has suffered from lack of precise definition and should be read with discretion.[3,5,15,21,24] For instance, terminological confusion has occasioned a widely held but inaccurate belief that nearly all forms of caudal blockade are associated with high rates of failure and toxic or other undesirable sequelae.

In this chapter *caudal blockade* denotes only blockade of coccygeal and sacral nerve roots by transhiatal injection but presupposes allowances for minor spillover of anesthetic solution to the lower lumbar epidural space and for occasional inadequate blockade of the first sacral nerves, both of which are unpredictable events of minor significance.

The previously popular although unreliable "high" and "mid" caudal techniques that preceded the introduction, in 1950, of safe epidural methods at higher spinal levels were essentially combinations of thoracolumbosacral or lumbosacral blockade, which involved serial injections of large volumes of local anesthetic solution to allow for inevitable leakages through intervertebral spaces and for the short duration of action of the then available drugs. Toxic reactions from drug absorption or accidental intravenous injection therefore unavoidably occurred. This resulted in the technique having few remaining adherents and being largely superseded by segmental epidural techniques. Continuous caudal techniques with fine polyvinyl catheters may still be a useful alternative if lumbar epidural puncture is not desirable or possible. In some units, catheters threaded to the lumbosacral region are used to provide lower abdominal and pelvic analgesia by injecting increments of local anesthetic. This is most satisfactory in children because leakage through sacral foramina is minimal; however, it has also been used in adults with the proviso that appropriate care be taken with drug concentration and volume (dosage). Agents with a marked tendency to cumulative toxicity are avoided (*e.g.*, prilocaine, mepivacaine). In most situations, continuous caudal techniques in adults yield the best safety to efficacy ratio for sacral analgesia, while if higher levels of blockade are required, lumbar epidural blockade is preferable.

History and Role

Because this chapter is based on departmental and personal experiences extending over 30 years, it must inevitably conflict with some established precepts and run counter to the views of some others. However, it does present changing attitudes that arise as experience is acquired and by the recognition that at least one in every five sacra was impossibly abnormal from the viewpoint of regional anesthesiologists.[12,13,17,18,20,30] It appeared reasonable to document the incidence of these prohibitive sacral anomalies as clinically diagnosed. Such a project was undertaken but as data were collected, it became evident that there was a changing pattern. With time, these anomalies became less and less frequent, and the project was, in retrospect, mistakenly abandoned. On reflection, increased competence in the use of caudal blockade was probably due to a number of factors including the use of narrow-gauge hypodermic or intravascular needles, improved identification techniques, and, with the introduction of long-acting local anesthetic agents, an ever-increasing preference for simplified single-dose methods.

The foremost role of caudal blockade (low) is to provide full anesthetic cover for obstetric and surgical operations and manipulations performed on organs exclusively innervated through the second, third, fourth, and fifth sacral and the coccygeal nerves or to serve as a component of balanced anesthetic techniques for surgery extending to the multiply innervated junctional pelviperineal organs and tissues.

Although restricted in anatomical ambit, the procedures that may be conducted under caudal blockade are extremely common in clinical practice and ideally suited to regional analgesic methods. Its particular advantages, which are not shared with alternative epidural techniques, are sparing of the nerve supply to the lower limbs, abdominal wall, and blood vessels; a low risk of accidental dural puncture; and, because of minimal physiologic and biochemical encroachment, its suitability for all categories of poor-risk patients.

The major disadvantages of caudal block are that blockade is technically exacting to perform in about 5 per cent of cases and that the skills necessary to overcome this initial barrier can be only acquired as a result of persistence in training and increasing familiarity with the variable features of sacral hiatal topography. In a teaching hospital in which caudal blockade is favored and extensively employed for most major pelvic and perineal surgery, it is anticipated that during a period of 6 months of extensive exposure, trainees will consistently reduce failure rates and the incidence of diagnosis of anatomical abnormality will be reduced to one per cent or less as experience is acquired. A similar trend has been noted by Rubin.[26]

Suggestions that blockade failures most often result from insurmountable anatomic barriers rather than from the anesthesiologist's level of expertise are disputable. As reported failure rates range from 3 to 20 per cent, it is reasonable to assume that significant allowances must be made for individual variations in experience, skill, and training as well as for the techniques employed.[2,6,8,22,26,28] Apart from initial difficulties in its performance, several reports of toxic sequelae and a small number of accidents have tended to dissuade many anesthesiologists from the practice of all forms of caudal blockade.[1,9,10,11,27] However, most of these reservations apply only to the high, mid, and intermittent blockade techniques and have little or no relevance to the low dose to low level blockade. With appropriate facility in its performance equal to that for midlumbar epidural blockade, there is little doubt that the caudal method would replace the former for a number of obstetric and surgical procedures such as forceps or breech delivery, circumcision, hemorrhoidectomy, episiotomy, and perineoplasty, for which extensive blockade is either unnecessary or undesirable.

The ease of single-dose administration and the frequent difficulties with catheter techniques are in sharp contrast. In approximately 7 per cent of subjects, the anterioposterior and, less comonly, the transverse apertures of the sacral canal are 1 mm or less in diameter, and thus insertion of even the finest-gauge catheters or introducers is impracticable; in a similar proportion, their introduction can be accomplished only with difficulty and a risk of local trauma.[19,29] This distinction between the two basic methods of administration is paramount to an understanding of the scope and problems of caudal blockade. In this chapter the primary emphasis is on matters of training, and technique, on which depend the ability to perform and exploit this useful, exceptionally safe, and elegant form of regional analgesia.

INDICATIONS AND CONTRAINDICATIONS

Caudal blockade should be considered as the most acceptable alternative to lumbar epidural or subarachnoid saddle blockade when it is desirable to avoid the consequences of dural puncture, hypotension from spread of solution to the thoracolumbar sympathetic outflow, or involvement of sensory or motor nerve supply to the abdomen or legs.

It should be noted that genuine subarachnoid saddle and caudal blockade are similar in the sensory cover provided, but although motor blockade is usual in saddle block, it is unusual in caudal block. However, because full passive relaxation of pelvic and perineal voluntary and sphincteric muscles follows sensory deprivation, their effects are similar in practice, apart from any sequelae that may arise from dural puncture.

A number of operations such as posterior colpoperineorrhaphy, urethral indwelling catheterization, circumcision, and hemorrhoidectomy and episodes such as the prolapse of hemorrhoids, strangury, and priapism are associated with considerable pain and restlessness; each can be effectively and dramatically controlled by caudal blockade. Caudal blockade can also be the means of avoiding the delirium frequently witnessed in the elderly after inadequate doses of narcotic analgesic drugs. Although these considerable practical benefits far outweigh most of the theoretical disadvantages of caudal blockade, they have not generally been exploited.

As with other forms of regional blockade, there are circumstances in which although surgical cover may be adequate, total patient comfort is not fully provided by caudal analgesia. This applies particularly to elderly or arthritic patients required to adopt strained positions (*e.g.*, lithotomy) for prolonged periods, and in such cases supplementary light general anesthesia or analgesia may be required (see also Chaps. 6 and 31).

Although most current indications are for procedures of brief duration, serial techniques still retain some usefulness, for example in the medium-term treatment of perineopelvic pain, be it postoperative or otherwise. However, as a general rule, catheter insertion should be undertaken only when specifically indicated and if it is anticipated that this can be atraumatically and easily performed. For similar reasons and in view of the many alternative methods of pain control now available, it is only in exceptional circumstances—when blockade is deemed essential but impracticable to perform at segmental levels (*e.g.*, in cases of spinal deformity or gross obesity—that the high complication and low predictability rates of high or mid levels of caudal blockade can be justified.[10,16]

It is appropriate to recall that when the high and mid techniques were in vogue as the only practical methods of epidural blockade, continuous or intermittent injection by means of indwelling needles or catheters was considered essential for operations performed in the dorsal decubitus and lithotomy positions because further access to the sacral region was not possible and most operations outlasted the duration of the then available local anesthetic agents.[1,4,20,30]

The applications of caudal blockade to pediatric surgery are discussed in Chapter 21. It is noteworthy that many of the considerations that prompt its use at the extremes of life are similarly based.

Obstetrics

In obstetrics the most rational use of caudal blockade is now restricted to instrumentation, examination, or repair procedures during the second and third stages of labor. It does not contribute to first-stage pain control and should not be initiated in early labor. It has particular relevance to circumstances in which women in labor having rejected or not needing predelivery pain control by blockade require anesthetic cover for instrumental or manipulative delivery.

A single-source report of four instances of injection of local anesthetic agent into the presenting part has occasioned undue alarm and has been overemphasized as a contraindication to blockade.[14,25,27] It has been correctly pointed out that in each case injection was performed when the presenting part was below the ischial spinous level.[25]

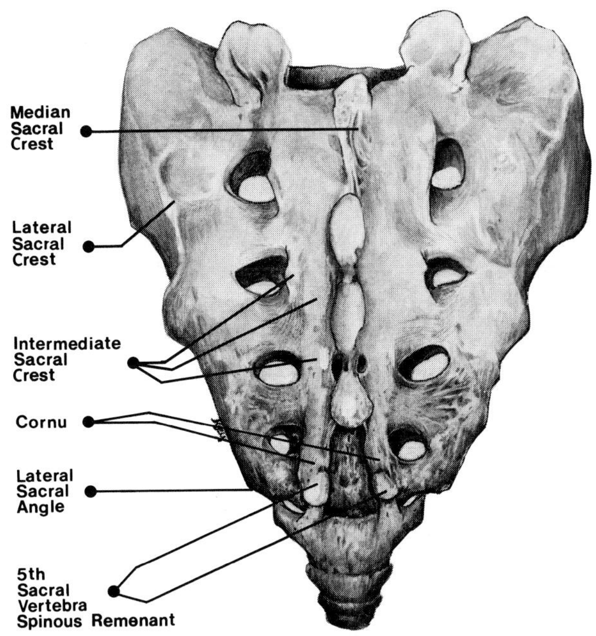

Fig. 9-1. The sacrum—dorsal aspect. This illustration shows the following important features. The median sacral crest is varyingly prominent and may extend throughout the total length of the roof of the sacral canal or be lacking at any or all segmental levels. When it is present the crest is always in line with the sacral hiatus and, as illustrated, usually terminates at or proximal to its apex. The indentations between the spines of S3 and S4 are inconstant features that may occur at any level and represent failures of laminar fusion (see Fig. 9-7). These various crevices are covered by the posterior sacral membranes and form sealed cavities that may be regarded as rather dubious decoys of the true hiatus. The intermediate sacral crest lies lateral to the sacral foramen and is seldom palpable *in vivo*. Inferiorly, it becomes much more prominent as it merges into the sacral cornua. The lateral sacral crest terminates distally at the lateral sacral angle and at this point may be prominent and occasionally palpable. The areas bounded by the lower borders of the sacrum, the lateral sacral angles, and the cornua form grooves in which are seated the fourth sacral foramen. When the hiatal outlines are difficult to feel on palpation *in vivo*, these grooves may frequently be mistaken for the hiatus, and injection is then performed through the foramen; all the signs of successful needle insertion can be elicited but blockade is patchy, usually unilateral, and slow in its onset. The sacral cornua are varyingly prominent, but, as in most of the illustrations in this chapter, are surmounted on each side by the remnants of the spinous process of S5, and these in over 90 per cent of patients are palpable and offer a guide to the lowest level of the sacral hiatus. Examination should always be regarded as incomplete if the lower extremities of the sacral cornua have not been palpated, if only to gain and store experience for future use in cases of difficulty.

tion, should the obstetric management require elimination of the bearing-down reflex. During the expulsive second stage of labor, it may also be used to eliminate expulsive reflexes in patients who suffer cardiac or respiratory failure or other conditions in which increased physical activity or acute rises of systemic arterial or venous blood pressures are undesirable. As noted above, this can be achieved with minimum physiologic disturbance in this group of high-risk patients.[16a]

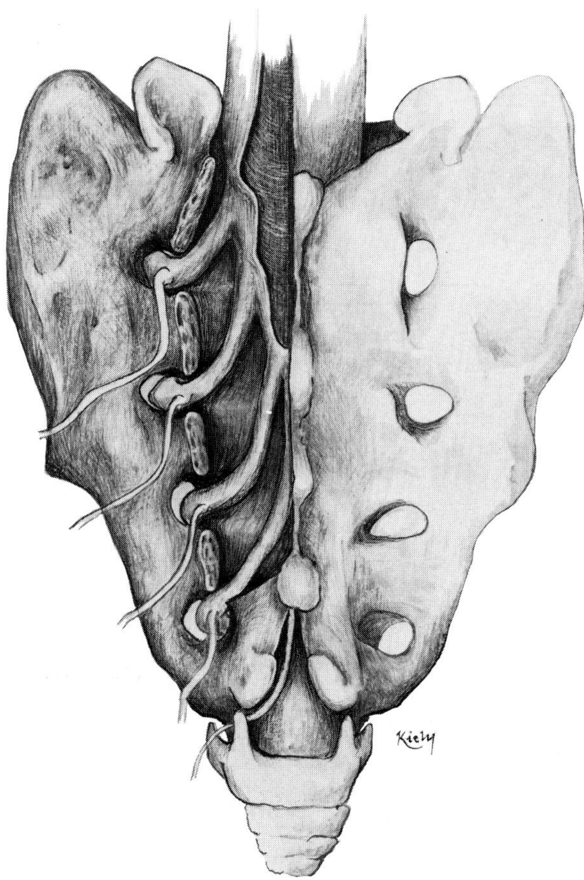

Fig. 9-2. The sacral canal. The following features are important to caudal blockade. The dura terminates at the lower border of S2 but may extend to S3. Dural sleeves accompany the sacral nerve roots to the sacral foramina and may be pierced by an exploring or injecting needle. Pivoting movements of the needle point within the sacral canal may damage the fifth sacral or coccygeal nerves and must be avoided. All needle movements within the sacral canal should be performed in its long axis. A line joining the posterior superior iliac spines serves as the surface marking for the termination of the dural sac.

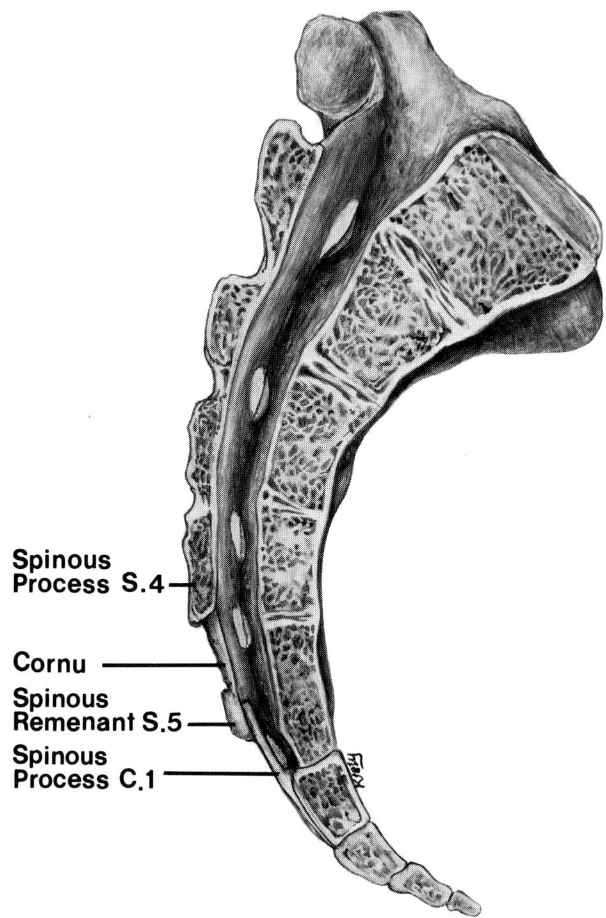

Fig. 9-3. The sacrum—transverse section. The sacral canal in its lower half is parallel to the contour of the dorsal wall of the sacrum, which, in turn, is a guide to the direction in which needle entry should take place. The cancellous bone of the vertebral bodies is covered by an eggshell layer of cortex, which is readily pierced by needles inserted at an angle to the anterior sacral wall. Since injection into the vertebral bodies is a proven complication of caudal blockade, the long-standing recommendation of angled needle insertion and subsequent repositioning is not fully acceptable.

The primary predelivery indication for caudal blockade is midcavity forceps application, and its use for head on perineum delivery cannot be recommended, because, apart from being unnecessary, the sacral outlines are so obscured by the bulging presenting part that they cannot always be identified with confidence. Caudal blockade is not an alternative to internal pudendal nerve blockade or local perineal infiltration for head-on perineum delivery. Caudal blockade is particularly appropriate to spontaneous breech delivery or breech extrac-

In my department there continues to be a longstanding preference for independent blockade of the separate thoracolumbar and sacral components of uterine pain, both during labor or subsequently for intrauterine manipulations such as removal of adherent placenta. This is satisfied by serial injections of 5 to 7 ml of anesthetic solution at the T11–12 or T12–L1 spinous levels and, later, when and if the indications for it arise, 8 to 10 mls by way of the sacral hiatus. Blockade thus follows the course of labor and, to a significant degree, permits sparing of the nerve supply to the legs and lower thoracic vasomotor efferents during the pre-expulsive stage of labor, as originally advocated by Cleland (1949).[5] Major advantages of this technique are full retention of patient mobility and a reduction in the incidence and degree of postblockade hypotension. The caudal injection is invariably single-shot, and there is no justification for insertion of both lumbar and caudal catheters, thus doubling the hazards associated with catheter insertion. As discussed in Chapter 18, many prefer to employ a single lumbar catheter and to allow analgesia gradually to descend to the sacral segments when epidural blockade is employed during the first stage of labor.

In a substantial minority of patients in labor, the difficulties of hiatal identification are greatly increased by turgidity of overlying soft tissues occasioned by edema or weight gain in pregnancy, and this problem is therefore most commonly associated with toxemic states. Thus, pregnancy may at the same time introduce the most pressing indications for caudal blockade and the most formidable hindrances to its performance. In such circumstances, recourse to identification by bidigital perrectal hiatal palpation and "walking"-the-needle techniques may be invaluable (see Fig. 9-12).

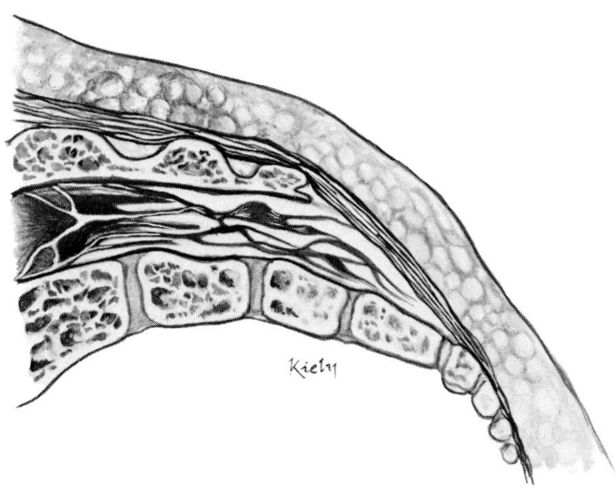

Fig. 9-4. The lower third of the sacral canal. The sacral venous plexus may extend to the level of S4 and may be traumatized on entry or by pivoting of needles. Needle movements must always be in the long axis of the sacral canal. The anatomy of this small area encompasses most of the difficulties of caudal blockade.

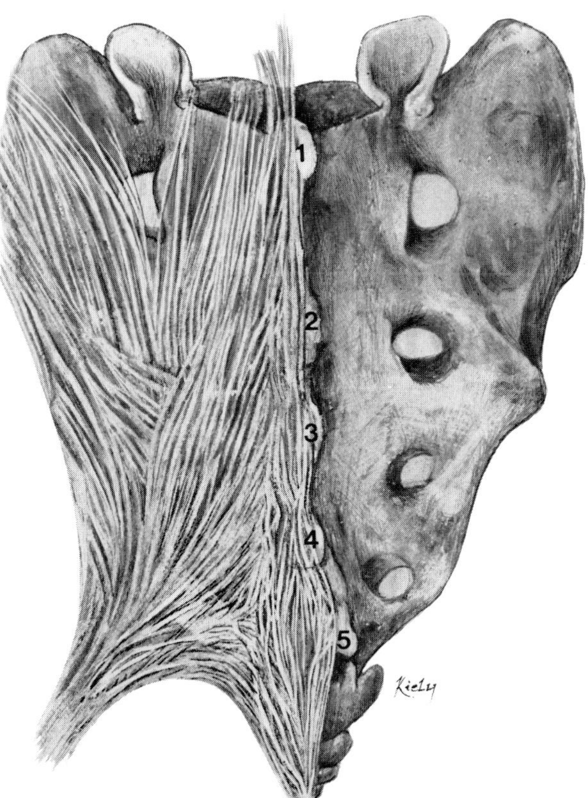

Fig. 9-5. The posterior sacral membranes are an amalgam of a number of aponeuroses of the sacrococcygeal ligaments and are at most points closely attached to the sacral bone. However, in areas such as illustrated in Figures 9-1 and 9-7, they may bridge indentations on the sacral surface and thus form cavities that may mimic the sacral hiatus.

ANATOMY

In order to implement caudal blockade successfully, it is important to understand the relationship of anatomic structure to technique. Figures 9-1 to 9-7, and their legends, present this relationship.

For complete details of sacral anatomy, the reader is referred to standard anatomical textbooks and the detailed studies of Black, Trotter, and Letterman.[2,19,28]

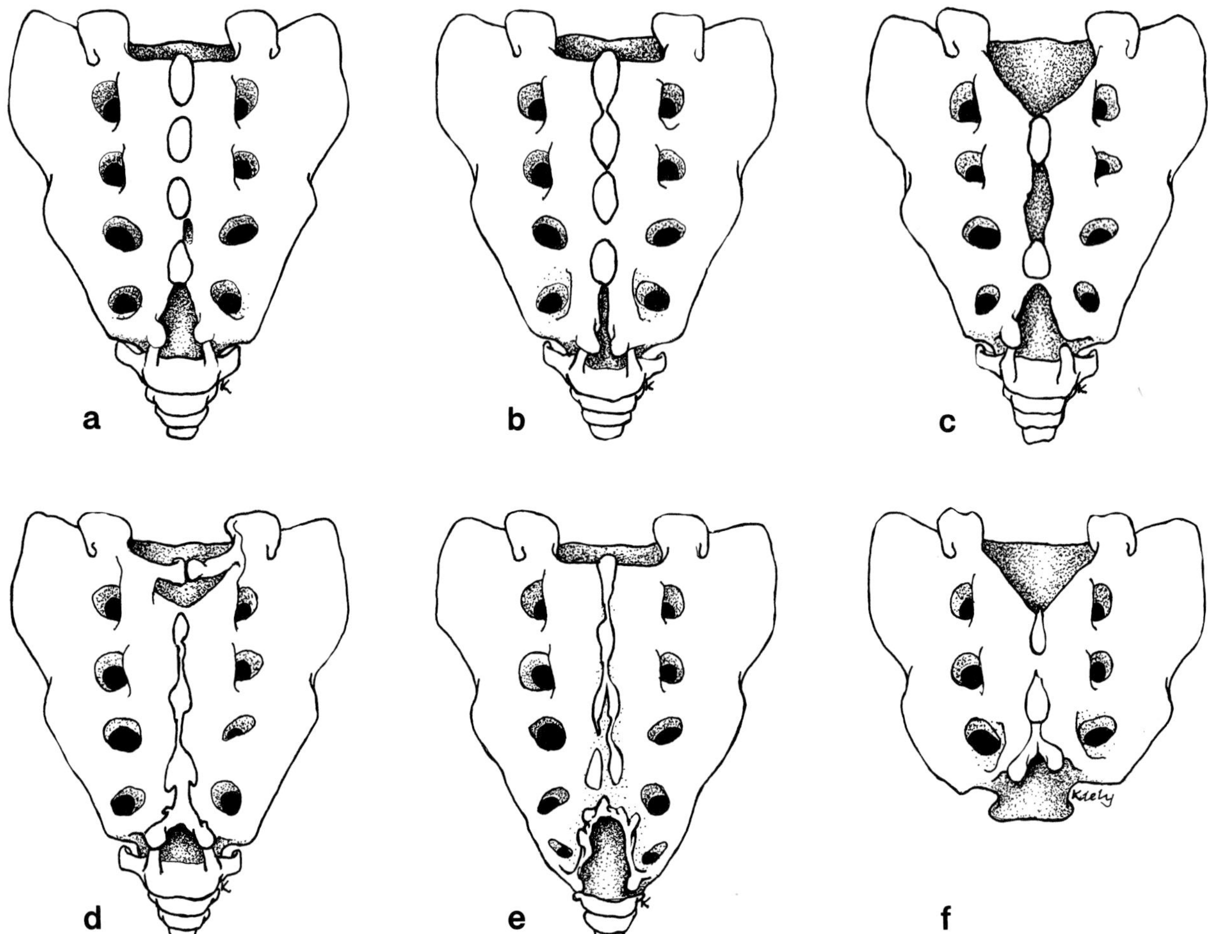

Fig. 9-6. The dorsal wall of the sacrum. Despite its many structural variations, the sacral canal is always open at the lower half of S5, and the hiatus is invariably in line with the median sacral crest. However, the median sacral crest does not always extend throughout the full length of the sacrum nor is it always palpable *in vivo*. In examining collections such as this, it should be remembered that since anatomical museums tend to collect an unusual number and variety of rare specimens, their representation of sacral anatomy often tends to be unduly discouraging.

Sacral Hiatus

Although the variations of sacral formation and abnormality are infinite, only a small number affect the performance of caudal blockade and of these the majority are genetic defects of the canal roof, which tend to facilitate rather than hinder blockade.

It is sometimes assumed that the hiatus is invariably an elongated opening conforming to the shape of an inverted V or U, and much of the literature on the subject fails to correct this error. In approximately 5 per cent of patients, it is represented by a transverse opening opposite the body of S5. It may even be that according to developmental biology it should be at this level only, and thus all extensions upward might well be regarded as anomalies! Be that as it may, S5 is the only level at which the hiatus is always present, although most often it extends upward a farther distance so that the hiatal apex is most frequently at the level of the lower half of S4 and least commonly at progressively higher levels. There is a convention of terminology that the level of S3 marks the highest point to which the hiatus extends and to regard failures of closure above this level as genetic defects of the canal roof. This convention is appropriate and relevant to caudal blockade because it also denotes the easily identifiable midsacral level, above which needle insertion

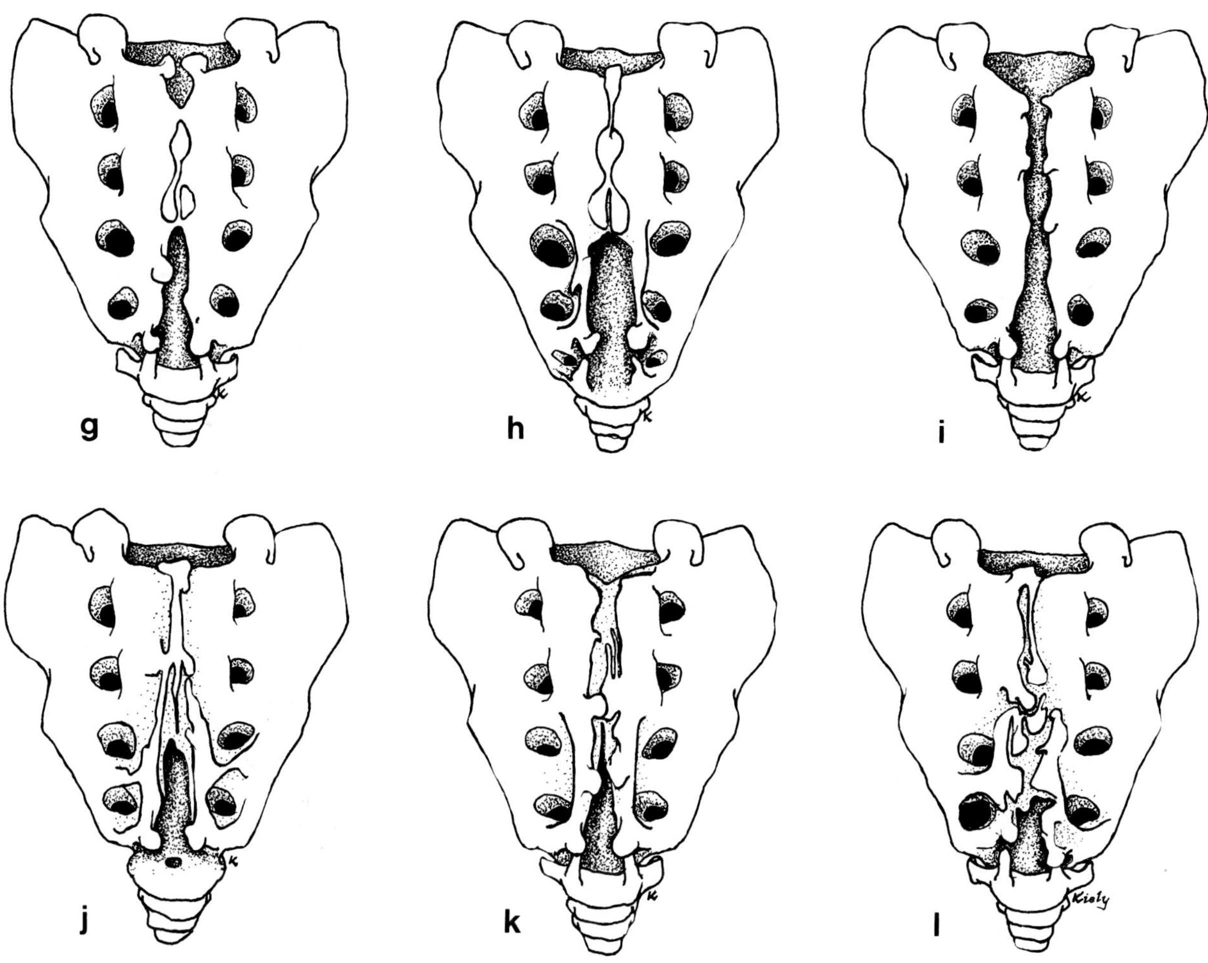

Fig. 9-6 (Continued).

should not be undertaken because of a prohibitive risk of dural puncture.

The focal points of caudal blockade are the sacral hiatus and the distal aperture of the sacral canal. Factors related to the anesthesiologist's ability to identify their variable outlines are the primary and commonest causes of failure to achieve successful blockade. All sacral landmarks, and particularly those of the cornua, are varyingly prominent and may differ in detail on opposite sides. For example, one may be robustly developed or easily palpable or may lie at a different angle to an underdeveloped and rudimentary counterpart, or the hiatal exit may be so distally sited that it presents as a narrow transverse slit hidden under a rim or ledge of bone formed from the remnants of the lower third of the S5 arch. In contrast, although they are usually widely separated from each other, the cornua may be so closely juxtaposed that the hiatus presents as a narrow longitudinal opening of varying length (Fig. 9-6). Even when readily identified and apparently conforming to a classical description on palpation *in vivo,* the genuine interval of separation of the cornua may be reduced to but a few millimeters as a result of their forward and medial shelving from their most prominent dorsal aspects (Fig. 9-7 *B,C*). Of importance to blockade, these variations and permutations of normal hiatal closure are more frequent and of much greater significance than significant defects of the sacral mass, few of which infringe on the patency of its canal or impede needle entry into it. When considering the problems of hiatal identification and needle placement, it is useful to imagine these and other variations as representing some of the difficulties and delays that na-

(*Text continued on p. 284.*)

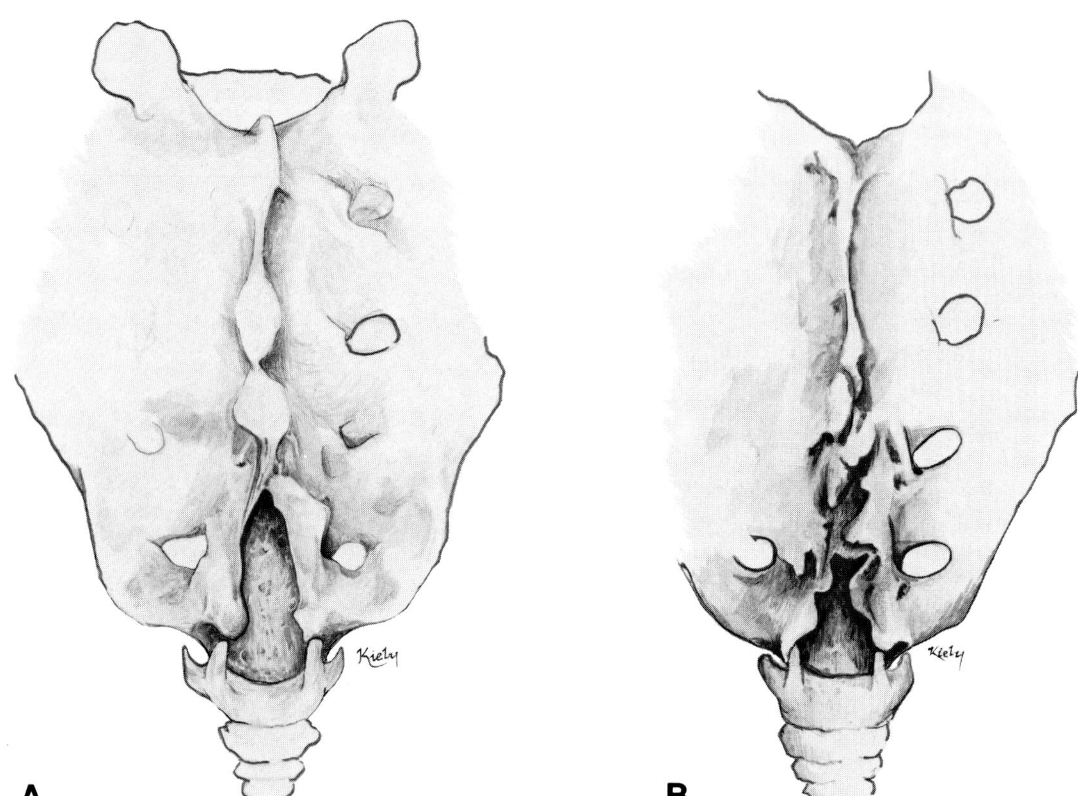

Fig. 9-7. Hiatal variants. The problems of hiatal identification are best solved by reference to anatomical specimens that should be handled, palpated, and examined for the possibilities of needle entry. (*A*) S4 surmounts the right sacral cornu. Should the overlying tissues be dense or turgid and the left cornu impalpable, the groove between the unduly prominent right cornu and the ipsilateral sacral margin could be readily mistaken for the sacral hiatus and lead to injection performed through the S4 foramen. This forms an effective decoy hiatus. (*B*) Although in line with the median sacral crest, the apex of this hiatus could be erroneously identified opposite S4; it would almost certainly be possible to inject solution under the sacrococcygeal membrane with little likelihood of its entering the sacral canal. As always, the canal is patent at the level of S5. *C* and *D* illustrate common variants to which comments similar to those describing *A* and *B* apply. To anesthesiologists who have complained, "I am certain I had the needle correctly placed but the block did not work," these illustrations may convey the message "do not wander too far from S5." (*E*) shows a transverse hiatus with two prominent proximal "decoys" for the unwary; again opposite the lower half of S5. (*F*) This dubiously palpable and low-lying hiatus would probably be felt as a transverse ridge. As seen end-on, the canal is narrow despite the prominence of the hiatal apex, and this again illustrates the advisability of injection in the line of the sacral canal rather than at an angle. The sacrococcygeal membrane may well have been separated into distinct anterior and posterior layers, thus to form between them another type of decoy hiatus.

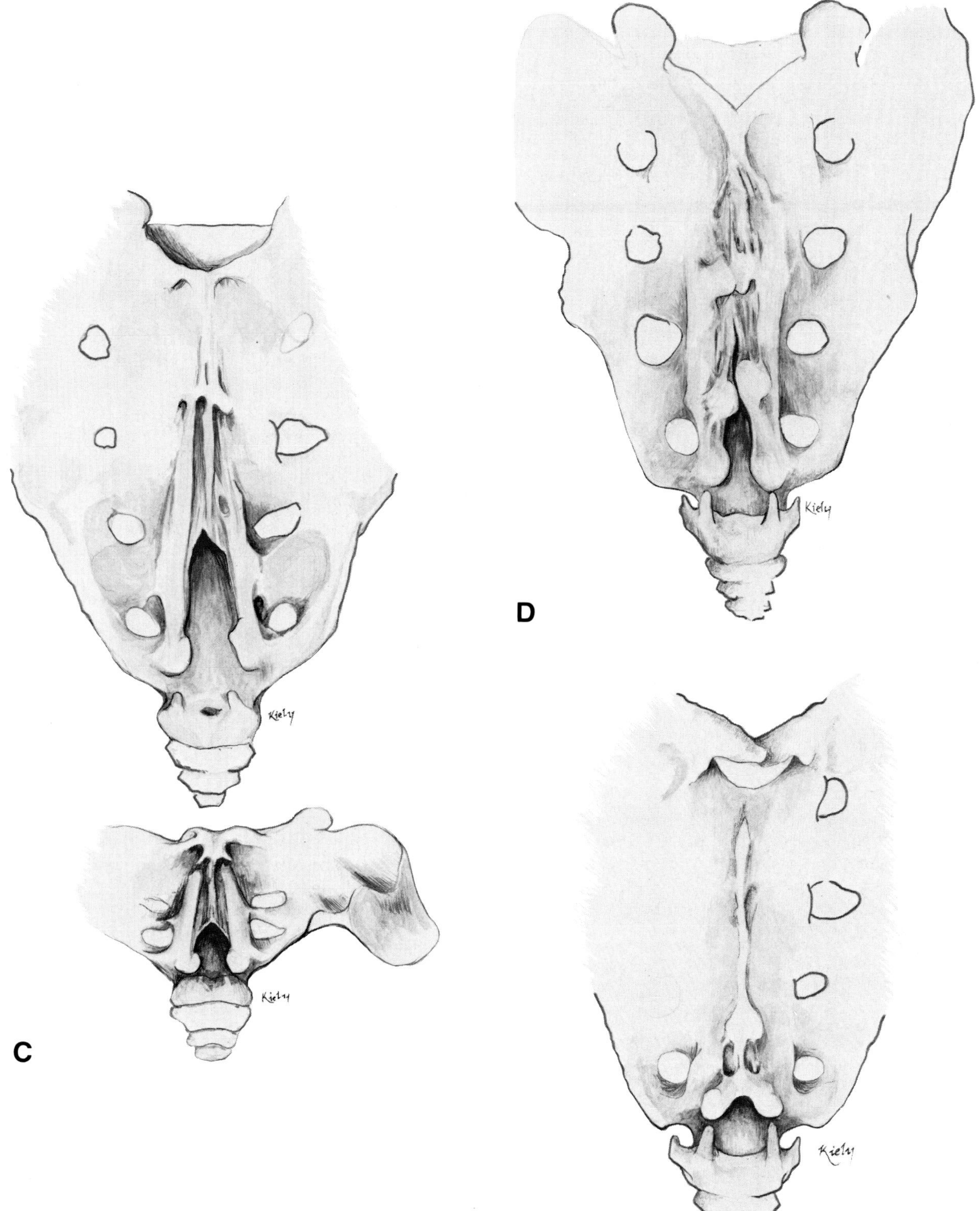

Fig. 9-7 (Continued).

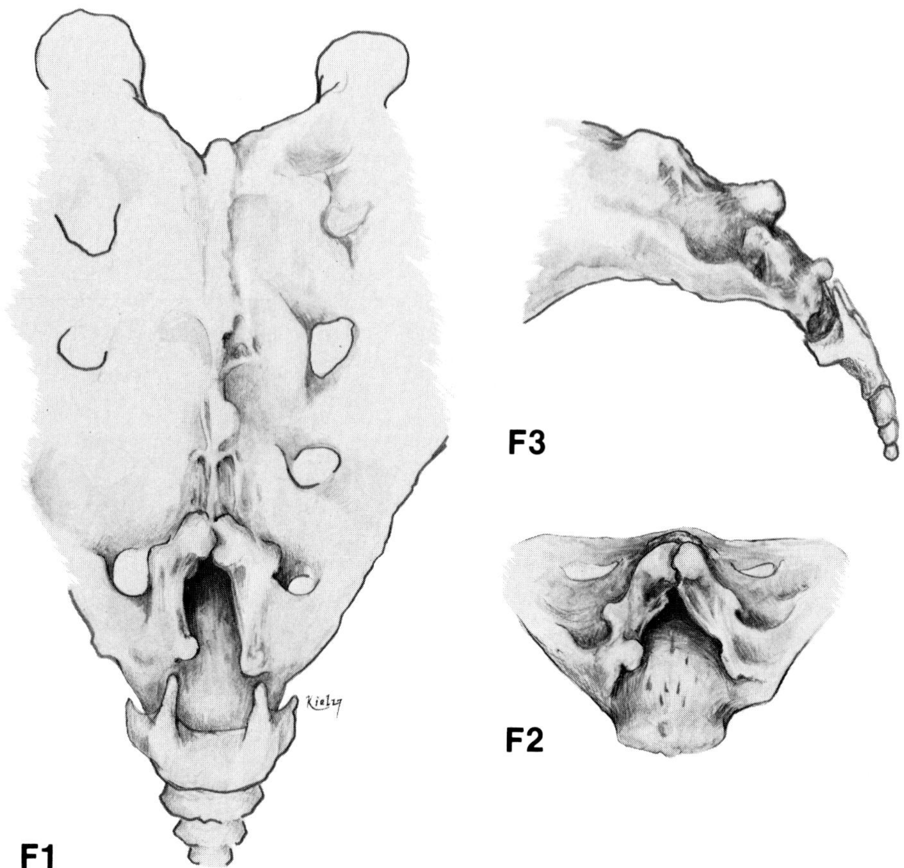

Fig. 9-7 (Continued).

ture experienced while attempting to close the sacral canal before birth. When hiatal outlines are impalpable or indeterminate, imagination may be a guide to their position as well as being helpful in relating the hiatal structure as palpated through overlying tissues to the possibilities of its genuine disposition at depth (Fig. 9-6).

Sacral Canal

Although the upper two-thirds of the sacral canal may be the site of total or partial agenesis, this, for the anesthesiologist, is of little more than passing interest. Such defects prohibit neither the injection nor the spread of introduced solutions nor should they encourage needle entry above the mid sacral level, which in adults is approximately at the level of a line joining the dimples over the posterior superior iliac spines.

Extreme narrowing of the lower third of the sacral canal above its aperture has been demonstrated and, although infrequent, must be regarded as favoring the leakage of injected solutions forward through the lowermost sacral foramina and hindering their spread upward. This is undoubtedly the commonest cause of blockade failure or patchy blockade following accurate solution placement deep to the sacrococcygeal ligament. The genuine incidence of this unwelcome problem has not been documented but may be in the region of 0.5 per cent.

Decoy Hiatus

The fourth sacral foramina lie in bilateral grooves bounded medially by the sacral cornu and the continuation of the intermediate sacral crest and laterally by the termination of the lateral sacral crest as it merges into the lower lateral sacral angle. With the tough membranous covering of the sacral foramen, a remarkably deceptive decoy hiatus is thus formed, which for the unwary invites injection through to the loose presacral tissues. This is probably the commonest cause of unexpected blockade failure and of unilateral or patchy caudal analgesia. Almost every trainee encounters this trap, and it cannot be overemphasized that once a site of needle entry is selected, rechecks should be made of position in the median sacral line. The cause of this error is failure to palpate the full extent of the lower third of the sacrum from the sacrococcygeal junction upward; this kind of decoy always has a companion on the opposite side and usually the true hiatus is at a lower level—but not invariably so—and is less conspicuous than the decoy. Every feature of successful caudal blockade—except success—is effectively mimicked.

Other kinds of decoy hiatus are found when large indentations on the sacral surface form sealed cavities with overlying elements of the posterior sacrococcygeal membranes, into which needle entry can be made (Figs. 9-1 and 9-7); however, in these instances resistance to injection of air or fluid is absolute and is confirmation of their presence.

Contents of Sacral Canal

The sacral canal contains the termination of the dural sac at the lower border of the second sacral body and its sleevelike prolongations that accompany the sacral nerves. Also, the sacral nerves as they transit to the sacral formina are located here. The fifth sacral nerves exit between the lower border of the sacrum and the upper edge of the coccyx. The coccygeal nerves pierce the sacrococcygeal ligament. The sacral canal contains, further, the sacral venous plexus; this usually terminates at the level of S4 but may extend throughout the canal. It tends to lie forward against the anterior wall of the canal, but this is an inconstant feature. Last can be found loose adipose tissues and the filum terminale.

NEUROANATOMY

The sacrococcygeal nerves relay total sensory input from the vagina, anorectal region, floor of the perineum, anal and bladder sphincters, urethra, and the perineal skin, excluding that covering the base of the penis and anterior extremities of the labia majora. A narrow band of skin extending from the posterior aspect of the gluteal region to the plantar and lateral surfaces of the foot are also innervated through the first sacral nerves.

Several organs on the pelvic floor and perineum have multiple innervation through preaortic and sacrococcygeal nerve groups. These include the uterus, bladder, testicles and scrotum, and the dorsal surface of the root of the penis. Although unsupplemented caudal blockade may not provide full pain control for operations on these structures, it can provide the primary component of a balanced anesthetic sequence.

In the elucidation of chronic pelvic pain that affects the multiply innervated structures and organs, caudal blockade provides a means to demonstrate or isolate any contribution through the sacral and coccygeal nerves. Further differentiation of somatic from other pain components is then effected by sequential blockade of the remaining afferent groups. Due to the management problems occasioned by total or partial denervation of the bladder, rectum, or sphincter muscles, caudal blockade cannot be recommended for prolonged or permanent neurolysis in the treatment of intractable pain other than for patients who have been subjected to permanent urinary and fecal diversion.

Sacral Membranes, Ligaments, and Foramina

The posterior sacral membranes are firmly attached to the dorsal surface of the sacrum and to the borders of the posterior sacral foramina, which are thus effectively sealed so that solutions injected into the sacral canal can diffuse only upward through the epidural space or forward through the unsealed anterior foramina. A number of irregularly placed indentations on the dorsal surface of the sacrum, most frequently adjacent to the median crest, may, when bridged by elements of the posterior sacrococcygeal ligaments, form sealed cavities that simulate the sacral hiatus on needle entry. However, total resistance to solution or air injection is diagnostic of their presence.

PHYSIOLOGIC EFFECTS

Cardiorespiratory Effects

Caudal blockade restricted to sacral segments with minor spillover to L5, as described in this chapter, results in minimal changes in cardiorespiratory function. To date, however, this has been documented only in the setting of obstetric analgesia.[16a] Nevertheless, large doses of local anesthetic may potentially result in cardiovascular effects described in Chapter 8 for epidural block. Similarly, the absorption of epinephrine may result in significant cardiovascular changes if large volumes of epinephrine-containing solutions are employed. The

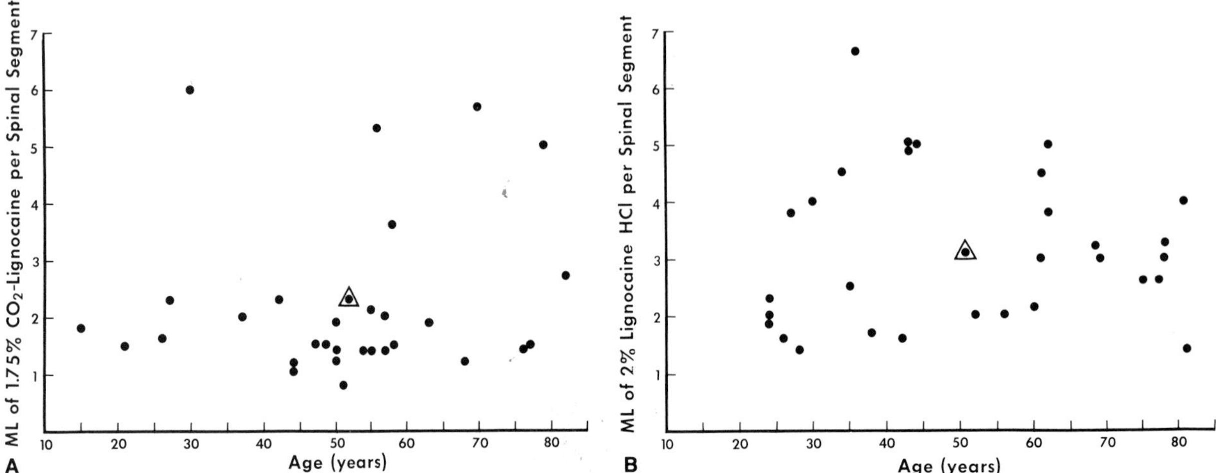

Fig. 9-8. Caudal blockade in adults: segmental spread of analgesia with advancing age. (*A*) 2 per cent lidocaine hydrochloride; (*B*) 1.75 per cent lidocaine carbonate. Dose requirements in milliliter per spinal segment are plotted against age, with the mean dose indicated by a dot in a triangle. There is no consistency in spread of analgesia at any age or any correlation between age and segmental spread. (Cousins, M.J., and Bromage, P.R.: Br. J. Anaesth. *43*:1149, 1971)

volumes and concentrations of local anesthetic recommended in this chapter minimize the potential for any cardiovascular changes following caudal blockade.

Nervous System

Convulsions. Rapid vascular absorption of large doses or direct vascular or marrow injection may result in local anesthetic toxicity.[10,11] The likelihood of this hazard is greatly reduced by the technique described in this chapter.

Horner's Syndrome. Caudal blockade with volumes of local anesthetic in excess of 12 ml (12–20 ml, 0.5% bupivacaine) has been reported to result in signs of paralysis of ophthalmic sympathetic fibers in 17 out of 20 consecutive caudal blocks for obstetric analgesia.[23] It should be noted that these doses of local anesthetic are larger than recommended in this chapter. However, many practitioners of caudal analgesia for surgery and obstetrics safely employ volumes of local anesthetic (up to 30 ml) without the aforementioned complication.

Endocrine Effects

Modification of the stress response to surgery has not yet been documented for caudal blockade. However, it is likely that complete "deafferentation" of the operative site would result in a similar modification of the neuroendocrine response to stress, which has been documented for lumbar epidural blockade (see Chap. 8).

ADMINISTRATION OF BLOCK

Drugs and Dosage

The general rules for drugs and dosage are the same as those for epidural blockade. In particular, it should be noted that segmental spread may be 30 to 40 per cent greater in obstetric patients, especially if injection is made by a catheter with the patient in the supine position. This explains why it is often not possible to block more than S2–5 in nonpregnant adults, whereas in the woman in labor it is not uncommon for blockade to reach T10 if 20 ml of solution is used. Both the volumes of the adult sacral canal and its contents are variable and unpredictable, and attempts to formulate precise schedules have been notably unsuccessful (Fig. 9-8). This is in contrast to the pediatric use of caudal block for which relationships between dose, age, and weight have been defined (see Chap. 21). However, in adults, it can be assumed that a volume of 10 ml of solution will fully cover the sacrococcygeal nerve roots in large adults. If adequate time is allowed for diffusion, this may be reduced to 7 or 8 ml. In fact, the use of 10 ml of solution for sacral analgesia in obstetric delivery has been described with a high success rate for complete analgesia.[5] As passive relaxation of pelvic voluntary and sphincteric muscles follows their sensory deprivation, upward adjustments of drug concentration to provide motor blockade is unnecessary for all procedures performed within the areas of sacrococcygeal innervation. The small volume and concentrations of solution required ensure that total dosage falls well within therapeutic range and that in the improbable event of accidental intrathecal injection, subarachnoid blockade is unlikely to be extensive or prolonged in duration. Similarly, any sequelae from rapid intravascular absorption tend to be mild and fleeting in appearance.

Blockade is usually effective within 5 minutes, but the sacral epidural space is relatively large so that for diffusion throughout it and its contained tissues, a lapse of 10 to 15 minutes should be allowed before commencement of surgery. Adherence to the recommended dose levels permits reinjection in the event of solution misplacement, and, except in obsese or edematous patients in whom there may exist physical barriers to solution spread, there are no substantial benefits from the use of highly concentrated solutions. Concentrations of solution that are adequate only to block sensory fibers are bupivacaine, 0.25 to 0.5 per cent; mepivicaine, 1 to 1.5 per cent; lidocaine, 1 per cent; prilocaine, 2 to 3 per cent; and chloroprocaine, 2 to 3 per cent. The effect of epinephrine is to increase the degree of motor block and improve onset time as well as decrease systemic toxity (see Chaps. 3 and 8 and Chap. 18 for effects on labor).

Carbonated solutions of lidocaine are preferred by some for caudal blockade because of their superior qualities of penetration (Fig. 9-9). Indeed, there is no other technique of neural blockade in which diffusion across voluminous lipid barriers is such a major obstacle to penetration of neural tissue. It is not surprising then that the more effective release of lipid-soluble base from lidocaine carbonate permits a much more rapid onset and more extensive blockade compared to lidocaine hydrochloride.[7]

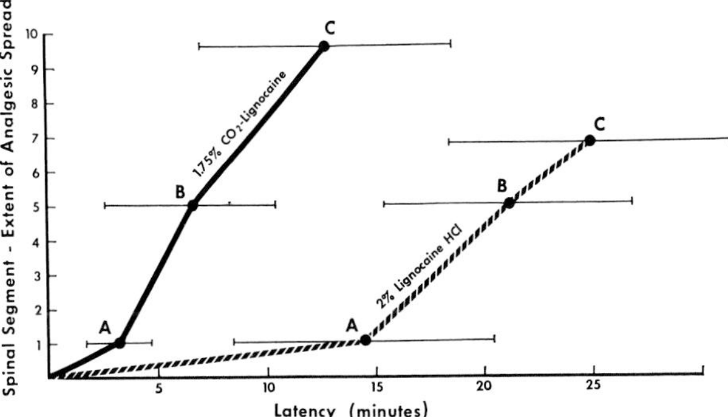

Fig. 9-9. Caudal blockade: latency of onset and spread of complete blockade (*i.e.*, "surgical" analgesia). Two per cent lidocaine hydrochloride is compared to 1.75 per cent lidocaine carbonate. Onset of blockade and complete loss of sensation is much more rapid with lidocaine carbonate. Even with the lidocaine carbonate solution, blockade of five segments may require close to 10 minutes, whereas with the lidocaine hydrochloride solution, this may require in excess of 20 minutes.

Training Methods

Until familiarity with the various types of hiatal anatomy has been acquired, unimpeded entry into the sacral canal should not be anticipated and failures should be accepted with some equanimity until at least some experience with the technique has been achieved. Because blockade can be a distressing experience for both patient and anesthesiologist when it is inexpertly performed, early training may be acquired on lightly anesthetized patients for whom caudal blockade may then form a component of a balanced anesthetic technique. The success of blockade in lightly anesthetized patients is readily determined by the disappearance of the anal reflex or by insensitivity to surgical stimulation.

Technique

Few descriptions of technique can substitute for practical experience, and, as in all forms of spinal blockade, previous successful administration becomes the guidepost. The accuracy of the needle's transit is usually best assessed by the sequence of sensations transmitted during its passage from skin through to the sacral canal. In order, these are the firmness and resilience of the sacrococcygeal membrane as it is contacted by the moving needle point; next, its firm grip on the needle during its passage through the membrane; and, finally, the sudden loss of resistance and sensation of space as the needle enters the sacral canal. The technique of insertion is illustrated in Figures 9-10 to 9-13, and the preference for insertion in the direction of the sacral canal should be noted. Equipment should be simple. Free-flowing glass or disposable syringes with Luer fittings and disposable hypodermic needles that range from 25-gauge to 22-gauge are suitable for single-injection techniques. For continuous or inter-

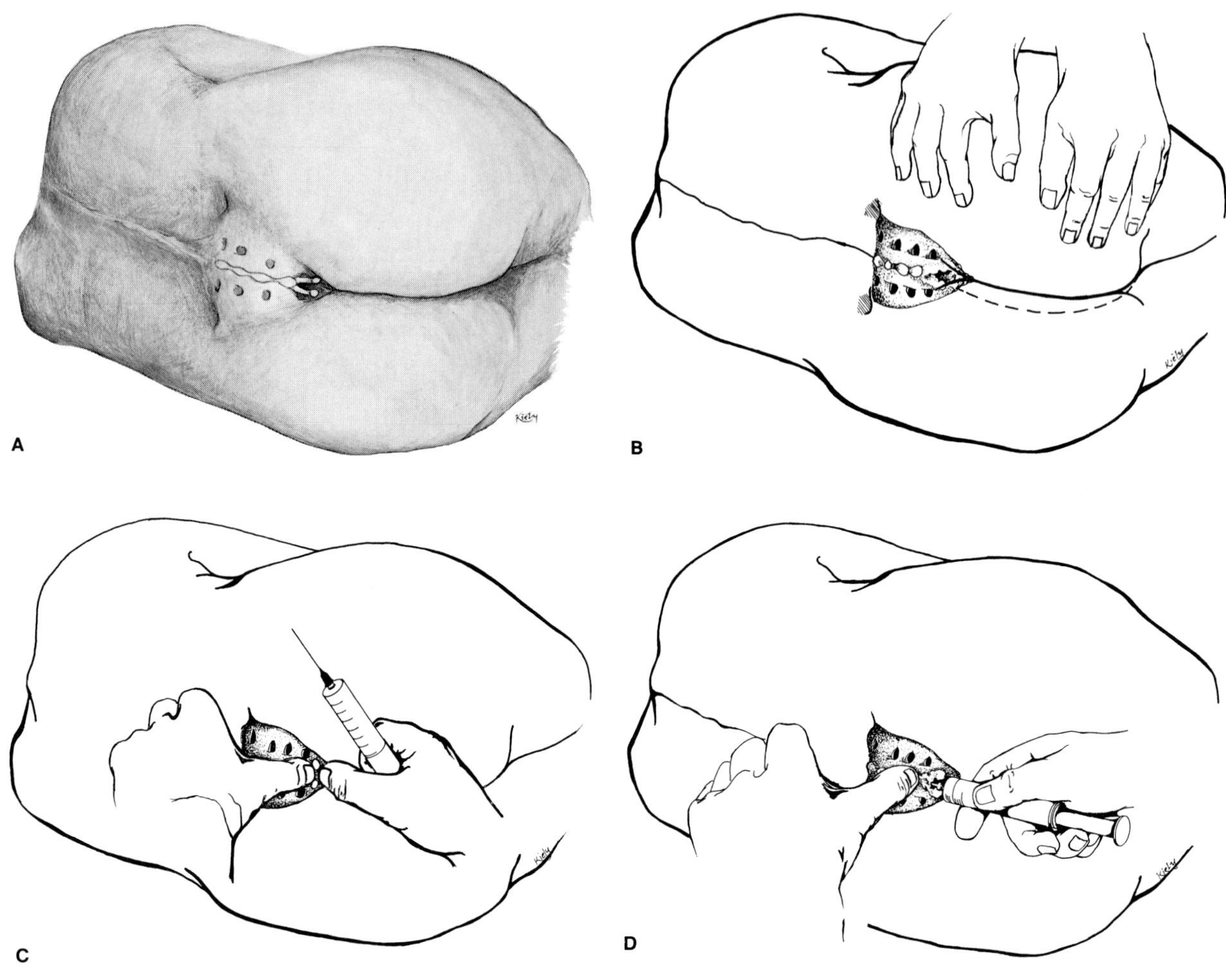

Fig. 9-10. Injection technique. (*A*) The left lateral or modified Sims's position is used for right-handed operators, the reverse if left-handed. (*B*) Following initial inspection and palpation, the natal cleft, if displaced from the midline, is repositioned by an assistant; this maneuver is necessary only in obese or wasted subject. (*C*) With syringe loaded and held as illustrated, palpation commences at the sacrococcygeal junction; the two-thumb method is recommended. (*D*) Once the landmark is located, the thumb of the left hand remains over the hiatal apex until needle insertion has been completed; the palm of the left hand may then be repositioned to monitor for development of an injection tumor.

mittent methods, standard epidural catheters with radiopaque markings may be inserted through 18-gauge Tuohy needles or Teflon intravascular cannulae. A further aid to correct needle placement for single-shot caudal block is the use of 22-gauge Teflon intravenous needle and cannula: the sacrococcygeal membrane is pierced as described above, then an attempt is made to thread the cannula over the needle into the sacral canal. Correct needle placement usually permits easy passage of the cannula, and injection is then made by way of the cannula before removing it or capping it until the anesthesiologist is certain that adequate blockade has been achieved. Needle entry into a decoy hiatus, or elsewhere, renders threading of the fine 22-gauge cannula impossible.

As illustrated in Figures 9-10 to 9-13 and for the following reasons needle insertion is best performed in the lateral (modified Sims's) position. It is aesthetically less objectionable and more comfortable for the patient than knee elbow or shoulder postures. It is fully applicable to women in labor

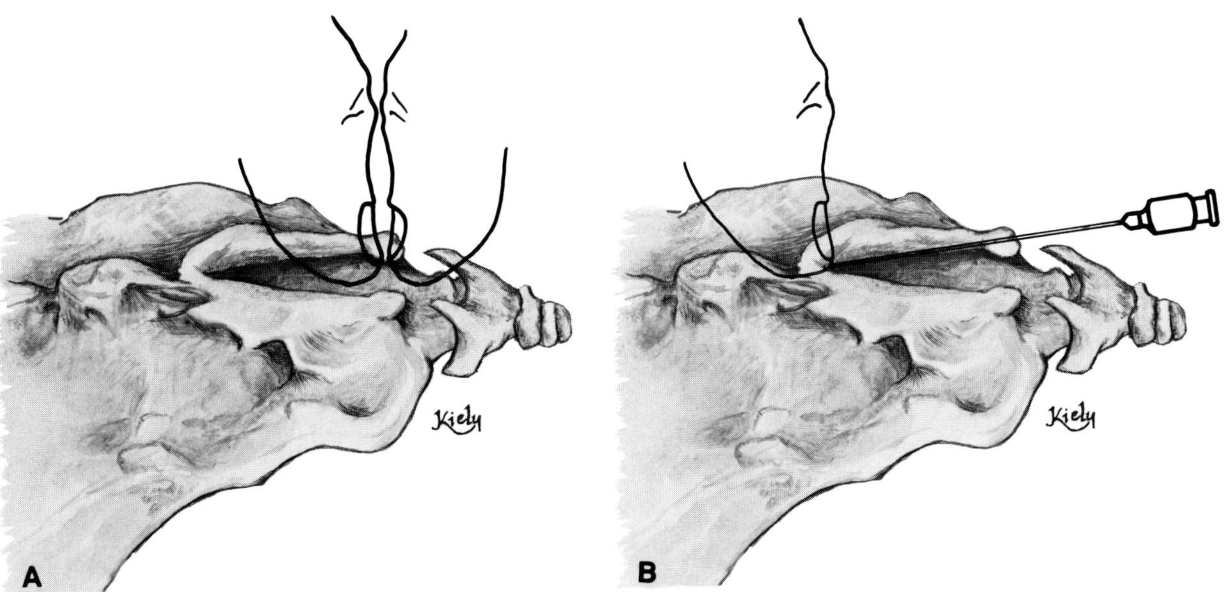

Fig. 9-11. Two thumb palpation. (*A*) The closely opposed thumbnails are moved firmly and with constant pressure across the mid sacral line from the sacrococcygeal junction cephalad until the cornual ridges or their remnants are identified. Sensation as transmitted through the tips and nails of both thumbs is a multiple of that from single finger palpation; the method requires practice and is strongly recommended. (*B*) When the landmark is identified, the left thumb should remain over the hiatal apex to act as a marker until needle insertion has been completed.

and to obese or disabled patients. It is not disturbing to patients under the influence of preanesthetic medication. For apprehensive patients, it permits the easy use of supplemental inhalational analgesia or light anesthesia during blockade without the necessity for endotracheal intubation. Also, it is ideal for the conduct of training, allows an unhurried approach to blockade, and facilitates repositioning to the dorsal position if and when required.

Following skin preparation, palpation is performed to identify hiatal outlines that, in over 80 per cent of patients, are easily felt deep to the proximal extremity of the natal cleft. Confirmation of hiatal position should be made by reference to the midsacral or midcoccygeal lines.

When outlines are obscured by density or mass of overlying tissues, the anesthesiologist should resort to the sensitive *two-thumb* palpation method (Figs. 9-10, 9-11). With the nails closely apposed, the thumbs are moved from side to side across the axis of the sacrum, commencing at the sacrococcygeal junction and proceeding proximally until the cornua are identified. The combined use of the tips and the nails of both thumbs imparts an unusual degree of sensitivity to this procedure.

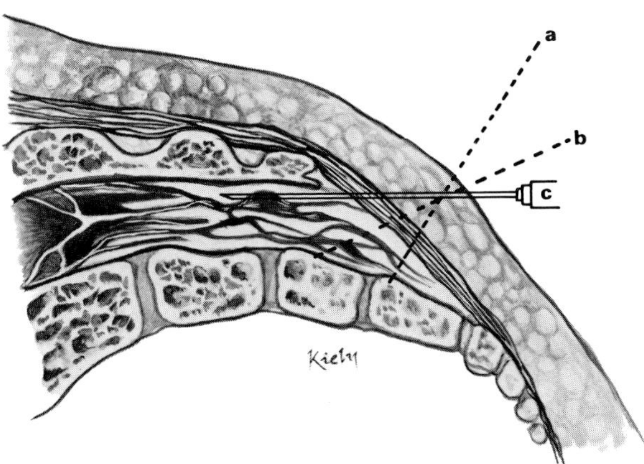

Fig. 9-12. Needle placement. The sacral venous plexus may extend downward to the hiatal opening and thus may be penetrated by an otherwise well-directed needle (*c*). The needle may be cleared from the vein by withdrawal or advancement until reaspiration of test solutions produces only light blood staining; injection may then be completed. In "walking"-the-needle techniques, there should be a single point of skin entry on which the needle is pivoted in the directions *a-b-c* until the sacrococcygeal membrane is identified and penetrated.

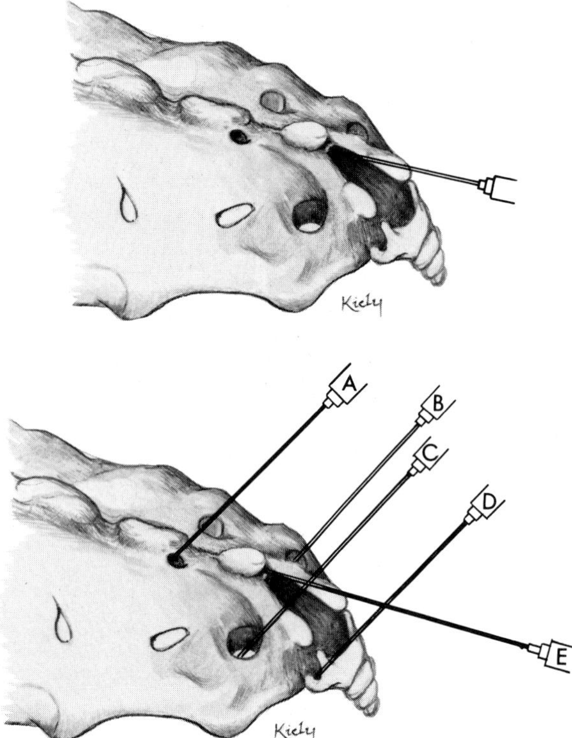

Fig. 9-13. Needle placement. (*I*) For correct placement, the needle is surrounded by sacral bone; that this is so is confirmed by index finger palpation in front of, behind, and to each side of the point of needle entry. (*II*) shows examples of incorrect needle placement. The needle *A* has entered a closed cavity and injection is resisted. Needles *B* and *C* have penetrated the fourth sacral foramen; this is probably the commonest cause of unilateral or patchy blockade, and all the signs of correct needle positioning can be elicited other than successful blockade. Needle *E* has impinged on S4 following its entry through the superficial layer of the sacrococcygeal membrane; the deep layer may not yet have been penetrated, and resistance to injection is absolute. Needle *D* has penetrated the sacrococcygeal junction.

When the landmark is identified, one thumb should remain firmly in position over the apex as a marker and guide until completion of needle entry.

Should identification of the hiatus be unusually difficult, as in obese or edematous patients during labor, bidigital palpation with one finger inserted rectally should be performed to verify landmarks and to select a point of needle entry through the skin. To facilitate rectal examination, a sterile second outer glove may be worn and discarded on completion of palpation.

When outlines cannot be palpated with ease or certainty, the hiatus may also be found by "walking" the needle along the midsacral or midcoccygeal line cephalad from the sacrococcygeal junction until the resilient sacrococcygeal membrane is identified and penetrated. Because this technique depends on recognition by touch, it should be employed only after reasonable familiarity with the feel of successful caudal blockade has been gained.

Signs of Correct Needle Placement. The following are the objective and subjective signs of accurate needle positioning, and those that appear appropriate should be elicited before completion of injection; the first four should be regarded as essential.

(1) Presence of sacral bone on each side of, in front of, and behind the needle at its point of insertion does not exclude the possibility of entry into a decoy hiatus but does protect against injection lateral to the sacral or coccygeal margins or into the presenting part of the fetus.

(2) The lack of CSF or free flow of blood on aspiration is important. Light blood staining is not uncommon and indicates that entry into the sacral canal has been achieved and that reaspiration should be attempted during the injection of solution.

(3) There should not be an injection tumor or superficial crepitus following injection of 2 or 3 ml of anesthetic solution or air.

(4) There should not be tissue resistance to injection; the force required to inject should not exceed that necessary to overcome syringe and needle resistances and should be constant throughout.

(5) There should not be local pain during injection of solution; pain indicates misplacement of the needle, and injection should cease.

(6) Paresthesia or a feeling of fullness that extends from the sacrum to the soles of the feet is common during injection but ceases on completion and portends successful blockade.

(7) The feeling of grating as the needle moves along the anterior wall of the sacral canal indicates accurate positioning but should not be purposefully elicited lest the sacral venous plexus be damaged.

(8) A useful test when substantial doubts about needle position cannot be resolved is slowly to inject 2 ml of air while listening with ear or stethoscope over the lumbar vertebrae for transmitted sound. Although I do not use this test, many trainees find it exceptionally useful during their initiation into the problems of blockade in obese or anatomically difficult patients.

(9) There should be ease of threading a short Teflon cannula over an intravenous needle, if the needle is used for caudal blockade.

The operator's free hand should remain in position over the sacrum in order to detect development of an injection tumor.

Catheter Techniques

There are few operative obstetric procedures suitable to performance under caudal blockade that outlast the duration of activity of long-acting local anesthetic agents. However, when extension of analgesia into the early postoperative period is desirable, a choice should be made between the practicabilities of repeated single-shot injections or catheter insertion (continuous intermittent fractional blockade). If not already performed, a preliminary exploration of the sacral canal with a normal needle technique should be undertaken to assess the practicality of introduction of 18-gauge needles or cannulae. The choice between Touhy or other epidural needles or intravascular cannulae depends on personal preference, but the principles of introduction are similar to those used for single-shot injections. The needle or cannula should be introduced in the previously determined line of the sacral canal, and progress should cease as soon as the sacrococcygeal ligament is cleared and aspiration and loss of resistance tests have been completed. Tuohy needles should be inserted with the shoulder anteriorly to avoid entry into or scraping along the anterior wall of the sacral canal and should remain in as close contact to the canal roof as is possible.

When intravascular cannulae are used, it is preferable that they be of radiopaque-marked Teflon and that their insertion cease on entry through to the sacral canal. Following withdrawal of the inner stylet and normal testing, a standard radiopaque-marked epidural catheter inserted for a short distance, not more than 3 to 4 cm, will discourage self-knotting. While caudal blockade is effective, normal bladder and rectal functions are in abeyance, and the insensitive saddle area is prone to trauma or pressure injury. Appropriate nursing measures must be instituted. The area of skin puncture should be protected from soiling, but liquid- or pressure-pack plastics must not be used for fear of catheter dissolution as a result of the solvents they contain.

COMPLICATIONS

Almost all published statistics on the complications of caudal blockade refer to the high, mid, continuous (intermittent) injection techniques or to a composite of all methods, and thus correct figures for simplified low-dose blockade are not available. The commonest problems are undoubtedly lack of success and pain on injection, and each bears, or should bear, a reciprocal relationship to experience and manipulative ability. Those who achieve high competence in hiatal identification are those most likely to perform injection with minimal trauma because each is a function of manual dexterity. As with many injection techniques, variations of technical ability are such that perhaps the best general advice is that caudal blockade is among the procedural activities best avoided by those who lack innate manual dexterity. Certainly, during the first 100 performances, failure rates should progressively decrease to less than 3 per cent, and in the ensuing 100 to less than 1 or 2 per cent; persistent high failure rates suggest a need for revision of technique and probably reference to a variety of anatomical specimens for contemplation and study of the possible causes of difficulty.

The second common problem, pain, is best eluded by the use of fine needles and by accurate identification of the hiatus in order to avoid multiple skin puncture. Twenty-two-gauge and 23-gauge needles are adequate for most patients, but for those with little subcutaneous tissue protection, 25-gauge is adequate. The use of subcutaneous infiltration to avoid pain during injection is usually unnecessary and tends to obscure landmarks. Intradermal injection is as painful as direct needle insertion. From the onset, a discipline should be adopted that needle puncture of the skin should be performed only once; this encourages the use of accurate identification techniques.

Infection

Infection is as frequently listed among the complications of caudal blockade as its lack is noted in clinical practice. This background fear of infection dates from the early use of indwelling needles and catheters for prolonged blockade during labor and often to their misplacement and the subsequent injection of epinephrine-containing solutions into the subcutaneous tissues. In the same historical context, other reported hazards such as fear of fecal contamination of the puncture site or of prolonged pressure on the anesthetized saddle area are not appropriate to modern single-dose injection techniques or to catheter insertion for brief periods.

Trauma to the presenting part during labor has been discussed in the section on obstetrics and it remains only to emphasize that this complication is totally avoidable if needle insertion takes place within the boundaries of the sacrum, which, when difficult to identify by percutaneous palpation, can always be defined by rectal examination.

Intraosseus Injection

Intraosseous injection was first described in 1971 by DiGiovanni and later by McGowan, who indicated an incidence of 0.6 per cent in 700 injections; it is reasonable to suggest that to a great extent this hazard is technique-dependent and probably favored by needle insertion in the direction of the anterior sacral wall and by the use of force (Fig. 9-12).[11,25a] The cancellous mass of sacral bone is covered by a wafer-thin, brittle layer of cortex that is easily damaged—even on prepared and hardened museum specimens. Intraosseus injection may be suggested by the appearance of a gritty aspirate of a small volume of apparently pure blood following a test injection of 2 ml of saline or anesthetic solution. This complication is best avoided by needle insertion in the line of the sacral canal, which, in its lower third, follows the curve of the posterior sacral wall; Tuohy-type needles should be inserted with the shoulder forward.[11]

Intravenous Injection

Intravenous injection is always a possibility and can be guarded against only by repeated aspiration following each needle movement or each reinjection through indwelling catheters. Though unwelcome, the aspiration of blood does at least indicate that the needle is within the sacral canal. A useful method of demonstrating its extravascular repositioning is to inject serially and reaspirate 2 to 3 ml of normal saline until blood staining is slight or lacking, at which point it may be assumed that injection with intermittent reaspiration may proceed.

Intrathecal Injection

The dural sac ends at the lower level of S2 on a line joining the dimples over the posterior superior iliac spines; the sacral canal is invariably patent at S5 and usually up to the mid S4 level. The midsacral level (*i.e.*, approximately 2–3 fingers' breadth distal to the posterior superior iliac spines) is the level below which needle passage within the canal should cease and above which entry should not be performed. Dural puncture is technique-dependent and its incidence should be nil, but it has been quoted within a range from 0 to 1.2 per cent. This suggests major technical deviations from those now recommended, particularly of the extent of needle insertion.

Misplaced Injections

The most frequent site of misplaced injection is into the subcutaneous tissues overlying the lower third of the sacrum, and the condition is readily diagnosed by the appearance or feel of an injection tumor. Injection deep to the sacrococcygeal ligament is probably less common than is frequently suggested because the rapid increase in resistance to injection serves as a warning. However, needle misplacement through the S4 foramina is probably the commonest cause of unilateral or patchy blockade. Other common areas for misplaced injection are lateral to the coccyx and sacrococcygeal junction (Fig. 9-11).

Breakage of Catheters and Needles

There have been occasions when spray plastics have been used to seal the skin puncture area, with subsequent dissolution of the catheter at the point of entry; some plastic sprays contain a solvent. Usual precautions pertain in avoiding needle breakage; in particular, needles should never be inserted to the level of the hub. Also, catheters should never be pulled back through needles lest they shear off.

Neurologic Complications

The neurologic sequelae of trauma to the lumbosacral plexus during descent or manipulation of the fetal presenting part include paresthesias, usually of one leg, or footdrop. Though often implicated, the nerve distribution for these infrequent occurrences is unrelated to sacral blockade. Postdelivery coccygodynia has similar causation, but its cause can usually be resolved by careful assessment of pain distribution to the site of needle entry or, as is more frequent, to trauma of the sacrococcygeal joint at the time of delivery.

REFERENCES

1. Adams, R.C., Langley, J.S., and Seldon, T.H.: Continuous caudal anesthesia or analgesia; a consideration of the technique, various uses and some possible dangers. J.A.M.A., *122*:152, 1943.
2. Black, M.G.: Anatomic reasons for caudal anesthesia failure. Anesth. Analg. (Cleve.), *28*:33, 1949.
3. Bonica, J.J.: Principles and Practice of Obstetric Analgesia and Anesthesia. Philadelphia, F.A. Davis, 1967.
4. Brown, P.R., Arthurs, G.J., and Glashan, R.W.: Epidural analgesia in the treatment of bladder carcinoma, a technique using two catheters. Anaesthesia, *29(4)*:422, 1974.
5. Cleland, J.G.P.: Continuous peridural and caudal analgesia in obstetrics. Anesth. Analg. (Cleve.), *28*:61, 1949.

6. Climie, C.R.: Epidural anaesthesia in obstetrics. N.Z. Med. J., *59*:331, 1960.
7. Cousins, M.J., and Bromage, P.R.: A comparison of the hydrochloride and carbonated salts of lignocaine for caudal analgesia in outpatients. Br. J. Anaesth., *43*:1149, 1971.
8. Cyriax, J.H.: Textbook of Orthopaedic Medicine. Vol. 1. pp. 469–486. London, Balliere Tindall, 1975.
9. Davies, A., Solomon, B., and Levene, A.: Paraplegia following epidural analgesia. Br. Med. J., *2*:654, 1958.
10. de Jong, R.H.: Anesthetic complications during continuous caudal analgesia for obstetrics. Anesth. Analg. (Cleve.), *40*:384, 1961.
11. DiGiovanni, A.J.: Inadvertant intra-osseus injection, a hazard of caudal anesthesia. Anesthesiology, *34*:92, 1971.
12. Edwards, W.B., and Hingson, R.A.: Continuous caudal anesthesia in obstetrics. Am. J. Surg., *118*:945, 1943.
13. _____: Continuous caudal anesthesia in obstetrics. Am. J. Surg., *57*:459, 1942.
14. Finster, M., *et al.*: Accidental intoxication of the fetus with local anesthetic drug during caudal anesthesia. Am. J. Obstet. Gynecol., *92*:922, 1965.
15. Flowers, C.E.: Obstetric Analgesia and Anesthesia. pp. 120–125. Harper & Row, Hagerstown, 1967.
16. Graham, J., and Saia, A.: Neurological complications of epidural analgesia. Br. Med. J., *2*:657, 1958.
16a. Hansen, J., and Ueland, K.: The influence of caudal analgesia on cardiovascular dynamics during normal labour and childbirth. Acta Anaesth. Scand. *23* [*Suppl.*]:449, 1966.
17. Hingson, R.A., Cull, W.A., and Benzinger, M.: Continuous caudal analgesia in obstetrics: combined experience of a quarter of a century in clinics in New York, Philadelphia, Memphis, Baltimore and Cleveland. Anesth. Analg. (Cleve.), *40*:119, 1961.
18. Hingson, R.A., and Southworth, J.L.: Continuous caudal analgesia. Am. J. Surg., *58*:93, 1942.
19. Letterman, G.S., and Trotter, S.M.: Variations of the male sacrum, their significance in continuous caudal anesthesia. Surg. Gynecol. Obstet., *78*:551, 1944.
20. Lewis, B., and Bartels, L.: Caudal anesthesia in genito-urinary surgery. Surg. Gynecol. Obstet., *22*:262, 1916.
21. Löfström, B.: in Illustrated Handbook in Local Anesthesia. pp. 129–134, Eriksson, E. (ed.). Copenhagen, Munksgaard, 1969.
22. Massey-Dawkins, C.J.: An analysis of the complications of extra dural and caudal block. Anaesthesia, *24*:554, 1969.
23. Mohan, J., and Potter, J.M.: Pupillary constriction and ptosis following caudal epidural analgesia. Anaesthesia, *30*:769, 1975.
24. Moore, D.C.: Regional Block. ed. 4. pp. 439–471. Springfield, Charles C Thomas, 1965.
25. Katz D., Moore, D.C., Stone W.J., Sinclair J.C.: Caudal Anaesthesia in Obstetrics. N. Engl. J. Med., *274*:749, 1966.
25a. McGown, R.G.: Accidental marrow sampling during caudal anaesthesia. Brit. J. Anaesth., *44*:613, 1972.
26. Rubin, A.P.: The choice between the lumbar and caudal route. *In* Doughty, A. (ed.): Proceedings of the Symposium on Epidural Analgesia in Obstetrics. pp. 19–100. London, H.K. Lewis, 1971.
27. Sinclair, J.C., Fox, H.J., and Lentz, J.F.: Intoxication of the fetus by a local anesthetic, a newly recognized complication of maternal caudal anesthesia. N. Engl. J. Med., *273*:1173, 1975.
28. Trotter, M.: Variations of the sacral canal, their significance in the administration of caudal analgesia. Anesth. Analg. (Cleve.), *26*:192, 1947.
29. Trotter, M., and Letterman, G.S.: Variations of the female sacrum, their significance in continuous caudal anesthesia. Surg. Gynecol. Obstet., *78*:551, 1944.
30. Tuohy, E.B.: Regional block for operations on the perineum, anus, genitalia and lower extremities. Anesthesiology, *2*:369, 1941.

PART TWO

Techniques of Neural Blockade

Section B: Extremities: Peripheral Blockade

10 The Upper Extremity: Somatic Blockade

F. R. Berry and
L. Donald Bridenbaugh

All of the deep structures of the upper extremity and the skin distal to the middle of the upper arm are rendered insensitive by blocking the nerves making up the brachial plexus. The nerves of the plexus may be blocked anywhere along their course—from their emergence from intervertebral foramina and entrance into the sheath between the anterior and posterior scaleni muscles until they terminate in the specific nerves in the hand. Techniques for blocking of the plexus involve infiltration at one of five anatomic areas—that is, paravertebral, supraclavicular, infraclavicular, in the axilla, and by blocking the specific terminal nerves. Thus, any surgical procedure on the arm—for example, reduction of fractures or dislocations, suturing of tendons, or repair of lacerations—is an indication for the use of this kind of anesthesia. However, frequently the primary indication for the choice of brachial plexus nerve block versus general anesthesia is the wish of the patient, the surgeon, or the skill of the anesthesiologist.

History

Brachial plexus nerve block was reportedly first accomplished by Halsted in 1884 when he "freed the cords and nerves of the brachial plexus—after blocking the roots in the neck with cocaine solution." In 1887, Crile disarticulated the shoulder joint after rendering the arm insensitive by blocking the "brachial plexus by direct intraneural injection of each nerve trunk with 0.5 percent cocaine under direct vision."[12] In 1911, Hirschel and Kulenkampff, working independently, were the first to inject the brachial plexus blindly through the skin without exposure of the nerves.[22,27] Subsequently, there have been many advocated modifications of these original techniques. These modifications vary mostly according to site and include the following; infraclavicular, supraclavicular, axillary, and perivascular infiltration and the sheath technique.[1–4,7,13,16,19,22,24,26,27,29,30,33,35,37,38,41,42,48,50] With the advent of barbiturates and cyclopropane, the enthusiasm for block anesthesia waned in the early 1940s. It has, in current years, however, enjoyed somewhat of a rejuvenation.

Each of the modifications previously noted has specific advantages and disadvantages. These will be discussed individually along with the techniques for performing each of the blocks.

Advantages

Brachial plexus block, like all other regional anesthetic procedures, offers certain advantages to the patient, surgeon, and anesthesiologist that may not be associated with general anesthesia. These include the following:

(1) *The anesthesia is limited to the restricted portion of the body upon which it is proposed to operate,* leaving the other vital centers intact. The physiology of the patient is taxed less than with general anesthesia because metabolism of the rest of the body is undisturbed. This consideration is important in the poor risk patient who cannot tolerate the stress imposed by general anesthesia. Patients who present complicating conditions such as heart, renal, and pulmonary disease; chest injuries; diabetes; and so forth are able to withstand surgery performed with brachial block anesthesia without aggravation of the disease. This should not, however, imply that this technique should be reserved only for poor risk patients. On the contrary, nearly all patients who present themselves for surgery of the upper extremity could be afforded the benefits of this form of regional anesthesia.

(2) *It is possible and desirable for the patient to remain ambulatory.* Outpatients may be sent home after procedures such as closed reduction of fractures or repair of lacerations. Brachial plexus block is also of great benefit in aged patients in whom early ambulation is necessary to prevent complications.

(3) *Whenever fluoroscopy is a necessary adjunct*

to the surgical procedure, brachial plexus block eliminates the potential general anesthesia dangers of explosions, respiratory depression, or obstruction in a darkened room in which the patient cannot readily be observed. It also permits the patient to cooperate with the surgeon or the radiologist.

(4) *Postanesthetic nausea, vomiting, and other complications of general anesthesia such as atelectasis, hypotension, ileus, and dehydration are reduced.* This allows the patient to maintain a regular diet and, thus, to benefit from oral feeding earlier in the postoperative period.

(5) *Prolonged operations on the upper extremity, if they are performed with general anesthesia, are sometimes followed by postoperative depression* because of the comparatively large doses of drugs required. Operations such as tendon repairs and plastic procedures can, therefore, have complications out of proportion to the surgical procedure.

(6) *Brachial block anesthesia allows patients who dread losing consciousness to be awake.* If it is properly performed, brachial plexus block provides a minimum degree of discomfort to the patient.

(7) *Patients who arrive at surgery in genuine or impending shock may improve as soon as the pain has been relieved by the block.* The improved circulation resulting from the sympathetic blockade may be a positive factor in the prognosis of the traumatized upper extremity, which has areas of severely compromised circulation and questionable tissue viability.

(8) *Any patient who arrives at surgery with a full stomach presents less danger of aspiration if he vomits.*

(9) *Ideal operating conditions can be obtained to meet surgical requirements.* Complete motor relaxation can be accomplished. If it is desirable to have the patient move and cooperate—such as for surgical repair of tendons—this can also be accomplished by using a weaker concentration of the local anesthetic drug.

(10) *If an anesthesiologist is not present, such as in rural regions or during wartime, brachial block anesthesia permits the maximum utilization of available personnel.* The surgeon can perform the block and then perform the operation, or one anesthesiologist can furnish anesthesia for more than one patient.

(11) *Ward nurses particularly appreciate the use of regional anesthesia.* Patients who return to the wards awake, without nausea and vomiting, and are able to help themselves immediately, enable the nursing staff to care for many more patients at one time.

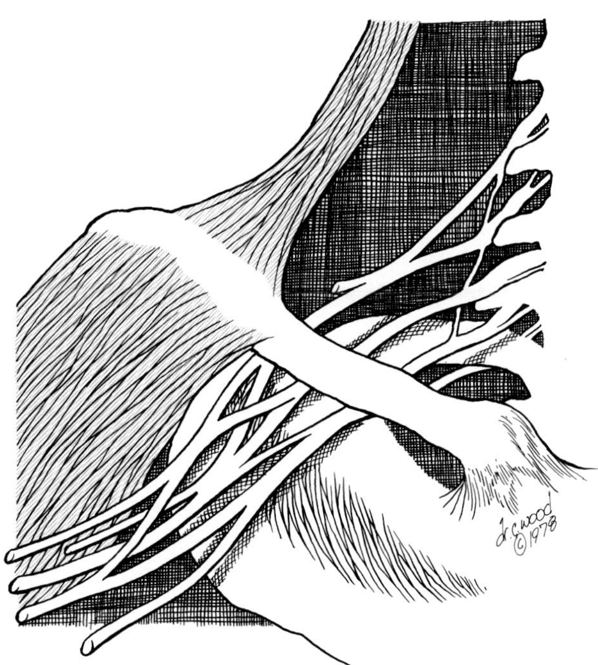

Fig. 10-1. Brachial plexus: Roots, trunks, divisions, and cords. Major branches are also shown.

Anatomy

The brachial plexus supplies all of the motor and almost all of the sensory function of the upper extremity. The remaining area—the skin over the shoulder—is supplied by the descending branches of the cervical plexus, and the posterior medial aspect of the arm extending nearly to the elbow is supplied by the intercostobrachial branch of the second intercostal nerve. The plexus is formed from the anterior primary rami of the fifth, sixth, seventh, and eighth cervical and the first thoracic nerves and frequently receives small contributing branches from the fourth cervical and second thoracic nerve (Fig. 10-1).

After these nerves leave their respective intervertebral foramina, they proceed anterolaterally and inferiorly to occupy the interval between the anterior and middle scalene muscles, where they unite to form three trunks—thus initiating the formation of the plexus proper. These trunks emerge from the interscalene space at the lower border of these muscles and continue anterolaterally and inferiorly to converge toward the upper surface of the first rib, where they are closely grouped. (It is to be noted that, as the newly formed trunks approach the first rib, they are arranged according to their designation "superior," "middle," and "inferior"—*i.e.,* one

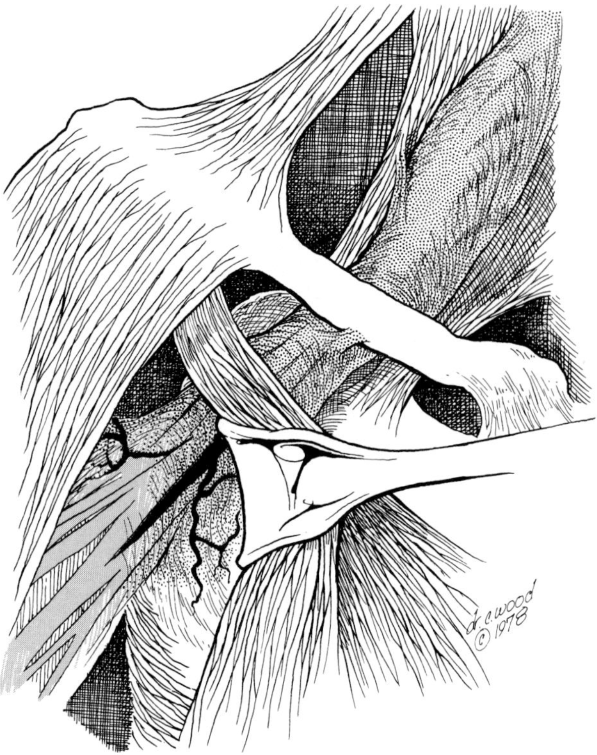

Fig. 10-2. Anatomical relationships of brachial plexus.

above the other vertically, not next to the others horizontally as is depicted in so many texts.) At the lateral edge of the rib, each trunk divides into an anterior and posterior division, which pass inferior to the midportion of the clavicle to enter the axilla through its apex. These divisions, by which fibers of the trunk reassemble to gain the ventral and dorsal aspect of the limb, reunite within the axilla to form three cords—the lateral, medial, and posterior—named because of their relationship with the second part of the axillary artery.

At the lateral border of the pectoralis minor, the three cords break up to give rise to the peripheral nerves of the upper extremity. The lateral cord gives off the lateral head of the median nerve and the musculocutaneous nerve; the medial cord gives off the medial head of the median nerve, the ulnar, the medial antebrachial, and the medial brachial cutaneous nerves; and the posterior cord terminates as the axillary and radial nerves (Fig. 10-2).

In its course, the brachial plexus is in close relationship to certain structures, some of which serve as important landmarks during the injection of the anesthetic. In its position between the anterior and middle scaleni muscles, the plexus lies superior and posterior to the second and third parts of the subclavian artery, which is also located between the two muscles. Anteromedial to the lower trunk and posteromedial to the artery lies the dome of the pleura.

Livingston originally pointed out, and Winnie has refocused our attention on, the fascial barriers that surround these structures.[30,48,50] The prevertebral fascia divides to invest the anterior and middle scalene muscles and then fuses at the lateral margins to form an enclosed interscalene space. Therefore, as the nerve roots leave the transverse processes, they emerge between the two walls of fascia that cover the anterior and middle scaleni muscles, and, in their descent toward the first rib to form the trunks of the plexus, the roots may be considered to be "sandwiched" between the anterior and middle scaleni muscles, the fascia of which serves as a "sheath" of the plexus (Fig. 10-3). As the roots pass down through this space, they converge to form the trunks of the brachial plexus and, together

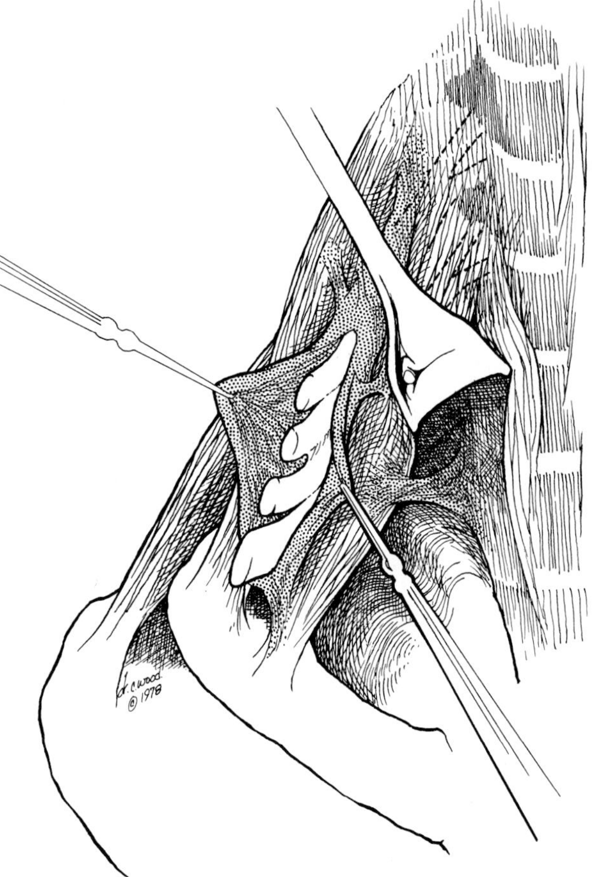

Fig. 10-3. Anatomy of interscalene sheath.

with the subclavian artery, invaginate the scalene fascia, which forms a subclavian perivascular sheath, which, in turn, becomes the axillary sheath as it passes under the clavicle (Fig. 10-4). It is important for the anesthesiologist to recognize a continuous fascia-enclosed space extending from the cervical transverse process to several centimeters beyond the axilla and enclosing the entire brachial plexus from the cervical roots to the great nerves of the upper arm. All the techniques for blocking the brachial plexus involve the location of the nerves and injection of the local anesthetic within the fascial sheath.

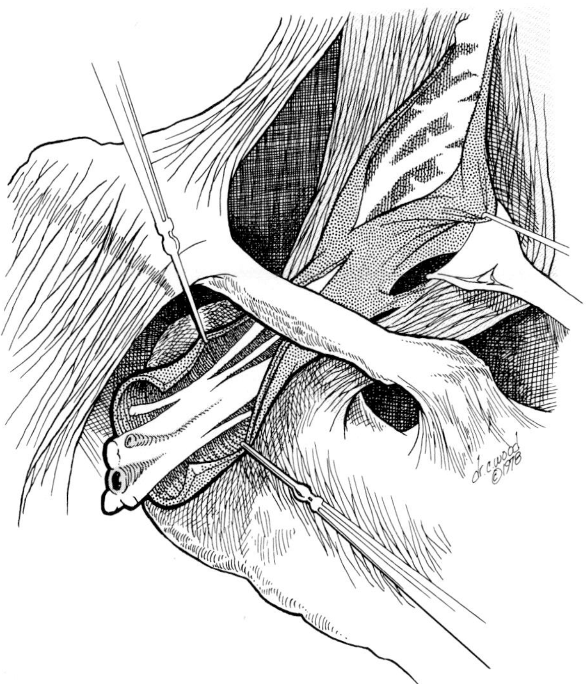

Fig. 10-4. Anatomy of interscalene–subclavian–axillary sheath.

PATIENT CARE, DRUGS, AND EQUIPMENT

Premedication

A high proportion of patients presenting for upper extremity block may be accident cases where opportunities for formal preparation and premedication may not be possible. Accordingly, the following points should be noted. First, the best way to achieve adequate pain relief is to insert a block as quickly as possible. Second, people who have suffered from injuries to their hands are especially anxious about the outcome. Third, fractures are most common in children and the elderly. Fourth, many patients can be treated as outpatients, and last, because paresthesias are sought to facilitate many upper limb blocks, cooperation of the patient is required.

For both elective surgery and, where practicable, with emergencies, premedication is strongly recommended, preferably a narcotic combined with a small dose (0.2–0.3 mg) of hyoscine or another mild sedative. It is important that the patient be alert and cooperative enough for the block procedure but not distressed by it.

Intraoperative Analgesia and Sedation

Requirements for intraoperative analgesia and sedation depend upon the patient's preference, the effects of premedication, the duration of the surgical procedure, additional stimuli such as a tourniquet, and the possibility of need for active tendon movement during stages of the operation. Even though complete analgesia is provided by nerve block, a narcotic and tranquilizer combination such as fentanyl and diazepam is recommended.

Postoperative Analgesia

Pain is not prominent following surgery on the upper limb. It is usually relieved by simple oral analgesics and the release of compression dressings if this is appropriate.

Except in a few cases of extensive surgery or trauma when stronger analgesics may be required for a short time, severe pain should be regarded as a sign of possible surgical complication. Because of this, the use of bupivacaine for nerve blocks may not be appropriate. However, many surgeons consider that following hand surgery, the prolonged period of immobility, together with functional sympathectomy and good pain relief from a long-acting block, outweighs the potential disadvantage of removing pain that might have indicated complications.

Posture of the Blocked Arm

Special care must be taken with the anesthetized limb. The arm must not be allowed to fall onto the face; this may occur when the patient attempts to move his half-paralyzed limb. Secondly, it is important that the arm should not be put into a position that would stretch the brachial plexus (*i.e.*, extended further than 90° or displaced posteriorly).[26] Thirdly, the ulnar nerve at the elbow should be properly padded, particularly if the forearm is pronated. Lastly, the arm should be properly supported during movement of the patient, transit from the operation table, and at all other times, until power and sensation return.

Local Anesthetic Drugs

At present, all upper extremity block techniques may be adequately performed with any of the local anesthetic drugs approved for peripheral nerve block (see Chap. 4). For emergency room use, practitioners may desire a short-acting drug with very rapid onset such as 2-chloroprocaine or lidocaine. As has been previously noted, a long-acting drug like bupivacaine or etidocaine will not only provide anesthesia for long operative procedures but will also ensure a prolonged period of postoperative analgesia and sympathetic blockade. In general, a short-acting drug, a drug of intermediate action, and a long-acting drug will suffice to meet the needs of most practitioners.

As in other peripheral nerve blocks, the use of epinephrine-containing solutions depends generally on the agent to be used, the total dose of drug being contemplated, and the duration of the block desired. Epinephrine-containing solutions should not be used on the digital nerves of the hands and feet.

Concentration of the drug required depends primarily on the size of the nerve trunk, the modalities required to be blocked (*i.e.*, fiber size), and the disposition of these fibers within the nerve trunk (see Chap. 2).

Muscle relaxation is important for shoulder surgery, particularly the reduction of dislocations. Although the brachial plexus trunks are quite large, the actual nerve fibers that supply the shoulder are thought to be distributed in their periphery as "mantle fibers," so that they are quickly and relatively easily blocked. In contrast, hand surgery requires little muscle relaxation but a profound degree of sensory anesthesia. The nerves to the hand at the brachial plexus level are centrally situated within the nerve trunks, thus they are more difficult to block and may require a stronger concentration of local anesthetic in spite of relatively small fiber size.

Equipment

In institutions where many regional blocks are performed and in which adequate preparation and sterilization can be assured, packs of appropriate syringes, needles, and other equipment can be assembled for various kinds of blocks. Finger control Luer-Lok glass syringes and stainless steel needles of appropriate length, bore, and bevel can be provided.

In other situations it may be better to rely on disposable syringes and needles, which are quite satisfactory for upper extremity blocks. However, there is not the same variety of needles available, and their long bevels may "spur" if contact with bony surfaces occurs.

For the nerve blocks described in this chapter, either 23-gauge, 32-mm or 25-gauge, 16-mm needles are suitable. Some anesthesiologists prefer stouter needles in order to be more certain of eliciting paresthesias and aspirating blood if the needle is within a vessel; others favor fine needles in the hope that they will do less damage.

SUPRACLAVICULAR BLOCK

Advantages

There are several advantages to the use of the supraclavicular block. The brachial plexus is blocked where it is most compactly arranged—at the level of the three trunks. A low volume of solution is required and quick onset is achieved. Also, the technique can be performed with the arm in virtually any position, and all of the brachial plexus is reliably blocked. There is no danger of missing peripheral or proximal nerve branches because of failure of local anesthetic spread.

Limitations and Problems

Supraclavicular block has certain drawbacks. A reliable quick-onset block is achieved only if paresthesias are elicited. Furthermore, the technique is rather difficult to describe and teach. (What is anterior, posterior, backward, above, below, the length not breadth of the rib, etc.?) Therefore, considerable experience is required to master it and this is best accomplished by personal observation of an experienced anesthesiologist or by time spent in the postmortem room. In addition, there is the risk of pneumothorax.

Contraindications

This approach to the brachial plexus is best avoided in the following patients: those who are uncooperative; those of difficult stature in which bony and muscular landmarks are not clear; the respiratory cripples in whom pneumothorax or even phrenic block would result in significant dyspnea. Patients who require bilateral block should not have both performed by this technique to avoid the risk of bilateral phrenic nerve paralysis, pneumothoraces or a combination of the two. In addition, supraclavicular block should not be performed by a person who is unfamiliar with the technique or has not performed the block under the supervision of an experienced colleague.

Anatomy

The following are important points in the descriptive and topographic anatomy (Fig. 10-5*A* and *B*). First, the component parts of the plexus unite in a bundle that lies inferior to the clavicle at about its midpoint, on the posterior and lateral aspect and of the subclavian artery. Second, the artery can often be palpated as a valuable landmark. Third, the first rib is a very important landmark to prevent the needle from passing medially and entering the pleural dome. The rib is short, broad, and flat. It slopes downward as it passes forward. Although it is deeply curved, that small portion in relation to the subclavian artery and the brachial plexus is primarily anteroposterior in the body plane.

Technique

The classical approach for supraclavicular block of the brachial plexus should be regarded as a combination of the early published techniques. It calls for a downward, backward, and inward direction for insertion of the needle from a point just (or 1 cm) behind the midpoint of the clavicle (Fig. 10-5*C*). This is generally very satisfactory; however, strict interpretation may not always be appropriate.

In some patients, beginning at a point just behind the clavicle results in a very backward (posterior) direction of the needle. A starting point 2 to 3 cm behind the clavicle may make it easier to locate the interscalene groove and the nerve trunks above the first rib.

If a point is taken directly behind the clavicle, it will almost certainly lie outside the lateral margin of the rib. Inward (medial) inclination of the needle can very easily penetrate the pleura. The more lateral the starting point, and the *more medial the inclination,* the more likely this is to occur.

"Rib walking" to achieve paresthesias, if they are not more simply obtained, is important for a satisfactory block. However, rib seeking or further "rib walking" after eliciting paresthesias would seem unnecessary and only increase the risk of pneumothorax.

The pulsation of the subclavian artery against the palpating finger or needle is the surest guide to the brachial plexus. It may not be felt if the clavicle is raised; if the platysma muscle is tense; or if the patient is obese.

An additional guide to locating the midpoint of the clavicle is finding the point where the straight portion of the external jugular vein, if continued, would cross the clavicle. Asking the patient to "blow out his cheeks" will frequently make the external jugular vein prominent.

Positions and Landmarks. The patient should lie supine without a pillow, arms at the side, and head turned slightly to the opposite side. The shoulder should be depressed downward (caudad) and posterior by gentle pressure on the relaxed shoulder and by asking the patient to touch his knee. This posterior displacement of the shoulder can be exaggerated by molding the shoulders over a roll placed between the scapulae. The patient is then instructed to raise his head approximately 20° from the table, putting strain on the neck muscles. This permits the clavicular head of the sternocleidomastoid muscle to be palpated and marked. The interscalene groove is palpated by rolling the finger back from the posterior border of the lower end of the identified sternocleidomastoid muscle and over the belly of the anterior scalene muscle. Because the brachial plexus makes its exit at the lateral border of the anterior scalene muscle, the skin is marked at this point immediately above the clavicle. Usually, this point lies approximately at the middle of the clavicle, 1.5 to 2 cm from the lateral border of the clavicular head of the sternocleidomastoid muscle. The subclavian artery can often be clearly palpated in the supraclavicular fossa because it also emerges from the lower end of the interscalene groove. This serves as a check on the other landmarks.

In spite of the multiple landmarks, this is one of the simplest of all blocks to perform if the subclavian artery can be palpated easily because the needle is inserted directly down from the tip of the palpating finger. If neither the artery nor the interscalene groove can be clearly felt, a point is taken approximately 2 cm along a line marked behind the mid point of and perpendicular to the clavicle (Fig. 10-5*B*). In a patient with a protuberant clavicle or in whom it is difficult to achieve adequate posterior displacement of the shoulder, this point should be taken nearer to 3 cm behind the clavicle.

Procedure. The area should be aseptically prepared and draped. The anesthesiologist stands at the side of the patient to be blocked, facing the head of the table, since this position allows better control of the needle. An intradermal wheal is raised at the previously determined point. If the anesthesiologist is right-handed, a filled 10 ml syringe with a 23-gauge, 32-mm needle attached, is held in the right hand and the patient is instructed to say "now" and

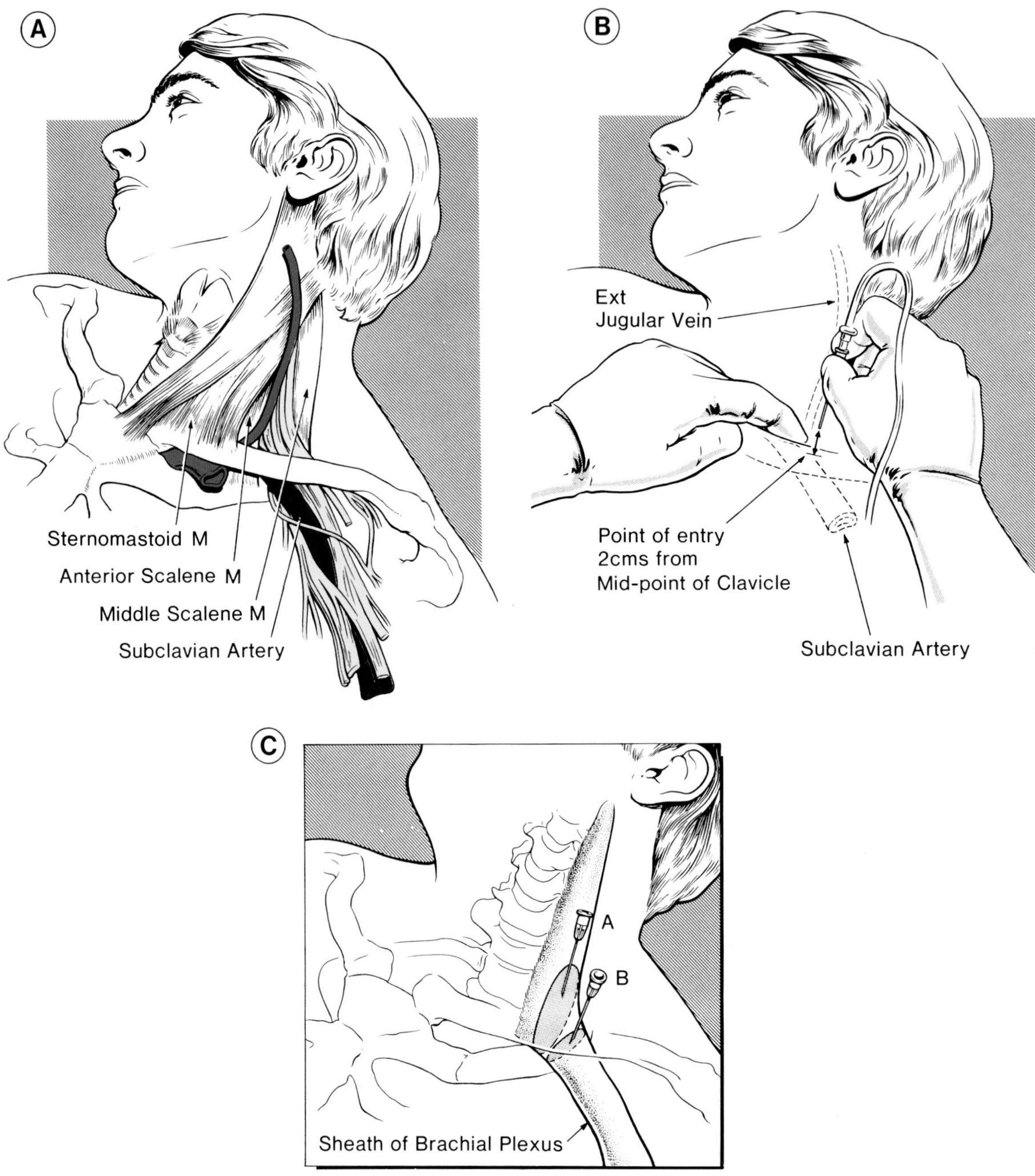

Fig. 10-5. (*A*) Supraclavicular block. Anatomical landmarks. (*B*) Supraclavicular block. Technique of needle insertion. (*C*) Supraclavicular block. Note that the brachial plexus sheath becomes deeper as one moves medially and further back from the clavicle (position A) than it is at the lateral margin of the first rib immediately behind the clavicle (position B).

not move as soon as he feels a "tingle" or "electric-like shock" going down his arm. This initial technique varies slightly depending on whether or not the subclavian artery is palpable. If the artery is palpable, the tip of the index finger is rested in the supraclavicular fossa directly over the arterial pulsation. The needle is inserted through the skin wheal and advanced slowly downward (caudad), rolled slightly inward (medially), and very slightly backward (posteriorly) so that the shaft of the needle and syringe are almost parallel to the patient's head (Fig. 10-5*B* and *C*). The index finger and thumb of the left hand firmly hold the hub of the needle and control the movement of the needle at all times.

Paresthesias will usually be immediately elicited. If so, the needle is fixed in position, and 15 to 25 ml of the local anesthetic drug is injected. If paresthesias are not immediately elicited, then one should proceed onto the rib and either deposit all the solution on or slightly superficial to the rib, in this position just behind the artery, or make further attempts to seek paresthesias by gentle reinsertions posteriorly for an estimated 2 cm along the length (not breadth) of the rib. After the rib is encountered, the anesthesiologist, by gently tapping it with the point of the needle, "walks" the needle forward (anteriorly) along the rib for approximately 1.5 cm, maintaining the initial plane of direction of the needle and seeking paresthesias. With each insertion of the needle, aspiration tests should be undertaken to see that the needle point is not in the subclavian artery. If it is, however, the anesthesiologist should not become alarmed; he has found a valuable landmark. By withdrawing the needle and reinserting it posterolaterally to the subclavian artery, paresthesias will usually be elicited as the needle is slowly advanced. If no paresthesias are elicited, but the rib is contacted, a barrage of solution between the skin and the rib behind the artery can be employed. This is the principle of the Patrick technique.

If the artery is not palpable and has not been located, the previously located point 2 cm behind the midpoint of the clavicle can be used and will more certainly be placed over the rib. The needle is inserted directly downward (caudad) until paresthesias are elicited or the rib is contacted, and again, if necessary, the needle should be "walked" anteroposteriorly along the rib to seek the plexus. In a robust patient, occasionally the rib cannot be contacted at the full depth of this needle. Under these circumstances, the anesthesiologist should make a sweep with gentle reinsertions posteriorly as before, each time to the depth of the needle, in an attempt to elicit paresthesias superficial to the rib. If no paresthesias or rib are encountered at full depth of the needle, it may be advisable to choose another method. If the patient is properly positioned and all of the available landmarks are utilized and checked against one another, the need to change techniques will be rare.

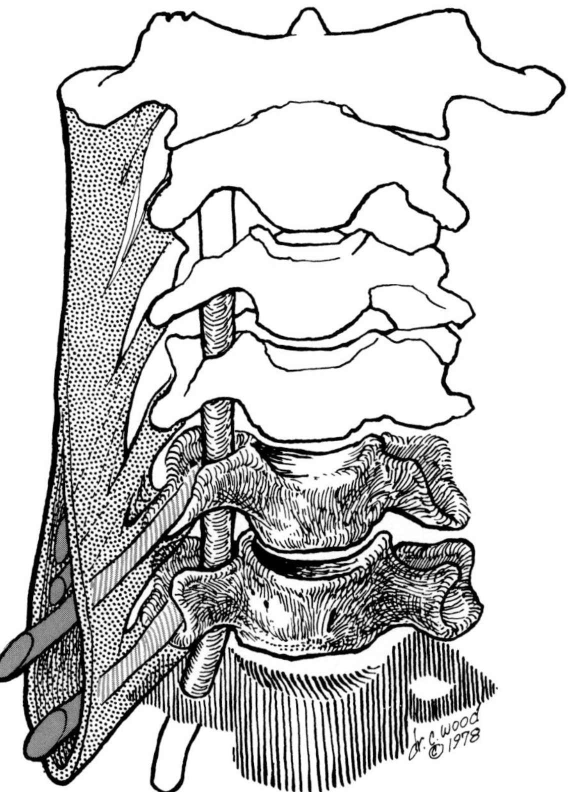

Fig. 10-6. Anatomical development of interscalene sheath.

Complications

Pneumothorax. Serious complications ensue very infrequently. The most specific complication of the supraclavicular approach for blocking the brachial plexus is pneumothorax. The frequency of occurrence is between 0.5 and 6 per cent and decreases as the anesthesiologist becomes more skilled. Tall, thin patients, who characteristically have a high apical pleura usually account for the greater number of these complications. Some authorities believe that the pneumothorax results from the piercing of the pleura, with air entering through the open needle. This is unlikely since many of the pneumothoraces seen following this block have not occurred for some hours following the procedure, and a syringe is kept on the end of the needle at all times. Most likely, the pneumothoraces are caused by the needle piercing the lung as exhalation occurs and the lung surface is torn by the needle point. The pneumothorax that results is then caused by air escaping from the lung. The risk of pneumothorax can be minimized by careful attention to detail, taking time, and being gentle; by the avoidance of multiple indiscriminate probings; and by the use of short and relatively fine needles. Fine needles limit the ability to elicit paresthesias and detect intravascular injections, but they are less damaging to the lung.

A pneumothorax must be suspected when there is dyspnea, cough, or pleuritic chest pain, but the diagnosis can only be confirmed by chest x-ray. It is important to realize in assessing the size of a pneumothorax that there is apparent exaggeration on a film taken in full expiration.

A minority of the pneumothoraces become obvious within a few hours. These are usually extensive and accompanied by symptoms. The majority of pneumothoraces take up to 24 hours to develop, are usually small to moderate in size, and may or may not cause symptoms so there is little point in routine x-rays in the hours immediately following the block. It is also encouraging to note that it is most unusual for a "brachial block" pneumothorax to get any larger after 24 hours.

The treatment of pneumothorax depends on the extent and symptoms. In the early, more extensive pneumothorax (*i.e.*, greater than 50%), the patient should be admitted to the hospital and the air removed. Under these circumstances, a continuous drainage system for 24 to 48 hours is preferable to simple aspiration.

With lesser degrees of pneumothorax, usually diagnosed the following day, the air should be removed only if it is causing symptoms. In this case, aspiration with a small catheter, syringe, and three-way stopcock is all that is required, provided that proper surgical sterility is observed.

Pneumothoraces that are asymptomatic and not extensive can usually be followed on an outpatient basis with suitable advice and warnings. Analgesics such as codeine and aspirin may be prescribed for pain and discomfort if indicated. Serial films of the chest should be taken to assure that expansion of the lung is proceeding. However, there is no point in daily films when it may take weeks for the air to absorb completely.

Other complications seen with the supraclavicular brachial plexus block include the following.

Block of the phrenic nerve occurs in 40 to 60 per cent of the cases and usually causes no symptoms. However, if a bilateral phrenic block occurs in a patient with underlying chest disease, signs of hypoxia may result. Ordinarily, no treatment is necessary for the unilateral phrenic nerve block. Symptoms, if present, clear as the block dissipates. If signs of hypoxia occur, oxygen should be given by bag and mask or by other forms of oxygen therapy.

Horner's syndrome (stellate ganglion block) occurs in approximately 70 to 90 per cent of the brachial plexus blocks when large volumes of solution (50 ml or more) of the local anesthetic drug are injected. The symptoms clear as the block is dissipated, and no treatment is necessary. These signs and symptoms should be explained to the patient, however, with assurance that they will disappear as the local anesthetic wears off.

Nerve damage or neuritis is a rare but possible complication of all peripheral blocks, including the supraclavicular technique for blocking the brachial plexus. When it occurs, the most frequent reason is faulty positioning of the anesthetized arm during surgery or in the immediate postoperative period rather than the block technique itself. Occasional trauma by the needle, prolonged ischemia of the nerve due to vasoconstrictor drugs, or too concentrated an anesthetic solution may also be potential offenders. Treatment usually consists of "tincture of time." These injuries may last days to months. Physiotherapy by trained technicians and exercise at home are invaluable to prevent muscle atrophy. A neurologic consultation should be obtained to establish the level, extent, and treatment of the lesion as well as to avoid and protect against medicolegal action.

Toxic Reactions due to High Blood Level of the Local Anesthetic Drug. The cause and treatment of toxic reactions to the local anesthetic drugs are discussed in detail in Chapter 4. The most common reason for its occurrence in supraclavicular brachial plexus block is an inadvertent intravascular injection of the local anesthetic drug or use of an excessive amount of solution. Properly treated, it should not be a serious complication.

Comments

It is strongly advised that paresthesias should be obtained since they denote contact with the plexus, assuring a successful block with quicker onset. Signs of injury following these blocks that could be attributed to paresthesias have not been observed.

On the other hand, promiscuous probing should be avoided. If, after five or six careful insertions, a paresthesia is not obtained, one of the other techniques should be used.

One of the most certain causes of presumed failure of the block is to commence the operation before the anesthesia has had time to become complete. This interval may be as brief as 5, or as long as 30, minutes. The custom with promiscuously sticking needles throughout the limb immediately after the injection for the purpose of testing the degree of anesthesia cannot be condemned too strongly. The patient's confidence is, too often, utterly destroyed by this method. An excellent rule is to keep the patient quiet for an interval of 15 minutes and to make the first tests for anesthesia no sooner than at the termination of this period.

Because the trunks of the brachial plexus are so compact at the point of crossing the first rib, 15 to 25 ml of solution is usually sufficient to produce a total brachial plexus block even in the robust patient. If no paresthesias are obtained larger volumes are often required and even then a delay in onset and possibly patchy anesthesia are likely.

A common error in locating the midpoint of the clavicle is to assume that the tip of the acromion is the lateral end. The "midpoint" will then be too far lateral. The accurately selected medial starting point and direct insertion towards the flat surface of the rib are important factors in avoiding missing the rib on either its *inner or outer* borders.

INTERSCALENE BLOCK

The interscalene block was developed and later described as an alternative to the supraclavicular approach to the brachial sheath.[29,30,48]

Advantages

Interscalene block is suitable when a proximal block is required, such as for shoulder surgery when it is often necessary also to block the cervical plexus. In addition, it can be performed with the arm in virtually any position, and the pneumothorax risk with conventional supraclavicular block is reduced. Last, the landmarks are usually clear even in patients of stout build.

Limitations and Problems

It is essential to elicit paresthesias. Also, unless large volumes are used, lower trunk anesthesia may be missed; supplementary ulnar block may then be required. Rare but potentially serious complications can occur.

Anatomy

The cervical nerves of the brachial plexus, after leaving their respective intervertebral foramen, pass laterally in a deep groove or "gutter" in the superior surface of the transverse process of the cervical vertebrae (Fig. 10-6). This groove separates the transverse process into anterior and posterior tubercles, which give origin to the scalenus anterior and scalenus medius muscles, respectively (Fig. 10-4). After leaving the transverse processes, the nerve roots of the brachial plexus pass immediately into a plane between the two scalene muscles—the paravertebral or interscalene space (Fig. 10-3). The direction of the "gutters" in the lower cervical vertebrae is primarily lateral but also slightly forward and almost 45° downward, as if they were drawn down by the scalene muscles.

Although transverse processes in this region tend to overlap, it must be remembered that they are quite short and offer little protection to the intervertebral foramina from a horizontally directed needle.

Before attempting this block, the anesthesiologist should closely examine the skeleton of the cervical vertebral column with particular regard to the intervertebral foramina and the shape and direction of the transverse processes.

Technique

Position and Landmarks. The patient lies supine with the neck straight but the head turned slightly to the side opposite to the side to be treated. The arm is placed by the side with the shoulder depressed as for supraclavicular block. The right-handed operator stands at the head of the table for a right arm block and by the patient's shoulder for left arm block.

The head is temporarily lifted in order to palpate the posterior border of the sternomastoid muscle. The interscalene groove is palpated by rolling the fingers back from the border of the sternomastoid over the belly of the scalenus anterior to the groove, which is then marked. A line is extended directly laterally from the cricoid cartilage to intersect the interscalene groove. The point of entry is at this intersection, which should be directly opposite the transverse process of C6. The external jugular vein may overlie this area (Fig. 10-7*A* and *B*).

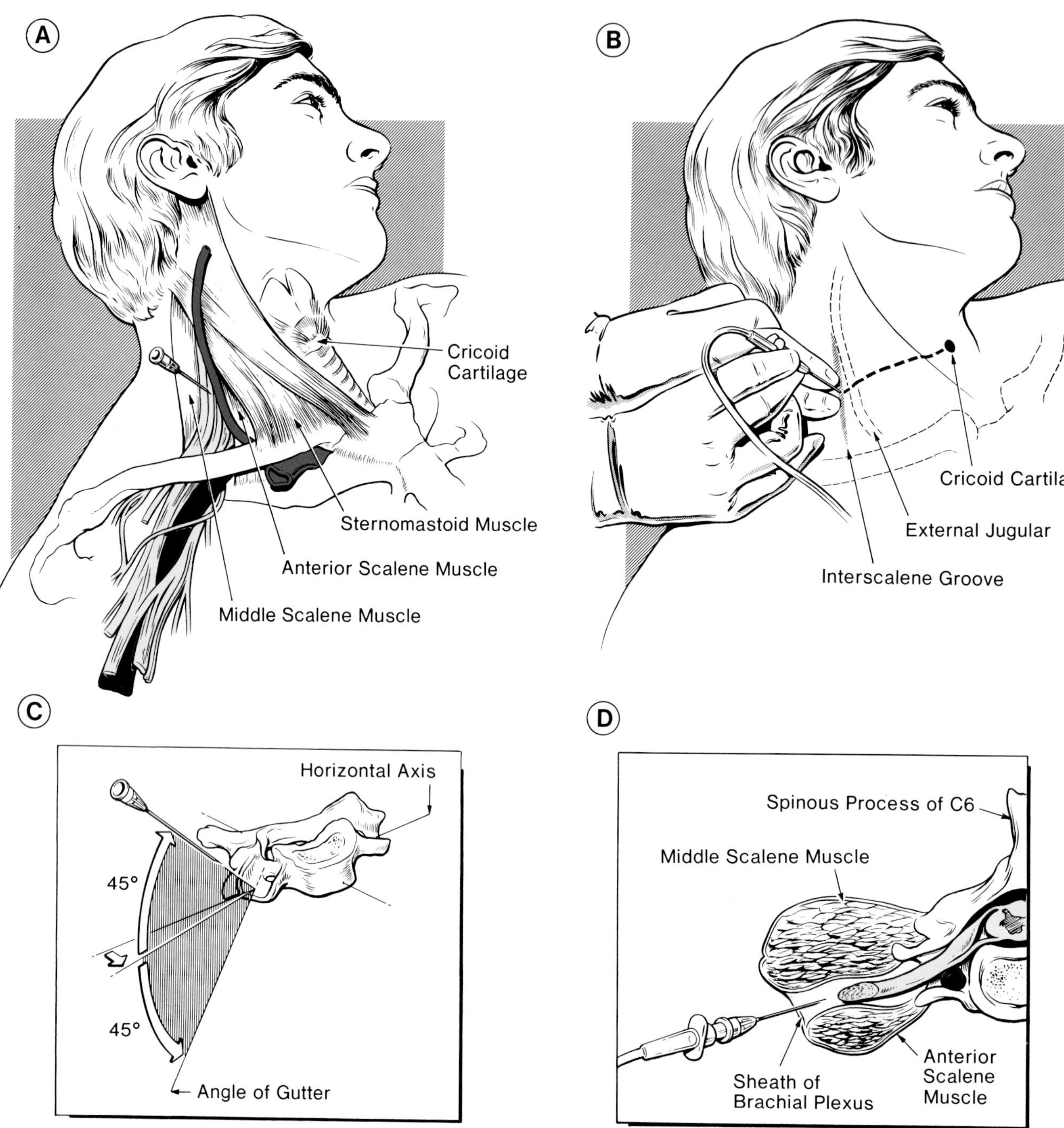

Fig. 10-7. (*A*) Interscalene block. Anatomical landmarks. (*B*) Interscalene block. Method of palpating interscalene groove and inserting needle. Note hand holding needle braced against clavicle. (*C–D*) Interscalene block. Needle direction in relation to spine from antero-lateral view (*C*), from above (*D*).

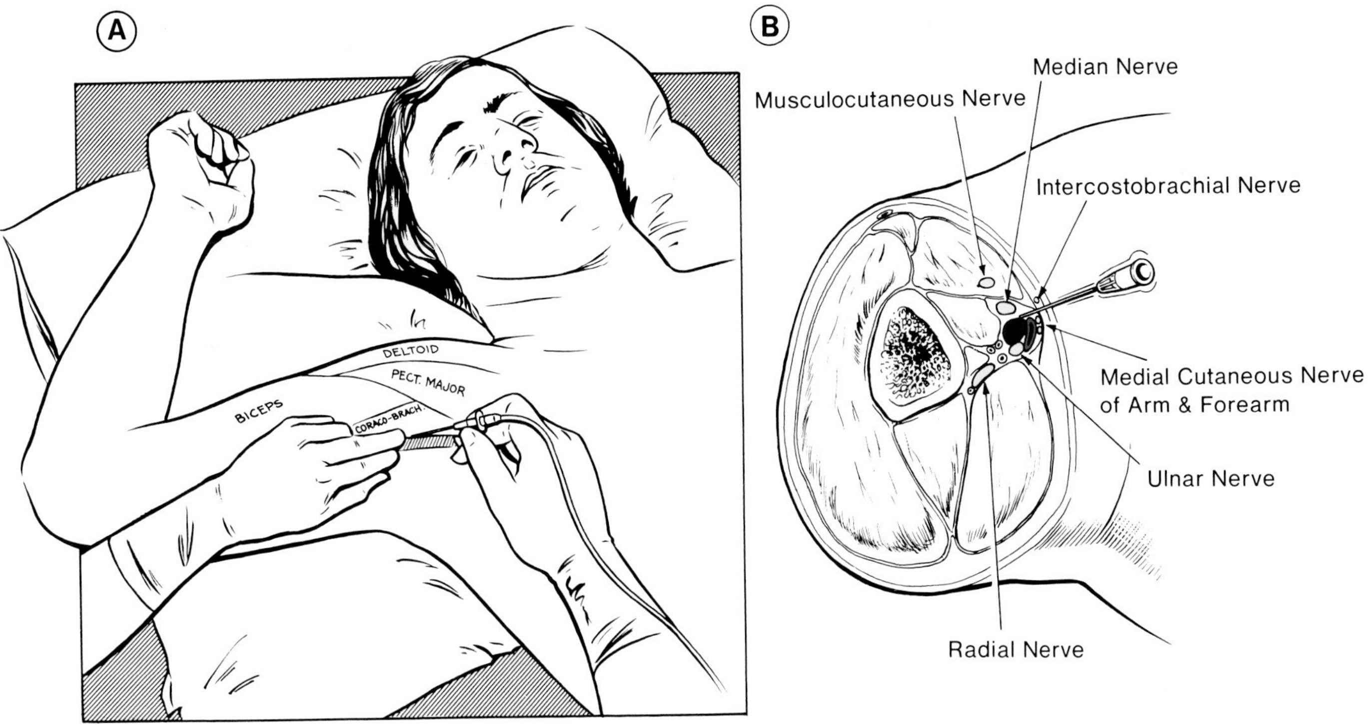

Fig. 10-8. Axillary block. (*A*) Technique of needle insertion. Index and middle fingers of left hand palpate immediately below sharp edge of coracobrachialis muscle. Fingers remain pressed against axillary artery during injection to help central spread of solution. Right hand holding needle is braced against patient and an assistant is used to aspirate and inject via extension tubing attached to needle. (*B*) Cross section of upper arm immediately below axilla.

Needle Insertion and Injection. After suitable preparation and the insertion of a skin wheal, with the index and middle fingers of the left hand still palpating the groove, a 23-gauge 32-mm needle is inserted in a direction almost perpendicular to the floor of the "gutter" on the superior aspect of the transverse process (Fig. 10-7*B*–*C*). The anesthesiologist should visualize the transverse process as being directed primarily laterally but also downward and slightly forward. The direction of the needle, therefore, is mainly inward but also 45° caudad and slightly backward.

The needle is advanced until paresthesias are elicited. Injection is then made of the full volume of solution. To avoid the problem of needle displacement, it should be held firmly by the hub during the period of injection. The transverse process is surprisingly superficial in the normal patient, no more than 1.5 to 2 cm. If bone is encountered at this depth but no paresthesias, one should "walk" the needle across the transverse process and thus across the path of the nerve.

If bony contact is made only on deep insertion, it is likely that the transverse process has been missed and what has been reached is the vertebral body. If no bony contact is made near full depth of the needle, the vertebral column has been missed, probably anteriorly, and a more posterior direction should be undertaken.[43]

In the vast majority of cases, paresthesias are easily obtained superficially. If a blunt bevel needle is used, the anesthesiologist may also feel the penetration of the fascia.

Ten to 40 ml of solution are injected, depending on the extent of the block required as well as the condition and stature of the patient. Volume to anesthesia relationships have been studied with radiopaque contrast, and these suggest that 20 ml of solution will anesthetize the lower cervical nerves and most of the brachial plexus; however, with this volume the lower trunk is often spared.[48] Forty ml of solution blocks all of the cervical and the brachial plexuses. Digital pressure during injection and massage following helps downward spread.

Comments

Anesthesia of the cervical plexus can also be readily obtained by this single injection into the interscalene groove.[51] The C4 level can be identified by extending a line laterally from the upper border of the thyroid cartilage. Injection of 10 to 15 ml is made in identical fashion to that for interscalene brachial plexus block.

Complications

As with any paravertebral technique, inadvertent epidural or spinal anesthesia is always possible and has been reported with this block.[28,40] Also, the vertebral artery is very close to the point of even a correctly placed needle.

The phrenic nerve must frequently be blocked because of either C4 root involvement or anterior spread under the prevertebral fascia in front of the scalenus anterior muscle, but this is rarely significant, at least in unilateral blocks. Vagus, recurrent laryngeal, and cervical sympathetic nerves are sometimes involved, but these are of no significance except that it may be very important to reassure the patient.

AXILLARY BLOCK

The perivascular axillary infiltration has become one of the most popular techniques for blocking the nerves of the arm.

Advantages

Axillary block provides excellent operating conditions for surgery of the forearm and hand with less risk of major complications than is associated with alternative supraclavicular methods. This makes it very suitable for emergency room and outpatient use. It is an easy technique to master and probably the safest and most reliable for the patient of stout build. It is not imperative to seek paresthesias, and fine needles are quite satisfactory. The block is, therefore, particularly useful in children (*e.g.*, for the reduction of fractures[10,21]).

Limitations and Problems

The axillary approach does have certain limitations, the first of which is that the arm must be abducted in order to perform the block. The extent of anesthesia also is insufficient for shoulder or upper arm surgery without using large volumes of solution. The circumflex and musculocutaneous nerves are sometimes missed because they have left the sheath proximal to the point of injection. The musculocutaneous nerve is most important because of its extensive area of innervation on the radial side of the forearm extending onto the thenar eminence.

Anatomy

A cross section of the arm at the level of anterior axillary fold demonstrates several anatomical points, including the compact, axillary neurovascular bundle (Fig. 10-8*B*). On its medial (superficial) aspect, the axillary sheath is covered only by connective tissue, being behind the biceps/coracobrachialis and in front of the triceps muscles. On its lateral or deep aspect, the sheath lies close to the neck of the humerus. In the sheath, the median nerve tends to lie anterior to the axillary artery (as did the musculocutaneous nerve higher up the sheath), the ulnar nerve, posterior, and the radial nerve, posterior and somewhat lateral. The medial antebrachial cutaneous nerve and the medial brachial cutaneous nerves are medial to the artery. The axillary vein overlies the artery on its medial aspect. The musculocutaneous nerve has already left the sheath and is now in the substance of the coracobrachialis muscle.

Technique

Position and Landmarks. The arm is abducted to 90° and externally rotated by resting the forearm comfortably back on a pillow near the head. The anesthesiologist should stand beside the patient, facing his axilla. For block of the left arm, the right-handed operator may be more comfortable standing by the patient's head, facing caudally and leaning over the arm.

The axillary artery is palpated and traced as far as possible toward the axilla. It is usually easy to palpate the vessel clearly up as far as the anterior axillary fold.

Point of Entry. The artery is fixed against the humerus by the index and middle fingers of the left hand, and a skin wheal is raised directly over the arterial pulse (Fig. 10-8*A*). The skin is then pierced with a 19-gauge needle in order to facilitate the entry of the smaller block needle.

Needle Insertion and Injection. A 23-gauge, 32-mm needle, either bare or attached to anesthetic-filled extension tubing or syringe, is inserted perpendicular to the skin and humerus and then directed to just miss the artery at its anterior aspect (Fig. 10-8*A*).

Evidence of entering the axillary sheath is sought by the feel of penetrating the fascia, parasthesias, blood flow back, or oscillation of a free needle.

The feeling of penetrating the sheath is facilitated

by the use of a short-bevel needle and the elimination of skin drag. The simple expedient of first puncturing the skin with a larger needle helps, but it can be further reduced by a needle-through-needle hole technique.[45]

The eliciting of paresthesias is encouraging and reliable evidence of correct position but is not essential for a satisfactory block, and it may be distressing.

The flow or aspiration of blood, particularly arterial blood, strongly suggests that the needle tip is within the sheath. The needle can then be either just withdrawn from the vessel or pushed on through to the other side before injection. Although it cannot be recommended, it is the practice of some anesthesiologists to set out deliberately to puncture the artery as their means of identifying the sheath.

Oscillation of the needle produced by arterial pulsation indicates that the needle is at least near the artery and thus probably within the sheath.

Single-Injection Technique. Following aspiration, which is particularly important in this site, the entire volume of local anesthetic may be injected. On the basis of sheath volume and assuming equal up and down spread, de Jong calculated that 42 ml of solution was necessary to fill the adult sheath sufficient to reach the coracoid process, which is the approximate level at which the musculocutaneous nerve leaves the sheath.[13] This kind of volume to anesthesia relationship has been confirmed with radiopaque contrast studies.[50]

Although the solution tends to spread up rather than down the sheath and measures can be taken to increase this central spread, 40 ml of solution is required to block, consistently, all of the brachial plexus. This, of course, is scaled downward in children and when other circumstances call for a reduction in dose.

Prevention of needle movement during injection may be a little awkward in the axilla but is absolutely essential with this technique. It can be aided by fixing the needle hub with the thumb and index finger of the left hand, if using direct syringe attachment, or the right hand if using needle attached to extension tubing. This "immobile needle" helps to prevent movement during syringe removal and reattachment.[49]

A few milliliters of solution are deposited in the subcutaneous tissue on withdrawal if required to block the intercostobrachial nerve and its communications with the medial cutaneous nerve of the arm (Fig. 10-8*B*).

Double-Injection Technique. Nearly all earlier descriptions of axillary block have employed the technique of injection on both sides of the artery.[7,13,19,34,44] However, if the first insertion was correct and the needle is not moved, this second injection should not be necessary, provided sufficient volume is used.

There are some advantages of a double-injection technique. If the anesthesiologist is prepared to disregard the musculocutaneous nerve or routinely to block it separately, the volume of solution can be significantly reduced—10 to 15 ml with each injection is quite sufficient to block the other nerves within the sheath. Also, there are two chances to enter the sheath. On rare occasions, the areolar septa within the sheath may act as a barrier to the spread of a single injection.[13]

The double injection technique can be performed with one or two needles. With a single needle, half the total volume is injected anterior to (above) the artery; the needle is then withdrawn from the fascia, redirected posterior to (below) the artery, and the remainder injected. Two needles are inserted through the same skin wheal, but one is directed anterior and the other, posterior to the artery, before injecting through each needle.[24] Again, subcutaneous injection on withdrawal may be indicated.

Promotion of Central Flow Within the Sheath. With the single-injection, high-volume technique, measures should be taken to promote proximal flow within the sheath. Digital pressure should be applied immediately distal to the needle with the index and middle fingers, both during and immediately following injection. If these fingers are required for fixation of the needle hub, pressure on the distal sheath can be applied with the ulnar side of the hand. The application of a distal tourniquet frees the left hand but is of doubtful effectiveness and causes some discomfort.[20] Directing the needle toward the apex of the axilla has also been used in an effort to gain more proximal spread and higher block. Winnie has suggested the use of a 37-mm needle directed centrally at approximately 20° to the artery.[47] Hopcroft uses a 21-gauge, 50-mm needle directed centrally along the axis of the artery.[23] These techniques no doubt achieve the desired goal, but, at some point, the pneumothorax problem must again arise. As soon as the injection is completed and while still applying some form of distal pressure, the arm should be adducted. This removes the effect of pressure of the humeral head, which may be a factor in limiting proximal spread.[46]

Comments. In children particularly, a standard 23-gauge or 25-gauge scalp-vein needle set is very useful. Paresthesias can, on some occasions, be an essential part of this method, particularly in a large arm with vague arterial pulsation and where there is difficulty in identifying the sheath.

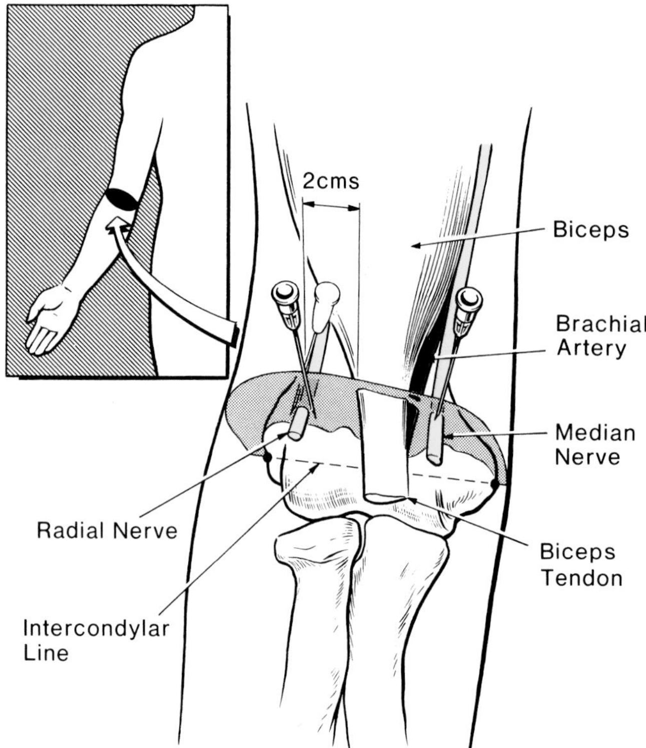

Fig. 10-9. Anatomical landmarks for median and radial nerve block at elbow.

Another method that has been described to be used when the sheath cannot be identified is to lay down a wall of anesthetic solution on each side of the artery from skin to humerus.

Complications and Contraindications

There are no complications or contraindications specific to this block; however, the risk of intravascular injection, particularly into the overlying vein, must always be kept in mind, and the patient with a bleeding diathesis is probably at an increased risk of incurring a hematoma with this approach.

PERIPHERAL BLOCKS

With safe and reliable brachial plexus anesthesia, and particularly with the more widespread use of axillary block, the need for distal nerve blocks has diminished; however, at times these can be of considerable value. Peripheral block can be useful when circumstances such as infection, difficult anatomy, bilateral surgery, or an anesthesiologist's inexperience may preclude the use of plexus blocks. Also, it can be used for surgery on the hand that is of limited extent and duration, when it is on a part supplied by individual nerves, or as an alternative to digital, particularly multiple digital, blocks.

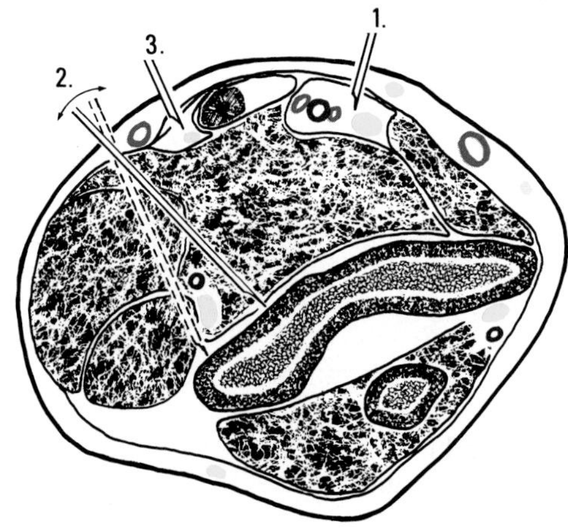

Fig. 10-10. Cross section of arm at elbow. (1) Median nerve block. (2) Radial nerve block. (3) Lateral cutaneous nerve block. (Note nerve under deep fascia and close to biceps tendon.)

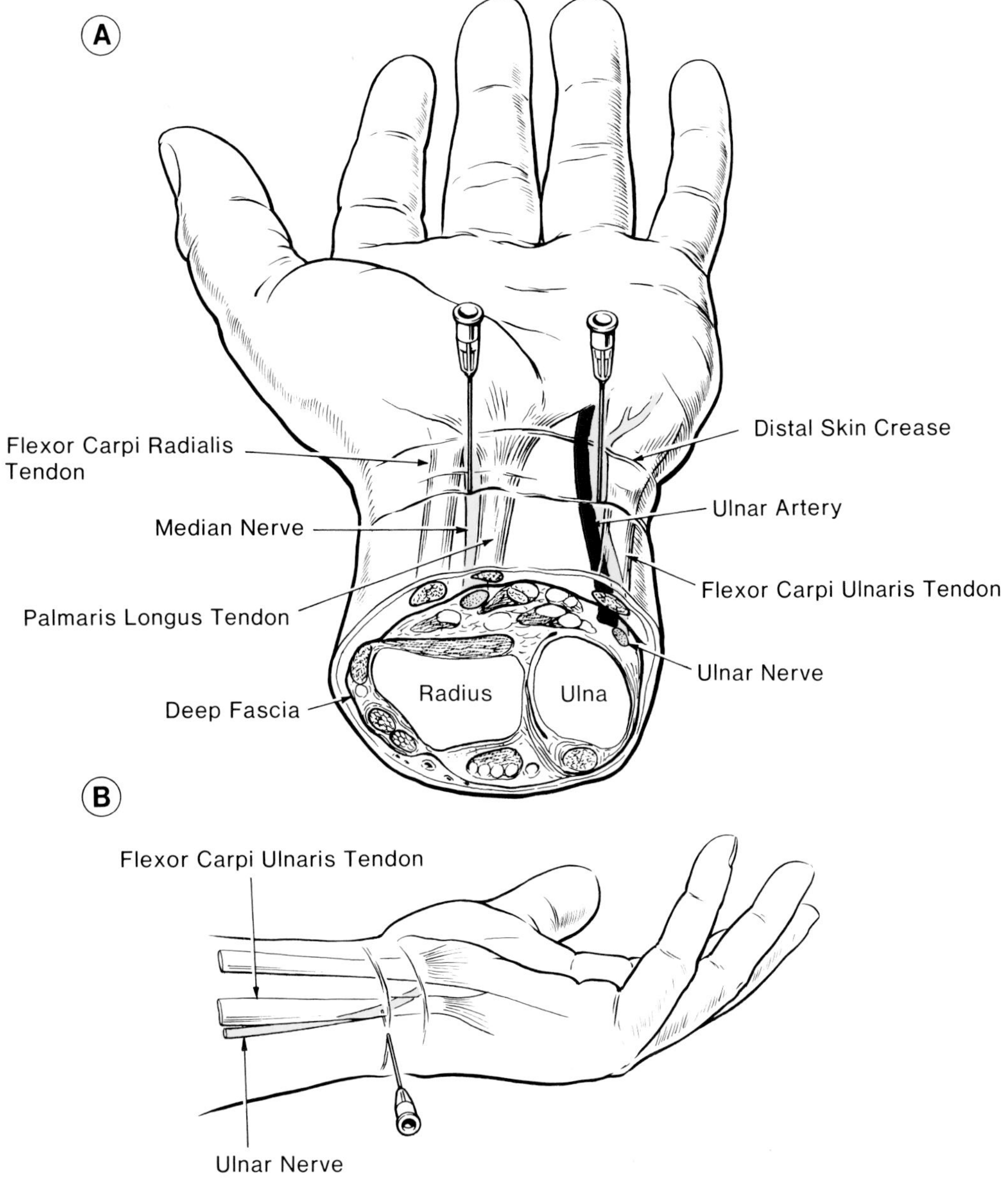

Fig. 10-11. (*A*) Landmarks and technique of needle insertion for median and ulnar nerve block at wrist. (*B*) Alternative method of ulnar nerve block, from ulnar side of wrist.

With nerve block at the wrist, long flexor motor power is retained and this is of considerable value in certain kinds of hand procedures such as tenolysis.[11,25] Peripheral block is always available to supplement patchy brachial plexus anesthesia and furthermore, the ulnar nerve is the most reliable model for testing local anesthetic drugs.[31]

GENERAL CONSIDERATIONS

Tourniquet

An upper arm tourniquet is usually applied before surgery on the limb, and this has often been said to contraindicate peripheral blocks as the method of anesthesia. Up to 30 minutes of tourniquet time is well tolerated by most patients even when they are unpremedicated, and this can easily be extended to an hour with suitable analgesic sedation.[17] A sterile Esmarch bandage should be available for the surgeon to apply *after* skin preparation and marking. The method of application of the tourniquet may also be a factor in patient tolerance.[18] The use of circumferential subcutaneous infiltration, although it is extensively used, would appear to be unnecessary and of very doubtful value.[34]

The Elbow or the Wrist?

There is little to be gained by blocking the nerves at the elbow as opposed to the wrist. Only hand anesthesia results from blocking the three major nerve trunks at the elbow because the forearm cutaneous nerves arise in the upper arm and are quite separate at this level. The wrist block is usually simpler to perform, but it is sometimes preferable to use a combination of the two levels (see Fig. 10-15 for areas of sensory supply of individual nerves of arm).

Paresthesias

As a general rule, anesthesia is quicker in onset and more reliable if paresthesias are sought when blocking the median and ulnar nerves at either elbow or wrist. Care should be taken, however, to avoid injecting the solution intraneurally. Intense paresthesias on injection of a small volume would tend to suggest intraneural placement, and the needle should be either advanced or withdrawn slightly (or both) as the injection is made.

Another method of avoiding intraneural injection is to keep moving the needle in and out while injecting; this will deposit solution superficial and deep to the nerve but has the potential disadvantage of greater needle trauma.[32]

Paresthesias, if they are not elicited on initial insertion, are sought by gentle fanwise insertions across the path of the nerve. If no paresthesias are found, the anesthesiologist should retrace the fan and inject as the needle is moved gently in and out, the aim being to lay down a wall of solution over an area of approximately 2 cm^2 across the path of the nerve.

MEDIAN NERVE BLOCK

Median nerve block is applicable for surgery on the radial side of the palm of the hand and radial three and one-half digits and for reduction of fractures, particularly the first metacarpal. It is usually combined with either ulnar or radial nerve blocks, depending on whether surgery extends to the ulnar side or to the back of the hand. There is also occasional variation in innervation, which may necessitate multiple blocks.

Technique for Block at the Elbow

The arm is abducted on a board with the elbow extended and the forearm supinated. One should stand beside the radial side of the forearm. The intercondylar line between medial and lateral epicondyles of the humerus is drawn across the cubital fossa and the brachial artery palpated and marked at this level (Fig. 10-9). A 23-gauge, 32-mm needle is inserted at a point just medial to the artery and directed perpendicular to the skin (Fig. 10-10). Three to 5 ml should be injected after eliciting paresthesias. If no paresthesias are obtained on initial insertion, the needle should be moved fanwise medially from the artery across the path of the nerve.

Technique for Block at the Wrist

The arm is abducted on a board with the elbow extended and the forearm supinated. One should sit beside the ulnar side of the hand for right arm block and radial side for left arm block.

The palmaris tendon should be made prominent by flexing the wrist against resistance with the fingers extended. The radial border of the tendon should be marked at a point approximately 2 cm proximal to the most distal wrist crease. If the tendon is absent, the point will be approximately 1 cm medial to the ulnar edge of the flexor carpi radialis tendon (Fig. 10-11).

With the wrist slightly extended, a 25-gauge, 16-mm needle is inserted perpendicular to the skin. The nerve is contacted on penetration of the deep fascia, usually at a depth of less than 1 cm (Fig. 10-12).

Three to 5 ml should be injected after eliciting paresthesias. If paresthesias are not obtained on initial insertion, they should be sought in a more ulnar direction under cover of the palmaris tendon. One ml of solution is deposited in the subcutaneous tissue on withdrawal to block the palmar cutaneous branch.

ULNAR NERVE BLOCK

This anesthetic technique is applicable for surgery of the ulnar side of the hand and one and one-half (usually) digits and reduction of fractures of the fifth digit, commonly the neck of the metacarpal. It is often used on its own but may be combined with median and radial nerve blocks. Block of the ulnar nerve at the elbow is often said to lead to residual neuritis. This is probably because where the nerve is palpable, it is well protected by fibrous tissue, and a total intraneural injection is required for success. This approach is quite satisfactory, provided it is performed with a fine needle and only a very small volume, such as 1 ml, is injected.[31] However, it may be preferable to block the nerve 2 to 3 cm proximal to the medial epicondyle with 5 to 8 ml of solution.

Technique of Block at the Elbow

With the patient lying supine, the elbow is flexed with the forearm across the chest. One should stand beside the patient on the side of the arm to be blocked. The medial epicondyle and ulnar groove are palpated and a point taken 2 to 3 cm proximal and along the line of the nerve. A 23-gauge, 32-mm needle is introduced perpendicular to the skin and advanced gently until a paresthesia is obtained or periosteum encountered (Fig. 10-13). Five to 8 ml should be injected following paresthesias. If no paresthesias are obtained on initial insertion, the needle should be moved fanwise across the path of the nerve until they are elicited. No paresthesias will probably result in a long delay or inadequate anesthesia.

Technique of Block at the Wrist

Ulnar block at the wrist is more reliable and carries less risk of complications than block of the ulnar nerve at the elbow. The arm is abducted on a board with the elbow extended and the forearm supinated. One should sit beside the ulnar side of the hand.

At the wrist, the ulnar nerve is blocked where it lies under cover of the flexor capri ulnaris tendon just proximal to the pisiform bone before the nerve bifurcates into its terminal deep (motor) and superficial (sensory) branches. At this point, the nerve lies on the ulnar side of, but deep to, the ulnar artery, and it has already given off its palmar cutaneous and dorsal branches (Fig. 10-12).

The nerve may be approached either from the volar aspect of the wrist, with the needle directed dorsally from the radial side of the flexor carpi ulnaris tendon, or preferably from the ulnar side of the tendon with the needle directed radially for a distance of approximately 1.5 cm (Fig. 10-11). A 25-gauge, 16-mm needle is again most suitable, and 3 to 5 ml is injected following eliciting of paresthesias. It is important to seek paresthesias with this second approach in case the needle comes into a plane anterior to the neurovascular bundle and thus anterior to a thick fascial layer. The approach from the side of the wrist is preferred because it is possible to block the cutaneous branches from the same site of entry. Also, there is probably less chance of damaging the ulnar artery.

If necessary, the two cutaneous branches may be blocked before completely removing the needle. The dorsal branch by subcutaneous infiltration of 2 to 3 ml back along the ulnar border of the carpus and the palmar branch by directing the needle onto the volar aspect of the wrist as far as the radial side of the flexor carpi ulnaris tendon and injecting 1 to 2 ml (Fig. 10-12).

RADIAL NERVE BLOCK

This is an easy and very useful block at the wrist to interrupt the terminal cutaneous branches that supply the radial side of the dorsum of the hand and proximal parts of the radial three and one-half (usually) digits. It is often combined with a median nerve block.

Block at the elbow is more difficult and uncertain and has limited application. It may be combined with block of the lateral cutaneous nerve of the forearm for arteriovenous fistula surgery at the wrist, and it may be needed to supplement inadequate plexus block, particularly when fractures of the radius are involved.

Technique of Block at the Elbow

The radial nerve is blocked as it passes over the anterior aspect of the lateral epicondyle, close to the bone (Fig. 10-9). The arm is abducted on a board with the elbow extended and the forearm supinated. One should stand beside the ulnar side of the arm for left arm block and the radial side for right arm block.

The intercondylar line is marked and the biceps tendon palpated at this level. From a point along the intercondylar line 2 cm lateral to the biceps tendon, a longer (4–5 cm) 23-gauge needle is inserted directly backward onto the bone of the lateral epicondyle towards its lateral margin (Figs. 10-9 and 10-10). The palpating index finger of the left hand on the posterior aspect of the epicondyle is used as a guide to direction. Two to 4 ml is injected as the needle is withdrawn 0.5 to 1 cm. The needle is withdrawn almost to the skin and redirected twice

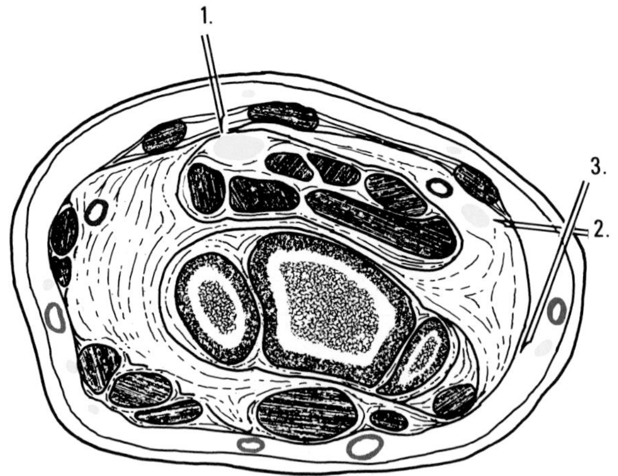

Fig. 10-12. Cross section of forearm at wrist showing alternative method of ulnar nerve block (2) from ulnar side of flexor carpi ulnaris tendon. The dorsal cutaneous branch of the ulnar nerve can also be blocked by redirecting the needle superficially in a dorsal direction (3). Median nerve block (1) is also shown. Note necessity to pierce the deep fascia. However median nerve lies less than 1 cm below the skin.

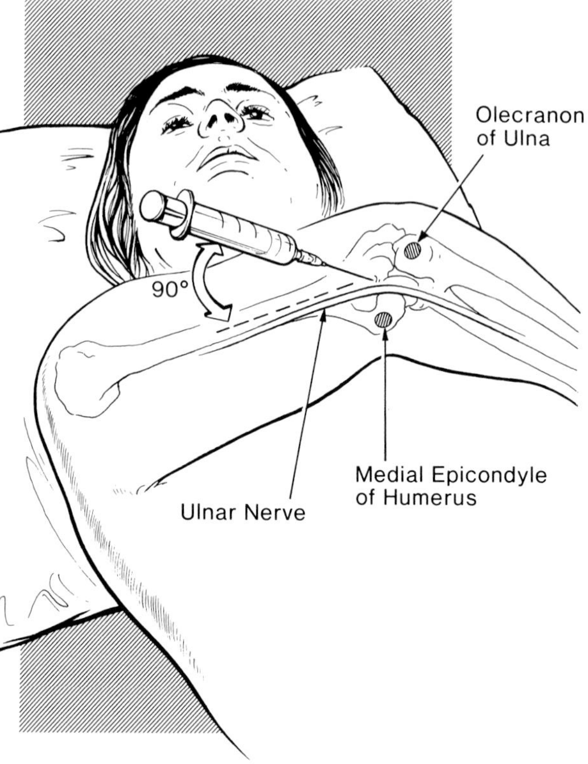

Fig. 10-13. Anatomical landmarks for ulnar nerve block at elbow. Note direction of needle at 90° to humerus.

slightly more medially each time, but again onto bone and further injections made in the same fashion.

Technique of Block at the Wrist

Radial nerve block at the wrist is a field block of the superficial terminal branches as they pass in a variable manner over the radial side of the carpus.

The anatomical "snuffbox" is made prominent by extension of the thumb. The extensor pollicis longus and brevis tendons are both marked. A point is taken over the extensor longus tendon opposite the base of the first metacarpal. A 23-gauge, 32-mm needle is directed proximally along the tendon as far as the dorsal radial tubercle as 2 ml is injected subcutaneously. The needle is withdrawn almost to the

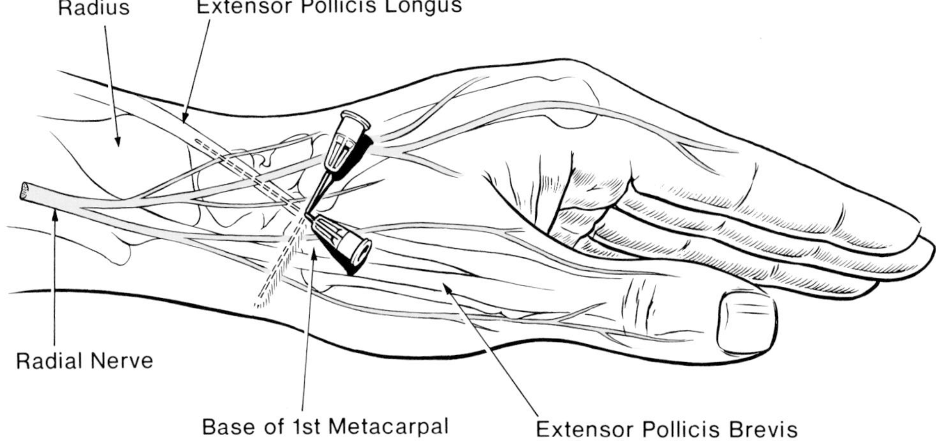

Fig. 10-14. Landmarks and method of needle insertion for radial nerve block at the wrist.

skin and redirected at a right angle across the snuffbox to a point just past the brevis tendon as a further 1 ml is injected (Fig. 10-14).

MUSCULOCUTANEOUS NERVE BLOCK

Block of the musculocutaneous nerve is usually performed as a supplement to axillary plexus block, but it may be indicated as an independent procedure or in combination with block of the radial nerve.

Firstly, it may be blocked as the main nerve trunk in the substance of the coracobrachialis muscle from the same point of entry as in the axillary block procedure.[14] Secondly, it may be blocked 5 cm proximal to the elbow crease where the terminal sensory lateral cutaneous nerve of the forearm is said to emerge from between the brachialis and biceps muscles.[14] Thirdly, a more recent technique has been described where the block is performed just lateral to the tendon of the biceps muscle at the level of the intercondylar line. Olson has shown in 64 cadaver dissections that the nerve, rather than emerging from the brachialis biceps groove and running down over the cubital fossa superficially and somewhat lateral to the biceps tendon, stays deep to the fascia and close in under cover of the lateral side of the tendon, before it becomes superficial at a variable distance distal to the elbow crease.[36] Lastly, the musculocutaneous nerve may be blocked as a subcutaneous field block.

Technique for Blocking Lateral to the Tendon of the Biceps Muscle. The arm is abducted on a board with the elbow extended and the forearm supinated; the intercondylar line and biceps tendon are marked. A 25-gauge, 16-mm needle is inserted at the point at which the intercondylar line crosses the lateral border of the biceps tendon, and 2 ml of anesthetic is injected deep to the fascia, just lateral to the tendon. Failures of block result from too deep an insertion (Fig. 10-10).

This method is more definitive than block in the biceps brachialis groove, much less solution is required, and it can be performed in a few seconds.

FIELD BLOCK OF THE CUTANEOUS NERVES OF THE FOREARM

The *lateral cutaneous nerve* often does not pierce the deep fascia until it is distal to the elbow crease (see above). Subcutaneous infiltration should begin from a point 5 cm distal to the crease and in line with the biceps tendon, thence directed laterally for a distance of 3 to 4 cm.

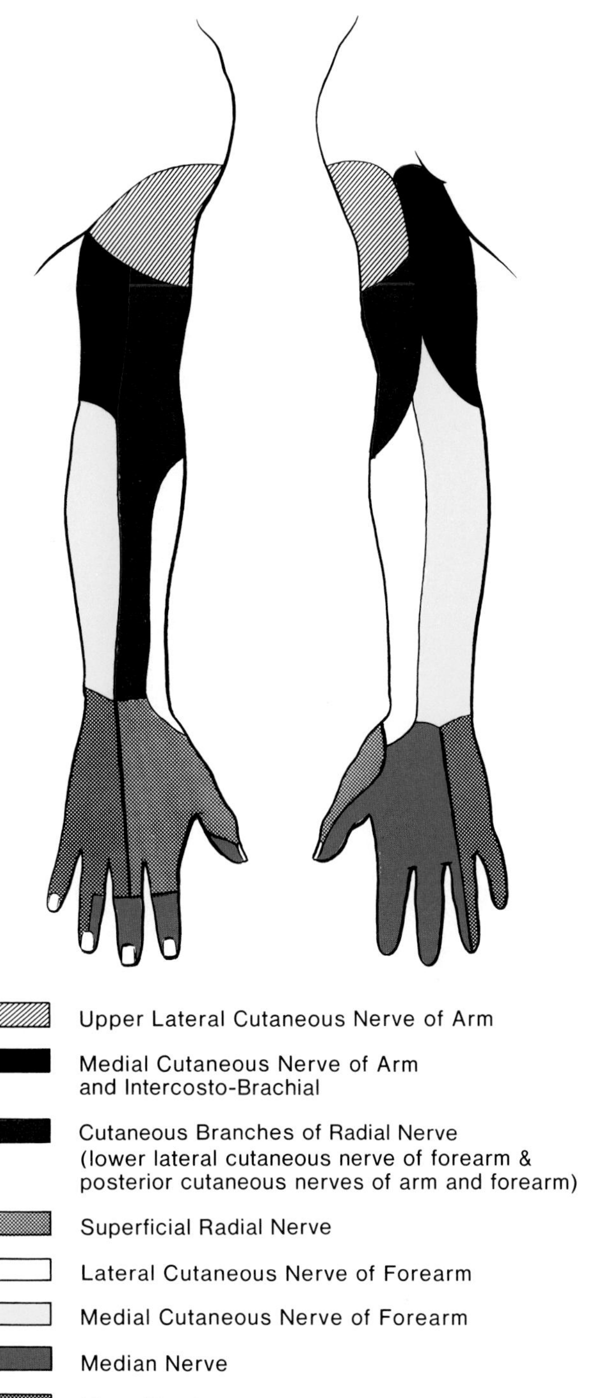

The *medial cutaneous nerve of the forearm* arises from the medial cord of the brachial plexus in the axilla. It pierces the deep fascia in company with

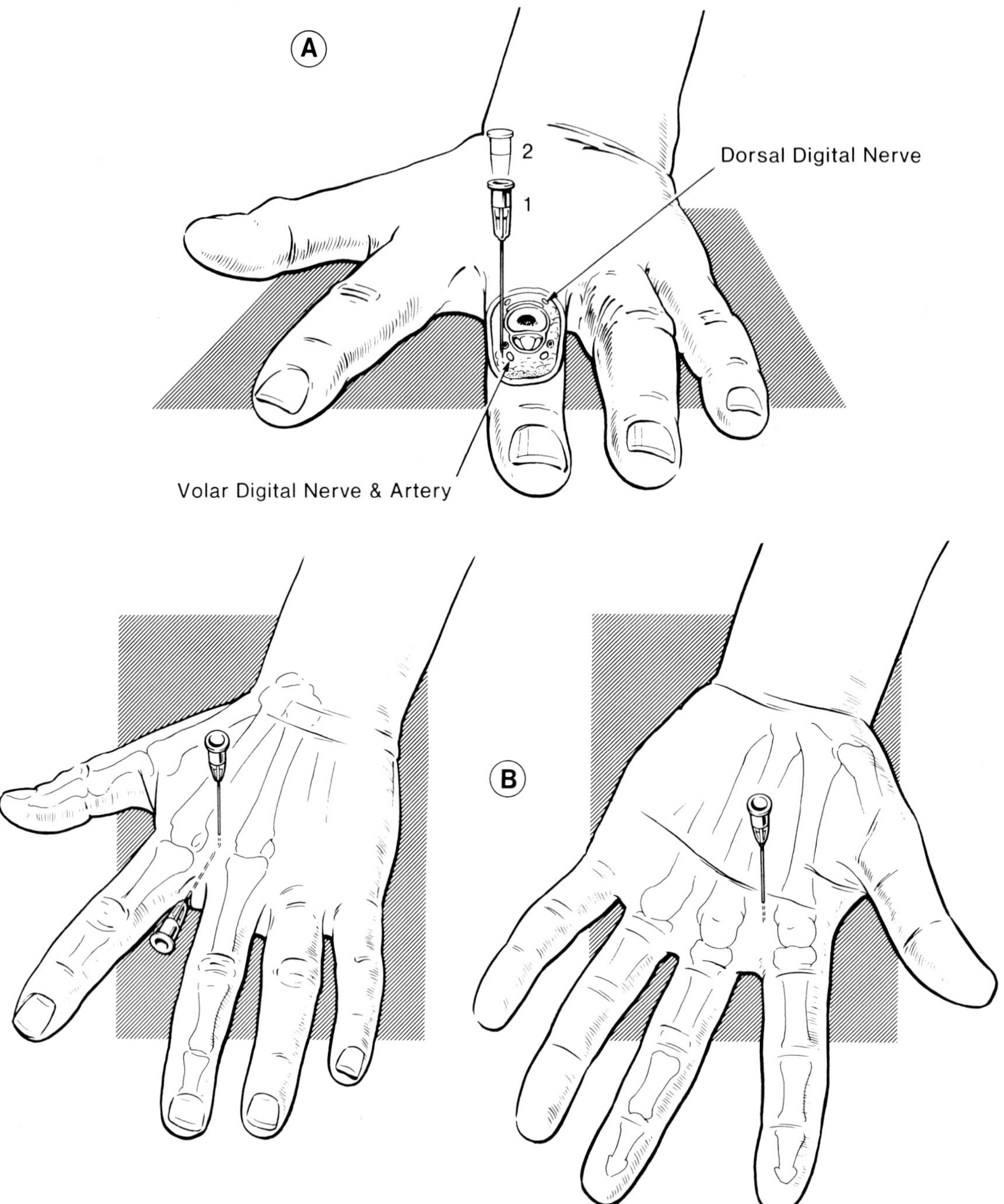

Fig. 10-16. (*A*) Technique of digital nerve block at base of finger. (*B*) Techniques of block of common volar digital nerves between metacarpal heads.

the basilic vein in the midarm and then bifurcates. Its anterior or volar branch passes down over the front of the cubital fossa medial to the biceps tendon to supply the anteromedial aspect of the forearm. The smaller posterior or ulnar branch passes downward farther back, just in front of the medial epicondyle to supply the posteromedial aspect (Fig. 10-15). Subcutaneous infiltration should extend from the biceps tendon to the medial epicondyle (Fig. 10-10).

The *posterior cutaneous nerve of the forearm* arises from the radial nerve and pierces the deep fascia above the elbow. It descends along the lateral side of the arm and then along the back of the forearm to the wrist. From a point directly over the lateral epicondyle of the humerus with the elbow slightly flexed, subcutaneous infiltration should extend for 3 to 4 cm toward the olecranon.

LOCAL ANESTHETIC BLOCK OF THE DIGITAL NERVES

Digital nerve block is a commonly used and very effective method of anesthesia for a wide variety of minor outpatient surgical procedures on the digits. However, because of the rare but serious complications of ischemia and necrosis, it should not be undertaken lightly; alternatives such as nerve block at the wrist should be considered, particularly when more than one digit is involved. When digital nerve block is used, certain aspects of technique must be strictly followed.

Anatomy

The common digital nerves are derived from the median and ulnar nerves and divide in the distal palm into the volar digital nerves to supply adjacent sides of the fingers, palmar aspect, tip and nail bed area. These main digital nerves are accompanied by digital vessels and run on the ventrolateral aspect of the finger beside the flexor tendon sheath. Small dorsal digital nerves derived from the radial and ulnar nerves supply the back of the fingers as far as the proximal joint. These run on the dorsolateral aspect of the finger.

Techniques

Block of Both Volar and Dorsal Digital Nerves at Each Side of the Base of the Finger. A 25-gauge, 16-mm needle is inserted at a point on the dorsolateral aspect of the base of the finger and directed anteriorly to slide past the base of the phalanx (Fig. 10-16*A*. The needle is advanced until the anesthesiologist feels the resistance of the palmar dermis or the pressure on a "protective" finger placed under the patient's finger and directly opposite the needle path. One ml of solution is injected as the needle is withdrawn 2 to 3 mm to block the volar nerve, and 0.5 ml is injected just under the point of entry to block the dorsal nerve. The volar digital nerves can also be approached from the side of the finger.

Block of the Common Volar Digital Nerves near Their Bifurcation Between the Metacarpal Heads. With the fingers widely extended, a 25-gauge, 16-mm needle is inserted into the web 2 to 3 mm dorsal to the junction of the web and palmar skin. It is directed straight back toward the hand in line with the extended fingers, and 2 ml of solution is injected when the needle almost reaches the hub (Fig. 10-16*B*).

Redirection from the same point of entry to the region of the dorsal nerves on each side can easily be performed, if necessary.

A metacarpal approach may also be performed either from the dorsal aspect and inserting the needles between the bones almost as far as the palmar skin or from the palmar aspect at the level of the distal crease and inserting a short fine needle just through the palmar aponeurosis.[8,9,39] (Fig. 10-16*B*). This second approach would seem to be unnecessarily painful. For these digital blocks, lower concentrations of local anesthetics are very satisfactory and *must be used without vasoconstrictors*.

INFILTRATION OF FRACTURE SITES

The principle of this technique is to render insensitive the periosteum in the region of the bony fracture. It has most commonly been applied in the treatment of Colles' fractures. The results under expert, careful, and patient hands would appear to be satisfactory.[15]

Technique. Under very strict aseptic conditions 10 to 15 ml (in the case of Colles) of 1 per cent lidocaine or prilocaine without adrenaline are injected into the periosteum at and around the fracture site from the dorsal aspect. At least 10 minutes must then elapse before the fracture is gently manipulated.

This technique is not recommended for routine use, not only because of the risk of infection and the possibility of rapid uptake of the local anesthetic, but also because it does not produce the satisfactory analgesia or muscle relaxation of appropriate nerve conduction anesthesia.

COMPLICATIONS AND CONTRAINDICATIONS

The only complication specific to these peripheral blocks, apart from those already mentioned, is vascular insufficiency and gangrene following digital nerve block. This catastrophe is a result of digital artery occlusion together with failure of adequate collateral circulation and a number of causative factors may be involved.

Epinephrine-Containing Solutions. Although not the only cause of gangrene, vasoconstrictor solutions in this region have undoubtedly been responsible for many cases in the past and should never be used.

Volume of Solution. The mechanical pressure effects of injecting solution in a relatively confined space should always be borne in mind, particularly in blocks at the base of the digit. Maximum volumes of 2 ml on each side should not be exceeded.

Tourniquets are commonly applied to produce a bloodless field (and perhaps in the hope that it would both hasten and prolong anesthesia). Bradfield, in a report on 44 cases of gangrene, could not exonerate the tourniquet but recommended that an upper limit of 15 minutes' duration could be set and that it never be used in patients with Raynaud's phenomena.[6] Bunnell has completely condemned the use of rubber-band type tourniquets at the base of the digit and has stated that whenever a tourniquet is to be required, a proper upper arm tourniquet should be applied.[5]

Peripheral Vascular Disease. In patients with small vessel disease, perhaps an alternative method should be sought in addition to avoidance of digital tourniquet.

Direct vascular damage by the needle may contribute to the complication.

The incidence of digital gangrene is unknown. Even in reported cases, the duration of the tourniquet and other important facts are often not recorded. With the present level of knowledge, it would seem wise to avoid vasoconstrictors; avoid a digital tourniquet or certainly limit its duration to 15 minutes; use small volumes of solution; avoid digital blocks in patients whose vessels may be suspect; and, as with all nerve blocks, be gentle and patient.

A source of infection in close proximity to the proposed site of injection is probably the main contraindication to nerve blocks on the upper limb.

REFERENCES

1. Accardo, N.J., and Adriani, J.A.: Brachial plexus block—a simplified technique using the axillary route. South. Med. J., *42*:920, 1949.
2. Babitski, P.: A New Method of Anesthetizing the Brachial Plexus. Zentralbl. Chir., *45*:215, 1918.
3. Bazy, L., and Blondin, S.: L'anesthesie du plexus brachial. Anesth. Analg. (Paris), *1*:190, 1935.
4. Bonica, J.J., Moore, D.C., and Orlov, M.: Brachial plexus block anesthesia. Am. J. Surg., 65, 1949.
5. Boyes, J.H.: Bunnell's Surgery of the Hand. Ed. 5. Philadelphia, J.B. Lippincott, 1970.
6. Bradfield, W.J.D.: Digital block anesthesia and its complications. Br. J. Surg., *50*:495, 1962.
7. Burnham, P.J.: Simple regional nerve block for surgery of the hand and forearm. J.A.M.A., *169*:109, 1959.
8. Burnham, P.J.: Regional block anaesthesia for surgery of the fingers and thumb. Industrial Medicine and Surgery, *27*:67, 1958.
9. Chase, R.A.: Atlas of Hand Surgery, Philadelphia, W.B. Saunders, 1973.
10. Clayton, M.L., and Turner, D.A.: Upper arm block anesthesia in children with fractures. J.A.M.A., *169*:99, 1959.
11. Conolly, W.B., and Berry, F.R.: Selective peripheral nerve blocks for reconstructive hand surgery. Med. J. Aust., *2*:94, 1974.
12. Crile, G.W.: Anesthesia of nerve roots with cocaine. Cleveland Med. J., *2*:355, 1897.
13. de Jong, R.H.: Axillary block of the brachial plexus. Anesthesiology, *22*:215, 1961.
14. ———: Modified axillary block. Anesthesiology, *26*:615, 1965.
15. Dinley, R.J., and Michelinakis, E.: Local anaesthesia in the reduction of Colles' fracture. Injury, *4*:345, 1972–1973.
16. Dogliotti, A.M.: Anesthesia: Narcosis, Local, Regional, and Spinal. [Authorized English translation by Scuderi, C.S.] Chicago, S.B. Debour, 1939.
17. Dupont, C. *et al.*: Hand surgery under wrist block and local infiltration anesthesia using an upper arm tourniquet. Plast. Reconstr. Surg., *50*:532, 1972.
18. Dushoff, I.M.: Letters to the editor. Plast. Reconstr. Surg., *51*:685, 1973.
19. Eather, K.F.: Axillary brachial plexus block. Anesthesiology, *19*:683, 1958.
20. Erikkson, E.: A simplified method of axillary block. Nord. Med., *68*:1325, 1962.
21. ———: Axillary brachial plexus anaesthesia in children with Citanest. Acta Anaesth. Scand. *16* [*Suppl.*]:291, 1965.
22. Hirschel, G.: Die Anasthesierung des Plexus Brachialis fur die Operationen an der oberen Extremitat. Munchen. Med. Wochenschr., *58*:1555, 1911.
23. Hopcroft, S.C.: The axillary approach to brachial plexus anaesthesia. Anaesth. Intensive Care, *1*:232, 1973.
24. Hudon, F., and Jacques, A.: Block of the brachial plexus by the axillary route. Can. Anaesth. Soc. J., *6*:400, 1959.
25. Hunter, J.M., *et al.*: A dynamic approach to problems of hand function. Clin. Orthop., *104*:112, 1974.
26. Jackson, L., and Keats, A.S.: Mechanism of brachial plexus palsy following anesthesia. Anesthesiology, *26*:190, 1965.
27. Kulenkampff, D.: Die anasthesierung des Plexus Brachialis. Zentralbl. Chir., *38*:1337, 1911.
28. Kumar, A., *et al.*: Bilateral cervical and thoracic epidural blockade complicating interscalene brachial plexus block. Anesthesiology, *35*:650, 1971.
29. Labat, G.: Brachial plexus block: Details of technique with lantern slides. Br. J. Anaesth., *4*:174, 1926–1927.
30. Livingston, E.M., and Werthein, H.: Brachial plexus block: Its clinical application. J.A.M.A., *88*:1464, 1927.
31. Löfström, J.B.: Ulnar nerve blockade for the evaluation of local anaesthetic agents. Br. J. Anaesth., *47*:297, 1975.
32. Löfström, J.B., *et al.*: Late disturbance in nerve function

after block with local anaesthetic agents. Acta Anaesth Scand., *10*:111, 1966.

33. Macintosh, R.R., and Mushin, W.W.: Local Anesthesia: Brachial Plexus. Oxford, Blackwell Scientific Publishers, 1944.
34. Moir, D.D.: Axillary block of the brachial plexus. Anaesthesia, *17*:274, 1962.
35. Neuhof, H.: Supraclavicular anesthetization of the brachial plexus. J.A.M.A., *62*:1629, 1914.
36. Olson, I.A.: The origin of the lateral cutaneous nerve of the forearm and its anesthesia for modified brachial plexus block. J. Anat., *105*:381, 1969.
37. Patrick, J.: The technique of brachial plexus block anesthesia. Br. J. Surg., *27*:734, 1939–1940.
38. Pitkin, W.M., Southworth, J.L., and Hingson, R.A.: Conduction Anesthesia. Philadelphia, J.B. Lippincott, 1953.
39. Rank, B.K., Wakefield, A.R., and Hueston, J.T.: Surgery of Repair as Applied to Hand Injuries. ed. 4. p. 88. Edinburgh, E. & S. Livingstone, 1973.
40. Ross, S., and Scarborough, C.D.: Total spinal anesthesia following brachial plexus block. Anesthesiology, *39*:458, 1973.
41. Sherwood-Dunn, B.: p. 242. Regional Anesthesia. Philadelphia, F.A. Davis, 1920.
42. Strachauer, A.C.: Brachial plexus anesthesia: A complete local anesthesia of upper extremities permitting all major surgical procedures. Lancet, *34*:301, 1914.
43. Ward, M.E.: The interscalene approach to the brachial plexus. Anaesthesia, *29*:147, 1974.
44. Webling, D.D.: Anaesthesia of the upper limb for casualty procedures. Med. J. Aust., *2*:496, 1960.
45. Wen–Hsien, W.U.: Brachial plexus block. J.A.M.A., *215*:1953, 1971.
46. Winnie, A.P.: Recent developments in anesthesia. Surg. Clin. North Am., *55*:878, 1975.
47. ———: The perivascular techniques of brachial plexus anaesthesia. A.S.A. Refresher Courses in Anesthesiology, *2*:151, 1974.
48. ———: Interscalene brachial plexus block. Anesth. Analg. (Cleve.), *49*:455, 1970.
49. ———: An "immobile" needle for nerve blocks. Anesthesiology, *31*:577, 1969.
50. Winnie, A.P., and Collins, V.J.: The subclavian perivascular technique to brachial plexus anaesthesia. Anesthesiology, *25*:353, 1964.
51. Winnie, A.P., *et al.*: Interscalene cervical plexus block. Anesth. Analg. (Cleve.), *54*:370, 1975.

11 The Lower Extremity: Somatic Blockade

Phillip O. Bridenbaugh

Although there are many anatomic similarities between the innervation and bony landmarks of the upper and lower extremities, there are fewer techniques for peripheral neural blockade of the lower extremity than for the upper extremity, and the enthusiasm for performing them is not as great. It is very probable that peridural or subarachnoid anesthesia, which provides rapid, complete, safe anesthesia of the lower extremities, is more easily accomplished by anesthesiologists than lower extremity peripheral neural blockade. Furthermore, although it is possible to accomplish complete anesthesia of the upper extremity with a single injection, that is still not the case with the lower extremity. Nonetheless, peripheral neural blockade of the lower limb is easily accomplished with a minimum of side-effects and should have a place in the armamentarium of the anesthesiologist who uses regional anesthesia as part of his overall practice.

Like other forms of peripheral neural blockade, lower extremity techniques are not new. Braun mentions that blockade of the lateral cutaneous femoral nerve was described by Nystrom in 1909.[2] Laewen expanded on this by describing the additional blockade of the anterior crural nerve, and Keppler improved both techniques by advocating the elicitation of paresthesias. Earlier than all of this—around 1887—Crile performed amputations by exposing the sciatic nerve in the gluteal fold and the femoral nerve in the inguinal fold and injecting cocaine intraneurally. Subsequently, no fewer than six others advocated percutaneous approaches to the sciatic nerve alone. Some of these same authors wrote about blockade of other nerves of the leg as well (see Chap. 1).

Not only is this old concept still valid today, but many of the techniques are nearly identical to the original descriptions. This emphasizes remarks made by Labat that "Anatomy is the foundation upon which the entire concept of regional anesthesia is built;" that "Landmarks are anatomic guideposts of the body which are used to locate the nerves;" that "Superficial landmarks are distinguishing features of the surface of the body which can be easily recognized and identified by sight or palpation. Bones and their prominences, blood vessels and tendons serve as landmarks. Deep landmarks can be defined only by the point of the needle. They are the only reliable guide for advancing the needle in attempting to reach the vicinity of the nerve;" and that "The anesthetist should attempt to visualize the anatomic structures traversed by the needle and utilize the tactile senses to determine the impulses transmitted by the point of the needle as it approaches a deep landmark (*e.g.*, bone)."[7]

Illustrative of the importance of bony landmarks are the many approaches proposed for blockade of the sciatic nerve. The course of the nerve through the pelvis and medial to the femoral head provides a plethora of bony landmarks, all at some time in the past 100 years having been advocated by someone in his favorite technique.

NERVE SUPPLY

The lumbar plexus is formed in the psoas muscle by the anterior rami of the first four lumbar nerves, including, frequently, a branch from the twelfth thoracic nerve and occasionally one from the fifth lumbar nerve. The sacral plexus is derived from the anterior rami of the fourth and fifth lumbar and the first two or three sacral nerves.

While the lumbosacral plexus as a whole contributes to the nerve supply of the lower extremities, the upper part of the lumbar division supplies the iliohypogastric and ilioinguinal nerves, which are in series with the thoracic nerves and innervate the trunk above the level of the extremity (see Chap. 14). Specifically, the iliohypogastric nerve provides cutaneous innervation to the skin of the buttock and the muscles of the abdominal wall. The ilioinguinal nerve supplies the skin at the base of the perineum and adjoining portion of the inner thigh. A third nerve, the genitofemoral, arises from the first and second lumbar nerves. It supplies filaments to the genital area and adjacent parts of the thigh. It also gives off a lumboinguinal branch, which supplies the skin over the area of the femoral artery and femoral triangle.

Caudad to these nerves are the major nerves that supply all of the lower extremity. Details of their course and distribution will be covered individually.

In brief, there are five major nerves to the lower extremity. The *lateral femoral cutaneous nerve,* the *femoral nerve* (sometimes called the *anterior crural nerve*), and the *obturator nerve* are derived from the lumbar plexus, along with minor contributions from the iliohypogastric, ilioinguinal, and genitofemoral. The two remaining nerves are the *posterior cutaneous nerve of the thigh* and the *sciatic nerve.* The posterior cutaneous nerve has sometimes been referred to as the "small sciatic" nerve. It derives from the first, second, and third sacral nerves, as does the larger sciatic nerve, which also receives branches of the anterior rami of the fourth and fifth lumbar nerves. Inasmuch as the two nerves course through the pelvis together and out through the greater sciatic foramen, they are considered together when techniques for blocking the sciatic nerve are discussed.

The sciatic nerve is really an association of two major nerve trunks. The first is the tibial, derived from the ventral branches of the anterior rami of the fourth and fifth lumbar and first, second, and third sacral nerves. The second is the common peroneal, derived from the dorsal branches of the anterior rami of the same five nerves. These two major nerve trunks pass as the sciatic to the proximal angle of the popliteal fossa, where they separate with the tibial portion passing medially and the common peroneal (lateral popliteal) laterally.

The smaller branches of these four nerves, which provide distal innervation of the lower extremity, are discussed in detail in conjunction with techniques for nerve block at the knee and ankle.

LUMBAR SOMATIC NERVE BLOCK

Anatomy

In considering neural blockade of the lower extremity at the lumbar level, the bony, muscular, and fascial relationships to the emerging nerves must be recalled. The spinal nerve that comes off the spinal cord at each level is formed by the union of a ventral motor root with a dorsal sensory root. This mixed spinal nerve gives off a dorsal ramus, a ventral ramus, and a ramus communicans, which contributes to the formation of the sympathetic ganglion and trunk. The lumbar plexus, as previously noted, is formed by the anterior (ventral) divisions of the first, second, third, and fourth lumbar nerves with about 50 per cent inclusion of a branch from the twelfth thoracic nerve and occasionally from the fifth lumbar. The lumbar plexus is formed in front of the transverse processes of the lumbar vertebrae into a series of oblique loops that lie deep in the substance of the psoas major muscle and at the medial border of the quadratus lumborum muscle. From here, the individual nerves form and course in the direction of their terminal innervation.

The relationship of the lumbar somatic plexus to the sympathetic chain should be remembered as each may be blocked separately but with a similar approach. The first and second lumbar spinal nerves, frequently the third, and sometimes the fourth, send communicating rami to form the lumbar portion of the sympathetic trunk. The sympathetic trunk lies on the ventrolateral surface of the lumbar and sacral bodies medial to the anterior foramina. It is apparent, therefore, that although these two nerve systems are separated by distance, muscle, and tissue planes, they have considerable intercommunication (Fig. 11-1).

Technique

The standard approach to blockade of the lumbar somatic nerves is paravertebral. The original writings of Labat and Pitkin advocate having the patient lying on the side opposite the one to be blocked. Additionally, a soft roll placed between the iliac crest and the costal margin will minimize the lateral spinal curvature. A preferred position, in the healthy patient, is that of having the patient lie prone over a soft pillow, which will flatten (or elevate) the lumbar curve. Regardless of position, the landmarks used are the spinous processes of the lumbar vertebrae. Skin wheals are raised opposite the cephalad aspect of the spinous processes, on a line 3 to 4 cm laterally from and parallel to the midline of the back (see Fig. 14-8). Depending upon the size of the patient, an 8- or 10-cm needle is inserted through each of the skin wheals and advanced perpendicular to the surface of the skin until its tip comes in contact with the transverse process of the vertebral body, usually at a depth of 4 to 5 cm. The needle is then partially withdrawn and reintroduced slightly more cephalad and medially, making an angle of about 25° with the saggital plane of the body. This should allow the needle to pass just tan-

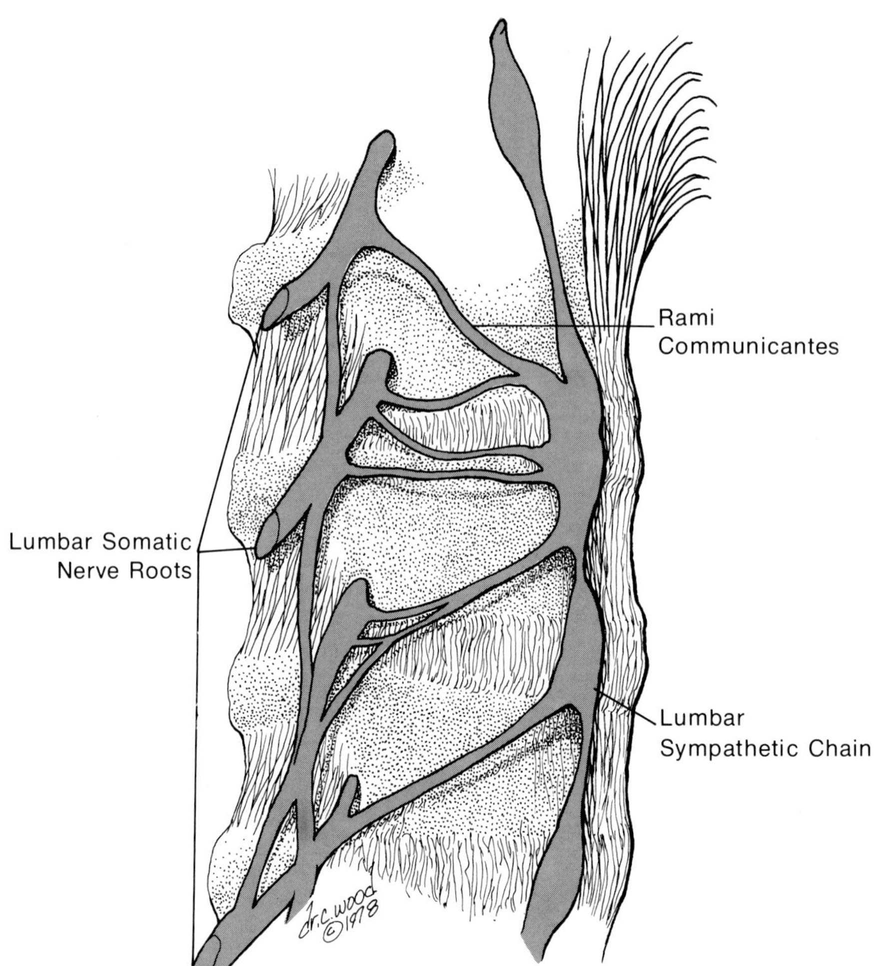

Fig. 11-1. Relationship of lumbar sympathetic chain to the somatic nerve roots. (Drawn by Dr. Charles D. Wood)

gential to the superior aspect of the transverse process and to be advanced an additional 2 to 3 cm. Paresthesias may frequently develop. If so, 8 to 10 ml of the selected local anesthetic solution should be injected. If no paresthesias are elicited, the solution is distributed in front of the transverse process while the needle is moved slightly in and out. It should be remembered that the spinous processes of the lumbar vertebrae do not slope downward as do the thoracic spines, their upper and lower borders being more nearly horizontal. Their average thickness is from 0.5 to 1 cm. The distance between the tip of the spine and its attachment to the vertebral lamina is approximately 3 to 4 cm. A horizontal line drawn tangential to the superior aspect of the spine will overlie the transverse process of that vertebrae. The transverse processes of the lumbar vertebrae are short, accounting for the paravertebral skin wheal being only 2 to 3 cm from the midline. The average depth of the transverse process to the skin is 5 cm, which varies with the size of the patient and the paraspinous musculature. The transverse processes of L4 and L5 are more deeply situated than those of the vertebrae above. When the needle passes superior to the transverse process, it is in close proximity to the somatic nerve of the preceding segment (*e.g.,* the needle passing over the transverse process of L1 injects the T12 nerve root, etc.; Fig. 11-2). The L5 root is blocked through the same skin wheal as L4, by redirecting the needle in a caudad direction until it passes from the lower border of the L4 transverse process and injecting the nerve root in a manner similar to the technique used in other roots (see Fig. 14-8).

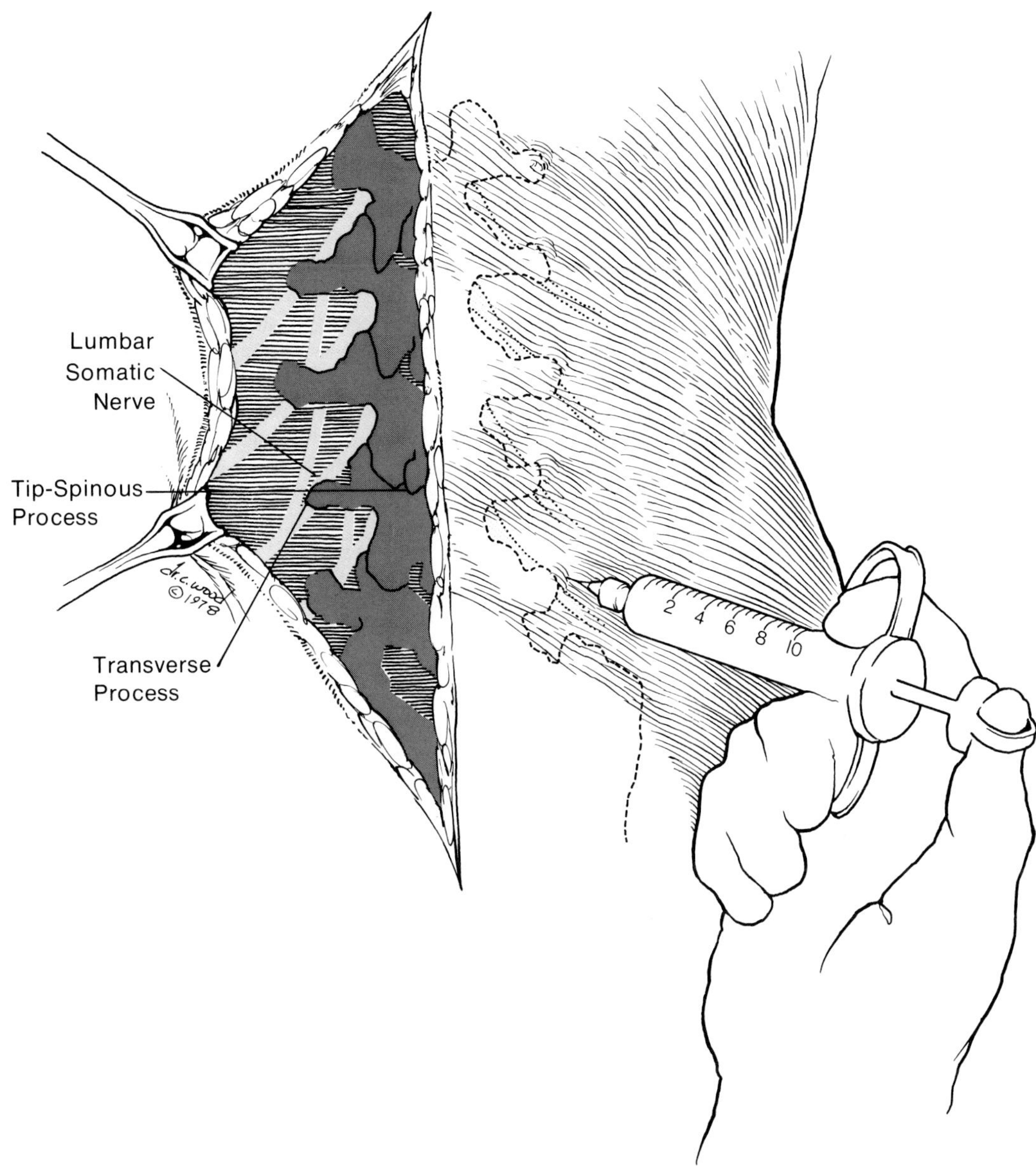

Fig. 11-2. Lumbar somatic nerves and surface landmarks. This drawing illustrates the spine of the vertebral body overlying the transverse process of the next inferior vertebrae. (Drawn by Dr. Charles D. Wood)

A more peripheral approach to the major branches of the lumbar plexus that supply the leg has been described by Winnie.[15] His *inguinal paravascular* technique of lumbar plexus block utilizes the fascial envelope around the femoral nerve as a conduit, which carries injected anesthetic superiorly to the level where the lumbar plexus forms (Fig. 11-3).

As previously noted, the lumbar plexus lies between the quadratus lumborum muscle posteriorly and the psoas major muscle anteriorly, being inverted, therefore, by the fasciae of those two muscles. Although the other nerves to the leg take divergent courses through the pelvis, the femoral nerve descends from under the psoas muscle and remains in the groove between the psoas and iliacus muscle. Superior to the inguinal ligament, the femoral nerve is then in a fascial sheath with the anterior covering being provided by the transversalis fascia.

Inguinal Paravascular Block

The technique for inguinal paravascular block is very similar to the technique for femoral nerve block. The patient lies supine with the anesthesiologist standing next to the side that is to be blocked. After careful palpation, a skin wheal is raised just lateral to the femoral artery where it emerges distal to the inguinal ligament. A short-bevel 22-gauge needle with translucent hub, connected by means of a short segment of plastic tubing to a syringe filled with anesthetic, is inserted just over the tip of the palpating finger in a cephalad direction. A paresthesia of the femoral nerve must be produced, as an indication that the tip of the needle is within the fascial sheath. The needle is then fixed, and the desired volume of local anesthetic is injected while firm digital pressure is applied just distal to the needle in an attempt to force the flow of local anesthetic proximally into the area of the lumbar plexus. The appropriate volume of local anesthetic to be injected may be calculated by dividing the patient's height in inches by a factor of 3.

Indication

The lumbar plexus and its somatic nerves supply not only the cutaneous nerves to the upper thigh but also to the lower abdominal area. (Analgesia for the abdomen is covered more completely in Chap. 14.) It should be kept in mind that lumbar paravertebral block alone or in conjunction with intercostal nerve block can provide somatic anesthesia of the lower abdominal wall in the poor-risk patient for whom it is necessary to avoid the side-effects of sympathetic block associated with spinal or lumbar epidural anesthesia. Lumbar somatic block is also indicated in patients who for some reason cannot be given a spinal or epidural anesthetic.

More important, branches of the first three lumbar nerves provide cutaneous distribution to the inner and outer aspects of the thigh and the anterior gluteal region along with adjacent perineal and suprapubic areas. With lumbar plexus block, it is possible to block these fibers. If the five major peripheral nerve blocks are performed, however, and procedures proximal to the midthigh are anticipated, then paravertebral blockade of the appropriate nerves is indicated. In contrast, lumbar somatic blockade alone will not be sufficient for complete anesthesia of the lower extremity, because this block cannot achieve blockade of the sacral roots that supply the sciatic nerve.

Side-Effects and Complications

For purposes of clarification, *side-effects,* as the word is used here, are physiologic occurrences that result from a particular technique or local anesthetic agent, which may not be desirable in a particular patient. The classic example is sympathetic nerve blockade. In theory, a carefully performed paravertebral lumbar somatic nerve block should not give rise to blockade of the lumbar sympathetic fibers. Nonetheless, in clinical practice, local anesthetic may reach the sympathetic chain, and the anesthesiologist should watch for such side-effects, especially in the hypovolemic patient in whom the magnitude of response (usually hypotension) may be exaggerated.

A rare complication of the parvertebral approach to neural blockade is that of subarachnoid injection. In a large patient with considerable soft tissue overlying the paraspinous area, a needle introduced at a slight medial angle can quite easily pass into the interspace and accomplish what is referred to in spinal anesthesia terms as a *paramedian approach* to the subarachnoid space (see Chap. 7).

Finally, anterior to the vertebral column are major blood vessels. If caution is not observed in recalling or marking the depth of the transverse process when the anesthesiologist is advancing the needle to the level of the lumbar plexus, it is quite possible to insert the needle too deeply and enter these vessels. Careful aspiration prior to injection of local anesthetic solutions should prevent the serious complication of direct intravascular injection, with a likely systemic toxic reaction. Mere needle entry into a normal blood vessel without injection of drug is usually of no consequence. The most frequently encountered vessel with the right paravertebral approach is the inferior vena cava—and on the left, of course, is the aorta.

SACRAL PLEXUS NERVE BLOCK

Since the derivation of the sciatic nerve comes in part from spinal roots S1–3, it is apparent that blockade of these roots must be combined with the aforementioned lumbar somatic block if complete anesthesia of the lower extremity is to be obtained by paravertebral blockade.

Anatomy

The sacral plexus is formed by the union of the first three sacral nerves and the fourth and fifth lumbar nerves. It also connects with the ascending division of the fourth sacral nerve. The sacral plexus is located on the anterior surface of the sacrum and is separated from the sacrum by the piriformis muscle. It is covered by the parietal portion of the pelvic fascia. In front of it lie the ureter, the pelvic colon, part of the rectum, and the iliac artery and vein. The plexus gives off two sets of branches—the collateral and the terminal. The collateral branches (anterior and posterior) supply the pudendal plexus, the hip joint, the gluteal structures, and the adductor and hamstring muscles. More pertinent to this discussion, the terminal branches supply the greater and lesser sciatic nerves.

The sacrum is the wedge-shaped, fused lower five sacral vertebrae attached by joints and ligaments to the iliac bones. On its posterior surface are two rows of openings—the posterior sacral foramina, present on each side of the fused spinous processes. The posterior divisions of the sacral nerves pass through these foramina to the soft tissues of the sacral region at the back. Although these rows of foramina are not exactly parallel, angling toward the midline, they are not as steeply angulated as the edges of the sacrum. This is an important point to bear in mind when surface landmarks are plotted (Fig. 11-4).

Another important anatomic relationship is that of the anterior sacral foramina to the homologous posterior foramina, thereby constituting the transsacral canal. The depth of the canal varies from 2.5 cm at the level of S1 to 0.5 cm, at S4. It is important to have these figures in mind when blocking the sacral nerves by the transsacral method; otherwise, the needle may be introduced into the pelvis.

Technique

For transsacral block, the patient is prone over a pillow placed under the hips. The posterior superior iliac spine and the sacral cornu are both palpated and marked. A skin wheal is raised immediately lateral to and above the sacral cornu, and another placed 1 cm medial to and below the posterior superior iliac spine of the side to be blocked. The distance between the wheals is divided into thirds, and two additional wheals are raised at these sites. Those four wheals thus identify the second, third, fourth, and fifth sacral foramina. The first sacral foramen is found by placing a wheal 2.5 to 3 cm above the second and on the same line as the others. The thickness of the soft tissues overlying the sacrum is greater superiorly—and, therefore, requires longer needles—than the lower segments. An 8- to 10-cm, 22-gauge needle is satisfactory for S1 and S2 and a 5-cm needle for the lower segments. The second foramen is often easiest to locate and thus usually attempted first. This helps in locating the others. The needle is inserted toward the posterior aspect of the sacrum, inclined slightly medially until striking bone. The needle is then withdrawn and reintroduced until it enters the respective transsacral canal. The needle is advanced approximately 2 to 2.5 cm into the first sacral canal and in 0.5 cm decrements for each succeeding canal. Similarly, 5 to 7 ml of solution should be injected into the first sacral foramen, the volume being reduced by 1 to 1.5 ml for each subsequent injection (Fig. 11-4).

Side-Effects and Complications

Since the sacral nerves represent the parasympathetic portion of the autonomic nervous system, sympathetic blockade and its potential for hypotension are not seen with transsacral block, unless excessive volumes of solution spread proximally to the lumbar sympathetic fibers. Loss of parasympathetic function to bowel, bladder, and sphincters may occur, however. Injection of local anesthetic through misdirected needles into the subarachnoid or vascular compartments is a remote risk. Classically, the dural sac is said to terminate at the lower border of S2. However, there are enough clinical reports of subarachnoid puncture with a 3-cm caudal needle to suggest the individual variations below this "classic" location. Finally, appreciation of the pelvic contents, especially colon, rectum, and bladder, should alert one to the risks of infection and contamination. Should a deeply inserted needle enter the colon or rectum and not be noticed, it could result in seeding fecal material into the sacral canals.

Indications

The combined lumbosacral paravertebral approach to neural blockade of the lower extremity conserves neither the number of needle insertions nor the total volume of solution used, compared to the more traditional "four-nerve block" approach to be described. It does offer the benefit of anesthesia over the upper thigh, hip, and perineum, which the peripheral nerve blocks do not. It may thus be used for high amputations and for the relief of sciatic pain. It is also useful when immediate access to

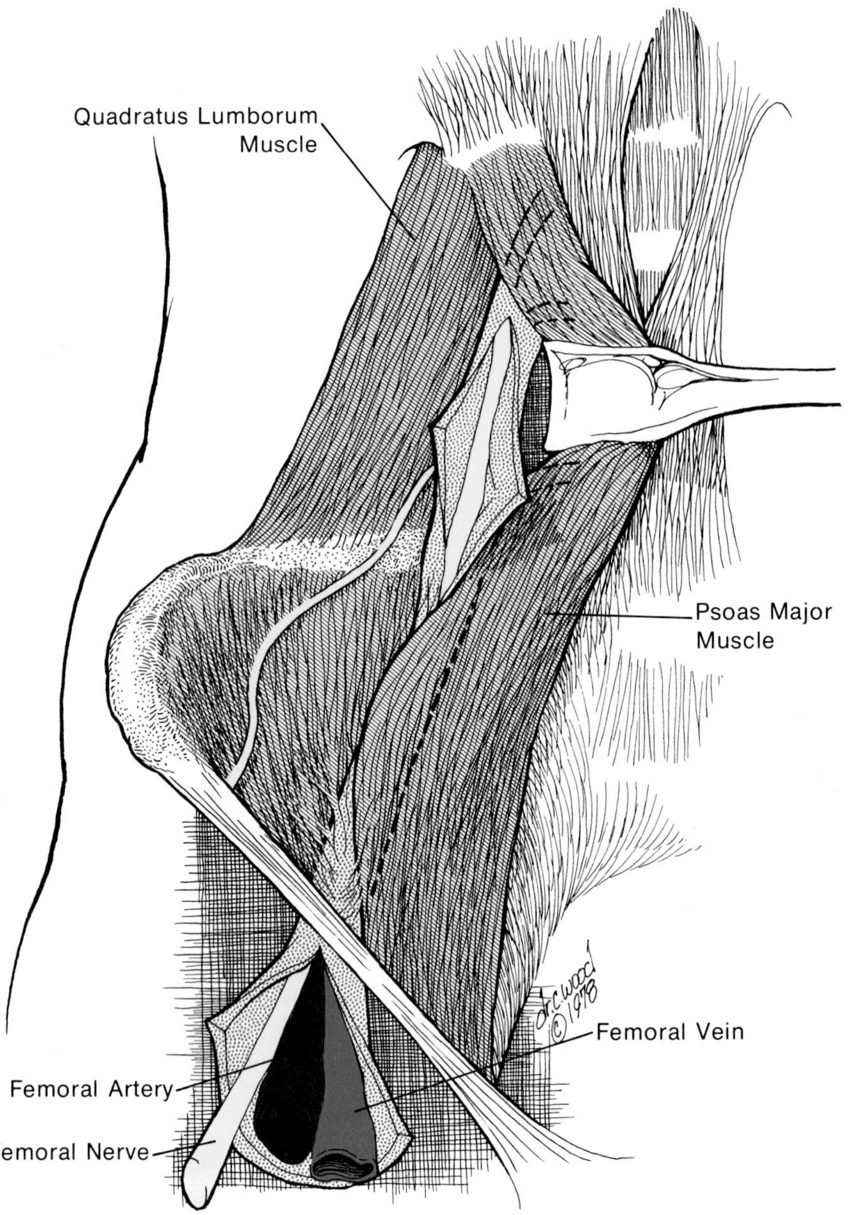

Fig. 11-3. Paravascular relationships of inguinal area. (Drawn by Dr. Charles D. Wood)

the nerves is not possible, owing to trauma, infection, and so forth.

SCIATIC NERVE BLOCK

Anatomy

The largest of the four major nerves supplying the leg is the sciatic nerve (L4–5, S1–3). The sciatic nerve, as previously noted, arises from the sacral plexus where it is nearly 2 cm in width as it leaves the pelvis in company with the posterior cutaneous nerve of the thigh. It passes from the pelvis through the sacrosciatic foramen beneath the lower margin of the piriformis muscle, and between the tuberosity of the ischium and the greater trochanter of the femur. The nerve becomes superficial at the lower border of the gluteus maximus muscle. From

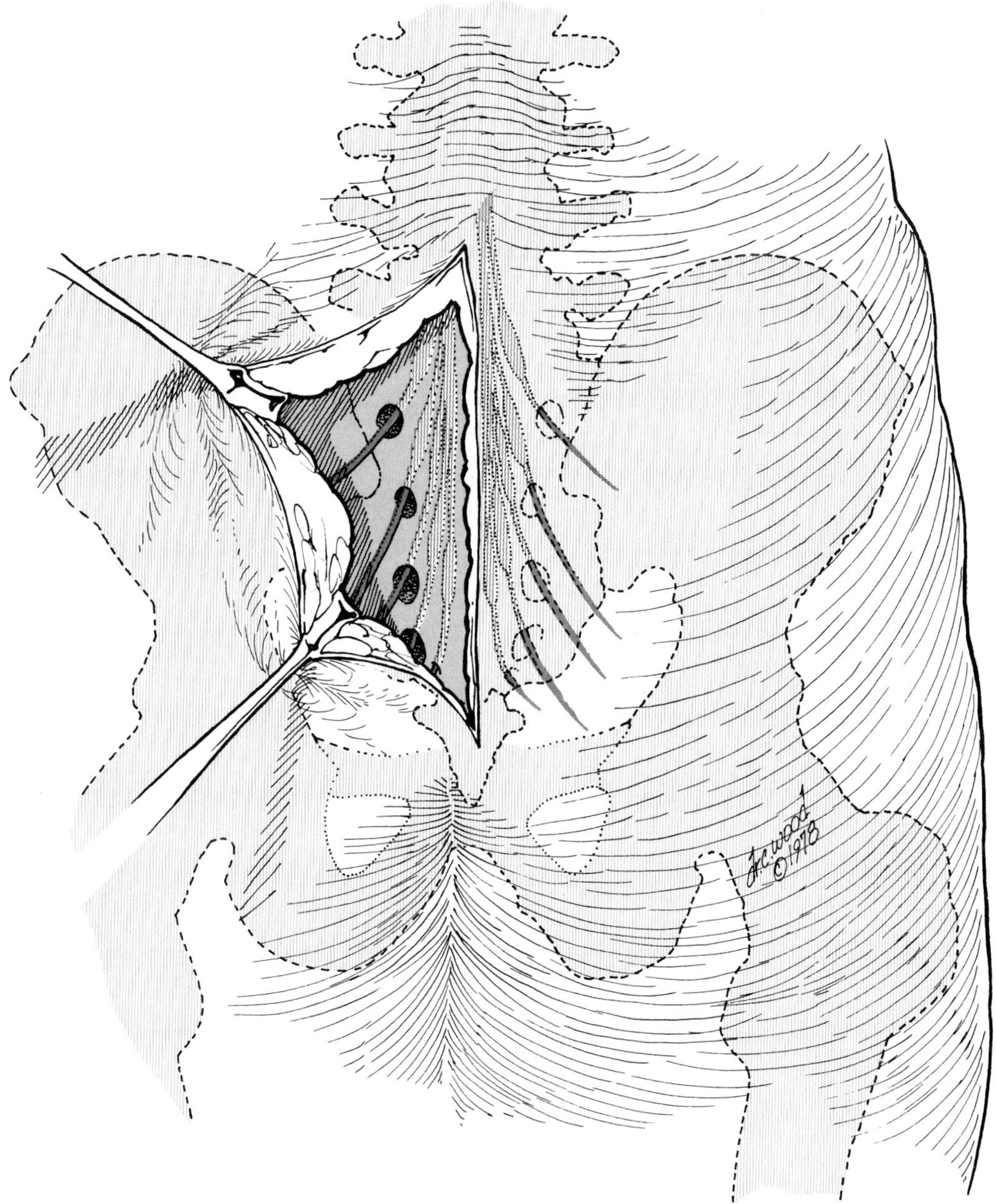

Fig. 11-4. Sacral foramina and sacral nerves. (Drawn by Dr. Charles D. Wood)

there, it courses down the posterior aspect of the thigh to the popliteal fossa, where it divides into the tibial and common peroneal nerves. Branches supplying the posterior thigh are given off during the descent of the nerve to the popliteal space. The sciatic nerve supplies sensory innervation to the posterior thigh and entire leg and foot from just below the knee.

Technique

Several approaches to blockade of the sciatic nerve have been proposed, primarily with the aim of avoiding positioning problems. The traditional lateral position is difficult for trauma patients and the elderly. Therefore, anterior and dorsal lithotomy approaches are also noted.

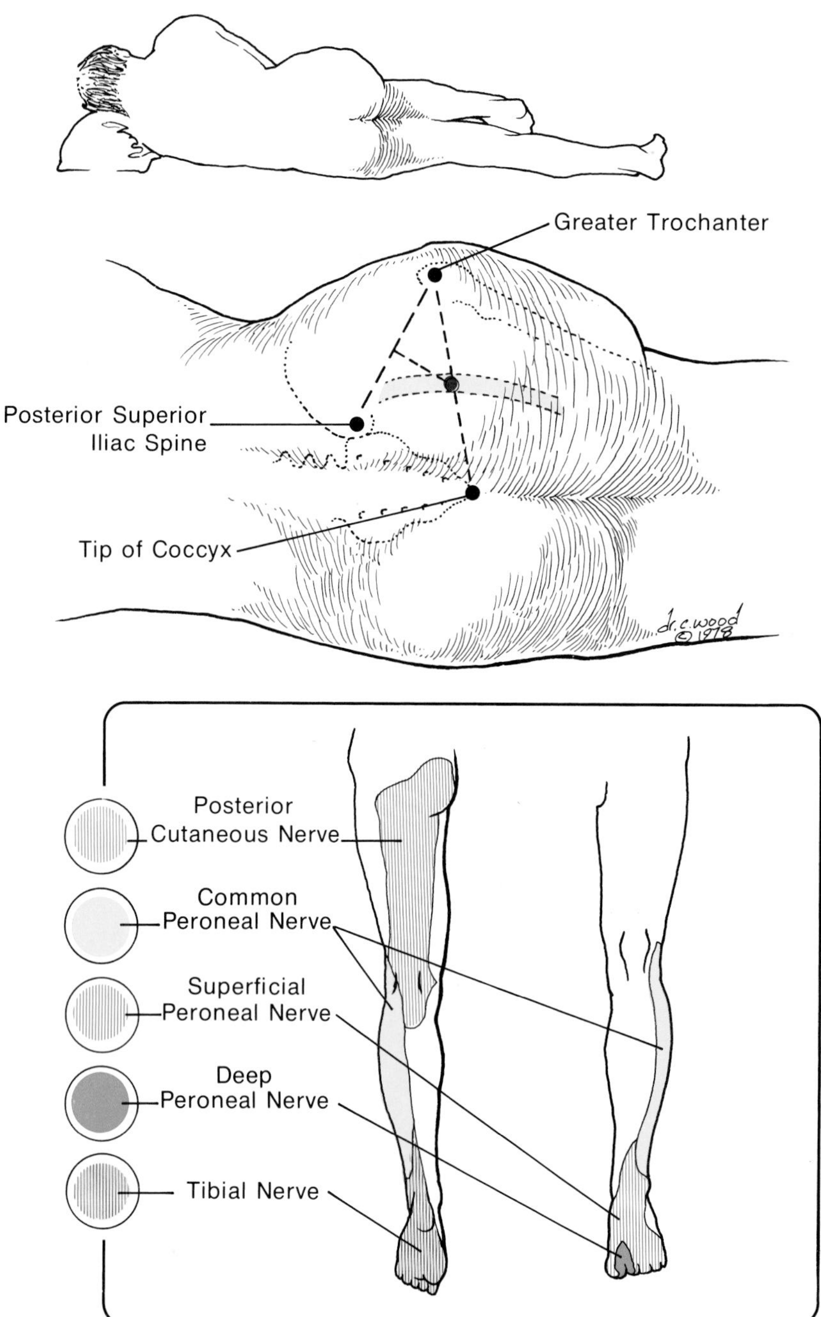

Fig. 11-5. Landmark anatomy and cutaneous distribution of sciatic nerve components. (Drawn by Dr. Charles D. Wood)

Classic Approach of Labat. The classic approach to the sciatic nerve block is with the patient lying on the side opposite the one to be blocked, rolled forward onto the flexed knee with the heel in opposition to the knee of the outstretched dependent leg (Fig. 11-5).

After careful palpation, a line is drawn between points made over the upper aspect of the greater trochanter of the femur and the posterior superior iliac spine. This line should coincide with the upper border of the piriformis muscle and also the upper border of the sacrosciatic foramen (sciatic notch). A line perpendicular and bisecting this is then drawn downward 3 cm and represents the point for injection. A second verification of this point may be made by projecting a line from the greater trochanter to the tip of the coccyx. This line crosses the perpendicular at about 3 cm and also represents a point overlying the sciatic nerve where it exits from the pelvis.

A 10- to 12-cm needle is inserted through a wheal made at this point in a direction perpendicular to the skin until it strikes bone. Usually this will occur at 6 to 8 cm in a patient of average stature. Occasionally, the needle will pass into the sciatic notch when it is first introduced. If this occurs, it should be withdrawn nearly to the skin, and the tip redirected more cephalad along the perpendicular line until bone is contacted. Determination of the depth of the bony pelvis assists in the correct evaluation of paresthesias, which must be elicited in the leg below the level of the thigh. A geometric-grid approach in searching the notch for sciatic paresthesias will also ensure greater success, compared to random thrusts up and down through the notch. Some also advocate the use of a nerve stimulator. Although successful blockade may be accomplished by injecting 10 ml of local anesthetic solution after one paresthesia, the sciatic is a large nerve, and it is often helpful to seek additional paresthesias and inject a total volume of 20 to 30 ml of solution. Conceivably, a single paresthesia at the edge of the nerve and injection there would not provide complete anesthesia over the entire nerve.

Other Approaches. Labat also describes an *anterior approach* to the sciatic nerve. The nerve passes from the lower border of the gluteus maximus, where it is bounded medially by the hamstring muscles. It runs down the thigh, lying on the medial surface of the femur. The posterior femoral cutaneous nerve sometimes branches away from the greater sciatic nerve above the level of blockade and may be missed with this approach.

The patient is placed supine with the lower extremity in a neutral position. A line that represents the inguinal ligament is trisected, and a perpendicular line from the junction of the middle and medial thirds of this line is extended downward and laterally on the anterior aspect of the thigh. The greater trochanter is located by palpation, and a line extended from its tuberosity medially across the anterior surface of the thigh parallel to the inguinal ligament. The point of insertion of this line and the perpendicular line from the inguinal ligament represents the point of injection (Fig. 11-6). A 10- to 12.5-cm needle is inserted through a wheal at this point and directed slightly laterally from a plane perpendicular to the skin. The needle is advanced until bone is contacted, then withdrawn and redirected more perpendicularly to pass 5 cm beyond the femur where it should be resting slightly posterior and medial to the femur within the neurovascular compartment (containing the sciatic nerve). After aspiration, a test injection should be made to determine ease of injection—whether the needle lies in a muscle bundle or fascial space. The former offers firm resistance to injection, and, the needle should be advanced until minimal resistance to injection indicates correct placement. Paresthesias, though not sought, would prove to be helpful. The use of a nerve stimulator would also assist in locating the nerve in this approach. Fifteen to 30 ml of local anesthetic solution should then be injected.

The lithotomy position has also been advocated to facilitate approaching the sciatic nerve.[12] The anatomy is nearly identical to that in the aforementioned anterior approach. After the sciatic nerve passes between the ischial tuberosity and the greater trochanter, it lies just anterior to the gluteus maximus muscle. The nerve is accompanied at this point by the sciatic artery and the inferior gluteal veins, but they are relatively small vessels and add little risk to the procedure.

The patient is placed supine and the extremity to be blocked is flexed at the hip as far as possible (90–120°). The extremity may be supported by stirrups, mechanical devices, or an assistant. In this position, the gluteus maximus muscle is flattened, and the sciatic nerve relatively more superficial. A line is drawn between the ischial tuberosity and the greater trochanter and a wheal raised at its midpoint. A 12- to 15-cm needle is inserted perpendicular to the skin and advanced until paresthesias are elicited. (A peripheral nerve stimulator has been advocated but is seldom necessary unless the patient is unable to respond to paresthesias.) Twenty to 25 ml of a local anesthetic solution are then injected.

Side-Effects and Complications

Sciatic nerve block is primarily a somatic nerve block. It does carry some sympathetic fibers to the extremity, however, and may, therefore, allow pooling of small quantities of blood—usually insufficient to cause significant hypotension. On some occasions, this sympathetic blockade may therapeutically be exploited. The effect of compensatory

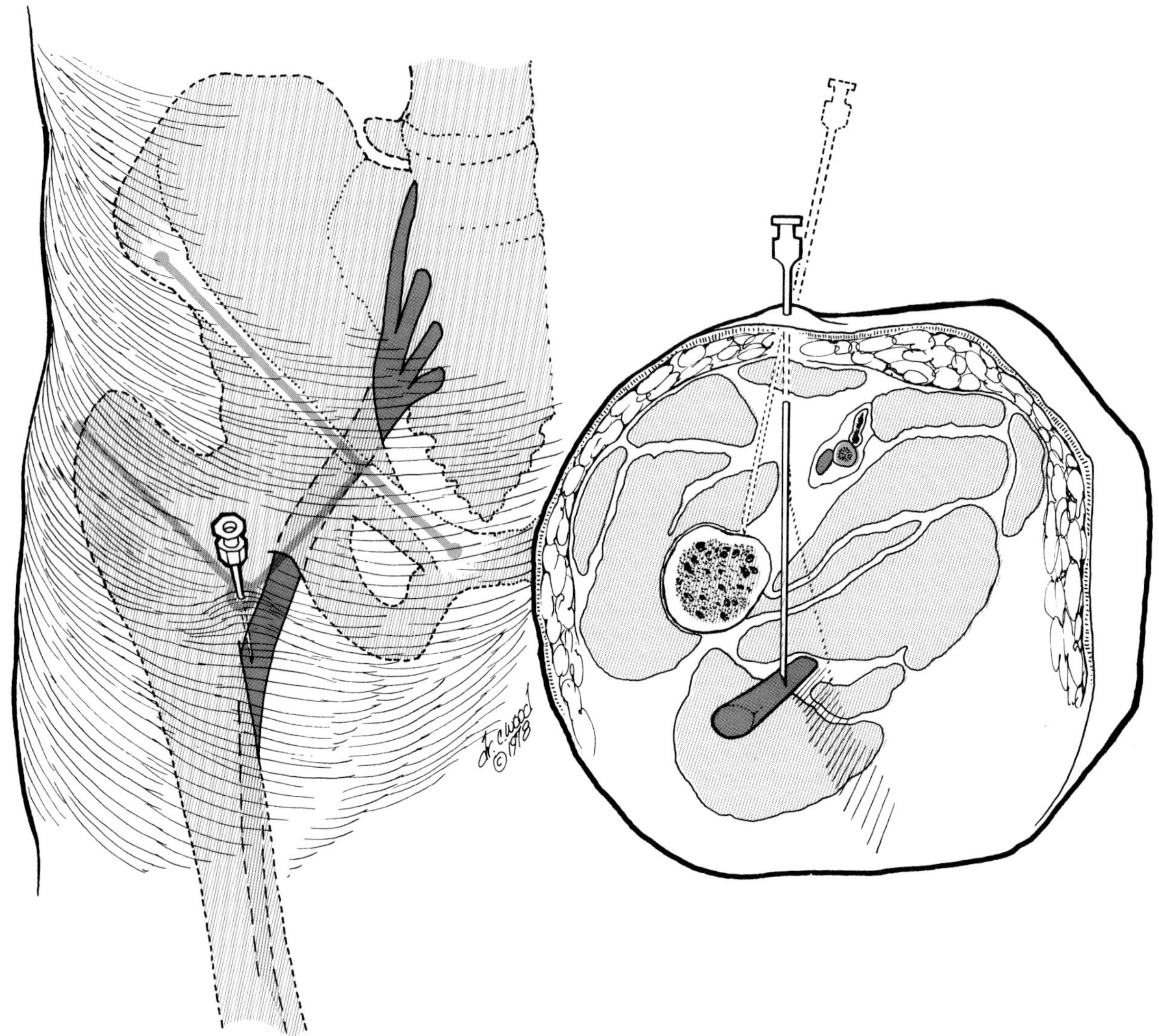

Fig. 11-6. Landmarks and anatomy for anterior approach to sciatic nerve. (Drawn by Dr. Charles D. Wood)

vasoconstruction on the opposite extremity should be considered, however. There is some evidence that tissue oxygenation may be further reduced during this period of compensation, although it is unlikely that this is of clinical significance.[3]

No significant complications secondary to this block have been documented. Residual dysesthesias for periods of 1 to 3 days are reported by some patients but are usually self-remitting.[13] It is reported that these minor problems may result from the use of long-bevel needles producing damage to nerve fascicles.

Indications

A few surgical procedures may be accomplished under sciatic nerve block alone. The block is, however, usually combined with femoral, obturator, or lateral femoral cutaneous nerve block to provide complete anesthesia of the lower extremity.

FEMORAL NERVE BLOCK

The femoral nerve (L2–4) proceeds from the lumbar plexus in the groove between the psoas major and iliac muscles, where it enters the thigh by passing deep to the inguinal ligament. At the level of the inguinal ligament, the femoral nerve lies anterior to the iliopsoas muscle and slightly lateral to the femoral artery (Fig. 11-7). It is important to remember that, at or even above the level of the inguinal ligament, the femoral nerve divides into an anterior and posterior bundle. The anterior branches innervate the skin that covers the anterior surface of the thigh along with the sartorius muscle; the posterior branches innervate the quadriceps muscles, the knee joint, and its medial ligament and give rise to the saphenous nerve, which descends over the medial side of the calf to supply the skin down to the medial malleolus. Another classification of the divided femoral nerve is into superficial and deep, which corresponds to the aforementioned anterior and posterior. It may be helpful to recall that, in general, the deep branches are chiefly motor in function with articular branches to the hip and knee joints. The superficial branches are chiefly sensory and cutaneous in their distribution. They supply the anterior, anteromedial, and medial aspects of the thigh, the knee, and the upper portion of the leg.

Technique

Classic Approach of Labat. The patient lies supine and may be sedated since paresthesias are not essential to this particular method. The femoral artery is palpated immediately below the inguinal ligament, and a wheal raised immediately lateral to the artery. A line drawn from the anterior superior iliac spine to the symphysis pubis will approximate the inguinal ligament, with the wheal adjacent to the femoral artery being approximately 1 to 2 cm below this line (Fig. 11-8). A 3- to 4-cm needle, without syringe, is advanced perpendicular to the skin until a paresthesia is elicited or the needle undergoes maximum lateral pulsation from its position adjacent to and at the level of the artery. It should be repositioned until one of these two indicators has been achieved. If paresthesias occur, 10 to 20 ml of local anesthetic solution should be injected, after careful aspiration, to ensure against intra-vascular injection. If no paresthesias occur, then 7 to 10 ml of local anesthetic are deposited fanwise lateral to the artery. The needle should then be carefully repositioned adjacent to the artery, and the injection repeated.

Paravascular Approach. An alternate technique for femoral nerve block has been noted in conjunction with blockade of the lumbar plexus (see Fig. 11-3).[15] This paravascular technique requires elicitation of paresthesias and a cooperative patient or, failing that, a nerve stimulator.

Complications and Side-Effects

As with the sciatic nerve block, some of the sympathetic fibers to the lower extremity are blocked with the femoral procedure. However, with femoral block this is more likely to be advantageous to blood flow without being of a magnitude likely to produce systemic hypotension. Inasmuch as the site of blockade is adjacent to a major artery and vein, hematoma at the site is a possibility. Although this probably occurs, it is seldom if ever a complication of clinical significance. With the advent of vascular surgery, the anesthesiologist should be alert to the presence of vascular grafts of the femoral artery, which would be a relative contraindication for elective femoral nerve block.

Residual nerve involvement—dysesthesias or paresis—is remotely possible, but trauma to the nerve from these techniques is minimal, and such complication, therefore, highly unlikely.

Indications

Femoral nerve block is indicated for the operation of the anterior portion of the thigh, both superficial and deep. Like sciatic nerve block, the femoral nerve block is usually performed in conjunction with lateral femoral cutaneous or sciatic nerve block to provide more complete analgesia of the lower extremity, especially for procedures below the knee. The block has also been advocated for analgesia in patients with a fractured shaft of the femur.[1]

LATERAL FEMORAL CUTANEOUS NERVE BLOCK

The lateral femoral cutaneous nerve (L2–3) emerges at the lateral border of the psoas muscle at a level lower than the ilioinguinal nerve. It passes obliquely under the iliac fascia and across the iliac muscle to enter the thigh deep to the inguinal ligament at a point approximately 1 to 2 cm medial to the anterior superior iliac spine. It then crosses or passes through the tendonous origin of the sartorius muscle and courses downward beneath the fascia lata. It emerges from the fascia lata at a point 7 to 10 cm below the anterior superior iliac spine where it branches into anterior and posterior branches. The anterior branch supplies the skin over the anterolateral aspect of the thigh as low as the knee.

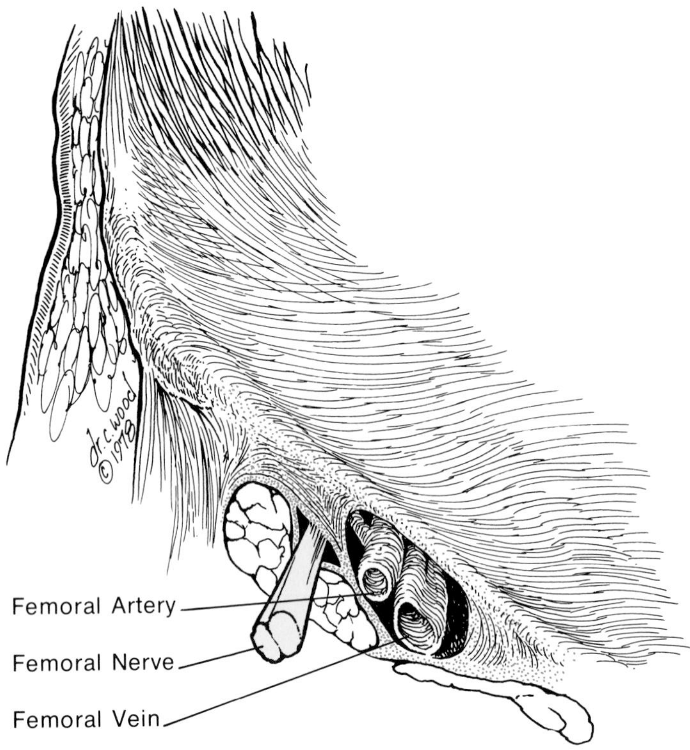

Fig. 11-7. Anatomical relationship of femoral nerve to the artery and vein. (Drawn by Dr. Charles D. Wood)

The posterior branch pierces the fascia lata and passes backward to supply the skin on the lateral side of the thigh from just below the greater trochanter to about the middle of the thigh (Fig. 11-8).

Technique

The patient is placed in the supine position. After palpation of the anterior superior iliac spine, a skin wheal is placed 2 to 3 cm inferior and medial to it. A 3- to 4-cm needle with syringe attached is then inserted through the wheal and perpendicular to the skin surface. Soon after passing through the skin, the firm fascia lata is felt and then a sudden release as the needle passes through. Ten ml of a local anesthetic solution should be deposited fanwise as the needle is moved upward and downward, depositing solution both above and below the fascia, most of it below (Fig. 11-8).

An alternate technique is to direct the needle through the skin wheal in a slightly lateral and cephalad direction to strike the iliac bone just medial and below the anterior superior iliac spine. Since the nerve emerges here, the deposition of 10 ml of local anesthetic solution in a medial fanwise fashion will also accomplish satisfactory blockade of the nerve. If the volume of the solution is of no concern to the total dose of drug administered, then the nerve could be blocked in both places on the same patient, to doubly ensure success.

Complications and Side-Effects

With the exception of a remotely possible dysesthesia or hypoesthesia, there are no known risks to this nerve block technique.

Indications

This block by itself is extremely suitable for anesthetizing the donor site prior to the removal of small skin grafts. Its primary indication as a supplement to the femoral and sciatic nerve blocks for operating on the lower extremity is the provision of analgesia for tourniquet pain. Since one of the terminal anterior branches forms part of the patellar plexus, it must be included with the other nerve blocks for operations on the knee, with or without tourniquet.

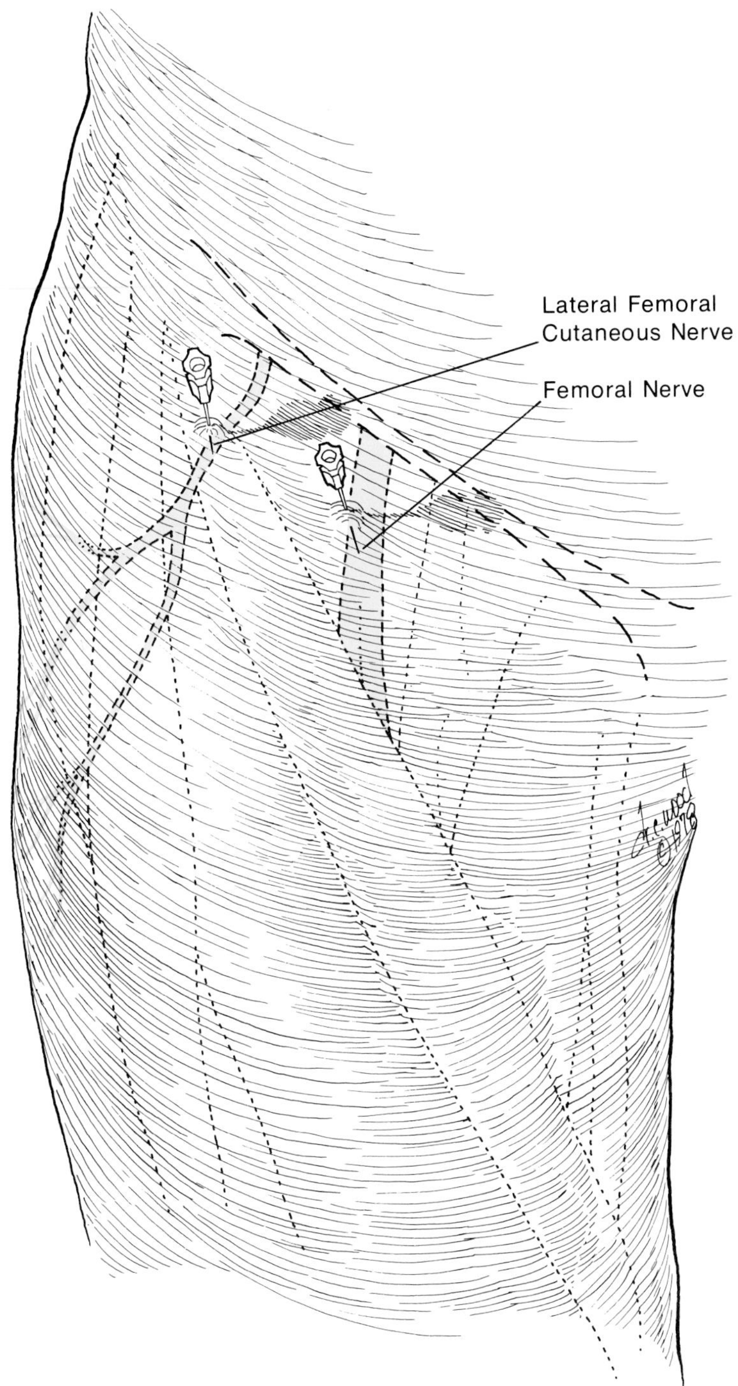

Fig. 11-8. Needle placement for lateral femoral cutaneous and femoral nerve blocks. (Drawn by Dr. Charles D. Wood)

OBTURATOR NERVE BLOCK

The obturator nerve (L2–4) derives its major source from L3–4—the portion coming from L2 is very small and sometimes even lacking. The nerve appears at the medial border of the psoas muscle, covered anteriorly by the external iliac vessels and passes downward in the pelvis. It continues with the obturator vessels along the obturator groove and passes through the obturator foramen into the thigh. As the nerve passes through the obturator canal, it divides into posterior and anterior branches. The anterior branch supplies an articular branch to the hip joint, the anterior adductor muscles and cutaneous branches, to the lower inner thigh. The size and/or existence of this cutaneous innervation is small and variable depending upon which anatomic reference material is quoted. The posterior branch innervates the deep adductor muscles and frequently sends an articular branch to the knee joint, which may be important in providing analgesia for knee surgery.

Technique

The patient is placed supine with the leg to be blocked in slight abduction. Caution should be taken to protect the skin of the genitalia from irritating antiseptic solutions used in preparing the area. It should not be necessary to shave the pubic area to be blocked.

The pubic tubercle is palpated and a skin wheal raised 1 to 2 cm below and 1 to 2 cm lateral to it. A 7- to 8-cm needle, without syringe attached, is introduced through the wheal in a slight medial direction to strike the horizontal ramus of the pubis. It is then withdrawn and redirected approximately 45° in a cephalad direction to identify the superior bony portion of the obturator canal. The depth at which the needle strikes bone in each direction should be noted. The needle is again withdrawn and the point redirected slightly laterally and inferiorly to bisect the previous angle and pass into the obturator canal. It should be advanced 2 to 3 cm beyond the previously noted depth of bone where, after careful aspiration to ensure the obturator vessels have not been entered, 10 to 15 ml of local anesthetic are injected. Only by identifying the two bony walls of the canal can the anesthesiologist be certain the needle has passed into the canal rather than into the soft tissues (*e.g.*, bladder or vagina) medially or superiorly (Fig. 11-9). Presence of successful obturator nerve block is determined by demonstrating paresis of the adductor muscles since the cutaneous distribution is small and inconstant.

Complications and Side-Effects

Obturator nerve block has vascular and neural complications and side-effects nearly identical to those of the femoral nerve. Similarly, these represent remote possibilities rather than clinically important considerations.

Indications

This is a valuable technique in diagnosing painful conditions of the hip and in the relief of adductor spasm of the hip. It is also necessary as a supplement to sciatic, femoral, and lateral femoral cutaneous nerve blocks for surgery on or above the knee.

NERVE BLOCKS ABOUT THE KNEE

There are three major nerve trunks that can be blocked at the level of the knee—the saphenous, the common peroneal, and the tibial.

Anatomy

The *saphenous nerve* is the cutaneous and terminal extension of the femoral nerve. It supplies the skin over the medial, anteromedial, and posteromedial aspects of the leg, extending from above the knee to as far distal as the ball of the great toe.

The common peroneal and tibial nerves are extensions from the sciatic nerve. The *tibial nerve* arises at the upper end of the popliteal fossa and is the larger of the two terminal branches of the sciatic nerve. It has both a muscular branch to the back of the leg and cutaneous branches in the popliteal fossa and down the back of the leg to the ankle. The *common peroneal nerve* is about one-half the size of the tibial nerve, being the other portion of the sciatic nerve when it bifurcates at the upper end of the popliteal space. It contains articular branches to the knee joint and cutaneous nerves to the lateral side of the leg, heel, and ankle.

Techniques

One of the unexplained phenomenon of regional blockade is the uniform lack of enthusiasm for—even less advocacy of—blockade of individual nerves at the level of the knee, by any of the authors of material on regional anesthesia (Braun, Labat, Pitkin, Sherwood-Dunn, Eriksson, and Moore). Some have, reluctantly, recommended circular in filtration at the thigh, and Löfström advocates only a block of the saphenous nerve, stating that ". . . tibial nerve block is difficult to perform and peroneal nerve block, though simple to carry out where the nerve winds round the head of the fibula, may carry a considerable risk of postanesthetic neuritis."[8] Documentation of these criticisms seems lacking in the literature, however. It would seem, therefore, that the anesthesiologist needing to obtain nerve block at the knee should, with full appre-

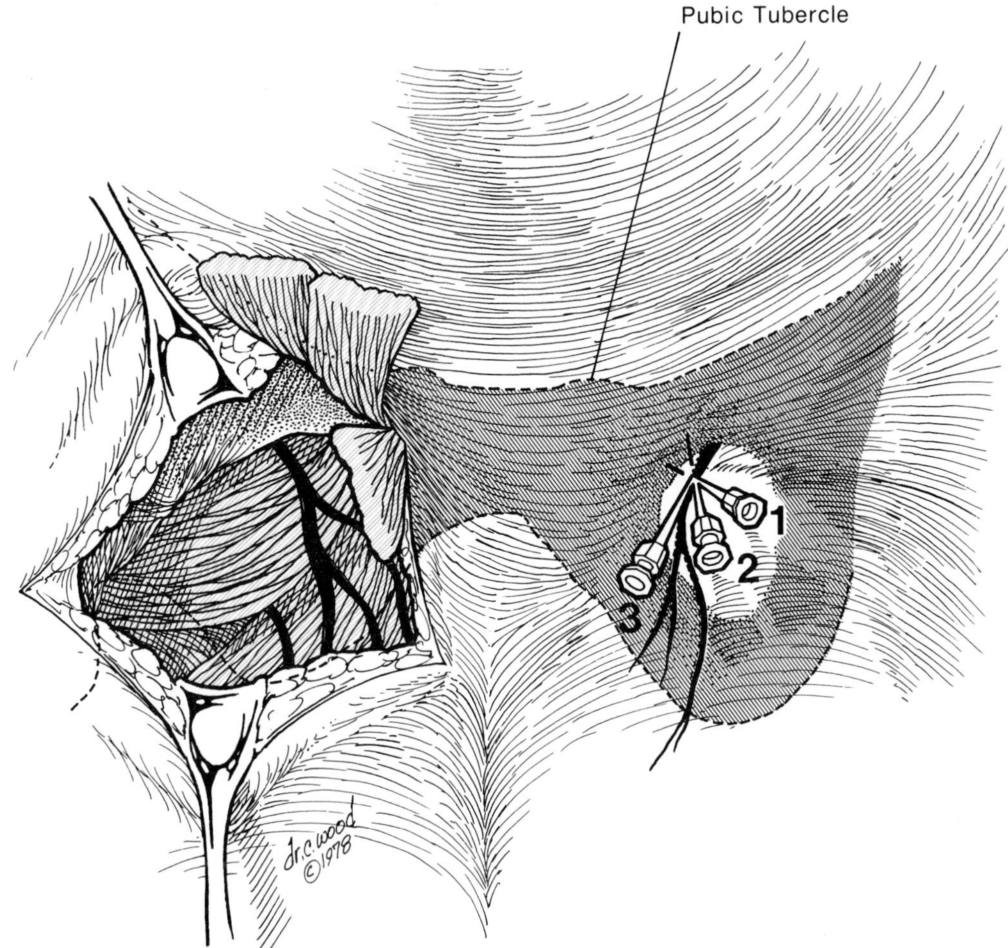

Fig. 11-9. Anatomy of obturator nerve, showing bony landmarks used in nerve block technique. (Drawn by Dr. Charles D. Wood)

ciation of the aforementioned reluctance, study the anatomy of the nerves about the knee and devise his own approach, keeping in mind all the fundamentals of regional blockade applied to other peripheral nerves.

Indications

The paucity of writing about nerve blocks at the knee may be due to a relative lack of need for doing such blocks. It is well appreciated that surgical procedures about the knee require blockade of the major nerves proximally. Furthermore, it will be seen that the terminal nerves may be approached easily at the level of the ankle. There remains only a need for nerve blocks about the knee to cover a surgical field distal to the knee and proximal to the ankle. Although there are some procedures performed here, certainly mastering nerve blocks proximally and distally would leave little reason to master techniques about the knee. This would be especially likely if, in fact, the risk of neuritis or dysesthesias were to be greater in that area.

NERVE BLOCKS AT THE ANKLE

There are five branches of the principal nerve trunks supplying the ankle and foot—posterior tibial, sural, superficial peroneal (musculocutaneous), saphenous, and deep peroneal (anterior tibial).[10] These nerves are relatively easy to block at the ankle (Fig. 11-10).

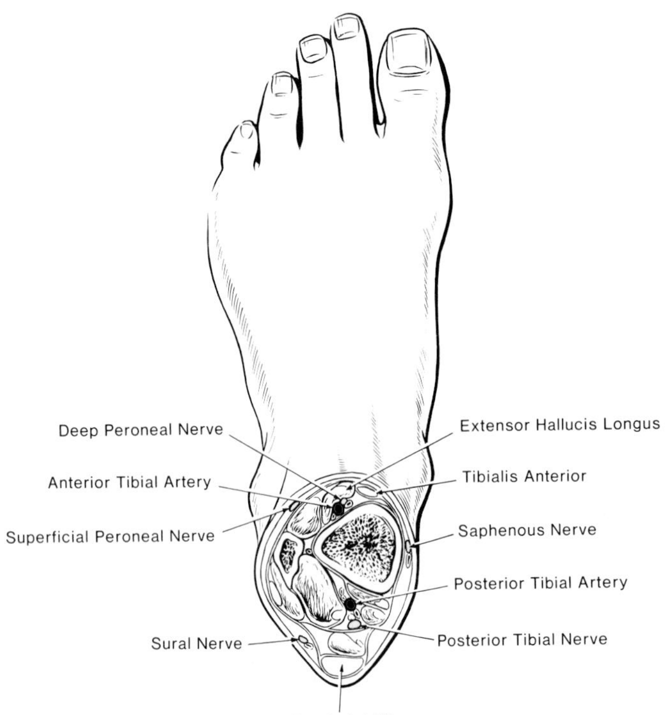

Fig. 11-10. Anatomic relationships of five nerves at the ankle.

Tibial Nerve Block

The tibial nerve (L4–5, S1–3), the larger of the two branches of the sciatic nerve, reaches the distal part of the leg from the medial side of the Achilles tendon, where it lies behind the posterior tibial artery. The nerve then gives off the medial calcaneal branch to the inside of the heel, after which it divides at the back of the medial malleolus into the medial and lateral plantar nerves, both under the abductor hallucis running to the sole of the foot. The medial branch supplies the medial two-thirds of the sole and plantar portion of the medial three and one-half toes up to the nail. The lateral branch supplies the lateral one-third of the sole and plantar portion of the lateral one and one-half toes.

The patient lies prone with the ankle supported by a pillow. A skin wheal is raised lateral to the posterior tibial artery, if the artery is palpable. If the artery is not palpable, then the wheal is placed to the medial side of the Achilles tendon, level with the upper border of the medial malleolus. A 1- to 3-cm needle is advanced through the wheal at a right angle to the posterior aspect of the tibia, lateral to the artery. Shifting the needle in a mediolateral position may elicit a paresthesia, and then 3 to 5 ml of local anesthetic solution should be injected. If paresthesias are not obtained, 5 to 7 ml of local anesthetic solution are injected against the posterior aspect of the tibia while the needle is withdrawn 1 cm (Fig. 11-11).

Sural Nerve Block

The sural nerve is a cutaneous nerve that arises through the union of a branch from the tibial nerve and one from the common peroneal nerve. It becomes subcutaneous somewhat distal to the middle of the leg and proceeds along with the short saphenous vein behind and below the lateral malleolus to supply the lower posterolateral surface of the leg, the lateral side of the foot, and the lateral part of the fifth toe.

With the patient in the same position as for tibial nerve block, a skin wheal is raised lateral to the Achilles tendon at the level of the lateral malleolus. A 1- to 3-cm needle is inserted through the wheal approximately 1 cm and angled toward the fibula, where paresthesias may be sought. If no paresthesias occur, then infiltration is accomplished from the Achilles tendon to the outer border of the lateral malleolus. Three to 5 ml of local anesthetic solution injected fanwise is usually sufficient to produce analgesia. Often the tibial and sural nerves are blocked at the same time with the same needles and equipment (Fig. 11-11).

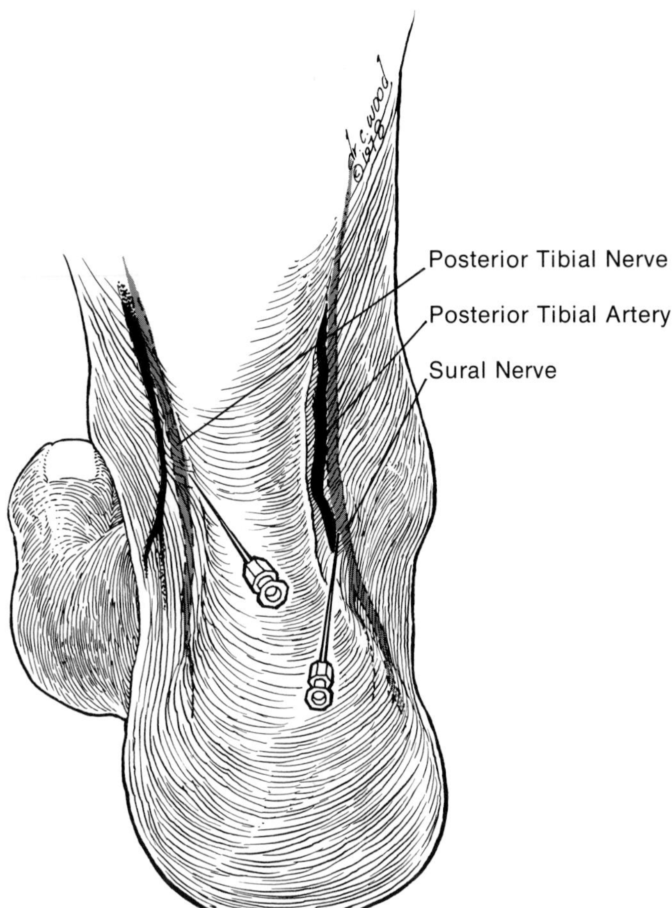

Fig. 11-11. Needle placement for blockade of posterior tibial and sural nerves at the ankle. (Drawn by Dr. Charles D. Wood)

Superficial Peroneal Nerve Block

The superficial peroneal nerve (L4–5, S1–2) perforates the deep fascia on the anterior aspect of the distal two-thirds of the leg and runs subcutaneously to supply the dorsum of the foot and toes, except for the contiguous surfaces of the great and second toes.

The superficial peroneal nerve is blocked immediately above and medial to the lateral malleolus. A subcutaneous infiltration of 5 to 10 ml local anesthetic solution is spread from the anterior border of the tibia to the superior aspect of the lateral malleolus (Fig. 11-12).

Deep Peroneal Nerve Block

The deep peroneal nerve (L4–5, S1–2) courses down the anterior aspect of the interosseus membrane of the leg and continues midway between the malleoli onto the dorsum of the foot. Here, it innervates the short extensors of the toes as well as the skin on the adjacent areas of the first and second toes. At the level of the foot, the anterior tibial artery lies medial to the nerve, as does the tendon of extensor hallicus longus muscle.

The deep peroneal nerve is blocked in the lower portion of the leg by placing a wheal between the tendons of the anterior tibial and extensor hallucis longus muscles at a level just superior to the malleoli. Often the anterior tibial artery may be palpated. If this is possible, the skin wheal and nerve should be just lateral to the artery. The needle is advanced toward the tibia, and 3 to 5 ml of local anesthetic solution are injected (Fig. 11-12).

Saphenous Nerve Block

The saphenous nerve, which is the sensory terminal branch of the femoral nerve, becomes subcutaneous at the lateral side of the knee joint. It then follows the great saphenous vein to the medial malleolus and supplies the cutaneous area over the me-

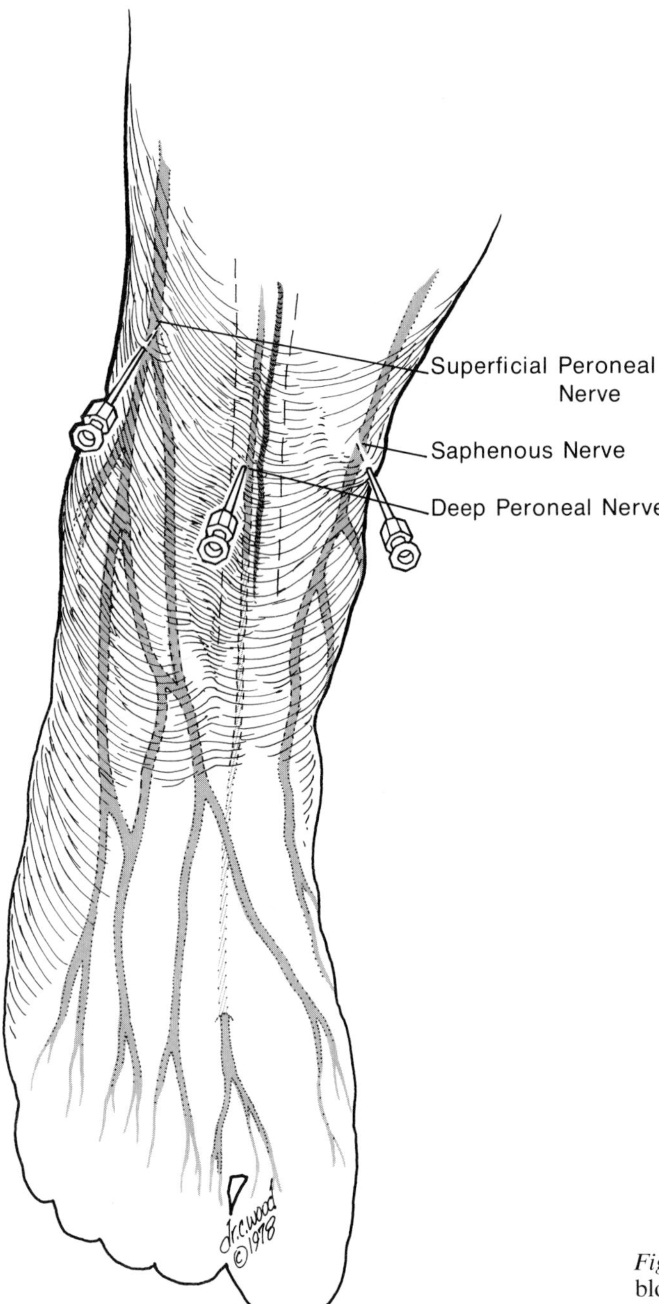

Fig. 11-12. Needle placement and relationships for blockade of superficial peroneal, deep peroneal, and saphenous nerves. (Drawn by Dr. Charles D. Wood)

dial side of the lower leg anterior to the medial malleolus and the medial part of the foot as far forward as the midportion. Occasionally, its innervation extends to the metatarsophalangeal joint.

To block the saphenous nerve, a skin wheal is raised immediately above and anterior to the medial malleolus, and 3 to 5 ml of local anesthetic solution are infiltrated subcutaneously around the great saphenous vein (Fig. 11-12).

It is apparent that all five nerve blocks at the ankle, undertaken simultaneously, would produce a ring of infiltration around the ankle at the level of the malleoli. Such an approach has, in fact, been advocated by more than one textbook of regional anesthesia; it is possible and usually successful at the distal extremes of all extremities and digits. Nonetheless, with circular infiltration there is the hazard of vascular occlusion if large volumes of anesthetic solutions are injected, especially if they contain epinephrine. In general, block to a specific nerve, such as one of those just described, with smaller quantities of non-epinephrine-containing solutions of local anesthetic agents have a higher success rate with less risk.

METATARSAL AND DIGITAL NERVE BLOCK

The relationship of the terminal nerves to the metatarsal bones and the toes is very similar to the structures of the hand, with the nerve fibers passing through the intermetatarsal space and alongside each toe, where they become the digital nerves.

Nerve block in the intermetatarsal space is very similar to the metacarpal block. Skin wheals are raised on the dorsum of the foot over the proximal aspect of each metatarsal space that bounds the toes to be blocked. Local anesthetic solutions are then infiltrated in a fanwise direction between the two wheals, taking care not to pierce the sole of the foot. Solution should carefully be injected around the plantar surface of the metatarsal bone as well. Digital block alone can be accomplished by injecting through the wheals at the webs of the toes, depositing 2 to 3 ml of local anesthetic solution along either side of the toes to be blocked. Use of epinephrine in the anesthetic solutions and excessive volumes should be avoided in these blocks (Fig. 11-13).

LOCAL ANESTHETIC AGENTS

Although patient selection and regional block equipment have been discussed in Chapter 6, there are some considerations of local anesthetic agents that apply specifically to regional blockade of peripheral nerves. Chapter 6 mentions only the volumes of local anesthetic agents necessary to bathe the nerves to be blocked for individual nerve techniques. The extremes of the volume–concentration relationships that provide satisfactory anesthesia depend upon the knowledge and technical expertise of the anesthesiologist.

Certain properties of the available local anesthetic agents must be exploited if the use of regional block of the lower extremity is to be maximally effective. Some of the more important of these properties are duration, concentration, toxicity, metabolism, and additives, such as epinephrine, carbon dioxide, and hyaluronidase (see Chap. 4).

Consideration of the appropriate agent, concentration, and, perhaps, an additive should allow the anesthesiologist to provide an optimal nerve block of the lower extremity. In general, since many of the surgical procedures on the lower extremity require little or no muscle relaxation, weaker concentrations of solutions may be used in the interest of reducing total dose while providing sufficient volume. For example, with the combined four-nerve block of the leg, it would be possible to use stronger concentrations on the sciatic and femoral blocks and dilute to a weaker solution for primary sensory blockade of the lateral femoral cutaneous and obturator nerves.

It is equally important that the duration of analgesia be selected according to need. For example, a short surgical outpatient procedure may well be performed with 2-chloroprocaine, which would restore the patient to early ambulation, whereas bupivacaine or etidocaine might well be used for a patient who would benefit from prolonged analgesia and the sympathetic block of a sciatic nerve block. Residual neurologic involvement (hypoesthesia and dysesthesia) is not uncommon after nerve block with the very long-acting agents. This should be kept in mind in certain orthopaedic procedures, especially those with plaster casts in which postsurgical neural involvement must be recognized.

Duration

The currently available local anesthetic agents may be separated into three general—albeit overlapping—categories: short-acting, intermediate-acting, and long-acting. The short-acting agents include procaine; 2-chloroprocaine, with or without epinephrine; lidocaine, without epinephrine; and prilocaine, without epinephrine. The intermediate group includes epinephrine-containing solutions of lidocaine and prilocaine; mepivacaine, with or without epinephrine; and, perhaps, tetracaine, without epinephrine. The long-acting agents cover a longer period of time. They include dibucaine and tetracaine, with epinephrine, having a relatively shorter duration, and bupivacaine and etidocaine, having a very long duration. It should be recalled that very weak concentrations of a local anesthetic agent have a much shorter duration and that the

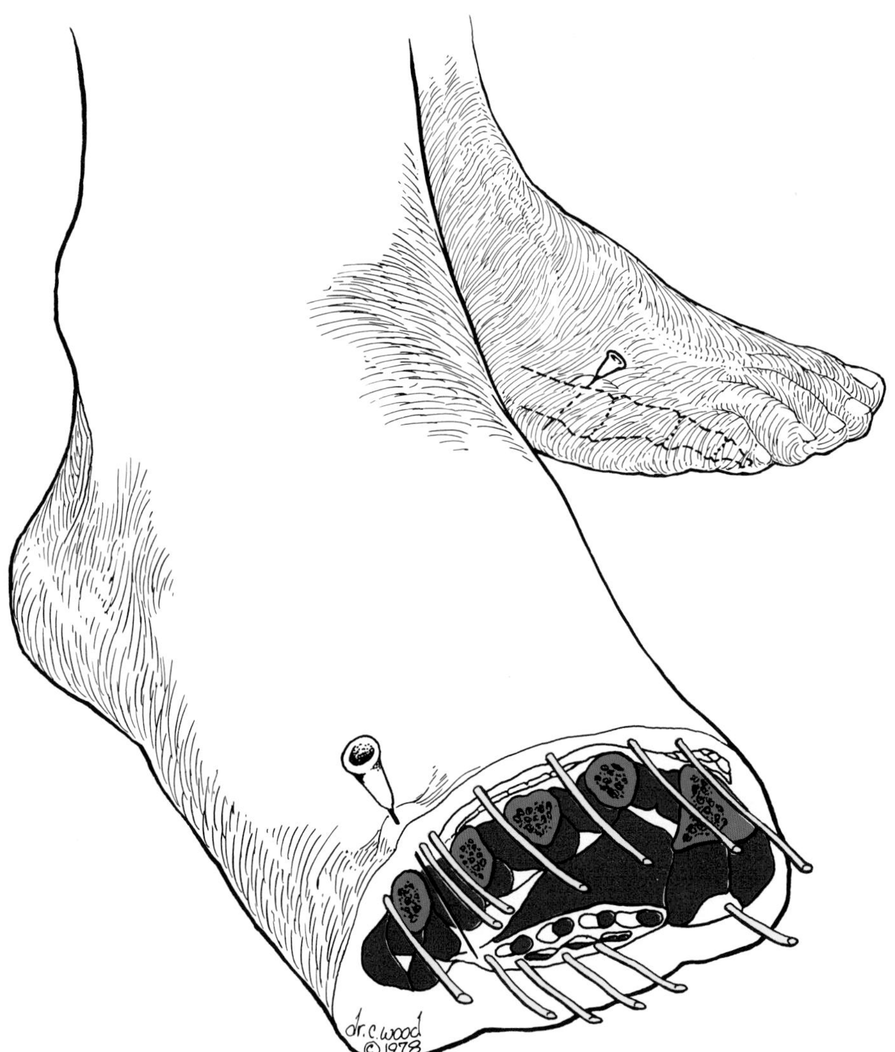

Fig. 11-13. Anatomic relationships and needle placement for metatarsal nerve block. (Drawn by Dr. Charles D. Wood)

very concentrated solutions have the longest duration of action.[6]

Perhaps the most complete data on peripheral nerve block, compiled by a single investigator, can be found in the work of Löfström, who used ulnar nerve blockade to evaluate the duration of local anesthetic agents.[9] Clinical studies from other investigators report longer durations of cutaneous hypoesthesia to pinprick or pinch with both bupivacaine and etidocaine. Wencker and colleagues report analgesia of 770 minutes with bupivacaine and 764 minutes with etidocaine for axillary nerve block.[14] This study also showed that motor anesthesia exceeded analgesia with both agents. It must be noted that duration of surgical anesthesia—or postsurgical pain relief, for that matter—will be considerably shorter than the analgesia to pinprick quoted in most studies. In general, 45 to 90 minutes of surgical anesthesia can be achieved with the short-acting agents, 90 to 120 minutes with the intermediate agents, and 120 to 748 minutes with the long-acting group—although, of course, individual patient variables contribute to this parameter in many situations.

Concentration

Traditionally, it was thought that the very weak concentrations would block only the smallest nonmyelinated fibers and provide mostly sympathetic nerve blockade or partial sensory analgesia and that the strongest concentrations provided blockade of major motor fibers, with excessive concentrations producing neuritis or other nerve toxicity. It is now appreciated, primarily through recent controlled studies with the newest long-acting agents, that this traditional concept of concentration effect is invalid. In spite of the difficulties inherent in arriving at clinically equipotent doses of local anesthetic agents, the work of Wencker, which noted differences in the motor blocking properties of bupivacaine and etidocaine, has been confirmed by many others.[14] Another observation by these investigators was that the sympathetic blockade by these agents varied, not only from agent to agent but also in degree of sensory and motor blockade—the sympathetic block with etidocaine apparently being of shorter duration than either its motor or sensory blockade.

Toxicity

In practice, the maximum recommended dose of most local anesthetic agents has been the dose that was, presumably, safe to administer to a patient without fear of central nervous system (CNS) toxicity (*i.e.*, seizures). This recommendation was based on animal studies. Advances in clinical chemistry, especially the advent of gas liquid chromatography, has enabled the measurement of blood levels of local anesthetics in humans. Although there is variability in the blood concentration at which seizures will occur, it is known that the site of administration does affect blood levels and, therefore, the hazard of toxicity (see Chap. 4). Many investigators have shown that levels are highest after intercostal nerve block, that levels after epidural block are 40 to 50 per cent lower, and that extremity blocks (arm and leg) produce intermediate levels. The risk of toxicity is especially increased after the combined nerve block of the lower extremity, chiefly through the relatively larger volumes of local anesthetic required to accomplish the block. That is why it is extremely important that the anesthesiologist initially determine the total volume required for the block, in conjunction with the maximum total dose recommended for the agent, and then dilute the concentration to comply with these requirements.

Metabolism

The metabolism of local anesthetic drugs has little specific application to nerve block of the lower extremity, other than the fact that certain conditions, such as hypercapnia and acidosis, have been shown to increase the likelihood of CNS toxicity for a particular dose of local anesthetic. Therefore, when maximum volume and total dose are determined, the systemic health of the patient should be carefully noted, and dosage reduced accordingly. A more detailed discussion of toxicity and metabolism may be found in Chapters 2, 3, and 4.

Additives

Epinephrine has been added to local anesthetic agents since the early 1900s because it was assumed that duration of action would be extended and the blood concentration of the local anesthetic would be reduced, owing to delayed absorption. Recent work indicates that the beneficial effects of epinephrine for both duration and blood concentration depend on which local anesthetic is being used. Certainly, epinephrine is not necessary to extend the duration of etidocaine and bupivacaine. On the other hand, etidocaine and bupivacaine are used in high total doses for leg blocks and, if epinephrine reduces blood levels at all, that is probably sufficient justification for its use.[4]

Hyaluronidase has been advocated to prevent large hematomas at the site of injection in arm and leg blocks.[11] Although no apparent problems have been reported from this use, there are also no reports of significant hematoma formation so that its benefit, if any, is difficult to evaluate. Also undocumented is the effect that this additive may have on blood levels of the administered local anesthetic agents. Since its action is to allow diffusion of blood (or drugs) through tissue planes, it is conceivable that this might increase vascular absorption of drug and further increase marginally safe blood levels of local anesthetics.

Bromage has been especially enthusiastic about the addition of carbon dioxide to solutions of local anesthetic in order to hasten their clinical effectiveness.[5] Although carbon dioxide has been advocated primarily in epidural anesthesia, it is effective for peripheral nerve block as well. Clinically, the speed of onset of nearly all of the local anesthetic agents, however, with the possible exception of 0.25 per cent bupivacaine, is sufficiently rapid to provide surgical analgesia within the usual surgical preparation time—10 to 15 minutes. Packaging of carbonated solutions is currently limited to Canada and, unless greater need is established, probably will not be extended.

REFERENCES

1. Berry, F.R.: Analgesia in patients with fractured shaft of femur. Anaesthesia, *32*:576, 1977.

2. Braun, H.: Local Anesthesia—Its Scientific Basis and Practical Use. ed. 2. p. 380. Philadelphia, Lea & Febiger, 1924.
3. Bridenbaugh, P.O., Moore, D.C., and Bridenbaugh, L.D.: Capillary P_{O_2} as a measure of sympathetic blockade. Anesth. Analg., *50*:26, 1971.
4. Bridenbaugh, P.O., *et al.:* Role of epinephrine in regional block anesthesia with etidocaine: A double-blind study. Anesth. Analg., *53*:430, 1974.
5. Bromage, P.R.: A comparison of the hydrochloride and carbon dioxide salts in lidocaine and prilocaine in epidural analgesia. Acta Anaesthesiol. Scand., *9*:55, 1965.
6. De Jong, R.H.: Physiology and Pharmacology of Local Anesthesia. pp. 132–136. Springfield, Charles C Thomas, 1970.
7. Labat, G.: Regional Anesthesia: Its Technic and Clinical Application. p. 45. Philadelphia, W.B. Saunders, 1924.
8. Löfström, B.: Nerve Block at the Knee–Joint. Illustrated Handbook in Local Anaesthesia. Chicago, Year Book Medical Publishers, 1969.
9. Löfström, B.: Ulnar nerve blockade for the evaluation of local anaesthetic agents. Br. J. Anaesth., *47*:297, 1975.
10. McCutcheon, R.: Regional anesthesia for the foot. Can. Anaesth. Soc. J., *12*:465, 1965.
11. Moore, D.C.: Regional Block. ed. 4. Springfield, Charles C Thomas, 1975.
12. Raj, P.P., Parks, R.I., Watson, T.D., and Jenkins, M.T.: New single position supine approach to sciatic–femoral nerve block. Anesth. Analg., *54*:489, 1975.
13. Selander, D., Dhuner, K.E., and Lundberg, E.: Peripheral nerve injury due to injection needles used for regional anesthesia. Acta Anaesthesiol. Scand., *21*:182, 1977.
14. Wencker, K.H., Nolte, H., and Fruhstorfer, H.: Brachial plexus blockade for evaluation of local anaesthetic agents. Br. J. Anaesth., *47*:301, 1975.
15. Winnie, A.P., Ramamurthy, S., and Durrani, Z.: The inguinal paravascular technic of lumbar plexus anesthesia. "The 3-in-1 block." Anesth. Analg., *52*:989, 1973.

12 Intravenous Regional Neural Blockade

C. McK. Holmes

Intravenous regional analgesia is a simple method of producing analgesia of the arm or the leg by the intravenous injection of a local anesthetic while the circulation is occluded.

HISTORY

The history of anesthesia of the arm has been reviewed in published reports.[29,30] Although both Halsted and Crile had produced block of the brachial plexus by infiltration under direct vision, the method of intravenous regional analgesia was the first method whereby analgesia of the arm could easily be achieved. This method was discovered by August Bier, in 1908.[5] Bier was Professor of Surgery in Berlin, and is best remembered as the first to make regular use of spinal anesthesia. His method of intravenous analgesia consisted of isolating a segment of the arm with tourniquets and injecting a solution of 0.5 per cent procaine into a vein in the isolated segment. Some of the details mentioned by Bier in his paper, many of which are still relevant are worth noting.

It is important to empty the blood from the region to be anesthetized. This is done by winding an Esmarch bandage proximally up the arm. The circulation is then occluded above the level of the operation by many turns of a soft rubber bandage. A similar bandage is applied below the site of the operation. A cannula is inserted in a suitable vein between the two tourniquets [Fig. 12-1]. A 0.25 per cent or 0.5 per cent procaine solution in physiologic saline is used. Using the 0.5 per cent strength, direct anesthesia (*i.e.*, between the 2 bandages) comes on very rapidly. In the distal part of the limb, below the distal bandage, one gradually obtains conduction (indirect) anesthesia.

After removal of the bandages, motor and sensory paralysis disappear within a few minutes. The onset of anesthesia in the deeper tissues is as rapid as in the skin, or sometimes more so. The procaine in physiologic saline passes rapidly through the vein walls and is absorbed (into the tissues); after reestablishment of the circulation it only slowly enters the general circulation. Only once was a slight reaction to procaine observed on removing the bandages. To minimize the risk of reactions one may loosen the proximal bandage to permit arterial inflow and thereby flush the procaine out by way of the wound [see also Chap. 1].

This method enjoyed wide popularity for a time, and somewhat similar intra-arterial and even intraosseous methods were also described. However, it was not long before simple and reliable techniques for brachial plexus block were developed, and the intravenous method declined in popularity. It was revived in 1963 by Holmes, who used lidocaine, which appeared to give more reliable anesthesia than procaine and is now regarded as one of the fundamental techniques of arm anesthesia.[28]

CRITERIA FOR USE

Advantages

Ease of Performance. The technique is simple and reliable and can be performed without any special training, provided the anesthesiologist can insert a needle in the vein. This is in distinction to methods such as brachial plexus block, for which definite skill is required. However, the same requirements for resuscitation skill and equipment apply.

Safety. The reported incidence of adverse side-effects is very low, and there is certainly no risk of complications, such as total spinal anesthesia or pneumothorax. The risk of grand mal seizure is genuine but less than with other arm block techniques, provided that correct procedures are followed.

Onset of analgesia is rapid, so that surgery or manipulation may begin almost at once.

Muscular relaxation is good, so that reduction of fractures and similar maneuvers are facilitated.

Controllable Duration of Action. The duration of action is governed not by the local anesthetic agent used, but by the time for which the tourniquet is kept inflated. Operations as long as 6 hours have been described.[33]

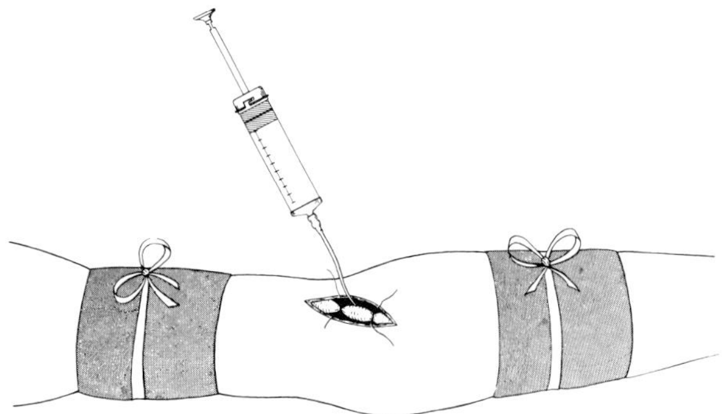

Fig. 12-1. Diagram of Bier's original method.

Controllable Extent. The extent of the analgesia is limited proximally by the position of the tourniquet. The closer the tourniquet is to the periphery, the smaller the quantity of analgesic solution required. Thus, in order to produce analgesia of only the hand or the foot, the tourniquet can be placed on the forearm or lower calf, respectively, and less solution used.

Rapidity of Recovery. Normal sensation and power return rapidly after cuff release, which enables reevaluation of neurologic signs after fracture reduction. This is also a valuable feature for outpatient surgery since a patient allowed to leave hospital with an anesthetized limb faces the hazards of accidental injury, cigarette burns, and the like.

Disadvantages

Tourniquet must be used. As a result, the method cannot produce analgesia of the entire limb but only of that portion below the tourniquet. The tourniquet must be kept inflated continuously; it is not possible to release it to enable bleeding vessels to be identified unless more local anesthetic is injected after reinflation.[8] The tourniquet may cause discomfort, though there are ways in which this may be minimized. The duration of the operation is generally limited by the time for which an arterial tourniquet may safely be left inflated.

Exsanguination. It is generally considered desirable to exsanguinate the limb as completely as possible. This cannot always be done by winding an Esmarch bandage up the limb because of a fracture or laceration. However, elevation for 2 to 3 minutes or use of an air-inflated splint will usually be satisfactory in such cases.[50]

Toxic Reactions. There is the possibility of a reaction to the local anesthetic agent when it is released into the general circulation. The risk will be greater when greater quantities are used, which, in turn depends on the size of the limb and the position of the tourniquet. For this reason, analgesia of the whole leg, with a thigh tourniquet, is not recommended because the quantity of solution would be too great, except in an amputation in which only a small amount remains to reenter the circulation.

Inability to Provide Bloodless Field. When analgesia of the hand is produced with a tourniquet about the forearm, there is likely to be a gradual engorgement of the hand, owing to intraosseous blood flow. This may be controlled by a second tourniquet on the upper arm.

Rapidity of recovery may be counted a disadvantage in major surgical cases, and parenteral narcotic analgesics may be required early in the postoperative phase.

Selection of Cases

Intravenous regional analgesia is most suited to surgery of the forearm and hand, including the manipulation of forearm fractures. It may be used for supracondylar fractures, but is less satisfactory because of the presence of the inflated cuff close to the fracture site. Similarly, other lesions much above the elbow are usually better managed with some type of brachial plexus block. The method is also not as suitable for the leg, because of the larger quantity of solution required; however, the foot may safely be anesthetized. The following description of the "standard" method for the arm includes the slight modifications necessary when only the hand or foot is to be anesthetized.

Other than patients with a known hypersensitivity to local anesthetic agents, there are no absolute contraindications to the technique, providing a tourniquet can be used. However, care must be exercised in patients with a history of epilepsy or cardiac disease. In particular, untreated heart block should be considered a relative contraindication, since sudden release of local anesthetic into the circulation may convert a partial heart block to a complete one or precipitate asystole. In practice, certainly, bradycardia has been recorded following cuff release if lidocaine is used for intravenous regional block, even in normal patients.[13,34]

TECHNIQUE

Standard Method for the Arm

Equipment. The anesthetic agent of choice for this technique is prilocaine, 0.5 per cent. Since up to 50 ml is required for the arm and larger quantities for the leg, the largest available ampules should be used. The solution must not contain epinephrine or any other vasoconstrictor. Usually a "butterfly" needle with a short extension tube is used for the venipuncture. A plastic cannula may be used and is perhaps less likely to be dislodged during the exsanguination. A long intravenous catheter should not be used, however, because there is at least one recorded case when the end of such a catheter was actually above the inflated cuff, which resulted in an injection directly into the general circulation.[1]

A disposable 50-ml syringe is convenient for the injection, though a smaller size (*e.g.*, 20-ml) may be used. An Esmarch-type rubber bandage is needed as well as a pneumatic tourniquet. The pneumatic tourniquet may be a conventional sphygmomanometer or an automatic gas-operated kind. Special cuffs, with two compartments, useful for relief of tourniquet discomfort in long operations, have been described.[27,32]

Preparation of the Patient. Having ascertained that the patient accepts this form of analgesia and has no history of allergic reactions to local anesthetic drugs, the anesthesiologist should explain the technique, and it is useful to check the blood pressure on the side of the operation, to demonstrate the sensation of the cuff to the patient. This also enables the cuff to be inflated to the correct pressure later, after exsanguination. After the blood pressure has been checked, the cuff may be left inflated above the diastolic pressure, in order to distend the veins for insertion of the needle. As with any anesthetic administration, it is a wise precaution to secure a route for intravenous fluids and supplemental drugs, usually in the nonoperated arm, and to place a blood pressure cuff on that side as well, so that the blood pressure can be monitored during the procedure.

Premedication. In emergency or outpatient cases, premedication may be omitted, particularly if the proposed operation is likely to be of short duration. However, for longer operations some form of sedation is desirable and may be a small dose of a narcotic or a benzodiazepine (preferably diazepam, see Chap. 2). Just prior to the performance of the block, an appropriate dose of a sedative, such as diazepam, or neuroleptanalgesia may be given intravenously. This will help to reduce the patient's reaction to the inflated cuff; small increments may be given during long operations.

Choice of Vein. Usually a vein on the dorsum of the hand is selected. However, if no veins are visible in this region, a vein on the forearm or even at the antecubital fossa may be chosen. There is, however, some evidence that failure, or "patchy" analgesia, is more likely to occur when proximal veins are used.[45] The butterfly or similar needle is placed in the vein and taped securely. Care must be taken not to dislodge the needle during the exsanguination or subsequent injection. As with any venipuncture, there should be careful palpation for superficial arteries to avoid intra-arterial injection.

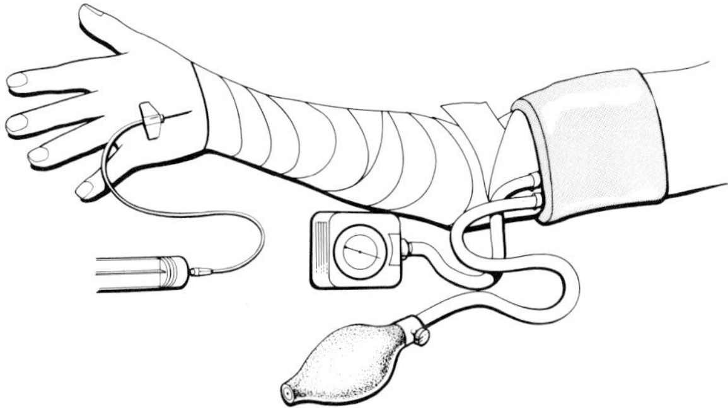

Fig. 12-2. Exsanguination with an Esmarch bandage prior to the injection.

Exsanguination. It has frequently been stated that exsanguination of the limb assists in the production of complete analgesia. However, not all writers agree on this point, at least two believing it to be unnecessary.[12,47] The usual method is to wind an Esmarch bandage snugly up the arm, starting, where possible, just proximal to the needle (Fig. 12-2). If this method is undesirable because of a fracture or wound, elevation or an air-inflated splint are acceptable alternatives.

The tourniquet is now inflated to a pressure above the patient's systolic value. The exact amount by which the tourniquet pressure should exceed the systolic cannot clearly be stated, for the patient's blood pressure may rise during the injection or during the operation. Some authors advise a tourniquet pressure of 200 to 250 torr, which should provide a margin of safety.[18,38] The practice of cross-clamping the tubing of the cuff after inflation is not recommended; should the cuff have a small leak, it might not be detected. It is better to observe the cuff pressure at all times on the aneroid dial (Fig. 12-3).

Injection. The quantity of drug injected is usually chosen according to the mass of tissue below the tourniquet and may not correlate well with the patient's weight. It may be necessary to use 50 ml for the muscular forearm of a slim man, whereas the slim forearm of an obese patient may satisfactorily be anesthetized with a smaller amount. As the drug

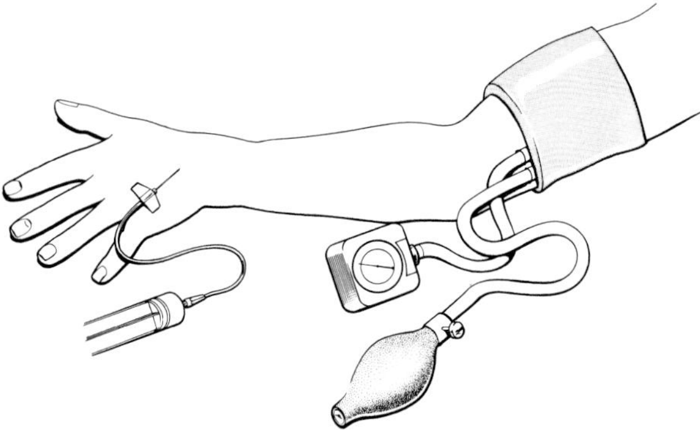

Fig. 12-3. The injection has been completed. The needle may be removed at this stage. Note the tourniquet tubing not clamped; the pressure is visible on the dial.

is injected, the skin usually becomes mottled, and analgesia develops rapidly. Muscular relaxation, usually quite profound, appears at the same time. If sufficient analgesia is not present 5 minutes after the injection of 40 ml, a further 10 ml should be given before removing the needle. Colbern[10] recommends injecting a "chaser" of 5 to 10 ml of normal saline after the local anesthetic, maintaining that it aids dispersion of the drug and not only hastens the onset of analgesia but also helps to avoid patchy areas of retained sensation.

Tourniquet Discomfort. During the operation, the tourniquet must be kept inflated above the systolic value. After a time, particularly in the unsedated patient, discomfort may develop. This may respond to a small intravenous dose of diazepam or an analgesic drug. An alternative, or additional, maneuver is to place another cuff below the first, and inflate it over the analgesic part of the arm, after which the upper cuff is deflated. This method is facilitated if the double-compartment cuff is available.[27,32] Another method, which is said to relieve tourniquet discomfort, is to apply a vibratory massager to the inflated cuff.[23]

Minimum tourniquet time is subject to some debate and is discussed further below. It is usually assumed that deflating the tourniquet soon after the injection would be equivalent to a rapid intravenous infusion of prilocaine and could produce a toxic reaction. Without any direct evidence to the contrary, therefore, it is recommended to keep the cuff inflated for a minimum of 15 minutes.

Tourniquet Release. At the end of the operation, and not before—because sensation returns rapidly, the tourniquet is released. It has been suggested that the cuff be released and reinflated immediately, to release a "test dose" of prilocaine into the general circulation. The effects of this procedure are discussed further below. However, pharmacokinetic data indicate that reinflation must occur within 30 seconds of deflation to have an appreciable effect.[48]

In any event, it is at the time of release that adverse reactions may occur, so pulse and blood pressure should be monitored closely during the first few minutes after tourniquet release (see Fig. 12-7). Appropriate resuscitation equipment should be available, and the patient should be warned to expect transient generalized paresthesias and, sometimes, tinnitus. There appears to be no risk of delayed after-effects.

Modified Method for the Hand

The cuff is placed on the forearm (Fig. 12-4). About 10 ml of solution will usually provide complete analgesia. A difficulty sometimes encountered with this method is that blood flow through the radius and ulna causes gradual congestion if the operation is other than quite short. Of course, since the quantity of solution is so small, the tourniquet could be released safely at any time, so a short procedure is quite feasible. For a longer operation, a second tourniquet on the upper arm may be needed.

Modified Method for the Foot

The same principles apply as apply for the hand (Fig. 12-5). The tourniquet should be well below the knee, to avoid compressing the peroneal nerve on the neck of the fibula.

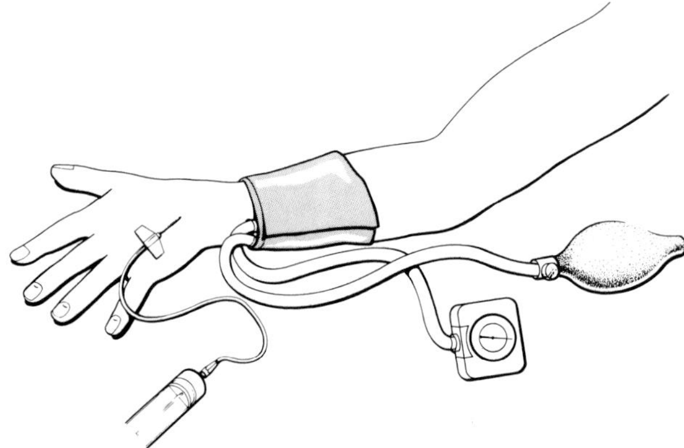

Fig. 12-4. The modified method for the hand. A second tourniquet might be placed on the upper arm, if necessary.

Prolonged Intravenous Regional Analgesia

Although intravenous regional analgesia is better suited to short procedures, it may be adapted for prolonged operations if the patient is well-sedated. The technique has been described by Brown and consists of inserting an indwelling plastic catheter in a suitable vein of the same arm but away from the operating site, and leaving it *in situ* during the operation.[7] After about 1 hour, the tourniquet is deflated, and during the short interval before sensation returns, bleeding vessels may be secured. The arm is then elevated, the tourniquet reinflated, and another dose of the local anesthetic injected. Brown found that this dose may be only one-half the volume of the first. The procedure may be repeated if necessary. If this intermittent method is not used, the governing factor in long operations is the time for which it is considered safe to leave a tourniquet inflated (see below).

Pediatric Use

The method is readily applicable to children, provided that they are old enough to comprehend a simple explanation of the procedure, and several authors have commented favorably on this use of the technique.[9,17,21] Because there does not have to be a delay in instituting treatment, even if the child has eaten recently, it is a valuable procedure for reduction of the common forearm fracture and similar lesions.

The standard method is used, making sure the tourniquet is an appropriate size for the child's arm. Elevation is used for exsanguination in preference to an Esmarch bandage, to avoid any discomfort. The dose of prilocaine may be calculated on the basis of 5 mg per kg.

CHOICE OF LOCAL ANESTHETIC AGENT

All the common local anesthetic agents have been used, including even cocaine. Procaine was, of course, the standard drug of the early researchers, but it is undoubtedly less effective than the modern agents. Lidocaine was used first by Holmes, and many large series have since been reported with this agent.[28]

Probably equally satisfactory analgesia has been obtainable with all the modern drugs. However, it should be noted that the duration of action does not depend on the drug but upon the time for which the tourniquet is kept inflated. Occasionally, a degree of patchy analgesia remains for a varying time after tourniquet release, and this analgesia has been shown to correlate well with the known duration of action of the agent used.[16]

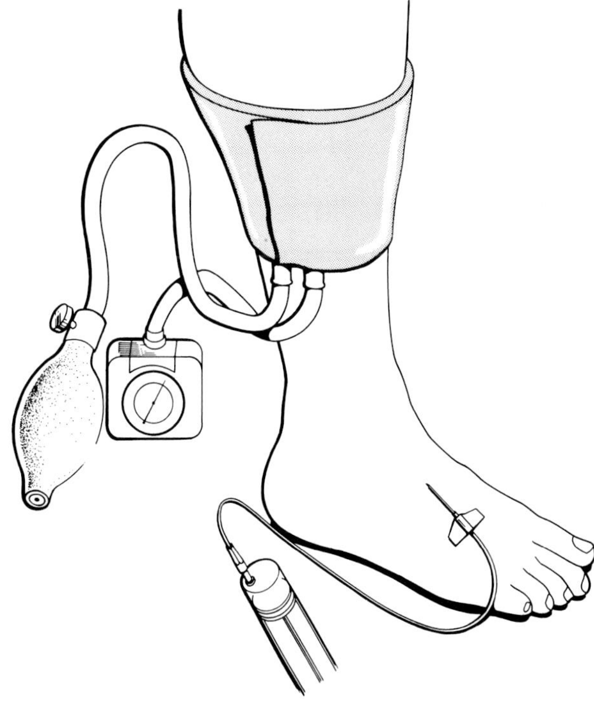

Fig. 12-5. The modified method for the foot.

It is also of interest to note that quite satisfactory analgesia can be obtained with 2-chloroprocaine, even though this agent is normally hydrolyzed rapidly in the blood. This agent is, of course, the least toxic agent and would, in theory, be the ideal choice. However, there is a higher incidence of thrombophlebitis with it, so it is not recommended.[25]

Prilocaine is the most rapidly metabolized of the amides and, given its efficacy by the intravenous route and its low incidence of thrombophlebitis, it appears to have most appeal of the drugs available (see Chap. 4).

Prilocaine was first used by Hooper in 64 cases and subsequently by many others.[31] In a double-blind trial, Kerr studied 22 patients who were given 0.5 per cent prilocaine and 20 who were given 0.5 per cent lidocaine.[35] Nearly half the patients who received lidocaine had neurologic side-effects (dizziness, tinnitus, muscular twitching), while there was only one minor episode of dizziness following prilocaine. Eriksson demonstrated that the effects on the electroencephalogram (EEG) with 200 mg of lidocaine (40 ml of 0.5%) were similar to but smaller in magnitude than those seen after direct intravenous injection of the same dose over a period of 2.3 minutes. Subjective symptoms could be correlated with the EEG changes and occurred in all subjects. With a similar amount of prilocaine, the EEG changes were considerably reduced, and there were no subjective symptoms. This could partly be explained by the lower plasma levels that occur after the administration of prilocaine and partly by its lower inherent toxicity. Eriksson also showed that when intravenous regional analgesia was produced with a mixture of 0.25 per cent lidocaine and 0.25 per cent prilocaine, the maximum plasma concentration of the prilocaine was less than that of the lidocaine. This effect has also been demonstrated by Thorn–Alquist.[46]

Prilocaine is therefore the drug of first choice for intravenous regional analgesia.

Concentration. Varying concentrations from 0.15 per cent up to 2 per cent have been used successfully. The governing factor is the total dose, and with the stronger solutions, a smaller volume would have to be used, which may result in rather patchy analgesia, although a dose-response study has not been performed. Twenty ml of 1 per cent prilocaine was recommended by Hooper, but most workers have favored the 0.5 per cent concentration, with a mean volume of about 40 ml, which may be varied slightly according to an estimate of the mass of tissue to be anesthetized.[31] This question of volume and, hence, of total dose of drug is discussed further in the next section.

COMPLICATIONS

The complications of intravenous regional analgesia are entirely those of systemic toxicity of the agent used (see Chap. 4). Local anesthetics affect principally the central nervous system (CNS), where they may be either stimulant or depressant, and the cardiovascular system, where they are depressant (see Chaps. 2 and 4).

A special problem with prilocaine is methemoglobinemia. Generally, with any drug, side-effects are proportional to the total dose administered but are modified by many factors, including individual susceptibility. It is noteworthy that no fatalities have been reported with this technique, even though at least 10,000 cases have been documented.[10]

Central nervous system symptoms and signs range from mild, transient giddiness, dizziness, or tinnitus to more serious phenomena such as muscular twitching, convulsions, and loss of consciousness. This second group is not common, however. In one series of 1400 patients, only 8 had CNS stimulation sufficient to require the administration of a barbiturate, and only 3 of these had frank convulsions.[49] All these patients had received a dose of lidocaine in excess of 5 mg per kg. Fleming records "5 or 6" convulsions in another large series, again after lidocaine.[18] No frank convulsions have been reported with prilocaine.

The highest frequency of minor CNS toxicity is recorded by Harris, 67.3 per cent with 5 mg per kg of prilocaine in a group of volunteers.[25] A 50 per cent incidence with lidocaine, 3 mg per kg, in a small group of volunteers was recorded by Bell, Slater, and Harris.[4] Most other workers report a lower incidence, 10 per cent or less. Dunbar and Mazze record an incidence of 2.1 per cent in 779 patients, with lidocaine or prilocaine.[13]

Cardiovascular system symptoms and signs are usually also mild and transient. In 779 patients, Dunbar and Mazze found no arrhythmias and only a slight drop in blood pressure or a slight bradycardia on release of the tourniquet.[13] This is in keeping with the observations of most other workers. By contrast, however, Kennedy, Duthie, Parbrook, and Carr, who monitored the electrocardiogram (ECG) in all their 77 patients, found a 15 per cent incidence of ECG changes, mostly of a minor nature, and recorded one cardiac arrest (successfully treated), preceded by bradycardia.[34] They did not feel justified in continuing to use the technique with lidocaine.

Methemoglobinemia is known to occur after the administration of prilocaine and may cause cyanosis (see Chap. 4). A significant rise in serum methemoglobin levels is not usually seen below a total dose of prilocaine of 600 mg, which is above the dose required for intravenous regional analgesia.[36] Harris, Cole, Mital, and Laver[26] studied 58 volunteers given 5 mg per kg of prilocaine for intravenous regional analgesia and found a small rise in methemoglobin from 0.33 ± 0.11 g per 100 ml (control) to 1.02 ± 0.33 g per 100 ml after tourniquet release. No cyanosis was observed.

Factors That Influence the Incidence of Toxic Reactions. It has been indicated earlier that the dose of prilocaine depends upon the mass of tissue below the tourniquet. This indicates the need for aproximately 40 ml of solution for an average-size arm with the tourniquet above the elbow. This quantity may be altered proportionately for large or small arms. However, the incidence of toxic reactions is related to blood level, and this, in turn, depends upon, among other factors, the dose given in proportion to the total body weight. For this reason, certain authors have recommended maximum doses (*e.g.*, lidocaine, 1.5 mg/kg or 3 mg/kg; prilocaine, 3 mg/kg or 4 mg/kg).[13,25]

Preinjection ischemia has been shown by Bell and colleagues and Harris to result in a significant reduction in the amount of solution required for satisfactory analgesia.[4,25] This modification involves inflation of the tourniquet 15 to 20 minutes before the injection. Without this ischemia, they found an average of 3 mg per kg of lidocaine was required, and this could be halved by the modified technique. Using prilocaine, Harris recommended 4 mg per kg with 15-minute preinjection ischemia. The mechanism of action of this maneuver is uncertain. In spite of the enthusiasm of these authors for this modification, it does not appear to have achieved widespread popularity, most researchers believing that it prolongs the procedure and subjects the patient to additional discomfort.

Plasma levels of local anesthetic after tourniquet release have been studied by several authors. Using 0.5 per cent lidocaine in a dose of 2.5 mg per kg and releasing the tourniquet in most cases after only 5 minutes, Hargrove, Hoyle, Parker, Beckett, and Boyes found maximum levels in venous blood from the other arm did not exceed 2 μg per ml.[24] A similar figure of 1.5 ± 0.2 μg per ml was found by Mazze and Dunbar following 3 mg per kg of 0.5% lidocaine.[37] They found considerably higher levels after axillary block and after lumbar epidural block (Fig. 12-6; Table 12-1).

Tucker and Boas, who studied plasma lidocaine concentration in the contralateral artery, observed that the peak levels were from 20 to 80 per cent lower than those found after direct intravenous infusion of the same dose over 3 minutes.[48] They also found the levels were lower (by about 40%) when the same dose was used for intravenous regional analgesia in a 0.5-per-cent solution, rather than a 1-per-cent solution. Pharmacokinetic calculations from this data, if a cuff time of 10 minutes is assumed, indicate that after cuff release the drug reaches the systemic circulation in the following biphasic manner: an initial fast release of 30 per cent of the dose, which is so rapid that reinflation of the cuff would only retard systemic uptake if it were performed within 30 seconds of cuff release and a slower washout of the remainder of the dose, so that up to 30 minutes after cuff release half the dose would still be retained in the arm.

These findings are supported by recent clinical data that indicate sustained high local anesthetic concentrations in the venous drainage from the blocked arm.[16] Thus, it is possible to reestablish anesthesia for approximately 10 to 30 minutes after

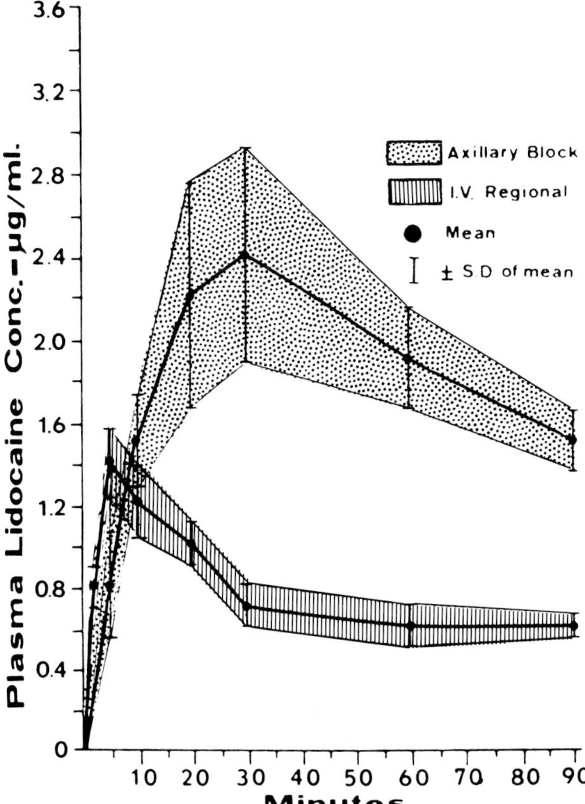

Fig. 12-6. A comparison of the blood levels of lidocaine after intravenous regional analgesia and axillary block. The horizontal axis refers to the time after tourniquet release for intravenous regional analgesia and time after injection of lidocaine for axillary block.

Table 12-1. Plasma Levels After Tourniquet Release

Block	*Dose of Lidocaine (mg/kg)*	*Mean Peak Plasma Level (μg/ml)*
Intravenous regional analgesia	3, 0.5%	1.5 ± 0.2
Axillary block	6–6.8, 1.5%*	2.5 ± 0.5
Lumbar epidural block	4.7–6.5, 1.5%*	3.1 ± 0.7
Caudal epidural block	5.8–7.5, 1.5%*	1.4 ± 0.6

* With 1:200,000, epinephrine

(Mazze, R. I., and Dunbar, R. W.: Plasma lidocaine concentrations after caudal, lumbar epidural, axillary block and intravenous regional anethesia. Anesthesiology, *27*:574, 1966)

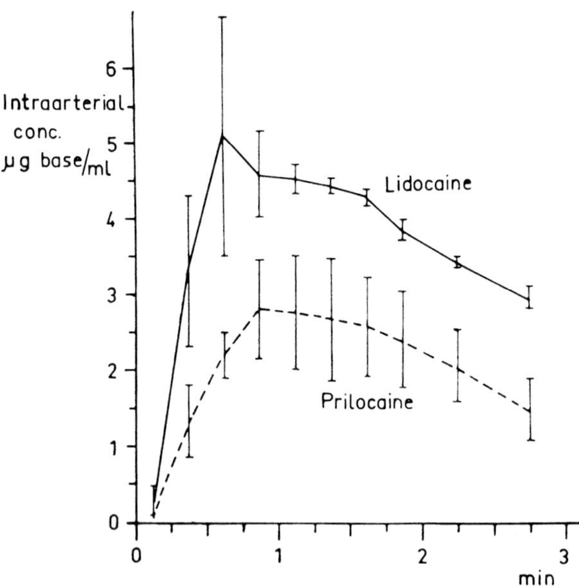

Fig. 12-7. The blood levels of lidocaine and prilocaine in the contralateral brachial artery after intravenous regional analgesia with a mixture of the two agents.

cuff release by injecting half the original dose, after reinflation of the cuff.

Eriksson studied 5 volunteers, who received intravenous regional analgesia on two occasions, once with prilocaine and once with lidocaine (40 ml of 0.5% in each case).[15] The tourniquet was left inflated for 30 minutes after all injections. Sampling was from the contralateral brachial artery. The results are shown in Figure 12-7, which demonstrates the consistently lower levels with prilocaine. These levels are less than those usually considered toxic. Englesson, Eriksson, Wahlqvist, and Ortengren found that symptoms were noted in awake patients who received intravenous infusions of lidocaine, at a mean plasma level of 4.4 µg per ml, while Foldes, Molloy, McNall, and Koukal supply a figure of 5.3 µg per ml.[14,20] In anesthetized patients, signs of toxicity were not seen below plasma levels of 10 µg per ml.[6]

The following factors may affect the peak blood level after tourniquet release: whether or not exsanguination is performed, time from injection to tourniquet release, mode of release of tourniquet, and arm movement after tourniquet release.

Exsanguination has been insufficiently studied. Adams, Dealy, and Kenmore suggested that the better the exsanguination the smaller would be the "reservoir" of lidocaine-containing solution to be flushed into the general circulation.[2] Eriksson, however, studied a few cases in which exsanguination had been performed with an Esmarch bandage, and found no difference in plasma lidocaine level, compared with those in which the arm had been elevated only.[15]

Time to tourniquet release has been studied by several workers, but their findings have been variable. Mazze and Dunbar found no correlation between peak venous levels and tourniquet time; indeed, the patient who had the longest tourniquet time had the third highest plasma lidocaine concentration (Fig. 12-8).[37] However, this may have related to errors inherent in venous sampling. Comparing tourniquet times of 15 and 30 minutes, Thorn-Alquist found no differences in peak levels when sampling from the contralateral artery.[46] By contrast, Tucker and Boas, again using arterial sampling, did find an inverse relationship between tourniquet time and peak plasma level (Fig. 12-9).[48]

Mode of Release of Tourniquet. Holmes suggested that release and rapid reinflation of the tourniquet several times would lessen the incidence of symptoms.[28] This maneuver has also been recommended by other workers. Merrifield and Carter found a mean peak venous lidocaine level of 5.9 ± 5.7 µg per ml when this procedure was performed, while with half the dose of lidocaine and without intermittent tourniquet release, the level was 4.7 ± 0.2 µg per ml, which indicates a definite protective effect.[39] This method is perhaps less important if prilocaine is used; however, since it is simple to perform, it is wise to employ it as a safety measure.

Arm movement immediately after tourniquet release should be discouraged because it has been

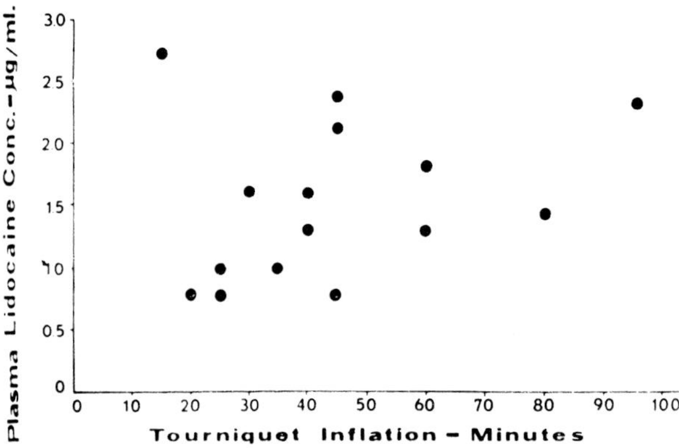

Fig. 12-8. Maximum plasma lidocaine concentration after tourniquet release, measured in venous blood, in relation to duration of tourniquet inflation.

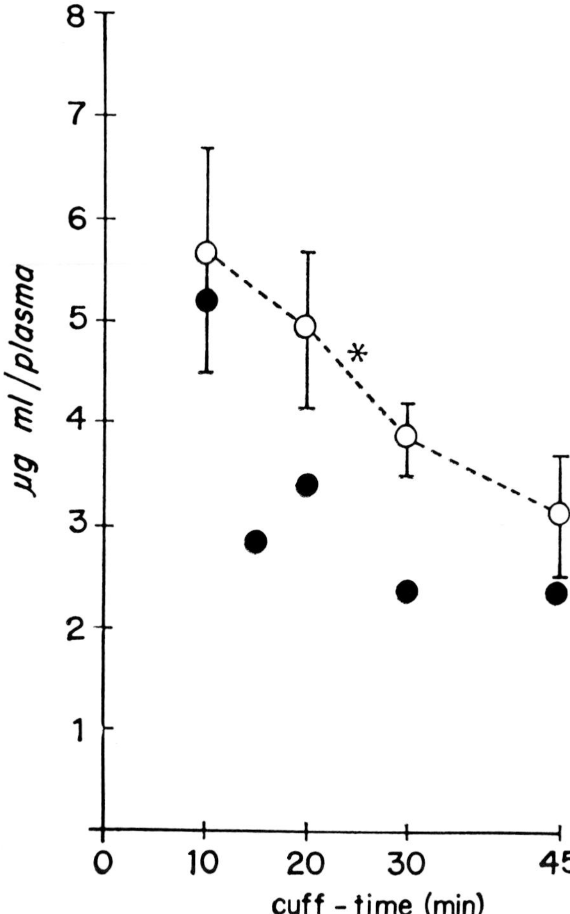

Fig. 12-9. Relationship between cuff time and arterial plasma level of lidocaine, 1 minute after tourniquet release. (Open circles represent mean data ± SD, solution; Asterisk represents the difference significant at P < 0.05; Closed circles indicate individual data with 0.5-% solution)

shown to result in increased plasma levels of the drug.[24]

Complications Related to the Use of a Tourniquet. When use of intravenous regional analgesia is considered, the fact that a tourniquet must be used for the entire duration of the operation must be taken into account. There may be operations in which this is undesirable or even impossible, so that other methods of regional analgesia might be more appropriate. There may be operations where the duration is considered too long for a tourniquet—though this is controversial—for there does not appear to be any clear relationship between tourniquet time and complications.

Middleton and Varian reviewed an estimated 630,000 tourniquet applications, and found an incidence of peripheral nerve damage of 1:8,000.[40] The incidence was higher in the upper limb (1:5,000) than the lower limb (1:13,000). In the upper limb, there were 27 patients with total palsy, eight following the use of a pneumatic tourniquet and 19 following the use of an Esmarch bandage. All recovered. The tourniquet time varied from 20 minutes to 2 and a half hours. There were 19 patients with radial nerve palsy, in whom the tourniquet applications varied from 15 minutes to 1 and a half hours. All but one of these recovered. In the lower limb, there were 30 patients with palsy, all following the use of an Esmarch bandage. The tourniquet time varied from 30 minutes to 4 and a half hours, and all but one had an eventual full recovery. These authors studied the pressures that could be produced with an Esmarch bandage and found them variable and usually higher than supposed. However, they were not able to draw definite conclusions about the etiology of tourniquet paralyses. There did not seem to be any common factor in any of their cases.

Moldaver believed that direct mechanical pressure was more likely to be a factor than ischemia and cautioned against using a tourniquet in any area where a nerve could be compressed against bony structures.[42]

The following general recommendations can therefore be made.

A pneumatic tourniquet is preferred to an Esmarch bandage, since the pressure will be known and can be checked throughout the operation.

The tourniquet should be applied where the nerves are best protected in the muscles.

Excessive tourniquet pressure should be avoided, by measuring the systolic blood pressure before and during the operation, and maintaining a tourniquet pressure of, for example, 50 torr above the systolic.

The tubing should not be clamped between the cuff and the gauge, for this would prevent a leaking cuff from being detected.

The duration of application of the tourniquet should be as short as possible. In prolonged operations the method of Brown could be used, though it is uncertain whether this really provides a greater safety margin.[8]

MODE OF ACTION

Mode of action has been the subject of much debate, and indeed there has been difficulty in separating the effects of the local anesthetic from those of ischemia alone. Direct pressure on nerves can cause anesthesia, and Miles, James, Clarke, and Whitwam and Shanks and McLeod found quite marked effects from ischemia alone.[41,44] In fact, the second group found that anesthesia, preceded by dysesthesia, usually developed in 15 to 30 minutes with ischemia alone, and there was variable muscle weakness. However, all agree that the onset of anesthesia is much more rapid and complete when a local anesthetic is added.

Miles and colleagues demonstrated that the action potential latency in muscle was increased 55 per cent by ischemia and 180 per cent by ischemia plus lidocaine.[41] They believed that their results indicated that lidocaine acts on the peripheral part of the neuron. They showed that the muscle weakness was not reversible by neostigmine.

Shanks and McLeod, however, using 1 per cent lidocaine, concluded that the block was in the nerve trunks.[44] They considered that the more pronounced effect of lidocaine on conduction in proximal segments of the nerve was the result of a greater concentration of the agent in the forearm, and would be in keeping with the radiographic studies of Fleming, Veiga-Pires, McCutcheon, and Emanuel and Sorbie and Chacha, who demonstrated that the local anesthetic proceeds rapidly in a proximal direction when it is injected on the dorsum of the hand.[19,45]

Cotev and Robin, in biopsy studies on dogs with C^{14}-labeled lidocaine, showed a selective accumulation of the agent in nerves and relatively little in muscle.[11] They noted a biphasic washout of the drug, which they attributed to reactive hyperemia.

In an elegant series of experiments, Raj, Garcia, Burleson, and Jenkins demonstrated, by means of a lidocaine-Renografin-60 mixture, that the contrast concentrated principally around the elbow.[43] No contrast was seen distal to the proximal phalanges. Anesthesia developed from the fingertips upward, reaching the elbow last. Contrast material confined to the hand, injected by way of the radial artery, did not produce anesthesia. When the block was established between two tourniquets, as in the original Bier method, nerve conduction above the block (median nerve in the axilla to thenar muscles) was decreased, whereas nerve conduction below the block (ulnar nerve at the wrist to hypothenar muscles) was unaltered. Anesthesia tended to develop earlier in the anteromedial aspect of the forearm and later in the posterolateral aspect.

The authors believe that these results show that the mode of action is on the larger nerve trunks. At the elbow, the median and ulnar nerves are fairly close together and surrounded by large venous channels. The radial nerve is posterolateral and has fewer large vessels near it. Histologically, the peripheral nerve shows a thick perineurium, but with many vascular channels in the core of the nerve in close proximity to the nerve fibrils. It would seem that these vascular channels take the drug to the core of the nerve, from which it would diffuse toward the periphery. The greater number of venous channels close to the median and ulnar nerves, compared with the radial nerve, would explain the earlier onset of analgesia on the anteromedial aspect of the forearm (Fig. 12-10).

Two difficulties remain insufficiently elucidated.[7] First, the speed of onset and, particularly, the rapidity of spread are not like those seen with the block of a major nerve trunk. Second, cases have been reported in which analgesia was complete everywhere but a digit, in which the local circulation was impaired; this does not support nerve trunk block.[3]

Perhaps Bier should have the last word: ". . . . [this] new method uses the vascular bed to bring the anesthetic agent to the nerve endings as well as the nerve trunks."[5]

INTRAVENOUS REGIONAL SYMPATHETIC BLOCK

Intravenous regional sympathetic block is similar to the intravenous regional analgesia technique. The method was devised, and is described in detail, by Hannington-Kiff.[22,23]

Premedication is usually unnecessary, but all the usual precautions should be taken. The blood pressure should be monitored, an intravenous infusion should be running, and the patient should be on a table capable of being tilted. The agent used is guanethidine, which is strongly bound to sympathetic nerve endings. The butterfly needle is placed in a hand vein, and the tourniquet on the upper arm. Elevation is used for exsanguination, and the tourniquet inflated to 50 to 100 torr above the systolic pressure. The solution consists of 10 to 20 mg of guanethidine and 500 of heparin in 25 ml of physiologic saline. (For the leg, 20 mg of the drug is used with 1000 IU of heparin and 50 ml of saline.) To reduce the discomfort of guanethidine injection, 25 ml of 0.5 per cent prilocaine may be substituted for the 25 ml saline.

The tourniquet is kept inflated for 10 minutes and then released and reinflated several times, while the

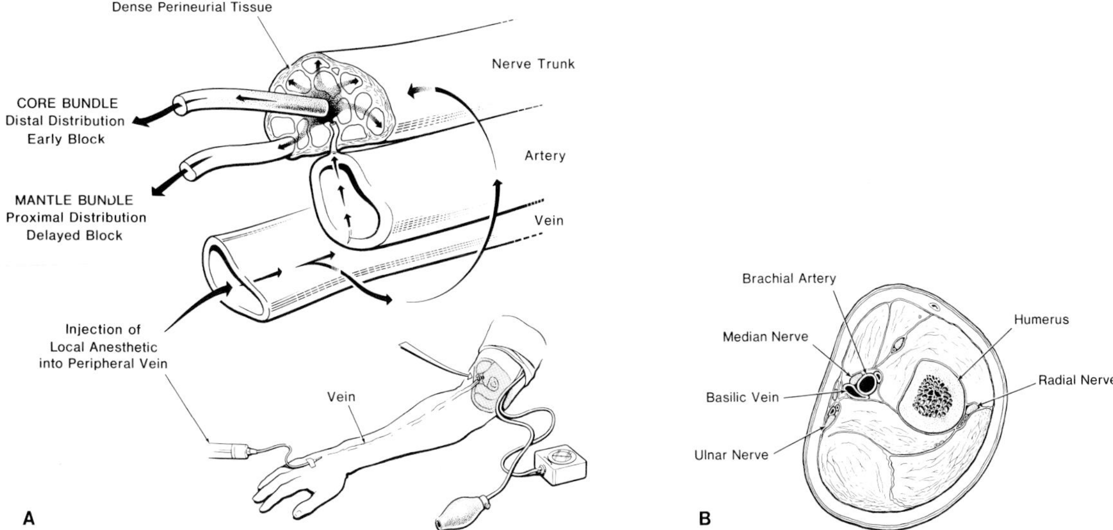

Fig. 12-10. Proposed mechanism of intravenous regional anesthesia. (*A*) Local anesthetic injected into a dorsal hand vein travels to the large venous channels at the elbow. Here, it is transferred by arteries through the thick perineurium into the core of the major nerve trunks. From here, it diffuses outward so that the core bundles are blocked, initially resulting in "early distal block," and the mantle bundles (supplying proximal areas) are blocked last, resulting in "delayed proximal block." (*B*) Note that, in a cross section of the arm at the elbow, the median and ulnar nerves on the anteromedial aspect have rich vascular channels nearby. The radial nerve, on the posterolateral surface, has less vascularity in its vicinity. This may explain the later onset of analgesia in radial nerve distribution.

blood pressure is monitored in the other arm. (A slight fall in blood pressure may occur.) The effectiveness of the sympathetic block may be checked with a temperature probe.

The advantages of this method are that it may be used after "post-sympathectomy escape," that it may be used in patients on anticoagulants, and that the potential complications of stellate ganglion block are avoided. Also avoided are the adhesions that can result from lumbar sympathetic block with phenol, which may render subsequent surgery difficult.

Hannington-Kiff describes several successful cases, with relief lasting for days or even months (see Chap. 13).

REFERENCES

1. Anesthesia Conference (Clinical), N. Y. State J. Med., *66*:1344, 1966.
2. Adams, J.P., Dealy, E.J., and Kenmore, P.I.: Intravenous regional anesthesia in hand surgery. J. Bone Joint Surg., *46A*:811, 1964.
3. Atkinson, D.I.: The mode of action of intravenous regional anaesthetics. Acta Anaesthesiol. Scand., *36* [*Suppl.*]:131, 1969.
4. Bell, H.M., Slater, E.M., and Harris, W.H.: Regional anesthesia with intravenous lidocaine. J.A.M.A., *186*:544, 1963.
5. Bier, A.: Ueber einen neuen Weg Lokalanasthesie an den gliedmassen zu Erzeugen. Verh. dtsch. Ges. Chir., *37*(*2*):204, 1908.
6. Bromage, P.R., and Robson, J.G.: Concentrations of lignocaine in the blood after intravenous, intramuscular epidural and endotracheal administration. Anaesthesia, *16*:461, 1961.
7. Brown, B.R.: Discussion on: The site of action of intravenous regional anesthesia. Anesth. Analg. (Cleve.), *51*:776, 1972.
8. Brown, E.M., and Weissman, F.: A case report: Prolonged intravenous regional anesthesia. Anesth. Analg. (Cleve.), *45*:319, 1966.
9. Carrell, E.D., and Eyring, E.J.: Intravenous regional anesthesia for childhood fractures. J. Trauma, *11*:301, 1971.
10. Colbern, E.C.: The Bier block for intravenous regional anesthesia. Anesth. Analg. (Cleve.), *49*:935, 1970.
11. Cotev, S., and Robin, G.C.: Experimental studies on intravenous regional analgesia using radioactive lidocaine. Acta Anaesthesiol. Scand. *36* [*Suppl.*]:127, 1969.
12. Dawkins, O.S., *et al.*: Intravenous regional anaesthesia. Can. Anaesth. Soc. J., *11*:243, 1964.
13. Dunbar, R.W., and Mazze, R.I.: Intravenous regional anesthesia. Anesth. Analg. (Cleve.), *46*:806, 1967.
14. Englesson, S., Eriksson, E., Wahlqvist, S., and Ortengren, B.: Differences in tolerance to intravenous xylocaine and ci-

tanest (L67) a new local anaesthetic. A double-blind study in man. Proc. First Eur. Congr. Anaesth., *2*:206.1, 1962.
15. Eriksson, E.: The effects of intravenous local anesthetic agents on the central nervous system. Acta Anaesthesiol. Scand. *36* [*Suppl.*]:79, 1969.
16. Evans, C.J., Dewar, J.A., Boyes, R.N., and Scott, D.B.: Residual nerve block following intravenous regional anaesthesia. Br. J. Anaesth., *46*:668, 1974.
17. Fitzgerald, B.: Intravenous regional anaesthesia in children. Br. J. Anaesth., *48*:485, 1976.
18. Fleming, S.A.: Safety and usefulness of intravenous regional anaesthesia. Acta Anaesthesiol. Scand. *36* [*Suppl.*]:21, 1969.
19. Fleming, S.A., Veiga–Pires, J.A., McCutcheon, R.M., and Emanuel, C.I.: A demonstration of the site of action of intravenous lignocaine. Can. Anaesth. Soc. J., *13*:21, 1966.
20. Foldes, F.F., Molloy, R., McNall, P.G., and Koukal, L.R.: Comparison of toxicity of intravenously given local anesthetic agents in man. J.A.M.A., *172*:1493, 1960.
21. Gingrich, T.F.: Intravenous regional anesthesia of the upper extremity in children. J.A.M.A., *200*:405, 1967.
22. Hannington-Kiff, J.G.: Intravenous regional sympathetic block with guanethidine. Lancet, *1*:1019, 1974.
23. ______: Pain Relief. ed. 1. p. 70. London, Heinemann Educational Books, 1974.
24. Hargrove, R.L., Hoyle, J.R., Parker, F.B.R., Beckett, A.H., and Boyes, R.N.: Blood lignocaine levels following intravenous regional analgesia. Anaesthesia, *21*:37, 1966.
25. Harris, W.H.: Choice of anesthetic agents for intravenous regional anesthesia. Acta Anaesthesiol. Scand. *36* [*Suppl.*]:47, 1969.
26. Harris, W.H., Cole, D.W., Mital, M., and Laver, M.B.: Methemoglobin formation and oxygen transport following intravenous regional anesthesia using prilocaine. Anesthesiology, *29*:65, 1968.
27. Hoffman, S., Simon, B.E., and Hartley, J.: A new tourniquet for intravenous regional anesthesia. Plast. Reconstr. Surg., *40*:243, 1967.
28. Holmes, C. McK.: Intravenous regional analgesia. Lancet, *1*:245, 1963.
29. ______: Anaesthetising the arm. N. Z. Med. J., *63*:24, 1964.
30. ______: The history and development of intravenous regional anaesthesia. Acta Anaesthesiol. Scand. *36* [*Suppl.*]:11, 1969.
31. Hooper, R.L.: Intravenous regional anaesthesia: A report of a new local anaesthetic agent. Can. Anaesth. Soc. J., *11*:247, 1964.
32. Hoyle, J.R.: Tourniquet for intravenous regional analgesia. Anaesthesia, *19*:294, 1964.
33. Ishibashi, T., Onchi, Y., and Okuda, T.: New method of local anaesthesia for operations on the upper extremity [in Japanese]. Jap. J. Anesthesiol., *15*:239, 1966.
34. Kennedy, B.R., Duthie, A.M., Parbrook, G.D., and Carr, T.L.: Intravenous regional analgesia: An appraisal. Br. Med. J., *1*:954, 1965.
35. Kerr, J.H.: Intravenous regional analgesia. Anaesthesia, *22*:562, 1967.
36. Lund, P.C., and Cwik, J.C.: Propitocaine (Citanest) and methemoglobinemia. Anesthesiology, *26*:569, 1965.
37. Mazze, R.I., and Dunbar, R.W.: Plasma lidocaine concentrations after caudal, lumbar epidural, axillary block and intravenous regional anesthesia. Anesthesiology, *27*:574, 1966.
38. ______: Intravenous regional anaesthesia—Report of 497 cases with a toxicity study. Acta Anaesthesiol. Scand. *36* [*Suppl.*]:27, 1969.
39. Merrifield, A.J., and Carter, S.J.: Intravenous regional analgesia: Lignocaine blood levels. Anaesthesia, *20*:287, 1965.
40. Middleton, R.W.D., and Varian, J.P.: Tourniquet paralysis. Aust. N. Z. J. Surg., *44*:124, 1974.
41. Miles, D.W., James, J.L., Clark, D.E., and Whitwam, J.G.: Site of action of 'intravenous regional anaesthesia'. J. Neurol. Neurosurg. Psychiatry, *27*:574, 1964.
42. Moldaver, J.: Tourniquet paralysis syndrome. Arch. Surg., *68*:136, 1954.
43. Raj, P.P., Garcia, C.E., Burleson, J.W., and Jenkins, M.T.: The site of action of intravenous regional anesthesia. Anesth. Analg. (Cleve.), *51*:776, 1972.
44. Shanks, C.A., and McLeod, J.G.: Nerve conduction studies in regional intravenous analgesia using 1% lignocaine. Br. J. Anaesth., *42*:1060, 1970.
45. Sorbie, C., and Chacha, P.: Regional anaesthesia by the intravenous route. Br. Med. J., *1*:957, 1965.
46. Thorn–Alquist, A–M.: Blood concentrations of local anaesthetics after intravenous regional anaesthesia. Acta Anaesthesiol. Scand. *13*:229, 1969.
47. Trias, A.: The use of intravenous regional anaesthesia in orthopedic surgery. Acta Anaesthesiol. Scand. *36* [*Suppl.*]:35, 1969.
48. Tucker, G.T., and Boas, R.A.: Pharmacokinetic aspects of intravenous regional anesthesia. Anesthesiology, *34*:538, 1971.
49. Van Niekerk, J.P., and Tonkin, P.A.: Intravenous regional analgesia. S. Afr. Med. J., *40*:165, 1966.
50. Winnie, A.P., and Ramamurthy, S.: Pneumatic exsanguination for intravenous regional anesthesia. Anesthesiology, *33*:664, 1970.

SUGGESTED READING

D'Amato, H., and Wiedling, S.: Intravenous regional anaesthesia: An international conference. Acta Anaesthesiol. Scand., *36* [*Suppl.*]:36, 1969.

Dundee, J.W., and Wyant, G.M.: Intravenous Anesthesia. Chap. 16. London, Churchill-Livingston, 1974.

Thorn-Alquist, A.M.: Intravenous regional anaesthesia. Acta Anaesthesiol. Scand., *40* [*Suppl.*]:40, 1971.

13 Sympathetic Neural Blockade of Upper and Lower Extremity

J. Bertil Löfström, J. W. Lloyd, and
Michael J. Cousins

HISTORY AND GENERAL CONSIDERATIONS

The effects of sympathetic nerves in maintaining normal constrictor tone in the blood vessels of the skin have been known since the classic work of Claude Bernard in 1852. The well-known observation of increased skin temperature of the foot after surgical lumbar sympathectomy was first made by Hunter and Royle.[14] Surgical sympathectomy has been performed at some clinics, as reported by De Bakey in 1950, to promote healing of ischemic cutaneous ulcers and to relieve pain in the foot at rest (*rest pain*).[73] However, at many vascular clinics today more emphasis is placed on vascular grafting procedures, and the refined surgical techniques undoubtedly have greatly improved the prognosis of the patient with occlusive vascular disease. Despite this movement away from sympathetic ablation, there is considerable potential benefit from sympathetic neural blockade as an adjunct to vascular surgery or as primary treatment for patients with rest pain who are not fit for, or not amenable to, vascular reconstruction. The large series of 1666 patients with neurolytic lumbar sympathetic blocks reported in 1970 by Reid and colleagues bear testimony to this, and it is surprising that many clinics have largely neglected this important option in the treatment of vascular disease.[60]

Mandl first described the technique of lumbar sympathetic neural blockade in 1926, and his technique was clearly very similar to that for celiac plexus blockade described by Kappis in 1919.[34,49] A similar neglect of celiac plexus block for upper abdominal cancer has been apparent (see Chap. 27). The classic "anterior" approach to stellate ganglion blockade was initiated by Leriche in 1934 and forms the basis of the technique described in this chapter; the use of this technique is still largely supported only by anecdotal information.

It is clear, then, that these techniques have all been available for well over 40 years. Surprisingly, precise documentation of their place in clinical medicine is only now becoming available, and much information remains to be obtained.

Sympathetic blockade is often produced as an accompaniment to motor and sensory blockade during regional block for operative surgery (*e.g.*, spinal and epidural anesthesia, brachial plexus block, etc). It is maintained that "differential" sympathetic blockade without sensory and motor block can be produced with low concentrations of local anesthetic by means of epidural or spinal subarachnoid block (see Chap. 28). This has its most common use in the diagnosis of chronic pain, although we believe that selective sympathetic ganglion block provides more reliable information (see Chap. 26). In the management of acute pain, sympathetic epidural block has been said to be capable of relieving labor pain and the pain of renal colic (see below and Chap. 8). However, the best application of sympathetic blockade appears to be in the use of selective blockade of the sympathetic ganglia.

Because the sympathetic ganglia are, except in the thoracic region, relatively safely separated from somatic nerves, it is possible to achieve sympathetic blockade without loss of sensory or motor function (see below). This offers the possibility of treating a variety of conditions in which reduced sympathetic activity might be beneficial. With careful technique, it is even possible to achieve permanent neurolytic blockade with essentially no loss of sensory and motor function. Thus, sympathetic blockade, at the three major levels indicated in Figure 13-2, is regarded as potentially one of the most rewarding series of techniques for diagnosis and management of acute and chronic pain syndromes and other conditions (see list on p. 363). Our clinical experience has been that, of all neural blockade techniques, lumbar sympathetic block for rest pain and celiac plexus block for upper abdominal cancer offer the most benefit at the lowest risk.

Celiac plexus blockade is described in Chapters 14 and 27, and lumbar sympathetic block and the remaining sympathetic ganglion blocks (stellate and thoracic) are described in this chapter. The new technique, intravenous regional sympathetic block is described in Chapter 12. At present, it is capable only of a duration of 2 to 3 weeks; however, often it is an attractive alternative to the higher-risk technique of thoracic sympathetic block or thoracic surgical sympathectomy. Current advances in producing "immune" lesions in the sympathetic nervous system may eventually make it possible to perform a selective intravenous regional immunosympathectomy.

The contribution of lumbar sympathetic blockade to the management of pain in the pelvic region requires further investigation. As outlined below, initial information indicates that it may be possible to employ either unilateral or bilateral lumbar sympathetic block for some kinds of pelvic pain (particularly urogenital). This, of course, poses a much lesser risk than the alternative of neurolytic subarachnoid block, with its possibility of loss of bladder function (see Chaps. 23 and 27).

In order to take full advantage of sympathetic neural blockade, it is essential to bear in mind the general features of the anatomy and physiology of the peripheral sympathetic nervous system, as described in the next section, and also the regional anatomy, as described with each of the techniques of sympathetic blockade. It is also important to use objective methods to evaluate the completeness of sympathetic blockade and its clinical effects, as shown in next column's list and described on pages 364 to 366.

Independent Tests of Sympathetic Function, Blood Flow, and Pain

Method of Evaluation
- *Sympathetic function*
  - Sympathogalvanic response (SGR)[44]
  - Sweat Test
    - Ninhydrin[19]
    - Cobalt blue[13]
    - Starch iodine
  - Skin plethysmography and "ice response"[13]
- *Blood flow*[26]
  - Plethysmography (muscle and skin)[52,53]
  - Xenon[133] clearance (muscle and skin)[27,31,71]
  - Sodium[24] clearance (muscle and skin)[30]
  - Antipyrine clearance[75]
  - Doppler technique (whole limb)[66,67]
  - Electromagnetic flow meter (whole limb)[14,15,39,61,72]
  - Pulse wave (skin)[1,35]
  - Temperature (skin)[47,48,55,56,68,70]
  - Size of ulcer (skin)[13]
  - Distal perfusion pressure[38,55,56,68–70]
  - Capillary oxygen tension (muscle or skin)[8]
  - Venous oxygen tension, saturation (muscle)[47]
  - Metabolism (muscle)[47]
- *Pain*
  - Pain score[13]
  - Analgesic requirements
  - Activity (*e.g.*, claudication distance)

SYMPATHETIC NERVOUS SYSTEM

Anatomy and Physiology

The peripheral sympathetic nervous system begins as efferent preganglionic fibers in the intermediolateral column of the spinal cord, passing in the ventral roots from T1 to L2 out of the spinal canal to run separately as white rami communicantes to the sympathetic chain, at the side of the vertebral bodies (Fig. 13-1). In the lower cervical region, the chain lies at the anterolateral aspect of the vertebral body and in the thorax is adjacent to the neck of the ribs, still relatively close to somatic roots (see Fig. 13-20). In the lumbar region, however, the chain angles forward to lie anterolateral to the body of the vertebra and is now separated from somatic roots by psoas muscle and psoas fascia (see Fig. 13-22). The preganglionic fibers pass a variable distance in the sympathetic chain to reach ganglia in the chain, or they may pass further to peripherally located ganglia (*e.g.*, in the gut; Fig. 13-1). The inconstant level of relay in the chain itself may be responsible for a number of disappointing results from an apparently technically successful block. Sympathetic ganglia are segmentally located in the chest (T1–11; T12). There are also three cervical ganglia, four to five lumbar ganglia, four sacral ganglia, and one coccygeal ganglion. The postganglionic fibers are widely distributed, partly to join peripheral nerves (the gray communicantes) and partly to join vessels in different organs. The sympathetic chain not only receives efferent preganglionic but also afferent visceral fibers, which conduct pain from head, neck, and upper extremity (cervicothoracic ganglia); abdominal viscera (celiac plexus); and urogenital system and lower extremity (lumbar ganglia; Fig. 13-2).

Sympathetic fibers are generally found in a deep fascial plane and are less accessible than segmental nerves. Interruption of sympathetic nerve fibers by neural blockade can be achieved in the following ways: intradurally or extradurally (blocking preganglionic fibers by subarachnoid or epidural blockade), at the sympathetic chain by a sympathetic blockade, at peripheral nerves by a nerve block, or at a vessel by perivascular infiltration. Sympathetic activity can also be blocked pharmacologically, by an alpha-receptor blocker (phentolamine, dibenzyline); by a blocker of norepinephrine activity in sympathetic nerve ending (guanethidine or reserpine); or by a beta-receptor blocker, propranolol ($beta_1$ and $beta_2$ receptors) or practolol (mainly $beta_1$ receptor).

Function

Vasoconstriction by Alpha Receptors. Arterioli (in the skin and in the splanchnic area), smaller arteries, and, in particular, peripheral veins are normally under moderate vasoconstrictor influence. Pain, anxiety, and blood loss can provoke a very marked increase in arteriolar vasoconstrictor tone, mediated by the sympathetic nervous system; this change results in increased resistance, particularly in skin vessels, and thus influences the distribution of blood flow. In addition, there is an associated increase in venous tone, which decreases the compliance of the venous system, reducing its blood content and increasing venous pressure. Blockade of efferent sympathetic outflow will produce the reverse of these effects with signs of increased capillary blood flow, such as reduced capillary refill time and signs of increased flow in arteriovenous anastomoses, as seen by increased skin temperature as well as a subjective feeling of warmth in the limb (Fig. 13-3; see also Fig. 13-6). Vasoconstrictor responses such as the "ice response" will be abolished.

Heart Muscle Activity (Chronotropic and Inotropic Effect). $Beta_1$ stimulation causes increased heart rate and increased cardiac contractility; thus high (T1–4) thoracic sympathetic blockade may cause a marked reduction in cardiac output.

Bronchial Tone. $Beta_2$ stimulation causes bronchodilation, so that it is theoretically possible for thoracic sympathetic blockade to cause bronchoconstriction, although this does not appear to be the case (see Chap. 8).

Vasodilatation. $Beta_2$ stimulation causes vasodilatation in some vascular beds (*e.g.*, muscle); however, this is a minor effect and is overridden by local metabolic effects (see below).

Smooth Muscle Tone (e.g., in the Gut and in the Bladder). $Beta_2$ stimulation causes smooth muscle relaxation and sphincter contraction. Thus, sympathetic blockade results in smooth muscle contraction (a small contracted gut) and sphincter relaxation. This provides excellent surgical access during procedures such as abdominoperineal resection.

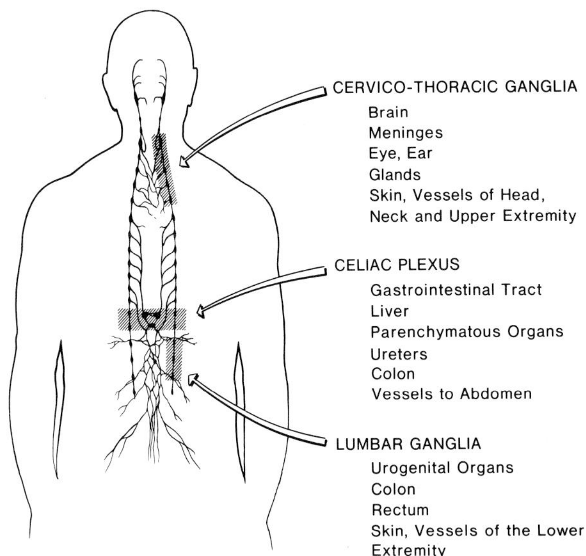

Fig. 13-2. An outline of the sympathetic nervous system. The three main levels of sympathetic blockade are shown together with major clinical uses. (Redrawn after Bonica, J.J.: The Management of Pain. Philadelphia, Lea & Febiger, 1953)

Metabolic. The sympathetic nervous system has a metabolic effect that is said to explain the relaxation of smooth muscle in vessels and in the gut and its effect on the heart muscle. This metabolic effect is widespread and also affects carbohydrate and lipoid distribution and utilization.[20]

Pain may be mediated through the sympathetic nervous system. Labor pain is transmitted by afferent fibers that traverse the lower thoracic sympathetic ganglia, while pain from upper abdominal viscera and the gut as far as the descending colon can adequately be relieved by celiac ganglion block. Pain from some pelvic viscera may be transmitted by the lumbar sympathetic ganglia (Fig. 13-2). Recent evidence suggests that sympathetic efferents may influence pain perception in the limbs.

PHYSIOLOGIC EFFECTS ON PERIPHERAL BLOOD FLOW

A regional sympathetic block has its primary and most obvious effect on vasomotor activity. In a normal subject, this leads to dilatation of veins, promoting an accumulation of blood in the veins, and dilatation of the arterial vessels, which leads to a fall in the regional resistance and, thus, if the perfusion pressure has not been altered, to an increased capillary blood flow.

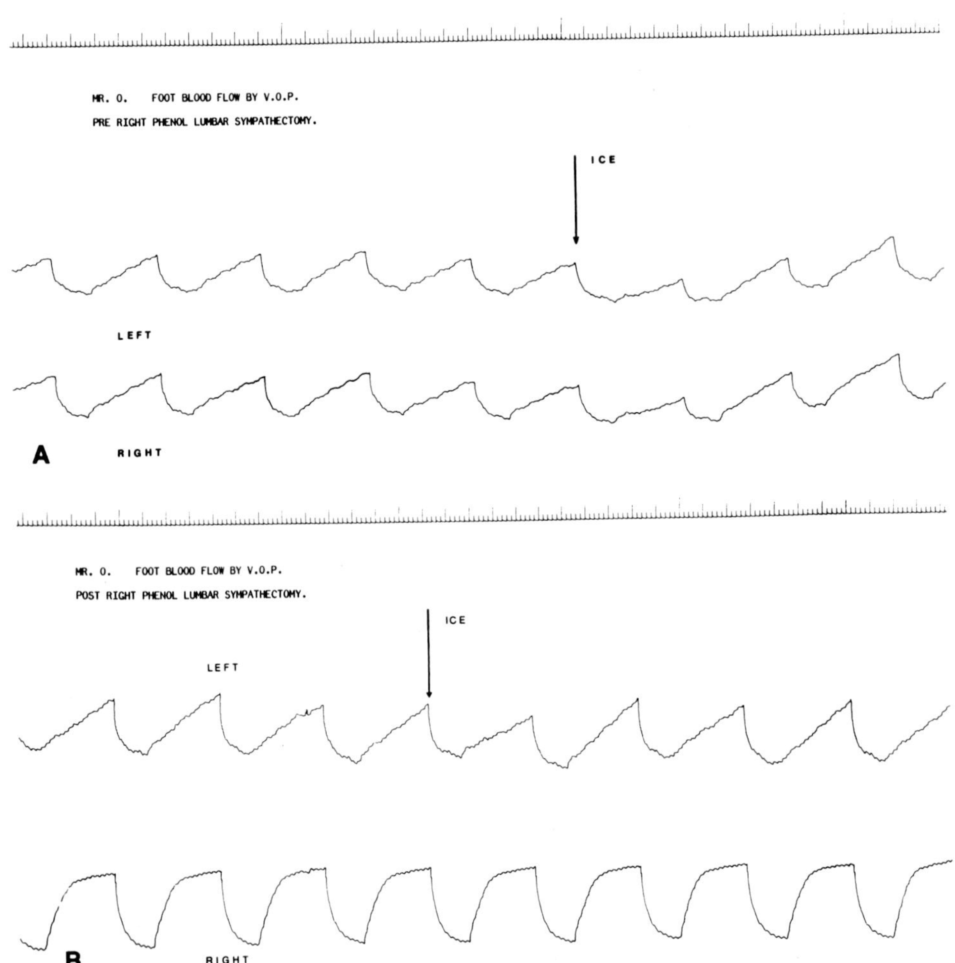

Fig. 13-3. Skin plethysmography and ice response: effect of sympathetic block. (*A*) Prior to sympathetic block. Skin blood flow is similar (2 ml/100 ml/min) in both limbs, and the response to ice (*arrow*) is a similar reduction in the height of the pulse wave in both limbs. (*B*) After sympathetic block. The blocked limb (*right*) shows a marked increase in the slope of the upward deflection of the pulse wave and an increase in height of pulse wave; this reflects a tenfold increase of skin blood flow to 22 ml per 100 ml per minute. There is no change in blood flow in response to ice. In contrast, the unblocked limb (*left*) shows the same shape and height of pulse wave, and there is a similar marked reduction in blood flow (40% decrease) in response to ice. (Cousins, M.J., Reeve, T.S., Glynn, C.J., Walsh, J.A., and Cherry, D.A.: Neurolytic lumbar sympathetic blockade: Duration of denervation and relief of rest pain. Anaesthesia and Intensive Care, 7:121, 1979)

In a normal subject, complete sympathetic block will be followed by visibly dilated veins or by increased blood flow, seen clinically in reduced capillary refill time or measured by plethysmography or xenon[133] clearance, which measures capillary blood flow accurately (see below). Oscillometrically recorded, the peripheral pulse waves will be enlarged. The blood flow increase will, to a large extent, be restricted to the skin, followed by an increase in skin temperature and a marked feeling of warmth in the extremity (Figs. 13-3 and 13-4).[73] Skin capillary oxygen tension and venous oxygen tension and saturation are also raised (see list on p. 356). A widespread block will cause a peripheral pooling of blood, diminishing the venous return and producing a fall in cardiac output and blood pressure, as seen in spinal blockade.

Muscle blood flow, being automatically regulated

SYMPATHETIC PATHWAYS

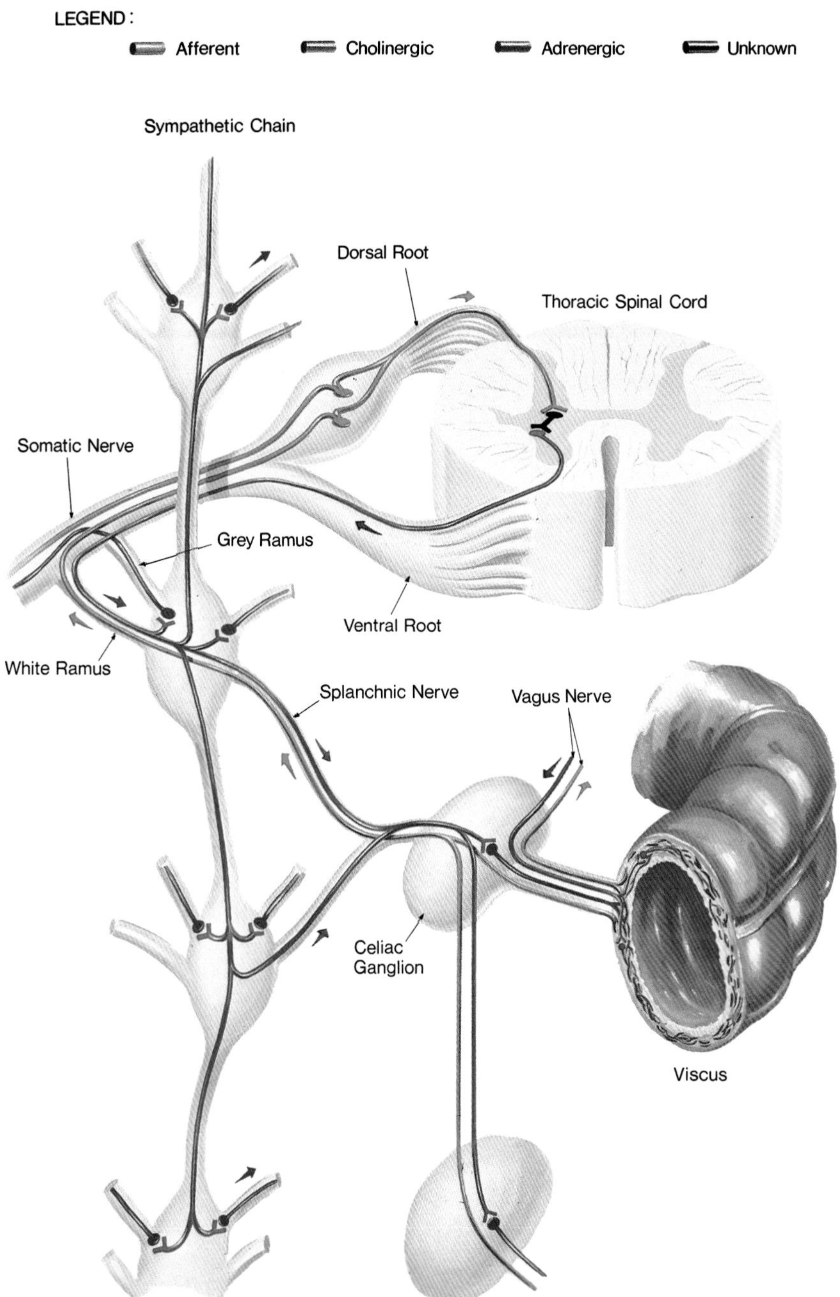

Fig. 13-1. Peripheral sympathetic nervous system. Cell bodies are located in the intermediolateral cell column of T1–L2 spinal segments. Efferent fibers (cholinergic) pass by way of the ventral root to a white ramus communicans and then to the paravertebral sympathetic ganglia or to more remotely located ganglia, such as the celiac ganglion. From each ganglion, they give rise to adrenergic fibers to supply viscera (celiac ganglion) or to join somatic nerves (from lumbar sympathetic ganglion). In the latter case, the adrenergic fibers swing backward by a grey ramus communicans to join the somatic nerve. Afferent fibers travel by way of ganglia, such as celiac and lumbar sympathetic, without synapsing and reach somatic nerves and then their cell bodies in the dorsal root ganglia. They then pass to the dorsal root and synapse with interneurons in the intermediolateral area of the spinal cord. These afferent fibers convey pain impulses from the viscera and possibly also from the limbs.

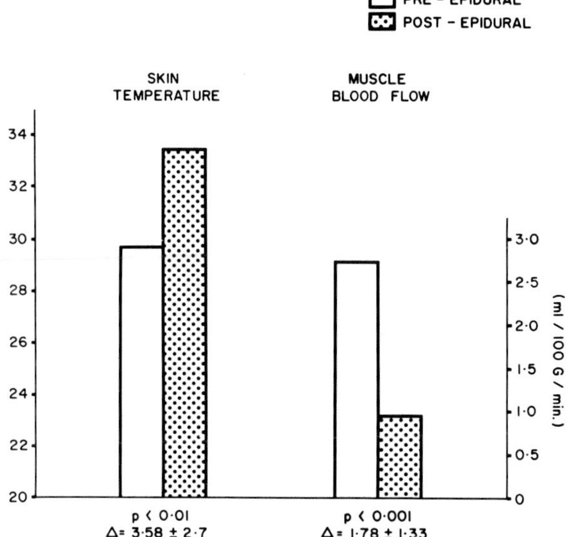

Fig. 13-4. Blood flow distribution following lumbar epidural sympathetic blockade in normal patients at rest. Note increased skin blood flow (skin temperature) but reduced muscle blood flow (xenon[133] clearance). (Wright, C.J., and Cousins, M.J.: Blood flow distribution in the human by following epidural sympathetic blockade. Arch. Surg., *105*:334, 1972 © 1972, American Medical Association)

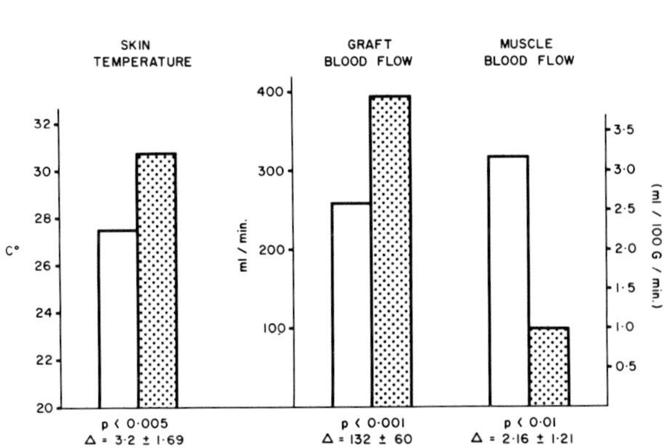

Fig. 13-5. Blood flow distribution following lumbar sympathetic blockade in arteriosclerotic patients at rest. Blood flow in the femoral artery (electromagnetic flow meter) is increased as is skin blood flow (skin temperature), however muscle blood flow (xenon[133] clearance) is reduced. Note, this is a widespread sympathetic block (both lower limbs). This may sometimes even reduce skin blood flow through diseased vessels (see Fig. 13-11). (Cousins, M.J., and Wright, C.J.: Graft muscle skin blood flow after epidural block in vascular surgical procedures. Surg. Gynecol. Obstet., *133*:59, 1971)

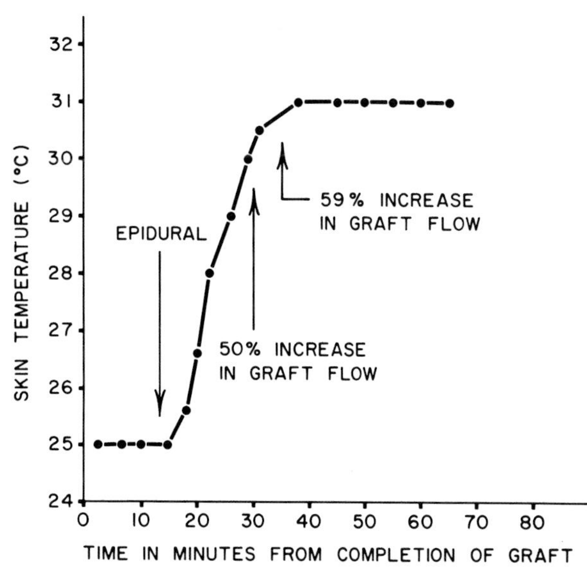

Fig. 13-6. Increased skin blood flow, following epidural sympathetic block, closely parallels increase in total limb blood flow on a vascular graft during vascular reconstruction. (Cousins, M.J., and Wright, C.J.: Graft muscle skin blood flow after epidural block. Surg. Gynecol. Obstet., *133*:59, 1971 by permission of the Franklin H. Martin Memorial Foundation)

according to muscle metabolism, should not be affected by a sympathetic blockade at rest, at work, or after ischemia.[14] Thus, reduced muscle flow (claudication) may not be helped by sympathetic block (Fig. 13-5). From what has been stated, it seems logical to use sympathetic blockade to improve the blood flow in a patient with insufficient peripheral skin blood flow because of vasospasm or arterial disease (*i.e.*, rest pain) (Fig. 13-6).[13,14] However, it is not possible to predict the effect of a sympathetic blockade in a patient with a diseased vascular system, as can be explained with the aid of the following illustrations. In Figure 13-7, an artery divides into two smaller branches. The total flow (Q_A) in the artery is proportionate to the perfusion pressure (P) and inversely proportionate to the peripheral resistance (PR). In each branch (*B* and *C*) the flows (Q_B and Q_C) are affected by the perfusion pressures, almost the same as in the artery (*A*) and inversely related to the regional resistance (RR_B and RR_C) in each branch. A blockade of the sympathetic fibers to branch B alone will have very little effect

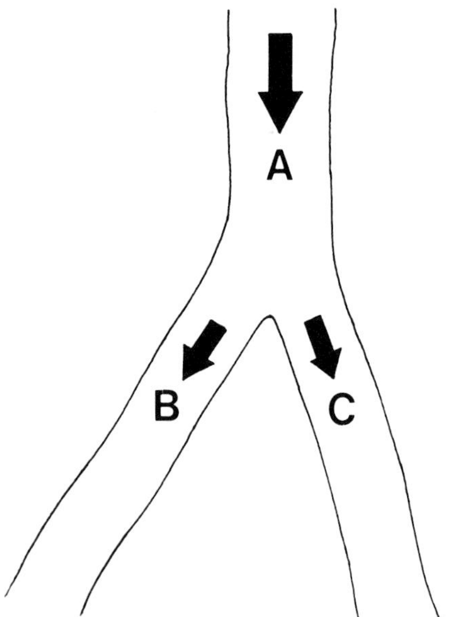

Fig. 13-7. The blood flows through an artery (*A*) or its branches (*B* and *C*) are proportionate to the perfusion pressures and inversely proportionate to total and regional resistances, respectively (see text).

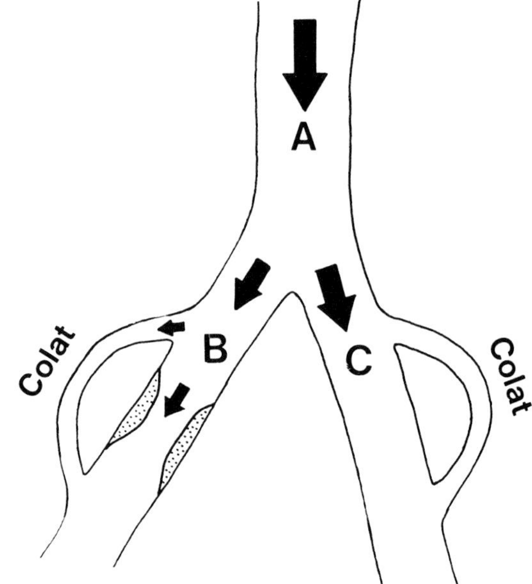

Fig. 13-9. A vasodilatation restricted to branch B and its collaterals and vessels beyond the arterial obstruction should increase blood flow to this region.

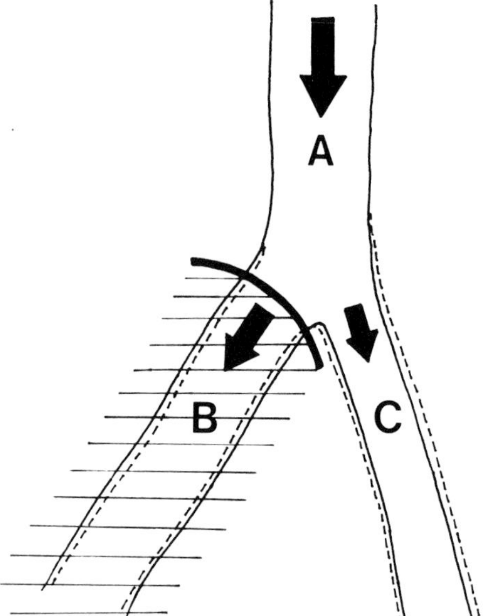

Fig. 13-8. A limited sympathetic blockade of fibers to branch B alone will little affect perfusion pressure. The flow in branch B will increase as the regional resistance is diminished. In branch C the flow will be slightly reduced as compensatory vasoconstriction occurs.

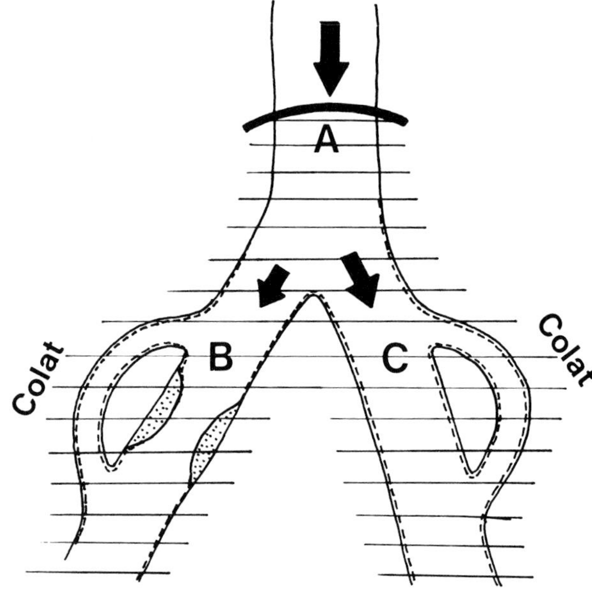

Fig. 13-10. An arterial obstruction in branch B will increase the resistance and thus hamper the blood flow. An increased flow through collaterals (*colat.*) may compensate for a fall in blood flow through the main channel (see text).

on the perfusion pressure (Fig. 13-8). As the regional resistance decreases in branch B, the flow through this vessel will increase. A unilateral sympathetic blockade (in humans) is generally followed by a slight increase in vasomotor tone in the contralateral side, thus increasing the regional resistance and reducing the blood flow through this part of the vascular system.

In Figure 13-9, an arterial obstruction in branch B is shown. Such an obstruction will in itself diminish the blood flow by mechanically increasing the regional resistance. However, this might at least be compensated by an increase in the collateral blood flow. A widespread sympathetic blockade, as illustrated in Figure 13-10, will diminish the regional resistance, mainly in branch C with its undamaged vessels. The blood flow will be diverted into this part of the vascular tree and thus blood will be stolen from the diseased part (*branch B*). Such stealing of blood is known to occur in patients with advanced arterial disease. In theory stealing can occur at three different levels: a generalized vasodilatation in the body will steal blood from, for instance, one extremity; increased blood flow around the hip and in the pelvis will diminish the blood flow to the peripheral part of the lower extremity; or increased skin blood flow might steal blood from the muscles (see Fig. 13-5).[14,17,75]

In contrast, a localized vasodilatation that affects the collaterals to branch B and vessels beyond the arterial obstruction should increase blood flow to this region (Fig. 13-11).

If a decrease in vasomotor tone in the collaterals cannot be achieved, the maintenance of a good perfusion pressure is essential, as stressed by Lassen and Larson.[41,42]

From this discussion, it is obvious that the clinical effect of a sympathetic block cannot easily be predicted. Only physiologic studies in patients and clinical experience will identify when a sympathetic block is indicated.

In patients with occlusive vascular disease, the prime indication for surgical or chemical sympathectomy is "rest pain in a limb not amenable to direct arterial reconstruction."[74] Because of associated coronary artery disease, pulmonary disease, and other physical conditions, many of these patients are poor candidates for surgery and are thus better candidates for neurolytic sympathectomy.[13] However, the clinical results of both surgical and neurolytic sympathectomy, as reported in the literature, are contradictory. This might be explained by a poor selection of patients or by a lack of use of independent assessment of successful sympathetic

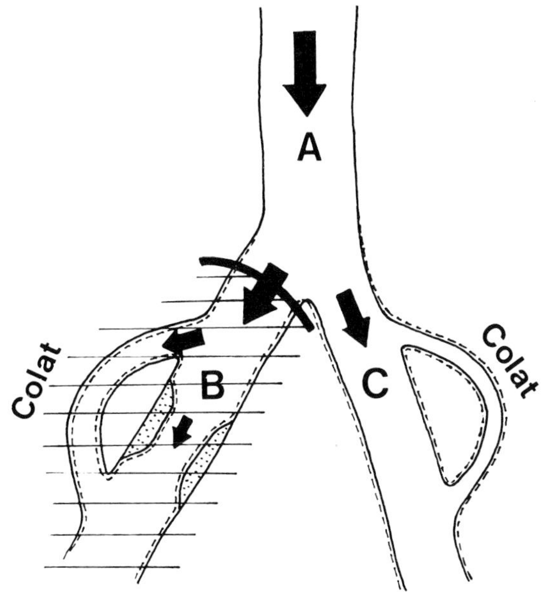

Fig. 13-11. A widespread sympathetic blockade of fibers to branches B and C will diminish resistance in undamaged vessels (*C*) and thereby potentially stealing blood from a diseased part (*B*) of the vascular tree.

ablation and its separate effects on blood flow and pain. This task may be simplified if one of the methods of evaluation in each category depicted in the list on page 356 is employed.

The detrimental effects of generalized vasodilatation in patients with arteriosclerotic vascular disease that causes rest pain or intermittent claudication have been well described and are generally accepted today.[75]

It has been suggested that an increased skin blood flow should always occur in the presence of regional vasodilatation. This has also been reported in patients with obliterative arterial disease.[39,52,68]

Although skin blood flow is markedly under the control of sympathetic activity, a decreased blood flow has been demonstrated in patients with severe arteriosclerosis and, in particular, patients with lower limb vascular disease who have a low ankle blood pressure before lumbar sympathetic blockade (below 60/20 torr).[38,55,56,68–70] In these patients, the vascular lesions in the periphery are so extreme that hypothetically a "proximal stealing" always occurs, and thus a fall in the perfusion pressure peripherally is followed by vasodilatation in vessels located proximally. Although rare, there are reports of worsening of pain and gangrene.[22] Remarkably enough, an increase in skin temperature is not always related to an increase in blood flow through the skin and may merely reflect venous pooling and local inflammatory changes.[70]

The blood flow through muscle is automatically regulated according to metabolic needs. Thus, in intermittent claudication, the muscle tissue hypoxia and accumulation of metabolites at exercise should be followed by maximal dilatation of the muscle blood vessels, and thus a sympathetic blockade should be of no value or even worsen the symptoms because of "stealing" blood flow to the skin.[14,23,71] However, this is not necessarily so. Pain is a primary factor in provoking increased sympathetic activity. Hypothetically, this could result in vasoconstriction in the collateral vessels that supply the affected muscle. Sympathetic blockade under these circumstances may improve blood flow to muscle and thus explain why a beneficial effect of sympathectomy is observed in some patients with intermittent claudication.[39,54,60] This assumption and the clinical experience of several investigators are supported by a metabolic study in which deep venous blood was drawn before and at the maximum of a one-leg bicycle ergometer test in patients with intermittent claudication.[47] In one group of patients with fairly high and segmentally located arterial lesions who received sympathetic block (Group I), the rise in femoral venoarterial lactate difference during exercise was not as marked as prior to their sympathetic block, indicating an improvement in nutrient blood flow. In contrast, in a group of patients with multiple vascular lesions (Group II), no improvement in nutrient blood flow was achieved by sympathetic blockade. In Group I, eight out of 10 also experienced less ischemic pain on exercise during the sympathetic blockade. No patients in Group II experienced such pain relief. The most important effect of sympathetic blockade in Group I seemed to be pain relief during exercise, at least partly because of an improved blood flow and also enhancement of the development of collateral vessels, which is known to occur over a period of time, providing opportunities for revascularization (see Table 13-3). It should be acknowledged that a placebo effect may occur, which has been reported with lumbar sympathetic blockade.[24]

Lumbar sympathetic blockade in connection with vascular surgery improves the flow through reconstructed vessels and should be of value in the immediate postoperative period.[15,37,39,61,72] Although less selective, this effect can also be achieved with epidural sympathetic block; however, the ganglion blockade is preferable, as discussed on p. 361.[14]

From the discussion above, it is obvious that a proper selection of patients for sympathetic blockade is of great importance. As the number of patients with vascular disease is very large, complicated and time-consuming physiologic studies are not always feasible. The use of continuous catheter sympathetic blockade that lasts for 5 days is one method of obtaining a clinical evaluation of the effect of the blockade, which should at least detect patients whose symptoms are exacerbated after blockade.[48] A selective alternative is intravenous regional sympathetic block, which can eliminate technical failure and is a useful preliminary test for whether surgical sympathectomy or permanent blockade by chemical sympathectomy will be successful.[29] The prolonged duration (1–3 weeks) of intravenous sympathetic block allows adequate time for clinical assessment. A third alternative is to perform diagnostic block with long-acting local anesthetic mixed with contrast medium and to check adequacy of coverage of sympathetic chain under image intensifier; however, this has proved the least reliable of the three.[13]

In a clinical series, Kövamees and Löfström, found that the most beneficial effect of sympathetic blockade was relief of rest pain (19:23, *i.e.*, 83%) with a somewhat lesser effect of improved healing of ulcers (23:55, *i.e.*, 42%) see Table 13-2.[38] Increased walking tolerance (7:16, *i.e.*, 44%) was of significant benefit in a small group of patients with intermittent claudication. It should be stressed that sympathetic blockade was part of a general treatment program that included mobilization and wound treatment and sometimes infusion of low molecular weight dextran. It was not possible to attribute an improvement to the sympathetic blockade alone. However, in a recent study, Cousins and colleagues reported that duration of relief of rest pain was similar to duration of lumbar sympathetic blockade, strengthening the relationship between pain relief and sympathetic denervation.[13] Good results with relief of rest pain in the lower limbs have been reported by others.[4,32,60] Very little data are available on upper limb vascular disease, although case reports indicate beneficial results with sympathetic block in vasospastic disorders such as those in the list on the next page.

Thus, it would appear that the primary benefits that result from sympathetic blockade are pain relief and improved healing of skin lesions. However, controlled studies of efficacy of sympathetic block are required to define better its role in the treatment of vascular disease of the lower and also upper limbs.

The pain-relieving effect of a sympathetic block in a patient with peripheral arterial disease is said to

Clinical Conditions That Sympathetic Blockade May Benefit

To produce pain relief
- Renal colic (lumbar sympathetic block)
- Obliterative arterial disease (lumbar sympathetic block)
- Acute pancreatitis and pancreatic cancer (celiac plexus block)
- Cancer pain from upper abdominal viscera (celiac plexus block)
- Cardiac pain (thoracic sympathetic or stellate ganglion block)
- Paget's disease of bone (stellate ganglion or lumbar sympathetic block)
- Reflex sympathetic dystrophy (stellate or lumbar sympathetic block)
  - *Major* causalgia, phantom limb, central pain
  - *Minor* post-traumatic syndrome, postfrostbite syndrome, shoulder/hand syndrome, Sudeck's atrophy

To improve blood flow in vasospastic disorders (stellate or lumbar sympathetic block)
- Raynaud's disease
- Accidental intra-arterial injections of thiopentone
- Early frostbite
- In obliterative arterial disease not suitable for vascular surgery
- In connection with vascular surgery to improve postoperative blood flow

To improve drainage of local edema (stellate or lumbar sympathetic block)

follow improved blood flow. However, good pain relief often occurs when no improvement in peripheral circulation can be noted; possible mechanisms are discussed below.

CONTRIBUTION OF PERIPHERAL SYMPATHETIC NERVOUS SYSTEM TO PAIN TRANSMISSION

The precise mechanism whereby the sympathetic nervous system is involved in the pain experience is as yet not fully elucidated. It has been suggested that the cutaneous pain threshold, by means of a negative feedback loop, is influenced by the sympathetic nervous system.[58] This may explain the often remarkable pain relief seen after sympathetic blocks in patients with threatening gangrene, despite a lack of improvement in skin blood flow. It is possible that increased efferent sympathetic activity increases activity in pain receptors by way of sympathetic fibers that are prevalent in close proximity to sensory receptors. This provides an explanation of pain relief that may follow stellate ganglion block in patients with arteriopathy (*e.g.*, associated with scleroderma) in the upper limb, despite the lack of change in blood flow.*

There are also clinical observations that early herpes zoster pain and skin vesicles respond favorably to sympathetic blockade (see list on p. 369.[12,50] That they also respond well to a block of the appropriate somatic nerve is well established, and it is doubtful whether there is any specific sympathetic involvement in this condition. The results of sympathetic block in the treatment of postherpetic neuralgia are uniformly disappointing.

It is, of course, well established that the pain of uterine contraction and cervical dilatation can be abolished by sympathetic blockade of afferents entering the spinal cord at T11–12. This is usually achieved by extradural sympathetic blockade (see Chap. 18). Also, in a small series of patients with renal colic treated with extradural sympathetic block at L1, nine out of 14 patients passed their stone in 10 days and all were pain-free from the commencement of treatment; this series has now been increased to 32, all of whom obtained complete pain relief.[46] This compares favorably with other methods, and it has been suggested that the relief of pain and reduction of ureteral spasm is brought about by sympathetic blockade of the first lumbar segmental outflow. Chronic pain from the urogenital tract has, in a few cases, been eliminated with chemical lumbar sympathectomy.[33] Cervicothoracic sympathetic blockade is also of value in the treatment of patients with severe angina pectoris, provided that the block extends down to the level of T4. However, the hazards may often outweigh the benefits (see Chap. 26).

In post-traumatic syndrome, a sympathetic blockade is often followed by relief of the burning pain in the injured extremity and a feeling of softening of the tissues, primarily around the joints.[2,18,62] The symptoms of post-traumatic syndrome might be caused by hyperactivity in the sympathetic nervous system, producing vasoconstriction, decrease in capillary surface area, redistribution of blood flow, fall in oxygen uptake (tissue hypoxia), increased vascular permeability, and lack of fluid mobilization.[45] A sympathetic blockade should then improve nutrient blood flow and decrease the accumulated fluid in the tissue, which explains the increased warmth and the rapid disappearance of tissue edema often seen during

* Cousins, M.J., *et al.:* Unpublished data.

this form of treatment. However, conclusive evidence is lacking.

TESTING THE COMPLETENESS OF SYMPATHETIC BLOCKADE

In a patient with a healthy vascular system, a sympathetic blockade produces clear-cut subjective and objective effects on the peripheral circulation, as have been discussed in the previous section. However, in a patient with severe arterial disease, a complete sympathetic blockade can have been achieved with little or no demonstrable effect on the peripheral circulation.

The venous circulation is generally not involved in the disease process, and swelling of the veins can be a valuable indication of a successful block. There are two objective tests that can be used to provide an assessment of completeness of sympathetic block.

SYMPATHOGALVANIC RESPONSE

The first test, the sympathogalvanic response, (SGR) tests not only efferent sympathetic activity but also afferent sensory activity and spinal interneurons.[44] Increased sympathetic activity, which in many people can be evoked by pinching the skin, is followed by a change in skin resistance that can be recorded with a simple electrocardiograph. One electrode is placed on the front and one on the back of the hand or foot (*i.e.*, where sweat glands are abundant). A third grounding electrode is placed anywhere on the body. In most patients, there will be a slow change in the baseline, which will come to rest after a few minutes. Pinching will now, with 1- to 2-second delay, be followed by a marked deflection that lasts for 4 to 5 seconds. This deflection does not occur if the sympathetic fibers of the extremity are blocked or if the patient is atropinized. It is preferable to perform separate tests on two limbs simultaneously, thus making it possible to compare the blocked side with the unblocked side. This is essential if the SGR deflections are to be measured (Fig. 13-12). It is well known that the baseline is far less stable and that the deflections much more marked in young patients than in the elderly. In elderly patients, it is also more difficult to provoke a sympathetic response. Therefore, verbal stimulation plus pinching is often necessary to obtain an acceptable response in elderly patients; for best quantitative results, a standard electrical stimulus should be used.

Ample experience with SGR has made it clear that it is not always possible to obtain a complete abolition of the SGR with a sympathetic blockade, even though the vascular response seems to be maximal. It has been suggested that SGR can be used to predict the value of a sympathetic blockade in patients with arterial disease.[7] In this study, most patients with a good to moderate deflection on stimulation benefited from a sympathetic block. This was not seen in patients with little or no deflection. The SGR has also been used by us to check the completeness of sympathetic denervation following local anesthetic or chemical sympathectomy. When a permanent sympathetic blockade is under consideration and no or only weak skin resistance deflections are seen following SGR, a continuous sympathetic blockade is unlikely to be followed by any improvement in the peripheral circulation, although in some cases it may offer pain relief.

Sweat Test

The second test of sympathetic activity is the sweat test. This is perhaps the most practicable test of sympathetic activity.

Ninhydrin Method. Fingerprints are taken (at intervals) before and after blockade.[19] After suitable preparation, which includes heating, the fingerprints are developed, and each functioning sweat gland can be seen and counted. This test is very accurate and, its results, reproducible; however, it is time-consuming and does not provide the clinician with an answer at the bedside.

Cobalt Blue Filter Paper Test. Filter papers are soaked in cobalt blue and then dried in an oven, following which they are kept in a dessicator until required. Two filter papers are removed from the dessicator with forceps and placed on a clean dry surface so that the patient can press both feet or hands onto the papers. Sweating is registered on the paper by a change in color from blue to pink. A limb with complete sympathetic block usually shows no color change (Fig. 13-13). Details for preparation of the filter papers are found in Appendix A of this chapter.

The starch-iodine test works on a principle similar to that of the cobalt blue test. It has the advantage that the material can be spread over a complete limb. However, it is a messy technique and not popular with patients.

Having ensured that sympathetic block is adequate, an independent assessment can then be made of the effect on blood flow. If this is combined with the ice test (Fig. 13-3), a further evaluation of sympathetic function is obtained and, if pain was present prior to blockade, pain relief can be independently assessed (see p. 356).

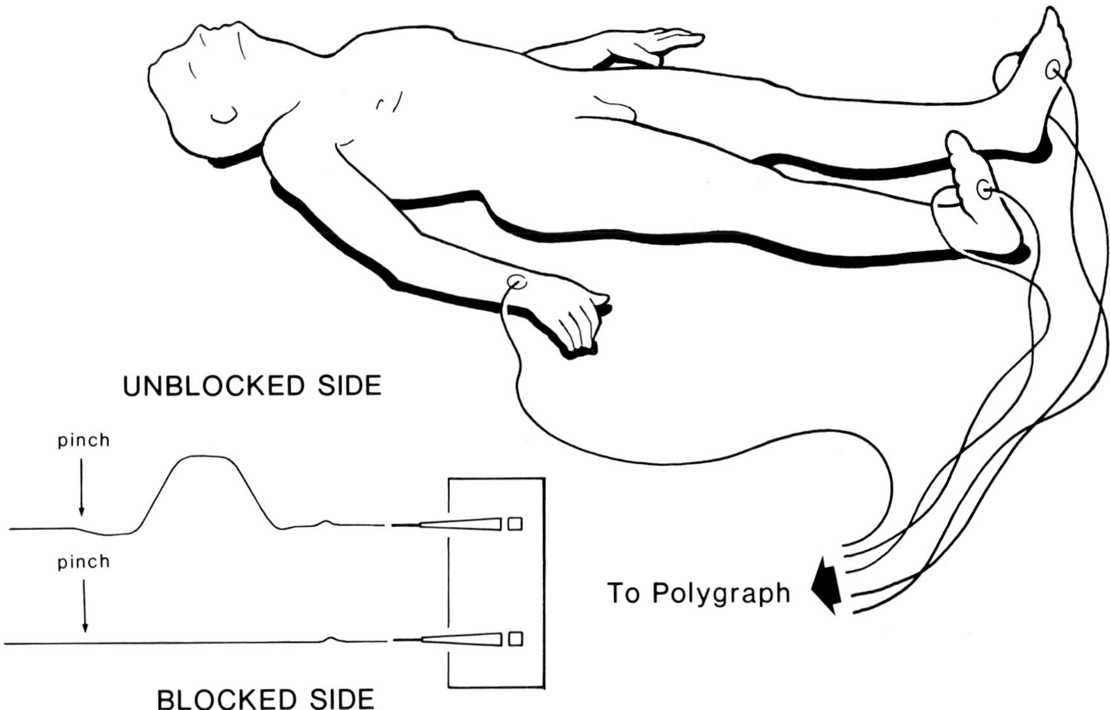

Fig. 13-12. Sympathogalvanic response (SGR). Electrodes are placed on the front and back of hands or feet and a ground electrode is placed elsewhere on the body.

ASSESSMENT OF BLOOD FLOW CHANGES

Whole Limb Blood Flow

Indirect. *Doppler Ankle/Brachial Index.*[74] An ultrasound probe is used to facilitate blood pressure measurement with a standard cuff at brachial artery and also at the ankle. An ankle to brachial index is then calculated

$$\frac{\text{ankle}}{\text{brachial}} = \frac{80/50}{120/80} = 0.65$$

This reading is then repeated after sympathetic block.

Impedance plethysmography is a new technique that attempts to correlate the changes in electrical impedance with blood flow. At this stage, it is not clear if it provides an accurate estimate of limb blood flow under the whole range of clinical conditions.

Direct. *Electromagnetic flow meter* can be applied either directly to the blood vessel during surgery or percutaneously using a "catheter tip" version.

Ultrasonic Flow Meter. Very small probes are now under development that can be placed on the vessel wall at operation and left *in situ* postoperatively.

Muscle Blood Flow

Venous occlusion plethysmography has been employed in the calf area under the assumption that the calf is mostly muscle with much less skin.

Clearance of radioactive substances after direct injection (*e.g.*, xenon[133]) provides one of the best measurements of nutritive blood flow (Fig. 13-14).[14]

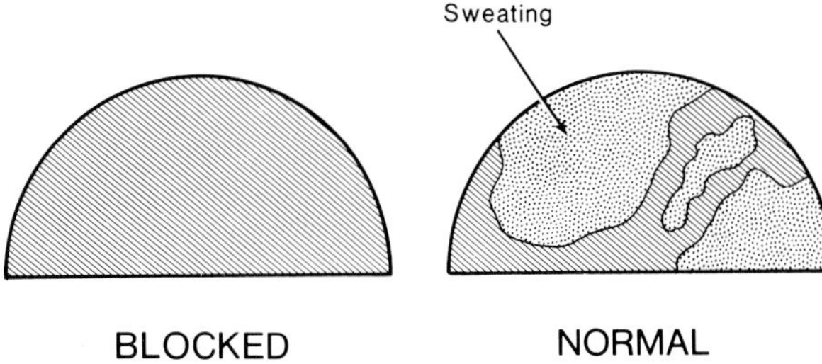

Fig. 13-13. Cobalt blue sweat test. The papers are blue (*shaded*) prior to the test. Sweating from the unblocked limb changes the color to pink (*stippled*).

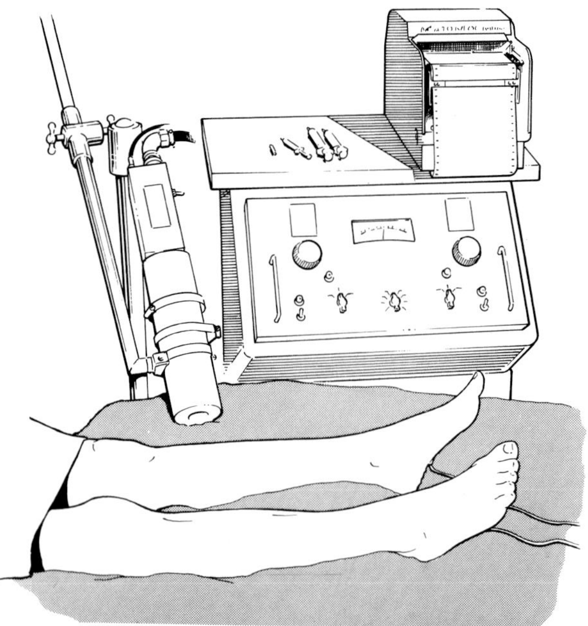

Fig. 13-14. Xenon[133] clearance technique for leg muscle blood flow. Xenon[133] is injected into the anterior tibial muscle and its clearance detected with a portable scintillation detector.

Arterial oxygen concentration in blood from deep calf veins has also been utilized for an indirect estimate to oxygen delivery to calf muscle.[47] Recently, a *mass spectrometer probe* has been developed to measure muscle tissue P_{O_2} directly.

Skin Blood Flow

Clearance of radioactive substances injected directly into the skin has been employed (*e.g.*, xenon,[133] sodium[124]).

Mass spectrometer microprobes and skin "cups" are also being utilized in this situation to measure changes in skin P_{O_2} with different forms of treatment.

Occlusion skin plethysmography has also been employed in the area of the foot, hand, and digits, as described above (see Fig. 13-3).[13]

Skin temperature measurements, using a telethermometer and thermistor or thermocouple skin probes, provide an indirect, but easily obtained, estimate of changes in skin blood flow (Fig. 13-15). Liquid thermal crystals and heat-sensitive papers are also available.

Optical Density Skin Plethysmography (or Pulse Monitor). Several quite sensitive finger "pulsemeters" are now available and employ several different wavelengths of light directed into the skin capillary bed. Capillary blood flow results in a cyclical change in optical density, yielding a wave form similar to that shown in Figure 13-3, and its amplitude is proportional to sympathetic activity.

Measurement of Size of Skin Ulcers. Progressive documentation of change in ulcer size is a very simple and practical method of checking progress after sympathetic block in patients with ischemic skin lesions.

PAIN ASSESSMENT

As discussed in Chapters 24 and 26, there is still no objective method of pain assessment. Indirect methods such as the pain score, analgesic requirements, and improved level of activity are employed; wherever possible these should be performed by an independent observer with a "triple-blind" study design (see Chap. 24).

It should be emphasized that a baseline measurement/assessment prior to sympathetic block should be made in each case for sympathetic activity, blood flow and pain score, by one of the methods described above. Following sympathetic blockade, this should then permit determination of the completeness of sympathetic block, its effect on blood flow, and then, finally, any associated effects on pain.

General Clinical Applications

The clinical situations in which sympathetic blockade may be considered are summarized in the

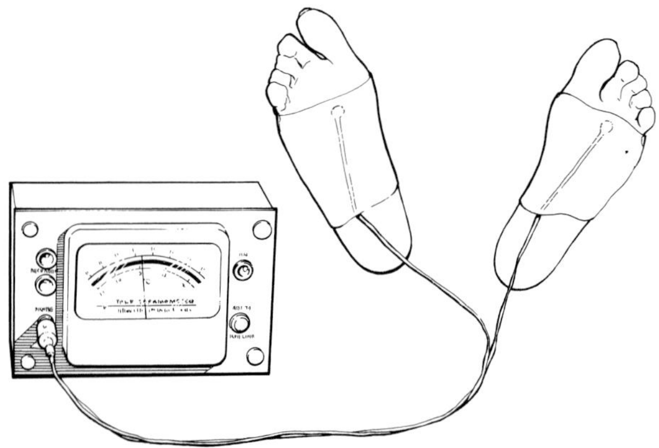

Fig. 13-15. Skin thermocouple probe and telethermometer. Simultaneous measurements are made on treated as well as untreated limb.

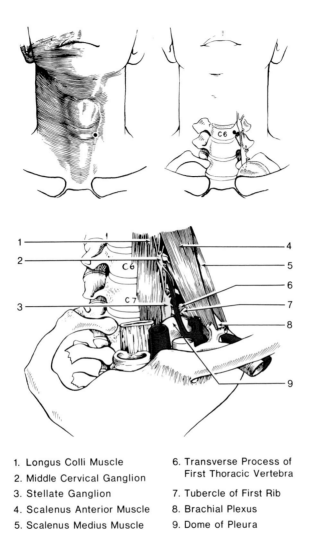

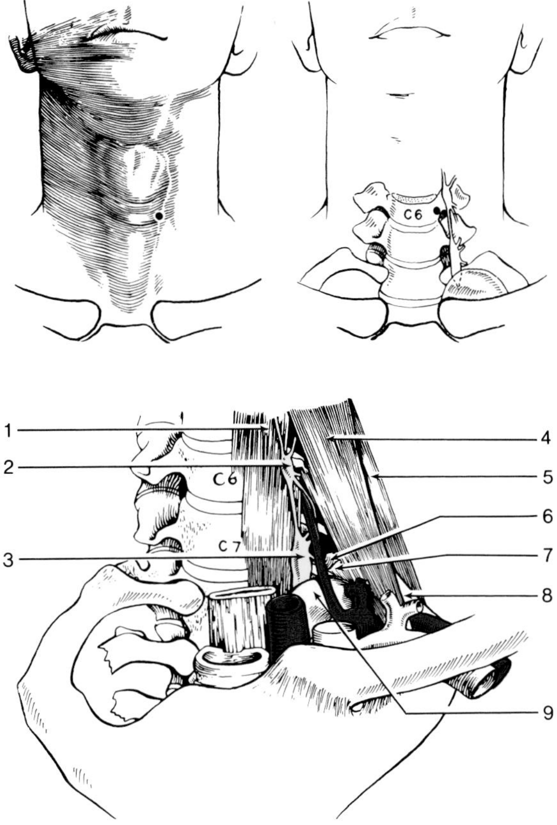

1. Longus Colli Muscle
2. Middle Cervical Ganglion
3. Stellate Ganglion
4. Scalenus Anterior Muscle
5. Scalenus Medius Muscle
6. Transverse Process of First Thoracic Vertebra
7. Tubercle of First Rib
8. Brachial Plexus
9. Dome of Pleura

Fig. 13-16. Cervicothoracic sympathetic chain: regional anatomy. (I) Anterior view. Note stellate ganglion on neck of first rib and extending up to transverse process of C7. At this level, the cervicothoracic sympathetic chain has the vertebral artery on its anterolateral aspect with the pleura covering the lower third of the stellate ganglion. At the level of C6, the vertebral artery has dived posteriorly into the foramen intertransversarium and the pleura is well below. Note also that even at C6, a large volume of solution may diffuse posteriorly between the slips of origin of scalenus anterior to the roots of the brachial plexus. (II) Cross section. Note the importance of lateral retraction of the carotid and extension of the neck to draw the esophagus medial to the needle path on the left side. It is necessary to withdraw the needle 2 to 5 mm after contacting the transverse process in order to clear the anterior aspect of the longus colli muscle. Correct needle direction onto the transverse process is very important, as is the avoidance of force with the risk of penetration of prevertebral fascia and intertransverse ligaments leading to entry into vertebral artery or dural cuff.

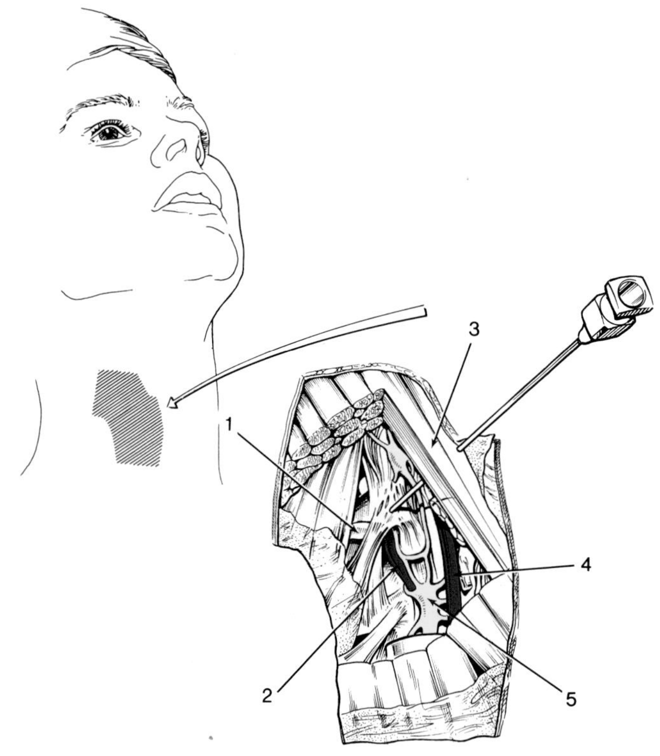

1. Transverse Process C6
2. Vertebral Artery
3. Sternocleidomastoid Muscle
4. Common Carotid Artery
5. Stellate Ganglion

Fig. 13-17. Landmarks for cervicothoracic sympathetic blockade (stellate ganglion). Note level of blockade is cricoid cartilage (C6).

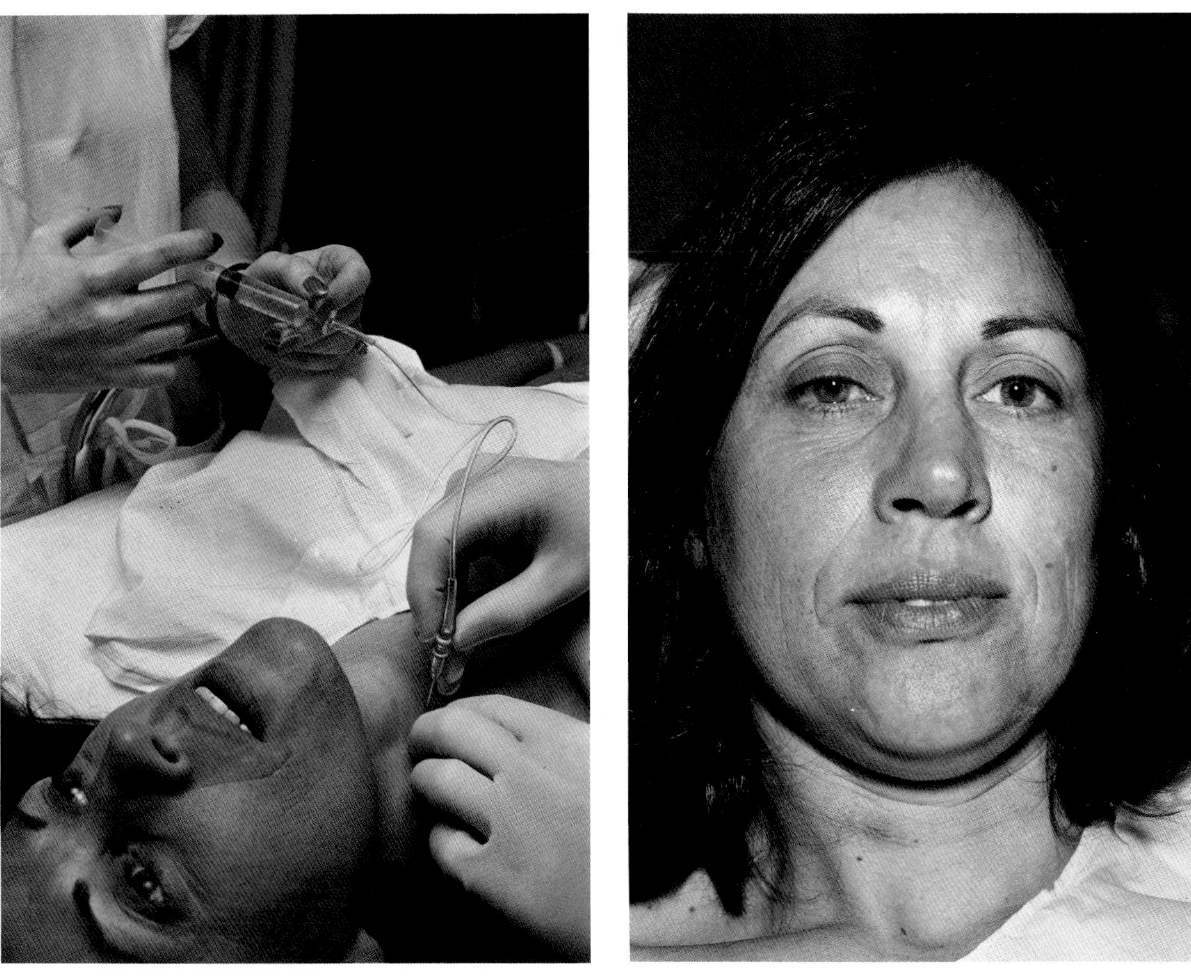

Fig. 13-18. (*A*) Stellate ganglion block needle correctly placed. Note palpating hand (*left*) retracting carotid sheath laterally and hand holding needle (*right*) braced against clavicle. An extension tubing is used so that an assistant may aspirate and inject. (*B*) Horner's syndrome (*right*). Note ptosis, miosis, and anhydrosis, also unilateral conjunctival engorgement.

list on page 363. It should be stressed that the present lack of definitive data makes it highly desirable to carry out a diagnostic block before considering permanent blockade. In addition, any the methods of independently assessing blockade, blood flow, and pain relief should be employed.

General Contraindications

Patients on Heparin. Severe bleeding has been observed, particularly after lumbar sympathetic blockade in a heparinized patient. The bleeding occurs within the psoas fascia, producing minimal symptoms until frank shock occurs. Early symptoms are pain in the groin or pain when the leg is actively lifted and rotated outward. A hematoma may also pass through an intervertebral foramen into the spinal canal, after stellate or lumbar sympathetic block, causing pressure on nerves and vessels followed by neurologic symptoms (see also Chap. 8). Hematoma after stellate block has been reported to interfere with carotid blood flow (see Chaps. 22 and 23).

Bilateral injection during one treatment session should probably be avoided. Dosage tends to be high, and vascular responses may be a significant problem for this class of patient. Various side effects may pose an increased hazard if both sides are blocked. For example, bilateral recurrent laryngeal block after stellate block may cause stridor (see Chap. 22).

Bilateral injection in the lumbar region for permanent blockade may cause loss of ejaculation and should be avoided in young persons. However, impotence does not occur, and the patient is not sterile.

AGENTS FOR SYMPATHETIC BLOCKADE

For short-term block, any of the conventional local anesthetics can be used. Addition of epinephrine to the local anesthetic solution will, to some extent, prolong the duration of action. However, the use of epinephrine in patients with severe vascular disease or vasospasm is questionable. Mepivacaine and bupivacaine, without epinephrine, have durations of 1-½ to 3 and 3 to 4 hours, respectively. These durations are only marginally influenced by the addition of epinephrine and therefore are the solutions of choice.[8,57] It is useful to add contrast medium (2 ml of Conray-420) since this allows confirmation of the adequacy of spread of solution (*e.g.*, over L2–4 ganglia; see Fig. 13-30).

The amount of local anesthetic agent needed in, for example, lumbar sympathetic blockade (1–5 ml, 0.5% mepivacaine or 0.25% bupivacaine at each level), even without epinephrine, poses a relatively small risk of a toxic reaction due to local anesthetic absorption. However, there is the ever present risk of acute intravascular injection and the other adverse effects of local anesthetic injection (see Table 4-8).

For a permanent block (chemical sympathectomy), 6 to 7 per cent phenol in water, 7 to 10 per cent phenol in Conray-420 contrast medium, or 50 to 100 per cent alcohol may be used. The last yields the highest incidence of neuralgia, and most authorities now prefer 7 to 10 per cent phenol in Conray-420 since it poses minimal resistance to injection, and its spread can be viewed under radiographic control.[4,13]

TECHNIQUES

STELLATE GANGLION BLOCK (Cervicothoracic Sympathetic Block)

Regional Anatomy

The cervical sympathetic chain lies in the fascial space, which is limited posteriorly by the fascia over the prevertebral muscles and anteriorly by the carotid sheath (Fig. 13-16).

Although the sympathetic preganglionic fibers for the head, neck, and upper limb leave the spinal cord from segments as widely separated as T1 to T6, pathways converge and pass anteriorly to the neck of the first rib. Here, the first thoracic and inferior cervical ganglion may be separated or fused to form the stellate ganglion. In the latter case, the ganglion lies over the neck of the first rib. The ganglion is covered anteriorly in its lower part by the dome of the pleura and in its upper part by the vertebral artery. Block of the stellate ganglion alone may provide disappointing results despite the correct anatomical placement of solution. This may be explained by the diverse origin of the sympathetic fibers in the thoracic cord and also the fact that some thoracic preganglion fibers lie in other sympathetic ganglia and may bypass the stellate ganglion completely on their way into the head, neck, and upper extremity.[51] For best results, the local anesthetic solution has to fill the space in front of the prevertebral fascia down to at least T4. This can be achieved by an injection of 15 to 20 ml of weak local anesthetic solution in front of the transverse process of C6 (see Fig. 13-19). It is obvious that there is

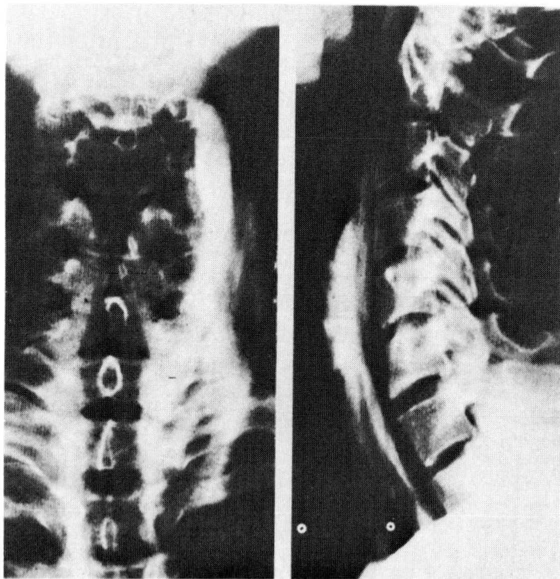

Fig. 13-19. The spread of 20 ml of local anesthetic solution injected in front of the prevertebral fascia at the 6th transverse process. (Courtesy of Eriksson, E., and Astra, A.B., 1969)

little advantage to be gained by needle placement at C7 and there is a greater risk of pneumothorax at this level. The term "cervicothoracic sympathetic block" thus seems more appropriate than "stellate ganglion block."

Procedure

A large number of techniques have been described. If the needle is aimed at the neck of the first rib, the risk of pneumothorax is considerable. On the other hand, the needle may be kept well above the pleura and reliance placed on the spread of a large volume of solution. This is the basis of the anterior approach first described by Leriche.[43]

"Paratracheal" (Anterior) Technique

The patient lies supine with the head slightly lifted forward on a thin pillow and tilted dorsally to stretch the esophagus away from the transverse process on the left side. The mouth should be slightly opened to relax the neck muscles.

The trachea and the carotid pulse are gently palpated by inserting two fingers between the sternocleidomastoid muscle and the trachea to find the most prominent cervical transverse process, C6—the Chassaignac tubercle, which lies at the level of the cricoid cartilage (Figs. 13-17–18). A skin wheal is raised with a fine needle over this transverse process. Two fingers are now gently pressed down to the C6 tubercle, pushing away the carotid artery laterally and the trachea toward the midline with the fingers slightly separated so that the tubercle lies just in between them (Fig. 13-18).

A 22-g, short-bevel, 4- to 5-cm-long needle, with a 20-ml syringe attached, is advanced through the skin and underlying tissues until it hits bone, that is, rests on the transverse process. The palpating fingers maintain their position; the hand holding the needle is kept braced against the patient, and the needle is withdrawn about 2 mm and fixed (Fig. 13-18).

An aspiration test is performed before and after turning the needle 90°. If no blood enters the syringe, a test dose of 2 ml is injected. Injection of even this small dose directly into the vertebral artery can result in a convulsion (see Chap. 4). A high resistance to injection may indicate periosteal injection, and a significant but lesser resistance indicates that the needle is still in prevertebral muscle. While the needle is *in situ,* it is important that the patient does not talk. If aspiration tests are negative and no sequelae follow, the full dose, 15 to 20 ml of local anesthetic, is injected (Fig. 13-19). In most instances, the patient will feel a lump in the throat and may often be temporarily hoarse, and should be warned beforehand of these events.

Continuous Technique

A continuous technique has been described. A thin intravenous plastic cannula with a stylet is introduced with the paratracheal technique described above. The stylet is withdrawn and the catheter properly fixed. It should be recognized, however, that movement of the catheter into proximity with vertebral artery, dural cuff, or other structures is a possibility.

Intravenous sympathetic block is a more attractive technique when prolonged effect is required (see Chap. 12).

Signs of a Successful Block

Horner's syndrome results if the cervical sympathetic fibers are successfully blocked: ptosis (drooping upper eyelid), myosis (small pupil), and enophthalmos (sinking of the eyeball). In addition, other features have been described, such as unilateral blockage of the nose (due to engorgement of nasal mucosa), flushing of conjunctiva and skin, anhydrosis (lack of sweating; Fig. 13-18*B*). It should be noted that these signs may be present without complete sympathetic denervation of the upper limb, which may receive sympathetic supply from as far down as T9. The cobalt blue sweat test or SGR is the most useful in this situation (see list on p. 356).

Indications

The clinical indications for cervicothoracic sympathetic blocks are listed in the following

Clinical Conditions That Cervicothoracic Sympathetic Blockade May Benefit

Circulatory insufficiency in the arm
- After embolectomy, traumatic or embolic vascular occlusion or impaired circulation
- Raynaud's disease, scleroderma and other arteriopathies, frostbite*
- Occlusive vascular disease: "acute or chronic" episodes

Pain
- Post-traumatic syndrome (causalgia)
- Herpes zoster
- Phantom limb
- Paget's disease
- Neoplasm
- Trophic changes in skin

Other
- Hyperhidrosis
- Shoulder/hand syndrome
- Miscellaneous conditions in head region: stroke, Meniere's disease

* All three of these conditions, at an early stage for "acute or chronic episodes."

(see also Chap. 26). It should be noted that these indications are based largely on anecdotal case reports so that an initial diagnostic blockade should always be accompanied by a separate assessment, by one of the methods in the list on page 356, for sympathetic ablation, blood flow, and pain.

The most controversial indications are stroke and other conditions in the cranial distribution of the sympathetic chain, such as Meniere's disease. At present, no definitive data are available to demonstrate any benefit from sympathetic blockade.

Complications

Intra-arterial as well as intradural injections are dangerous complications. (See next column.) It should be firmly stated that the negative aspiration test, as described above, does not exclude an intra-arterial or an intra-dural injection. To prevent

Complications of Cervicothoracic (Stellate Ganglion) Sympathetic Blockade

Common
- Temporary hoarseness and feeling of a lump in the throat
- Unpleasant effects of Horner's syndrome
- Hematoma may occur
- Neuritis along chest wall and inner aspect of upper arm

Uncommon
- Brachial plexus, rarely affected
- Pneumothorax
- Osteitis—transverse process

Severe
- Injection into the vertebral artery—immediate CNS effects
- Intradural injection—slow onset of symptoms

the occurrence of these complications, it is of the utmost importance to realize that the needle should not meet any resistance after it has passed through the skin until it rests on what is obviously plain bone. If the needle is pushed through the prevertebral fascia and the ligaments connecting the transverse processes (this fascia and the ligament can usually be felt), the tip of the needle might be in or close to the vertebral artery or the dural sheath enclosing the cervical nerve roots. Spinal analgesia follows dural sheath injection.

An injection of local anesthetic solution into the paravertebral fascia may also spread along the fascial plane to involve the brachial plexus.[11] Bilateral injection is inadvisable since inadvertant bilateral recurrent laryngeal nerve block may result in airway problems (loss of laryngeal reflex). Also, loss of cardioaccelerator activity may result in bradycardias and hypotension.

If a hematoma occurs, it might be necessary to inject below C6. This can usually be accomplished as it is possible to feel the prevertebral fascia and the ligaments over C7, after which the needle should be withdrawn several mm and the block completed as described above; the risk of pneumothorax increases.

Osteitis of the transverse process has been described after a stellate ganglion block.* This may have been because the needle traversed the esophagus before it reached the transverse process.[51]

Chemical Stellate Ganglion Block

An injection of 1 to 2 ml of 6 per cent aqueous phenol or 10 per cent phenol in Conray dye (see

* Nilson, E., Lund, P.: Personal communication.

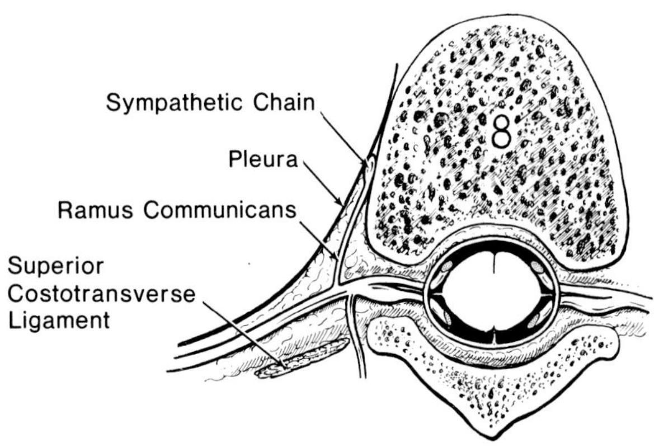

Fig. 13-20. Thoracic sympathetic chain. Note proximity of somatic nerves, dural cuff region, and pleura (redrawn after Macintosh).

below) at C6 will interrupt the cervical chain but not produce a complete cervicothoracic sympathetic blockade. The arm may partially escape, and, in these cases, an injection of the sympathetic chain at T2 and T3 may be used as a supplement; however, this technique is uncommonly practiced because of the proximity of pleura and somatic nerves (see also Chap. 27).

THORACIC SYMPATHETIC BLOCK

Regional Anatomy

As noted on page 356, the sympathetic chain in the thoracic region lies close to the neck of the ribs, and, thus, it is very close to the somatic roots (Fig. 13-20). In the cervical region, the sympathetic chain is separated from somatic roots by longus colle and anterior scalene muscles and, in the lumbar region, by psoas major. In contrast, no such muscle is present in the thoracic region, and the proximity of the pleura to the sympathetic chain adds a second hazard (Fig. 13-20).

Technique

A 10-cm needle is introduced three fingers breadth (6 cm) from the midline opposite the T2 spinous process. As the needle is advanced, it either strikes rib or passes through the intercostal space and continues until it is held up by the body of the vertebra in the true para-vertebral space (Fig. 13-21). It is generally easy to decide whether the bone encountered is rib or vertebral body as the rib is more superficial and transmits through the needle a feeling of smoothness in contrast to the gritty roughness of the vertebral body; because of the anatomic problems outlined above, confirmation of position by radiograph is highly desirable. When the needle reaches the vertebra, it is angled to pass less than 1 cm behind the crest of the vertebral body (Fig. 13-21). An injection of 2 ml of local anesthetic or, for permanent block, 6 per cent phenol or alcohol is made at this point, and a successful result is indicated if the patient has a warm dry hand and no evidence of Horner's syndrome. The use of image intensifier and injection, under direct vision, of 10 per cent phenol dissolved in Conray-420 greatly increases the safety of this technique.

Indications

Some possible indications for permanent neurolytic sympathectomy for the upper limb syndromes are given in the list on page 369. Many clinics still prefer surgical sympathectomy, although a transaxillary (thoracic) approach is necessary to obtain complete sympathetic denervation of the upper limb. The results and complications of the neurolytic technique with an image intensifier remain to be assessed. Intrathoracic pain, such as status anginosus, has been treated by sympathetic block (by either stellate or thoracic approach). However, the availability of beta-blockers has diminished the appeal of sympathetic block since the potential complications are very serious in a patient with severe myocardial disease.

Complications

The two principle complications of this technique are pneumothorax and intrathecal injection by way

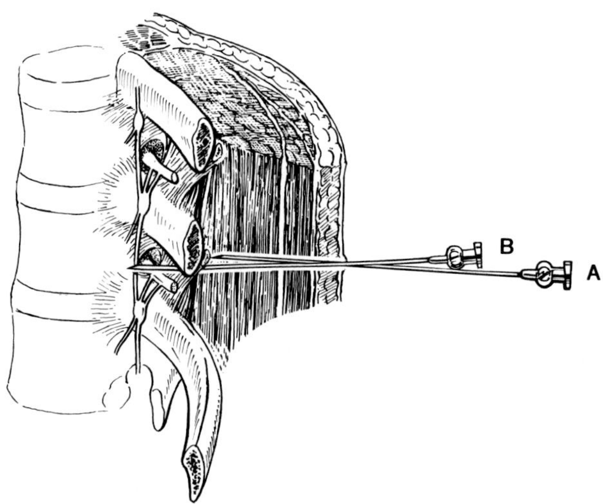

Fig. 13-21. Thoracic sympathetic blockade (see text).

of the intervertebral foramen. Because of these two complications, this technique was used only minimally, until recent application of image-intensifier techniques permitted direct viewing of needle placement and appropriate spread of solution.

LUMBAR SYMPATHETIC BLOCK

Regional Anatomy

The lumbar part of the sympathetic chain and its ganglia lies in the fascial plane close to the anterolateral side of the vertebral bodies, separated from somatic nerves by the psoas fascia and psoas muscle (Fig. 13-22). An injection of a large volume of fluid (*e.g.*, 25 ml) anywhere in this space will, in most instances, fill the whole space. Theoretically, one injection at L2 or L3 should be enough to achieve adequate longitudinal spread. However, in order to obtain a complete block, injections are performed at different levels, particularly with a neurolytic agent such as phenol to limit lateral spread at any one level since this poses a risk of spread across psoas to the genitofemoral nerve, perhaps by a fibrous tunnel to a somatic nerve, or, worse still, to a dural cuff region and thence to subarachnoid space (Figs. 13-23; 13-24).[10] When continuous blockade with catheters is used, it is also preferable to have

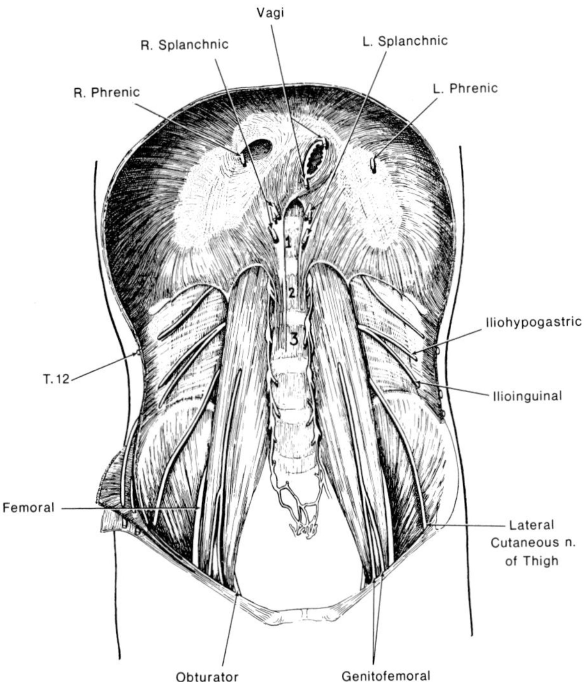

Fig. 13-23. Posterior abdominal wall, genitofemoral nerve. Note its course anterior to psoas major, thus being more vulnerable to neurolytic solution spreading laterally from the sympathetic chain.

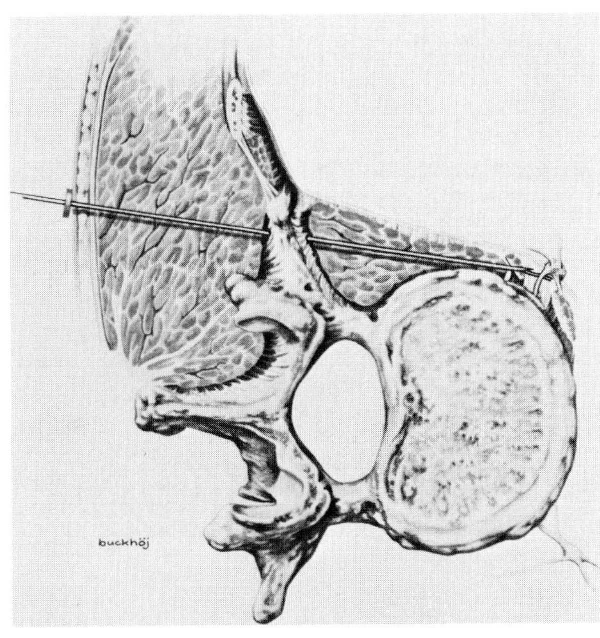

Fig. 13-22. Lumbar sympathetic block. The correct position of the needle close to the lumbar sympathetic trunk. (Courtesy of Eriksson, E., and Astra, A.B., 1969)

two catheters because there is a tendency for one of the catheters to slide dorsally out of position.

Technique (Mandl)

The method of blocking the lumbar sympathetic chain was first introduced by Mandl in 1926 and was similar to that used by Kappis for injecting the celiac plexus.[34,49]

The spinous processes of L2 and L4 are marked. L1 is level with the line between the two points where the lateral side of the erector spinae muscles meet the twelfth ribs; a line joining the posterior superior iliac crests passes through the lower part of the spine at L4 (Fig. 13-25).

A subcutaneous wheal is raised about 8 cm laterally to the spinous processes of L2, L3, and L4. Local anesthetic solution is injected subcutaneously and also, with an intramuscular needle, against the transverse process above or below the site of injection by directing the needle 45° cranially or caudally and in between the transverse processes.

A 19- to 20-gauge needle of approximately 12 cm in length (or an 18-gauge needle for continuous

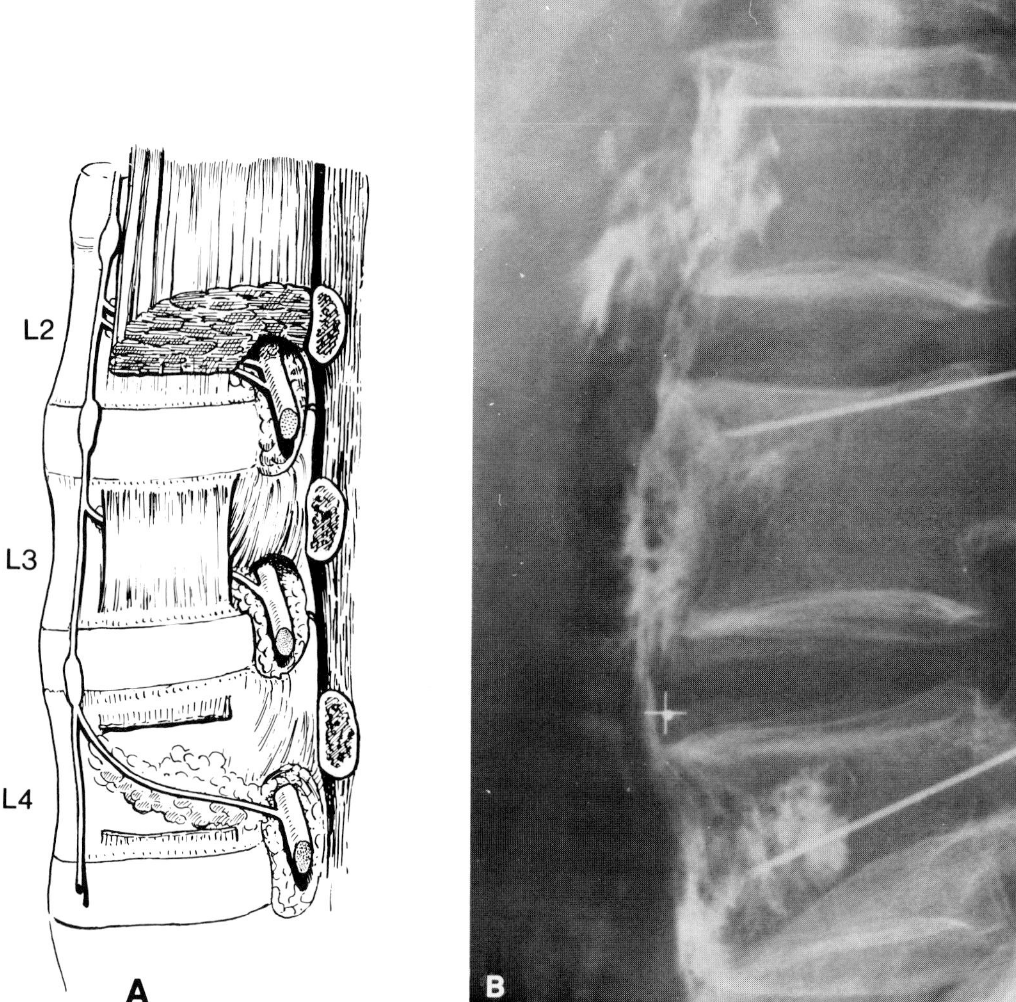

Fig. 13-24. (*A*) Possible mechanisms of somatic neuralgia due to solution spread by fibrous arch. (*B*) Contrast medium injected too close to side of vertebral body, spreading via fibrous arch (see text; Macintosh).

blockade) with a rubber marker is introduced through the skin until the tip of the needle has reached a transverse process. The marker is pushed down to the skin and the needle is withdrawn. The distance from the skin to the transverse process is, in the normal adult, roughly half the distance from the skin to the lateral side of the vertebral body (10 cm). This may be a shorter distance if the patient has thin back muscles, longer if the muscles are thick. The marker on the needle is moved toward the hub of the needle so that the distance from the tip to the marker is roughly twice the first marked distance.

The needle is reintroduced and directed slightly medially to pass between the transverse processes. When bone is reached, the marker should be almost flush with the skin, the bevel of the needle being directed toward the lateral side of the vertebral body. A slight change in angle of the needle will allow the tip of the needle to slide off the vertebra and to reach the sympathetic chain on the ventrolateral aspect of the vertebral body (see Fig. 13-22).[21] Correct position can be verified by using a loss-of-resistance test with a syringe filled with air or saline. Penetration of the psoas fascia gives a resistance change not dissimilar to that of epidural block. A loss of resistance, at a shallower level, is often obtained between psoas and quadratus lumborum in

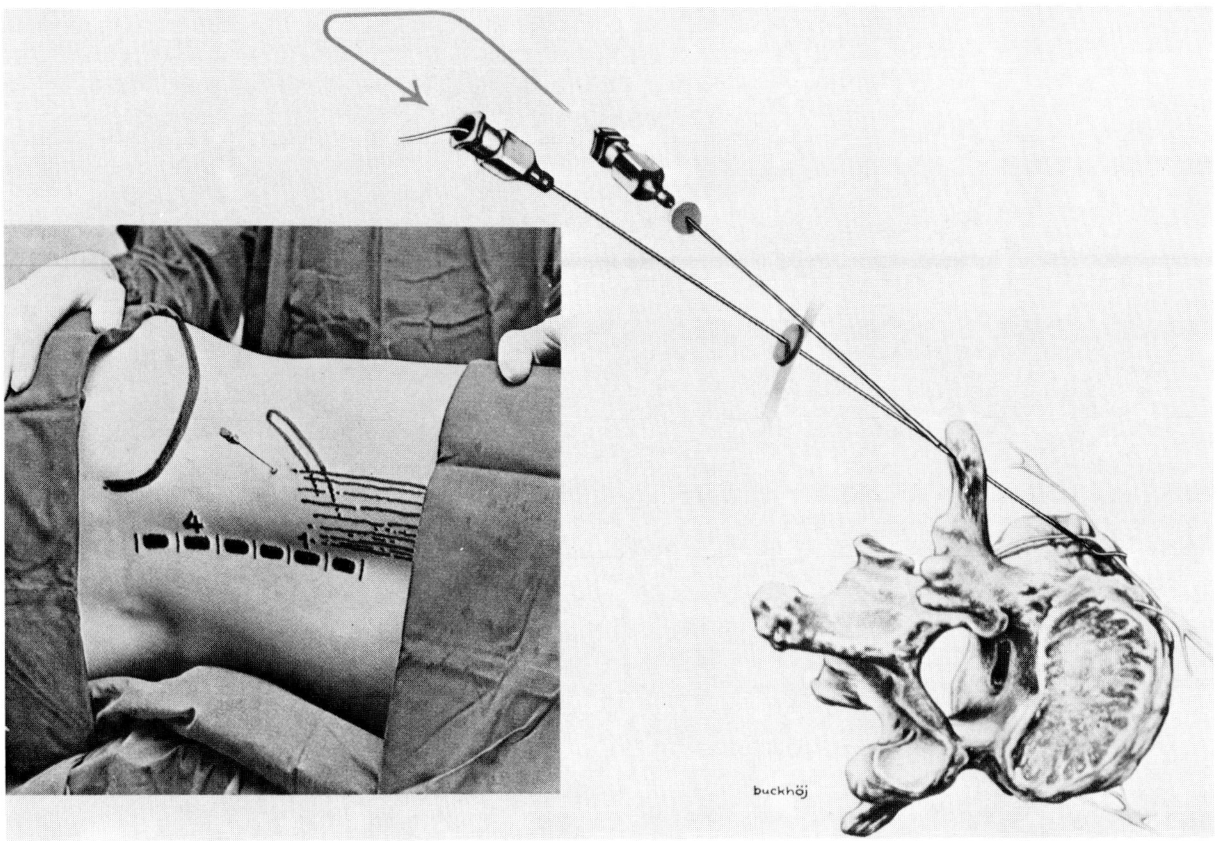

Fig. 13-25. Illustrates the technique used in lumbar sympathetic blocks (see text). (Courtesy of Eriksson, E., and Astra, A.B., 1969)

the region of the transverse process. Placement of solution at this level would result in lumbar plexus block—highly undesirable if a neurolytic solution is employed.

In clinical practice, the anesthesiologist often starts at L2 and, in a second step, introduces the needle at L4. When the needle is correctly placed at L2, the part of the needle outside the skin should be measured and the marker for L4 properly placed. In most patients, owing to the lumbar lordosis at L4, the distance from the skin to the vertebral body is usually a little greater than at L2. It is vitally important to aspirate to ensure that neither blood nor cerebrospinal fluid (CSF) is present and to check that there is no resistance to injection; resistance could be due to the needle being in the wall of aorta or vena cava, an abdominal viscus, or an intervertebral disc. Once again, radiographic confirmation (local anesthetic mixed with contrast medium) and injection under direct vision increases safety.

In the most simple cases (*e.g.*, renal colic), one injection of 20 to 30 ml, preferably of 0.25 per cent bupivacaine with epinephrine, 1:200,000 (5×10^{-6} g/ml), at L2 will completely eradicate pain. In patients with obliterative arterial disease, a diagnostic block with 1 to 5 ml of local anesthetic mixed with contrast medium may be made at L2, L3, and L4, under radiographic control. The continuous blockade technique is also very useful; needles are placed at L2 and L4, and after the proper positioning of each needle, catheters are passed through the needles, which are then withdrawn over the catheters. The catheters are fixed along the erector spinae muscles. The cranial ends of the catheters, each with a needle and a Millipore filter, are placed in a sterile sponge in the supraclavicular fossa. The time interval between injections may be increased to 6 hours if bupivacaine is used. The continuous blockade is maintained for 5 days, during which the clinical effects of the blockade should be evaluated. In the case of the single-shot diagnostic block, the volume of local anesthetic in contrast

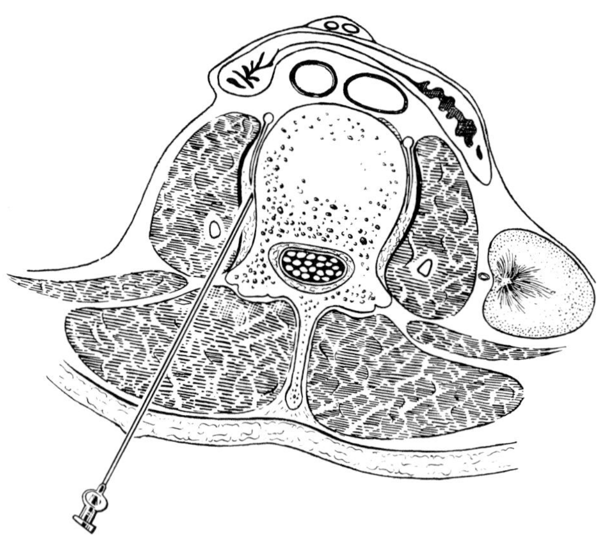

Fig. 13-26. Alternative technique for local anesthetic lumbar sympathetic block (see text).

medium should be the same as that proposed for neurolytic block. Also, a method of assessment from each category on the list on page 356 should be employed immediately after the block. Often, diagnostic blocks are repeated if there is any doubt about results.[6]

In most instances, the procedure is short (< 30 min) and fairly free of pain. Heavy premedication or general anesthesia is not necessary. However, now and then, a needle may pass close to a segmental nerve, provoking "lightening" pain. The needle should always be advanced slowly and redirected slightly if paresthesia should occur. The needle should not be directed too much toward the midline. We believe that it is better to be able to detect that the needle is close to a nerve in a lightly medicated patient than to accept the risk of laceration of the nerve with a fairly large needle. One case of severe segmental neuritis, most likely the result of a nerve injury, supports this view.

Technique of Bryce–Smith

A simpler approach to local anesthetic lumbar sympathetic blockade has been described by Bryce–Smith (1951).[9]

Regional Anatomy

Because of the anterolateral position of the ganglia in the lumbar region, the course of the rami communicantes is long and winds around the vertebral body in a fibrous tunnel. This arch forms one of the origins of the psoas muscle and provides indirect access to the lumbar sympathetic chain (Fig. 13-26).

Technique

A wheal is raised three-fingers breadth lateral to the tip of the spinous process of L3, a 12-cm needle is introduced at 70° and advanced toward the body of the vertebra; when the point of the needle reaches the body of the vertebra, it lies within the fibrous tunnel (Fig. 13-26). Fifteen to 20 cm of solution are deposited here, and this tracks forward to reach the sympathetic chain. This approach should not be used when neurolytic solutions are employed as some of the fluid backtrack and set up a neuritis of the third lumbar nerve or enter a dural cuff and cause paraplegia.

Since this technique frequently leads to somatic block and does not provide a selective sympathetic block it is also not indicated for diagnosis of pain syndromes.

LUMBAR SYMPATHECTOMY WITH NEUROLYTIC AGENT

Neurolytic lumbar sympathectomy should never be used for the treatment of vascular disease without consultation with a vascular surgeon. It is clear that even a successful sympathetic block in a patient with rest pain may result sometimes in demarcation of a nonviable area, such as a distal phalanx of a toe. This will require appropriate surgical treatment and should be viewed as a disappointing side-effect of the block but as a necessary part of a rational treatment regimen.

The sensible use of lumbar sympathetic block with proper collaboration offers the following very considerable advantages:

Symptoms can be ameliorated without risk of surgery and anesthesia in a group of patients with a high incidence of severe ischemic heart disease, pulmonary disease, and other problems of old age. In the series reported by Reid et al there was a mortality of 1:1666 injections (less than 0.1%); this compares favorably with surgical sympathectomy, which has a mortality rate of at least 6 per cent and as much as 20 per cent in patients with severe vascular disease.[60] In a recent series of 386 blocks, there was only 1 death within 1 week of blockade, and this patient had severe ischemic heart disease with congestive cardiac failure prior to blockade.[13]

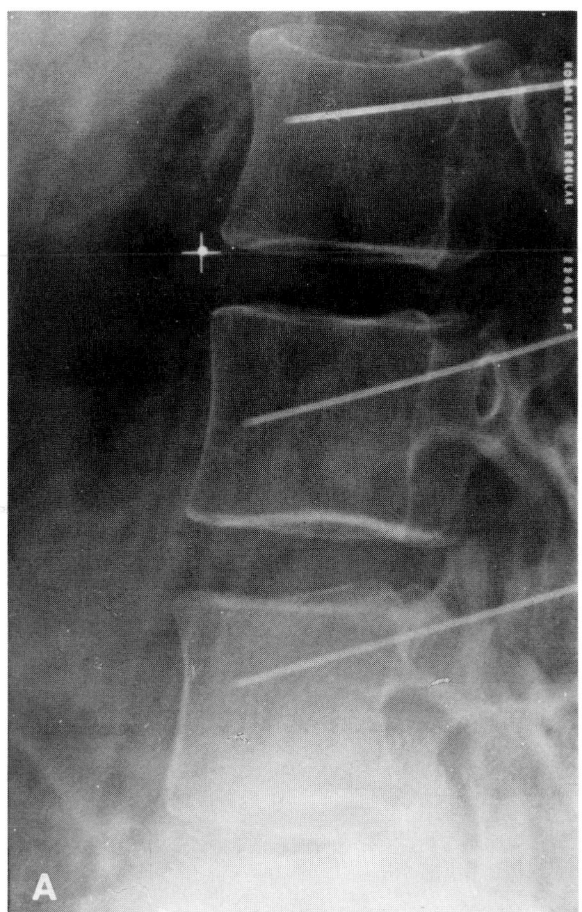

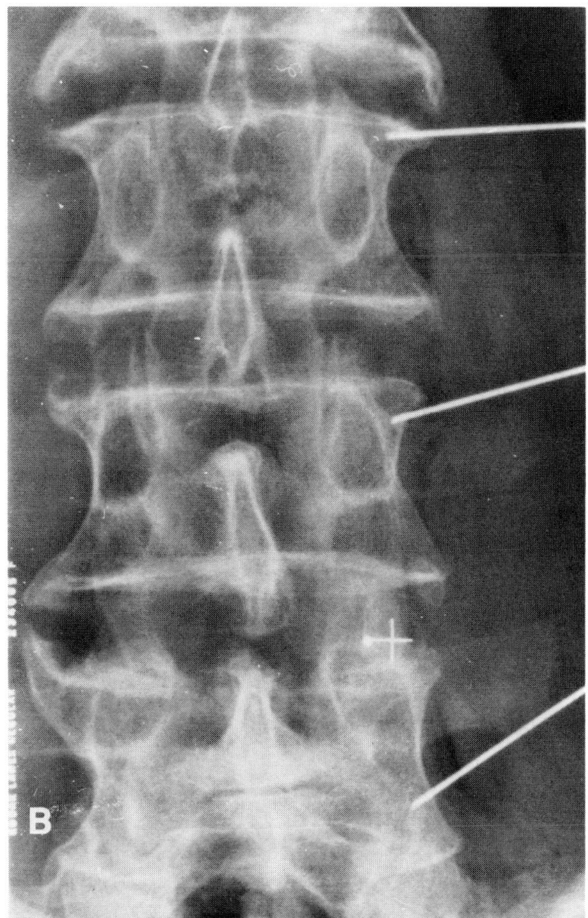

Fig. 13-27. (*A*) Lateral view. Three needles are placed so that they lie in the center of L2, L3, and L4 bodies, well clear of the disc space. (*B*) The anteroposterior view shows that all needles are beside the lateral aspect of the vertebral body.

Outpatient Treatment. Treatment may be performed on an outpatient basis, and elderly patients (usually 65–70 years) can be released after a short stay. This allows for considerable economy in hospital-bed use; surgical sympathectomy often requires 6 to 10 days in the hospital when there are no complications.

Fewer Postoperative Thrombotic Phenomena. Reduction in the elderly since an operation and bed rest are avoided.

A large turnover of patients is possible (as many as 8–10 procedures in a single-day session).

If necessary a bilateral procedure can be performed, with the second side blocked 1 week later, also on an outpatient basis.

Duration. Since the duration of sympathetic ablation is similar with surgical or neurolytic sympathectomy (mean, 6 months), the neurolytic technique offers an advantage. It can be repeated with very minimal morbidity. Nevertheless, the natural history of occlusive vascular disease is such that in one series only 5 per cent required repeated blockade.[13]

Agents

Absolute alcohol has been employed by several groups; however, it has a higher incidence of L1 neuralgia (see Chap. 27).[13] Seven per cent phenol in water was employed by Reid and colleagues in a very large series because of the low viscosity of the solution and ease of injection.[60] Seven to 10 per cent phenol in Conray-420 dye has a similar low resistance to injection and has the added advantage of

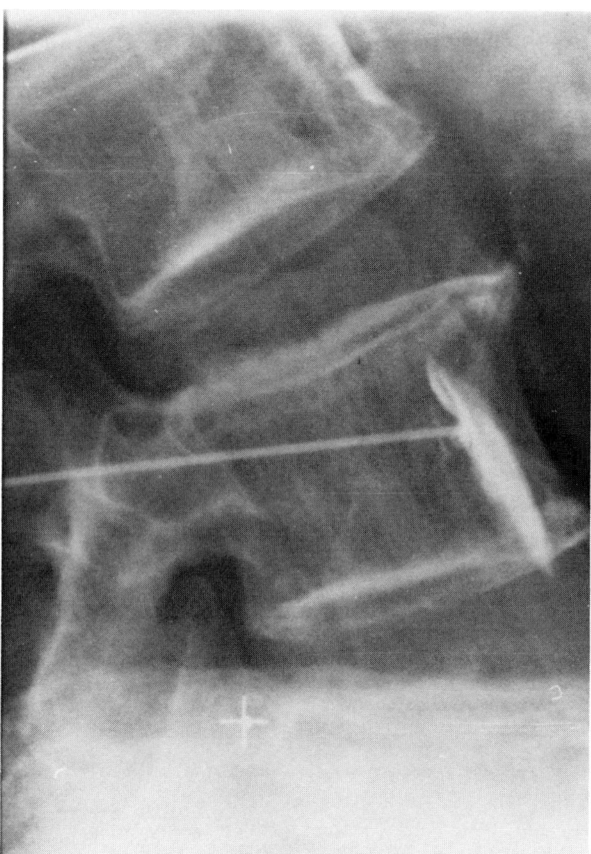

Fig. 13-28. Injection of 0.1 ml of contrast medium, showing correct linear spread along anterior aspect of psoas fascia.

Lateral, Center. Needle position in the center of L2, L3, and L4 vertebral bodies is checked with a lateral view (see Fig. 13-27). Proximity of the needle to the disc space is avoided.

Lateral, Anterolateral. Needle position at the anterolateral angle of the L2, L3, and L4 bodies is also checked in the lateral view (Fig. 13-27). Lack of movement of the needle during deep inspiration and expiration is carefully checked. With correct placement in psoas, needle tips should be immobile. Movement on respiration indicates placement lateral to psoas—possibly in the kidney.

Anteroposterior, Lateral. An anteroposterior view is taken to check that each needle is close to the lateral aspects of the vertebral bodies (Fig. 13-27).

Lateral. Neurolytic solution is injected under direct vision, lateral view (see Fig. 13-28).

Initially, 0.1 ml of contrast medium is injected and confirmation obtained that a sharp linear spread being visible under image intensifier (see Fig. 13-28).[4,13] When the patient is placed on his side under a vertical radiographic beam, it is also of value to tilt the patient slightly ventrally and dorsally to check that the needle is fairly close to the vertebral column. If a biplanar image intensifier is available, then both lateral and anteroposterior views should be obtained (Figs. 13-27; 13-28). A convenient way to determine the spread is to dissolve phenol in an aqueous radiographic contrast medium (Conray-420) and to inject it under direct radiographic control. This often permits confirmation of complete coverage of the lumbar sympathetic chain with as little as 3 to 4 ml of solution (see Fig. 13-30).

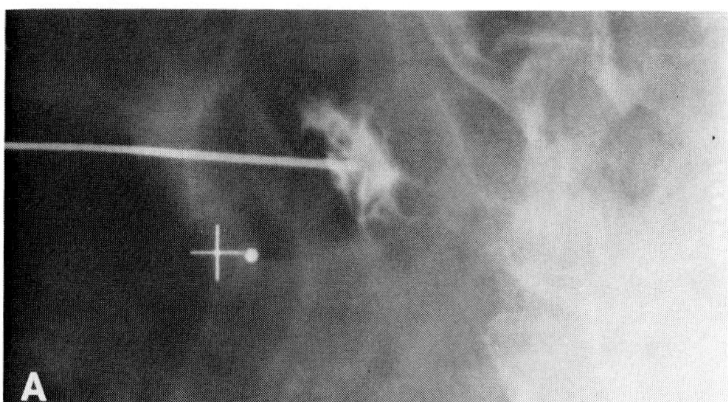

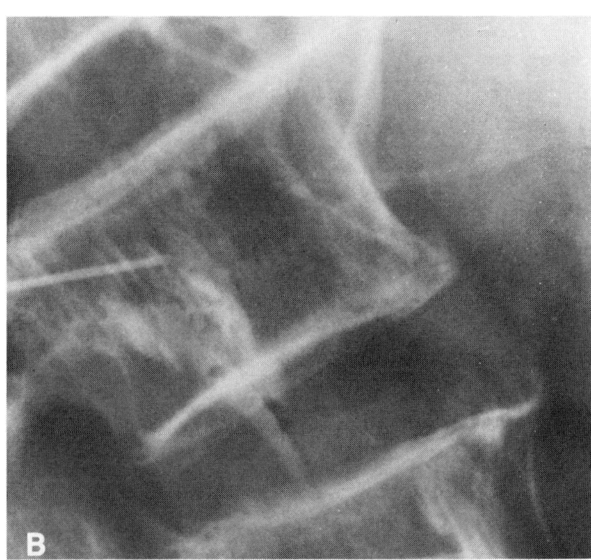

Fig. 13-29. Incorrect spread of 0.1 ml of contrast medium to produce a "fuzzy blob," indicating needle tip has been displaced, probably back into psoas major.

Technique

The following modifications of local anesthetic blockade are advisable when neurolytic agents are used.

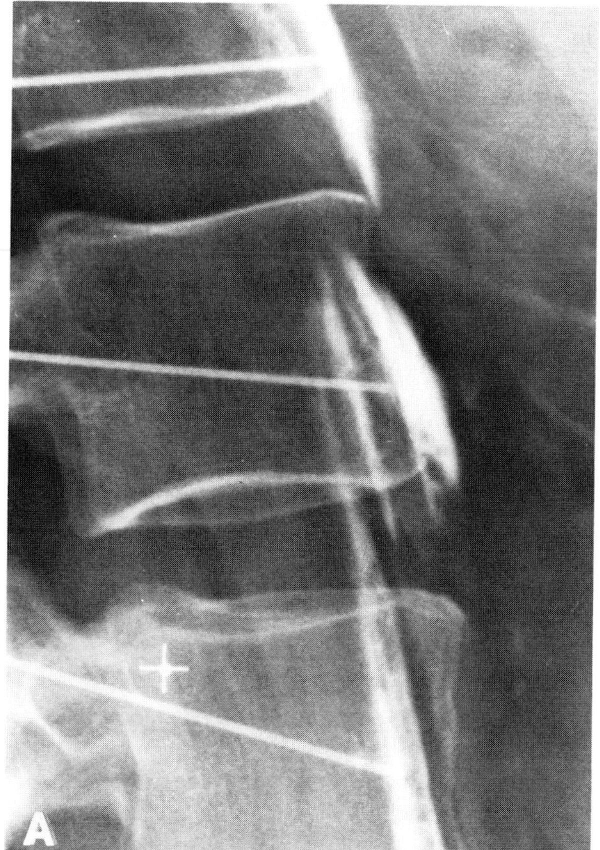

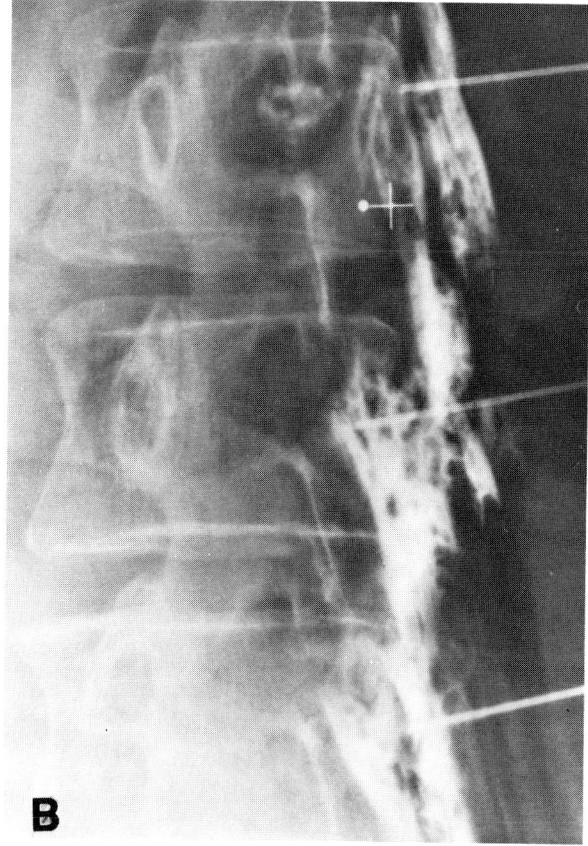

Fig. 13-30. (*A*) Lateral view. Complete coverage of L2, L3, and L4 vertebral body levels with injection of only 1 ml of 10 per cent phenol in Conray 420 at each level. (*B*) Anteroposterior view to show spread of solution following line of psoas muscle. Note limitation of lateral spread to reduce risk of genitofemoral nerve involvement.

is occurring (Fig. 13-28). Resistance to injection and the appearance of a "blob" or fuzzy patch of contrast medium indicates injection into muscle or fascia, and injection is ceased (Fig. 13-29). As soon as linear spread is obtained, the injection is continued with neurolytic solution until each level has linear coverage. In most instances this requires no more than 2 ml and often as little as 1 ml of solution (Fig. 13-30).

Anteroposterior. At the completion of the injection, an anteroposterior view is taken to confirm the spread of solution along the line of the psoas muscle (Fig. 13-30).

For All Modifications. With all three solutions, .5 ml of air is injected immediately prior to removing each needle to prevent the needle's depositing neurolytic solution on somatic nerve roots during removal.

Patients are kept on the side for 5 to 10 minutes to attempt to prevent the solution from spreading laterally toward the genitofemoral nerve or posteriorly between the slips of origin of the psoas major and along the fibrous tunnel occupied by the rami communicantes, toward somatic nerve roots.[9,10]

Patients are then turned supine but instructed not to raise their heads for 1 hour.

Observations of skin temperature, blood pressure, and pulse are continued.

Recovery Procedure

Observations are continued for 1 hour in a recovery room and, if stable, patients are permitted to sit to 45° and commence oral intake again. After another hour, blood pressure is checked sitting and then standing, and, if unchanged, patients are allowed to ambulate and the intravenous line is removed. Patients with highly unstable cardiovascular disease are maintained on an observation chart for at least 24 hours post block.

Table 13-1. Lumbar Sympathetic Examples of Block in Three Clinical Series

*Study**	*Number of Cases*
After vascular surgery ("continuous" local anesthetic lumbar sympathetic block)	70
Arterial embolism—no surgery	13 (7 improved)
Cytostatic perfusion (melanoma)	4
Frost bite	2
	89
Obliterative arterial disease (local anesthetic block followed by chemical sympathectomy in 72 cases)	122 (see Table 13-2)
Diagnostic Local Anesthetic Followed by Neurolytic Agent†	
Rest pain and ischemic ulcers	386 (80% relieved)
Gangrene of lower extremity (pain relief and speeding up demarcation)	50 (55% relieved)
Raynaud's disease	4 (all temporary relief only)
Reflex sympathetic dysfunction	12 (50% relieved—those treated early)
Claudication	12 (50% relieved; only those with response to local anesthetic block received neurolytic block)
Neurolytic Agent over 10-Year Period‡	
Rest pain	194 (80% relieved)
Gangrene of lower extremity	40 (50% relieved)
Raynaud's disease	16 (Only 20% had long-term relief)
Reflex sympathetic dysfunction (post-traumatic)	42 (45% relieved—those treated early)
Phantom limb	19 (60% relieved)

* Data from Löfström, B., and Zetterquist, S.: Lumbar sympathetic blocks in the treatment of patients with obliterative arterial disease of the lower limb. Int. Anesthesiol. Clin. 7:423, 1969.
† Data from Cousins, M.J., Reeve, T.S., Glynn, C.J., Walsh, J.A., and Cherry, D.A.: Neurolytic lumbar sympathetic blockade: Duration of denervation and relief of rest pain. Anaesthesia and Intensive Care, Vol. 7, No. 2, 121–135, May, 1979.
‡ Unpublished data from Lloyd, J.W., *et al.*

Indications

The most common clinical indications for lumbar sympathetic blocks are listed in the following.

Clinical Conditions in That Lumbar Sympathetic Blockade May Benefit

Circulatory insufficiency in the leg
- Arteriosclerotic disease, severe pain +++, gangrene ++; intermittent claudication* ++ in selected cases; diabetic gangrene +, Buerger's disease +
- After reconstructive vascular surgery
- Arterial embolus

Pain
- Renal colic
- Post-traumatic syndrome, causalgia†
- Herpes zoster
- Intractable urogenital pain in selected cases
- Sudecks Atrophy†
- Phantom limb†
- Amputation stump pain†
- Chilblains

General
- Hyperhidrosis—reduced sympathetic activity employed to reduce sweating
- White leg phlegmasia alba dolens‡
- Trench foot‡
- Erythromelalgia‡
- Acrocyanosis‡

* Aortoiliac (small percentage responding) and femoropopliteal (higher percentage responding)
† See Chapter 26
‡ Miscellaneous conditions in which reduced sympathetic activity may help to correct an abnormality in nutritive blood flow or venous or lymphatic drainage

Only patients who have received diagnostic sympathetic block or continuous technique blockade should be considered for a chemical sympathectomy. As discussed in the section on physiologic effects of sympathectomy, the best rationale for the use of lumbar sympathectomy in arterial disease is to obtain improved skin blood flow. Tables 13-1 to 13-3 summarize available clinical data on the use of lumbar sympathectomy for pain and skin ulcers as well as other conditions in which its efficacy is more difficult to determine except by diagnostic block in each case.

Complications

Complications of lumbar sympathetic blocks are extremely rare; however, a needle directed too far medially may pass into a intervertebral foramen, causing paraplegia. This may be recognized by the flow of cerebrospinal fluid, but it is not always the

Table 13-2. Results of Lumbar Sympathetic Blockade in Patients With Obliterative Arterial Disease

Primary Symptoms	*Number of Patients*		*Results of Initial Continuous Local Anesthetic Block Relief*				
			2+		*1+*	*0*	–
Gangrene arteriosclerotic	55	L.A.		28		27	0
			∴ 28 phenol blocks				
			14 ↓		9	5	0
Diabetic	28	L.A.		14		14	
			∴ 14 phenol blocks				
			8 ↓		4	2	0
Severe rest pain	23	L.A.	19		4	0	0
				23			
			∴ 18 phenol blocks (5 resolved with LA)				
			18 ↓		0	0	0
Intermittent claudication	16	L.A.	7		6	2	1
				12			
			∴ 12 phenol blocks (1 resolved with LA)				
				7		9	

(Kövames, A., and Löfström, B.: Continuous lumbar sympathetic blocks in the treatment of patients with ischemic lower limbs. Tenth Congress of Int. Cardiovascular Soc., 1971)

case. Thus, confirmation of correct placement by radiography is highly desirable (see also Chap. 23).

Complications of Lumbar Sympathetic Blockade*

Puncture of major vessel or renal pelvis
Subarachnoid injection
Neuralgia—genitofemoral nerve (5–10% pain in the groin)
Somatic nerve, damage—neuralgia (1%)
Perforation of a disc
Stricture of the ureter after phenol or alcohol injection
Infection from catheter technique. (extremely rare)

* Pain in the groin following injection is the commonest untoward sequel. Subarachnoid tap is occasionally seen but easily recognized and should not constitute a hazard. The remaining complications are very rare.

After surgical as well as after chemical sympathectomy, a pain or discomfort in the groin is often seen, hypothetically attributed to a genitofemoral nerve neuritis. The discomfort may last 2 to 5 weeks.[4,13,16,59] This is so-called L1 neuralgia and is characterized by hyperesthesia in L1 distribution and a burning pain. The patient often says that it is unbearable even to have clothes touch the thigh and may also describe the leg as "feeling as though it will explode." The condition responds well to transcutaneous electrical stimulation. The incidence is much higher with alcohol and appears to be least when the volume injected at any one level is the minimal amount necessary to achieve coverage of sympathetic ganglia, as checked by image-intensifier.[13]

Table 13-3. Percentage of Patients With Occlusive Vascular Disease Who Responded to Lumbar Sympathetic Block

Rest Pain (%)	*Skin Lesions (%)*	*Claudication (%)*	*References*
	55	13	25, 26
	60	41	65
	64		3
57	45		36
71	55	20	28
62	100 (5/5)		52
63–51	35		64
48 (some)	33		23
57	43		63
	6		22
49 (Complete relief)	50		13
80 (Complete or partial relief)			
		0	24
		0	53

Appendix A

COBALT BLUE SWEAT TEST

*General Requirements

Whatman No. 41 Filter papers 5.5 cm (halved) × 100
Cobalt chloride crystals (500 g)
Silica-gel crystals
Thermometer (and antiseptic)
Distilled water
Dressing forceps
Oven and tray
Blankets
Infrared lamps × 2 (or heat cradle)

Filter Paper Preparation

Dissolve 10 g cobalt chloride in 100 ml distilled water
Dip and drain halved filter papers, using forceps
Place on tray in oven at approximately 150° for 20 minutes (avoid excessive drying)
Remove with forceps from oven when pink color changes to bright blue
Seal in airtight jar with silica-gel crystals.

Procedure

Record patient's oral temperature
Apply lamp for 30 minutes to trunk and arms (take care not to burn patient or heat face excessively)
Using forceps, place filter paper on firm dry surface and apply both palms or plantar surfaces of feet, ensuring application as airtight as possible
Rerecord oral temperature, aiming to increase oral temperature by 0.3°F
Cease heat application if the above is recorded or if frank sweating is present

COMMENTS

The procedure should be performed pre- and postblock as some patients have decreased sweating preblock (not including diabetic patients).

Ideally an area is also needed whereby the patient may bathe after treatment because a profuse sweating reaction is desired to ensure that adequate heating of the patient has been achieved before adequate denervation exists.

* Available from any large chemical supplyhouse.

Response	*Filter Paper*
Normal response (profuse sweating)	blue → pink
Slight reduction (moderate sweating)	blue → mottled pink/blue small area
Moderate reduction (slight sweating)	blue → mottled pink/blue large area
Complete reduction (no sweating)	remains blue

Appendix B

Name of Preparation
10% Phenol in Conray-420
Ingredients
100 g Phenol A.R. (crystals)
1L Conray-420
Equipment
1-liter glass measuring cylinder with stopper
1-liter vacuum flask
Scintered glass filter
Tufryn 0.45μ 7-mm (Gelmann HT-450) membrane filter mounted in a millipore swinnex 47-mm holder
Sterile disposable 50-ml syringe
Connector tube (about 9-in) for outlet of filter
Identity number
All washed with pryogen-free water for injections filtered through a 0.2μ filter, and then dried in hot air oven, with all exposed outlets covered with aluminium foil.
Method of manufacture
Weigh phenol into 1-liter measuring cylinder
Remove outer seals of Conray-420 bottles, leaving stoppers in place
Rinse exterior of these bottles with filtered water for injections
Place bottles in laminar flow cabinet after rinsing, and allow to dry in air stream
Remove stoppers with rinsed forceps
Pour Conray-420 into graduated cylinder containing phenol
Shake to dissolve phenol; make to volume and mix
Container/closure description
Container, 20-ml antibiotic vial
Stopper, red merco lacquered to suit
Crimp cap, gold aluminium long skirt to suit
Packing—equipment and method
Laminar flow cabinet
Filter through scintered glass into 1-liter vacuum flask
Pour into pyrex dish and load 50-ml syringe

Filter from syringe through 47-mm Tufryn filter with connector tube attached to outlet of filter holder and leading to vials

Pack 20-ml per vial; insert stoppers and seal

Example label

Injection Solution: PHENOL 10% IN CONRAY 420

20 ml PROTECT FROM LIGHT

Prepared by:

Flinders Medical Centre Pharmacy, Bedford Park,

South Australia, 5042., Australia.

Batch:

Expiry: (6 months from manufacture)

REFERENCES

1. Beene, T.K., and Eggers, G.W.N., Jr.: Use of the pulse monitor for determining sympathetic block of the arm. Anesthesiology, *40*:412, 1974.
2. Bergan, J. J., and Conn, J., Jr.: Sympathectomy for pain relief. Med. Clin. North Am., *52*:147, 1968.
3. Blain, A., Zadeh, A.T., Teves, M.L., and Bing, R.J.: Lumbar sympathectomy for arteriosclerosis obliterans. Surgery, *53*:164, 1963.
4. Boas, R.A., Hatangdi, V.S., and Richards, E.G.: Lumbar sympathectomy—A percutaneous chemical technique. Advances in Pain Research and Therapy, *1*:685, 1976.
5. Bonica, J.J.: The Management of Pain. Philadelphia, Lea & Febiger, 1953.
6. ———: Clinical Application of Diagnostic and Therapeutic Nerve Blocks. Oxford, Blackwell Scientific Publications, 1958.
7. Boucher, J.R., Falardeau, M., Plante, R., Audet, J., and Jannard, A.: Le reflexe sympatho-galvanique (*RSG*) et la sympathectomie. Can. Anaesth. Soc. J., *17*:504, 1970.
8. Bridenbaugh, P.O., Moore, D.C., and Bridenbaugh, L.D.: Capillary P_{O_2} as a measure of sympathetic blockade. Anesth. Analg. (Cleve.), *50*:26, 1971.
9. Bryce-Smith, R.: Injection of the lumbar sympathetic chain. Anaesthesia, *6*:150, 1951.
10. Bryce-Smith, R., and Macintosh, R.R.: Local Analgesia: Abdomen. Edinburgh, Livingstone Press, 1962.
11. Carron, H., and Litwiller, R.: Stellate ganglion block. Anesth. Analg. (Cleve.), *54*:567, 1975.
12. Colding, A.: Treatment of pain. Organization of a pain clinic: Treatment of acute herpes zoster. Proc. R. Soc. Med., *66*:541, 1973.
13. Cousins, M.J., Reeve, T.S., Glynn, C.J., Walsh, J.A., and Cherry, D.A.: Neurolytic lumbar sympathetic blockade: Duration of denervation and relief of rest pain. Anaesthesia and Intensive Care, Vol. 7, No. 2, 121–135; May, 1979.
14. Cousins, M.J., and Wright, C.J.: Graft muscle skin blood flow after epidural block in vascular surgical procedures. Surg. Gynecol. Obstet., *133*:59, 1971.
15. Cronestrand, R., Juhlin-Dannfeldt, A., and Wahren, J.: Simultaneous measurements of external iliac artery and vein blood flow after reconstructive vascular surgery: Evidence of increased collateral circulation during exercise. Scand. J. Clin. Lab. Invest., *31*[*Suppl. 128*]:167, 1973.
16. Dam, W.H.: Therapeutic blockade. Acta Chir. Scand., *343*[*Suppl.*]:89, 1965.
17. De Bakey, M.E., Burch, G., Ray, T., and Ochsner, A.: The "borrowing-lending" hemodynamic phenomenon (hemometakinesia) and its therapeutic application in peripheral vascular disturbances. Ann. Surg., *126*:850, 1947.
18. Detakats, G.: Sympathetic reflex dystrophy. Med. Clin. North Am., *49*:117, 1965.
19. Dhunér, K.G., Edshage, S., and Wilhelm, A.: Ninhydrin test—An objective method for testing local anaesthetic drugs. Acta Anaesthesiol. Scand., *4*:189, 1960.
20. Dollery, C.T., Paterson, J.W., and Conally, M.E.: Clinical pharmacology of beta-receptor-blocking drugs. Clin. Pharmacol. Ther., *10*:765, 1969.
21. Eriksson, E.: Illustrated Handbook in Local Anaesthesia. Copenhagen, Munksgaard, 1969.
22. Froysaker, T.: Lumbar sympathectomy in impending gangrene and foot ulcer. Scand. J. Clin. Lab. Invest., *31*[*Suppl. 128*]:71, 1973.
23. Fulton, R.L., and Blakeley, W.R.: Lumbar sympathectomy: A procedure of questionable value in the treatment of arteriosclerosis obliterans of the legs. Am. J. Surg., *116*:735, 1968.
24. Fyfe, T., and Quin, R.O.: Phenol sympathectomy in the treatment of intermittent claudication: A controlled clinical trial. Br. J. Surg., *62*:68, 1975.
25. Gillespie, J.A.: Future place of lumbar sympathectomy in obliterative vascular disease of lower limbs. Br. Med. J., *2*:1640, 1960.
26. ———: Late effects of lumbar sympathectomy on blood flow in the foot in obliterative vascular disease. Lancet, *1*:891, 1960.
27. ———: An evaluation of vasodilator drugs in occlusive vascular disease by measurement. Angiology, *17*:280, 1966.
28. Haimovici, H., Steinman, C., and Karson, J.H.: Evaluation of lumbar sympathectomy in advanced occlusive arterial disease. Arch. Surg., *89*:1089, 1964.
29. Hannington-Kiff, J.G.: Pain Relief, p. 68. London, Heinemann Press, 1974.
30. Herman, B.E., Dworecka, F., and Wisham, L.: Increase of dermal blood flow after sympathectomy as measured by radioactive sodium uptake. Vasc. Surg., *4*:161, 1970.
31. Hoffman, D.C., and Jepson, R.P.: Muscle blood flow and sympathectomy. Surg. Gynecol. Obstet., *127*:12, 1968.
32. Hughes-Davies, D.J., and Redman, L.R.: Chemical lumbar sympathectomy. Anaesthesia, *31*:1068, 1976.
33. Johansson, H.: Chemical sympathectomy with phenol for chronic prostatic pain. A case report. European Urology, *2*:98, 1976.
34. Kappis, M.: Sensibilitat und lokale Anasthesie im chirurginchen Gebiet der Bauchhohle mit besonderer Berucksichtigung der Splanchnicus-Anasthesie. Beitr. Z. Klin. Chir., *115*:161, 1919.
35. Kim, J.M., Arakawa, K., and von Linter, T.: Use of the pulse-wave monitor as a measurement of diagnostic sympathetic block and of surgical sympathectomy. Anesth. Analg. (Cleve.), *54*:289, 1975.
36. King, R.D., Kaiser, G.C., Lempke, R.E., and Shumacker, H.B.: Evaluation of lumbar sympathetic denervation. Arch. Surg., *88*:36, 1964.
37. Kövamees, A.: Skin blood flow in obliterative arterial disease of the leg. Effect of vascular reconstruction examined with xenon and iodine antipyrine clearance and skin temperature measurements. Acta Chir. Scand. [*Suppl. 397*], 1968.
38. Kövamees, A., and Löfström, B.: Continuous lumbar sympathetic blocks in the treatment of patients with ischemic lower limbs. Tenth Congress of Int. Cardiovascular Soc., 1971.

39. Kövamees, A., Löfström, B., McCarthy, G., and Aschberg, S.: Continuous lumbar sympathetic blocks used to increase regional blood flow after peripheral vascular reconstruction. Eighteenth Congress Eur. Soc. Cardiovascular Surg., 1974.
40. Langer, J., and Matthes, H.: Blockaden mit Lokalanasthetika im Bereich der Sympathikuskette. Z. Prakt. Anaesth. Wiederbeleb., *8*:93, 1973.
41. Larsen, O.A., and Lassen, N.A.: Medical treatment of occlusive arterial disease of the legs. Walking exercise and medically induced hypertension. Angiologia, *6*:288, 1969.
42. Lassen, N.A., *et al.*: Conservative treatment of gangrene using mineralocorticoid-induced moderate hypertension. Lancet, *1*:606, 1968.
43. Leriche, R., and Fontain, R.: L'Anesthesie isolee du ganglion etoile: Sa technique, ses indications ses resultatas. Presse Medicale, *42*:849, 1934.
44. Lewis, L.W.: Evaluation of sympathetic activity following chemical or surgical sympathectomy. Anesth. Analg. (Cleve.), *34*:334, 1955.
45. Linde, B.: Studies on the vascular exchange function in canine subcutaneous adipose tissue with special reference to effects of sympathetic nerve stimulation. Acta Physiol. Scand., *433*[*Suppl.*] 1976.
46. Lloyd, J.W., and Carrie, L.E.S.: A method for treating renal colic. Proc. R. Soc. Med., *58*:634, 1965.
47. Löfström, B., and Zetterquist, S.: The effect of lumbar sympathetic block upon nutritive blood-flow capacity in intermittent claudication. A metabolic study. Acta Med. Scand., *182*:23, 1967.
48. ______: Lumbar sympathetic blocks in the treatment of patients with obliterative arterial disease of the lower limb. Int. Anesthesiol. Clin., *7*:423, 1969.
49. Mandl, F.: Die Paravertebrale Injektion. Vienna, Springer-Verlag, 1926.
50. Masud, K.Z., and Forster, K.J.: Sympathetic block in herpes zoster. Am. Fam. Physician, *12*:142, 1975.
51. Moore, D.C.: Stellate Ganglion Block. Springfield, Charles C Thomas, 1954.
52. Myers, K.A., and Irvine, W.T.: An objective study of lumbar sympathectomy. II. Skin ischaemia. Br. Med. J., *1*:943, 1966.
53. ______: An objective study of lumbar sympathectomy. I. Intermittent claudication. Br. Med. J., *1*:943, 1966.
54. Nielsen, J.: Thrombangiitis obliterans (Buerger's disease). A study of the prognosis. Ugeskr. Laeger., *131*:1740, 1969.
55. Nielsen, P.E., Bell, G., Augustenborg, G., and Lassen, N.A.: Reduction in distal blood pressure by sympathetic nerve block in patients with occlusive arterial disease. Scand. J. Clin. Lab. Invest., *31*[*Suppl. 128*]:59, 1973.
56. Nielsen, P.E., Bell, G., Augustenborg, G., Paaske–Hansen, O., and Lassen, N.A.: Reduction in distal blood pressure by sympathetic block in patients with occlusive arterial disease. Cardiovasc. Res., *7*:577, 1973.
57. Nolte, H., Ahnefeld, F.W., and Halmagyi, M.: Die lumbale Grenzstrangblockad zur Beurteilung der Wirkungsdauer von Lokalanaesthetika. Acta Anaesthesiol. Scand., *23*[*Suppl.*]:618, 1966.
58. Procacci, P., Francini, F., Zoppi, M., and Maresca, M.: Cutaneous pain threshold changes after sympathetic block in reflex dystrophies. Pain, *1*:167, 1975.
59. Raskin, N.H.: Levinson, S.A., Hoffman, P.M., Pickett, J.B.E., III, and Fields, H.L.: Postsympathectomy neuralgia. Amelioration with diphenylhydantoin and carbamazepine. Am. J. Surg., *128*:75, 1974.
60. Reid, W., Watt, J.K., and Gray, T.G.: Phenol injection of the sympathetic chain. Br. J. Surg., *57*:45, 1970.
61. Scheinin, T.M., and Inberg, M.V.: Intraoperative effects of sympathectomy on ipsi- and contralateral blood flow in lower limb arterial reconstruction. Ann. Clin. Res., *1*:280, 1969.
62. Sternschein, M.J., Myers, S.J., Frewin, D.B., and Downey, J.A.: Causalgia. Arch. Phys. Med. Rehabil., *56*:58, 1975.
63. Strand, L.: Lumbar sympathectomy in the treatment of peripheral obliterative disease. An analysis of 167 patients. Acta Chir. Scand., *135*:597, 1969.
64. Szilagyi, D.E., Smith, R.F., Scerpella, J.R., and Hoffman, K.: Lumbar sympathectomy. Current role in the treatment of arteriosclerotic occlusive disease. Arch. Surg., *95*:953, 1967.
65. Taylor, G.W., and Calo, A.R.: Atherosclerosis of arteries of lower limbs. Br. Med. J., *1*:507, 1962.
66. Thulesius, O.: Beurteilung des schwergrades arterieller Durchblutungsstorungen mit dem Doppler-Ultraschallgerat. Angiologie, *13*. Hans Huber, Bern, 1971.
67. Thulesius, O., and Gjöres, J.E.: Use of Doppler shift detection for determining peripheral arterial blood pressure. Angiology, *22*:594, 1971.
68. Thulesius, O., Gjöres, J.E., and Mandaus, L.: Distal blood flow and blood pressure in vascular occlusion: Influence of sympathetic nerves on collateral blood flow. Scand. J. Clin. Lab. Invest., *31*[*Suppl. 128*]:53, 1973.
69. Uhrenholdt, A.: Relationship between distal blood flow and blood pressure after abolition of the sympathetic vasomotor tone. Scand. J. Clin. Lab. Invest., *31*[*Suppl. 128*]:63, 1973.
70. Uhrenholdt, A., Dam, W.H., Larsen, O.A., and Lassen, N.A.: Paradoxical effect on peripheral blood flow after sympathetic blockades in patients with gangrene due to arteriosclerosis obliterans. Vasc. Surg., *5*:154, 1971.
71. Verstraete, M.: A critical appraisal of lumbar sympathectomy in the treatment of organic arteriopathy. Angiologia, *5*:333, 1968.
72. Weale, F.E.: The hemodynamic assessment of the arterial tree during reconstructive surgery. Ann. Surg., *169*:484, 1969.
73. Wright, C.J., and Cousins, M.J.: Blood flow distribution in the human leg following epidural sympathetic blockade. Arch. Surg., *105*:334, 1972.
74. Yao, J.S.T., and Bergan, J.J.: Predicting response to sympathetic ablation [quoted in editorial]. Lancet, *1*:441, 1974.
75. Zetterquist, S.: Muscle and skin clearance of antipyrine from exercising ischemic legs before and after vasodilating trials. Acta Med. Scand., *183*:487, 1968.

PART TWO

Techniques of Neural Blockade

Section C: Thorax and Abdomen: Peripheral and Autonomic Blockade

14 Celiac Plexus, Intercostal, and Minor Peripheral Blockade

Gale E. Thompson

In 1953, Sir Robert Macintosh introduced his book *Local Analgesia: Abdominal Surgery* with the following paragraph: "A local analgesic can provide ideal operating conditions when used alone; a fortiori it will afford ideal conditions if a general anesthetic is given at the same time. Local analgesia, alone or combined with light general anesthesia, is therefore theoretically justified in every abdominal operation." [17] Now, nearly 3 decades later, there is even better justification for the use of regional analgesia in nearly every abdominal or thoracic operation. It is hoped that it will soon become common practice—not merely a good recommendation. There are several reasons for the tendency to pay "lip service" to regional anesthesia and then fail to use it. First, there is prevalent among many anesthesiologists, surgeons, and patients an element of bias and emotion that has some of its origin in fact but is perpetuated by fallacy. This leads to a halting and lame conceptual approach to regional anesthesia. Second, there are very few training environments in which to develop expertise in performing nerve blocks. Regional anesthesia is not just a medical curiosity, and it is not to be practiced only infrequently and then on the high-risk patient. To be performed well, it must be used routinely. Thus, each time a surgical anesthetic is being selected, the anesthesiologist should consider what kind of regional anesthetic technique would be adaptable to this case. Last, there has been a trend to think of survival following an anesthetic or surgical procedure as the only important end point. Indeed, the issue is of basic importance, but there are a variety of routes to any goal. The patient may perceive only that he went to sleep and later awakened. However, this time asleep can be rendered immeasurably less stressful if the value and physiologic soundness of peripheral (or central) nerve blocks are realized.

There are certain basic factors that are pertinent to the successful use of the regional nerve blocks described in this chapter. These are the following: a personal conviction on the part of the anesthesiologist that he would prefer this kind of anesthesia for himself (*i.e.*, that it is indeed the safest and best anesthetic available for a given surgical procedure); a thorough knowledge of anatomy; a thorough knowledge of the pharmacology and physiology of local anesthetic drugs; adequate training in the use of regional anesthesia; frequent practice in regional anesthetic techniques; a philosophy of using supplemental drugs at appropriate times and in adequate amounts; a perceptive awareness of the possible side effects and complications of regional anesthesia (side effects are not complications); and finally an enlightened patient who has been counseled on the benefits and nature of regional anesthesia.

RATIONALE

There are some fundamental arguments that support the use of peripheral nerve block in surgery of the abdomen and chest. First, it is a basis for the ideal form of "balanced anesthesia." Second, it provides an attractive method of protecting against the stress of surgery, and third, it provides excellent analgesia during the postanesthetic recovery period.

Balanced Anesthesia

Balanced anesthesia has many connotations. In essence, it implies accomplishing the various anesthetic requirements by using a number of different drugs in relatively small amounts. The term was introduced by Lundy in 1926, although elements of the concept were emphasized as early as 1915 by Crile.[16] The general tendency today is to consider only inhaled or intravenous drugs in balanced anesthesia. It is certainly just as reasonable (albeit uncommon) to consider regional anesthesia as one of the components of balanced anesthesia. Peripheral nerve block of the abdomen and chest may be deemed the basis for the development of a more complete anesthetic. The addition of appropriate and complementary doses of either inhaled or intravenous drugs would be dictated by the nature and duration of the surgical procedure, the patient's safety and desires, and the operating room environment (*e.g.*, noise, temperature, teaching, conversations). With few exceptions, it is possible to achieve most of the analgesic and muscle-relaxant objectives by using standard dosages of local anesthetic drugs. The risks are minimal and the benefits are maximal compared to other groups of drugs used in anesthesia.

Many anesthesiologists immediately react negatively to the concept of combining regional nerve block with light general anesthesia. "Why give two anesthetics when one will do?" "It takes too much time," "It's not worth it." These are frequently heard criticisms. Surprisingly, though, the same comments are not expressed about the potpourri of drugs used to accomplish general anesthesia. Often, these expressions merely reflect a lack of expertise or inclination to use regional anesthesia. The best way to solve the problem of lack of expertise is by putting a much greater emphasis on regional anesthetic techniques during specialty training. However, there are additional factors currently tending to promote greater use of regional anesthesia. For instance, there is an increasing focus on the potential dangers of general anesthetic drugs. Ecologic hazards, renal and hepatic problems, induced enzyme changes, and the possibilities of increased malignancies have already been acknowledged.[4,29] Until the fabled "ideal" or complete anesthetic agent is found, a variety of drugs will continue to be used to produce anesthesia. In practical terms, the local anesthetic drugs ought to play a primary role in providing genuinely balanced anesthesia for many patients.

Protection from Surgical Stress

A third rationale for using peripheral nerve blocks comes from an area of medicine still poorly documented. Much of the basic reasoning can be found in Crile's theory of anociassociation. Unfortunately, specific definition of many aspects of this phenomenon is not possible, owing to the inability to define or measure stress accurately. Crile's book, published in 1915, contains many ideas which were based upon rudimentary knowledge.[6] Although much more is now known about humoral influences, nerve transmission, drug action, and cellular response, there are still some glaring deficiencies in the understanding of shock and stress. Since stress cannot be quantitated, we tend to form clinical impressions of the degree of physiologic insult to patients during surgery. Many patients appear "washed out" or "beaten down" by the experience. This may be due to the anesthetic, the surgical technique, or other factors. There are many noxious impulses against which the patient must consciously or unconsciously defend. Whatever the stimulus and the response, it is important to consider possible ways of reducing the insult.

An important feature of the theory of anociassociation is that blocking nerve pathways between the site of surgical stimulation and the spinal cord would protect the central nervous system (CNS) from bombardment by noxious impulses. General anesthesia allows such impulses to penetrate the CNS but obtunds the body's ability to respond. Nonetheless, intense central neuronal activity occurs. Indirect evidence that regional anesthesia prevents significant noxious impulses from reaching the spinal cord or brain is provided by the pronounced changes in hydroxycorticosteroid secretion and blood glucose, which are modified or lacking with regional anesthesia.[1,18,21,22] As a result of this reduced stress during the recovery period the patient appears less fatigued and therefore better suited to deal with other postoperative stresses. Many anesthesiologists favor regional anesthesia for surgery performed on themselves, no doubt because of clinical experience.[14] It is likely that the concepts of protection from stress play a significant if unwitting role in shaping such opinions.

Analgesia in the Postanesthetic Recovery Period

The recovery rooms of various hospitals can suggest the different approaches to anesthesia. Some recovery rooms are filled with patients who are relatively quiet and seemingly comfortable. Others are filled with patients who are moaning and in anguish. The patients who experience pain are usually treated with parenteral narcotics. This process is medically acceptable but necessitates judgment about what dosage of narcotic will be adequate to provide analgesia. Too much narcotic may essentially reanesthetize the patient and may lead to ventilatory depression, airway obstruction, hypoxia, and loss of consciousness. Too little narcotic will not resolve the patient's complaints. The balance between adequate pain relief and oversedation is especially critical immediately after the operation and is of particular significance in the elderly patient with cardiovascular and respiratory disease.

The capacity of narcotics to compound the action

Table 14-1. Anatomic Sites at Which Peripheral Nerve Block May Be Performed to Produce Sensory Anesthesia of Abdomen and Thorax

Component Portion of Nervous System	*Specific Nerves*	*Possible Site of Block*
Parasympathetic	Vagus	Neck, esophageal hiatus, celiac plexus
	S2,3,4	Pudendal, transsacral
Sympathetic	Thoracolumbar Sympathetic chain	Stellate ganglion Paravertebral sympathetic chain, celiac plexus
Somatic	T1–12 intercostal	Posterior angle of rib
	Lumbar somatic	Paravertebral

of residual inhaled or intravenous anesthetic drugs is progressively lessened after surgery. However, during any portion of the postsurgical period, the ideal means of providing pain relief may not be narcotics but rather peripheral nerve blocks. There are no better candidates for this therapy than patients who have had surgical procedures on the abdomen or thorax. Whereas the risks and dangers of narcotics are potentially troublesome, the deep breathing, good cough, and mental alertness, which are possible with peripheral nerve blocks, can be most beneficial.

It is just as important to achieve freedom from pain in the postoperative period as it is to control pain during surgery. Patients have many fears about their operations, but they also dread the thought of pain following surgery. They can be reassured to an amazing degree if the anesthesiologist would visit before surgery, to offer them a basic regional anesthetic technique whereby immediately after surgery they will be able to regain consciousness but remain relatively pain-free. Although effects of the nerve block will eventually wear off, a dangerous period can be bypassed before either narcotic sedation or additional nerve blocks are indicated. With presently available local anesthetic drugs, only 10 to 12 hours of analgesia can be achieved. It is hoped that drugs will be developed with durations of action of 24 to 48 hours and with the characteristic of preferentially blocking only sensory nerves. The slight pain and time involved in performing repeated blocks in the postoperative period would be more than offset by the benefits and duration of pain relief. This offers not only the benefit of greater duration than that of narcotics but also avoids the problems of hypotension, immobility, tachyphylaxis, fear of subarachnoid injection, and urinary retention encountered with repeated epidural injections by catheter.[25] With presently available drugs, intercostal blocks have been repeated as many as 14 times in the postoperative period. Despite the discomforts of turning to the lateral position and the multiple needle-sticks involved in this procedure, patients consistently prefer repeated blocks rather than sedation with narcotics. There is no doubt that analgesia is more profound and pain therapy more specific with intercostal blocks than with narcotics. Pao_2 values are slightly better in patients treated with repeated blocks, and the ability to cough and move about is especially impressive. The total hospital stay has been shortened in patients who received blocks as compared to those who were treated with narcotics for pain relief.[2]

PAIN PATHWAYS

Noxious stimuli from the thoracic and abdominal cavities are transmitted by nerve impulses carried along afferent fibers of the somatic, sympathetic, and parasympathetic divisions of the nervous system. The afferent somatic and sympathetic pain fibers converge on cells of secondary afferent neurons in the posterior horn of the spinal cord. After synapsing, they ascend in the spinothalamic tracts. Afferent vagal impulses from the abdominal viscera pass through the celiac plexus and by way of the vagus nerve to the medulla. Complete sensory anesthesia of thoracic and abdominal contents can be achieved only by blocking all afferent impulses from each of these three divisions of the nervous system. This is a formidable task to achieve with regional anesthesia alone. Table 14-1 lists some of the anatomic sites at which peripheral nerve block might be attempted for deafferentation of the thorax and abdomen.

It is technically easier to block somatic nerve fibers, which are anatomically precise, as compared to the autonomic pain fibers which are diffuse, often ill-defined, and more difficult to isolate. It is also important to appreciate that there may be significant side-effects from blocking autonomic nerves. When the balance between sympathetic and parasympathetic tone is upset, the ensuing functional changes in heart, lung, and gut may be quite disturbing. Therefore, bilateral vagus nerve block or major sympathetic nerve blocks are better avoided or at least undertaken with caution.[23] For abdominal surgery, intercostal nerve block may be combined with blockade of the visceral pain pathways at the level of the celiac plexus. Although celiac plexus blockade of sympathetic fibers may result in pooling of blood in the mesenteric vessels, it avoids interference with cardiac and pulmonary autonomic fibers.

There is little doubt that pain from the abdominal viscera can be perceived through the sympathetic, vagus, and sacral nerve fibers. Physiologists and anatomists have difficulty in precisely locating or describing such fibers, but the clinical response of many patients demonstrates their existence. For instance, patients may respond to surgical manipulation of abdominal viscera even though they have spinal anesthesia to upper thoracic levels. Similarly, female patients may respond to uterine manipulation while under an epidural anesthetic that is perfectly adequate for skin incision and abdominal wall relaxation. Vagal afferent nerves must convey many of these impulses to brain stem levels and thence to the cerebral cortex. Although pain defies description, there appear to be some differences in pain perceived by the autonomic nervous system[13] from the perception by the somatic nervous system. The following list provides a way to characterize these differences.

Differences in Pain Experienced by the Somatic and Autonomic Divisions of the Nervous System

Somatic
- Precisely localized
- Sharp and definite
- Hurts where the stimulus is
- Associated with external factors
- Represented at cortical levels
- Increases with increasing intensity of stimulus (*e.g.*, cut or burned skin will produce pain)

Autonomic
- Poorly localized
- Vague (may be colicky, cramping, aching, squeezing, etc.)
- May be referred to another part of the body
- Associated with internal factors
- Primarily reflex or cord levels
- Intensity of stimulus important but quality of stimulus also important (*e.g.*, cut or burned bowel will produce no pain—distended bowel produces pain)

No matter what kind of pain a patient perceives or what neural pathway is involved, the anesthesiologist must respond to a patient's surgical pain on a moment-to-moment basis. It is often difficult to identify precisely which nerve or nerves are transmitting noxious impulses to the patient's level of perception. Regional anesthetic techniques may leave certain pain pathways open, either by design or by default. Only by close observation and anticipation of difficulties can the basic regional anesthetic be properly complemented with some form of supplementary drug.

PREMEDICATION AND SUPPLEMENTATION

The anesthesiologist who routinely advocates regional anesthesia will tend to use heavy premedication. He realizes the importance of having a relaxed, analgesic, and amnesic patient during the performance of the nerve block. Likewise, he realizes that most patients desire to sleep during the course of operation. Sights, sounds, and conversations in the surgical suite that escape the attention of medical personnel may leave vivid impressions in the mind of a wide-eyed alert patient. There is a definite need to create an operating room environment where teaching and other professional conversation can take place without unduly alarming patients.

All of the peripheral nerve block procedures for thoracic and abdominal analgesia utilize bony or vascular anatomic landmarks and, hence, require no patient participation for proper execution of the block. In contrast, performance of these blocks may elicit significant skin and periosteal stimulation, necessitating sedation during administration of the block. This is not to say that these nerve blocks cannot be performed without sedation. In fact, that may be mandatory when their purpose is diagnostic, when these blocks are performed on seriously ill surgical patients, or for postoperative analgesia. However, for routine surgery, the nerve blocks described in this chapter are best performed on patients who will not be able to recall the event. It is a challenge to achieve the proper degree of sedation for execution of the block while maintaining the patient in a stable condition.

For premedication, surgical patients may be given a combination of narcotic and anticholinergic drug 1 hour prior to performance of the nerve block. In healthy patients below age 60, this consists of 10 to 15 mg of morphine sulfate and 0.4 to 0.6 mg of scopolamine hydrobromide. Scopolamine is generally omitted in patients over 60 and the morphine dosage appropriately decreased. Atropine may be substituted for scopolamine in a patient of any age or added intravenously should vagal reflexes be evidenced during surgery. The state of calmly detached consciousness produced by scopolamine is an ideal complement to regional anesthesia. The occasional disturbing central side-effects of this drug can readily be controlled with physostigmine.[10]

Following the patient's arrival in the operating suite, an intravenous line should be established. This supplies fluid and caloric requirements but, in addition, serves as a means of titrating supplementary sedative drugs. These may be indicated to accentuate premedication effects, to briefly produce loss of awareness during completion of the nerve block, or to produce sleep during the operation. Some drugs commonly used for these purposes are diazepam, fentanyl, droperidol, and the barbiturates. The clinical situation dictates which one or ones should be used, depending upon the need for hypnosis, analgesia, tranquilization, or some combination of effects. A wide variety of other drugs may be used, but it is important to titrate them in small intravenous doses while observing closely for the desired action.

The drugs and techniques used to produce loss of consciousness during completion of intercostal and celiac plexus nerve block deserve special comment. Ideally, these blocks should be performed in an induction or other room that is separate from the noise and confusion of the operating room and equipped with appropriate monitors and resuscitation material. Ordinarily, they are performed during a brief period for which the patient is rendered unaware. Upon completion of the nerve block, the patient will usually quickly regain awareness, which permits questioning and testing of the block while initiating additional monitoring equipment. A most satisfactory drug for patient sedation during this block is methohexitone. When it is prepared in 0.2-per-cent solution and administered intravenously, it affords a convenient means of titrating sedation to an appropriate level. The effects are rapidly reversible. It is helpful to have an assistant administer the drip and observe the patient's vital signs during performance of block. Ketamine, diazepam, althesin, droperidol, and fentanyl have also been used for the same purpose.[27] Intravenous diazepam is doubly effective: first, as a sedative and amnesia-producing agent and, second, as a prophylactic against toxic effects of local anesthetic drugs. Large dosages of local anesthetic drugs are used for the blocks described in this chapter. de Jong has shown that the threshold for toxic effects of local anesthetic drugs can be raised by pretreatment with diazepam. In cats pretreated with 0.25 mg per kg of intramuscular diazepam, the mean convulsant dose of intravenous lidocaine was raised from 8.4 mg per kg to 16.8 mg per kg.[8] In later work, he also demonstrated a protective effect of nitrous oxide on the lidocaine seizure threshold. Seventy per cent nitrous oxide raised the threshold from 7.6 mg per kg to 11.4 mg per kg intravenous lidocaine.[9]

Inhalation agents must be used intraoperatively to supplement regional anesthesia used for thoracic and intra-abdominal surgery. In the great majority of patients, a combination of nitrous oxide and oxygen will ensure toleration of the endotracheal tube, adequate ventilation, oxygenation, and loss of consciousness. The anesthesiologist should not be chagrined at having at times to administer low, supplementary concentrations of more potent inhalation agents or neuromuscular blocking drugs. This is rarely necessary and should not detract from the advantages to the patient of the nerve block and still avoids the need for large doses of relaxants or high concentrations of the inhalation agents and their subsequent reversal. Thus, regional nerve block must be considered a component of balanced anesthesia with the required supplementation varying on a case basis.

LOCAL ANESTHETIC DRUGS

There are many ways to classify local anesthetic drugs. For instance, they may be viewed from a perspective of history, chemical structure, metabolism, dosage, or duration of action. The last is of utmost importance for the nerve blocks discussed in this chapter. The lack of effective long-acting local anesthetic drugs has been a major deterrent to the usefulness and application of many of the more important peripheral regional anesthetic techniques. A local anesthetic agent with a predictable duration of action of 48 to 72 hours would be especially desirable. However, there are problems in developing such drugs, primarily neurotoxicity. Another feature of the long-acting local anesthetic drugs is the widespread variation of duration of block, and the problems of tachyphylaxis must also be evaluated.[3] However, once such difficulties are overcome, anesthesia, which includes the postoperative as well as the intraoperative period, can be seriously considered.

At present, there are short- (*e.g.,* procaine), intermediate- (*e.g.,* lidocaine), and long- (*e.g.,* bupivacaine) acting local anesthetic drugs. When ultra-long-acting drugs come into widespread use, the clinical role of the nerve blocks described here will be greatly enhanced.

Prior to beginning any regional anesthetic, the anesthesiologist must consider a variety of issues. The

Table 14-2. Some Possible Drug Combinations for Peripheral Nerve Blocks of Abdomen and Thorax

Drug	*Duration (hrs)*	*Volume (ml)*	*Concentration (%)*	*Amount of Epinephrine to Be Added (mg)*
Bupivacaine	9–11	60	0.5	0.25–0.3
Bupivacaine	8–10	60–100	0.25	0.25–0.4
		(will allow celiac block as well)		
Etidocaine	8–10	60–80	0.5	0.25–0.3
Tetracaine	6–8	60–100	0.2	0.25–0.3
Mepivacaine	3–4	60	1	0.25–0.3

aim or purpose of the block must be determined by asking questions such as the following: "Do I want profound motor block or is sensory anesthesia adequate?" "How many nerves are to be blocked?" "Is the patient going to be further anesthetized following the block or will no supplementary drugs be given?" "Does the patient have major cardiovascular, respiratory, hepatic, or renal disease?" "What is the patient's size, body build, and age?" "Are there any special demands of this surgeon or of the surgical procedure?" Only when these questions have been answered, can the anesthesiologist determine the proper volume, concentration, and dosage of local anesthetic drug to be used. For instance, in preparing a solution of local anesthetic for bilateral intercostal and celiac plexus nerve block, the anesthesiologist must determine the following: total volume of solution needed, effective concentration of drug, total dosage of drug, volume of epinephrine to be added, effective concentration of epinephrine, and total dosage of epinephrine. There are safe or ideal limits for each of these factors. It is obvious that all are related. Volume multiplied by concentration determines total dose. Excesses of volume or concentration may possibly be tolerated by a particular patient, but toxic effects are more likely to occur. On the other hand, small volumes or low concentrations of drug will result in an ineffective regional anesthetic. The block might be inadequate in area, inadequate in duration, or inadequate in extent of motor or sensory fiber blockade. The drug must be tailored to the block, which requires more than just a vague knowledge of local anesthetic drug dosages and effective concentrations.

Choice and Dosage of Drug

The total volume of drug necessary for bilateral intercostal nerve block varies from 40 to 70 ml of solution. This allows for a deposit of 4 to 5 ml of solution under each of the lower ribs. The effective concentration will depend primarily on the drug used and the desired degree of motor nerve blockade. Some commonly used combinations are provided in Table 14-2.

For each of the local anesthetic drugs, there are approved recommendations on maximum total dosage and effective concentrations. The anesthesiologist should select the lowest concentration and dose needed to provide effective anesthesia. Many regional anesthetic techniques (*e.g.*, subarachnoid block) involve drug dosages that do not even begin to approach the maximum recommended dose. However, to perform the nerve blocks considered in this chapter, the anesthesiologist will often need to use the maximum recommended dose, but he needs to be aware of the variables that affect blood levels of local anesthetic agents and CNS toxicity (see Chaps. 3 and 4).

Systemic Absorption

Blood levels of the local anesthetic drug are higher following intercostal nerve block than for any other of the commonly used regional anesthetic procedures. Tucker compared arterial plasma levels following epidural, caudal, intercostal, brachial plexus, and sciatic/femoral nerve block with a single injection of 500 mg of mepivacaine. These blocks were performed with both 1 and 2 per cent mepivacaine, with and without epinephrine. The highest plasma concentrations (5–10 μg of base/ml) were observed following intercostal nerve blocks without epinephrine. When a 1:200,000 concentration of epinephrine was added to the injected solution, plasma levels fell to the range of 2 to 5 μg base per ml. These levels were comparable to those seen with all the other regional anesthetic procedures.[28]

Systemic absorption of epinephrine may have significant effect on both alpha- and beta-receptors and result in tachycardia, hypertension, and arrhythmias. These are infrequent in healthy patients if the total dose of epinephrine does not exceed 0.3 mg. In patients with coronary artery disease and hypertension, the dose should be limited to less than 0.25 mg or avoided completely. The blood levels of bupivacaine and etidocaine are minimally reduced with the addition of epinephrine. If cardiac patients would benefit from intercostal block, consideration should be given to using these drugs (see Chap. 3). Epinephrine may be added to the local anesthetic solution just prior to the time of injection. This ensures optimum *p*H of the final solution. Commercial preparations of local anesthetics that contain epinephrine are strongly acidic, owing to the addition of sodium bisulfite as an antioxidant. Acidity promotes the ionized form of local anesthetic drugs[7] and inhibits passage into the nerve cell membrane where block occurs.

METHODS OF BLOCK

There are specific techniques of performing peripheral nerve blocks to produce anesthesia of the thorax and abdomen. Proper technique begins with a thorough knowledge of anatomic relationships. To this foundation is applied the technical expertise required to do the block. The need to tailor the choice of local anesthetic drug to the contemplated nerve block has previously been emphasized. In a similar manner, the anesthesiologist can use various combinations of peripheral nerve blocks to adapt the anesthetic to the appropriate needs of the patient and surgeon. The most useful combination for upper abdominal surgery is that of intercostal block combined with celiac plexus block. However, it is possible to mix the following blocks together in any manner suited to the anesthetic goal—be it surgical or nonsurgical. The imaginative anesthesiologist will recognize many different situations in which one or more of these blocks might be of value.

INTERCOSTAL NERVE BLOCK

Anatomy

The intercostal nerves are the primary rami of T1 through T11. In the most accurate sense of the word, T12 is not an intercostal nerve, although it will be considered as one here. Since it does not run a course between two ribs, it would be more appropriately termed a *thoracic* or *subcostal* nerve.[11] Some of its fibers unite with other fibers from the first lumbar nerve and are terminally represented as the iliohypogastric and ilioinguinal nerves. Many fibers from T1, at the opposite end of the thoracic group, become united with fibers from C8 to form the lowest trunk of the brachial plexus. These fibers leave the intercostal space by crossing the neck of the first rib, while a smaller bundle continue on a genuine intercostal course. The only other notable variation in intercostal nerves is the contribution of some fibers from T2 and T3 to the formation of the intercostobrachial nerve. Terminal distribution of this nerve is to the skin of the medial aspect of the upper arm.[12]

A typical intercostal nerve has four significant branches. First is the gray rami communicans, which passes anteriorly to the sympathetic ganglion. The second branch arises as the posterior cutaneous branch. This nerve supplies skin and muscles in the paravertebral region. The third branch is the lateral cutaneous division, which arises just anterior to the midaxillary line. This branch is of primary concern to the anesthesiologist because it sends subcutaneous fibers coursing posteriorly and anteriorly to supply skin of much of the chest and abdominal wall. The fourth and terminal branch of an intercostal nerve is the anterior cutaneous branch. In the upper five nerves, this branch terminates after penetrating the external intercostal and pectoralis major muscles to innervate the breast and front of the thorax. The lower six anterior cutaneous nerves terminate after piercing the sheath of the rectus abdominis muscle to which they supply motor branches. Some final branches that continue anteriorly become superficial near the linea alba and provide cutaneous innervation to the midline of the abdomen.

Medial to the posterior angles of the ribs, the intercostal nerves lie between the pleura and the internal intercostal fascia. This fascial layer is also known as the *posterior intercostal membrane*. In the paravertebral region, there is only fatty tissue between nerve and pleura. At the angle of the rib, the nerve comes to lie between the internal intercostal muscle and the intercostalis intimus muscle. The nerve is accompanied by an intercostal vein and artery, which lie superior to the nerve in the inferior groove of each rib. The location of these vessels explains the tendency to high blood levels of local anesthetic agents following intercostal block.

Technique

Intercostal nerve block may be performed at several possible sites along the course of the nerve. The most common site is in the region of the angles of the ribs just lateral to the sacrospinalis group of muscles. For technical ease of performance, the patient is best placed in a prone position. However, when nerve blocks are being performed postoperatively or for diagnostic purposes, a lateral or supine

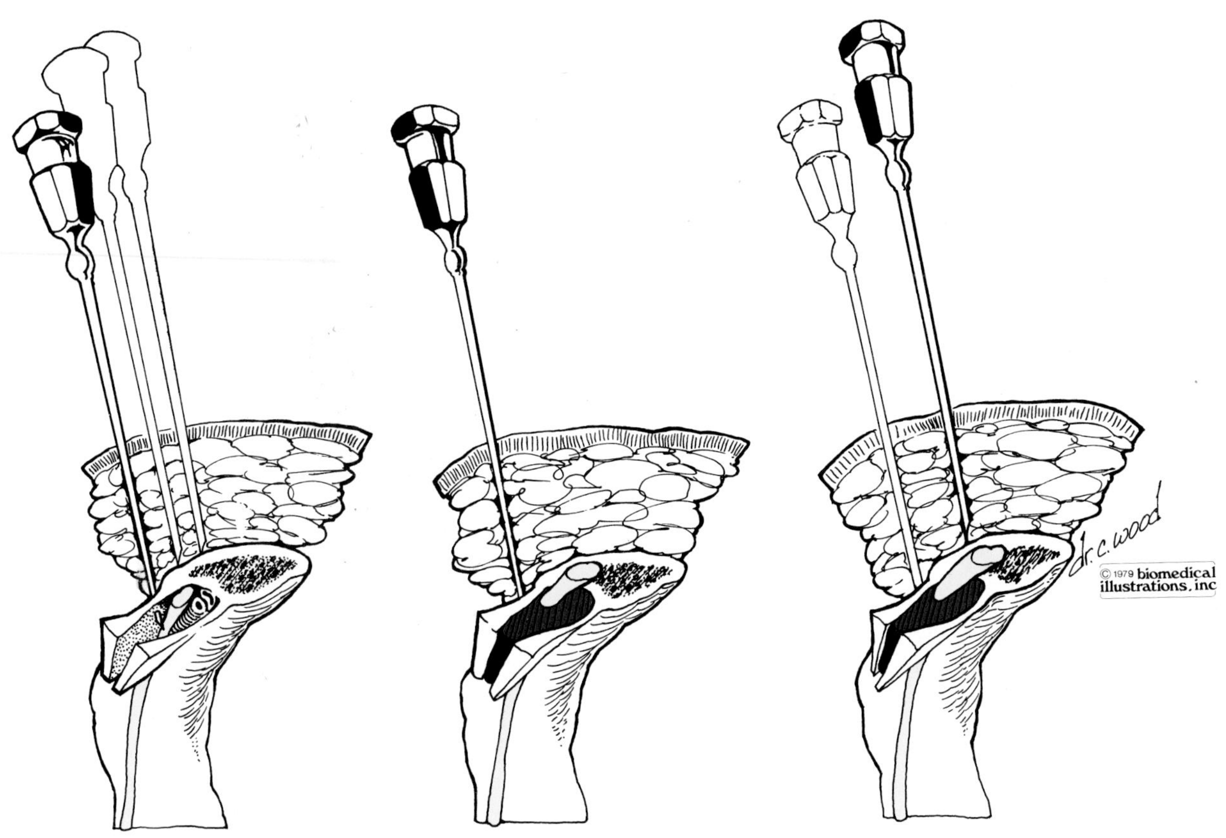

Fig. 14-3. Method of "walking" needle off inferior margin of rib and vertical movement while injecting solution for intercostal nerve block.

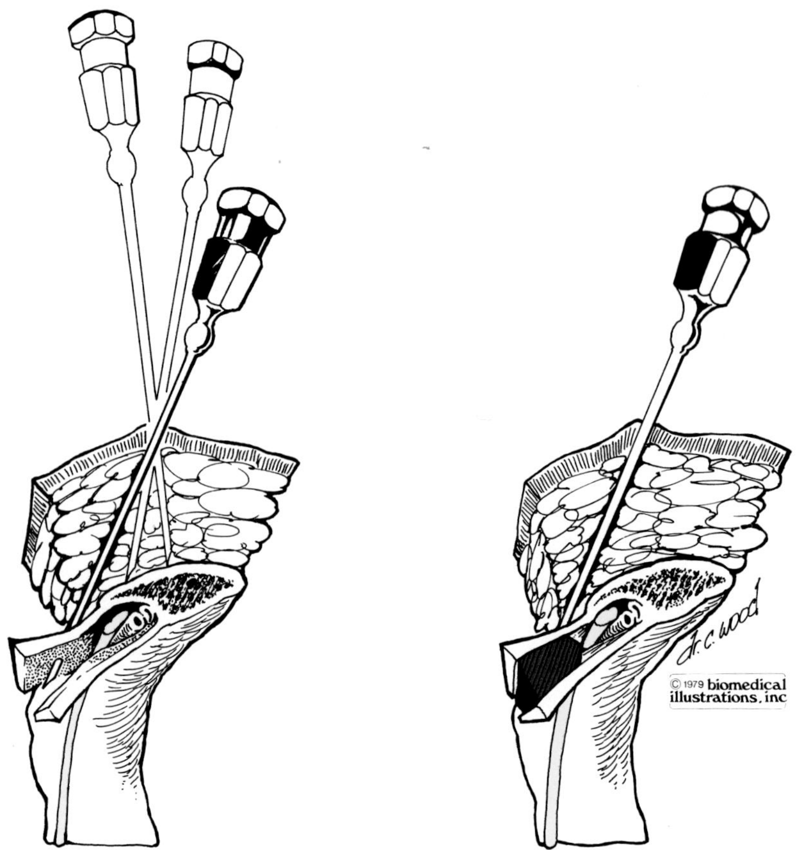

Fig. 14-4. Illustration of the incorrect way to ''walk'' the needle off the rib in intercostal nerve block.

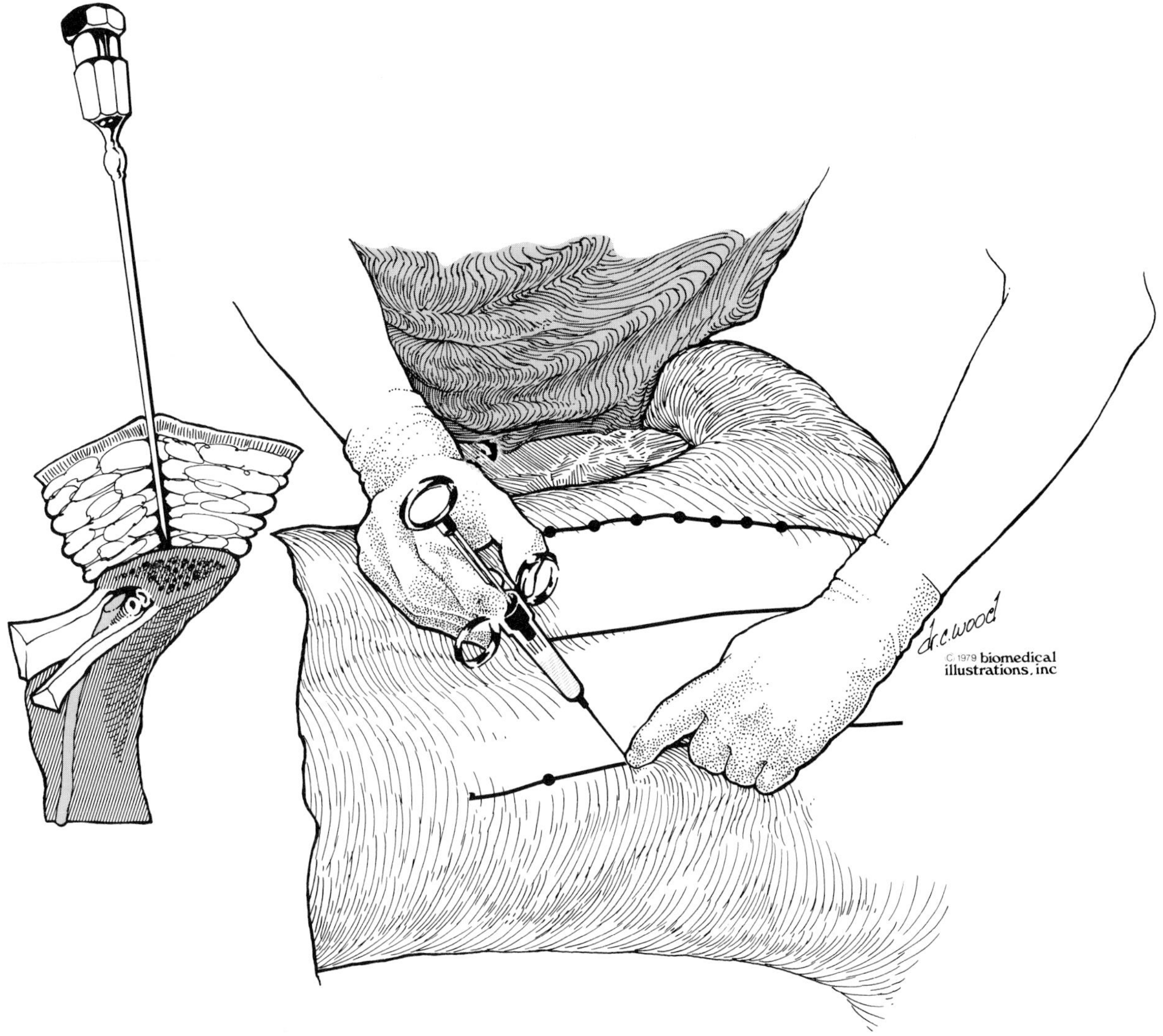

Fig. 14-1. Landmarks for intercostal nerve block. Note that the hand holding the syringe rests on the patient as the index finger of the opposite hand retracts skin wheal over rib surface.

position can be used. The supine position prevents predictable blocking of the lateral cutaneous branch of the nerve. Optimal analgesia and muscle relaxation for surgical procedures is achieved by a posterior block. The prone position facilitates performance of celiac plexus block, which is frequently combined with bilateral intercostal nerve block for abdominal surgery. The premedicated patient is turned to a prone position after establishment of an intravenous infusion. A pillow or roll of some kind is placed under the midabdomen to straighten the lumbar curve and to increase the intercostal spaces posteriorly.

The next step greatly facilitates nerve blocking but is often neglected. This is the process of using skin markings on the patient's back (Fig. 14-1). One of the primary values of skin marking is that it forces the anesthesiologist to pay specific attention to anatomic details. It also serves as a map to illustrate the next space to be blocked and thus speeds performance of the block. First, a vertical line should be drawn along the posterior thoracic vertebral spines. Next, the anesthesiologist should palpate laterally to the edge of the sacrospinalis group of muscles where the ribs are most superficial. This distance is somewhat variable depending on body

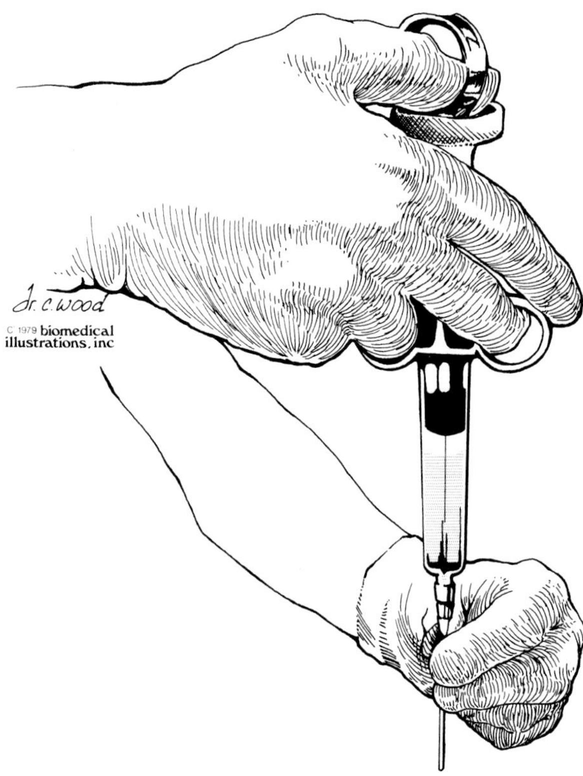

Fig. 14-2. This illustration of intercostal nerve block technique shows the left hand, which rests on the patient, controlling the needle movement as right hand stabilizes the syringe and injects the solution.

size, muscle mass, and physique, but is usually 8 to 10 cm from the midline. Vertical lines are drawn somewhat parallel to the first line, but with a tendency to angle medially at the upper levels as to avoid the scapulae. The anesthesiologist should ensure that the caudal end of the line crosses the end of the shortened 12th rib. Then, by successively palpating the inferior edge of each rib along these lines, the diagram is completed. For abdominal surgery, six or seven ribs on each side are marked. For thoracic or other unilateral chest wall surgery, only the appropriate side and ribs are marked.

Following positioning and marking of the patient, the local anesthetic solution is prepared (Table 14-2). The usual volume injected under each rib is 5 ml. Smaller volumes will decrease the number of successful blocks but afford some protection from high blood levels of absorbed drug if that should be of major concern. Epinephrine should be added to achieve a final concentration of 1:200,000. The final solution is best prepared in a large mixing cup to afford ready access and refilling of the syringe during performance of the block.

Prior to starting the block, intravenous sedation should be given to the level required for patient comfort. At that time, skin wheals are raised at each of the previously marked sites of injection. A 2- to 3-cm, disposable 27- to 30-gauge needle is ideal for raising these wheals. For maximal patient comfort, procaine or lidocaine might be chosen since these drugs, injected subcutaneously, cause less pain than do the long-acting local anesthetics.

A 3- to 4-cm, 22-gauge, reusable security Lok needle attached to a 10-ml Luer-Lok syringe is used to inject each intercostal nerve. Disposable needles are less satisfactory because the tip is easily bent with repeated bony contact and soon becomes a barb, which can increase bleeding or cause nerve damage. Hand and finger position is of utmost importance in performing this nerve block. Beginning at the lowest rib, the index finger of the left hand is used to pull the skin at the lower edge of the rib up and over the rib. The needle is then introduced to the rib as the anesthesiologist holds the syringe in his right hand and with the right hand resting on the patient's back (Fig. 14-1). Should there be difficulty in reaching the rib, the palpating left index finger is used to redefine its depth and position. Obviously, care should be taken not to allow the needle to penetrate beyond this palpated depth because it would enter pleura. While the right hand maintains firm contact between needle and rib, the left hand is shifted to hold the hub and shaft between thumb, index, and middle fingers (Fig. 14-2). Of utmost importance is the firm placement of the left hypothenar eminence against the patient's back. This allows firm control of needle depth as the LEFT hand now "walks" the needle "off" the lower edge of the rib. At this point, it is then advanced about 2 to 3 mm and a slight jiggling motion is begun and controlled by the left hand while with the right hand 5 ml of solution is injected (Fig. 14-3). The jiggling motion decreases the risk of significant intravascular injection and ensures proper spread of solution between the internal intercostal and the intercostalis intimus muscles. This process is repeated for each of the nerves to be blocked. In certain patients with severe barrel chest deformity and neurasthenic habitus, the intercostal injection can best be done with a short 23- or 25-gauge needle. If it is disposable, the needle should be changed after each four to five ribs so it will not develop a barbed point.

Figure 14-4 is included to demonstrate improper

technique for intercostal block. If the needle and syringe are rotated around a point on the skin as the needle is "walked off" the rib, the tip will be considerably displaced from the nerve after it has left the rib. It will also lead to a tendency to deposit the anesthetic solution in a superficial plane since penetration from the rib is being measured in a horizontal rather than a vertical direction. The novice tends to use this rotary motion mechanically in performing his first intercostal blocks. It results from a failure to pull the skin up over the lower edge of each rib before inserting the needle through the skin (see Fig. 14-1). When this technique is performed correctly, the retracted skin will tend to pull the needle off the rib and facilitate accurate placement of the local anesthetic agent.

Surgical Applications

Relatively few surgical procedures can be performed under intercostal nerve block alone. It is possible to perform minor procedures on the chest or abdominal wall, but, in general, some degree of supplemental anesthesia must complement the block. For intra-abdominal procedures, celiac plexus block may be added to provide visceral anesthesia. Intercostal block may be combined with brachial plexus block for operations on the breast, upper extremities, and axilla. Pain from pelvic structures is not relieved by intercostal block, and operations primarily on such organs might better be performed under spinal, caudal, or lumbar epidural anesthesia.

Nonsurgical Applications

There is no method of pain relief more effective for fractured ribs than intercostal nerve block. Chest wall contusion, pleurisy, and pain from flail chest can also readily be relieved. Blockade of two or three nerves is a simple way to prepare for insertion of thoracostomy tubes. Herpes zoster pain may be relieved and even treated in this way. Intercostal nerve block can be helpful in the differential diagnosis of visceral *versus* abdominal wall pain. The most effective but least exploited use of this block is for postoperative control of pain (see Chap. 25).

Complications

The most frequent complication of intercostal nerve block is pneumothorax. The actual incidence is extremely low, but many physicians avoid this block because of an imagined high frequency. However, the gross abuse of proper technique will indeed lead to such a complication. The most common technical error that leads to pneumothorax is improper positioning of hands while the anesthesiologist finds and injects the nerves, but the dictum, "When all else fails, follow directions," can lessen the risk.[19] Physicians in all stages of training performed over 10,000 individual nerve blocks with a reported incidence of pneumothorax of only .073 per cent.[20] An earlier study in which silent pneumothorax was studied by obtaining routine postoperative chest films showed a 0.42 per cent incidence. Treatment of pneumothorax by needle aspiration or just careful watching is usually all that is necessary, although reabsorption of a small pneumothorax is aided by administration of oxygen. Chest drainage should be performed only if there is failure to resolve or an increase in the size of the pneumothorax.

A second problem arises from the toxic effects of absorbed local anesthetic and epinephrine following intercostal block. As previously mentioned, blood levels of the anesthetic drug are higher for this block than for any other regional anesthetic procedure. Systemic toxic reactions rarely occur in patients having diagnostic or therapeutic blocks because smaller volumes of more dilute solution of drug are used. Greater amounts of more concentrated drug are injected to provide complete motor and sensory block in the surgical patient. These greater doses may result in delayed systemic toxicity, so that patients should be monitored very closely for at least 30 minutes after administration of the block.

Any regional anesthetic procedure, especially intercostal blocks, can lead to complications if the anesthesiologist becomes so involved in the mechanics of administering the nerve block that total patient care is neglected. The beginning practitioner of regional anesthesia tends to become so engrossed by technique and methods that he fails to see the patient as more than a portion of anatomic detail through which a needle is being inserted. Vital signs may not be heeded, which is especially dangerous when depressant drugs are administered prior to the nerve block. The complications from this would not be those of the nerve block *per se* but rather hypoventilation, apnea, or cardiocirculatory collapse. Recognition of this hazard is the first step in prevention. Consequently, making periodic inspections of the whole patient or having a vigilant assistant is mandatory for effective use of intercostal nerve block.

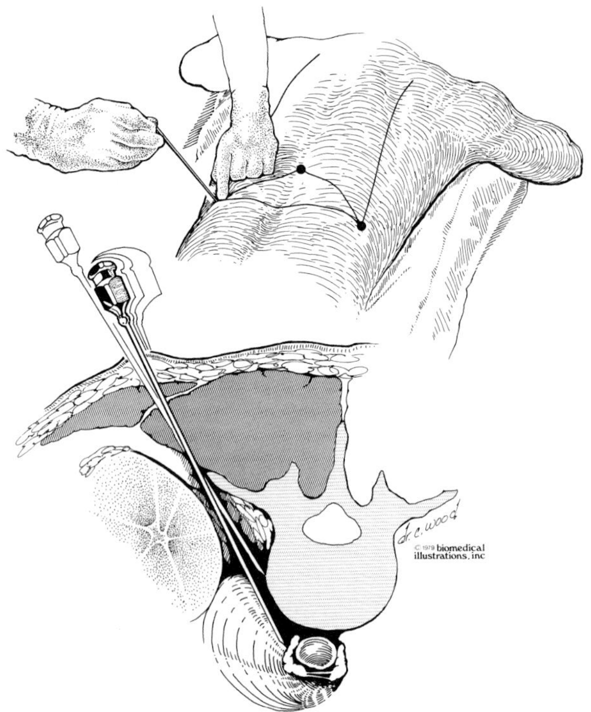

Fig. 14-5. Landmarks and technique for celiac plexus block. The apex of the triangle is the inferior aspect of T_{12} spine. The base passes through the inferior border of the L_1 spine.

CELIAC PLEXUS NERVE BLOCK

Anatomy

The celiac plexus is the largest of the three great plexuses of the sympathetic nervous system: the cardiac plexus innervates thoracic structures; the celiac plexus innervates abdominal organs; and the hypogastric plexus supplies pelvic organs. All three contain visceral afferent and visceral efferent sympathetic fibers. In addition, they contain parasympathetic fibers that pass through these ganglia after originating in cranial or sacral divisions of the spinal cord. Although both types of autonomic fibers can be found in each of these plexuses, they are primarily considered to be sympathetic nervous system structures.

The celiac plexus surrounds the axis of the celiac artery and overlaps the aorta at this level, which is directly anterior to the body of L1. It is possible to subdivide the celiac plexus into a variety of secondary structures, and terminology may become confusing. Different texts have used terms such as *solar plexus, semilunar ganglia, celiac ganglia,* and *splanchnic plexus* to refer to part or all of this great sympathetic nerve center. Although the terms *plexus* and *ganglia* are often used almost interchangeably, it is important to realize that *plexus* is a more inclusive term. A plexus is composed of a number of ganglia and nerve fibers that converge in a fairly well defined anatomic location. The greater (T5–10), lesser (T10–11), and least (T12) splanchnic nerves feed into the two semilunar or celiac ganglia, which in reality are the major right and left portions of the celiac plexus. The right celiac ganglion lies medial and posterior to the inferior vena cava. It intertwines anterior to the aorta with a dense network of fibers from the left ganglion. The left ganglion lies posterior to the pancreas and medial to the upper pole of the kidney and adrenal gland. Superiorly, both ganglia lie flattened against the crura of the diaphragm. They are readily identified in the dissection necessary for an abdominal approach to hiatal herniorrhaphy. As mentioned earlier, this great nerve center is also referred to as the *solar plexus,* but this term might better be used to refer to all of the sympathetic nerves, ganglia, and plexuses of the upper abdomen.

Technique

Celiac plexus nerve block is of special interest in that both bony and vascular landmarks can be utilized to best advantage in the performance of this block. As with any nerve block, it is advisable to mark out a diagram on the skin that, when projected mentally, yields three-dimensional perspective for the ultimate placement of the needle. This block can be performed by means of a posterior or lateral percutaneous, or by an anterior approach during laparotomy. The easiest and most useful approach, however, is the posterior. The patient is placed in a prone position with pillow under his abdomen, head turned flat to the table or cart, and arms dangling down at each side. The primary external topographic features are the 12th ribs and the inferior aspects of T_{12} and L_1 spinons processes (Fig. 14-5). The figure formed by connecting the spine of T-12 and L_1 with points 7–8 cm lateral at the lower edges of the twelfth ribs is that of a flattened isosceles triangle. The equal sides of this triangle serve as directional guides for the two needles that are passed under the edge of each of the twelfth ribs to approach the midline anterior to the body of L1. A 10- to 15-cm, 20-gauge needle is preferable, although the length may be varied for the extremely frail or massively obese patient. The block can be performed on an awake, unsedated patient. Commonly, it is performed under the same sedation and at the same time as intercostal block in the patient on whom a laparotomy is being performed. Skin wheals are raised 7 to 8 cm from the midline at the inferior edge of the 12th rib. Infiltration with a small amount of local anesthetic solution can then be carried deeper for 1 to 3 cm. If the patient is awake, he should be warned that he may feel brief twinges of pain, which result from the needle coming in contact with the periosteum or lumbar nerves.

Initially, the needle is tilted about 45° from the horizontal so that contact can be made with the lateral body of L1 at an average depth of 10 to 12 cm. Bony contact at a more superficial level indicates that a vertebral transverse process has been contacted. This must be recognized for what it is, and the physician should not be deceived about the depth of the celiac plexus because an incorrect judgment might lead to injection of anesthetic solution just 2 to 3 cm deep to the transverse process. The ensuing epidural or psoas injection might result in a widespread somatic nerve paralysis. This point is of special importance when neurolytic solutions are to be used. An experienced anesthesiologist who can mentally project a three-dimensional view will be able initially to identify the lateral surface of L1 at a depth of 8 to 10 cm. This is dependent on the patient's size, as well as on the location on the vertebral body at which contact is made (*i.e.*, posterolateral or anterolateral). Once the body is identified, the needle is withdrawn to subcutaneous levels and the angle increased to allow the tip of the needle to pass roughly 2 to 3 cm beyond the point of original contact. This angle may have to be changed two or three times until the needle slides off the anterolateral side of the vertebral body. The process can be painful to the awake patient but is readily tolerated if the anesthesiologist manifests a calm and authoritative manner, coupled with reassurances to the patient.

The precise depth to which the needles are to be advanced is best determined by a subtle but accurate means of locating the depth of the plexus; that is, by locating the depth at which aortic pulsations can be sensed by the fingertips holding the advancing left-sided needle. For this reason, it is advisable to perform the left-sided needle insertion first. As the needle is felt to slide anterior to the vertebral body, it should be advanced very slowly, and soon the vibrating periaortic structures will herald the precise location for effective injection (Fig. 14-5). Once the aortic depth is discovered, the right-sided needle can be inserted and advanced to a similar depth. Problems due to bleeding from penetration of either aorta or inferior vena cava have not been encountered. The well-accepted and common clinical performance of lumbar aortography would serve to confirm this point.

Once the needles have been positioned in the periaortic region, other confirmatory tests of needle placement should be performed to rule out improper position of the needle tip. For instance, leakage of blood, urine, or cerebrospinal fluid (CSF) will sometimes be spontaneous. If not, aspiration should be gently performed in four quadrants. Should this prove negative, a 2 ml-test dose of anesthetic solution is injected. This will provide additional confirmation of needle placement since paralysis will rapidly follow subarachnoid injection, and intravascular injection may be heralded by a ringing in the ears or restlessness. The final confirmatory test depends on the "feel" to the anesthesiologist of injecting the larger final volume of anesthetic solution. As a result, the difference between a 20- and a 22-gauge needle can be very pronounced. A 12-cm, 22-gauge needle requires such firm pressure during injection that it is difficult to appreciate whether resistance is due to the small-needle bore or whether the site of injection is subperiosteal, intratumor, or otherwise abnormal. On the other hand, injection of 20 to 25 ml of solution through a 20-gauge needle offers little resistance to the injecting thumb. This is to be expected if the injection is being properly performed in the loose retroperitoneal area where nerve fibers of the celiac plexus are located. The question has been raised whether intraperitoneal injections might not occur. This is conceivable but would require overly lateral and overly deep placement of the needles. However, whether or not this has occurred has not been documented from any reports of untoward results (Fig. 14-6).

Surgical Applications

The combination of intercostal and celiac plexus nerve block is ideal for any surgery of the upper abdomen. Usually, these blocks are supplemented with light general anesthesia since celiac block does not provide total anesthesia of upper abdominal viscera. One advantage to the surgeon is the diminution in the size of the bowel that results from block of sympathetic fibers.

As with spinal or epidural anesthesia, there is a tendency for the sympathetic block of celiac plexus anesthesia to produce a fall in blood pressure. This is neither as frequent nor as severe as the hypotension following high spinal anesthesia. However, the tendency can persist into the postoperative period if

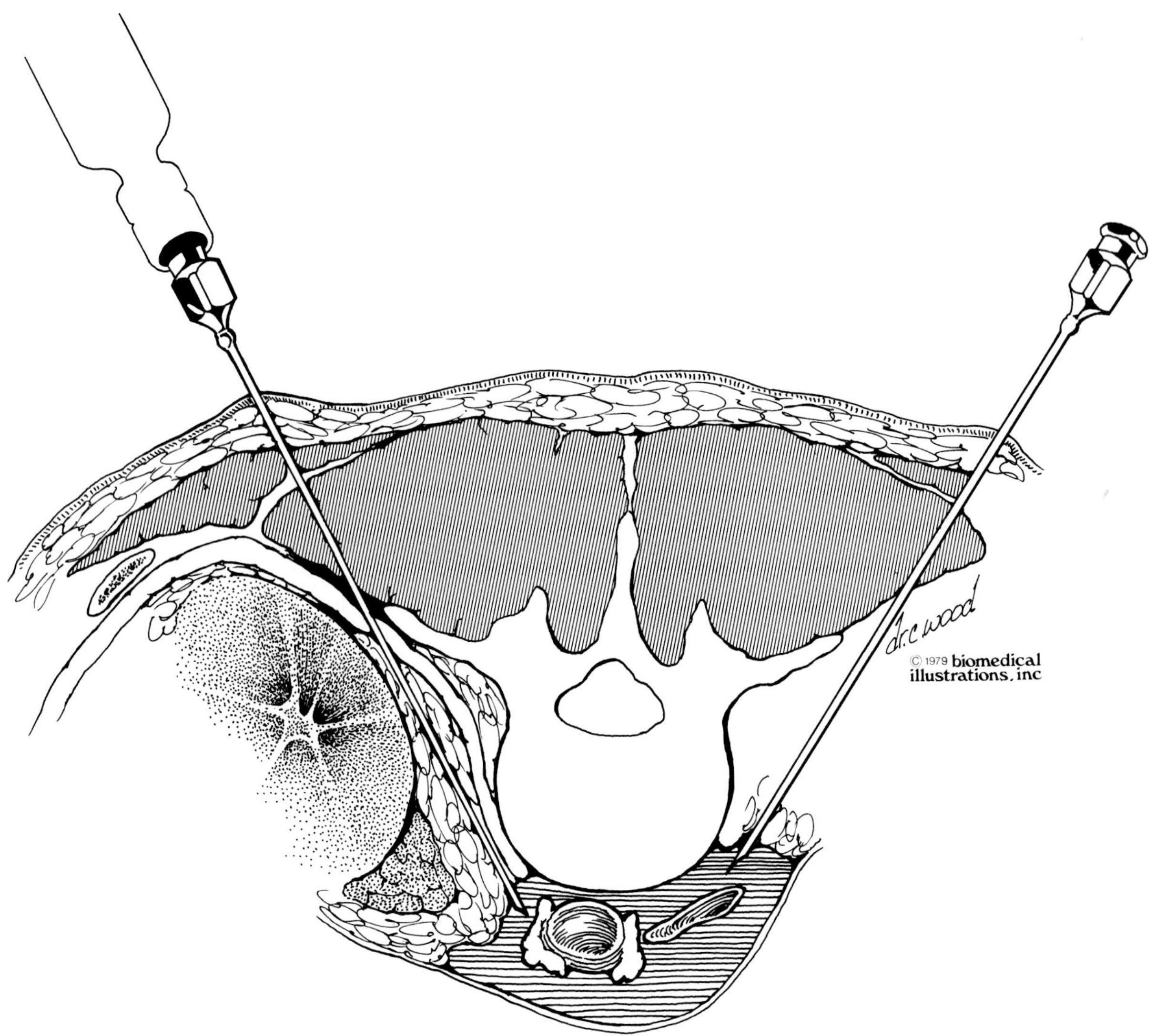

Fig. 14-6. Illustration of final needle position for bilateral celiac plexus block with relationship to surrounding anatomic structures.

long-acting local anesthetic drugs are used. This problem can be treated by using a shorter-acting local anesthetic for the celiac block than for the intercostal block, by adequate replacement of blood and fluid losses during surgery, by small doses of vasopressors such as ephedrine and by vigilance with close monitoring of the patient. In general, the supine patient will be asymptomatic and physiologically preserved even at pressures as low as 70 torr systolic. Rollason's report on hypotension following spinal anesthesia is illustrative of this point.[24] At present, extrapolation from such studies for patients with severe cerebral, cardiac, or renal disease must be cautious, but even in these patients, there is a far greater tendency to treat numbers (*i.e.*, the chart, the manometer, or the blood pressure tracing) than to treat the patient.

Nonsurgical Applications

Celiac plexus block can be used alone or in various combinations with intercostal block to help in the differential diagnosis of visceral *versus* abdominal wall pain. The block can be of therapeutic value in acute pancreatitis by relieving spasm of ducts and sphincters in the pancreatic system. Alcohol celiac plexus block is the most effective of all therapeutic blocks used in the treatment of pancreatic cancer pain.[26]

Complications

The possible complications of celiac plexus block include the following: hypotension; subarachnoid, epidural, or intrapsoas injection; intravascular injection; retroperitoneal hematoma secondary to bleeding from aorta or vena cava, and puncture of viscera, abscess, or cysts.

Hypotension may occur in 30 to 60 per cent of patients, depending on blood volume and physical status. It is not abrupt in onset and does not always require treatment. Misplaced injections are best prevented by experience, drawing the proper skin markings, and having the patient fully prone for the injection. Although celiac block can be performed on a patient in a lateral or semiprone position, these positions make it more difficult to ensure proper orientation to anatomic details. Initial aspiration plus the use of a test dose of local anesthetic solution are satisfactory precautionary measures against the complications of misplaced injections.

PARAVERTEBRAL LUMBAR SOMATIC NERVE BLOCK

Anatomy

When lumbar somatic nerve block is performed paravertebrally, it has many similarities to intercostal nerve block. However, instead of using the ribs as bony landmarks, the primary bony guide becomes the transverse process of the lumbar vertebral body—a "rudimentary" rib. The lumbar nerves exit their respective intervertebral foramina just inferior to the caudad edge of each transverse process. These nerves immediately divide into anterior and posterior branches. The posterior branches supply the skin of the lower back and the paravertebral muscles. Of primary interest, however, are the anterior branches of the first four lumbar nerves. These nerves, together with a small branch from the (12th thoracic nerve) form the lumbar plexus. This plexus is largely conceived within the substance of the psoas major muscle. Most of the peripheral branches exit laterally in a plane between the psoas and quadratus lumborum muscles.

The major branches of the lumbar plexus (*i.e.*, the iliohypogastric, ilioinguinal, and lateral femoral cutaneous nerves) continue laterally around the rim of the pelvis. Their terminal branches approach and pass near the anterior superior iliac spine. The femoral nerve passes almost directly caudad after emerging from the lateral edge of psoas major. The obturator nerve emerges from the medial edge of psoas major, descends under the common iliac vessels, and finally emerges from the pelvis through the obturator foramen. The ultimate cutaneous distribution of each of these nerves is quite variable in the groin and anterolateral leg. There is also considerable overlap of cutaneous branches of individual nerves. The primary peripheral branches of the lumbar plexus are listed in Table 14-3 and illustrated in Figure 14-7.

Table 14-3. Origins and Distribution of the Lumbar Plexus

Peripheral Nerve	*Root Segments*
Iliohypogastric	T12, L1
Ilioinguinal	L1
Genitofemoral	L1, L2
Lateral femoral cutaneous	L2, L3
Femoral	L2, L3, L4
Obturator	L2, L3, L4

It is apparent from Figure 14-7 that paravertebral nerve block L1–L4 will result in sensory and motor block of the groin, as well as of much of the leg. For intra-abdominal, pelvic, or groin operations, it is necessary to block only the upper two lumbar segments. In general, the lumbar nerves tend to slope sharply caudad as they emerge from the intervertebral foramina. In doing so, they tend to course anterior to the tips of the transverse processes of the next lower lumbar vertebral bodies. A needle placed at the inferior edge of a transverse process will be close to nerves from two lumbar segments: medially, it will be the nerve exiting the vertebral foramen; laterally, it will be the nerve from the next most cephalad vertebral level, which is now coursing inferiorly at a distance of several centimeters from where it left the vertebral canal. Local anesthetic solution injected at the proper depth inferior to one lumbar vertebral process can actually result in nerve block of two or more root segments.

Similarly, anesthesiologists can take advantage of the passage of lumbar nerves between the quadratus lumborum and psoas major muscles. There are two approaches to lumbar plexus anesthesia that capitalize on this anatomy. One is the inguinal paravascular technique, and the other is the lumbar paravertebral approach.[30] Both techniques depend on spread of anesthetic solution along fascial planes or within the fascial compartment of muscle (see Chap. 11).

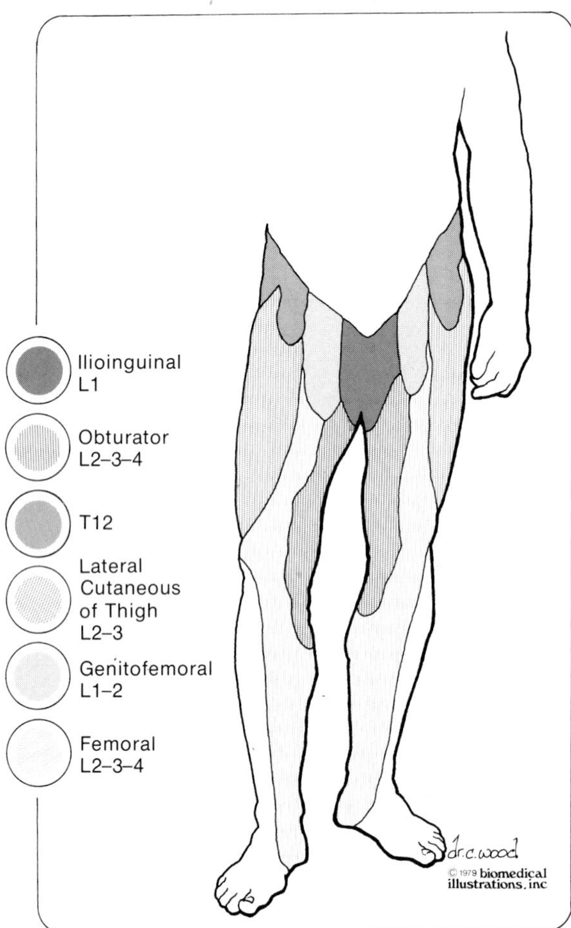

Fig. 14-7. Branches of the lumbar plexus showing their associated cutaneous distribution.

Technique

The patient's position is unchanged from that described for intercostal and celiac plexus nerve block. The injection sites are marked while keeping in mind that "the cephalad edge of a lumbar posterior spinous process lies opposite the caudad edge of its homologous transverse process." [19]

The distance between any two lumbar transverse processes is about 2 cm. A bony landmark that can be palpated and marked is the spinous process. The bony landmark that must be visualized in this block is the transverse process. Locating the transverse process is fundamental to a successful block. After palpating and marking each of the lumbar vertebral spinous process, horizontal lines are drawn at the cephalad edge of each one and projected laterally. Two vertical lines should then be drawn parallel to and 4 to 5 cm lateral from the midline. The points of intersection of the vertical and horizontal lines mark the sites where skin wheals are raised (Fig. 14-8). In surgical patients, the block is performed under the same sedation used for intercostal and celiac plexus block. A 8-cm, 22-gauge needle is inserted perpendicular to the skin until it contacts the transverse process at a depth of 3 to 5 cm. The needle should then be withdrawn to a subcutaneous level and redirected to slide off the caudad edge of the transverse process. As the needle is advanced 1 to 2 cm beyond the point where it previously made contact with bone, 6 to 10 ml of local anesthetic solution is injected. This process is repeated at each of the lumbar levels at which anesthesia is desired. The concentrations of local anesthetic drug are the same as that used for intercostal block (Fig. 14-8).

Surgical Application

Only infrequently would lumbar paravertebral nerve block be used as the sole anesthetic for surgery. It effectively complements intercostal and celiac plexus block for intra-abdominal and pelvic procedures. Groin operations such as herniorrhaphy can be performed with lumbar block, but supplementation with local infiltration or intravenous drugs may be necessary.

Nonsurgical Application

When the block is diagnostic, it is preferable to use small volumes of local anesthetic solutions to limit spread centrally or to adjacent lumbar nerves. Some physicians utilize fluoroscopy to locate precisely the needle tip and then inject only .5 to 1 ml of drug. This technique may be especially helpful in evaluating patients with back pain, in which a small branch known as the *recurrent meningeal nerve* may play a role. This branch is highly variable but tends to arise from the main nerve root just before separating into anterior and posterior parts. Another diagnostic use of paravertebral lumbar block is in evaluating groin or genital pain, such as the nerve entrapment syndromes that sometimes follow herniorrhaphy.

Complications

It is possible to inject into intravascular, epidural, or subarachnoid spaces during performance of this block. Should the needle point be inserted too far medially, it could enter a vertebral foramen or penetrate a dural sleeve to produce spinal anesthesia. There would be rapid onset of sensory and motor paralysis. Likewise, there could be perineural spread of solution into the epidural space with a consequent variable degree of anesthesia. Intravascular injection can be minimized by aspiration tests and use of the slight jiggling motion during injection. The lumbar sympathetic chain may be anesthetized either from local block of gray and white rami communicantes or by deeper penetration of local anesthetic drug to involve directly the sympathetic chain. Intra-abdominal injection or puncture of retroperitoneal or intra-abdominal organs is possible, although only as a result of gross errors.

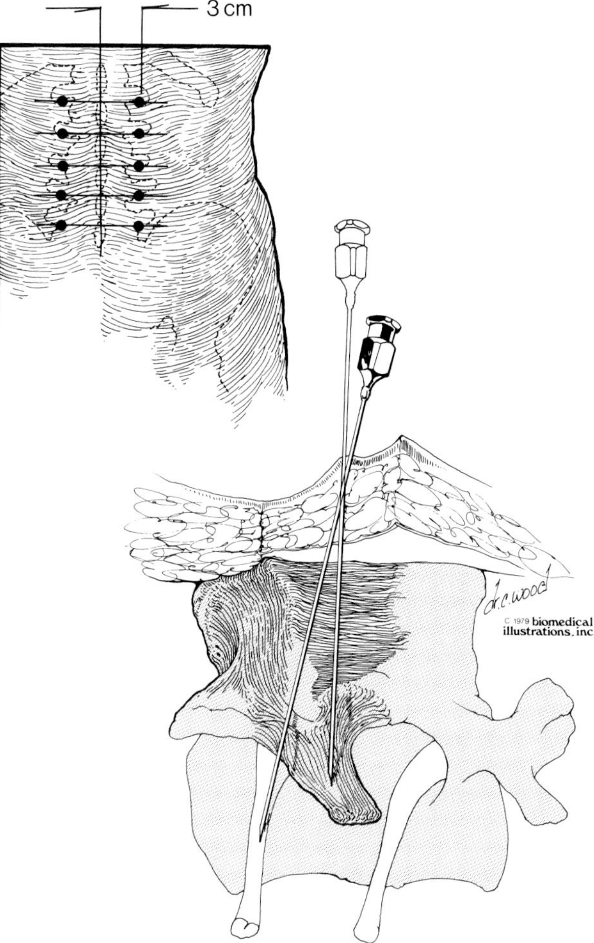

Fig. 14-8. Landmarks and technique for lumbar somatic nerve block. Right lateral view.

MISCELLANEOUS NERVE BLOCKS OF THE ABDOMEN AND CHEST

The three nerve blocks previously described in this chapter are performed at anatomic sites near the central neuraxis. There are multiple more peripheral sites along these nerve pathways for nerve block, but it must be remembered that all are merely variations and that the more distal the site on a peripheral nerve, the greater are the chances for incomplete block. This is due to factors such as spatial distribution, overlap of nerve territories, and the inability to reach each of the multiple branches of an arborizing nerve with injected local anesthetic solution. These factors can be partially overcome by using large volumes of solution, by using multiple injections, and by selecting local anesthetic agents with high penetrability. However, it is easier to hit the trunk of a tree than to touch each of its branches. A small amount of anesthetic drug injected at a primary nerve trunk will provide the most effective anesthesia. The following blocks are described primarily for the sake of completeness of information, historical perspective, and to improve appreciation of anatomic detail of nerve distribution.[15] They are of very limited use compared to the blocks previously discussed.

Rectus Block

Anatomy

As the lower five intercostal nerves course anteriorly, they eventually surface and terminate after penetrating the rectus abdomonus muscle. These nerves enter the rectus sheath at the posterolateral border of the body of that muscle. The tendinous intersections of the rectus tend to create segmental distribution of individual intercostal nerves, but there is much overlap and communication of adjacent fibers. Anteriorly, the rectus sheath is tough and fibrous from ospubis to xiphoid. Posteriorly, it is strong and readily identifiable down to the level of the umbilicus, but then it fades into a thin sheath of transversalis fascia, which is closely adherent to peritoneum below the semicircular line of Douglas. The posterior rectus sheath above the umbilicus is quite substantial and can serve as a "backboard" for injecting local anesthetic solution. This solution will be confined by the tendinous intersections but within those limits will spread up and down to anesthetize the peripheral branches of the intercostal nerves.

Technique

The patient lies supine, and the anesthesiologist may stand at either side. Usually four to six sites are injected, depending on the location and size of surgical incision (Fig. 14-9). Skin wheals are raised at the middle of each segment of the rectus muscle body that can be palpated between tendinous inter-

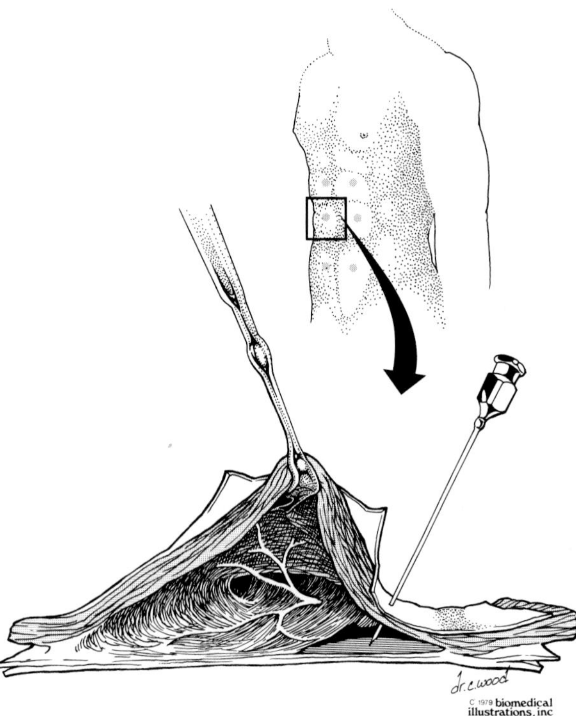

Fig. 14-9. Landmarks and technique for rectus sheath block.

sections. A reusable 5-cm, 22-gauge needle is passed through skin and subcutaneous tissue until it meets the firm resistance of the anterior rectus sheath. The block should be discontinued unless this sheath can be convincingly demonstrated by pushing on the needle. With controlled steady pressure, the needle is pushed to penetrate this sheath with a definite snap and then passed on through the softer belly of the muscle. As the needle approaches the posterior rectus sheath, a firm resistance will again become apparent, and, at this point, 10 ml of local anesthetic solution is injected. The process is repeated at each injection site. Blocks above the umbilicus should be performed first and needle depth noted before completing any additional blocks below the umbilicus.[19]

Surgical Application

The block may be used for surgical pain from a midline incision. It requires supplementation if the abdominal cavity is to be explored.

Nonsurgical Application

This block may be useful in diagnosing abdominal nerve entrapment syndromes or localized myofascial problems (see Chap. 26).

Complications

Near the xiphoid and ospubis, it is difficult to identify the posterior rectus sheath. Attempting this block at these levels may result in penetration of peritoneum and underlying organs such as intestine, bladder, or uterus. In the patient with a distended abdomen, the thinly stretched rectus may prevent clear identification of anterior and posterior sheaths. A visable bulge in the abdominal wall upon injection indicates that the needle is too superficial, and a poor block will result. The block is difficult in the obese, cachectic, or elderly patient with poor abdominal muscle tone.

Iliac Crest Block

The peripheral extensions of the ilioinguinal, iliohypogastric, and 12th thoracic nerves follow a circular course that is somewhat determined by the bowl-like shape of the ilium. In sweeping around anteriorly, these branches pass near the anterior superior iliac spine—a prominent landmark even in the obese patient. At or near the level of the anterior superior iliac spine, all three of the nerves lie between the internal and external oblique muscles. They continue anteromedially and become superficial as they terminate in branches to skin and muscles of the inguinal region. Using the anterior superior iliac spine as a primary point of orientation, the anesthesiologist can perform an infiltration block known as *iliac crest block.* Success depends on spreading a large volume of anesthetic solution between several abdominal-wall muscle layers. The block is inadequate to provide total anesthesia for inguinal herniorrhapy because structures that enter the inguinal canal through the internal inguinal ring will not be anesthetized.

Technique

The anesthesiologist or surgeon stands on the side opposite that which is to be blocked. The patient lies in the supine position. A point is marked on the skin roughly 3 cm medial and 3 cm inferior to the anterior superior iliac spine. A skin wheal is raised, and an 8-cm, 22-gauge needle inserted and directed almost horizontally to contact the inner surface of the ilium. Ten ml of local anesthetic solution is injected as the needle is slowly withdrawn. Then the needle should be reinserted at a somewhat steeper angle to ensure penetration of all three lateral abdominal muscles. The injection is repeated. In the obese or heavily muscled patient, a third injection may be necessary at an even steeper angle. Subcutaneous infiltration superior to the skin wheal will give a broader area of skin anesthesia as it catches some cutaneous branches of the last two or three intercostal nerves (Fig. 14-10).

If herniorrhaphy is to be performed, a second skin wheal should be raised 2–3 cm above the midinguinal point. A 5-cm needle is inserted, perpendicular to the skin, to a depth of 3 to 5 cm. Ten to 20 ml of local anesthetic solution should be injected during insertion and withdrawal of this needle. It will produce anesthesia of the genitofemoral nerve, sympathetic fibers, and peritoneal sac.

Surgical Application

This block is an excellent first maneuver for the surgeon or anesthesiologist who performs infiltration anesthesia for inguinal herniorrhaphy. Although the two injection sites described above may be adequate for herniorrhaphy,[11a] it is quite possible that additional direct local infiltration may be required to have a completely pain-free operation. It is especially difficult to anesthetize completely all the structures in the internal ring with a percutaneous injection.

Nonsurgical Application

This block may be useful in diagnosing nerve entrapment syndromes following herniorrhapy.

Complications

Fairly large volumes of local anesthetic solution can be injected with this block, and the anesthesiologist must watch for signs and symptoms of systemic toxic reactions. It is possible to penetrate peritoneum, intestine, or blood vessels. This is unlikely but may not be apparent when the block is performed. Aspiration should be performed prior to each injection. The solution often spreads to provide some anesthesia of the lateral buttocks and thigh. Although this is not likely to interfere with a patient's ability to walk, it may be necessary to offer the patient an explanation or a word of caution.

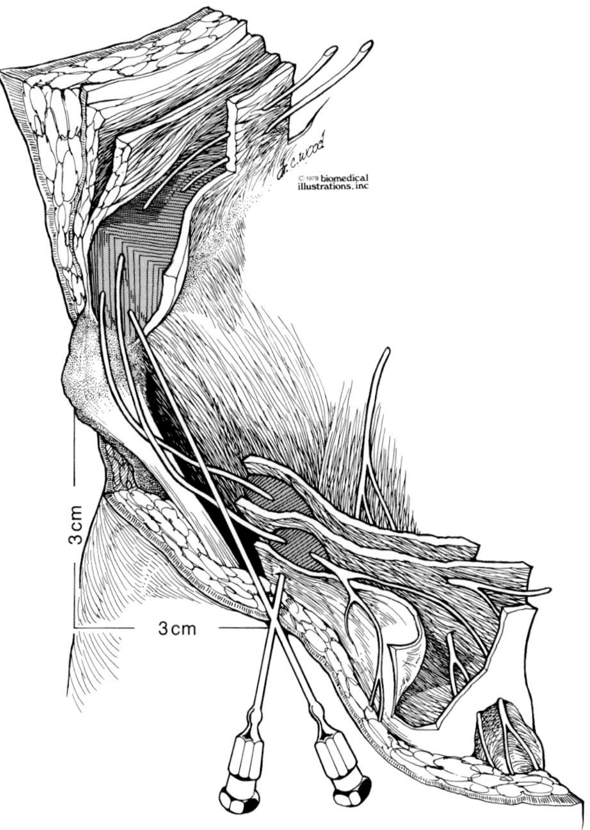

Fig. 14-10. Anatomy and technique for iliac crest block.

Cave of Retzius Block

Anatomy

The variable space located between urinary bladder and symphysis pubis is known as the *cave of Retzius*. This space contains a great venous plexus, as well as many terminating nerve fibers of the sacral plexus. An infiltration block of this area can be a useful adjunct to anesthesia for prostatectomy or bladder procedures. It will provide analgesia, decrease bleeding if vasoconstrictors are used, and facilitate the surgical dissection.

Technique

A skin wheal is raised 2.5 cm superior to the pubic symphysis. Subcutaneous infiltration can be performed laterally in the line of skin incision for retropubic prostatectomy. A 7 to 8-cm needle is then directed to the posterior aspect of the ospubis and anterior to the bladder. Ten ml of local anesthetic solution is injected as the needle reaches its maximum depth and is slowly withdrawn. This process is repeated with two lateral injections made through the same skin wheal (Fig. 14-11).

Surgical Application

The block may be combined with rectus block and infiltration of the incision in the poor-risk patient who undergoes prostatectomy.

Nonsurgical Application

There are few useful nonsurgical applications.

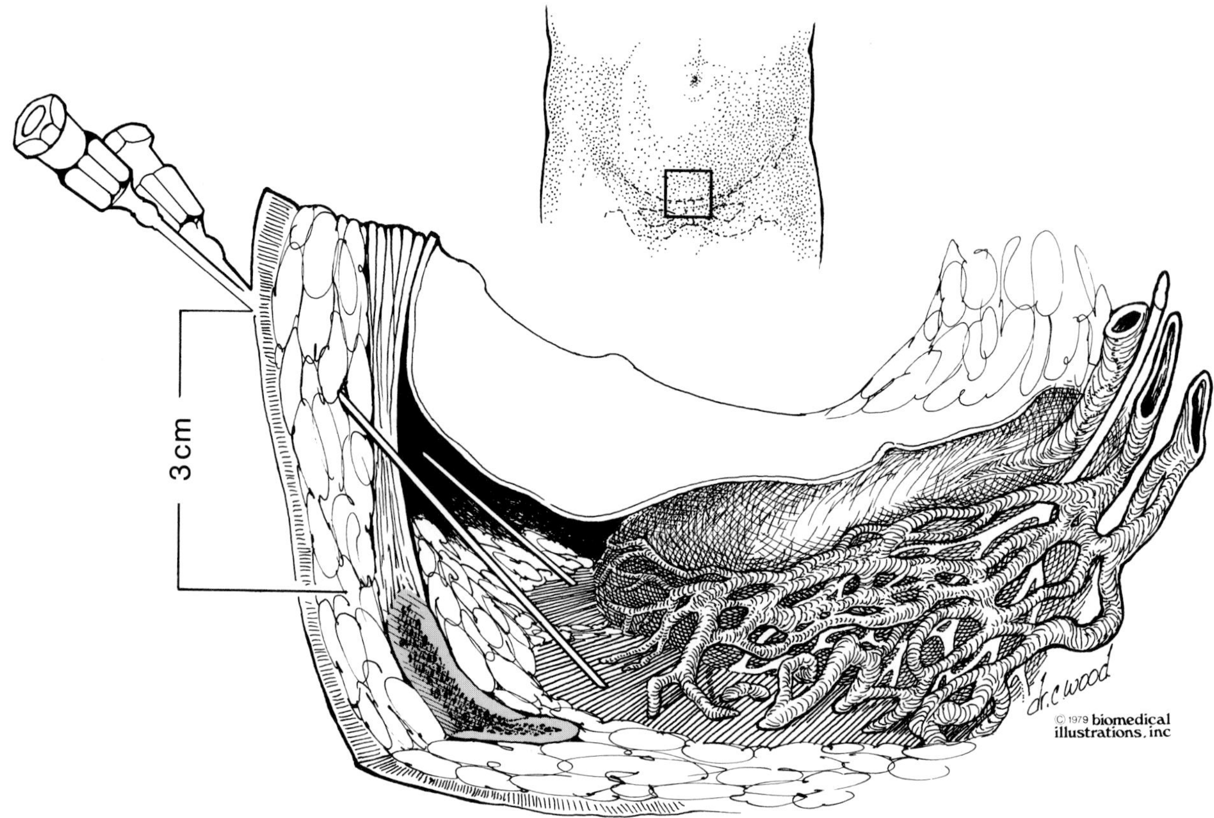

Fig. 14-11. Sagittal view of retropubic area showing anatomy and technique for cave of Retzius block.

Complications

The chief concern is for excessive intravascular injection, which is avoided by periodic aspiration. Bladder puncture may occur, but it is unlikely unless the block is performed in a patient with a distended bladder.

INTRA-ABDOMINAL NERVE BLOCK

Many anesthesiologists become frustrated with regional anesthesia for intra-abdominal operations because the patient experiences pain from manipulation of viscera or from the surgeon's exploring hands. This can occur even if the patient has evidenced no response to skin incision or dissection through the anterior abdominal wall. Once the peritoneal cavity is entered, there are additional pathways over which pain is transmitted. As previously discussed, these are the afferent pain fibers of the sympathetic and parasympathetic nervous systems. Light general anesthesia, heavy intravenous sedation, and rapid delicate surgical technique are measures calculated to offset the problem. In addition, the surgeon might conceivably be persuaded to use additional amounts of local anesthetic solution to provide the necessary anesthesia. Major drawbacks, though, are that the surgeon must now inject; this consumes time when there seems an almost irresistible urge to proceed with the operation; potentially toxic amounts of local anesthetic can be used; this may be painful; and there is no guarantee of pain relief. Despite these objections, the following three procedures might prove useful during the course of laparotomy.

Peritoneal Lavage

Local anesthetic solutions are readily absorbed from mucosal surfaces. Lavage of the peritoneal cavity with large volumes of local anesthetic solution will result in analgesia. However, it is difficult to lavage completely all peritoneal surfaces. One hundred ml of solution (*e.g.*, 0.5% lidocaine, 0.25% bupivacaine, 1.0% procaine) are instilled through a slight nick in the peritoneum or into the opened peritoneal cavity. Slight jostling of the abdomen may aid distribution. The Trendelenberg position aids flow of the solution over the celiac area and often improves analgesia. Some authors have apparently observed marked shrinking of the intestine following this maneuver. Use of a laparoscope also provides an additional port of entry for the lavage solution and might be a useful adjunct when laparoscopy is being performed.

Vagus Nerve Block

The familiar abbreviation LARP (left anterior, right posterior) indicates that the left vagus is anterior and the right vagus is posterior at the esophageal hiatus. It is possible for the surgeon to infiltrate these nerves directly from the inferior side of the diaphragm. They are deep within the abdomen, and access is not simple. However, infiltration of 10 to 20 ml of dilute anesthetic solution at or near the level of the hiatus will provide marked diminution of sensation from the abdominal cavity.

Celiac Plexus Block

Numerous reports and observations have been made of the celiac plexus reflex during laparotomy. Burstein has vividly described the clinical picture of this reflex and its tendency to produce hypotension.[5] It is possible to infiltrate the celiac plexus directly with local anesthetic solution (20–40 ml). The surgeon may not always find this technically easy. Tumor masses, obesity, and the high posterior location of the celiac plexus in the abdomen make direct visualization a challenge. However, in this situation, infiltration of a large volume of solution near the plexus may result in an adequate nerve block. A variation is to wash 40 to 60 ml of anesthetic solution into the upper posterior abdominal cavity. Dilute concentrations of local anesthetic are quite adequate and should be used as previously described.

REFERENCES

1. Bonica, J.J.: Regional anesthesia with tetracaine. Anesthesiology, *11*:606, 1950.
2. Bridenbaugh, P.O., DuPen, S.L., Moore, D.C., Bridenbaugh, L.D., and Thompson, G.E.: Postoperative intercostal nerve block analgesia versus narcotic analgesia. Anesth. Analg. (Cleve.), *52*:81, 1973.
3. Bridenbaugh, P.O., Tucker, G.T., Moore, D.C., Bridenbaugh, L.D., and Thompson, G.E.: Etidocaine: Clinical evaluation for intercostal nerve block and lumbar epidural block. Anesth. Analg. (Cleve.), *52*:407, 1973.
4. Brown, B.R., Jr.: Hepatic microsomal enzyme induction. Anesthesiology, *39*:178, 1973.
5. Burstein, C.L.: Fundamental Considerations in Anesthesia. Ed. 2. New York, Macmillan, 1955.
6. Crile, G.W., and Lower, W.E.: Anoci-Association. W.B. Saunders, Philadelphia, 1915.
7. deJong, R.H., and Cullen, S.C.: Buffer-demand and *p*H of local anesthetic solutions containing epinephrine. Anesthesiology, *24*:801, 1963.
8. deJong, R.H., and Heavner, J.E.: Diazepam prevents local anesthetic seizures. Anesthesiology, *34*:523, 1971.
9. deJong, R.H., Heavner, J.E., and deOliveira, L.F.: Effects of nitrous oxide on the lidocaine seizure threshold and diazepam protection. Anesthesiology, *37*:299, 1972.
10. DuVoisin, R.C., and Katz, R.C.: Reversal of central anticholinergic syndrome in man by physostigmine. J.A.M.A., *206*:1963, 1968.
11. Ellis, H., and McLarty, M.: Anatomy for Anesthetists. Philadelphia, F.A. Davis, 1963.

11a. Glasgow, F.: Short-stay surgery (shouldice technique) for repair of inguinal hernia. Ann. Surg. *58*:134, 1976.

12. Gray, H.: Anatomy of the Human Body. ed. 29. Philadelphia, Lea & Febiger, 1973.
13. Haugen, F.P.: The Autonomic Nervous System and Pain. Anesthesiology, *29*:785, 1968.
14. Katz, J.: A survey of anesthetic choice among anesthesiologists. Anesth. Analg. (Cleve.), *52*:373, 1973.
15. Labat, G.: Regional Anesthesia—Its Technic and Clinical Application. Philadelphia, W.B. Saunders, 1924.
16. Lundy, J.S.: Balanced Anesthesia. Minn. Med., *9*:399, 1926.
17. Macintosh, R.R., and Bryce Smith, R.: Local Analgesia: Abdominal Surgery. Edinburgh, E & S Livingston, 1953.
18. Moore, D.C.: Pontocaine solutions for regional analgesia other than spinal and epidural block: An analysis of 2500 cases. J.A.M.A., *146*:803, 1951.
19. ______: Regional Block. ed. 4. Springfield, Charles C Thomas, 1971.
20. Moore, D.C., and Bridenbaugh, L.D.: Pneumothorax: Its incidence following intercostal nerve block. J.A.M.A., *174*:842, 1960.
21. Moore, D.C., Bridenbaugh, L.D., Bridenbaugh, P.O., and Thompson, G.E.: Bupivacaine hydrochloride: A summary of investigational use in 3274 cases. Anesth. Analg. (Cleve.), *50*:856, 1971.
22. Moore, D.C., Bridenbaugh, L.D., Thompson, G.E., Balfour, R.I., and Horton, W.G.: Factors determining dosages of amide-type local anesthetic drugs. Anesthesiology, *47*:263, 1977.
23. Mushin, W.W.: Bilateral vagal block. Proc. R. Soc. Med., *38*:308, 1945.
24. Rollason, W.N., Robertson, G.S., Cordiner, C.M., and Hall, D.J.: A comparison of mental function in relation to hypotensive and normotensive anesthesia in the elderly. Br. J. Anaesth. *43*:561, 1971.
25. Simpson, B.R., Parkhouse, J., Marshall, R., and Lamberts, W.: Epidural analgesia and the prevention of postoperative respiratory complications. Br. J. Anaesth. *33*:628, 1961.
26. Thompson, G.E., Artin R., Bridenbaugh, L.D., and Moore, D.C.: Abdominal pain and alcohol celiac plexus nerve block. Anesth. Analg. (Cleve.), *56*:1, 1977.

27. Thompson, G.E., and Moore, D.C.: Ketamine, diazepam and Innovar: A computerized comparative study. Anesth. Analg. (Cleve.), *50*:458, 1971.
28. Tucker, G.T., Moore, D.C., Bridenbaugh, P.O., Bridenbaugh, L.D., and Thompson, G.E.: Systemic absorption of mepivacaine in commonly used regional block procedures. Anesthesiology, *37*:277, 1972.
29. Walts, L.F., Forsythe, A.B., and Moore, J.G.: Critique: Occupational disease among operating room personnel. Anesthesiology, *42*:608, 1975.
30. Winnie, A.P., Ramamurthy, S., and Durrani, A.: The inguinal paravascular technic of lumbar plexus anesthesia: The "3-in-1" block. Anesth. Analg. (Cleve.), *52*:989, 1973.

PART TWO

Techniques of Neural Blockade

Section D: Head and Neck

15 Somatic Blockade

Terence M. Murphy

The status of regional anesthesia for surgery of the head and neck improved dramatically prior to the introduction of endotracheal intubation. However, with the widespread use of intubation, its popularity waned, and it is now used much less frequently for surgical procedures. Nevertheless, there are still many occasions when it can provide an optimal form of anesthesia, either alone or as a complement to general anesthesia, and it can afford excellent analgesia for postoperative recovery and for chronic pain.

Because of the very compact anatomy and the close relationship of cranial and cervical nerves to many vital structures, meticulous placement of the needle and small discrete doses of the anesthetic agent are usually required for accurate and safe regional anesthesia in this area. Perhaps more so than in other parts of the body, the landmarks for regional anesthesia in the head and neck are relatively constant, easily located, and, for anesthesiologists prepared to acquire the skills necessary in utilizing these techniques, predictable, so that satisfactory regional anesthesia can be attained.

The trigeminal nerve and the cervical plexus provide cutaneous sensory innervation to the face, head, and neck. In addition, the glossopharyngeal and vagus nerves supply the pharynx and larynx. This chapter is concerned mainly with nerve blocks of these cranial nerves and the cervical plexus to provide anesthesia for surgery, endoscopic procedures, and endotracheal anesthesia, as well as the use of such blocks in pain states. For the sake of completeness, block of the 11th cranial nerve, the accessory nerve, is also described.

Although the pharmacology of the agents used has considerable affect on regional anesthesia in any region of the body, probably the greatest reason for failure is incorrect placement of the needle, which can be ensured only by a thorough understanding of the anatomy of the area in which the needle is inserted. Applied anatomical knowledge is of vital importance for success in regional anesthesia, in general, and particularly in regional anesthesia of the head and neck. The anesthesiologist who wishes to become skilled in these techniques would do well to consult the reading suggested at the end of the chapter and, most important, to familiarize himself with the anatomy by dissecting the cadaver or reviewing prosected specimens whenever possible.[1–8] Frequent recourse to a skull is advisable when learning how to perform these blocks and even as a means of review just prior to such procedures.

ANATOMY

Face

The anatomy and complexity of the nerve supply of the face in the adult is perhaps best understood in light of its development in the embryo, as the face forms around the primitive mouth (the stomodeum). Initially, the stomodeum is surrounded caudally by the mandibular arch (which is supplied by the mandibular nerve), laterally on each side by the maxillary processes (which are supplied by the maxillary division of the trigeminal nerve), and rostrally by the forebrain capsule, from which develops the frontonasal process (which is supplied by the first division of the trigeminal nerve, the ophthalmic nerve). The frontonasal process grows down into the primitive stomodeum from the forebrain capsule, and this will eventually form the nose of the mature embryo (Fig. 15-1). The two maxillary processes grow inward from either side and join together below the primitive nose, as shown, and they then form the rostral margin of the primitive mouth. Thus, in the mature face, the forehead, eyebrows, upper eyelids, and nose are supplied by the first division ophthalmic branch of the trigeminal nerve. The lower eyelid, cheek, and upper lip are supplied by the second division (*i.e.*, the maxillary nerve), and the lower lip and chin and mandibular and temporal regions are supplied by the third divi-

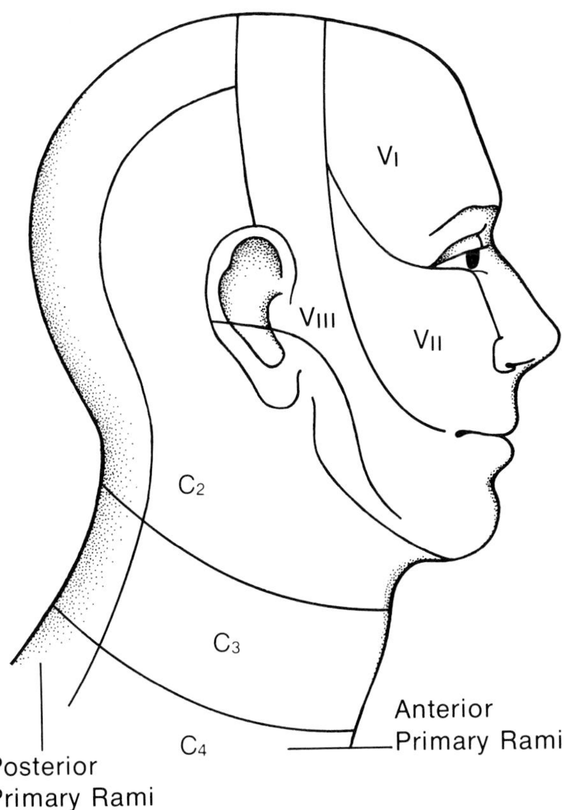

Fig. 15-2. Dermatome innervation of head and neck.

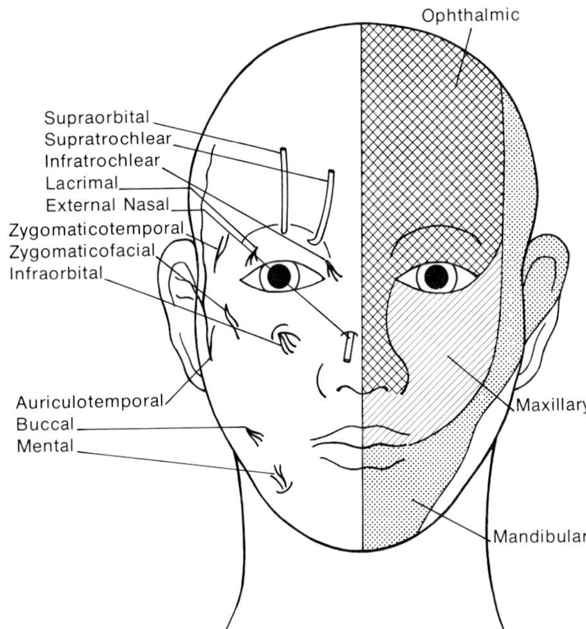

Fig. 15-3. Cutaneous and dermatome innervation of face. Note the five terminal cutaneous divisions of the opthalmic nerve (V_I), that is, supraorbital, supratrochlear, infratrochlear, lacrimal, external nasal. The terminal divisions of the second division (V_{II}) are the infraorbital, zygomaticofacial, and zygomaticotemporal. The three terminal divisions of the mandibular nerve (V_{III}) are auriculotemporal, buccal, and mental. Note that the supraorbital, infraorbital, and mental nerves all lie in the same vertical plane as the pupil, with the eye looking straight forward.

Innervation of Nose

External nose
- Infratrochlear and anterior ethmoidal branches of nasociliary nerve (V_1)
- Infraorbital branch of maxillary nerve (V_2)

Nasal cavity
- Anterior ethmoidal branch of nasociliary (V_1): to anterior one-third of septum and lateral walls; also to roof of nose
- Long and short sphenopalatine nerves and greater palatine nerve from sphenopalatine ganglion (V_2): to posterior two-thirds of septum and lateral walls; also to roof of nose
- Anterior superior dental nerve from V_2 in infraorbital canal: to anterior end of floor of cavity

←

Fig. 15-1. Frontal and lateral views of development of dermatomes of the head and neck. (*A*, *B*) The primitive stomodeum (mouth) is surrounded by the three parts of the developing face. (*C*, *D*) The frontonasal process (supplied by the ophthalmic nerve) grows in from above, the maxillary processes (maxillary nerve) grow in from each side, and the mandibular process (mandibular nerve) forms the caudal margin. (*E*, *F*) The frontonasal process forms the brow, eyebrows, upper eyelid, and nose in the fully developed face. The maxillary process forms both cheeks, lower eyelid, and upper lip. The mandibular process gives rise to the lower lip and the chin and a strip of skin extending up the side of the face, often to the vertex, including the superior anterior two-thirds of the anterior surface of the ear. The cervical plexus derivatives of the second, third, and fourth cervical nerves supply the posterior part of the head and neck from the vertex down. Note in *F* that the skin over the angle of the jaw and the lower part of the auricle on the anterior surface and all of its posterior surface are supplied by cervical plexus dermatomes (C_2).

Thus, the external nose requires blockade at two sites: above the inner canthus of eyelid and at infraorbital foramen. The nasal cavity is also conveniently blocked at two primary sites: the sphenopalatine ganglion and the point of entry of the anterior ethmoidal nerve at the anterior end of the cribriform plate. Fortunately, both of these sites are high in the nasal cavity in the region known as the *sphenoethmoidal recess*. If the skull is turned upside down, local anesthetic solution instilled by way of the nose pools in this area. Thus, both sites of innervation can be blocked simultaneously. The small remaining area on the floor of the nasal cavity requires local application by holding the nares together after instilling local anesthetic or by direct application (see below).

Innervation of Nasal Sinuses

Maxillary sinus
  Maxillary nerve (V_2) and sphenopalatine ganglion
Ethmoidal sinus
Nasociliary nerve (from V_1) by way of anterior and posterior ethmoidal branches
Frontal sinus
  Frontal nerve (from V_1)

Thus, drainage of the maxillary sinus by an oral approach (Caldwell–Luc) under neural blockade requires maxillary nerve block. Infiltration of the line of the incision over the canine fossa with epinephrine solution improves hemostasis. Sometimes, the operation of Caldwell-Luc extends to the ethmoidal sinus so that anterior ethmoidal block is also necessary.

Cervical Plexus

The cervical plexus contributes to the supply of both the deep and superficial structures of the neck, and blockade of the deep cervical plexus is essentially a paravertebral block in which the needle is inserted and adjusted in relation to the transverse processes of the appropriate cervical vertebrae. Because of the obliquity of the transverse processes of the cervical vertebrae, it is important to direct the needle in a caudad fashion. To do otherwise risks entering the spinal canal at this site and thereby, perhaps, producing profound epidural or spinal anesthesia or even worse damage to the spinal cord (see Fig. 15-11).

Because of the course of the vertebral artery—through the foramina transversaria in each transverse process—it is especially at risk and a potential site for inadvertent intravascular injections. Even a very small amount of local anesthetic agent (0.2 ml) injected into this vessel can produce profound toxic effects of convulsions, presumably because of high cerebral blood levels.

Cutaneous Innervation of Head and Neck

The cutaneous supply of the head and neck derives from the three divisions of the trigeminal nerve and from the cervical plexus (see Figs. 15-3; 15-10).

In the region of the scalp, the nerves of supply have long superficial upward courses. Four sensory nerves pass in front of the ear to the scalp (supratrochlear and supraorbital from V_1; zygomaticotemporal from V_2; auriculotemporal from V_3), and four pass behind the ear (great auricular and greater, lesser, and least occipital nerves from cervical plexus). All eight nerves converge toward the vertex of the scalp and are effectively blocked if a band of local anesthetic is infiltrated from the glabella, above the ear to the occiput. Infiltration is made with 0.5 to 1 per cent lidocaine immediately beneath the skin in the subcutaneous tissue. It is useful to inject some solution into the temporalis muscle to prevent undue movement of the muscle during procedures on the scalp. Injection next to the periosteum is required only if bone is to be removed.

In the face, cutaneous branches are short and radiate. Thus, in this area blockade of individual branches is more satisfactory than "barrage" block. For example, the skin below the eye as far as the upper lip can be anesthetized by infraorbital block (see below).

In the neck, all of the cutaneous supply derives from the cervical plexus and can be blocked by a single injection of the superficial cervical plexus at the midpoint of the posterior border of the sternomastoid muscle or by single injection blockade of the deep cervical plexus (see Figs. 15-10 and 10-7). The latter has the advantage of also blocking the branches of the posterior primary rami if analgesia is required toward the back of the neck; however, it is associated with phrenic nerve palsy.

Styloid Apparatus—Glossopharyngeal Nerve

The structures of the styloid process are involved in blocking the glossopharyngeal nerve. The styloid process is the calcified rostral end of the stylohyoid ligament, and it varies considerably in length from patient to patient. Its tip lies approximately halfway between the angle of the mandible and the mastoid process and, therefore, provides a bony landmark to identify when blocks of the glossopharyngeal nerve are planned (see Fig. 15-7). This nerve emerges from the jugular foramen posterior and medial to the styloid process. It exits from the foramen in very close relationship with the 10th and 11th cranial nerves and sweeps down parallel with the posterior border of the styloid process and at a slightly deeper plane. Therefore by "walking" the needle until it just slips off the posterior aspect of the styloid process, the ninth cranial nerve can be blocked (usually along with the 10th and 11th as well). The large vascular conduits of the internal jugular vein and internal carotid artery are very closely related to this nerve at this point, and care must be exercised to avoid injecting into these vessels.

The glossopharyngeal nerve supplies the posterior third of the tongue and the oropharynx from its junction with the nasopharynx at the level of the hard palate. It supplies the pharyngeal surfaces of the soft palate and the epiglottis, the fauces, and the pharyngeal wall as far down as the pharyngoesophageal junction at the level of the cricoid cartilage (C6).

Innervation of the Larynx—Vagus Nerve

The vagus nerve supplies sensation to the larynx. The undersurface of the epiglottis and the laryngeal inlet down to the vocal folds are supplied by the internal laryngeal branch of the vagus. This nerve reaches the larynx by piercing the thyrohyoid membrane, which joins the thyroid to the hyoid cartilages. By blocking its parent nerve (the superior laryngeal branch of the vagus) below the tip of the greater cornu of the hyoid bone, the laryngeal inlet can be rendered insensitive down to the vocal cords. Below the cords, the larynx and trachea are supplied by the recurrent branch of the vagus that ascends in the neck in the groove between the trachea and esophagus. Although the nerve can be blocked in this groove (and frequently is as a complication of stellate ganglion block), usually anesthesia of the trachea is effected by spray techniques, either transorally or by percutaneous puncture at the cricothyroid membrane. The recurrent laryngeal nerve also supplies motor function to all the intrinsic muscles of the larynx (except the cricothyroid), and bilateral motor block produces loss of phonation and loss of ability to close the glottis.

Innervation of Mouth and Pharynx

A detailed description of the innervation of teeth and mouth is given in Chapter 17, together with appropriate neural blockade techniques.

Innervation of Tonsil

The tonsil and its surroundings are innervated by the lesser palatine nerve (from V_2), the lingual nerve (from V_3), and by way of the glossopharyngeal nerve by way of the pharyngeal plexus.

Thus, it is most practical to denervate the tonsillar fossa by infiltration around the tonsil rather than blocking individual nerves. This is usually preceded by requesting the patient to suck viscous local anesthetic solutions.

TRIGEMINAL NERVE BLOCK

Gasserian Ganglion Block

Gasserian ganglion block results in extensive anesthesia of the ipsilateral face over the area shown in Figure 15-2. It was once used extensively for surgery of the head and neck. However, with the advent of endotracheal intubation and more sophisticated techniques of general anesthesia, its appeal as a primary surgical anesthetic declined. However, it is still used diagnostically and therapeutically for neuralgias of the trigeminal system. It has merit as a diagnostic block, a permanent neurolytic block, and as a means of introducing heated probes for the new technique of thermogangliolysis.[9]

Anatomy

Lying at the apex of the petrous temporal bone at the junction of middle and posterior cranial fossa, the ganglion is situated in a fold of dura mater that forms an invagination around the posterior two-thirds of the ganglion. This invagination is in continuity with the CSF and bears the name of Meckle's cave or the cavum trigeminale. It is reached with a needle by traversing the infra-temporal fossa and entering the middle cranial fossa by way of the foramen ovale. Medially, the gasserian ganglion is bounded by the cavernous venous sinus, which contains the carotid artery, and the third, fourth, and sixth cranial nerves. Superiorly, there is the inferior surface of the temporal lobe of the brain, and posteriorly, the brain stem. Any of these structures might be damaged by the introduction of the needle through the foramen ovale. Also, because the ganglion is partially bathed in CSF, injections into the area might spread into the spinal fluid and, hence, produce a remote effect on other parts of the central nervous system (CNS). (See Fig. 15-5.)

Technique

An 8- to 10-cm, 22-gauge needle is required for gasserian ganglion block. The point of introduction

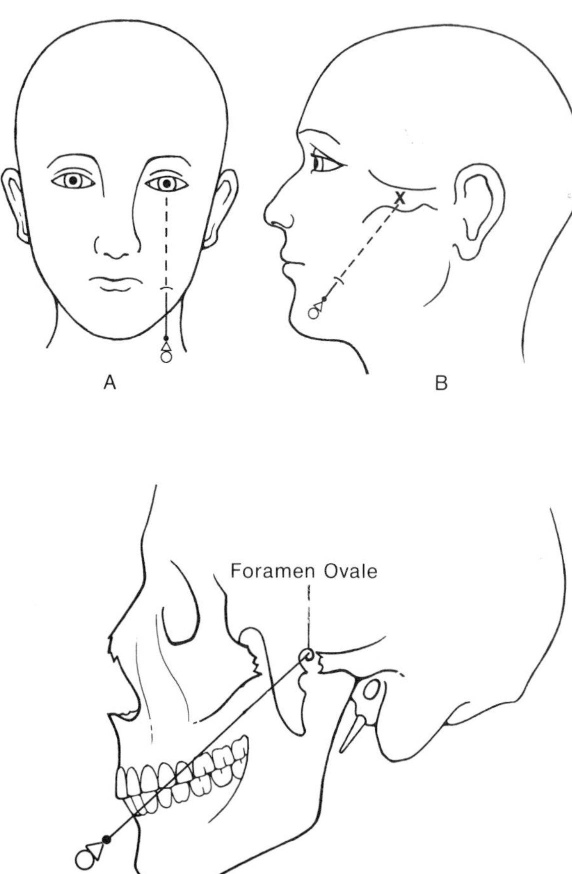

Fig. 15-4. Gasserian ganglion nerve block. Note that needle is directed toward the pupil in the anterior plane (*A*) and toward the midpoint of the zygoma in the lateral plane (*B*). This should result in the needle's entering the foramen ovale, as shown in *C*.

of the needle is approximately one finger's breadth posterior to the lateral margin of the mouth, next to the medial border of the masseter muscle. In edentulous patients, this landmark may not permit a sufficient angle of approach to the foramen ovale, and therefore a point of insertion more caudad is needed. The direction of the needle is both rostral and medial to a point that coincides with the midpoint of the zygomatic arch from the lateral aspect and the pupil from the anterior view (with the eyes looking straight forward), as in Figure 15-4. It is important to keep a guiding finger in the oral cavity, palpating the cheek to ensure that the needle does not enter the mouth and thereby potentially introduce contaminating bacteria into deeper structures. Such an approach will usually result in impingement of the needle on the roof of the infratemporal fossa (*i.e.*, the base of the skull, which is also the floor of the middle cranial fossa). The needle is then adjusted until it slips through the foramen ovale; usually just prior to this, a mandibular nerve paresthesia is obtained in the lower jaw or lip. This maneuver should be performed under radiographic control, so that the needle and its path through the foramen ovale can be visualized.

Having entered the foramen ovale, the needle should not be advanced more than 1 cm, and usually its advance is guided by the appropriate paresthesia. Initially, there will be a third division mandibular paresthesia, but this can occur while the needle is still in the infratemporal fossa. It is necessary to obtain a second division or first division paresthesia to the upper jaw or frontal area of the face, respectively, to confirm that the needle is in fact in the immediate vicinity of the gasserian ganglion. A stimulating device can be used to confirm the place of the needle in patients who are unable to locate the paresthesia accurately. This is, of course, a painful procedure, and it is not inappropriate, perhaps, to administer some intravenous analgesic, for example, .05 mg of fentanyl, as a preoperative medication. For diagnostic blocks, however, it is better not to cloud the sensorium with any analgesics whatsoever in order to obtain a more nearly accurate assessment of the block. Prior to injection, aspiration tests are, of course, mandatory to ensure that the needle has not entered a blood vessel or, more likely, Meckle's cave with its CSF contents. If these aspiration tests are negative, then the anesthetizing agent, either a local anesthetic (1% lidocaine or the equivalent) or neurolytic agent is injected in small aliquots (*e.g.*, 1/4 ml at a time) until the desired analgesic effect is obtained. If injection affords evidence of analgesia in only one of the divisions, then adjustment of the needle can sometimes affect spread to the other divisions—in patients in whom the needle is in the same vertical axis as the ganglion. However, there appear to be some patients in whom the ganglion lies at a more horizontal axis, and in these patients it is sometimes difficult, if not impossible, to obtain a first division paresthesia.

Complications

Depending upon the manipulations needed to produce satisfactory block, the patient's face will quite frequently be painful for the following few days, and there is often bruising at the injection site. This usually responds well to treatment with systemic analgesics. Probably the most serious side-effect is injection of local anesthetic or neurolytic agent into the CSF contained within Meckle's cave and its resulting spillover into the circulating CSF of the cranial cavity. In our clinic, injections of as little as ¼ of a ml of 1 per cent lidocaine have resulted in unconsciousness and profound paralysis of the ipsilateral cranial nerve system, albeit temporary, but the patient needed cardiorespiratory support for a brief period (10 min). If a hyperbaric solution is used (*e.g.*, lidocaine with epinephrine or phenol in glycerine), then the drug that emerges from Meckle's cavity will tend to flow over the free margin of the tentorium cerebelli to affect immediately the sixth, eighth, ninth, 10th, 11th, and 12th cranial nerves and usually consciousness also. With neurolytic agents, there is a potential hazard of spread to these nerves, so that meticulous attention to aspiration tests and perhaps even a test injection of a small dose of local anesthetic is appropriate prior to the injection of any neurolytic substances. If hypobaric solutions are used (*e.g.*, lidocaine without epinephrine, or alcohol), then the flow will tend to be cephalad, involving probably the trochlear and oculomotor nerves initially and almost certainly affecting consciousness to some extent.

OPHTHALMIC NERVE BRANCHES: SUPRAORBITAL AND SUPRATROCHLEAR NERVES

Ophthalmic nerve block is a very simple block that can effect excellent analgesia of the forehead and scalp back to the vertex (Retrobulbar block is described in Chap. 17). It is a simple and safe form of anesthesia for minor surgical procedures in this area (*e.g.*, repair to lacerations, removal of cysts, etc.). The terminal divisions of the ophthalmic branch of the trigeminal nerve involved are the supraorbital and supratrochlear branches, which emerge from within the orbit. The supraorbital branch, like the infraorbital and mental nerves, lies in the same vertical plane as that of the pupil when the patient is looking straight ahead (see Fig. 15-3). A block of this nerve is best effected above the eyebrow after the nerve has emerged from the orbit through the supraorbital notch. A small dose of 2 to 4 ml of local anesthetic infiltrated between the skin and frontal bone will usually produce satisfactory anesthesia. The other terminal branch that supplies the forehead is the supratrochlear nerve, which emerges from the superomedial angle of the orbit and runs up on the forehead parallel to the supraorbital nerve, a finger's breadth or so, medial to it. This nerve is blocked as it emerges above the orbit or can be involved by a medial extension of the anesthetic wheal used to block supraorbital nerve.

Combined Infratrochlear and Anterior Ethmoidal Nerve Block

The nasociliary nerve divides into its terminal branches, anterior ethmoidal and infratrochlear, on the medial wall of the orbit 2.5 cm from the orbital margin. Both branches are blocked by inserting a 5-cm, 25-gauge needle 1 cm above the inner canthus. The needle is directed backward and slightly medially to pass just lateral to the inner wall of the orbit and medial to the eyeball and medial rectus muscle. Depth of insertion is 2.5 cm, and at this point 1 ml of 2 per cent lidocaine, or equivalent, is injected as the needle is slowly withdrawn (see Chap. 17). Orbital veins are easily damaged, resulting in proptosis; thus, small-gauge needles should be used, and repeated insertion should be avoided. The infratrochlear nerve can be blocked by infiltrating at the superomedial border of the orbit and along its medial wall with 2 to 4 ml of local anesthetic. The external nasal branch of the anterior ethmoidal nerve can also be blocked by infiltration at the junction of nasal bone with cartilage, as shown in Figure 15-3. Anterior ethmoidal and infratrochlear nerve blocks accompanied with an infraorbital nerve block can be very effective when they are performed bilaterally for plastic surgical procedures and reduction operations on the nose.

If the mucous membrane of the nose is likely to be stimulated, as in reduction of fractured nose, then branches of the anterior ethmoidal nerve and sphenopalatine ganglion that supply the septum and lateral wall of nose should be blocked by topical application of local anesthetic.

Topical Analgesia of Nasal Cavities

As noted in the description of nerve supply, only two main sites require blockade: the sphenopalatine ganglion and the anterior ethmoidal nerve, both located in the region of the sphenoethmoidal recess.

Applicators. Macintosh described a technique with 25 per cent cocaine paste applied with nasal probes or applicators.[6] Prior spraying of the nasal cavities with 0.5 ml of 5-per-cent cocaine solution on each side provides some shrinking of the mucous membrane and makes the insertion of the applicators more comfortable for the patient. The anesthesiologist then employs a headlight and nasal speculum and gradually applies cocaine paste upward and backward in the nasal cavity. Insertion should ini-

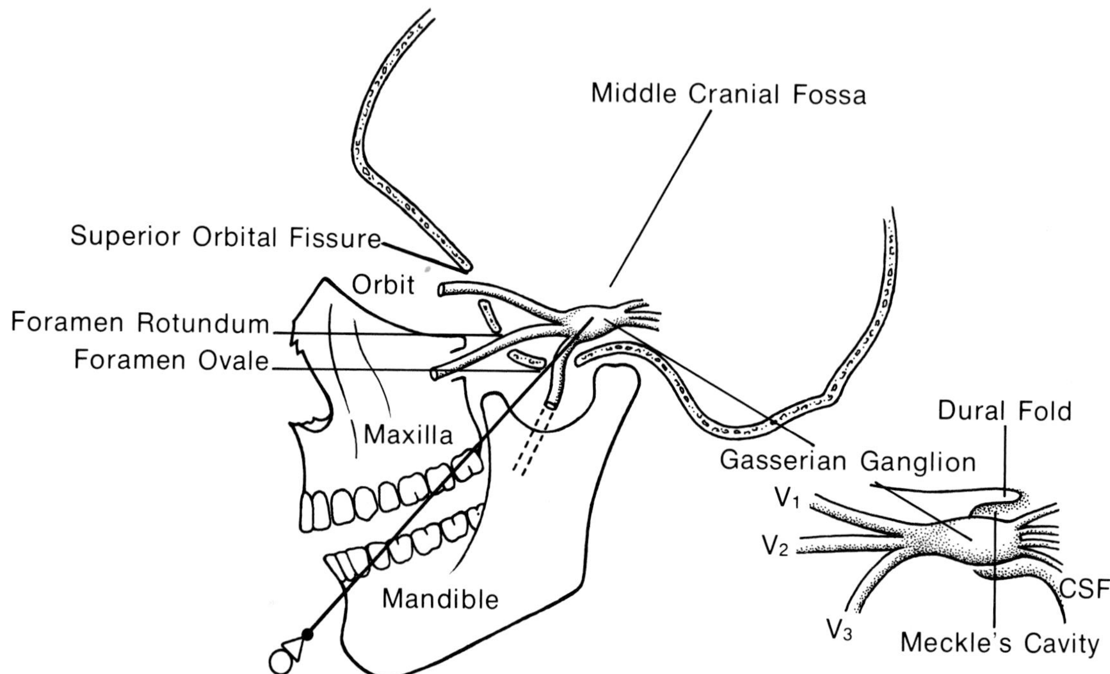

Fig. 15-5. Gasserian ganglion and distribution of its three main branches to the orbit, upper jaw, and lower jaw, respectively. In this diagram, the needle has traversed the foramen ovale, situated in close proximity to the gasserian ganglion. Note relationships of dura to gasserian ganglion, producing Meckle's cavity and bathing the posterior part of the ganglion in cerebrospinal fluid.

tially be close to the septum to avoid injuring the lateral wall. Finally, one applicator is inserted parallel to the anterior border of the nasal cavity until it reaches the anterior end of the cribriform plate at a depth of approximately 5 cm. A second applicator is inserted at an angle of about 20° to the floor of the nose until bone is felt at a depth of approximately 6 to 7 cm. The end of the applicator should now lie close to the sphenopalatine foramen. The two applicators are left in place for 10 to 15 minutes, and the patient is asked to breathe through the mouth. Cocaine pastes of 10 per cent are also available and are preferable if bilateral blocks are to be performed. It should be noted that the total administered dose of solution and paste should not exceed 200 mg (*e.g.,* 1 ml 5-% solution [50 mg]; 1.5 ml 10% paste [150 mg]).

Because of the danger of overdose, some now prefer to use a 10 per cent lidocaine spray for initial anesthesia (20 mg/puff) and then 5 to 10 per cent lidocaine solution up to a maximum dose of 500 mg.

Instillation into sphenoethmoidal recess is unsatisfactory if the mucous membrane is grossly thickened or other pathology exists. Also, it requires the patient to lie with the head upside down, which is distressing to many patients.

Technique. The mucous membrane is initially sprayed with local anesthetic solution, as is described under Applications. The patient is then placed supine with a pillow under the shoulders and the neck extended so that the skull is upside down. The patient is told to breathe through the mouth. A blunt-nosed 10-cm cannula with a 120° angle at its midpoint is inserted through the nares until the angle lies at the external nares. The cannula is now swiveled, keeping close to the septum, until the end reaches the roof of the nose. Local anesthetic (*e.g.,* 2 ml 5% cocaine or 2 ml 10% lidocaine) is injected. The procedure is repeated on the other side. The position is maintained for 10 minutes, and then the patient rolls supine, while holding the nares pinched, and lets the solution run out of the external nares.

MAXILLARY NERVE

Block of Main Division in Pterygopalatine Fossa

As it crosses the pterygopalatine fossa, the maxillary nerve is usually blocked by a lateral approach. The resulting block will produce profound anesthesia of the upper jaw and its teeth on the ipsilateral side of the face (Fig. 15-6).

Technique. The nerve is approached by way of the infratemporal fossa, and the needle is inserted in the skin at a point below the midpoint of the zygomatic arch overlying the coronoid notch of the mandible. Location of the point of needle insertion is aided by asking the patient to open the mouth wide and palpating the condyle of the mandible as it moves anteriorly to the midpoint of the zygoma. When the mouth is closed, the condyle leaves a clear entry path through the coronoid notch. An 8-cm 22-gauge needle is inserted through the skin and subcutaneous tissues, which contain the parotid gland and possibly some of the rostral portions of the "pes anserinus" branches of the facial nerve, destined for the orbicularis oculi muscles. An extensive subcutaneous infiltration of local anesthetic at this site may result in some temporary weakness of these muscles. Having traversed the coronoid notch of the mandible, the needle is directed medially until it reaches the medial wall of the infratemporal fossa, where it will strike the lateral surface of the lateral pterygoid plate, usually at a depth of about 5 cm. The needle is now "walked" anteriorly from the lateral pterygoid plate until it enters the pterygopalatine fossa, where it is advanced a further quarter of an inch into the fossa. Usually, a paresthesia is not obtained or sought, and 5 ml of local anesthetic is injected into this fossa to produce anesthesia of the maxillary nerve.

Complications. Because of the highly vascular nature of the contents of this fossa—containing as it does the five terminal branches of the maxillary artery with all their venae comitantes plus the veins that drain the orbit by way of the inferior orbital fissure—a hematoma is frequently a sequel to this block. Such a hematoma can spread into the orbit and produce a profound black eye. The treatment of this is symptomatic since it usually resolves in several days. Spread of local anesthetic to the optic nerve may occur, producing temporary blindness. The patient should, of course, be forewarned. This approach is not favored for neurolytic blockade because of proximity to the orbit. If maxillary division neurolytic blockade is required, it is common practice to employ the approach described under Gasserian Ganglion Block. Alternatively, some favor neurolytic blockade of the infraorbital nerve if pain is confined to infraorbital nerve territory.

Alternate Approach by way of the Orbit. An alternative approach for blocking the maxillary nerve involves traversing the inferolateral borders of the orbit and depositing the local anesthetic in the pterygopalatine fossa superolaterally. A 6 cm 22-gauge needle is inserted at the junction of the inferior and lateral borders of the orbit and, keeping close to the bone, is advanced for a distance of 4 cm. It will then have entered the inferior orbital fissure, and its tip lies in the pterygopalatine fossa. No attempts are made to seek a paresthesia, and 5 ml of local anesthetic is injected at this site. This approach may also be complicated by hematoma

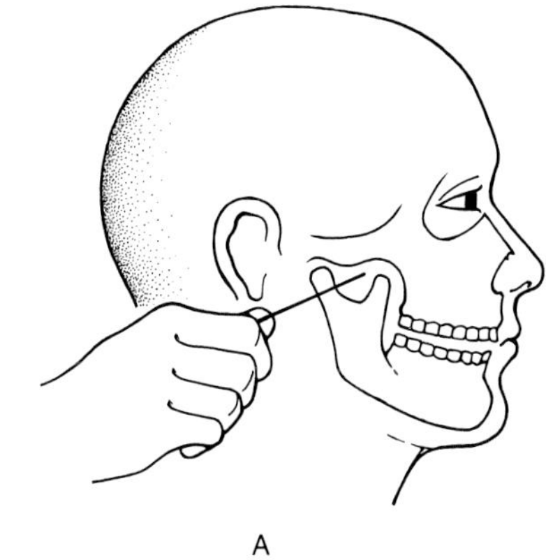

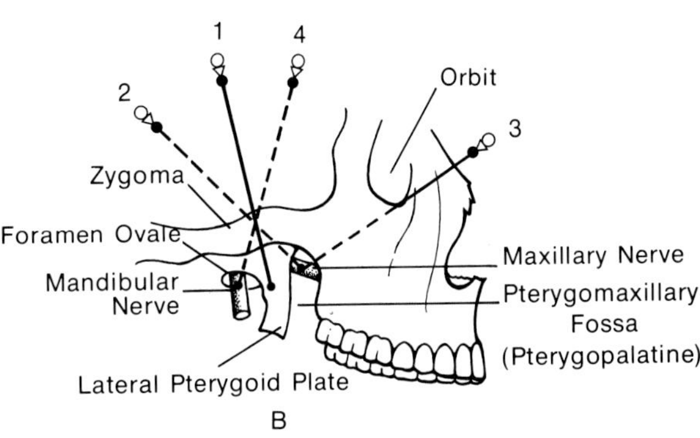

Fig. 15-6. Maxillary and mandibular nerve block. (*A*) Approach to the infratemporal fossa is by way of the coronoid notch of the mandible below the midpoint of the zygoma. (*B*) The needle is positioned in relationship to deeper structures. Upon introduction, the needle strikes the lateral pterygoid plate (*needle 1*) and is then positioned for the chosen block. For maxillary nerve block, the needle is "walked" anteriorly from the lateral pterygoid plate into the pterygomaxillary fossa (*needle 2*). An alternative approach to the maxillary nerve in this situation is by way of the inferiolateral aspect of the orbit, as shown by *needle 3*. For mandibular nerve block, the needle is "walked" posteriorly from *position 1* to *position 4*, where it will encounter the mandibular nerve emerging through the foramen ovale immediately posterior to posterior edge of the lateral pterygoid plate.

production or spread of local anesthetic to the optic nerve, producing temporary blindness. The eyeball itself does not encroach directly upon the path of the needle in this block.

Although this is not recommended as a first choice for second division trigeminal block, it is an alternative when local conditions may preclude the conventional approach by the infratemporal fossa.

Alternate Approach by Way of the Infratemporal Fossa. Yet another alternative approach to the maxillary nerve is by way of the anterior aspect of the infratemporal fossa.[6] The needle is introduced anterior to the coronoid process of the mandible at a point below the anterior aspect of the zygomatic arch. This permits a medial approach toward the pupil of the eye, passing posterior to the posterior surface of the maxilla directly into the pterygopalatine fossa. The needle should not be inserted to a depth greater than 5 cm because this approach can be used to proceed unchecked into the optic nerve and by way of its foramen into the cranial cavity.[6] In contrast, the approach by way of the coronoid notch involves an anterior direction so that if the needle is advanced too deeply it will impinge on the posterior surface of the maxillary or palatine bones and thereby be prevented from damaging deeper structures.

Block of Branches of Maxillary Nerves

Extraoral block of infraorbital nerve is accomplished below the junction of the medial and middle thirds of the lower border of the orbit. This point lies in the same vertical plane as the pupil and the supraorbital and mental foramina (see Fig. 15-3). It is important to appreciate that the infraorbital foramen emerges in a caudad and medial direction and actually to enter this foramen it is important to direct a 4-cm 22 to 25-gauge needle laterally and cephalad. However, to block the nerve, infiltration of 1 to 2 ml of 1 per cent lidocaine or the equivalent at its exit from the foramen is usually all that is needed, and it is not essential actually to enter the foramen. Block of this nerve will afford satisfactory anesthesia of the skin of the cheek medially to, and only partially including, the nose, which is also supplied by terminal branches of the first division of the trigeminal (*i.e.*, infratrochlear and external nasal nerves). It will provide analgesia of the upper lip to the midline except in patients whose philtrum is derived from first division dermatomes; in them, this middle portion of the upper lip will be supplied by the first division of the trigeminal nerve. This block is useful for superficial surgery in the dermal distribution of the nerve but will not, of course, produce any analgesia of deeper second division structures, such as the teeth, unless the injection is made directly into the canal (see Chap. 16).

The two remaining branches of the maxillary division, zygomaticotemporal and zygomaticofacial, can be anesthetized by infiltration at the sites of emergence from the zygomatic bone, as shown in Figure 15-3. The indications for these are infrequently encountered.

MANDIBULAR NERVE

Block of Main Division in the Infratemporal Fossa

The approach for blocking the main division in the infratemporal fossa is initially the same as that described for the maxillary nerve; that is, a 6 cm, 22-gauge needle is introduced below the midpoint of the zygomatic arch and passes through the coronoid notch of the mandible, directed medially across the infratemporal fossa until it impinges upon the bony medial wall (*i.e.*, the lateral aspect of the lateral pterygoid plate) (Fig. 15-6). At this stage, the directions differ from those for a maxillary nerve block; for here the needle is "walked" posteriorly from the lateral pterygoid plate until a third division paresthesia is obtained. If a paresthesia is not obtained, the needle, once it leaves the posterior aspect of the lateral pterygoid plate, can pierce the attached superior constrictor muscle and enter the pharynx.

Third division block here produces analgesia of the skin over the lower jaw, except at the angle, of the superior two-thirds of the anterior surface of the auricle, and of a strip of skin that often extends up to the temporal area (see Fig. 15-2). If sufficient concentration of local anesthetic is injected to result in motor blockade (1% lidocaine or equivalent), then the muscles of mastication will also be anesthetized, resulting in some incoordination of ipsilateral movements of the jaw. This is well tolerated after temporary blocks but is a long-term complication of permanent blockade. The otic ganglion lying in such intimate connection posterior to the mandibular division just below the foramen ovale is inevitably blocked. This nerve supplies secretomotor fibers to the parotid gland, which pursue a peripatetic course from the inferior salivary nucleus, and thus permanent impairment of secretion of this gland is a possible sequel of neurolytic blockade of the mandibular nerve.

Block of Branches

Extraoral Block of Mental Nerve. The mental foramen, as mentioned above, lies in the same vertical line as the supraorbital and infraorbital foramen and the pupil, with the pupil in the midposition (Fig. 15-3). The position of the mental foramen varies with age, being more caudal on the mandibular ramus in youth and much nearer the alveolar margin of the mandible in the endentulous aged person. Although this nerve can be blocked by the intraoral route, it is possible to accomplish blockade extraorally (see Chap. 16). To enter the mental foramen, it is necessary to direct the needle anteriorally and caudad. However, it is not necessary actually to enter the foramen, and an infiltration over the midpoint of the mandible in the vertical line, is usually ample to produce analgesia of the lower lip and chin and is effective anesthesia for operative procedures there.

Auriculotemporal nerve can be blocked as it ascends over the posterior root of the zygoma behind the superficial temporal artery, and infiltration of 3 to 5 ml 1 per cent lidocaine or the equivalent results in anesthesia of the upper two-thirds of the temporal fossa.

GLOSSOPHARYNGEAL NERVE BLOCK

The ninth cranial nerve emerges by way of the jugular foramen in very close relationship to the vagus and accessory nerves along with the internal jugular vein. It is blocked just below this point, and therefore both temporary and permanent blocks usually involve these other two cranial nerves, all three of which lie in the groove between the internal jugular vein and the internal carotid artery (Fig. 15-7*B*). These two large vascular conduits may well be punctured during attempts to block these nerves at this site, resulting in either intravascular injection or hematoma. Even very small amounts (*e.g.*, ¼ ml of local anesthetic injected into the carotid artery at this point) can produce quite profound effects of convulsion and loss of consciousness.

Therefore, as always, aspiration tests must be meticulous. The landmarks for this block involve locating the styloid process of the temporal bone. This osseous process represents the calcification of the cephalic end of the stylohyoid ligament. This fibrous band, which passes from the base of the skull to the lesser cornu of the hyoid bone, ossifies to a different extent in different patients. Although it is relatively easy to identify in people with a large styloid process, if ossification has been limited, then the styloid process sometimes cannot be located with the exploring needle.

Technique

A 5-cm, 22-gauge needle is inserted at a point midway on a line joining the angle of the mandible to the tip of the mastoid process of the occipital bone (Fig. 15-7). The needle is advanced directly medially until it locates the styloid process. In the event that the styloid process is not located, it is inserted to a depth of 3 cm. In patients who have had a radical neck dissection and therefore are often candidates for this kind of block, the removal of the sternomastoid muscle places the styloid process and its adjacent nerves and vessels at a much more superficial location. In fact, in these patients, the styloid process can often be palpated in the interval between mastoid process and the posterior border of the mandible. The needle will need to be inserted only 1–2 cm. Ideally, the styloid process is located as a bony endpoint and the needle adjusted posterior to this at the same depth as the process. An injection of 1 to 2 ml of 1 per cent lidocaine or the equivalent will produce anesthesia of the glossopharyngeal and the vagus and accessory nerves as well. It is not possible at this site to block selectively one of these three nerves.

Glossopharyngeal nerve block is utilized most frequently for inoperable carcinomas that invade the distribution of the nerve in either the posterior third of the tongue or the pharyngeal areas. Such patients are often quite willing to undergo additional unilateral blockade of the accessory nerve with resulting weakness of the sternomastoid and trapezius muscles and with numbness of the laryngeal inlet and trachea, and paralysis of the ipsilateral vocal cords (with resulting hoarseness).

The injection of neurolytic agents at this site so close to the large vascular carotid and jugular conduits is cause for concern because of the possibility of damage to the walls of these vessels, which might result in slough and necrosis with potentially disastrous sequelae. However, such a complication has not yet been reported.

An alternative approach for intraorally blocking the glossopharyngeal nerve has recently been reported by DeMeester.[3] This technique involves injecting local anesthetic into the midpoint of the posterior pillar of the fauces. This appears to offer considerable promise as a means of blocking the glossopharyngeal nerve distribution to the oropharynx and, in combination with laryngeal nerve

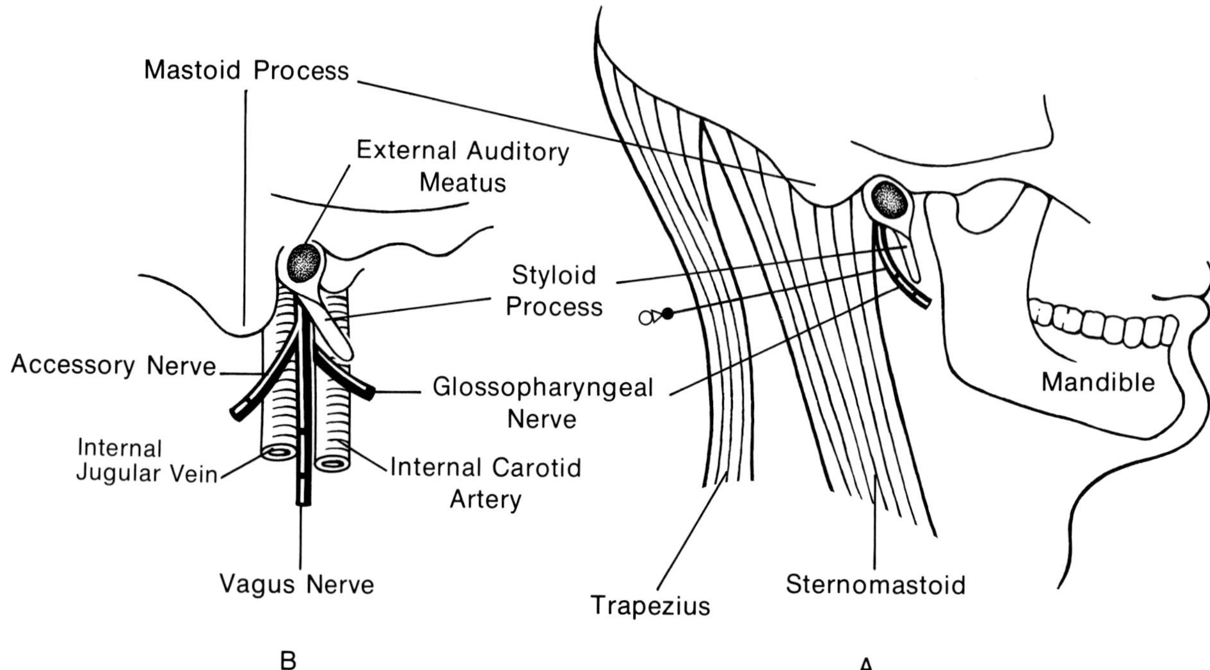

Fig. 15-7. Glossopharyngeal nerve block. (*A*) The glossopharyngeal nerve is shown curving posterior to the styloid process and is blocked approximately halfway between the mastoid process and the angle of the jaw. (*B*) shows the close relationship of the vagus and the accessory cranial nerves with the internal carotid artery and jugular vein. Any or all of these structures may be involved in attempts to block the glossopharyngeal nerve at this point.

blocks (see below) and topical anesthesia, poses great potential for endoscopic procedures under regional anesthesia.

VAGUS NERVE BLOCK

The main trunk of the vagus nerve is rarely, if ever, blocked as a primary procedure. However, the branches of sensory distribution to the larynx can be blocked simply and efficiently, thereby rendering the laryngeal inlet and trachea insensitive to pain. This is very useful for intubations performed on conscious patients and other endoscopic procedures. These branches can also be blocked permanently for pain relief in terminal neoplastic disease in the area.

Superior Laryngeal Nerve Block

This branch of the vagus nerve is easily blocked as it sweeps around the inferior border of the greater cornu of the hyoid bone, which is readily palpable even in the most obese patients. By pressing on the opposite greater cornu of the hyoid bone, the laryngeal structures can be displaced toward the side to be blocked (Fig. 15-8). A small 2.5-cm, 25-gauge needle is usually all that is required. It is "walked" from the inferior border of the greater cornu of the hyoid near its tip, and 3 ml of local anesthetic is infiltrated both superficially and deep to the thyrohyoid membrane. Penetration of this membrane is felt as a slight loss of resistance. The procedure is repeated on the other side. This will produce anesthesia over the inferior aspect of the epiglottis and the laryngeal inlet as far down as the vocal cords. It will also produce motor blockade (if the concentration of lidocaine exceeds 1% or the equivalent for other drugs) of the cricothyroid muscles.

To produce anesthesia below the cords, the simplest and most useful method is transtracheal puncture. Here, a relatively wide-bore needle (*i.e.*, 20- or 22-gauge) is used so that air can be aspirated. The needle is introduced in the midline through the cricothyroid membrane. Entry of the needle into the trachea is identified by aspiration of air, and the patient will usually cough slightly at this stage.

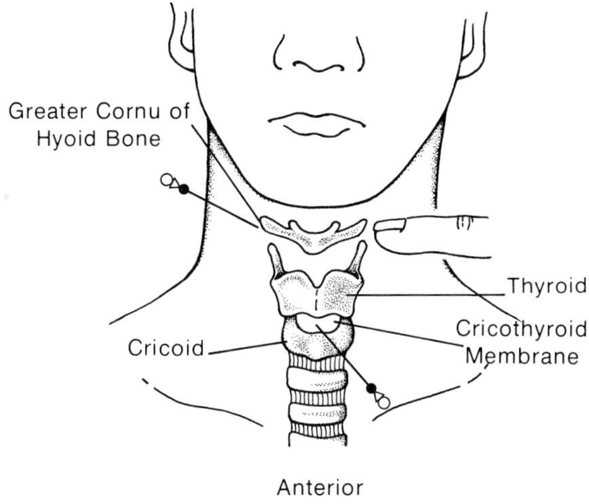

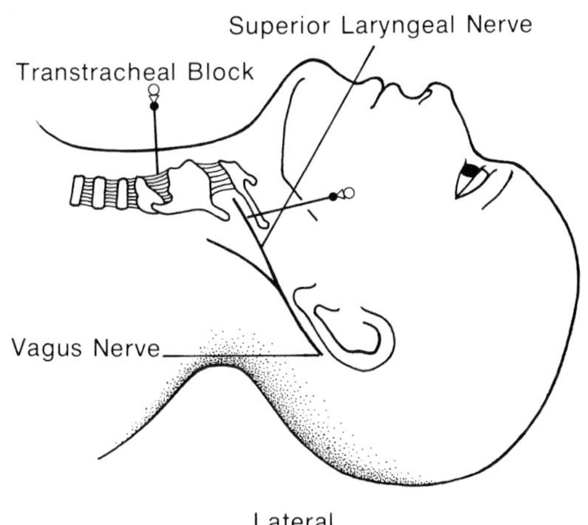

Fig. 15-8. Block of vagal nerve distribution to larynx and trachea. The superior laryngeal nerve and, therefore, both its internal and external branches are blocked below the apex of the greater cornu of the hyoid bone. This affects analgesia of the laryngeal inlet as far down as the vocal cords. Anesthesia below the vocal cords is best affected by a transtracheal spray, in which the needle is introduced through the cricothyroid membrane as shown.

Rapid injection of 3 to 5 ml of local anesthetic will produce a dramatic cough in all but the most obtunded patients, and this spreads the local anesthetic up and down the trachea and yields satisfactory topical anesthesia. It is usually necessary to use a higher concentration for this topical anesthesia than for nerve block, and 4 per cent lidocaine is frequently chosen, although 2 per cent lidocaine will produce adequate blockade but will take a little longer.

The nerve that supplies the wall of the trachea below that of the vocal cords is the recurrent laryngeal nerve. Although it is possible to block this nerve specifically (and in fact block of this nerve frequently occurs as a complication of stellate ganglion blocks), there is usually no need to block this nerve per se. In the event that blockade of the recurrent laryngeal nerve was ever required (*e.g.,* for a possible neurolytic block for cancers of the vocal cords or below), then the nerve, which lies, in the groove between esophagus and trachea can be blocked at any cervical level below the cricoid cartilage. Attempts at this block would, of course, demand meticulous technique to avoid involvement of brachial plexus with an overly deep insertion of the needle.

ACCESSORY NERVE (11TH CRANIAL NERVE) BLOCK

There are very few indications to block the accessory nerve. It may be useful for trapezius block as an adjunct to interscalene nerve blocks of the brachial plexus for surgery on the shoulder. With interscalene block alone, the patient has adequate analgesia of the operative site, but motor power is maintained in the trapezius muscle. He can, by shrugging his shoulders, inadvertently interfere with the procedure.

By also blocking the accessory nerve in the posterior triangle of the neck, the trapezius muscle is paralyzed and the surgery often facilitated. The posterior triangle of the neck is a compartment bounded anteriorly by the posterior border of sternomastoid muscle, laterally by the anterior border of the trapezius, and inferiorly by the middle third of the clavicle. The accessory nerve traverses this triangle in a very superficial location (Fig. 15-9). It emerges from the substance of the sternomastoid muscle at the junction of the superior and middle thirds of the posterior border of the muscle and proceeds in a downward and lateral course across the triangle to enter the trapezius muscle at the junction of the middle and inferior third of its anterior border. Anywhere along this course, it can successfully be blocked. The accessory nerve lies superficial to the prevertebral fascia and therefore is lying deep only to skin, platysma, and deep cervical fascia. Therefore, if a needle is introduced at the junction of the middle and superior thirds of the sternomastoid muscle at its lateral border and an infiltration of 10 ml or so of local anesthetic is used, block can be

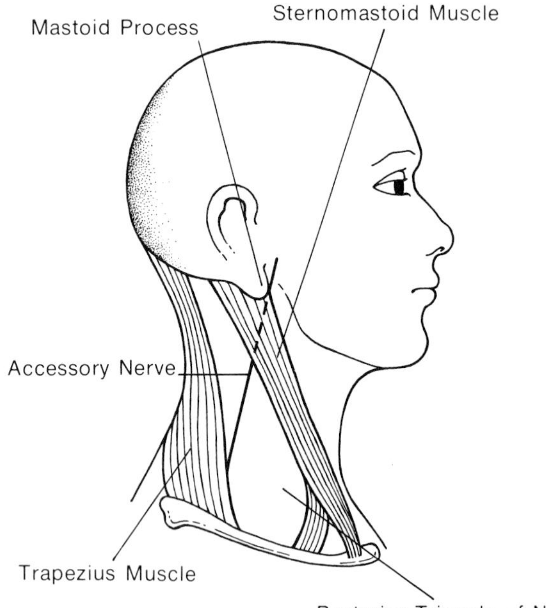

Fig. 15-9. Accessory nerve block. The path of the accessory nerve is shown after its exit from the jugular foramen through the substance of the sternomastoid muscle and in the posterior triangle of the neck. It is blocked as it enters the posterior triangle at the junction of the superior and middle thirds of the posterior border of the sternomastoid muscle. It is also possible to produce block of this nerve by infiltration of the sternomastoid muscle below the mastoid process.

accomplished. Accuracy can be increased if a stimulating device is used to locate the nerve. This nerve is not infrequently inadvertently blocked when a superficial cervical plexus block is performed, and vice versa.

Ramamurthy has recently described a technique for blocking this nerve as it lies within the sternomastoid muscle.[8] This is accomplished by infiltrating the substance of the muscle with 10 to 20 ml of local anesthetic below its attachment to the mastoid process. It is used for the therapy of spasms and painful conditions of the sternomastoid muscle itself.

CERVICAL PLEXUS BLOCK

The cervical plexus is formed by loops between the anterior primary rami of the upper four cervical nerves. Its muscular branches are distributed to the prevertebral muscles, strap muscles of the neck, and, of course, the contributions to the phrenic nerve.

Superficial Cervical Plexus Block

Block at the Midpoint of the Posterior Border of the Sternomastoid. The cutaneous distribution of the cervical plexus is to the skin of the anterolateral neck by way of the anterior primary rami of C2–4. These emerge as four distinct nerves from the posterior border of the sternoidmastoid at approximately its midpoint, just below the emergence of the accessory nerve. The first branch radiates upward and backward as the lesser occipital nerve to supply part of the posterior surface of the upper part of the ear and skin behind the ear; the second branch runs upward and forward as the great auricular nerve, which supplies skin over the posterior surface of the ear and the anterior lower third of the ear, as well as over the angle of the mandible; the third branch, the anterior cutaneous nerve of the neck, supplies skin from the chin to the suprasternal notch; the fourth branches, the supraclavicular nerves, supply the skin over the inferior aspect of the neck and the clavicle and down as far as the area overlying the second rib, while laterally, these supraclavicular nerves supply the skin over the deltoid muscle and posteriorly as far as the spine of the

Fig. 15-10. (*A*) Superficial cervical plexus block is performed in the posterior triangle of the neck at the midpoint of the posterior border of the sternomastoid muscle (note how close this is to the accessory nerve as shown in Fig. 15-9, and therefore block of either of these nerves can involve the other). Note also greater occipital branch of posterior rami, which is blocked at midpoint of superior nuchal line between the mastoid process and greater occipital protuberance. (*B*) Results of blockade of cutaneous nerves of head and neck. The approximate areas of denervation resulting from blockade of individual cutaneous nerves are shown. The area of complete analgesia varies considerably when only peripheral branches are blocked. In the scalp, the ascending nerves are effectively blocked by a band of local anesthetic injected from glabella to occiput, immediately above the ear (see text). In the face, individual nerves, such as the infraorbital and external nasal and infratrochlear, may be blocked for restricted areas of denervation. In the neck, either the superficial or deep cervical plexus may be blocked to achieve complete denervation of the neck.

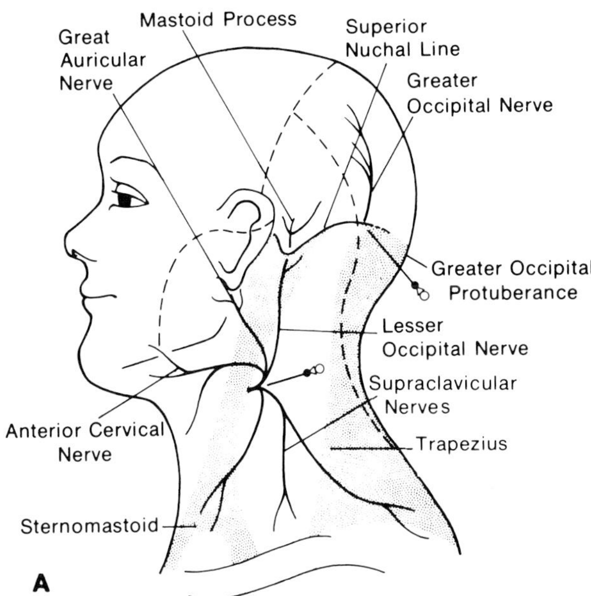

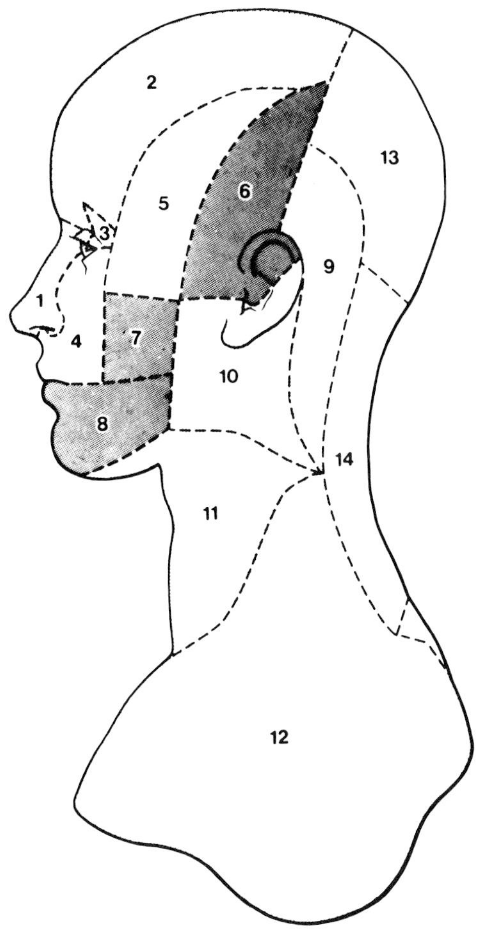

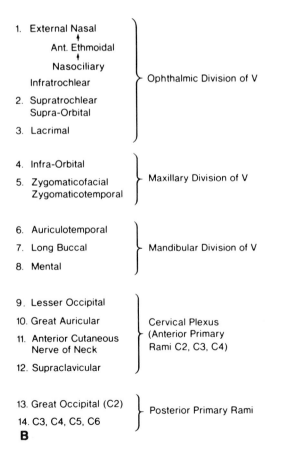

1. External Nasal
   ↑
   Ant. Ethmoidal
   ↑
   Nasociliary
   Infratrochlear
2. Supratrochlear
   Supra-Orbital
3. Lacrimal

} Ophthalmic Division of V

4. Infra-Orbital
5. Zygomaticofacial
   Zygomaticotemporal

} Maxillary Division of V

6. Auriculotemporal
7. Long Buccal
8. Mental

} Mandibular Division of V

9. Lesser Occipital
10. Great Auricular
11. Anterior Cutaneous Nerve of Neck
12. Supraclavicular

} Cervical Plexus (Anterior Primary Rami C2, C3, C4)

13. Great Occipital (C2)
14. C3, C4, C5, C6

} Posterior Primary Rami

B

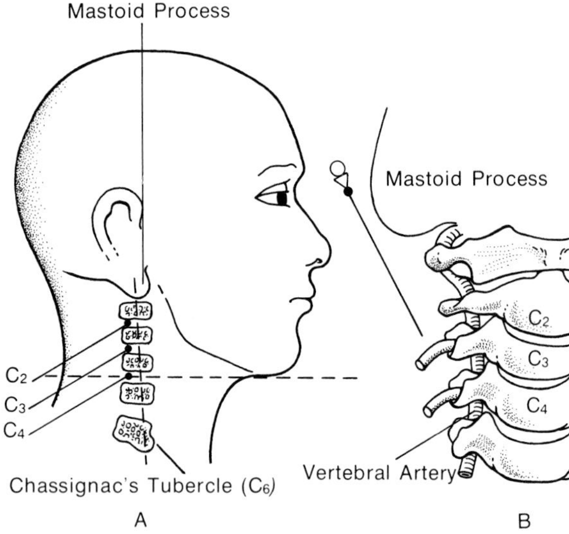

Fig. 15-11. Deep cervical plexus block. (*A*) Note that C2–4 cervical nerves lie in a plane just posterior to a line joining the mastoid process to Chassaignac's tubercle on C6. A horizontal line drawn through the chin intersects this vertical line approximately at the level of the C4 nerve. (*B*) Note the caudal direction of the needle. This is to prevent its entering the neuraxis, as might occur with a more horizontal or cephalad direction. Note also the proximity of the vertebral artery as it traverses the foramina transversaria in the transverse processes.

scapula. All four nerves can be blocked by infiltration at the midpoint of the posterior border of the sternomastoid (Fig. 15-10). Lidocaine, 1 per cent (5–10 ml), or the equivalent (5 ml–10 ml), infiltrated at this area will produce analgesia of the neck from the mandible to the clavicle, both anteriorly and laterally.

Block of Greater Occipital Nerve

The skin over the posterior extensor muscles of the neck and extending up over the occiput as high as the vertex is supplied by the posterior rami of the cervical nerves. Of these, the greater occipital nerve is perhaps the most clinically significant. It is best blocked as it crosses the superior nuchal line, approximately midway between the external occipital protuberance and the mastoid process. It is located at this site by palpating the occipital artery that lies adjacent to it. Infiltration of 5 ml of 1 per cent lidocaine or the equivalent around the artery will usually effect satisfactory block of this nerve and result in a band of anesthesia from the occiput to the vertex. This block is used along with blocks of the supraorbital, supratrochlear, auriculotemporal, and lesser occipital nerves to render the scalp anesthetic for operative procedures. It is also a useful block in both the diagnosis and treatment of occipital tension headaches. The mechanisms whereby such a block would relieve these headaches have not been elucidated.

Deep Cervical Plexus Block

Deep cervical plexus block is, in effect, a paravertebral nerve block of C2–C4 spinal nerves as they emerge by way of the foramina in the cervical vertebrae. Each nerve lies in the sulcus in the transverse process of these vertebrae (Fig. 15-11*B*). Usually, three needles are used, being inserted at the levels of C2, C3, and C4. The sites of insertion are located by reference to a line that joins the tip of the mastoid process with Chassaignac's tubercle of C6, which is readily palpated at the level of the cricoid cartilage. A further line is drawn parallel and posterior to this at a distance of 1 cm. The C2 transverse process is usually located approximately one finger's breadth caudad to the mastoid process on this line, and C3 and C4 are at similar intervals caudally on the same line. A horizontal line through the lower border of the ramus of the mandible intersects this line at C4 (Fig. 15-11*A*). Five cm, 22-gauge needles are directed medially and caudad. The reason for the caudad direction is to avoid inadvertently entering the intervertebral foramen and producing a peridural or spinal block. The endpoint is the bony landmark of the transverse process, and paresthesias are obtained. Injection of 3 to 4 ml of 1 per cent lidocaine or the equivalent on each nerve is usually adequate for anesthesia. Fortunately, the paravertebral space communicates freely in the cervical region, and the anesthetic solution can spread easily to adjacent levels. Deep cervical plexus block can quite often be obtained with injections at just one level with a larger volume, that is, 6 to 8 ml (see also Chap. 10).

This block is sometimes useful for such procedures as thyroidectomy and tracheostomy under local anesthesia and is also used effectively for carotid endarterectomy or for removal of cervical lymph nodes. A significant complication of the block is due to the proximity of the vertebral artery, so that direct intra-arterial injection may produce the profound and very rapid toxic side-effects of convulsions and unconsciousness; therefore, aspiration tests are of great importance. Extension of the anesthetic into the epidural or subdural spaces is theoretically possible by either dural sleeves or leakage through intervertebral foramen; thus patients who undergo such procedures must be observed very carefully.

When the block is performed bilaterally, bilateral phrenic nerve block is a serious hazard. Because the deep cervical plexus lies deep to the deep cervical fascia, spread to the cervical sympathetic chain should not occur. If, however, infiltration has spread anterior to the prevertebral fascia, then the cervical sympathetic chain will be involved, with resultant Horner's syndrome and also spread to the recurrent laryngeal nerve, resulting in hoarseness. Both of these complications in a failed block will indicate that, in fact, the anesthetic has been injected at a site too superficial to the deep cervical fascia.

PRACTICAL APPLICATIONS

Regional anesthesia of the head and neck can be very useful for surgical anesthesia, for the diagnosis and therapy of various pain states, and for postoperative pain relief.

This anesthesia is eminently suited for minor plastic and other procedures on superficial structures in patients in whom general anesthesia may well constitute a greater than normal risk (*e.g.*, elderly patients, patients with full stomachs or cardiorespiratory failure, etc.). It is well suited for outpatient surgery. It is also very useful as a supplement to light general anesthesia for many of the surgical procedures around the oral cavity, particularly since regional block of the second or third division of the trigeminal nerve with a long-acting local anesthetic agent can afford excellent postoperative analgesia for patients who have had their jaws wired together and, because of the threat to the airway, effective doses of narcotics are usually being withheld.

Some surgical procedures in the neck lend themselves well to regional anesthesia. Thyroidectomy does constitute a risk to the recurrent laryngeal nerve and, rarely, may be performed with an awake, cooperative patient so that the patient's voice can act as an excellent monitor to the integrity of the nerve however, as noted above, bilateral deep cervical plexus block is required. The patient's state of wakefulness is such a good indication of cerebral perfusion that some vascular surgeons prefer performing their carotid arterial surgery this way. This can be accomplished with deep cervical plexus block.

It is perhaps in the field of endoscopy that regional anesthesia of the oral, pharyngeal, and laryngeal compartments has its most frequent application. There are a significant number of instances in anesthesia in which it is desirable to ensure intubation of the trachea prior to obtunding the patient's normal protective reflexes. This "awake" intubation can be executed admirably with either spray or nerve blocks. Such "awake" intubations are often necessary on patients with an unstable neck, secondary to cervical fracture, and a combination of spray or laryngeal nerve blocks will permit oro- or nasotracheal intubation without the necessity of risking undue flexion or extension movement in the neck, as occurs in routine laryngoscopy. Also, with the patient awake, the integrity of his CNS can be monitored during this maneuver. In cases in which there may be difficulty with intubation, such as facial fractures, intubation under local analgesia does not preclude the use of any alternatives if it fails. Such analgesia also lends itself well to diagnostic endoscopies of the pharynx, larynx, and even trachea for investigative and biopsy purposes (see also Chap. 16).

For patients with pain problems in the head and neck, regional analgesia permits elucidation of the pathway of the noxious stimulus, if any, and by an appropriate combination of different long- and short-acting local anesthetics, with placebo blocks, it is often possible to predict the effect of nerve section or neurolysis. In patients with cancer of the head and neck, blocks of the trigeminal, glossopharyngeal, laryngeal, or cervical plexus, either alone or in combination, can often afford excellent pain relief (see also Chap. 27).

Skill in regional anesthesia of this area of the body is not only a challenging and technically satisfying addition to the anesthesiologist's repertoire, it also provides optimal anesthesia for certain kinds of surgical procedures, can provide long lasting postoperative pain relief, and is important in pain-unit work.

In order to acquire the required level of expertise, it is useful to begin learning these techniques on anesthetized patients. Successful blockade then permits reduction, or deletion, of doses of supplemental anesthetics. If long-acting local anesthetics, such as bupivacaine or etidocaine, are employed, then the patient also receives the benefit of excellent postoperative analgesia in situations in which effective analgesic doses of narcotics are contraindicated (*e.g.*, surgery in close proximity to the airway).

The majority of operations in the head and neck area can be performed under the effects of some form of supplementary neural blockade. Only by routine supplementation of light general anesthesia by neural blockade in such cases can the success rate gradually improve. Unless this approach is used, the anesthesiologist will find it difficult to provide an acceptable success rate for patients who have strong indications for head and neck procedures under neural blockade alone. It should be recognized that selection of the appropriate peripheral nerves for blockade can permit very effective and efficient analgesia for a wide range of plastic surgery procedures. Volumes of local anesthetic as small as 1 ml can be employed for individual nerves and then supplemented by minimal infiltration of the incision line, which is marked on the skin preoperatively. In one large plastic surgery unit, virtually all major plastic surgery of the face in elderly patients is carried out with peripheral neural blockade.*

* Grey, W.: Personal communication.

REFERENCES

1. Adriani, J.: Labat's Regional Anesthesia: Techniques and Clinical Applications. ed. 3. Philadelphia, W.B. Saunders, 1967.
2. Bonica, J.J.: The Management of Pain. Philadelphia, Lea & Febiger, 1953.
3. DeMeester, T.R., and Benson, D.W.: Glossopharyngeal block for endoscopy. Clinical Trends in Anesthesiology, *6*:2, 1976.
4. Ericksson, E.: Illustrated Handbook in Local Anesthesia. Chicago, Year Book Medical Publishers, 1969.
5. Last, R.J.: Anatomy: Regional and Applied. ed. 5. Edinburgh, Churchill Livingstone, 1973.
6. Macintosh, R.R., and Ostlere, M.: Local Analgesia, Head and Neck. ed. 2. Edinburgh, E & S Livingstone, 1967.
7. Moore, D.C.: Regional Block. ed. 4. Springfield, Charles C Thomas, 1975.
8. Ramamurthy, S., Akkinemi, A., and Winnie, A.P.: A simple method for spinal accessory nerve block. *In* Abstracts of Scientific Papers—Annual Meeting. Chicago, American Society of Anesthesiologists, 1976.
9. Sweet, W.T., and Wepsic, J.G.: Controlled thermocoagulation of trigeminal ganglion and rootlets for differential destruction of pain fibers, Part I: Trigeminal neuralgia. J. Neurosurg., *39*:143, 1974.

PART TWO

Techniques of Neural Blockade

Section E: Specialized Surgical Applications

16 Neural Blockade for Dental, Oral, and Adjoining Areas

Jeffrey G. Garber

Regional anesthesia of the oral cavity and adjoining tissues can be achieved by either extraoral or intraoral techniques. Anesthetic techniques that involve extraoral routes have traditionally been utilized by the medical profession, while the dental profession has mainly relied on intraoral methods to achieve its anesthetic goals. In an attempt to reform this practice, this chapter is an initiation into methods of intraoral regional anesthesia. It is hoped that readers already familiar with extraoral techniques will utilize the techniques presented here to expand their anesthetic armamentarium, enabling them to offer a wider range of clinical skills.

Dental and surgical operations on the maxilla and mandible may be performed using intraoral nerve block techniques. Selective use of these blocks may also aid the practitioner in defining and treating various facial pain problems. Careful attention must be paid to details of technique, as well as to selection of the least toxic drugs and vasoconstrictors, if complications and unpleasant side-effects are to be avoided.

The area around the mouth is psychologically very sensitive. Care must be taken to alleviate anxiety produced by the thought of anesthesia and surgery. In most cases, informing the patient in advance about what is to happen will encourage cooperation. With a gentle, caring approach and adherence to technique, the patient and anesthesiologist will find these various injections to be performed easily and with little or no discomfort. With this in mind, members of both the medical and dental community will find ever increasing use for these techniques.

Learning to block sensory pathways of the oral cavity and its surrounding tissues requires a mastery of the anatomical features that serve as guides for delivering local anesthetics to sites within close proximity to specific nerves or nerve fibers.[1–6] Consequently, the anatomical descriptions of the oral cavity and its associated structures attempt to focus attention on particular landmarks that will be most helpful in establishing good technique.

The oral cavity and adjoining structures are organized into regions according to innervation. The fifth cranial nerve, the trigeminal nerve, serves as the major source of sensory innervation to this area. This chapter discusses two of its three major sensory nerve divisions (ophthalmic, maxillary, and mandibular), the maxillary and mandibular nerves with their peripheral branches, for regional anesthesia. Anesthesia of these subdivisions is examined from a central to a peripheral site.

CLASSIFICATION OF TECHNIQUES

As with other techniques of regional anesthesia, intraoral regional anesthesia can be accomplished through nerve block, field block, or local infiltration or topical administration. The choice of these techniques is dependent upon the existent need for anesthesia (*i.e.*, surgical procedure, diagnostic testing, or pain relief), the anatomical location of the procedure, and the duration and profoundness of anesthesia required.

According to this classification of intraoral techniques, a *nerve block* is the deposition of local anesthetic around the main nerve trunk; a *field block* is the deposition of local anesthetic around main terminal branches of the larger nerve trunk; and a *local infiltration* is the deposition of local anesthetic around the smallest and most terminal branches and nerve endings of the larger nerve groups. This usually involves the direct deposition of local anesthetic solution in the area in which surgery is to be performed. For blockade of sensory impulses from the teeth in the oral cavity, the terms *field block* and *local infiltration* may become interchangeable.

Field block and local infiltration in the oral cavity, particularly in the maxilla, result from "supra" or "paraperiosteal" injections. In these injections, local anesthetic solutions are deposited "above" or "next to" the periosteum opposite the root apices of certain teeth. The anesthetic solution is allowed to diffuse through the periosteum and the bony plate penetrating the nerve fibers of the teeth, alveoli, and periodontal membranes. This procedure is most useful in the maxilla because of the relatively thin buccal or labial bony cortical plate found, allowing for easier diffusion of the local anesthetic solution.

Nerve block for intraoral regional techniques allows local anesthetic solution to be deposited at the major nerve root sites as they leave and enter the bony canals of the face. Anesthesia from intraoral nerve block injections has several advantages. The resultant anesthesia usually covers a wider anatomical area, is usually more profound, and can often be used when the more local supraperiosteal field blocks and infiltrations are contraindicated. This last advantage is particularly useful when local oral infection of dental or nondental origin requires surgical treatment.

PREPARATION

As with all other kinds of local anesthesia, certain requirements must be met prior to induction. It is, of course, important to procure an adequate medical and dental history, with particular emphasis on previous reactions (allergic and nonallergic) to local anesthetics. Because of the similarity of metabolic pathways, a history of postanesthesia apnea should be obtained if the ester-type local anesthetic agents are to be used (see Chap. 3). In addition, the preparation of the oral mucosa prior to injection of a local anesthetic should be thoroughly understood.

Although preparation for a regional anesthetic at extraoral sites involves disinfection of the area with some kind of scrubbing solution, draping, and gloves for the operator, it would seem desirable to apply the same rules of sterility to procedures within the oral cavity. However, in practical terms, they are impossible to achieve.

Certain basic principles of sterility and safety can be applied to minimize the chance of infection and mishap. First, the mucosa, at the site of injection, should be wiped with a disinfectant or at least made dry with a sterile cotton swab. Wiping the mucosa with a disinfectant reduces the number of bacterial colonies cultured from these sites, but experience seems to indicate that even without disinfection, clinically significant infection does not occur. Second, it is absolutely necessary that a sterile needle and anesthetic solution be used. As a result, the use of disposable needles, syringes, and anesthetic cartridges are recommended. Third, anesthetic cartridges (or Carpules) should never be used for more than one patient. Fourth, injection into infected tissue should be avoided because spread of infectious material and infection along needle tracts is not uncommon. Fifth, aspiration, to prevent intravascular injection, must be performed wherever local anesthetic solution is to be deposited. Sixth, the needle should not be placed directly into a bony foramen because injury to the neurovascular bundle may occur.

Preparation of the patient is also important. In order to perform both the anesthetic and operative technique under optimal conditions, the patient should be comfortably positioned and cooperative. For most intraoral procedures, the patient sits in a reclining chair. This not only provides optimal technical position but also affords the opportunity to place the patient nearly supine should complications such as fainting or seizures occur. Some extremely anxious patients will benefit from a light oral dose of a sedative agent, such as diazepam (5–10 mg) 30 to 60 minutes prior to the procedure.

EQUIPMENT

Although the equipment required for neural blockade is standard without regard to the area of the body being blocked, the intraoral approach to nerve blocks does benefit from some special equipment.

The anesthesiologist cannot obtain the best results with inadequate or inferior equipment. Makeshift material usually results in haphazard analgesia. Furthermore, safety is often sacrificed when the dentist compromises by using equipment not adaptable to a particular procedure. The equipment needed can be divided into two categories: that used to obtain regional anesthesia and that used in the treatment of complications and emergencies.

Basic Apparatus

Equipment for regional analgesia briefly, includes needles, syringes, and cartridges.

Needles. For intraoral techniques, needles should range from 22- to 27-gauge and vary from 1 to 10 cm in length. Although it has been the practice to use platinum-alloy needles that can rapidly be sterilized by flaming, at present disposable needles are usually used. These needles may be stainless steel

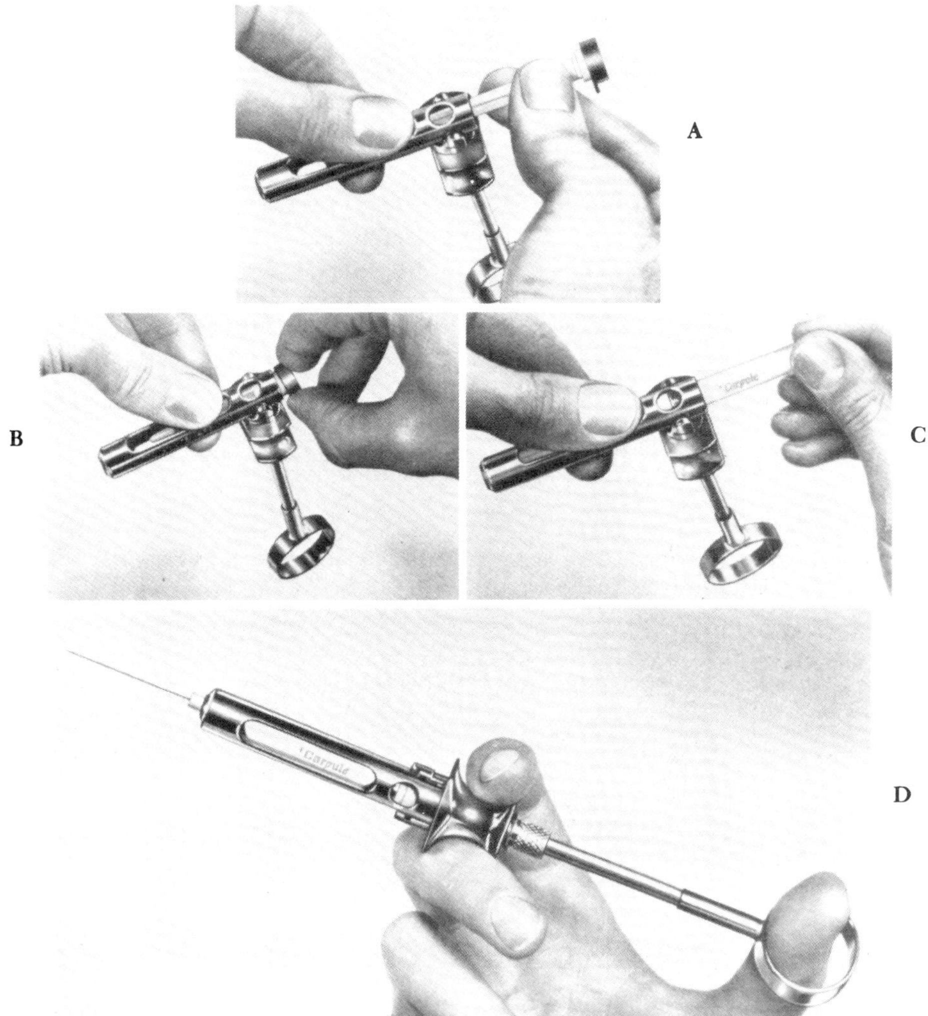

Fig. 16-1. A, Breech-loading metal cartridge syringe. Presterilized needle is inserted into syringe barrel. *B,* Colored protective cap is removed. *C,* Cartridge is inserted after plastic hub drops into barrel. *D,* Syringe is ready for injection. (Bennett, C.R.: Monheim's Local Anesthesia and Pain Control in Dental Practice, 5th edition, p. 272. St. Louis, C.V. Mosby, 1974)

and have the advantages that they are reasonably rigid, have a sharp point, are always sterile, and are relatively inexpensive. In general, a short-bevel needle is preferable for these blocks because the tip is less apt to "spur."

The 27-gauge, 1-cm needle is ideal for infiltration of wheals in which tissue is extremely sensitive. Otherwise, needles should be of sufficient length that no more than one-half to two-thirds of the shaft is inserted. This is a safety measure should the needle break (it can be retrieved) and allows for handling the proximal shaft of the needle with less tissue contamination.

In dental practice, there are two hub-types necessary. The first is threaded hubs for attachment to the cartridge-type syringe. This is the interchangeable long or short hub through which the needle is inserted. The second is the Luer-Lok hubs for attachment to the Luer-Lok glass or disposable syringes. These are indicated for deep injections or when venipuncture is required.

Syringes. The most commonly used syringe for intraoral nerve block, at least in dental offices, is the breech-loading metal cartridge syringe (Fig. 16-1). A hermetically sealed glass cartridge (or Carpule) fits into the breech of the syringe. The length of the needle, which extends into the breech, penetrates a rubber stopper or metal cap and extends into the anesthetic solution that the glass cartridge contains. A plunger rod is then forced into the breech of the syringe against the rubber stopper at the plunger-end of the cartridge. Gentle pressure with the thumb on the plunger rod forces the rubber plug at the plunger-end of the cartridge to be pressed into the glass cartridge, expelling the liquid contents through the needle, which has previously penetrated into the cartridge from its distal end.

This particular arrangement is adequate for infiltration but does prevent aspiration, an essential part of many nerve block techniques. Therefore, manufacturers have adapted the syringe to enable positive aspiration. By means of a barb or a screwlike tip on the plunger rod, the rubber stopper in the top of the cartridge may be engaged (Fig. 16-2). This allows the plunger to be either advanced or retracted.

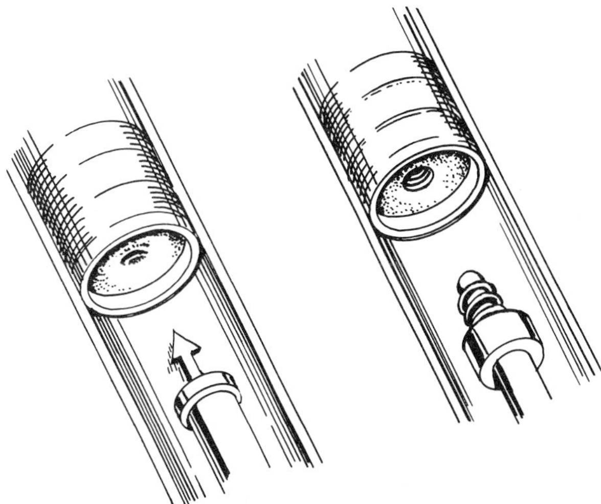

Fig. 16-2. Barb and screw tip plungers for aspiration before infiltration. (Bennett, C.R.: Monheim's Local Anesthesia and Pain Control in Dental Practice, ed. 5. St. Louis, C.V. Mosby, 1974)

Aspirating syringes of the Luer-Lok type, glass or disposable, should be available in 2-, 5-, and 10-ml sizes as well.

Cartridges. Glass cartridges (or Carpules) of local anesthetic agent have become extremely popular for dental anesthesia. The major advantage of the cartridge is that a single-dose of ensured sterility and uniformity of concentration is delivered. The cartridge is a glass tube sealed at one end by a rubber stopper that can be forced into the tube by the plunger of the cartridge-type of syringe. The other end is sealed by a metal cap or rubber diaphragm that is punctured by the cartridge end of the needle.

The ingredients of the cartridge vary to meet the individual requirements of the patient and anesthetist. Each contains the following: the local anesthetic drug or combination of drugs; the vasoconstrictor in various concentrations per millimeter; a preservative, usually sodium metabisulfite; sodium chloride to make the solution isotonic; and distilled water in sufficient amount to equal the desired volume.

The cartridges are usually vacuum-packed in groups of 50 in a metal container to prolong shelf life. Once the container is opened, the cartridges should be used in approximately 60 days. This is well within limits of deterioration, but light and temperature do hasten this process.

Emergency Instruments

Just as all anesthesiologists who perform neural blockade use the same basic anesthesia equipment, so should all who practice neural blockade be equipped to treat any ensuing complications. These may range from the fainting of hypotension to a grand mal seizure.

An emergency tray containing the necessary syringes, needles, tourniquet, and drugs should be immediately available to every anesthesiologist. In addition, oxygen and a suitable means of administering it should be available. This varies from a simple insufflating mask for patients to hold to a self-inflating bag (*i.e.*, Ambu) through which positive pressure ventilation may be administered. A laryngoscope, endotracheal tube, and an adequate suction device are also essential to complete the emergency equipment of every anesthesiologist's office.

LOCAL ANESTHETIC DRUGS AND VASOCONSTRICTORS

A wider variety of local anesthetic drugs have been available for dental use than for neural blockade elsewhere. Among the factors to be considered in the correct selection of a local anesthetic agent are induction of action, toxicity, allergies, and vasoconstrictor concentration. For intraoral anesthetic use, duration may be defined as follows: short-acting anesthetic—45 to 75 minutes; medium-acting anesthetic—90 to 150 minutes; and long-acting anesthetic—180 minutes or longer.

Although the common ester- and amide-type local anesthetic agents are discussed extensively in Chapters 3 and 4, there are other groups of drugs,

Table 16-1. Chemical Groups of Injectable Local Anesthetics Used in Denistry

Drug Type	*Generic Name*	*American Trade Name*
Esters		
Benzoic acid esters	Piperocaine	Metycaine
	Meprylcaine	Oracaine
	Isobucaine	Kincaine
Para-aminobenzoic acid esters	Procaine	Novocain
	Tetracaine	Pontocaine
	Butethamine	Monocaine
	Propoxycaine	Ravocaine
	2-Chloroprocaine	Nesacaine
	Procaine and butethamine	Duocaine
Meta-aminobenzoic acid esters	Metabutethamine	Anacaine
	Primacaine	Primacaine
Paraethoxybenzoic acid ester	Parethoxycaine	Intracaine
Anilides	Lidocaine	Xylocaine
	Mepivacaine	Carbocaine
	Pyrrocaine	Dynacaine
	Prilocaine	Citanest
	Bupivacaine	Marcaine
	Etidocaine	Duranest
Other		
Cyclohexylamino-2-propyl benzoate	Hexylcaine	Cyclaine

chemically related, which are unique to dental anesthesia. For practical purposes, they may be divided into three main groups; to include the hydroxy compounds, they may be divided further chemically into the following: benzoic acid esters, para-aminobenzoic acid esters, meta-aminobenzoic acid esters, para-ethoxybenzoic acid esters, cyclohexylamino-2-propyl-benzoate, and amide (anilide, nonester).

Seventeen separate local anesthetic agents have been developed for dental use in these six chemical groups (Table 16-1). Furthermore, since duration is as much a function of concentration of vasoconstrictor as type of drug and since most drugs are prepackaged in cartridges, the number of marketed products has been expanded significantly. The most common drugs in use are probably lidocaine and mepivacaine.

Topical anesthesia has a definite value in intraoral techniques. Its judicious use and the employment of the smallest, sharpest needle possible can make any needle insertion painless. Of the drugs in the groups just mentioned, lidocaine (5%) and tetracaine (1–2%) are most active topically. In addition to lidocaine and tetracaine, the most commonly used topical anesthetics are ethylaminobenzoate (benzocaine) and benzyl alcohol. Benzocaine is related to the other ester drugs because it is an ester of aminobenzoic acid. It is irritating to tissues when it is injected. It is poorly soluble in water, accounting for its slow absorption from the area of topical application. This is beneficial in prolonging its duration and reducing its toxicity. Benzyl alcohol is an aromatic alcohol that is soluble in water. It possesses anesthetic properties, but it is very irritating upon injection into tissues. It is used in 4- to 10-per-cent solutions for topical anesthesia and is shorter-acting and less toxic than benzocaine.

Vasoconstrictors are valuable adjuncts to local anesthetic solutions by serving four useful purposes: they slow absorption and thereby reduce toxicity; they prolong the action of the local anesthetic agent; they permit use of smaller volumes of solution; and they increase the efficiency of the anesthetic solution.

Most local anesthetics in dental use today are vasodilators and, as such, are rapidly absorbed into the systemic circulation. In fact, the stronger the concentration, the greater is the vasodilating effect. This was dramatically proven when 4 per cent procaine was introduced. Its vasodilating properties became so marked that its action was shorter than lower concentrations. Vasoconstrictors have frequently been maligned in dental practice for the following reasons: first, they are used in greater than necessary concentrations; second, repeated injections increased the volume of vasoconstrictors to toxic or near toxic levels; and third, the occasional intravascular injection resulted in toxic manifestations. All too often, it has been these symptoms of vasoconstrictor excess, relative or absolute, that has led patients to believe that they were allergic to the local anesthetic agent being used.

The four vasoconstrictors most commonly used in dental local anesthetic solutions are epinephrine, norepinephrine (Levophed), nordefrin (Cobefrin), and phenylephrine (Neo-Synephrine). The vasoconstrictors are unstable in solution and therefore contain a preservative, usually sodium metabisulfite, to prevent the oxidation of the sympathomimetic amine. The preservative, being more active, successfully competes with the vasoconstrictor for the available oxygen in the cartridge and is oxidized to sodium bisulfate.

The dosage for the vasoconstrictors varies by both concentration and total dose. It is preferable to plan the total dose and alter the concentration according to the volume of local anesthetic solution needed. Conclusive data are lacking about the relative efficacies of a 1:10,000 concentration and a 1:200,000 solution. Most authorities today believe that the 1:200,000 concentration of epinephrine offers optimal safety and efficacy.

A more flexible dosage guide is to establish 0.2 mg as the total dose for a healthy outpatient. This translates to 10 ml of a 1:50,000 concentration, 20 ml of a 1:100,000, and so forth. Norepinephrine should be used as judiciously as epinephrine and on a similar dosage schedule. A further consideration with norepinephrine is its local ischemic effect. It is suggested that not more than 3 to 4 ml of a norepinephrine-containing solution be injected at one time. Nordefrin is rated one-fifth as vasoactive as epinephrine and has a similarly reduced toxicity. It is commonly used in 1:10,000 concentrations and should be limited to a 1-mg total dose. It is said to hold an advantage over the other drugs because of its reduced effect on the central nervous system (CNS). Phenylephrine is used in an even stronger concentration than the other vasoconstrictors, 1:2,500 being the usual concentration. Its vasoconstricting properties are less pronounced than the other drugs that have been mentioned. However, because of its increased stability, it is longer-lasting. Its systemic effects, especially on the heart and CNS, are also reduced, making it the preferred drug in patients with preexisting cardiovascular disease. Dosage should be limited to 4 mg of the 1:2,500 concentration (10 ml).

All of the vasoconstrictors are effective, but, as has been seen, with a diminishing efficiency. It is important to remember that dosage must be kept within safe limits. Each milliliter of local anesthetic solution injected increases, independently, the relative toxicity of the local anesthetic agent and the vasoconstrictor. One drug may well be within the safe range at a time when the other is approaching toxic levels, and vice versa.

NERVE BLOCKS OF THE MAXILLA

Interruption of neural transmission to the oral cavity by way of the maxillary nerve (second division of the trigeminal nerve) may be accomplished by intraoral blocks of the maxillary nerve itself, the infraorbital nerve (anterior superior alveolar nerve), the posterior superior alveolar nerve, the greater palatine nerve, or the nasopalatine nerve. Interruption of the smaller terminal branches of these nerves can also be accomplished within the oral cavity by field block or local infiltration of the appropriate areas. Because anesthetic solutions can diffuse through the thin maxillary cortical plate, anesthetizing the terminal branches can often be more easily accomplished than the more central nerve block.

Maxillary Nerve

Anatomy. The maxillary (second) division of the fifth cranial nerve (trigeminal) is entirely sensory. It leaves the skull through the foramen rotundum and enters into the pterygopalatine fossa, from where it progresses forward, entering the inferior orbital fissure to pass into the orbital cavity. Here, it turns slightly laterally in a groove called *the infraorbital groove* on the orbital surface of the maxilla. As it continues forward, it becomes covered by a thin plate of bone and then passes through the infraorbital canal. Continuing forward, the second division emerges on the front of the maxilla by the infraorbital foramen. While still in the pterygopalatine fossa, the maxillary nerve gives origin to the *posterior superior alveolar nerves* and the small *zygomatic nerve* and sends branches to the pterygopalatine ganglion. Because the maxillary nerve lies in the infraorbital fissure, it is renamed the *infraorbital nerve*. Near the center or end of the canal, it gives origin to the *anterior superior alveolar nerve*.

Areas Anesthetized. Since the maxillary nerve is purely a sensory nerve, blockade will provide anesthesia over all its components, distal to the point of injection. This includes the maxillary teeth (incisors to molars) on the affected side, the alveolar bone with overlying gingiva and mucosa, the hard palate and portions of the soft palate and the upper lip, cheek, side of nose, and lower eyelid.

Technique. The nerve can be approached intraorally from behind the tuberosity of the maxilla or through the greater palatine canal. The tuberosity approach is identical to the approach to the posterior superior alveolar nerve and is accomplished with the patient in a semireclining position so that the occlusal plane of the maxilla is at a 45° angle to the floor. After drying the mucosa and preparing the site with antiseptic solution and topical anesthetic, the anesthesiologist, using his forefinger, palpates posteriorly along the mucobuccal fold of the maxilla until he reaches the posterior surface of the zygomatic process. This will be felt as a concavity in the mucobuccal fold, slightly distal to the maxillary second molar (see Fig. 16-3).

With the tip of his forefinger maintaining contact with this concave surface, the hand and finger are positioned so that they are pointing at right angles

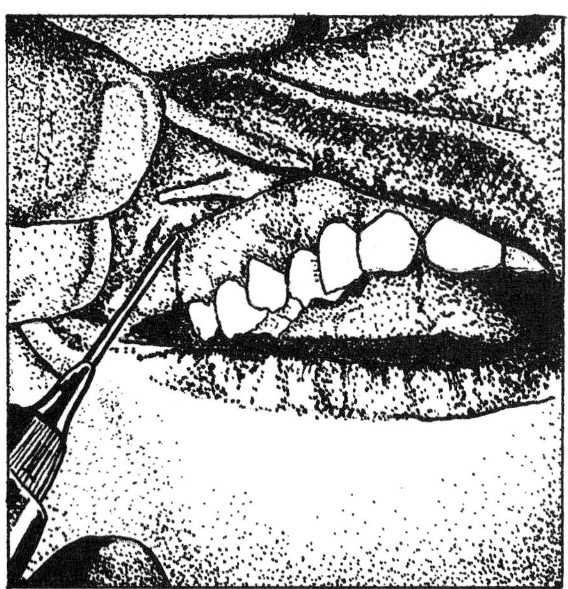

Fig. 16-3. Tuberosity approach to the maxillary and superior alveolar nerves is shown with insertion of needle into the mucobuccal fold, slightly distal to the maxillary second molar. (Final position of needle for superior alveolar nerve block is 1.5–2 cm)

to the maxillary occlusal plane and at a 45° angle to the patient's sagittal plane. Thus positioned, the hand and forefinger serve as a guide to the insertion of the needle. Using a dental aspirating syringe with a 4-cm (1⅝-in), 25-gauge needle, insertion is made parallel along the guiding finger to a previously marked needle depth approximately 3 cm (1¼ in). Following this guide will allow the needle to be advanced close to the maxillary tuberosity in an inward, backward, and upward direction. The needle should be advanced slowly, with intermittent aspiration, along the premarked course. At the desired position, 1 to 2 ml of local anesthetic solution should be deposited.

Adherence to the anatomical landmarks will allow the needle to reach a point posterior to the posterior surface of the maxilla, anterior and lateral to the anterior margin of the external pterygoid muscle, and anterior to the pterygoid venous plexus. This last position is close to the vascular plexus so that the hazard of intravenous deposition of local anesthetic solution is obvious; therefore, the injection must be performed after careful aspiration.

The other approach to the maxillary nerve is through the greater palatine canal. The greater palatine foramen, the opening to this canal, lies between the maxillary second and third molars on their palatal side, approximately 1 cm from the palatal gingival margin toward the midline of the palate. It is sometimes possible to feel a slight depression with the tip of the forefinger over this foramen. If it is difficult to palpate, it may usually be located by gentle probing of the needle in the generalized area between the two molars.

After preparation of the mucosa, a 25-gauge 4-cm (1⅝-in) needle attached to an aspirating syringe is placed in the palatal mucosa where a few drops of local anesthetic solution are deposited prior to locating the greater palatine foramen. The palatal mucosa is impressively sensitive to pain, and local infiltration must precede the block procedure if patient comfort and cooperation are to be maintained. The greater palatine foramen and canal are approached from the opposite side with the needle as near to a right angle with the curvature of the palatal bone as possible. When the canal is found by gentle probing, it is entered slowly and carefully. Once within the canal, the needle should be passed to a precisely premarked distance of 4 cm (1½ in). At this point, the local anesthetic solution should be deposited following aspiration. Redirection of the needle during its passage through the canal may be necessary if any undue resistance is met. At no time should force be used to overcome the resistance to passage of the needle to its desired depth. Should repositioning not allow further movement of the needle, this approach may have to be abandoned.

Indications. Greater skill and care are required for both the tuberosity and greater palatine canal approaches than are required for other intraoral blocks. These approaches are, however, quite useful when extensive surgery over the second division is contemplated and other types of anesthesia are contraindicated or less desirable, particularly for oral surgical and plastic surgical procedures in which local infection may prevent blocking terminal branches of the nerve in which anatomical distortion with local anesthetic solution is undesirable. The anesthesiologist may find that a complete block of the second division is useful as either a diagnostic or therapeutic tool in patients with orofacial pain. Repetitive blocking of the maxillary nerve may break pain patterns established with typical and atypical neuralgias of this division of the trigeminal nerve.

Posterior Superior Alveolar Nerve

Anatomy. The posterior superior alveolar nerves (2 or 3) arise from the maxillary nerve before it has passed the inferior orbital fissure. The infraorbital nerve then descends through the pterygomaxillary fissure on the posterior surface of the maxilla. The branches enter small canals in the bone to run horizontally around the maxillary sinus. They communicate with each other and with the anterior superior alveolar nerve.

Areas Anesthetized. Block of the posterior superior alveolar nerve will provide anesthesia for the maxillary molars of the blocked side, with the exception of the mesiobuccal root of the first molar. Also anesthetized will be the buccal alveolar process of the maxillary molars, including overlying structures—periosteum, mucous membranes, and the buccal gingiva (Fig. 16-4).

Technique. A technique identical to that described for the maxillary nerve is used, except that the needle is inserted to a depth of only 1.5 to 2 cm (see Fig. 16-3). The same care and skill taken with the maxillary nerve block must be exhibited in approaching the posterior superior alveolar nerve, or else the unpleasant sequelae of intravascular injection and hemorrhage in the pterygoid venous plexus may occur.

Indications. Dental procedures that involve the maxillary molars, buccal alveolar housing, and gingival and mucosal tissue may be performed under this block. For surgical procedures in which manipulation of the palatal tissue is likely, this block must be supplemented with a greater palatine nerve block. Also necessary is supplementation by local infiltration of the innervation of the mesiobuccal root of the first molar when procedures on this tooth are anticipated. Anesthesia of this area can be achieved by local infiltration in the buccal alveolar mucosa above the buccal roots of each of these molars. This is considerably easier and less hazard is associated with it than the foregoing block techniques. The block technique should be used only when surgery that requires prompt and profound anesthesia for prolonged periods is necessary or when local infection prohibits local infiltration over the root tips.

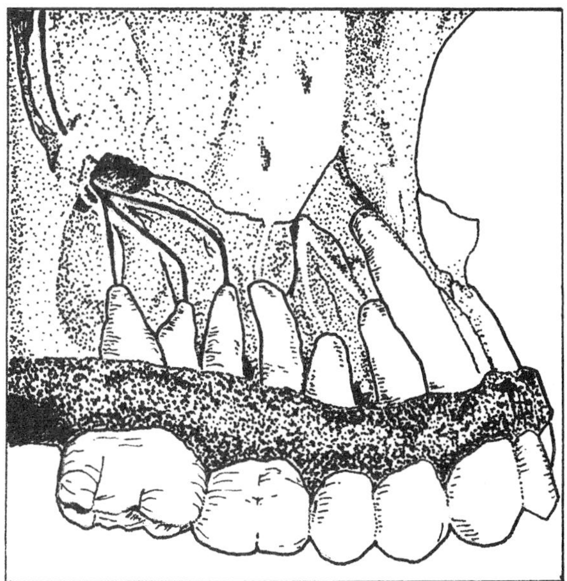

Fig. 16-4. The posterior superior alveolar nerve, a branch of the maxillary nerve.

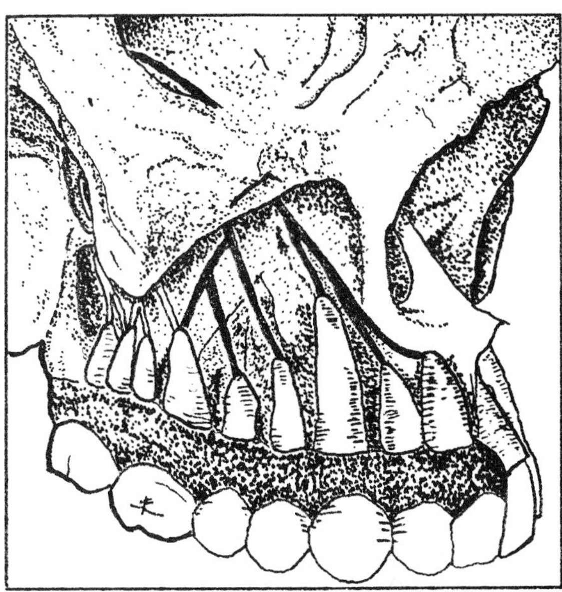

Fig. 16-5. The infraorbital nerve forms the anterior and middle superior alveolar nerves.

Infraorbital Nerve

Anatomy. The infraorbital nerve appears as a direct continuation of the maxillary nerve. It passes through the inferior orbital fissure into the orbital cavity, traveling along the floor of the orbit through the infraorbital canal and emerging through the infraorbital foramen (Fig. 16-5). While still in the infraorbital canal, it gives off, first, the middle superior alveolar nerve and, later, the anterior superior alveolar nerve. Here, the nerve divides to form the inferior palpebral, lateral nasal, and superior labial nerves.

Areas Anesthetized. Block of the infraorbital nerve induces anesthesia of the maxillary incisors, cuspids, bicuspids, and mesiobuccal root of the first

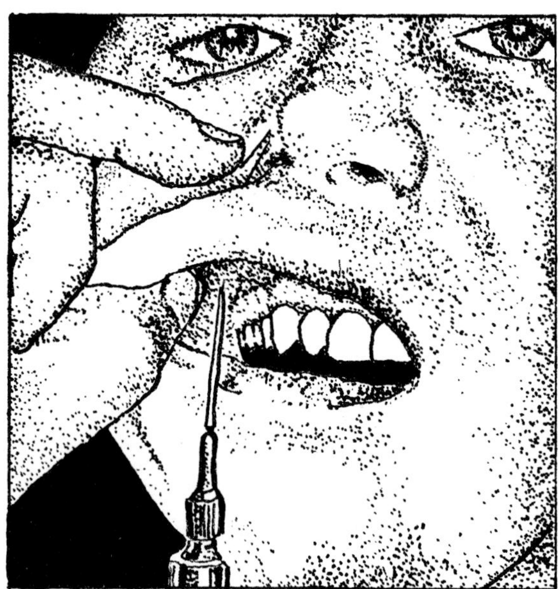

Fig. 16-6. The depression of the infraorbital foramen is fixed with the index finger, while the thumb is used to retract the lip upward and outward in order to expose the mucobuccal fold over the bicuspid teeth.

molar on the side injected. Anesthesia also extends to the bony alveolar supporting structure as well as the soft tissues (gingiva and mucosa). Other areas affected by this block are the upper lip and its mucosa, the lower eyelid, and part of the nose on the blocked side.

Technique. The intraoral approach to the infraorbital nerve uses the supraorbital notch, infraorbital notch, pupil of the eyes, and the second bicuspid tooth as landmarks to achieve proper needle placement. With the patient looking straight ahead, the supraorbital notch and the infraorbital notch are palpated. An imaginary straight line passing through these notches and the pupil of the eye will pass through the infraorbital foramen and the second bicuspid tooth. Having palpated the infraorbital notch, the anesthesiologist moves his finger approximately 0.5 cm below the notch along the imaginary straight line and should be able to discern a depression in which the infraorbital foramen is located. It is probably easiest to palpate the necessary bony landmarks using an index finger. When the depression has been located, it is fixed with the index finger while the thumb of the same hand is used to retract the lip upward and outward, in order to expose the mucobuccal fold over the second bicuspid tooth (Fig. 16-6). Using a dental aspirating syringe with a 3-cm (1⅝-in), 25-gauge needle, the mucosa (previously dried and prepared) is entered at a distance of approximately 0.5 cm away from the alveolar plate in order to pass over the canine fossa. The needle is aligned parallel to the straight line created by connecting the supraorbital notch, pupil, infraorbital notch, and long axis of the second bicuspid tooth. The needle is passed along this line, the tip being guided by the index finger over the infraorbital foramen. The distance necessary for the needle to travel to reach this location is usually not more than 3 cm (¾ in). Care must be taken at all times to prevent the needle from entering the orbital cavity. Limiting the depth of needle penetration and use of the index finger as a guide are likely to prevent this complication.

When the point of the needle is in contact with the boundaries of the infraorbital foramen, approximately 2 ml of local anesthetic solution is slowly deposited. While the injection is being completed, the index finger is maintained in its position above the foramen. Some authorities recommend inserting the needle a distance into the canal in order to achieve satisfactory block. Alternatively, placement of the needle in contact with the entrance of the foramen leads to a highly successful block. The continuous pressure from the index finger tends to promote diffusion of the anesthetic solution into the canal and prevent its escaping into the infraorbital fossa.

Indications. Indications for this block include surgical or operative (dental) procedures of the five anterior maxillary teeth, differentiation of trigger zones of trigeminal neuralgias in this area of the nerve, intraoral flap and alveolar surgery, and excision of root cysts and granulomas in the anesthetized area. This technique is useful when more distal approaches to the nerve branches provide incomplete anesthesia or are contraindicated because of infection. The infraorbital block does not provide anesthesia for palatine structures. Supplementary blocks are necessary for surgery on these structures.

Distal branches of the infraorbital nerve that may be blocked by other intraoral techniques include the middle and anterior superior alveolar nerves (see Fig. 16-5). Local infiltration of anesthetic solution in the mucolabial fold above the maxillary incisors, canines, bicuspids, and mesialbuccal root of the first molar will usually achieve anesthesia of these distal branches. At the midline, it is often necessary to infiltrate areas across the midline to affect crossing-over terminal branches.

The need to anesthetize the palatal structures in order to achieve a complete block for most intraoral surgical procedures on the maxilla has been mentioned. Intraoral blocks to achieve anesthesia of the anterior and posterior regions of the hard palate are directed at the nasopalatine nerve and the anterior palatine nerve.

Nasopalatine Nerve

Anatomy. The pterygopalatine (sphenopalatine) nerves are two short nerve trunks from the maxillary nerve that unite at the pterygopalatine (sphenopalatine) ganglion and are then redistributed into a number of branches. These branches, by distribution, are divided into orbital branches, nasal branches, palatine branches, and pharyngeal branches. The nasal branches, in turn, pass medially and enter the upper posterior nasal cavity by way of the sphenopalatine foramen. In the nasal cavity, the branches divide into the posterior or superior lateral branches (the *short sphenopalatine nerves*) and the medial or septal branch, usually referred to as the *nasopalatine* (or *long sphenopalatine*) *nerve*.

This nerve branches downward and forward between the periosteum and the mucous membrane of the nasal septum in a groove on the side of the vomer bone. As it continues farther downward, it reaches the floor of the nasal cavity, giving off branches to the septum and floor of the nose, finally descending into the anterior portion of the hard palate through the incisive canal. The incisive canal

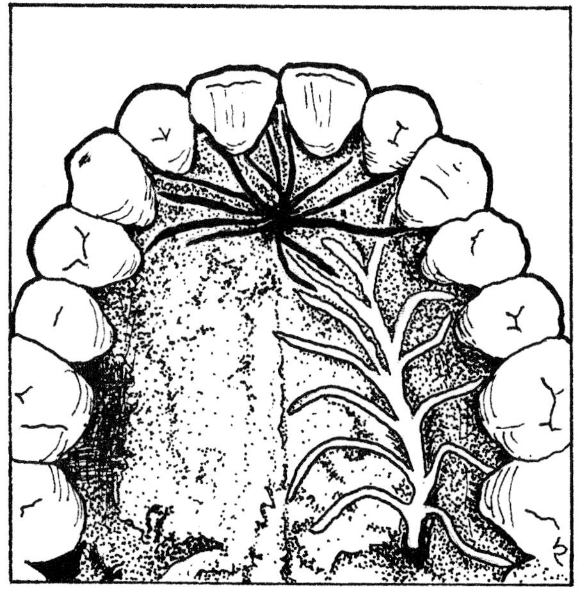

Fig. 16-7. Distribution of the nasopalatine nerve.

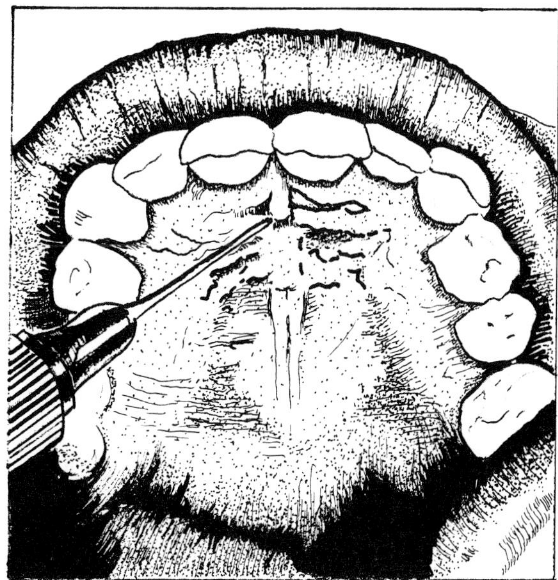

Fig. 16-8. Insertion of a 25-gauge, 2-cm needle into the crest of the incisive papilla will achieve anesthesia of the nasopalatine nerve.

lies underneath the incisive papilla, being in the palatine midline directly behind the maxillary central incisor teeth (Fig. 16-7).

Areas Anesthetized. Blockade of the nasopalatine nerve will anesthetize the anterior portion of the hard palate and its overlying structures back to the bicuspid area, where branches of the anterior palatine nerve coursing forward create a dual innervation. Some debate exists whether this block will anesthetize the four or six anterior maxillary teeth. Apparently, the number of teeth is a function of number of injections and whether operative dentistry is required, that is, the profoundness of the block over the last two maxillary teeth.

Technique. The procedure for blocking the nasopalatine nerve is relatively simple. Unfortunately, insertion of the needle into the incisive papilla is quite painful and may well increase already raised anxiety levels in the patient. It is therefore desirable to make a preparatory injection prior to the actual block attempt (Fig. 16-8).

With the 25-gauge, 2.5-cm (1-in) needle at a right angle to the maxillary labial plate, the labial septal tissue between the maxillary central incisors is penetrated. Resistance by the labial intraseptal plate is felt, and a small amount (<0.5 ml) of local anesthetic solution is deposited. Now, insertion into the incisive papilla will be considerably less painful, and the needle can then be slowly and care-

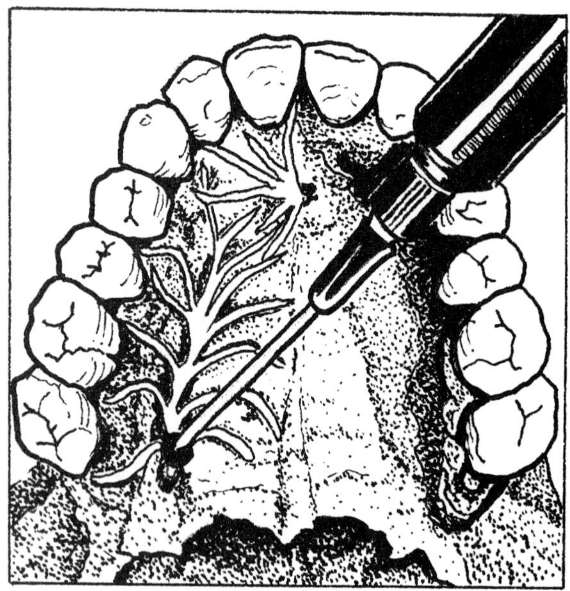

Fig. 16-9. The anterior palatine nerve entering through the greater palatine foramen.

fully advanced into the incisive foramen where a small amount of the local anesthetic solution (<0.5 ml) may be deposited, care again being taken not to inject the anesthetic solution forcefully or rapidly in order to prevent damage to the tightly bound palatal tissues.

Indications. The nasopalatine nerve block is useful as a supplement to the block of the anterior and middle superior alveolar nerves. It is used to provide or augment anesthesia to the six maxillary incisors and to provide complete anesthesia of the nasal septum.

Anterior Palatine Nerve

Anatomy. Just as the nasopalatine nerve derives from the pterygopalatine ganglion through its nasal branches, the anterior palatine nerve is derived from its palatine branches (Fig. 16-9). The palatine branches descend in the pterygopalatine canal where the fibers divide into three strands: greater or anterior palatine, middle palatine, and posterior palatine. The anterior palatine nerve emerges onto the hard palate by passing through the greater palatine foramen and continues in an anterior direction between the osseus hard palate and the mucoperiosteum to divide into numerous branches. It extends as far forward as the premaxillary palatine mucosa, which is also supplied by terminal branches of the nasopalatine nerves. The greater palatine foramen lies between the maxillary second and third molars approximately 10 mm above the palatal gingiva toward the palatal midline.

Areas Anesthetized. The anterior palatine nerve block anesthetizes the posterior portion of the hard palate and its overlying structures up to the first bicuspid on the injected side. At the first bicupsid area, branches of the nasopalatine nerve will be overlapping. The area affected will extend from the tuberosity of the maxilla to the canine region.

Technique. The approach to the greater palatine foramen is made across the arch (*i.e.,* from the opposite side). Again, a 2.5-cm (1-in), 25-gauge needle is used. Puncture is made at a right angle to the curvature of the palate between the second and third maxillary molar teeth, approximately 5 to 10 mm above the gingival margin (Fig. 16-10). When bone is reached, the needle is withdrawn 1 mm, and less than 0.5 ml of anesthetic solution is deposited slowly. It may be advantageous to inject the solution so that the anterior palatine nerve will be anesthetized anterior to the foramen. If the bicuspid area is to be anesthetized, it is helpful also to deposit solution in the palatal curvature opposite those bicuspids. This will ensure anesthetizing the area that overlaps from the nasopalatine nerve fibers extending posteriorly.

It must be emphasized that palatal injections are quite painful and the use of a topical anesthetic or

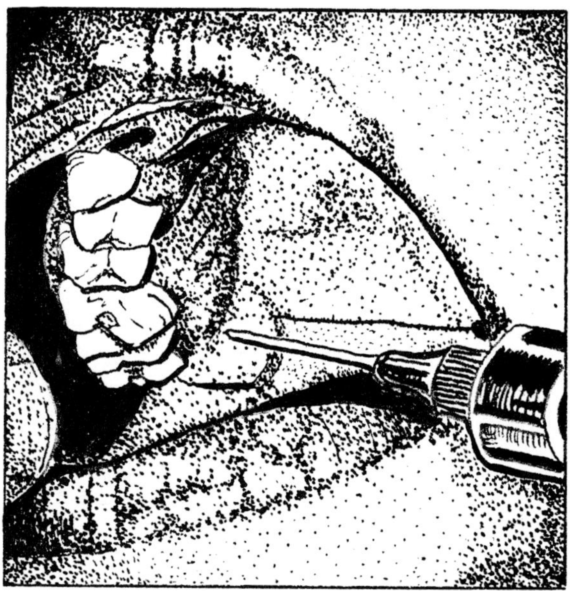

Fig. 16-10. Placement of the needle between the maxillary second and third molars for the anterior palatine nerve block.

gently placed wheal on or in the mucosa will be helpful. Slow injection of the anesthetic solution to prevent distortion of the tightly bound palatal tissues is essential. Forceful injection into these tissues may lead to hematoma formation.

Indications. The anterior palatine nerve block is necessary to provide anesthesia of the palate in conjunction with the posterior or middle superior alveolar nerve block. It is especially beneficial for surgical procedures on the posterior portion of the hard palate.

NERVE BLOCKS OF THE MANDIBLE

The mandibular nerve, or third division of the trigeminal nerve, consisting of both motor and sensory branches, can be approached by intraoral block techniques that allow access only to its major branches, such as the inferior alveolar nerve. In contrast to nerve block of the maxilla in which terminal branches are easily reached by anesthetic solutions diffusing through the thin maxillary plate, terminal branches of the mandibular nerve generally cannot be reached by diffusion through the much thicker mandibular plate.

Mandibular Nerve

The branches of the mandibular nerve accessible to intraoral block include the inferior alveolar nerve, the lingual nerve, the mental nerve, and the long buccal (buccinator) nerve. Blockade of these branches will eliminate the need for local infiltration to achieve anesthesia of the smallest terminal branches. As an example, blockade of the inferior alveolar nerve will affect the distribution of the mental nerve, which is a distal branch of the major nerve trunk.

Anatomy. Understanding the anatomy of the mandibular nerve is most important if successful blocks of its branches are to be achieved. The mandibular division contains both sensory and motor nerves, although most of the nerves are sensory. After passing through the foramen ovale and down into the infratemporal fossa, motor nerves to the muscles of mastication branch. These nerves include the external pterygoid, the masseter, and the temporalis.

Along with these motor nerves, a solitary sensory nerve, the long buccal, branches to innervate the skin and mucous membrane of the cheek, mucosa and gingiva of the buccal molar area, and the mucosa of the retromolar triangle region (Fig. 16-11). The long buccal nerve crosses the anterior ramus at about the level of the occlusal plane of the molar teeth. It arrives at this point, having passed downward anteriorly and laterally between the external pterygoid muscles, to travel underneath the anterior border of the masseter muscle. Crossing to a position lateral to the anterior border of the ramus, it becomes accessible to intraoral block.

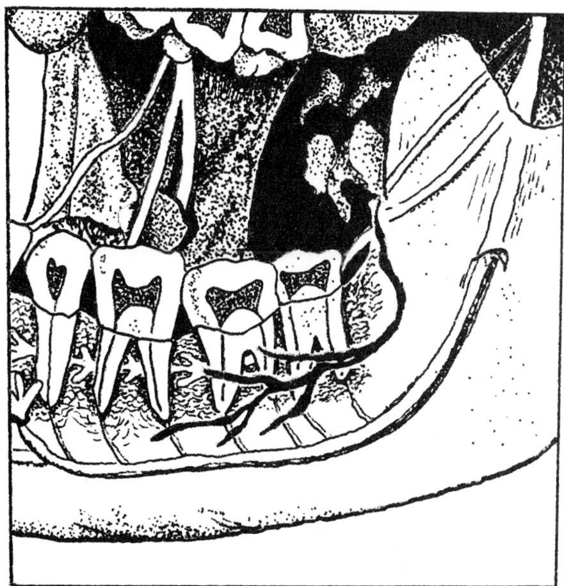

Fig. 16-11. Distribution of the long buccal nerve.

The mandibular nerve, in addition to having this anterior group of nerve branches, has a group of branches that constitute a posterior division. These include the auriculotemporal nerve and the lingual nerve. The former is sensory and has terminal branches innervating the parotid gland, temporomandibular joint, anterior portion of the ear, external auditory meatus, tympanic membrane, and the scalp over the temporal region.

Intraoral block techniques are incapable of anesthetizing this nerve. Only with extraoral block of the entire mandibular division is block anesthesia of this nerve possible. In contrast, the lingual nerve branch is commonly anesthetized by intraoral pathways. The lingual nerve runs downward medial to the external pterygoid muscle and lateral to the internal pterygoid muscle but between it and the ramus of the mandible in what is referred to as the *pterygomandibular space* (Fig. 16-12). It is here that it is most accessible to local anesthetic block. From this point, the nerve runs deeply to a position beside the base of the tongue (below and behind the third molar), from which it passes anteriorly and

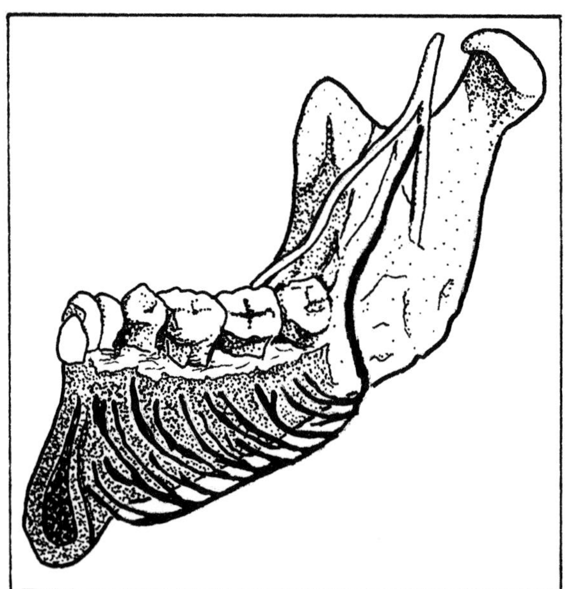

Fig. 16-12. The lingual nerve and its distribution, along with the inferior alveolar nerve entering the mandibular canal and the long buccal nerve crossing the anterior border of the ramus.

medially. Its distribution is sensory to the anterior two-thirds of the tongue, the mucosa of the floor of the mouth, and mucosa and the gingiva on the lingual surface of the mandible.

The continuing mandibular nerve proceeds in its downward direction, reaching the pterygomandibular space where it lies between the sphenomandibular ligament and the medial surface of the ramus. At this point, it enters the mandibular foramen to the bony mandibular canal, where it becomes the inferior alveolar nerve. Just prior to entering this canal, the nerve gives off two motor branches that innervate the mylohyoid muscle and anterior belly of the digastric muscle.

Areas Anesthetized. Extraoral blockade of the mandibular nerve provides sensory anesthesia of the following seven areas. First, it affects the mucous membrane and the skin of the cheek and the buccal gingiva of the mandibular molar region. Second is the skin over the muscles supplied by the facial (seventh) nerve (*i.e.*, zygomatic, buccal, and mandibular areas). Third, it affects the parotid gland and fourth, the temporomandibular articulation. Fifth, it anesthetizes the skin lining the external auditory meatus and the lateral and external surface of the tympanic membrane. Sixth is the skin and scalp over the upper part of the external ear and the side of the head up to the vertex of the skull, and seventh, the mucous membrane covering the anterior two-thirds of the tongue, the floor of the mouth, and the lingual side of the mandibular gingiva and the submandibular and sublingual glands and their ducts.

Technique for the mandibular nerve is essentially the same as that used for the blockade of the maxillary nerve. After the needle contacts the lateral pterygoid plate, it is withdrawn (just as in the maxillary block), only, in this case, it is reinserted in a direction upward and slightly posterior so that the needle will pass posterior to the lateral pterygoid plate. Usually a paresthesia manifest as tingling and numbness of the lower lip and anterior two-thirds of the tongue will result. The needle should not be inserted to a depth greater than a premeasured 5 cm.

Indications. Although blockade of the entire mandibular nerve will produce sufficient anesthesia, as would blockade of any of its various branches, it is a major nerve block better reserved for when it is specifically desirable to anesthetize all subdivisions of the nerve with one needle insertion and a minimum of anesthetic solution. It is also indicated when infection or trauma renders intraoral blockade of its branches difficult or impossible.

Inferior Alveolar Nerve

Anatomy. The inferior alveolar nerve is the largest of the branches of the posterior division of the man-

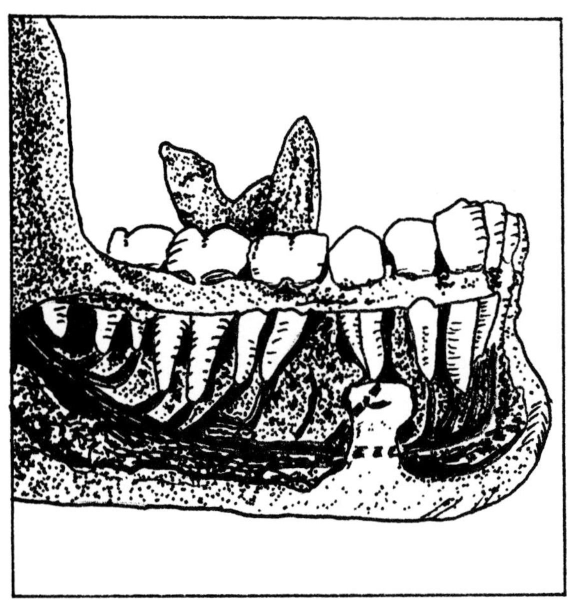

Fig. 16-13. Distribution of the inferior alveolar nerve within the mandibular canal.

dibular nerves (Fig. 16-13). It descends between the pterygoid muscles, passes between the mandible and the sphenomandibular ligament, and gives rise to the *mylohyoid nerve* before entering the mandibular foramen. The inferior alveolar nerve, in company with the inferior alveolar artery and vein, enters the mandibular foramen and runs forward in the mandibular canal. Here, it gives rise to a dental plexus to the premolar and molar teeth and part of the gum. Near the mental foramen, the inferior alveolar nerve divides into a mental nerve and a small incisive branch, which, continuing through the bone, supplies the lower canine tooth and the incisor teeth and labial gingiva.

There is some evidence that the mylohyoid nerve contains some sensory fibers that continue forward toward the chin region. These fibers may supply the skin on the inferior, and possibly the anterior, surfaces of the mental protuberance. It is suggested that a twig of sensory fibers of the mylohyoid nerve may enter the mandible in the area of the chin to aid in the sensory nerve supply to the mandibular incisors.

Areas Anesthetized. Blockade of the inferior alveolar nerve provides anesthesia of the body of the mandible and an inferior portion of the ramus. It also anesthetizes the mandibular teeth, as well as the mucous membranes and underlying tissues anterior to the first mandibular molar. This includes the lower lip, both skin and mucosa.

Technique. Proper placement of a needle to achieve a block of the inferior alveolar nerve is a position superior to the inferior alveolar nerve and blood vessels, superior to the insertion of the internal pterygoid muscle, superior to the nerve (while being medial to the inner ramus of the mandible), and lateral to the lingual nerve, internal pterygoid muscle, and the sphenomandibular ligament. In order to achieve such a position, anatomical landmarks such as the anterior border of the ramus, external and internal oblique ridges, retromolar triangle, and pterygomandibular ligament and space must be recognized (Fig. 16-14).

From a position in front and to the side of the patient, the anesthetist, using his index finger, palpates, posteriorly from the mucobuccal fold, the external oblique ridge and the anterior border of the ramus.

Palpating the anterior border of the ramus, the anesthesiologist locates the coronoid notch. This is an indentation indicating the greatest depth of the anterior border. At this level, the thumb or index finger is then moved medially across the retromolar pad onto the internal oblique ridge. The opposing digit is then moved laterally, again tensing the tissue of the retromolar pad across the anterior border of the ramus, giving a clearer exposure to the internal oblique ridge and pterygomandibular raphe. With an aspirating dental syringe and a 3-cm (1⅝-in), 25-gauge needle directed from the bicuspid (premolar) teeth of the opposite side of the jaw, the needle is inserted at the level of the retracting finger or thumb (Fig. 16-15). The injection site lies approximately 1 cm above the occlusal surfaces of the molars, medial to the retracting finger and lateral to the pterygomandibular raphe. The needle is advanced posterolaterally along the medial surface of the ramus. The syringe should be held in the horizontal position at all times. When the needle comes in contact with the middle portion of the ramus, it should be withdrawn slightly and aspirated to ensure that it is not intravascular, and the local anesthetic solution (1–2 ml) slowly deposited. Contact along the middle medial surface of the ramus should place the needle in close proximity to the mandibular sulcus, which funnels into the mandibular foramen. Placement of the needle too far posteriorly will result in anesthetic solution being deposited at the posterior margin of the ramus, which may result in anesthesia of branches of the facial nerve. If the needle is withdrawn one-half its inserted depth and 0.5 to 1 ml of the remaining anesthetic injected, the anesthesiologist can doubly ensure blockade of the lingual

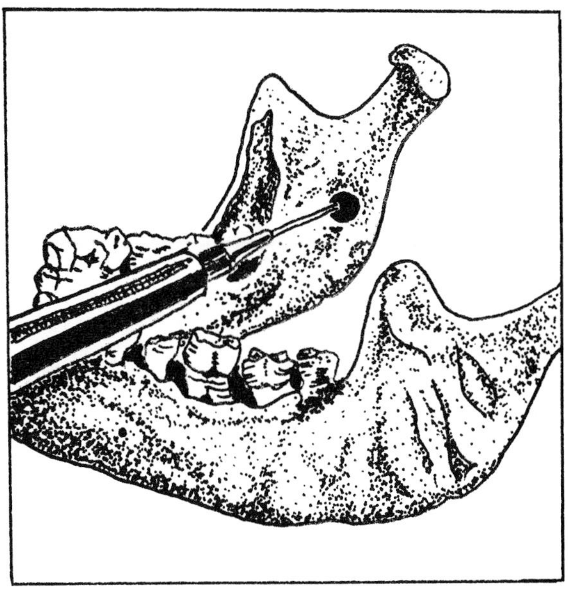

Fig. 16-14. Proper placement of needle on medial surface of the ramus of the mandible for block of the inferior alveolar nerve.

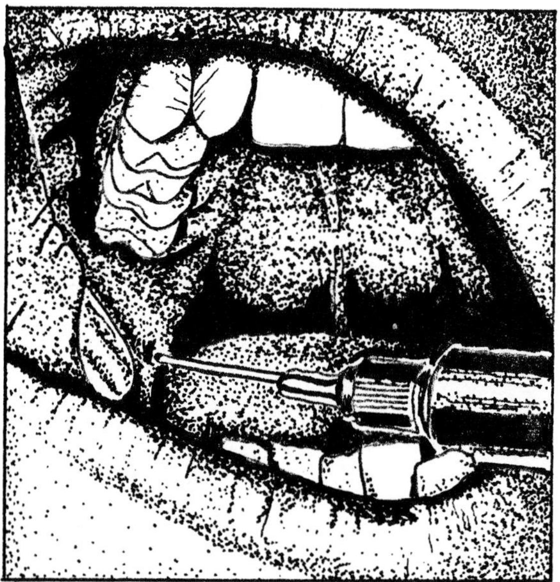

Fig. 16-15. Placement of the needle between the pterygomandibular raphe and retracting finger or thumb for block of the inferior alveolar nerve.

nerve, which is frequently accomplished, otherwise, by diffusion from the original injection site.

During the mandibular block procedure, it is helpful to have the patient's mouth open at all times. Access and definition of the anatomical landmarks are greatly enhanced.

Successful block of the inferior alveolar nerve will result initially in a tingling of the lower lip on the affected side, rapidly progressing to a numbness of the lip. This numbness is often described by patients as "a feeling of a fat lip." In most cases, the lingual nerve is also anesthetized during the block of the inferior alveolar nerve and subjectively feels as if one-half of the tongue is numb.

Indications. There are many uses for the inferior alveolar nerve block. One use includes anesthesia for operative dentistry on all the mandibular teeth. Surgical procedures, likewise, may be accomplished on mandibular teeth and supporting structures anterior to the first molar if the block is supplemented by anesthesia of the lingual nerve. Similar surgical procedures posterior to the second bicuspid may also be performed with this block if both lingual and buccinator nerves are blocked. This block may also be used for the diagnosis or treatment of pain.

Lingual Nerve

Anatomy. The lingual nerve is the smaller of the two terminal branches of the posterior division of the mandibular branch of the trigeminal nerve. As it descends, it lies between the internal pterygoid muscle and the ramus of the mandible in the pterygomandibular space. It gives off small branches to the inferior alveolar nerve, which pass as sensory fibers to part of the tonsil and mucous membrane of the posterior oral cavity.

In the pterygomandibular space, the lingual nerve lies parallel but medial and anterior to the inferior alveolar nerve. It then passes below the mandibular attachment of the superior constrictor of the pharynx to reach the side of the base of the tongue a short distance behind and below the mandibular third molar. In the lateral lingual sulcus, it lies just below the mucous membrane, at the side of the tongue separated from it by the alveolingual groove. As it passes forward, it loops downward and medially beneath, and on the hyoglossus muscle medial to the submandibular duct.

Areas Anesthetized. The lingual nerve provides sensory fibers to the mucous membranes of the floor of the mouth and to the gingiva on the lingual and sublingual salivary glands and their ducts. It occasionally supplies sensory fibers to the bicuspids and first molar teeth. Blockade of the lingual nerve will provide anesthesia over the anterior two-thirds of the tongue and the floor of the oral cavity. Also anesthetized will be the mucosa and mucoperiosteum on the lingual side of the mandible.

Technique. The lingual nerve block is achieved when local anesthetic solution is deposited at a point approximately midway between the injection site for the inferior alveolar nerve block and the medial surface of the ramus. Local anesthetic solution may be deposited as the needle enters along the pathway to the inferior alveolar nerve or as the anesthesiologist is withdrawing the needle from the area of the mandibular foramen. At all times, it is imperative to aspirate prior to injection of local anesthetic, so that intravascular injection can be prevented (Fig. 16-16).

During intraoral block of the inferior alveolar and lingual nerves, occasionally a sharp paresthesia of the tongue will occur as the needle contacts the lingual nerve during approach or withdrawal.

Indications. Block of the lingual nerve is useful for surgical procedures of the anterior two-thirds of the tongue, the floor of the oral cavity, and mucous membranes on the lingual side of the mandible. With block of both the inferior alveolar nerve and lingual nerve, anesthesia to one-half of the lower jaw is nearly complete. Innervation from the long buccal nerve and accessory fibers crossing over the midline must be blocked to assure complete anesthesia.

Buccal Nerve

Anatomy. The anterior division of the mandibular nerve, the buccal nerve, is smaller than the posterior division and is primarily motor in function. The buccal nerve passes downward between the pterygoid muscles to emerge from beneath the anterior border of the masseter muscle. At about the level of the occlusal plane of the mandibular second and third molars, it crosses the anterior border of the mandibular ramus, where it divides into a number of branches to the buccinator muscle. Although the nerve penetrates this muscle, it has no motor fibers. The motor supply to the buccinator comes from the seventh cranial nerve. From here, the nerve sends many terminal fibers to its final sensory distribution.

Areas Anesthetized. Sensory fibers from the buccal nerve supply the mucous membrane and skin of the cheek. Other branches provide sensation to the buccal gingivae about the mandibular molars and the mucous membrane of the lower part of the buccal vestibule. Occasionally, the buccal nerve contributes to the sensation of the second bicuspid and the first molar of the lower jaw. The sensory supply may not cover the posterior superior area of the cheek (gingival branch of posterior superior alveolar nerve), but it may extend a short distance into the mucous membrane of the upper and lower lips near the corner of the mouth.

Technique. The terminal branches of the buccal nerve may be blocked by entering the mucosa above the buccal fold of the first mandibular molar (Fig. 16-17). A 2.5-cm (1-in), 25-gauge needle is advanced in a horizontal position, distally under the cheek toward the ramus of the mandible, depositing approximately 0.5 ml of anesthetic solution along the way.

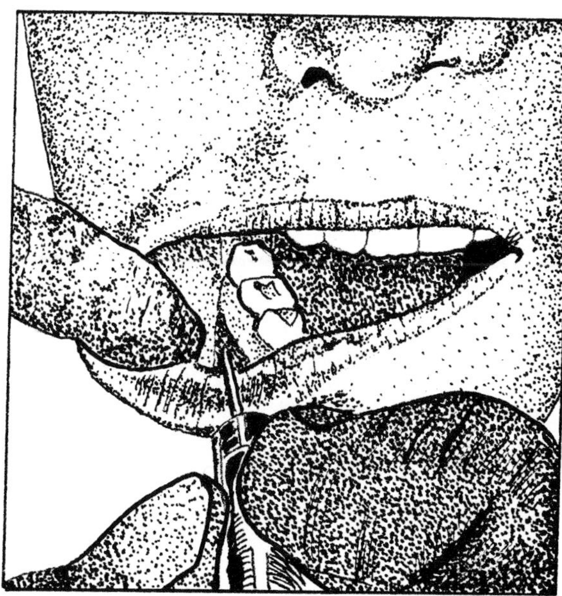

Fig. 16-17. The approach to the long buccal nerve and its branches in the mucobuccal fold below the mandibular first molar.

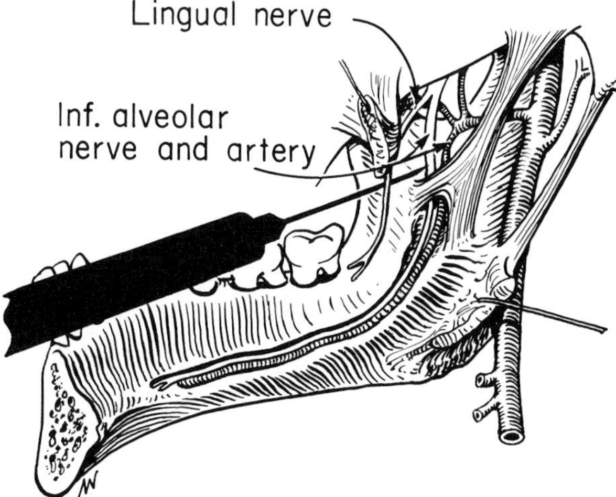

Fig. 16-16. Approach to inferior alveolar and lingual nerve block. (Bennett, C.R.: Monheim's Local Anesthesia and Pain Control in Dental Practice. ed. 6. St. Louis, C.V. Mosby, 1978)

An alternate method is to block the buccal nerve itself. This is accomplished by injecting into the buccal mucosa in the retromolar fossa approximately on line with the occlusal surface at the maxillary level of the third molar. The patient should hold his jaw wide open while 0.5 ml of local anesthetic solution is injected.

Indications. Block of the buccal nerve is used for surgery on the mandibular buccal mucosa and to supplement the inferior alveolar nerve block.

Mental Nerve

Anatomy. It will be recalled from the descriptive anatomy of the inferior alveolar nerve that the mental nerve is one of its two terminal branches. Near the mental foramen of the mandible, the inferior alveolar nerve divides into the mental nerve and a small incisive branch. The mental nerve, having emerged through the mental foramen, sends a few fine twigs to form a delicate plexus on the surface of the bone. The mental foramen usually lies at the apex and just anterior to the second bicuspid root.

Areas Anesthetized. The mental plexus provides innervation for the incisor teeth of the mandible, as well as for the skin of the chin and lower lip and the

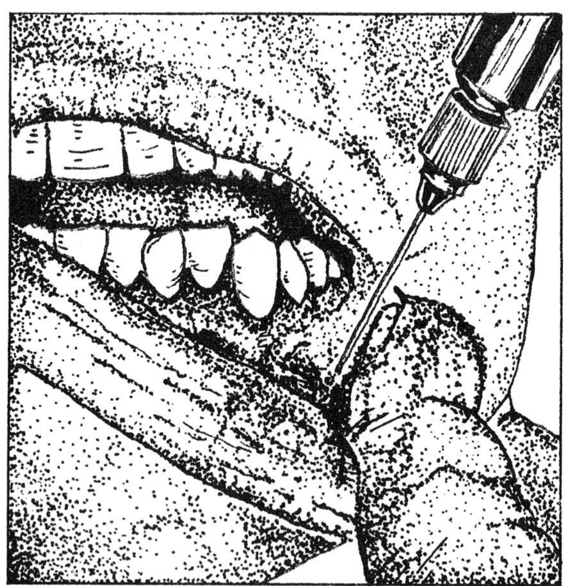

Fig. 16-18. Retraction of lower lip and placement of needle into the buccal labial fold between the bicuspid teeth for block of the mental nerve.

mucous membrane of the lower lip. Because block of the mental nerve usually anesthetizes the incisive nerve as well, anesthesia of the anterior portion of the mandible from the bicuspids to the incisors, including the overlying labial structures anterior to the mental foramen, usually results.

Technique. When a mental block is to be performed, the lower lip and cheek are pulled to the buccal side and a 2.5-cm (1-in), 25-gauge needle is inserted into the labial fold, directed toward the periosteum of the mandible to a point between the bicuspid teeth at a level just below their root apices (Fig. 16-18). It is often helpful to palpate the foramen with an index finger before insertion of the needle. The needle is "walked" gently along the periosteum until it enters the mental foramen. Following aspiration, 0.5 to 1 ml of local anesthetic solution is deposited.

If penetration of the foramen is inadequate, the anterior portion of the inferior alveolar nerve will be poorly anesthetized, with resulting poor anesthesia on the incisor and canine teeth. Supplementation by infiltrating local anesthetic solution around the root areas of the anterior teeth and periosteum of the bone may be required. However, this concomitant method of securing anesthesia is, as a rule, not highly successful in the mandible, although it will on occasion be successful with the anterior teeth.

Indications. Block of the mental nerve is highly effective for surgery on the lower lip or mucous membrane in the mucolabial fold anterior to the mental foramen when, for some reason, the inferior alveolar block is not indicated. If the incisive nerve is blocked as well, then procedures on the mandible may also be accomplished.

REFERENCES

1. Adatia, A.K.: Regional nerve block for maxillary permanent molars. Br. Dent. J., *140*:87, 1976.
2. Bennett, C.R.: Monheim's Local Anesthesia and Pain Control in Dental Practice. ed. 6th. St. Louis, C. V. Mosby, 1978.
3. Eriksson, E.: Illustrated Handbook in Local Anesthesia. Chicago, Year Book Medical Publishers, 1969.
4. Haglund, J., and Evers, H.: Local Anesthesia in Dentistry. ed. 2. Sodertalje, Sweden, Astra Lakemedel, 1975.
5. Sicher, H., and DuBaud, E.L.: Oral Anatomy. ed. 5. St. Louis, C. V. Mosby, 1970.
6. Manual of Local Anesthesia in General Dentistry. ed. 2. New York, Cook-Waite Laboratories, 1947.

17 Neural Blockade for Ophthalmologic Surgery

Jorn Boberg–Ans and
Soren S. Barner

The eye and its surroundings are usually considered to be the most sensitive part of the entire body. The suggestion of surgery in this area usually arouses anxiety, not only in the patient but also frequently on the part of the inexperienced surgeon. Most patients do not know that the anatomy of this region renders it accessible and also susceptible to the effect of local anesthetics in small quantities. The most sensitive parts of the region, the cornea and conjunctiva, are completely anesthetized in less than 60 seconds by just one drop of a proper topical anesthetic agent.

It is, of course, a basic presumption that either the surgeon or anesthesiologist is thoroughly familiar with the anatomy of the region, as well as the detailed technique of achieving complete anesthesia. This is obtained by using as little volume of anesthetic agent as necessary with the smallest possible degree of trauma to the ocular tissues.

Unique to eye surgery and especially eye microsurgery is the need for complete immobilization of the region and of the patient himself. The complications that most often spoil the results of intraocular operations are caused by displacement of the ocular contents, especially the iris or vitreous, and by extensive bleeding from the iris or choroid. Since the eye is a spherical organ, any change in its shape is bound to cause a reduction of volume. Deformation may arise from pressure behind the globe, contraction of the ocular or facial muscles, or from congestion of the vascular bed. All these changes are predispositions for iris or vitreous displacement forward into the wound. Through effective akinesia of the extraocular and surrounding muscles and by proper preoperative preparation of the patient and of the surgical team, these complications are effectively obviated.

It requires no unusual skill to prepare a patient for ocular surgery. The induction of local anesthesia is frequently performed by the ophthalmic surgeon or by an anesthesiologist with a special interest in this field. This chapter contains the necessary practical information that should enable surgeons and anesthesiologists to carry out these rather simple procedures.

LOCAL VERSUS GENERAL ANESTHESIA

A variety of extraocular and intraocular surgical procedures are possible with local anesthesia. In intraocular surgery and especially intraocular microsurgery, a basic requirement is that the eye is completely immobile and also that the intraocular tension and retrobulbar pressure are as low as possible during the entire procedure. The patient should, therefore, be well sedated. This can be achieved through local, as well as general, anesthesia.[1,3–10,12–18]

Advantages of Local Anesthesia

With well-planned preanesthetic preparation of patients capable of cooperative understanding (*i.e.*, not below 14–15 years of age), the selection of local anesthesia will lead to limited anxiety (Table 17-1).[11] The patient should be convinced that he will feel only two or three needle sticks and will relax as soon as the injections are completed. Sometimes, the patient may feel that the draping over the face is unpleasant, but this is easily alleviated by administering oxygen.

Local anesthesia entails little risk and is therefore less dependent on the patient's general health. Local anesthesia is preferable in diabetic patients because it does not interfere with their usual treatment or food intake. Even though the patient is conscious during the operation, the procedure does not feel too unpleasant to him, and he is often pleased to be able to keep informed about the proceedings of his own treatment. Local anesthesia has a rapid onset, and with the available anesthetic agents, it can be dispensed to last for a sufficiently long period of time to alleviate immediate postoperative

Table 17-1. Advantages and Disadvantages of Local and General Anesthesia

Advantages	*Disadvantages*
Local Anesthesia	
Possible in patients above age 15	Impossible in children
Independent of the patient's general health condition	Risk of intravascular injection
Limited patient anxiety	Risk of oculocardiac reflex
Low intraocular tension	Limited duration—may have to be supplemented in long procedures
Manageable dilated pupil	Distortion of the regional anatomy by
Effects lasts long enough to avoid postoperative pain	Fluid volume injected
Only three injections	Hemorrhage, edema
Easy; usually sufficient	Immediate allergy and postoperative allergy
Rapid in effect	Local hemorrhage subcutaneously, subconjunctivally, and retrobulbarly
Inexpensive	Scar tissue curtails effect
	Patient is awake
	Dryness of the mucous membranes, due to preoperative atropine
	Physically unpleasant to lie still for more than 90 minutes
General Anesthesia	
Indispensable with children	Unsatisfactory general health condition increases risk
Indispensable in cases of major trauma with perforating lesions of the eyeball	Risk of vomiting or coughing upon awakening
Patient is unconscious	Intubation/extubation complications
Responsibility rests entirely with the anesthesiologist	Patient anxiety
No disturbance of the local anatomical condition	No food or fluid for 6 hours prior to surgery
Duration of surgery of little importance	Unpleasant upon awakening
Control of intraocular tension by controlled manual hyperventilation	Availability of the anesthetic team
Narrow pupil, which is preferable in glaucoma and graft surgery	Surgical field close to the working area of the anesthesiologist
	Narrow pupil, which is not preferable in cataract extractions and insertion of pupillary lenses
	Additional personnel needed
	Expensive
	Additional time needed

pain.[4] Local-anesthesia-induced akinesia creates a low intraocular tension advantageous for intraocular surgery and an immobile eye and permits the surgeon to manage the size of the pupil, which is usually somewhat dilated, owing to paralysis of the ciliary ganglion.

Disadvantages of Local Anesthesia

It is extremely difficult to administer local anesthesia to children (see Table 17-1).[18] Due to preoperative atropine administered to prevent the oculocardiac reflex, uncomfortable dryness of oral mucous membranes develops. This can be alleviated to some degree by permitting the patient to wet his lips during the operation. The duration of the local anesthesia is usually limited to 2 to 3 hours. If the effect wears off too early, the subconjunctival anesthesia can be supplemented, but it is difficult and risky to supplement retrobulbar anesthesia when the eyeball is open. The volume of injected fluid, edema, and hemorrhage may distort the original anatomy. With ester-type drugs, unexpected immediate allergy may cause complications. Additionally, local subcutaneous hemorrhage of the skin and lids or subconjunctival or retrobulbar hemorrhage may cause such complications that the surgery may have to be postponed. Sudden movements if the patient dozes and awakens may also induce complications.

It is physically unpleasant for the patient to lie still for more than 90 minutes, especially elderly patients.

Scar tissue, which poses a problem in operations being performed again, lessens the effect of the anesthetic agent, and the often increased number of blood vessels curtails the duration of the anesthetic effect.

Advantages of General Anesthesia

General anesthesia has the definite advantage of relieving the eye surgeon and his assistants of the responsibility for the patient's general condition during surgery (see Table 17-1).[18] This responsibility is transferred to the anesthesiologist, making it possible for the surgical team to concentrate their attention exclusively on the surgery.

General anesthesia is definitely indicated for all children under 12 years of age, as well as any patient physically or mentally unable to cooperate reasonably.

It causes no distortion of the local anatomical condition, making it much easier for the surgeon to achieve satisfactory plastic surgical corrections and also allows the operation to be independent of any time limitation.

Intraocular tension can be controlled for short periods by manual hyperventilation. General anesthesia usually causes a narrow pupil, which is preferable in treating glaucoma and in graft surgery.

Disadvantages of General Anesthesia

As most or all extraocular and intraocular interventions may be performed under local anesthesia, the drawbacks and complications of general anesthesia, therefore, weigh more heavily than the advantages in deciding which to use (see Table 17-1).

General anesthesia involves some extra cost, and surgery has to be planned according to the availability of the anesthesiologist and his staff.

The patient is forbidden food or fluid for several hours prior to surgery. An unsatisfactory general health condition of the patient increases the hazards associated with general anesthesia. Postanesthesia complications, such as coughing or even vomiting, may be harmful to the surgical result.

General anesthesia yields a small pupil, which renders cataract surgery and implantation of an artificial lens more difficult. This can, of course, be altered by the topical installation of mydriatic drugs. Also, the nearness of the surgical field to the working area of the anesthesiologist is undesirable.

The choice of general or local anesthesia may be based on the facilities available and left to the discretion of the surgeon and the anesthesiologist. For instance, if a patient is blind in one eye, whether general or local anesthesia is used for an operation on the other eye is dependent upon the psychological condition of the patient, as well as that of the surgeon.

ANATOMY OF THE EYE AND THE ORBIT

A thorough knowledge of the anatomy, especially of the nerve supply to the orbital structures and surroundings, is essential to obtain effective neural blockade. The numerous anatomical textbooks should be consulted for their comprehensive surveys.[2,5,12,15–17]

Eye

The eyeball measures 24 mm, weighs about 7 g, and consists of three concentric layers; an outer fibrous layer (the cornea and sclera), a middle vascular layer (the iris, the ciliary body, and the choroid), and an inner nervous layer (the retina). Within the globe are the refracting media (aqueous humor, lens, and vitreous).

At the posterior aspect is the optic nerve, which traverses the orbit from the optic foramen to the eyeball. It is ensheathed in the meningeal layer of the dura of the brain. The diameter is 1.5 mm, the intraorbital length, 30 mm. It pierces the globe 3 mm nasal to the posterior pole.

The extraocular striated muscles are small, band-shaped structures approximately 4 cm long. Six muscles control the movements of the globe: the four recti and the two oblique muscles. A seventh striated muscle is the levator of the upper eyelid. The four rectus muscles arise from a common tendon ring that encircles the optic foramen (annulus of Zinn), and the insertions form a spiral around the limbus of cornea. The superior oblique muscle arises from the orbital apex above and medially to the superior rectus muscle, runs medially to the trochlea, then bends backward to insert beneath the superior rectus muscle. The inferior oblique muscle arises medially from the periosteum of the lacrimal bone, runs beneath the inferior rectus muscle, and

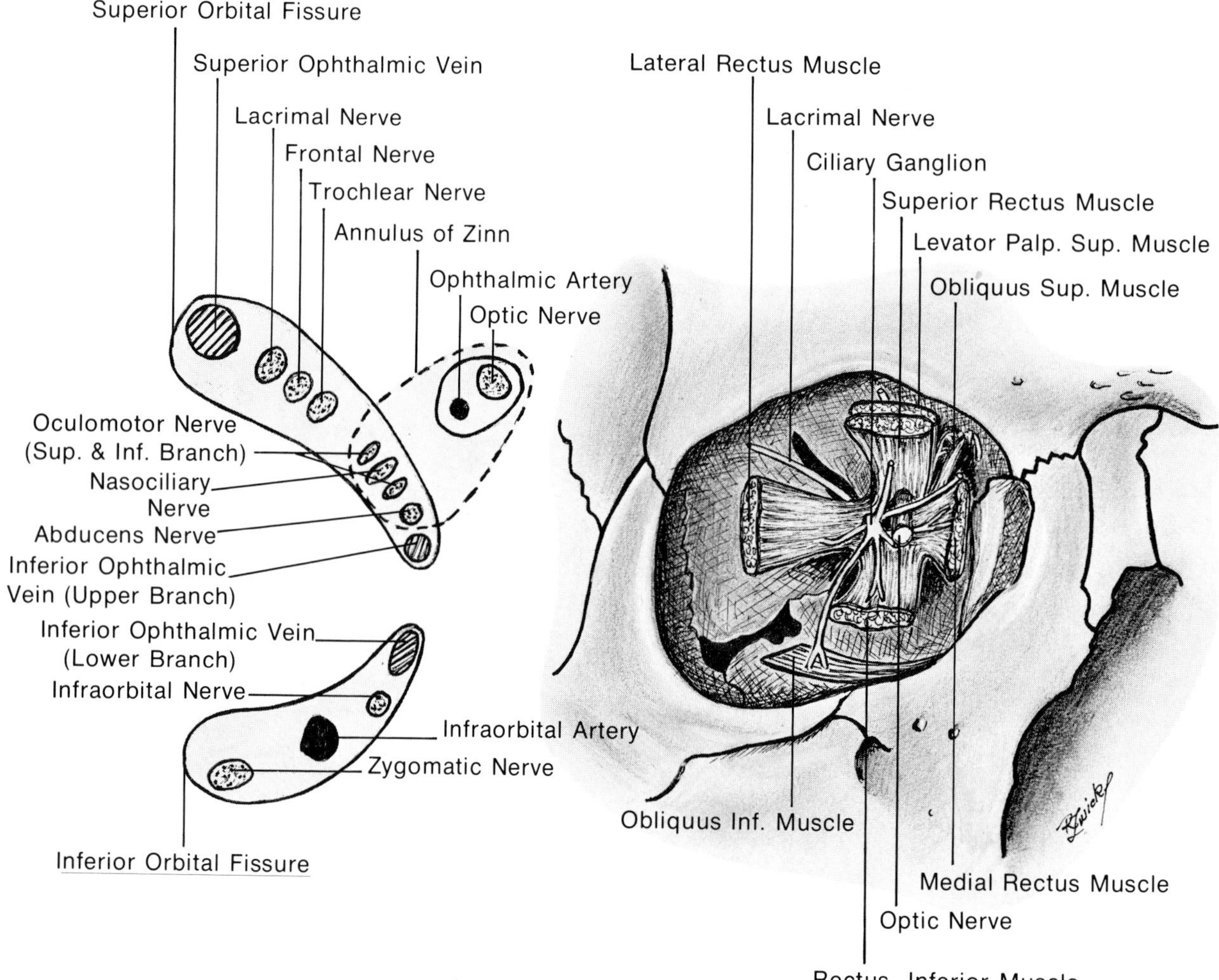

Fig. 17-1. Superior and inferior orbital fissure at apex of the muscle cone.

inserts on the posterolateral aspect of the eyeball. The levator muscle originates from the periosteum of the apex of the orbit above the superior oblique muscle. It runs forward between the roof of the orbit and superior rectus muscle and spreads out into an aponeurosis to insert to the skin of the upper eyelid and the tarsal plate.

Orbit

The orbit is a bony cavity that is in the shape of a pyramid with its apex at the optic foramen and its base at the orbital margin. The volume is approximately 29 ml. The bony orbit is covered by the outer periosteal layer of the dura mater (periorbita). The roof of the orbit is formed by the anterior cranial fossa. The floor of the orbit is related to the maxillary sinus and its medial wall to the nasal cavity and ethmoidal air cells. Adjacent to the lateral wall are the temporal and the middle cranial fossae. There are nine canals and fissures in the orbit, the most important being the optic foramen, the superior and inferior orbital fissures, and the supraorbital and infraorbital foramina (Fig. 17-1).

The orbital contents include the eyeball and the optic nerve, the seven extraocular muscles and their three motor nerves, sensory nerves including the ciliary ganglion, blood supply to the globe and adnexa through the ophthalmic artery and veins, muscular sheaths and bulbar fascia (Tenon's capsule), and adipose tissue (Fig. 17-2).

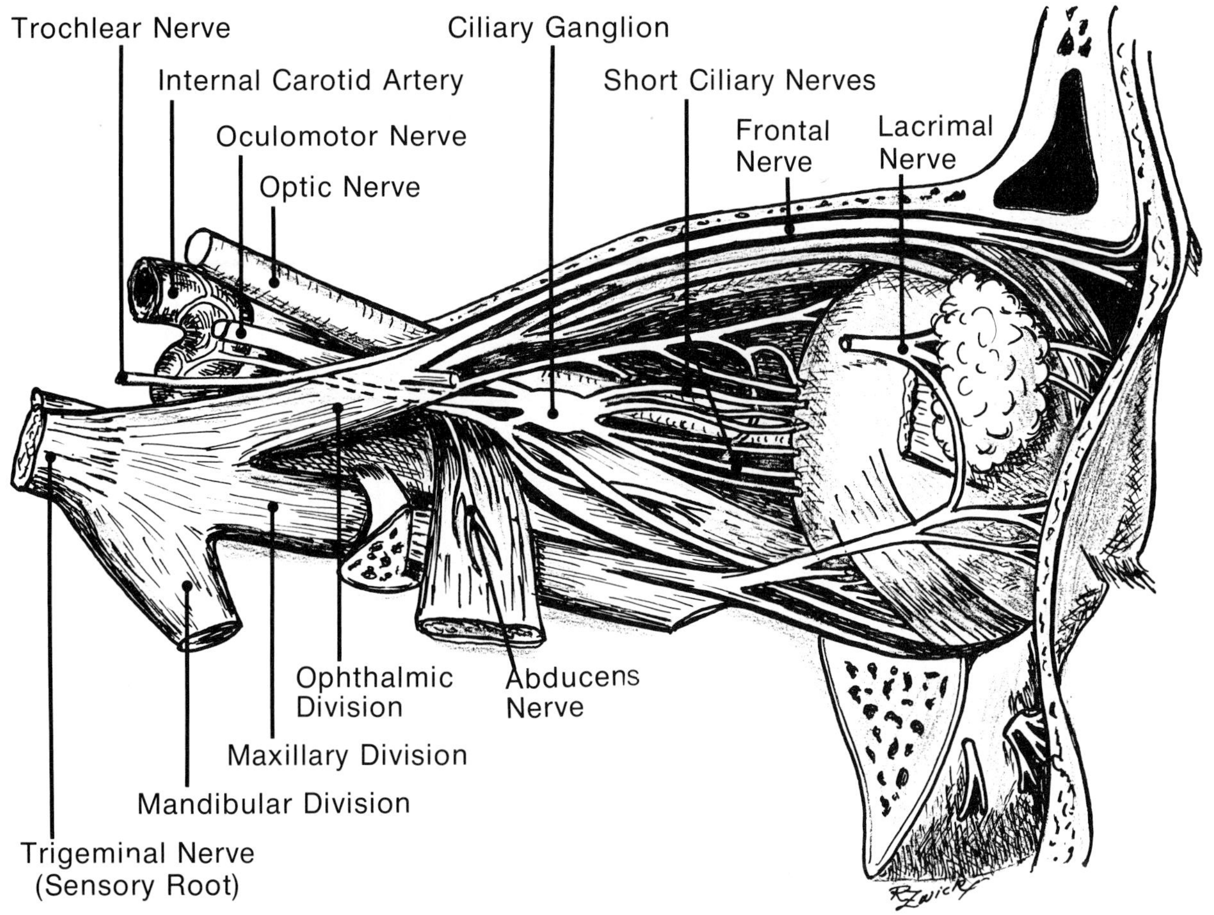

Fig. 17-2. Lateral view of the orbital contents.

Sensory Nerves from the Eye

The nuclei in the central nervous system (CNS) and the intracranial course of the various cranial nerves are not included in this presentation, which includes only nervous distribution to pertinent structures. The sensory nerve supply to the eye and its surroundings derive from the fifth cranial nerve (*trigeminal;* Fig. 17-3). This is a mixed nerve that consists of a large sensory part and a small motor part. The sensory portion of the nerve divides at the trigeminal ganglion into three branches: ophthalmic, maxillary, and mandibular.

The ophthalmic division is entirely sensory. Entering the orbit through the superior orbital fissure it divides into three branches: lacrimal, frontal, and nasociliary.

Lacrimal nerve travels to the lateral part of bulbar conjunctiva, lacrimal gland, and lateral canthus.

Frontal nerve divides into the *supratrochlear nerve* to the skin over the medial part of the upper eyelid and lower part of the forehead and the *supraorbital nerve* to the skin and palpebral conjunctiva of the upper eyelid.

Nasociliary nerve is the sensory nerve to the entire eyeball. It gives off two *long ciliary nerves* to the cornea, iris, and ciliary muscle and the *infratrochlear nerve* to the medial bulbar conjunctiva, inner canthus, and the lacrimal sac. The *ciliary ganglion* contains sensory fibers from the long sensory root, deriving from nasociliary nerve. The sensitive innervation is mainly from the cornea, the iris, and the ciliary body through the short ciliary nerves to the ganglion.

The maxillary division is also entirely sensory. As the *infraorbital nerve,* it traverses the floor of the orbit and emerges through the infraorbital foramen, giving off branches to the lower eyelid, lacrimal sac,

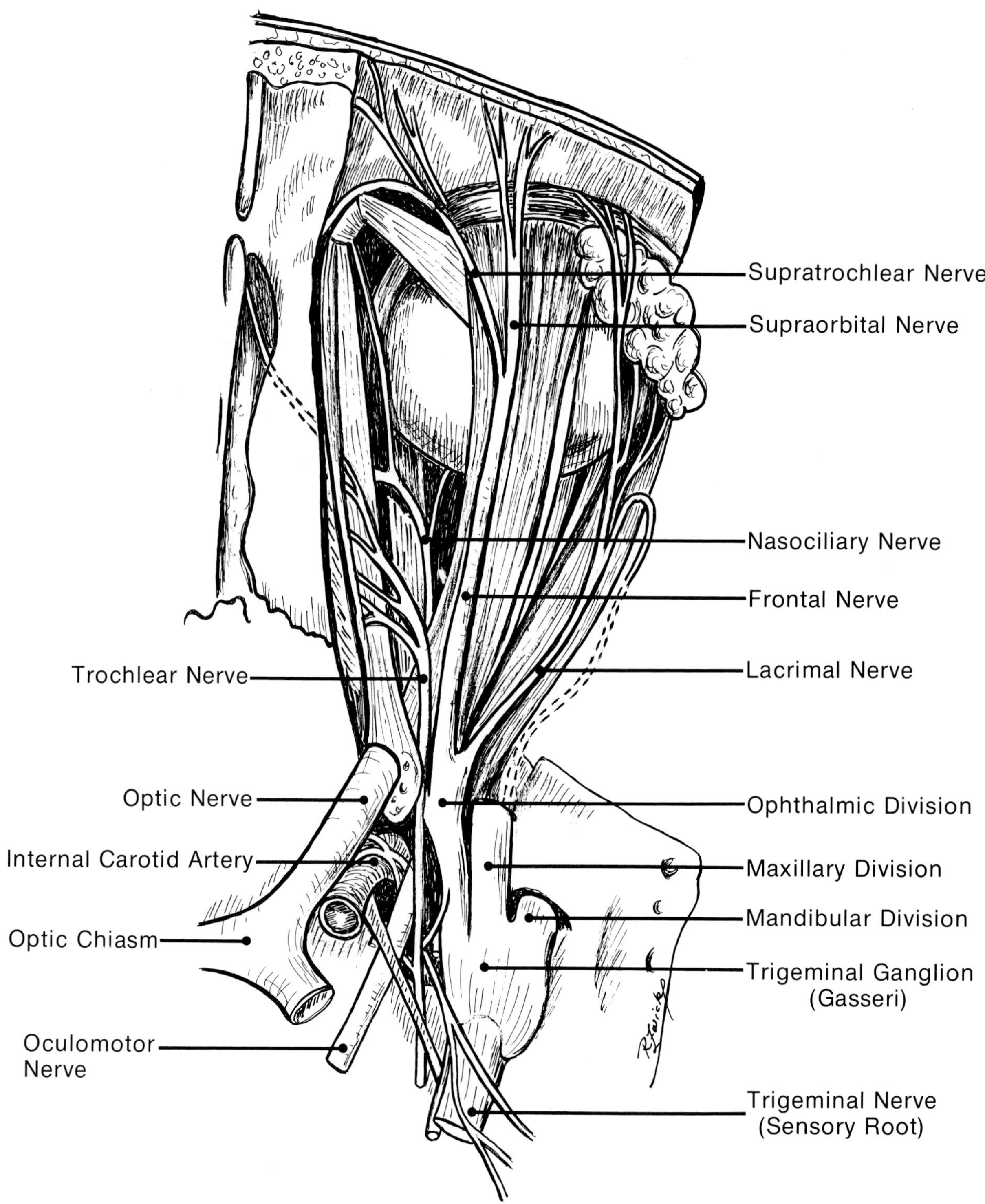

Fig. 17-3. Superior view of trigeminal nerve and distribution of branches.

Sensory Innervation of the Eye and Surrounding Structures

Forehead
- Supratrochlear nerve (frontal nerve)

Upper eyelid
- Supratrochlear nerve (frontal nerve)
- Infratrochlear nerve (nasociliary nerve)
- Lacrimal nerve

Lower eyelid
- Supraorbital nerve (frontal nerve)
- Infraorbital nerve (maxillary nerve)
- Supraorbital nerve (frontal nerve)

Medial canthus
- Infratrochlear nerve (nasociliary nerve)
- Supraorbital nerve (frontal nerve)

Lateral canthus
- Lacrimal nerve

Eyeball
- Long ciliary nerves (nasociliary nerve)
- Short ciliary nerves (nasociliary nerve)

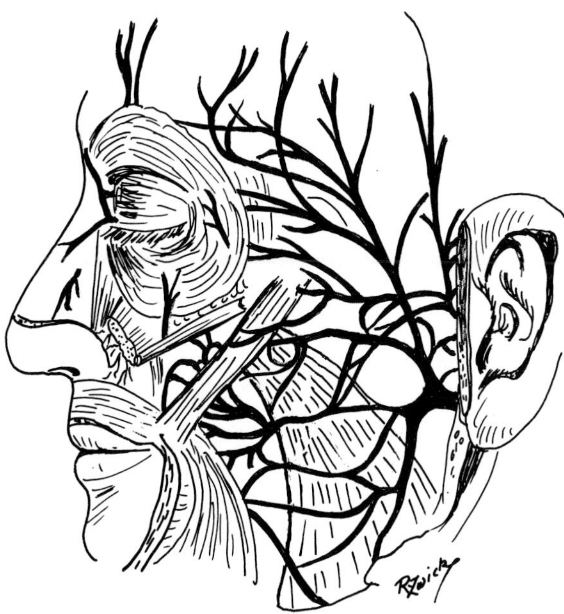

Fig. 17-4. Facial nerve and distribution of branches.

nasolacrimal duct, and the upper lip (see Chap. 16).

The mandibular division consists of two roots, of which the sensory part is the larger. It does not supply any of the ocular structures (see Chap. 16).

Motor Nerves to the Eye

The six extrinsic eye muscles and the levator palpebrae muscle are supplied by four cranial nerves: oculomotor (third), trochlear (fourth), abducens (sixth), and facial (seventh).

The oculomotor nerve enters the orbit through the superior orbital fissure, having first divided into two branches, a "superior" and an "inferior." The "superior" division supplies the levator palpebrae superioris muscle and the superior rectus muscle. The "inferior" division innervates the medial rectus, the inferior rectus, and the inferior oblique muscles.

The trochlear nerve has a long intracranial course before entering the orbit through the superior orbital fissure, where it crosses the third nerve before entering the superior oblique muscle.

The abducens nerve runs through the cavernous sinus and appears in the orbit through the superior orbital fissure to supply the lateral rectus muscle.

The facial nerve supplies all the muscles of expression, including the orbicularis oculi in the eyelids. During its passage through the facial canal of the temporal bone, it gives off several branches to the ear. Through the stylomastoid foramen, it emerges just below the osseus part of the outer ear, now containing only motor fibers. Turning forward, it enters the parotid gland superficial to the neck of the mandible, where it divides into five branches (temporal, zygomatic, buccal, mandibular, and cervical). The temporal division supplies the upper part of the orbicularis oculi, the corrugator supercilii, and the frontalis muscle. The zygomatic branch supplies the lower part of the orbicularis oculi muscle (Fig. 17-4).

Autonomic Innervation of the Eye

The autonomic nervous system supplies the eye through the sympathetic and parasympathetic system.

The sympathetic postganglionic fibers arise from the superior cervical ganglion and reach the eyeball by way of the ciliary ganglion either through the two long ciliary nerves or through the multiple short ciliary nerves. They supply the vascular system of the choroid, ciliary body, and iris as vasoconstrictors and carry the motor impulses to the radial dilator pupillae muscle in the iris.

The parasympathetic nerve supply arises from the oculomotor nerve as preganglionic fibers, entering the parasympathetic ciliary ganglion situated inside the orbit. They then leave the ganglion as postganglionic axons and are the main constituents of the short ciliary nerves. They pierce the eyeball in a circle around the optic nerve and supply the circular sphincter pupillae muscle and the ciliary muscle. In-

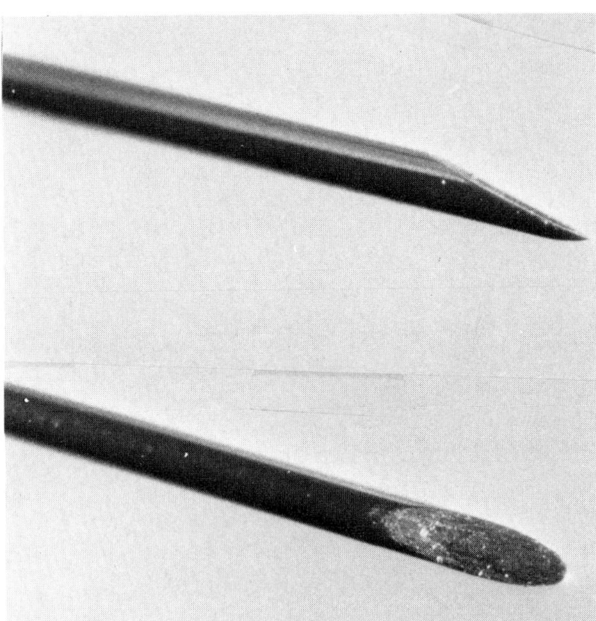

Fig. 17-5. Frontal and lateral views of the Atkinson needle.

terruption of the parasympathetic innervation lessens the secretion from the ciliary body.

INSTRUMENTS AND ANESTHETIC AGENTS

Instruments

A 2-ml Luer-Lok syringe usually suffices because rarely more than 2 ml is injected at one time.

The Atkinson needle—a 35-mm long, 23-gauge needle with the point ground off to a specially rounded, sharpened tip, is most widely employed for ophthalmic anesthesia. This needle is indispensable for retrobulbar injection and is suitable for subconjunctival injection, as well as for facial nerve block. The advantage of this needle is the diminished risk of piercing a vessel, a genuine concern in some kinds of ophthalmic surgery (Fig. 17-5).

If the anesthesiologist prefers the shorter, fine, disposable needle, a 25-mm, 23-gauge may be used for subconjunctival injections or injections along the muscles in squint surgery. Long pointed needles should be avoided.

Supplementary Equipment

The personnel in the operating theater should have available and be acquainted with the monitoring and resuscitation equipment necessary for neural blockade (Fig. 17-6; see also Chap. 4).

Anesthetic Agents

Agents to be injected for local anesthesia in ophthalmic surgery are basically the same as those used in other peripheral nerve blocks (see Chap. 4).

Complications

The toxic symptoms of local anesthesia in ophthalmologic surgery are usually increased CNS excitability secondary to accidental intra-arterial or intravenous injection (see Chap. 4).

Stimulation of the parasympathetic system, the vagal reflex, may cause bradycardia or, rarely, laryngospasm. This condition can be alleviated by atropine, 0.5 mg intravenously. In order to prevent this reaction, atropine can be administered intravenously immediately before the operation.

Coughing and vomiting can also be indirect complications of local anesthesia for eye surgery. Preoperative antiemetic and sedative medication, such as promethazine or diazepam, may be used. Other sedatives and tranquilizers may cause hypotension, which may manifest as dizziness when the patient leaves the operating table.

PREANESTHETIC PREPARATION

Often, too little attention is paid to the preanesthetic preparation of the patient, particularly when the surgery is performed in the office or in a casualty room. Careful preanesthetic preparation combined with adequate anesthesia and akinesia is responsible for saving many eyes.

The preanesthetic factors to be considered are the psychological preparation of the patient and premedication.

Psychological Preparation

The psychological preparation of the patient is of great importance in intraocular surgery. It includes careful explanation of the nature of the surgery, reassurance that the procedure will not cause undue pain, and establishment of sound cooperation between the surgeon and the patient during the operation.

Because modern ocular surgery is frequently performed under a microscope, small movements of the head, a cough, a sneeze, or conversation during delicate stages may be serious to the outcome. This

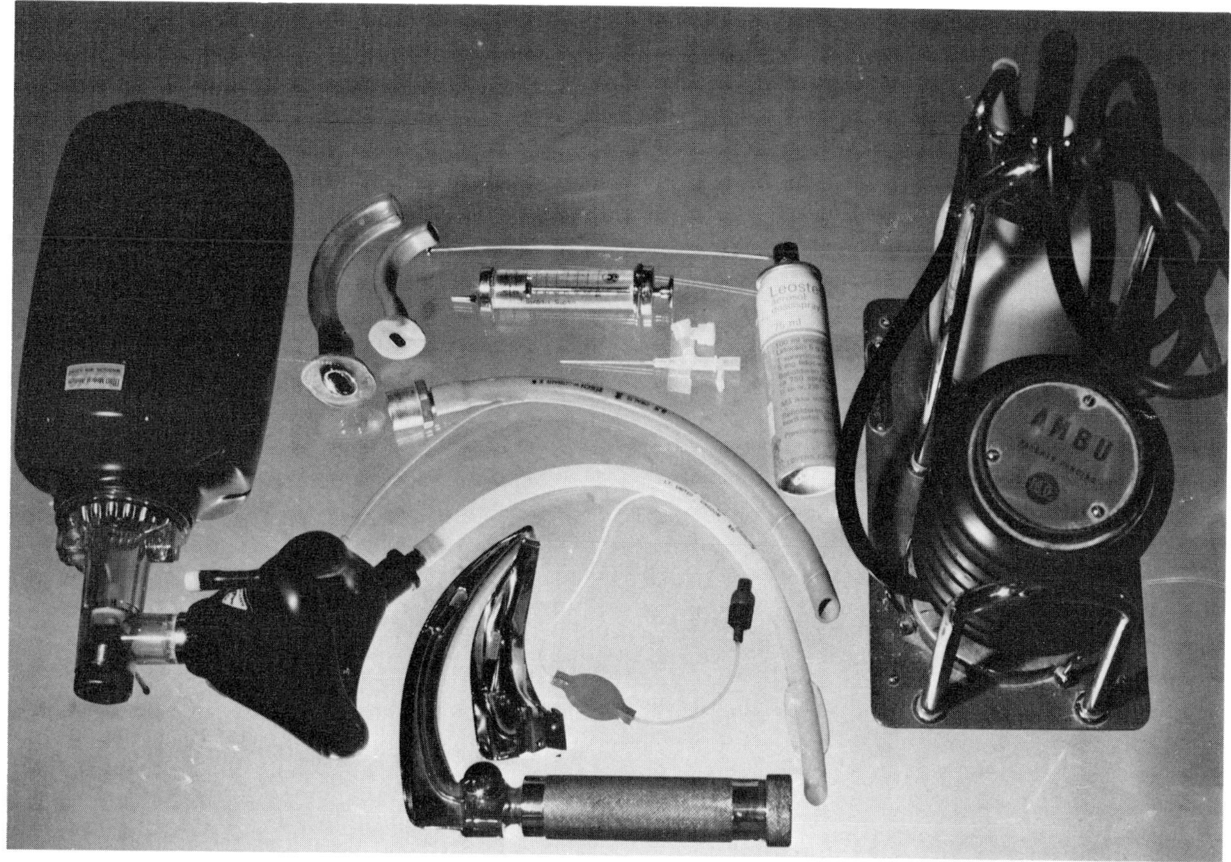

Fig. 17-6. Resuscitating instruments.

must be explained prior to surgery in a quiet manner, and the patient should never be blamed if the procedure is not successful. This point seems obvious, but it is nevertheless too often neglected.

Premedication

Premedication is largely a matter of specific requirements and of the experience and habit of the anesthesiologist.[3,9,13] Usually, a sedative and an analgesic are used together in order to make the patient quiet, comfortable, and calm. In apprehensive patients the administration of an oral sedative the night before the operation is recommended. Additionally, drugs may be administered before surgery to obtain a certain degree of depression of the CNS, to eliminate or diminish untoward autonomic reflexes, and to minimize pre- or postoperative nausea and vomiting. The amount of premedication is dependent on the status of the patient (age, sex, weight, and physical and psychological condition) and the nature of the surgery (extent, duration). The aim is to administer enough to obtain the required effect, but not more than necessary.

Timing of the administration of the premedication is also important. With the usual combinations, it is recommended that drugs be given approximately 30 to 45 minutes before surgery. Because of the annoying increased diuresis, routine use of ocular hypotensive drugs preoperatively should be avoided.

Operating Room

Consideration should be given to the atmosphere in the operating room. With patients under local anesthesia, it is important to avoid unnecessary noise and conversation. A spirit of willing cooperation, in combination with good surgical discipline, is desirable. The technical preparations of the surgical procedure should be completed before the patient is brought to the theater. The operating table should be comfortable without being too soft. The operating lights need not be turned on before the anesthesiologist and surgeon are ready. All manipulations with the patient are best explained to him before they are carried out to avoid unwanted reactions. When the face is covered with a drape, the feeling of suffocation or claustrophobia can be reduced by insufflating oxygen under the drape.

Intraocular surgery is unique in that it demands complete immobility of the patient during the entire procedure. If the preanesthetic preparations for some reason cannot be accomplished within the framework described, general anesthesia should seriously be considered.

SURFACE ANESTHESIA

The indications for surface anesthesia are numerous because most surgical interventions in or on the eye require complete elimination of corneal and conjunctival reflexes. Although solutions of most local anesthetic agents may be used on the eye, their effectiveness depends on their ability to penetrate the mucous surfaces. This usually requires increased concentrations of local anesthetics, and, for this reason, such preparations should not be used for injection.

Drugs

Clinical use of local anesthetic agents was first reported in Kohler's report on cocaine for ophthalmologic surgery (see Chap. 1). The cornea can be anesthetized with solutions of 0.25 to 0.5 per cent. There is an accompanying constriction of the conjunctival vessels, and the sclera is blanched. Mydriasis also occurs. The pupil of the cocainized eye responds to light, and pilocarpine and physostigmine will still produce miosis. Cocaine in high concentration is capable of causing cycloplegia. With the usual anesthetic concentrations, however, loss of accommodation is only partial. Cocaine has variable effects on intraocular pressure. In most cases, it will reduce the pressure through its vasoconstricting properties. Occasionally, however, it may precipitate an attack of acute glaucoma thought to be due to the mydriasis exerting a mechanical block of drainage from the anterior chamber.

In anesthetic concentrations, cocaine has a deleterious effect on the cornea, causing it to become clouded and pitted and sometimes ulceration ensues. Because of the drawbacks of mydriasis and corneal injury, cocaine should be abandoned except for special procedures.

In addition to dibucaine, piperocaine, and tetracaine, which are used not only for surface anesthesia but also for infiltration and injection, there are agents whose use is restricted to the production of corneal anesthesia. Their main advantage is that they produce little or no mydriasis and, in small doses, are not injurious to the cornea.

Benoxinate (Dorsacaine) is an ester related to procaine, with the same toxicity index as tetracaine, compared to procaine. It is used primarily for tonometry, in which a single instillation of .075 to 0.1 ml of a 0.4-per-cent solution will provide sufficient anesthesia in approximately 60 seconds.

Proparacaine hydrochloride (Ophthaine) is a benzoic ester chemically distinct from procaine, benoxinate, and tetracaine. Thus, it is said to be free of cross-sensitization with the other local anesthetic agents. It is about as potent as tetracaine but, unlike many of the other agents, produces little or no initial irritation. It is available in a 0.5-per-cent solution for topical application.

Phenacaine hydrochloride (Holocaine, Tanicaine) was one of the earliest topical anesthetics introduced. It is a derivative of phenetidin and not an ester. It is more toxic than cocaine, both systemically and after subcutaneous injection. It is used solely for topical anesthesia in a 1-per-cent solution and is said to cause "smarting" or irritations prior to onset of anesthesia.

The absorption or duration of these agents is not influenced by the addition of vasoconstrictor drugs. Some commercially available eye-soothing preparations contain a small amount of highly viscous agents. These drugs are contraindicated prior to intraocular surgery as the macromolecules may enter the globe.

Cornea

For measuring the intraocular tension, for removal of superficial foreign bodies, for suture removal, and for irrigation of the tear ducts, 1 to 2 drops of a topical anesthetic agent will suffice. It should be remembered that it is not the number of drops but the number of instillations that is important. Thus, repeated instillations with intervals of a few minutes are usually satisfactory, even in an inflamed eye.

As noted, the use of cocaine should be abandoned except for special diagnostic or therapeutic procedures. It has a pronounced toxic and a desiccating effect on the corneal epithelium, eventually leading to erosions. Furthermore, the sympathomimetic effect that causes dilation of the pupil is often undesirable.

It should also be noted that instillation of a sur-

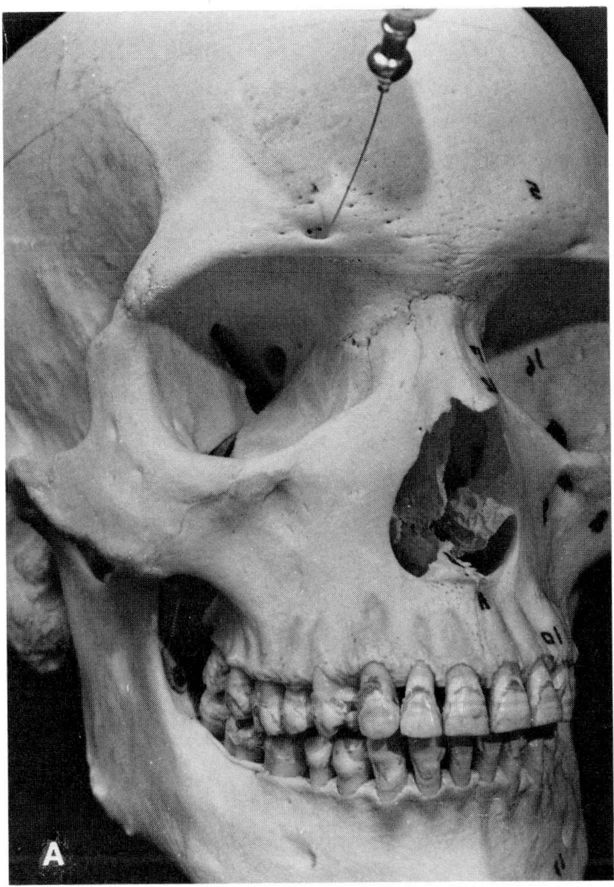

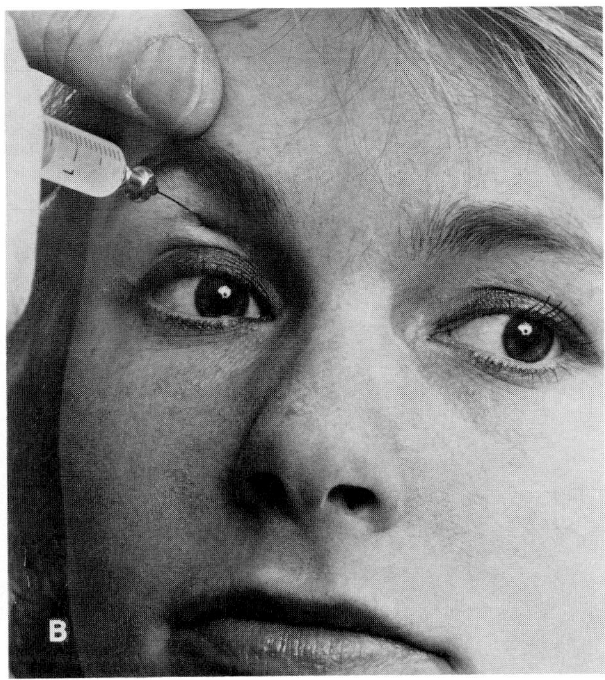

Fig. 17-7. Anatomical and clinical aspects of supraorbital nerve block.

face anesthetic temporarily alleviates the pain caused by corneal erosions, making it possible for the patient to neglect the corneal trauma for a lengthened time. This practice is unwise, however, because repeated instillation of surface anesthetics has a pronounced toxic effect and may, in a few hours, cause a complete denudation of the cornea, which may require a prolonged period to heal.

Conjunctiva

Due to the rich vascular supply and the unique innervation of the conjunctiva, it is not uncommon that the surface anesthetic effect wears off prematurely during surgery. To obtain reliable surface anesthesia, it is recommended that the instillations be repeated at short intervals, up to ten times over a period of 10 minutes. Primary exploration and suturing of small lacerations can easily be performed with this anesthesia, as can removal of minor foreign bodies and sutures. If more extensive surgery is required, a subconjunctival injection of a proper anesthetic agent is indispensable.

ANESTHESIA FOR EXTRAOCULAR SURGERY

Orbital Surroundings

Infiltration. For minor interventions of the eyelids, it is sufficient to give a small amount of subcutaneous infiltration injection, 0.25 to 2 ml of an anesthetic solution. This small amount of anesthetic solution causes no complications and requires no special preoperative preparation of the patient.

For more extensive interventions on the eyelids, a field block is advisable. A long fine needle is inserted just under the skin at the center of the superior or inferior orbital margin and introduced farther to each side along the bony margin of the orbit, beyond the line of the palpebral fissure.

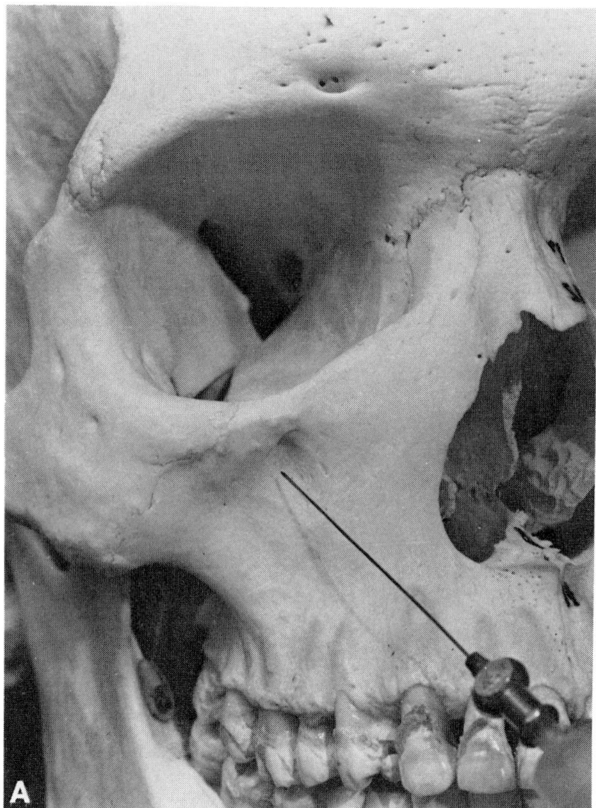

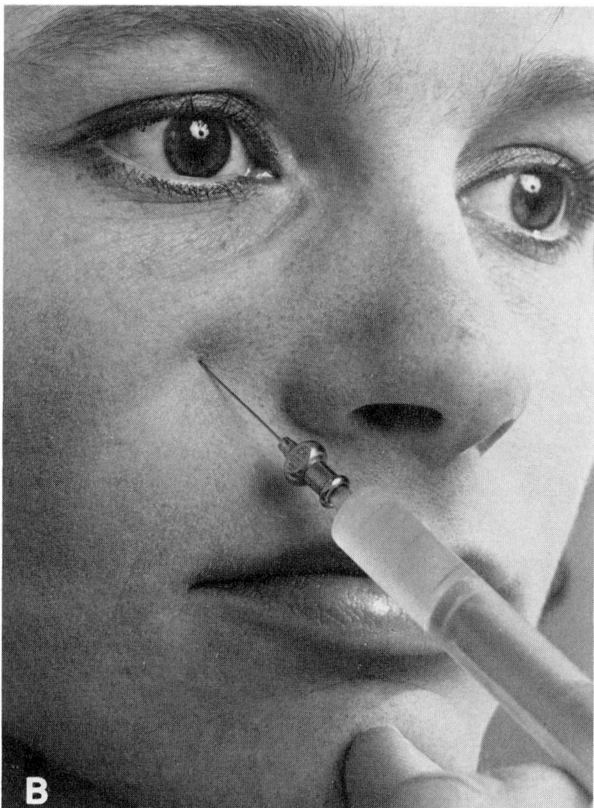

Fig. 17-8. Anatomical and clinical aspects of infraorbital nerve block.

Three-fourths of 1 ml of anesthetic solution is injected as the needle is carried forward. When this technique does not yield satisfactory anesthesia, topical anesthesia of the conjunctiva followed by subconjunctival injection of anesthetic solution along the cul-de-sac that corresponds to the part of the lid that is the object of surgery should be a satisfactory supplement. Sometimes, it may be easier for the surgeon to inject percutaneously instead of through the conjunctiva because the conjunctival approach often causes more anxiety in sensitive patients.

For yet more extensive surgical intervention of the eyelids and surroundings, larger quantities of anesthetic solution are required. This will distort the appearance and disturb the anatomical condition.

Nerve Blocks. The notch of the supraorbital nerve or foramen is easily found by palpation along the supraorbital border. When the supraorbital notch or foramen is found with the tip of the needle (Atkinson or some short fine needle), the syringe is raised, and the point of the needle is introduced along the supraorbital nerve for 3 to 4 mm. A deposit of 1 to 2 ml of anesthetic solution injected (Fig. 17-7).

Although it is safe to introduce the needle into the supraorbital notch, the anesthesiologist should be more careful when anesthetizing the *infraorbital nerve,* which supplies the skin of the lower eyelid and that of the face down to the upper lip.

Technique. By palpation 4 to 6 mm below the nasal part of the midpoint of the infraorbital margin, the infraorbital foramen is easily felt (Fig. 17-8). While he is palpating the small depression of the opening of the canal, the anesthesiologist directs the needle from the lower outer corner of the nostril, aiming toward the outer canthus. When the tip of the needle is felt at the infraorbital foramen, it should not be introduced, but rather the anesthetic solution deposited just outside the foramen. If the injection occurs inside the foramen, the pressure exerted may damage the nerve, causing a more permanent anesthesia of the area involved. If the infraorbital nerve or foramen cannot be found, the anesthesia can be administered in the inferior orbital fissure, where it is possible to block both the infraorbital and *anterior superior alveolar nerve*. This is necessary in operations on the lacrimal sac.

Technique. The needle is introduced percutaneously at the middle of the outer third of the infraorbital margin, or rather at the most inferior point of the infraorbital margin, as if aiming for a retrobulbar injection at the apex of the orbital pyramid (Fig. 17-9). The needle is moved along the orbital floor for about 20 mm, where the inferior orbital fissure should be felt. After aspiration, 1.5 ml of anesthetic solution is injected.

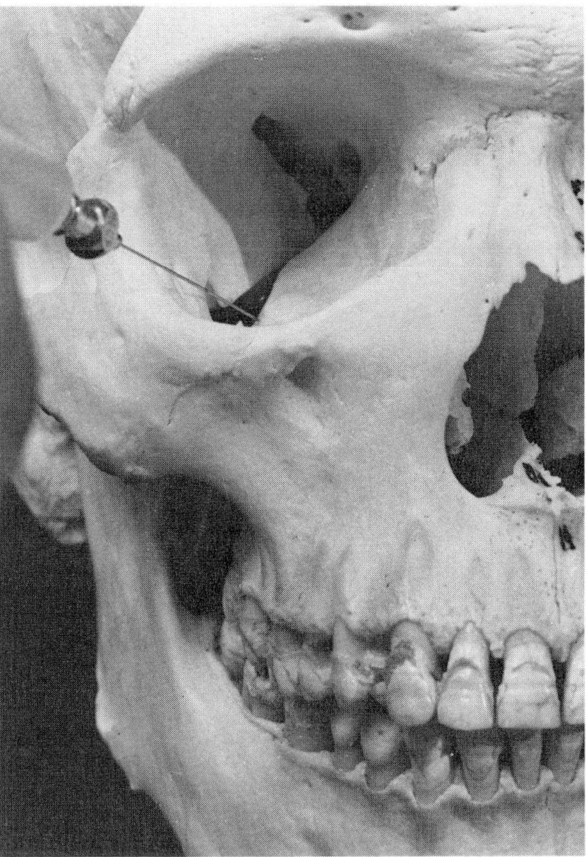

Fig. 17-9. Intraorbital technique for infraorbital nerve block.

Ocular Adnexae

Examination of the tear duct is considered rather unpleasant but can be performed without causing too much discomfort to the patient. A 23-gauge (0.4-mm) curved needle with a completely rounded "soft" end can be introduced in the upper and lower lacrimal ducts. Touching the cornea or conjunctiva when the "lacrimal needle" is introduced often causes undue anxiety in the patient. A few drops of surface anesthesia are therefore advisable prior to the introduction of the tear duct cannula into the punctum. The lacrimal system is washed with a local anesthetic solution. This usually yields sufficient anesthesia for examination with a narrow, blunt-ended probe. If it is necessary to probe farther and, especially, to probe the nasolacrimal duct, it may be advisable to anesthetize the nasolacrimal duct through block anesthesia.

Anesthesia for surgery on the lacrimal sac requires blocking the *nasociliary* and *infraorbital nerves*. The needle is introduced percutaneously at the most nasal part of the orbit (1 cm above the inner canthus), following the nasal wall of the orbit for about 25 mm, where the injection of 1.5 to 2 ml of anesthetic solution will anesthetize the nasociliary nerve and its more important branches, the infratrochlear and anterior ethmoidal nerves. A small deposit in the lacrimal fossa, which is easily felt by palpation, will decrease the bleeding and may add to the anesthesia for the operation of dacryocystorhinostomy (Fig. 17-10).

To anesthetize the nasal mucosa further, a small piece of gauze soaked in anesthetic solution, (*e.g.*, 5% cocaine), is deposited inside the nostril.

Extraocular Muscles

Most surgery of the extraocular muscles under local anesthesia involves adult squint surgery. Different techniques may be applied. Usually, topical anesthesia, combined with 1 to 3 ml of local anesthetic solution injected in Tenon's capsule along the muscle on which the operation will be performed, will suffice. When an operation is being performed again, a retrobulbar block is advisable because the dense adhesions of the perimuscular membranes, sequelae from previous surgery, may prevent proper local anesthesia.

Akinesia of the orbicularis oculi muscle is not mandatory but renders the patient more comfortable during the surgery and avoids the patient's involuntary squeezing.

Because retrobulbar anesthesia by experienced anesthesiologists entails very few complications and demands only one injection, it is as effective and much less unpleasant for squint surgery than repeated injections along the extraocular muscles. For squint operations in nervous adults, a retrobulbar injection followed by subconjunctival anesthesia is recommended because this last injection is not

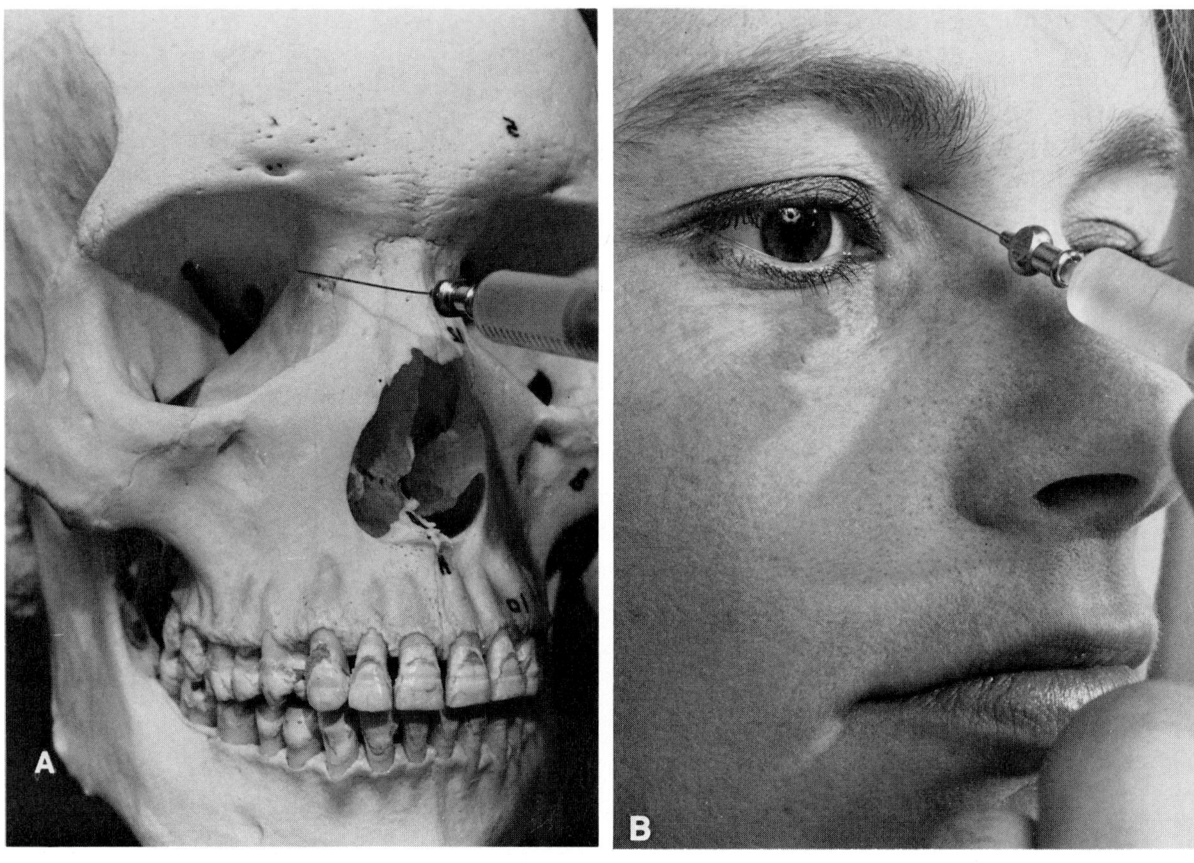

Fig. 17-10. Anatomical and clinical aspects of nasociliary nerve block.

felt by the patient. However, because most squint surgery is performed in children under the age of 15, general anesthesia is preferred.

Retinal Detachment Surgery

Retinal surgery can be, and often is, performed with local anesthesia. Since primary retinal surgery with cryotherapy and diathermy and, possibly, some kind of infolding technique may often be planned to last less than an hour and a half, local anesthesia is useful. The technique of anesthesia is the same as with intraocular surgery, that is, retrobulbar cone injection, subconjunctival injection, and akinesia. Additionally, it is often necessary to supplement the anesthesia during the operation, for instance, with an injection along the muscles or subconjunctivally.

However, because retinal detachment surgery may often be a procedure of long duration, general anesthesia is frequently preferable. In repeated operations for retinal detachment, extensive scar tissue is usually present, and local anesthesia is therefore often insufficient. Thus, general anesthesia is indispensable.

Orbit

For surgery of orbital tumors, local anesthesia is often contraindicated, even though it is possible to remove many tumors that are apparently easily accessible. Local anesthesia not only distorts the anatomy but may tend to spread the tumor cells if they are malignant.

Removal of the eye by either *enucleation* of the bulb or *exenteration* of the contents of the eyeball has usually been considered an indication for general anesthesia because it has been thought that the patient under local anesthesia may suffer psychologically when the eye is removed. In our opinion, this is not true. A thorough retrobulbar anesthesia is sufficient to render the operation completely painless under local anesthesia. The optic nerve is usually anesthetized to such a degree that the pa-

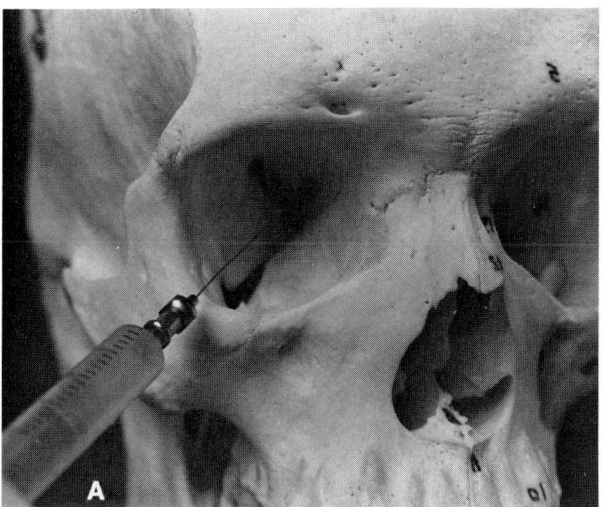

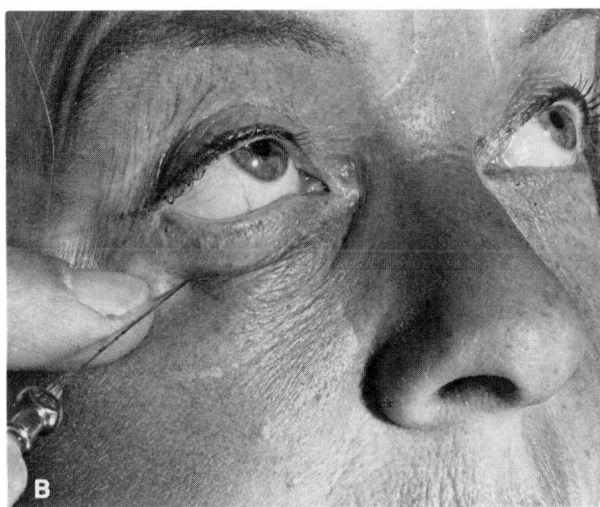

Fig. 17-11. Anatomical and clinical aspects of retrobulbar injection.

tient does not feel the cutting of the nerve and therefore is unaware of the actual removal of the eye. Bleeding rarely causes problems. Because the surgical procedure is rather short, retrobulbar anesthesia lasts long enough to insert a prosthesis if this is required.

It is also possible under local anesthesia to exenterate the contents of the bulb and insert an intrascleral prosthesis before the anesthesia disappears. Exenteration of the orbit is an extensive procedure and is best performed under general anesthesia.

ANESTHESIA FOR INTRAOCULAR SURGERY

Anesthesia for intraocular surgery involves retrobulbar anesthesia, subconjunctival anesthesia, and block of the facial nerve (*i.e.*, akinesia of the orbicularis oculi muscle). A detergent may be used to clean the skin of the eyelids and surroundings, while the conjunctival sac is washed with 1:1,000 solution of mercury chloride followed by washing with normal saline. The site for retrobulbar injection (*i.e.*, the skin of the outer canthus of the eye) is dabbed with antiseptic solution, as is the skin area in front of the ear. After proper washing, cleaning and irrigation of the eye, and cleaning of the skin of the eyelids, the patient is ready for injection.

Retrobulbar Injection

The anesthetic solution is usually 2 ml of local anesthetic solution with epinephrine. Hyaluronidase may be added to this solution if desired. A special needle is important, preferably 25-gauge and 35-mm long. The needle for retrobulbar injection should have a rounded point in order, as mentioned earlier, not to pierce a vessel. In order also to avoid piercing a vessel, it is advisable to inject solution slowly while the needle is being advanced.

If the eye is deeply set in the socket, it is simpler to inject through the eyelid. If the eye is normally set in the socket or there is some proptosis, it is just as simple for the surgeon and less unpleasant for the patient to carry the injection through the lower conjunctival fornix.

Ready for injection, the patient lies supine on the operating table with the head in fixed position and the nose pointing toward the ceiling. The patient is asked to look to the side opposite to the side of the eye to be injected and, at the same time, to keep the head still. The patient should look straight to the side, slightly up—never down. The surgeon, using his left index finger, palpates the inferior orbital margin at its lateral and most inferior aspect. This is the site of the injection (Fig. 17-11). The needle is directed from this point toward the top of the orbital pyramid just skirting below the ball of the eye. Because the eye has been rotated, the inferior oblique muscle has been turned out of the field of the route of the injection needle; therefore, the needle should only penetrate the orbital fat (Fig. 17-12). The needle should be introduced slowly and cautiously until the shoulder of the needle presses against the skin (Fig. 17-13). Often, there is no resistance felt although the penetration of a fine fascia

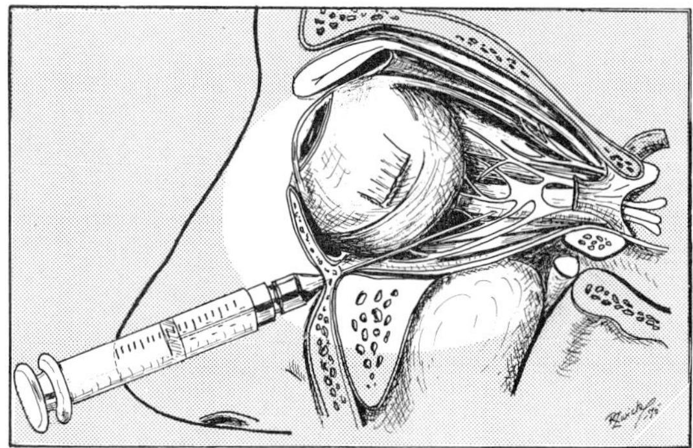

Fig. 17-12. Direction of the needle in the orbit.

may just barely be felt. If a more "tough" feeling is experienced—that is, if the tip is engaged into the substance of a muscle, the wall of the eye, or the optic nerve—the introduction should immediately be stopped, and the needle should be withdrawn a short distance and reinserted in a more vertical direction. If the patient happens to turn his eye away from the extreme adducted position, the needle may more easily be engaged in or penetrate the inferior oblique muscle. This may cause bleeding.

Before the solution is injected, the anesthesiologist should aspirate to be certain that the needle is not inside a vessel. If it is, the needle should be withdrawn a few millimeters, redirected, reinserted, and its position retested. A small amount of solution (0.5 ml) should slowly be injected, after which additional injection will cause no pain. As mentioned before, the injection will be completed in about 20 seconds.

When the needle has been withdrawn, the eye is watched a few seconds for proptosis, and a rather firm digital pressure is exerted over the closed eyelids for about 2 to 4 minutes. The pressure should be intermittent, more like a massage than constant. It is advantageous to cover the eye with a pad of cotton before the pressure or massage is applied.

The eye should be watched, making certain that retrobulbar hemorrhage has not occurred. If it has, an increasing proptosis will be seen and felt. The retrobulbarly injected anesthetic solution causes some proptosis, which by the less experienced may be mistaken for a beginning retrobulbar hemorrhage. As this should always be presumed possible, pressure and massage should be started, as described. After a few minutes, a retrobulbar hemorrhage will usually betray itself by appearing subconjunctivally, usually in the inferior fornix, but it may, of course, present itself anywhere around the eyeball. Many surgeons are disconcerted by a retrobulbar hemorrhage and postpone the intraocular surgery for a few days. Others believe that this is not necessary. The retrobulbar hemorrhage usually stops after early, firm pressure and massage. If the eye feels soft, if the hemorrhage has stopped, and if the retrobulbar resistance feels normal, it is generally safe to continue the planned surgical procedure.

When the eyelids are opened, some of the fluid may have escaped from the retrobulbar site into the subconjunctival space, making the eye look as if a subconjunctival injection had already been given. The patient then does not feel the subconjunctival supplementary injection.

Subconjunctival Injection

In subconjunctival injection, the upper eyelid is lifted with the surgeon's left thumb and forefinger. The same needle as is used for the retrobulbar injection is introduced subconjunctivally. The conjunctiva is pierced with a quick jerk just at the bulbar side of the upper fornix, to either one or the other side of the superior rectus. When 1 ml of anesthetic solution is injected, the conjunctiva is ballooned. An additional 1 or 2 ml may be injected if the ballooning spreads evenly. If, as in repeated operations, there are scar adherences that prevent the spreading of the subconjunctival solution, the needle is withdrawn and reinserted subconjunctivally in one or two places, where the surgeon may find enough loose subconjunctival tissue to permit the diffuse spreading of the injected solution. Care should be

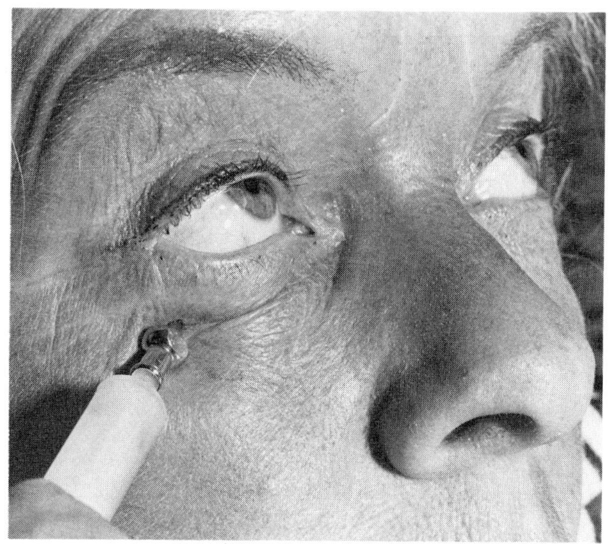

Fig. 17-13. Retrobulbar injection completed.

taken not to pierce the conjunctiva haphazardly, creating holes in the conjunctiva that later prove undesirable. Some attention should be given to the injection at the superior rectus in order to avoid pain when the bridle suture is inserted under this muscle.

If the surgeon prefers to use special holding sutures in the lids instead of a speculum, a small depot of anesthetic solution should, at this time, be injected into the lid.

Akinesia. While the eye is massaged, the injection for akinesia of the orbicularis oculi is performed.[14] This is the proper time because the patient is concentrating his attention upon the slightly unpleasant feeling around the eye caused by the retrobulbar injection and is usually feeling relieved that the procedure was not at all as unpleasant as he had expected. Therefore, at this time, the patient will be less conscious of the injection for the block of the facial nerve.

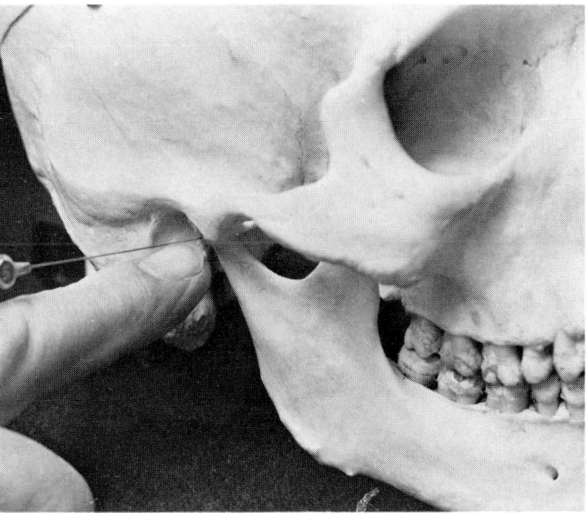

Fig. 17-15. Anatomical aspect of O'Brien method for akinesia of the orbicularis oculi muscle.

AKINESIA OF THE ORBICULARIS MUSCLE

In all major ocular operations and especially in intraocular interventions, motor paralysis of the orbicularis oculi muscle is mandatory. If the akinesia is insufficient, the patient may squeeze the eyelids, thus forcing out the speculum or, even more serious, the intraocular contents. The paralysis is achieved through blocking of the facial nerve or its divisions at various sites.

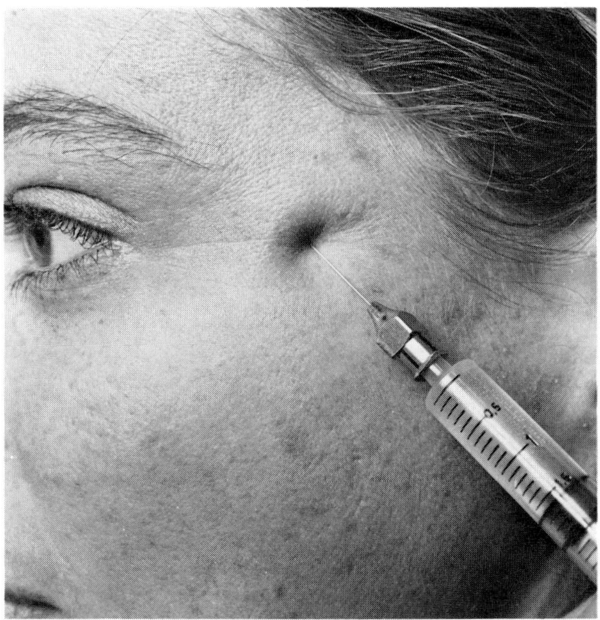

Fig. 17-14. van Lint method for akinesia of the orbicularis oculi muscle.

van Lint Method

The van Lint technique (1914) was modified several times (Villard, Wright), but was generally performed as a nerve block close to the outer canthus (*i.e.*, 20–30 mm lateral to the orbital margin; Fig. 17-14). The needle is introduced through the skin while simultaneously injecting and carried 30 to 33 mm subcutaneously, first being aimed at the lateral end of the supercilium. The needle is then partially withdrawn and redirected, being aimed at a point 1 or 2 mm above the infraorbital foramen, the anesthetic solution being injected while the needle is carried forward.

O'Brien Method

In 1927, O'Brien suggested paralyzing the facial nerve proximally just in front of the condyloid process (*i.e.*, just anterior and a little below the tragus of the ear; Fig. 17-15).[14] The short needle is carried straight inward, and the bony condyloid process is struck at a depth of about 1 cm. Two ml of anesthetic agent is injected while gradually withdrawing the needle. Because the course of the facial nerve varies, sometimes crossing the mandible at a lower point, the block is frequently incomplete and has to be supplemented.

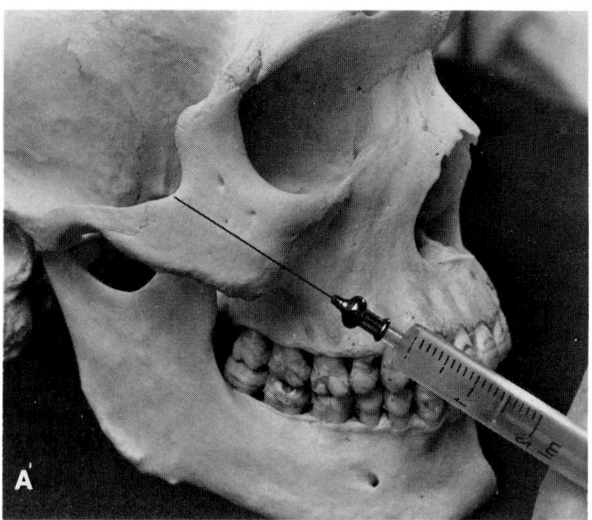

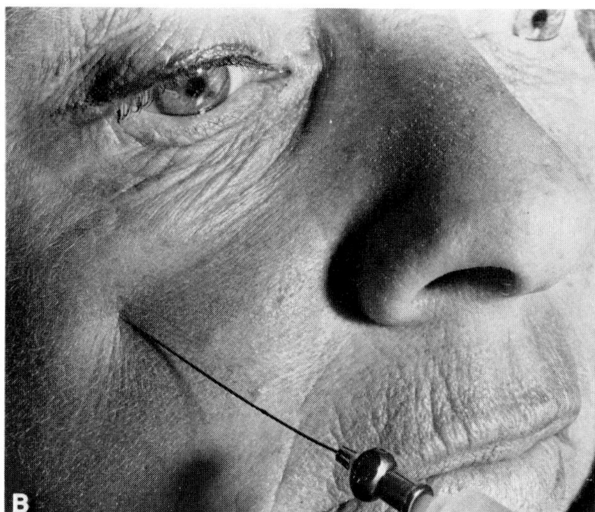

Fig. 17-16. Anatomical and clinical aspects of Atkinson method for akinesia of the orbicularis oculi muscle. Resuscitation equipment.

Atkinson Method

Atkinson prefers a modification with one injection, starting with an intradermal wheal at the inferior edge of the zygomatic bone in line with the lateral orbital margin (Fig. 17-16).[1] The needle is directed upward and posteriorly, being aimed just to the laterial side of the midpoint of a line between the tragus and the lateral orbital margin.

Boberg–Ans and Barner Method

We prefer a combination of the O'Brien and van Lint methods (Fig. 17-17). The condyloid process is located in front of the tragus. If it is difficult to locate, it will easily be felt when the patient is asked to open and close his mouth. Using a 2-ml syringe with the 35-mm, 23-gauge Atkinson needle, the skin is pierced perpendicular to the surface, and the needle is introduced for 5 to 7 mm until there is bony resistance. Three-quarters to 1 ml of local anesthetic solution is injected. The needle is slightly withdrawn, reinserted subcutaneously, and directed toward the lateral canthus superficially to the zygoma. When the needle is completely inserted, the remaining contents of the syringe (*i.e.,* 1–1.5 ml) is injected. The depot caused by the injected fluid is easily felt with the surgeon's left index finger, which is pressed firmly against the underlying bone, thus

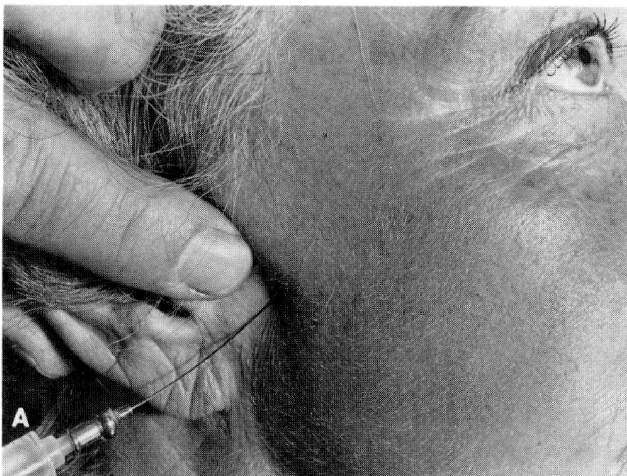

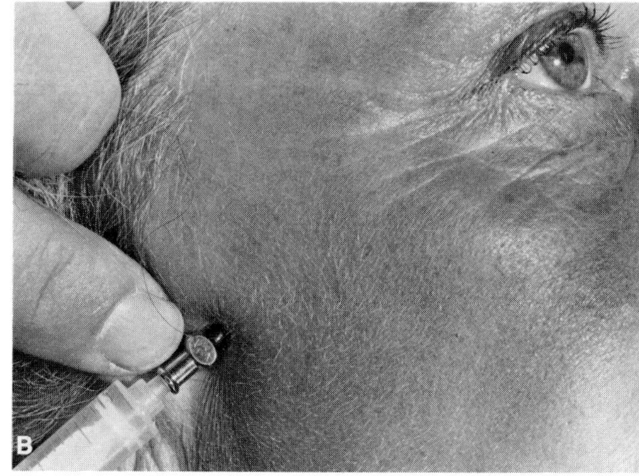

Fig. 17-17. Beginning and completion of injection in Boberg–Ans and Barner method for akinesia of the orbicularis muscle.

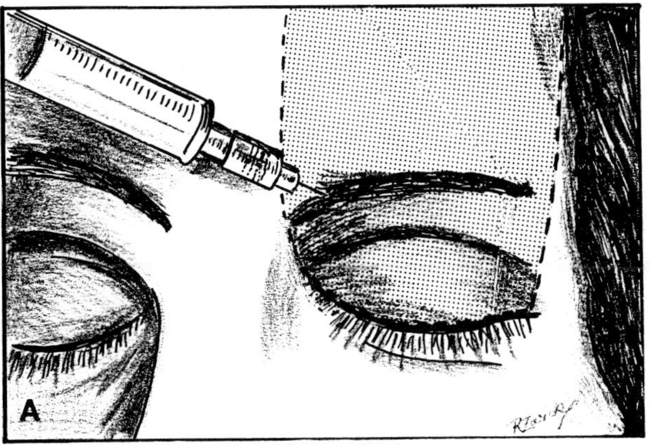

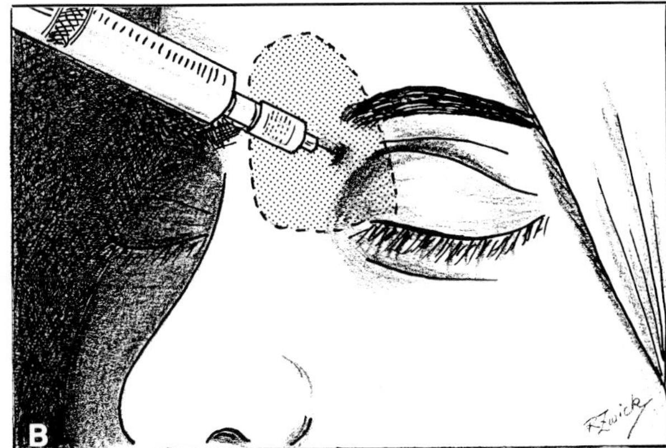

Fig. 17-18. (*A*) Supraorbital nerve block. (*B*) Supratrochlear nerve block.

causing the anesthetic fluid to diffuse to each side. Within a few minutes, the orbicularis muscle is paralyzed. The patient is unable to close the lids and should also, at this time, be unable to open them. If the patient can still squeeze or blink, the local anesthetic may be supplemented, preferably by another injection following the technique suggested by either van Lint or Atkinson.

THERAPEUTIC ANALGESIA

Retrobulbar Block

The technique described for retrobulbar block, as used for intraocular surgery, may be of value in cases of medically intractable attacks of painful glaucoma, in either essentially acute glaucoma or secondary cases of high intraocular tension. The pain, nausea, and vomiting usually associated with this condition are extremely distressing to the patient. Furthermore, a high tension for any length of time may choke the optic nerve and blind the eye. A retrobulbar block by the technique described may in seconds change the condition, lower the intraocular tension to acceptable values, relieve the pain, and provide a few hours' respite for trans-

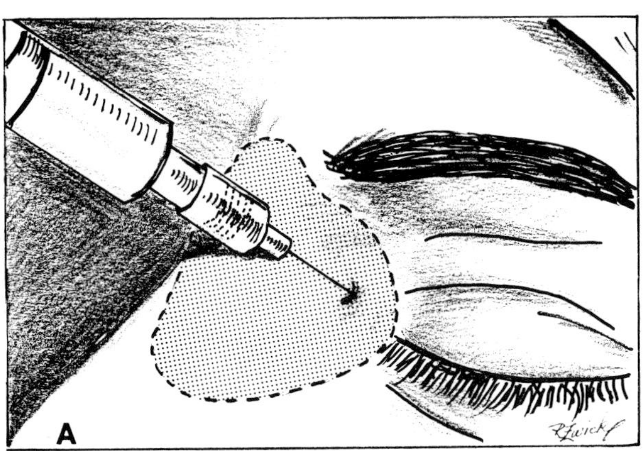

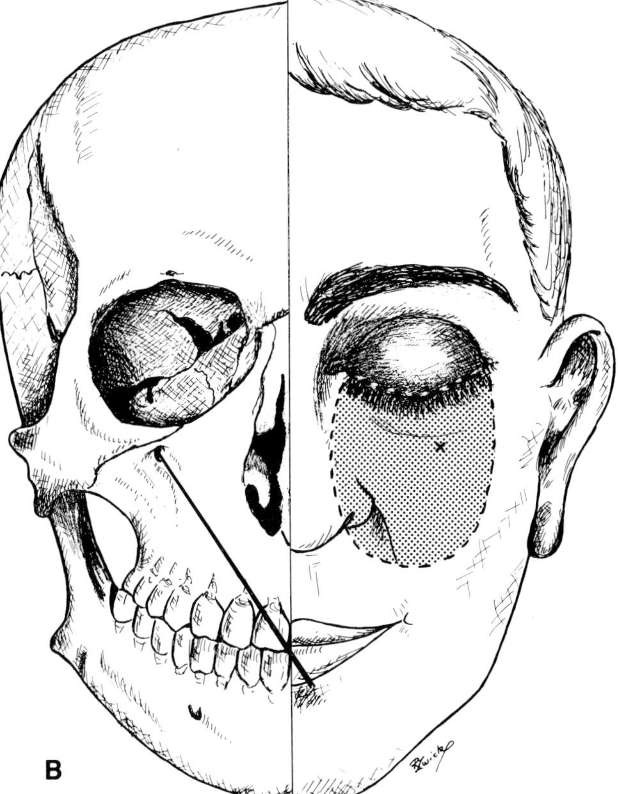

Fig. 17-19. (*A*) Infratrochlear nerve block. (*B*) Infraorbital nerve block.

Dosage (mg) for IM Premedication

Concentration (mg/ml)*
  Meperidine (injectable), 50
  Promethazine (injectable), 25
Dosage (mg/kg)
  Children
    As required for general anesthesia
  Young adults
    Meperidine, 1
    Promethazine, 0.2
  20–50 years
    Meperidine, 2
    Promethazine, 0.5
  50–60 years
    Meperidine, 1.5
    Promethazine, 0.4
  60–70 years
    Meperidine, 1
    Promethazine, 0.2
  Over 70 years
    Meperidine, 0.5
    Promethazine, 0.1

* Given intramuscularly 45–60 minutes before surgery

Dosage (mg) for Oral Premedication

Evening before the operation
  Acetazolamide, 250
  Diazepam, 5
  Promethazine, 10
One hour before operation
  Acetazolamide, 250
  Diazepam, 5
  Promethazine, 10
  Theophylline, 300
Just before operation
  Atropine (injectable; IV), 0.5
Postoperatively
  Salicylate preparation, 1000(1g)
  Propoxyphene, 65
  Katobemidone, 30

porting the patient and for preparing further treatment.

Also, for more intense treatment of inflammations or allergic conditions in the posterior part of the eye, as in uveitis or in case of more intensive steroid therapy, steroids may be injected retrobulbarly or subconjunctively. Retrobulbar injection of steroids has been reported beneficial in thyroid exophthalmos.

Supraorbital Nerve Block

Occasionally, the ophthalmic surgeon must treat neuralgic pain in the areas supplied by the trigeminal nerve (Fig. 17-18).[12] The trigger zone may be either around the two branches of the *supraorbital* nerve or the *supratrochlear* nerve (see Chap. 15).

Infraorbital Nerve Block

Neuralgia of the trigeminal nerve may also arise through the second division, the maxillary nerve, and its terminal branches (Fig. 17-19). The infraorbital nerve may act as a trigger zone. The nerve may be blocked either by the extraoral route or through the intraoral route (see Chaps. 15 and 16).[12]

When treating neuralgic pain by nerve block, steroid injections may often enhance and prolong the effect of the local anesthetic. If the painful conditions are caused by malignancy, then consideration should be given to the use of neurolytic solutions (alcohol) in these nerve block techniques (see Chap. 27).

REFERENCES

1. Atkinson, W.: Anesthesia in Ophthalmology. ed. 2. Springfield, Charles C Thomas, 1965.
2. Bedrossian, E.H.: The Eye. Springfield, Charles C Thomas, 1958.
3. Burn, R.A., *et al.:* Sedation for ophthalmic surgery. Combination of chlorpromazine, promethazine and pethidine. Br. J. Ophthalmol., *39*:333, 1955.
4. Castren, J.A., and Tammisto, T.: A clinical evaluation of a new local anaesthetic (Marcain-Adrenalin) in ocular surgery. Acta Ophthalmol. (Copenh.), *44*:837, 1966.
5. Duke-Elder, S., and Wybar, K.C.: System of Ophthalmology. vol. 2. (Copenh.) London, Henry Kimpton, 1961.
6. Duncalf, D., and Rhodes, D.: Anesthesia in Clinical Ophthalmology. Baltimore, Williams & Wilkins, 1963.
7. Eriksson, E.: Illustrated Handbook in Local Anaesthesia. Copenhagen, Munksgaard, 1969.
8. Gills, J.P., and Rudisill, J.E.: Bupivacaine in cataract surgery. Ophthalmic Surg., *5*:67, 1974.
9. Havener, W.H.: Ocular Pharmacology. ed. 2. St. Louis, C.V. Mosby, 1970.
10. Jaffe, N.S.: Cataract Surgery and Complications. St. Louis, C.V. Mosby, 1972.
11. Katz, J.: A survey of anesthetic choice among anesthesiologists. Anesth. Analg. (Cleve.), *52*:373, 1973.
12. Macintosh, R., and Ostlere, M.: Local Analgesia, Head and Neck. ed. 2. London, E. & S. Livingstone, 1967.
13. Nutt, A.B., and Wilson, H.L.J.: Chlorpromazine hydrochloride in intraocular surgery. Br. Med. J., *1*:1457, 1955.
14. O'Brien, C.S.: Akinesia during cataract extraction. Arch. Ophthalmol., *1*:447, 1929.
15. Philps S., and Foster, J.: Ophthalmic Operations. ed. 2. London, Bailliere & Cox, 1961.
16. Sorsby, A.: Modern Ophthalmology. ed. 2. vol. 4. London, Butterworth & Co., 1972.
17. Stallard, H.B.: Eye Surgery. ed. 4. Bristol, John Wright & Sons, 1965.
18. Wolf, G.L., *et al.:* Intraocular surgery with general anesthesia. Arch. Ophthalmol., *93*:323, 1975.

18 Neural Blockade for Obstetrics and Gynecology

Peter R. Brownridge, Gordon Taylor and D. H. Ralston

Part 1: Neural Blockade for Obstetrics

Neural blockade in general (and epidural analgesia in particular) has been central to major developments in obstetric anesthesia and analgesia for several reasons:

The analgesia provided by parenteral narcotics and by inhalational agents is limited and unlikely to improve. These approaches impair maternal awareness of birth—sometimes completely—and may spoil the initial contact between the mother and her infant. Neural blockade, on the other hand, offers high quality of pain relief while enabling full maternal awareness of the birth. This ill-defined yet apparently important experience is made possible by neural blockade and is most obvious during a cesarean section.

Despite a steady overall reduction in maternal and perinatal mortality in developed countries, the rate of maternal deaths from anesthesia has remained fairly constant. In most cases, these deaths have followed general anesthesia. From 1973 to 1975 in the United Kingdom, general anesthesia accounted for 21 per cent of maternal deaths following cesarean section and for seven deaths following forceps delivery or manual removal of the placenta.[54] It is possible that the increased use of neural blockade in obstetrics will reduce the rate of maternal death and permanent disability.

Apart from efficient pain relief, neural blockade has produced beneficial effects on the progress of labor and on several biochemical parameters that are adversely affected during labor and delivery.

Under certain conditions (*e.g.*, prematurity, preeclampsia, vaginal breech delivery and cesarean section), the neonate has been shown to benefit from neural blockade in comparison to other methods. New developments in neonatal assessment and further studies on drug elimination in the newborn will shed further light on the relative merits of neural blockade in obstetrics.

While the general principles of modern obstetric neural blockade are widely accepted, there are differences in approach among different countries and major medical centers. These differences are exaggerated by current national differences in the prohibition of certain drugs (*e.g.*, 2-chloroprocaine, etidocaine 1.5%, bupivacaine 0.75%, and heavy tetracaine) that have properties attractive to obstetric anesthesia.

The efficiency, flexibility, and remarkable safety of epidural analgesia would seemingly "be appealing to the laboring parturient." Yet, many mothers do not seek (and some may even resent) pharmacological pain relief. Unfortunately, the anesthesiologist may be tempted to assume the traditional role of technician by failing to ascertain whether the patient actually desires pain relief. An inadequately prepared patient may well feel resentful, especially if analgesia does not reach her expectations, or if the potential side-effects have not been adequately discussed. Further dissatisfaction may occur when the anesthesiologist is summoned to relieve pain in an already demoralized mother undergoing a prolonged labor—especially when she has been totally unprepared.

A satisfactory rapport between physician and patient and sensitivity to the patient are necessary not only in obstetric practice but in anesthesiology as well. In no other field is patient teamwork, discussion, and cooperation as important. When these requirements are met, neural blockade falls naturally into place and becomes satisfying to the patient and her attendants.

PERIPHERAL PAIN PATHWAYS DURING LABOR

The peripheral pain pathways involved during labor are now firmly established, following observations by Cleland[32] and detailed studies in patients by

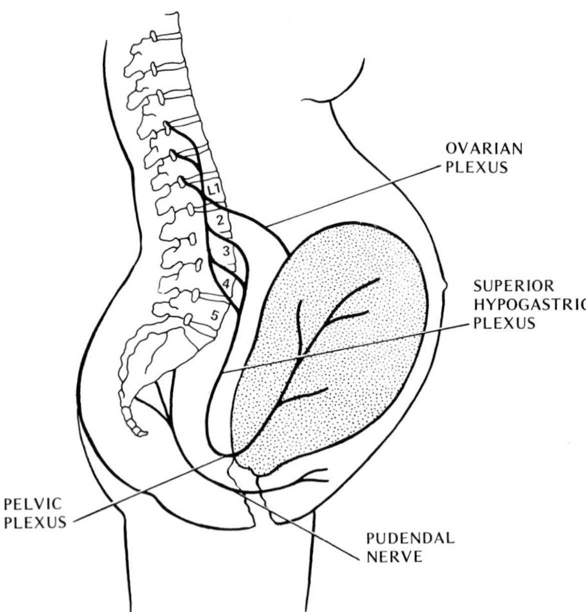

Fig. 18-1. Neuroanatomy of pelvic and perineal structures.

Bonica.[14,15] However, there are still some misconceptions.[15] It is convenient to discuss separately the pain associated with the first and second stages of labor, as originally proposed by Cleland, since these pathways are quite different (Fig. 18-1).

First Stage of Labor

Pain in the first stage of labor primarily results from dilation of the cervix and lower uterine segment, and distention of the body of the uterus from uterine contractions. The intensity of pain is related to the strength of the contraction and pressure thus generated. Noxious impulses from the cervix and uterus are transmitted by afferent nerves that accompany sympathetic pathways through, in turn, the pelvic, inferior, middle, and superior hypogastric plexuses; the lumbar sympathetic chain; the white rami of the spinal nerves of T10, T11, T12, and L1; and the posterior roots of these nerves to the cord. In early labor only the nerve roots of T11 and T12 are involved, but as contractions become more intense, segments T10 and L1 also become involved.

Low backache during the first stage of labor is almost certainly referred pain, to the dorsal rami of T10 to L1, the lateral branches of which descend before becoming superficial and supplying the skin some 10cm caudal to their spinal origin.[15,214]

Second Stage of Labor

In addition to the pain of contraction, descent of the fetal head into the pelvis causes distention of the pelvic structures and pressure on roots of the lumbosacral plexus to produce referred pain by way of segments L2 and below. Thus, pain may be felt in the region of L2 low in the back and also in thighs and legs (L2–S1). Pain produced by stretching of the perineum is transmitted by way of the pudendal nerve. This nerve is derived from the second, third, and fourth sacral nerves and passes posteriorly to the junction of the ischial spine and the sacrospinous ligament, and anteriorly to the sacrotuberous ligament. The ischial spine is the bony landmark for pudendal nerve blockade. The analgesia accomplished by a successful pudendal block affects the posterior two-thirds of the labia and the rest of the perineal area including the anus (Fig. 18-2). The anterior third of the labia majora is supplied by the genitofemoral nerve, which can be blocked effectively by local infiltration.

APPLIED PHYSIOLOGY

Changes in respiratory, cardiovascular, and gastrointestinal function during pregnancy apply particularly to obstetric neural blockade and have been summarized in Chapter 8. The most significant changes are highlighted further below.

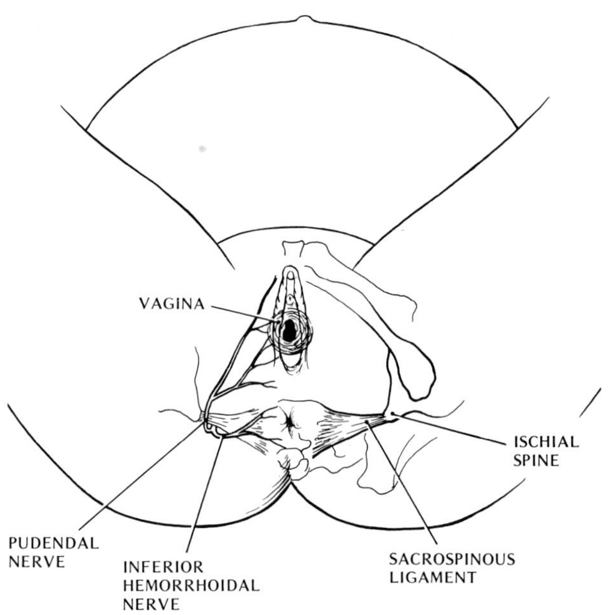

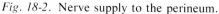

Fig. 18-2. Nerve supply to the perineum.

Respiratory Changes

The 70-per-cent increase in alveolar ventilation[51] more than compensates for the 20-per-cent rise in oxygen consumption at term,[178] as a consequence of which maternal $Paco_2$ falls to 30 to 32 torr. During labor, considerable hyperventilation may occur in response to pain,[72] with a further exaggeration of hypocapnia ($Paco_2$ < 20 torr in 24% of mothers),[188] and respiratory alkalosis. Oxygen consumption also rises to 400 ml per minute or more during labor.

As a result of these changes, hypoventilation leads to a more precipitous onset of hypoxemia.[14] It is important to recall that the degree of change in Pao_2 with ventilation follows a series of hyperbolic curves depending on oxygen consumption (Fig. 18-3).[161] Thus, at levels of oxygen utilization of 400 ml per minute, Pao_2 shows a progressive decline when alveolar ventilation falls below approximately 7L per minute.

Particular care is therefore required to ensure full preoxygenation prior to a short period of apnea (*e.g.*, at induction of general anesthesia). Caution should also be taken whenever regional analgesia is performed following the failure of other methods of pain relief. On these occasions, efficient analgesia may unmask the depressant effects of parenteral and inhalational agents. Extra vigilance is also required to ensure that major or profound neural blockade does not depress ventilation by motor involvement. Oxygen supplementation under these circumstances is mandatory, as are facilities to support ventilation quickly and safely.

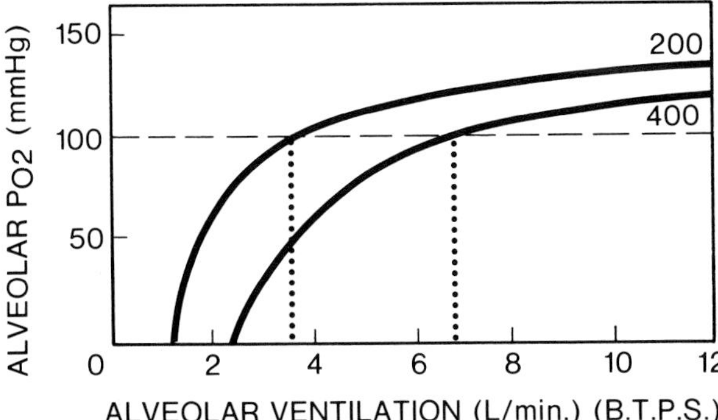

Fig. 18-3. The relationship between alveolar ventilation and alveolar Po_4 for values of oxygen consumption of 200 ml/min and 400 ml/min for a patient breathing air at normal barometric pressure. Note the alveolar ventilation required to maintain alveolar Po_4 above 100 mmHg at the higher oxygen consumption in labor. (Modified from Nunn 1971.) By kind permission of the Editor, 'Anaesthesia and Intensive Care'.

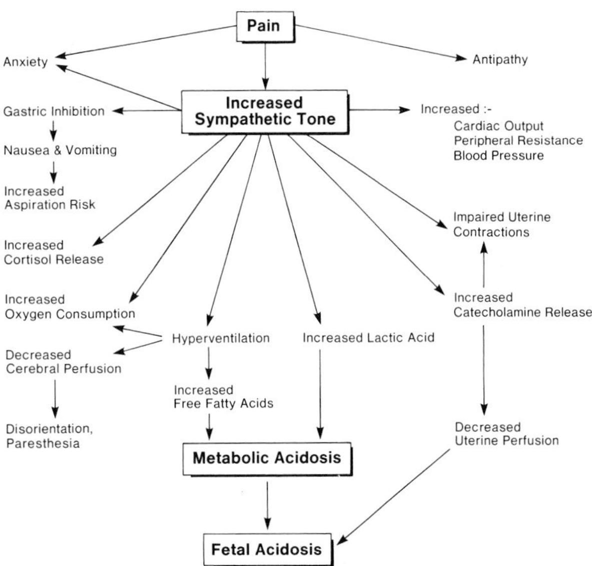

Fig. 18-4. Physiological sequelae of unrelieved pain in labor.

Hyperventilation and hypocapnia during labor not only reduce cerebral blood flow, thereby potentiating disorientation and paresthesia, but also may reduce uterine blood flow and contribute to maternal and fetal metabolic acidosis. All of these changes are inhibited by epidural analgesia (Fig. 18-4).[72,166,167]

The rapid induction of hypoxemia owing to hypoventilation that is possible in pregnancy is further compounded by the concomitant reduction in functional residual capacity (FRC).[51] In 50 per cent of mothers at term, this reduction is sufficient to cause some airway closure during normal tidal ventilation,[10] and therefore it creates an increased pulmonary venous admixture. Obesity and recumbency may aggravate this effect further—as may hypotension, hypovolemia and reduced venous return—each of which can complicate pregnancy.

Cardiovascular Changes

Pregnancy produces a "dynamic circulation"; there is a 30- to 50-per-cent increase in cardiac output and a similar rise in blood volume in association with a fall in peripheral resistance.[117] These changes are such that blood pressure is normally unaltered, or slightly reduced. Because placental perfusion at term depends upon a uterine blood flow of 500- to 700 ml per minute,[6] it is important to ensure that this level of perfusion is maintained. Accordingly, myocardial depression, reduced venous return, hypovolemia, and hypotension must be avoided or promptly treated if they do occur. This requirement for a high level of uterine perfusion may be compromised by neural blockade and, therefore, requires constant surveillance in order to ensure maternal and fetal well-being.[24]

One of the most important (yet easily avoided) causes of sudden falls in venous return, cardiac output, and therefore, placental perfusion is aortocaval compression by the gravid uterus which occurs with the patient in the supine position. Despite a great deal of evidence to support undesirable consequences of the supine position,[11,64,66,114,194,215] the obvious remedy, complete avoidance of the supine position, is commonly ignored. Perhaps this apparent lack of concern occurs because most patients "tolerate" the supine position without symptoms and without significant falls in blood pressure; in these cases aortocaval compression is "concealed" by a compensatory increase in peripheral resistance.[44] Only in 2 to 3 per cent of mothers in late pregnancy[97] are the compensatory mechanisms unable to maintain adequate cerebral perfusion—and then the symptoms of the supine "hypotensive syndrome" occur.

Aortocaval compression is of particular importance to the anesthesiologist, because after central neural blockade the ability to compensate for a fall in cardiac output by increasing peripheral resistance is considerably diminished. Therefore, hypotension with its associated symptoms (pallor, sweating, nausea, faintness) is very likely to occur: Aortocaval compression is then "revealed." It is clear that the supine position should be avoided in all patients in labor, including those in the lithotomy position.

The serious consequences of the supine position are most evident when cesarean section is performed under central neural blockade. Indeed, it is a very likely that several "unexplained" deaths have been precipitated by a reduction in cardiac output owing to reduced venous return or to vagal arrest.[96,146] Therefore, suitable tilt of uterine displacement is a mandatory requirement during cesarean section.

The interest in the effect of aortocaval compression on the fetus is more than academic. Using intrapartum monitoring, several studies have shown the deleterious effects of the supine posture on neonatal status both in labor[79,99,193] and at cesarean section.[3,46,62,80,212] Clinical studies that have ignored aortocaval compression are of dubious significance. For example, some investigators have attributed changes in fetal heart rate (FHR) during labor and following neural blockade to the local anesthetic agent per se, or to "hypotension"[13,125,177,222]; yet, the patients studied were treated in the supine position. That aortocaval compression was a significant causative factor in these cases is supported by a separate study that invariably showed improvement occurred in FHR once the patient was turned from a supine to a lateral position.[193] A five-fold increase in FHR late decelerations associated with epidural analgesia occurred in another study, when patients were treated in the supine position instead of the lateral position.[100] When patients remained in a tilted or lateral position (providing uterine hypertonia and dehydration were avoided) FHR changes during epidural analgesia were minimal (5% or less) and of no pathological significance.[9,110,179]

The limited ability of the circulatory system to vasoconstrict in a patient with a central neural blockade is important during the second stage of labor. In this period of active bearing down, the patient exercises a series of valsalva maneuvers. Since peripheral compensation for reduced cardiac output secondary to the raised intrathoracic pressure is obtunded, there is a greater fall in blood pressure when pushing and "overshoot" is much smaller.[216] These responses may have a deleterious effect on placental perfusion. This may explain why fetal deterioration is greater in mothers receiving epidural analgesia who push compared with those who do not.[169] The second stage of labor may be prolonged under the influence of epidural analgesia. In view of the popular adoption of the supine position for delivery, it is important to monitor the fetus carefully and expedite delivery when appropriate. As a result of popular trends toward "normal deliveries," some physicians persevere unduly with active pushing which only prolongs the second stage of labor, to the detriment of the fetus.

Gastrointestinal Changes

Acid aspiration is the most common cause of maternal death related to anesthesia and is aggravated by several physiological changes: a raised intra-abdominal and intragastric pressure, an increased tendency to esophageal reflux, a decreased gastric emptying time, and increased gastric acidity. Nausea and vomiting are further exacerbated by labor pain, stress, and the administration of narcotics. The importance of narcotic administration has recently been supported by a study on stomach content volumes prior to cesarean section.[91] The largest volumes were found in patients who had received meperidine during labor and the smallest volumes in those who had received either epidural analgesia or no analgesia.

Hypotension subsequent to aortocaval compression with central neural blockade and hypoxia are also causes of vomiting. After delivery, ergometrine frequently precipitates vomiting.[147,152]

These physiological changes indicate that surveillance by experienced staff and facilities for rapid and skilled intubation are necessary for anesthetized patients in labor. The administration of oral antacids during labor has been shown to raise the gastric *p*H[171,202] and to reduce morbidity in the event of regurgitation.[49] They should therefore be a part of the normal treatment given to patients in labor.

Changes Secondary to Pain

Several physiological and biochemical changes occur during labor largely as a result of pain itself; they can be reversed partially or completely by efficient neural blockade. These sequelae are summarized in Figure 18-4.

The emotional burden of pain and suffering of women in labor has been described over the centuries. Although anxiety and fear were viewed as the major causes of pain during labor by Dick-Read,[55] experience suggests that the converse is closer to the truth. Indeed, relaxation and relief following neural blockade is the most notable and earliest feature of efficient analgesia. A woman's feelings concerning future pregnancies following a painful labor should not be underestimated. A consumer study revealed that antipathy toward a future pregnancy occurred most often in women who received inadequate analgesia.[34]

Increased autonomic activity consequent to pain in labor can be demonstrated in several ways, and all are inhibited by central neural blockade. A rise in plasma cortisol is also more pronounced when labor is conducted without analgesia or with narcotics, compared to epidural blockade.[108] The increased oxygen consumption during labor also returns to normal when either epidural or paracervical block is instituted.[189]

The inhibition of efficient uterine contractions, or inertia, which can occur in prolonged labor, is probably induced primarily by the adrenergic response to pain,[129] although biochemical changes are also contributory. Epidural analgesia in patients with uterine inertia allows a substantial increase in the rate of cervical dilatation,[149] and a less abnormal type of uterine action has been confirmed by uterine manometry. Experimental evidence suggests that catecholamine release not only impairs uterine contractility but may also reduce uterine perfusion.[15]

Hyperventilation is induced by pain with subsequent hypocapnia. Apart from contributing to disorientation and paraesthesia, oxygen consumption is increased, uterine perfusion may be reduced,[157] and progressive metabolic acidosis may be aggravated. Hyperventilation usually does not occur in labor conducted under epidural blockade.[166]

During the first stage of labor conducted without neural blockade, a progressive maternal acidosis occurs.[166,206] Blood concentrations of free fatty acids increase steadily to reach a peak at delivery.[131] Similarly, lactate accumulation occurs.[107,132,166] In contrast, these researchers have demonstrated normal maternal acid-base status during the first stage when labor is conducted under epidural analgesia.

During the second stage of labor a maternal metabolic acidosis occurs under epidural analgesia which is directly related to active pushing.[107,167] This further supports the view that active pushing should not be encouraged as soon as full cervical dilatation occurs. Provided the patient is in the lateral position, and there are no signs of fetal distress, it is preferable to allow fetal descent to the perineum by the uterine contractions alone. Active intervention should be performed whenever there is evidence of fetal deterioration.

It now seems clear that in terms of acid-base balance, the infant closely follows the changes seen in the mother,[168] and that the fetus is less acidotic at the onset of the second stage of labor, when neural blockade is utilized. This may be significant in the outcome of "at risk" pregnancies.

Placental Circulatory Changes

The uterine circulation can be regarded as a system of low resistance grafted in parallel with other maternal vascular beds.[6] In some respects, it behaves like an arteriovenous shunt. The increase in maternal cardiac output is more than sufficient to supply the uteroplacental circulation (about 500–700 ml/min at term). Unlike the cerebral circulation, animal studies have shown that autoregulation of flow in response to changes in arterial pressure does not occur,[6] and therefore placental perfusion is probably dependent on, and directly related to, systemic arterial pressure in the clinical range.

Measurement of intervillous and myometrial blood flow in patients after intravenous injection of ^{133}Xe[183] may shed further light upon the influence of labor and analgesia—although the method shows a

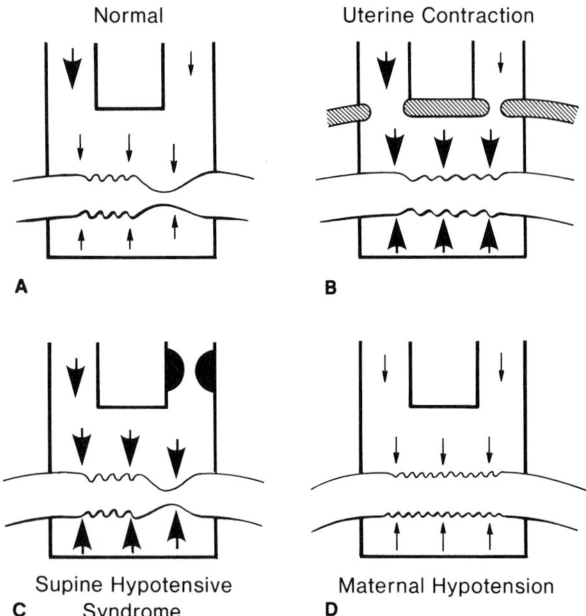

Fig. 18-5. Diagram of clinical conditions that may affect umbilical circulation by sluice mechanism. Size of arrows illustrates changes in vascular pressures relative to normal (left upper panel). Diagram for uterine contraction (right upper panel) is meant to suggest that uterine venous outflow is restricted by either (a) direct action of myometrial muscle fibers on uterine veins or (b) squeeze of increased intrauterine pressure on veins as they exit from uterus. Rise in fetal intrauterine pressures is also shown. Diagram for supine hypotensive syndrome (left lower panel) is meant to suggest collapse of inferior vena cava. By kind permission of the authors, Power and Longo, 1973, and the editor, Amer. J. Physiol.

wide variation and standard deviation in values of intervillous flow. Using this technique, Jouppila and colleagues were able to demonstrate decreases in uterine flow that accompanied periods of hypotension during cesarean section under epidural blockade.[111] During labor, however, the same investigators found no significant change in placental blood flow after institution of epidural analgesia, if hypotension was avoided.[110]

These studies further emphasise the importance of maintaining maternal cardiac output and blood pressure to ensure placental perfusion and fetal well-being. Uterine flow is also reduced during uterine contractions, which accordingly represent intermittent stressful hypoxic stimuli to the fetus.[7] This relationship is, incidentally, the basis of changes in fetal heart rate, which are now commonly demonstrated using modern monitoring methods during labor. The anesthesiologist must ensure that overstimulation of uterine contractions with oxytoxic agents or tetanic contractions do not lead to fetal asphyxia. Efficient analgesia provided by neural blockade may mask the occurrence of excessive uterine contractility. Constant attention to the frequency and strength of contractions is required, either by manual palpation or intrauterine manometry, in conjunction with monitoring of fetal heart rate.

Animal studies have also shown that maternal pressure within the placental cotyledon (*i.e.*, intervillous pressure) may influence fetal blood flow through the villi by a "sluice" flow mechanism, analogous to that which occurs in the lungs.[176] It is suggested that normal fetal flow through the placenta is a function of fetal artery pressure minus the surrounding maternal intervillous pressure. Several clinical implications arise from this interesting study (Fig. 18-5).

In animal studies, an increase in intervillous pressure produced by a uterine contraction, or caval occlusion, was found to reduce fetal flow as well as maternal flow within the placenta—a result which indicates an additional compromise in gaseous interchange. On the other hand, an increased fetal flow occurred in the presence of aortic occlusion and may therefore be regarded as a compensatory effect in the presence of hypotension. This study indicates that fetal flow may be altered directly as a result of undesirable changes in maternal arterial, venous, and intrauterine pressures.

APPLIED PHARMACOLOGY

The fate and significance to the fetus of local anesthetics administered to the mother prior to delivery have received much attention in the 1970s and has been the subject of several reviews.[56,118,121,142,170,174,181,190,208] It is clear that rapid equilibration of these agents occurs between the two circulations and is governed largely by their physicochemical properties (see Chap. 3). Certain techniques of neural blockade and certain individual agents are more likely to achieve toxic blood levels than others. Direct fetal injection has occurred following attempted paracervical, caudal,[71] and pudendal blocks, and even during perineal infiltration. Local anesthetic toxicity is potentially lethal and the predisposing factors, recognition and treatment (see Chap. 4) must be well understood by all staff who practice and supervise neural blockade in obstetrics.

The significance of lower, nontoxic concentrations of local anesthetics to the ultimate well-being of the newborn is less certain. Despite an acceptable status at birth, neurobehavioral examinations performed some hours afterward have detected changes that are seemingly related to effects of local anesthetics or their metabolites. The neonate may be more "sensitive" to local anesthetics than adults, although only mepivacaine and lidocaine have been incriminated in neurobehavioral assessment studies. The significance of neurobehavioral changes remains debatable; in comparison to other drugs administered during labor, (*e.g.*, narcotics, barbiturates, sedatives, and tranquilizers), even mepivacaine and lidocaine have a much shorter duration of measurable depression.[17,35] Nevertheless, it seems sensible to apply pharmacological principles and to use techniques of neural blockade that have been shown to produce the least fetal accumulation compatible with therapeutic efficacy.

Before discussing the role of individual neural blockade techniques in modern obstetric practice, it is necessary to outline these pharmacological principles in an attempt to "set confidence limits on the safety of different agents and regional block techniques."[134]

RELATIVE MERITS OF LOCAL ANESTHETIC AGENTS IN OBSTETRICS

Ester-Linked Agents

2-Chloroprocaine has by far the shortest plasma half-life of all local anesthetics. In neonatal blood, half-life is about 43 seconds, or double the value for adult blood.[70] Fetal blood levels following neural blockade are therefore negligible, and it is not surprising that neonatal depression has not been detected following clinical use. Cumulative toxicity does not develop on account of its rapid esterification. For these reasons, it has been recommended for use in women in labor,[89] especially if there is fetal distress,[2] and for paracervical block.[74] Its shorter duration of action, however, might make 2-chloroprocaine less attractive for continuous epidural analgesia when more frequent top-up doses are required, although tachyphylaxis has surprisingly not been reported. Despite its attractive properties, 2-chloroprocaine is not available in many countries.

Tetracaine is the most commonly used intrathecal agent in North America but is not currently available in the United Kingdom or Australasia. A major advantage of subarachnoid anesthesia is the negligible blood level it produces, regardless of the agent used. Coupled with the profound degree of neural blockade and the rapidity of onset, the intrathecal route is attractive for certain obstetric procedures (*e.g.*, cesarean section, forceps delivery, placental removal, and perineal surgery).

Amide-Linked Agents

All local amide-linked anesthetics depend primarily upon hepatic metabolism prior to elimination. Since transfer of the unbound, undissociated form rapidly occurs across the placenta to the fetus, the physicochemical properties of each agent are of crucial importance in the total dose received and distribution within the fetus.

The fetal to maternal ratio (U/M) of local anesthetic plasma levels varies widely following local administration of amide anesthetics; prilocaine has a ratio close to unity, whereas lidocaine and mepivacaine have values of 0.5 to 0.7. These characteristics favor placental transfer.[209] Bupivacaine and etidocaine, on the other hand, have a U/M of 0.2 to 0.3 (see Fig. 3-30 and Table 3-10).[124,173]

Protein binding in maternal blood limits the proportion of local anesthetic that is transferable to the fetus,[209] and therefore it can be regarded as a desirable property. However the U/M does not itself reflect the magnitude of transfer or of fetal distribution, and the values for different agents mainly reflect differences in fetal tissue uptake rather than protein binding.[174] Thus, the low U/M for etidocaine reflects its high lipid solubility and large volume of distribution, and the greater degree of protein binding does not necessarily limit placental transfer.[156] Therefore, both binding and lipid solubility play important roles in placental transfer and neonatal tissue distribution.

Differences in *p*H between maternal and fetal blood also influence local anesthetic uptake by the fetus. Thus, an elevated U/M has been reported with both lidocaine and mepivacaine in the presence of fetal acidosis,[22] owing to "trapping" of the ionic dissociated form. When there is fetal distress, the anesthesiologist should exercise caution in dosage administration.

Although elimination half-life of lidocaine is greater in the newborn compared with the adult as a result of the larger volume of distribution,[139] metabolic clearance is very similar on a weight-for-weight basis.[69] The plasma half-life of mepivacaine (9 hours) is, however, considerably longer than that of lidocaine (3 hours). Lidocaine is therefore more suitable for obstetric use.[134] Plasma half-life of bupivacaine in the neonate is comparable with that in the adult (2 hours).[23]

Toxic effects of local anesthetic agents in a fetus, as in an adult, or neonate are manifested by central nervous and cardiovascular changes. Gross CNS toxicity following maternal toxicity has led to perinatal death or serious morbidity.[181] More subtle CNS changes have been revealed by the application of neurobehavioral assessment techniques,[19] and the effects of local anesthetics have been reviewed by Ostheimer.[163] Using a modified and simpler assessment, Scanlon reported an increased incidence of hypotonia, reduced muscle strength, and lowered habituation to certain repetitive stimuli in infants 2 to 8 hours old following delivery using epidural analgesia with lidocaine and with mepivacaine.[191] Palahniuk and colleagues also reported some decrease in neonatal muscle tone at 6 hours following cesarean section using epidural lidocaine.[164] These infants have been described as "floppy but alert."[191]

Tronick and colleagues, using the more complex Brazelton Neonatal Behavioural Assessment Scale up to 10 days after delivery, reported that the diminished neonatal muscle tone following lidocaine and mepivacaine administered epidurally to the mother had disappeared within 12 hours of birth.[207] These workers concluded that the observed changes were of little consequence.

Neurobehavioral depression, however, has not been detected following epidural bupivacaine during labor,[36,192] or epidural etidocaine for cesarean section.[123] Indirect effects of neural blockade (*e.g.*, hypotension) may also be important; one study has shown significant correlations between hypotension following epidural blockade for cesarean section and depression of some neurobehavioral reflexes.[95] Pathological factors are probably even more important, because the same study showed a higher incidence of abnormal neurological activity in infants of high-risk obstetric patients, regardless of anesthetic regime—general or epidural.

Reduced muscle tone in neonates following delivery using lidocaine and mepivacaine may reflect the sensitivity of the neuromuscular junction to these agents.[192] The lack of these effects following delivery with bupivacaine and etidocaine may be the result of their rapid disappearance from the blood and therefore from the neuromuscular junction.

Circulatory depression in vivo is of late onset and is related to high circulatory levels in the neonate, as it is in the adult (see Chap. 3).[75,181] A transient loss of fetal beat-to-beat variability following epidural blockade is of no known significance. Hypotension and aortocaval compression are far more likely to produce changes in fetal heart rate than direct effects of local anesthetics per se, with the exceptions of paracervical block.

Lidocaine is commonly used for all techniques of neural blockade. A choice of varying doses, used with or without epinephrine, provides useful versatility in obstetric anesthesia. Development of tachyphylaxis occurs frequently with continuous epidural analgesia,[150] and use of lidocaine in parturients has been superseded by bupivacaine. Despite some neonatal neurobehavioral depression, 2-per-cent lidocaine (with epinephrine, 1:200,000) provides excellent conditions for cesarean section under epidural block, and is an agent of choice for this procedure in countries where chloroprocaine is unavailable. Epinephrine should be added in all types of blocks.

Mepivacaine. Transplacental transfer of mepivacaine is greater than that of lidocaine, and neonatal metabolism of this agent is much slower.[23] Neonatal neurobehavioral depression is more common, and frank toxicity makes this agent unattractive for obstetric use.[155] Other agents are preferable from all points of view.

Prilocaine has the highest U/M, which may indeed exceed unity.[86,175] Although less toxic than lidocaine, methemoglobinemia has been reported in degrees bearing a direct relation to the duration of exposure in both mother and neonate.[4] In some instances more than 10 per cent of fetal hemoglobin has been converted and has produced neonatal cyanosis that is not improved with oxygen. These factors outweigh any advantages of prilocaine, except possibly for pudendal block or perineal infiltration, when delivery is imminent.[145]

Bupivacaine is currently the amide agent of choice for epidural analgesia in parturients. In concentrations of 0.25 per cent or less, effective analgesia can be provided with minimal motor blockade (see Fig. 4-3). Tachyphylaxis has not been a problem, and the duration of action is convenient for use in women in labor. Neonatal blood and urine concentrations are so low following epidural block as to cause "a problem of identification,[56] and neurobehavioral depression has not been reported.

For cesarean section, 0.5-per-cent bupivacaine may be insufficient to ensure adequate spread, and muscle relaxation may not be ideal for surgery. Time to onset is also longer than that of lidocaine or etidocaine. A concentration of 0.75 per cent may be more satisfactory for surgery, but this strength is not available in many countries.

Etidocaine provides motor blockade out of proportion to its sensory block. Therefore, it is not as suitable as bupivacaine for epidural analgesia during labor. However, the rapid onset, excellent speed, and good muscle relaxation, coupled with a very low U/M, make 1-per-cent etidocaine attractive for use in cesarean section.[122] Unfortunately, this agent is unavailable in some countries and many anesthesiologists will be obliged therefore to turn to lidocaine or bupivacaine.

Effects of Local Anesthetics on the Uterus

Clinical studies on the effect of neural blockade on uterine activity have produced divergent results. It is most unlikely that a direct effect on myometrial contraction will ever be observed in practice.[174] Isolated human uterine muscle only begins to show a significant dose-related depression of contractility at levels in excess of 25 μg per ml[158]—a level unlikely to be attained except in the event of gross toxicity or following paracervical block.

In vitro studies have demonstrated a *vasoconstricting* effect on uterine vessels, but again only at blood levels in excess of 20 μg/ml.[77] Clinical uterine effects of neural blockade are therefore more likely to be related to other factors (*e.g.*, hypotension[174]) and the addition of epinephrine.

Effects of Epinephrine Added to Local Anesthetics

The addition of epinephrine reduces drug absorption and thereby enhances the spread and quality of neural blockade; it also lowers peak blood levels—particularly those of lidocaine and mepivacaine (see Figs. 3-13 and 3-17). Because these two agents are also likely to cause fetal depression, it would seem that epinephrine administration (5 μg/ml) should be a part of all neural blockade techniques in obstetrics. However, the action of epinephrine on uterine tone, contractility, and uterine flow is currently controversial.

Several studies have shown greater reduction in uterine activity following epidural blockade when epinephrine has been added, an effect that may last for up to 60 minutes.[38,110,133,180,211,220] Although other factors are known to inhibit contractions (*e.g.*, hypotension, aortocaval compression[28] and, possibly, interruption of Ferguson's reflex), it appears that epinephrine contributes to inhibition.

Diminished contractions have also been reported following pudendal block when epinephrine is added to lidocaine,[221] which further supports a direct uterine effect. Some investigators have accordingly recommended avoidance of the use of epinephrine,[1,170] while others do not regard the addition of 5 μg per ml to significantly affect the progress of labor.[14,145]

The addition of epinephrine to epidural bupivacaine or etidocaine prolongs duration of action only marginally,[37,185] and it has little effect on reducing peak blood levels at the low doses required for analgesia during labor.[184] There is therefore no advantage in adding epinephrine to bupivacaine for epidural analgesia.

In contrast, the significant reduction in blood levels achieved by the addition of epinephrine to lidocaine or mepivacaine neural blockade outweighs the doubtful disadvantage of diminished uterine contractility. Toxicity is a frequent cause of maternal death related to local anesthesia—especially lidocaine[92] and epinephrine (5 μg/ml) should be added to all neural blockades using lidocaine.[21] Lidocaine is ideal for infiltration, pudendal block, and caudal block prior to delivery—all circumstances in which the uterine effects of epinephrine are of little practical importance—and yet some obstetricians and midwives are reluctant to use the preparation containing epinephrine. This concentration (*i.e.*, 5 μg/ml or 1:200,000) is ideal and should not be exceeded, particularly for infiltration in the perineal area.

The addition of epinephrine is required when larger doses of lidocaine are used for cesarean section under epidural blockade. Epinephrine-induced uterine depression is of no practical importance during a cesarean, but the greatly reduced anesthetic uptake and the circulatory effects of epinephrine (see Chap. 8) are wholly beneficial.

ERGOMETRINE AND OXYTOCIN

Ergometrine and oxytocin are invariably administered either singly or in combination at delivery in order to contract the uterus and reduce blood loss. Both drugs have cardiovascular effects and sequelae that are important, especially in patients with central neural blockade.

Both ergometrine (0.5 mg) and oxytocin (10 units) are equally effective in reducing hemorrhage when given as an intravenous bolus at delivery.[147,152] The cardiovascular effects are quite different. Ergometrine increases peripheral resistance, including venoconstriction, and produces systemic hypertension, a raised central venous pressure, and coronary artery vasoconstriction.[106] These effects can last for several hours. Postpartum hypertension

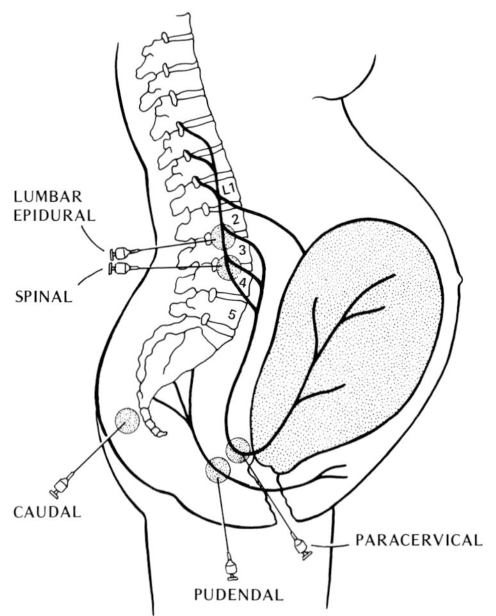

Fig. 18-6. Types of regional blocks that may be used to provide analgesia during obstetric and gynecological surgery.

may have serious effects in the patients with essential hypertension, preeclampsia, valvular heart disease, pheochromocytoma or thyrotoxicosis.[145] Simultaneous vasoconstrictor administration to a patient with severe hypertension may result in cerebrovascular accident[29] or pulmonary edema.[106]

Oxytocin given as an intravenous bolus, on the other hand, produces a transient fall in peripheral resistance and blood pressure, with compensatory increase in cardiac output.[106,218] The severity of hypotension is also posture-dependent, and it is not usually demonstrated when oxytocin is administered as an infusion rather than a bolus.[106]

Another major difference between intravenous oxytocin and ergometrine lies in their emetic actions. Ergometrine was associated with vomiting or retching in 13 per cent of mothers following normal vaginal delivery,[147] and 46 per cent following forceps delivery and epidural analgesia.[152] In contrast, no emetic actions were observed in the same circumstances following intravenous oxytocin (5 units). At cesarean section under epidural analgesia, vomiting was reduced in another study from 40 to 2 per cent when ergometrine was replaced by oxytocin.[141]

For these reasons, it seems that intravenous ergometrine should not be used except possibly in the event of atonic uterine postpartum hemorrhage that is unresponsive to oxytocin. Despite theoretical concern about cardiovascular collapse following oxytocin in the presence of central neural blockade,[218] in practice hypotension is not noticeable.[147] Ergometrine should be reserved for intramuscular use, and only then in patients without medical and obstetric complications.

ATROPINE AND VASOPRESSOR AGENTS

Atropine and vasopressors are used in the supportive role when systemic hypotension occurs. In many patients, significant hypotension is due to a block up to or higher than T4 and may be associated with a sinus bradycardia. This is evidence of relative vagal overaction in the absence of sympathetic activity that has been blocked. Atropine given intravenously (0.4–0.6 mg) in divided doses is indicated to restore the heart rate to normal (see Chap. 8), provided severe reductions in venous return have been excluded (see Fig. 8-21 and Table 8-9).

The vasopressor agent of choice in obstetrics is ephedrine, which is capable of cardiac stimulation as well as peripheral vasoconstriction, which combine to treat hypotension.[198] The effect of ephedrine upon uterine blood flow appears to be small in comparison with vasopressors such as methoxamine.[182]

TECHNIQUES OF NEURAL BLOCKADE

The blockade techniques which are commonly used are conveniently divided into two groups, central and peripheral (Fig. 18-6). Description of the applied anatomy and methods for the central techniques are found elsewhere (see Chaps. 7–9).

The following peripheral techniques are frequently used in obstetric surgery: local infiltration; pudendal block; paracervical block.

LOCAL INFILTRATION

Local infiltration is frequently used during a delivery that requires an episiotomy. Infiltration subcutaneously is carried out along the episiotomy incision, followed by deposition of the local anesthetic solution in the ischiorectal fossa in a fan-shaped pattern.

Following pudendal blocks, the genitofemoral and ilioinguinal nerves that supply the anterior one-third of the labia majorum are not blocked. Local bilateral infiltration subcutaneously in this area provides adequate analgesia. One of the disadvantages of extensive local infiltration is related to the large volumes of local anesthetic that may be used. Dilute solutions, such as 0.5-per-cent lidocaine or 1-per-cent chloroprocaine, are more than adequate and should be used with epinephrine (1:200,000). A total of 30 ml of these solutions should suffice to provide adequate analgesia.

Analgesia by infiltration of the lower abdomen, groin, and lumbar region has been advocated in the past but has no place in modern obstetrics; it has been superseded by epidural analgesia.

Infiltration analgesia has also been described for cesarean section, but large volumes of local anesthetic are required and toxicity is therefore a risk. Bonica has described a modified technique involving separate injections of subcutaneous, intrarectus, parietal peritoneal, visceral peritoneal, and paracervical tissues.[14] However, central neural blockade has rendered infiltration methods obsolete in most clinical situations.

PUDENDAL BLOCK

Pudendal block is primarily used during vaginal obstetric procedures. The pudendal nerve in its neurovascular bundle passes just posterior to the junction of the sacrospinous ligament and the ischial spine (Fig. 18-6). There are two basic techniques used in pudendal block: transvaginal and transperineal. The transvaginal technique has a higher success rate, probably owing to its simplicity.[116] In addition, it is less painful for the patient and produces a low incidence of complications. The transperineal pudendal block is now used infrequently and only when the fetal head is fully descended onto the perineum.

Transvaginal Pudendal Block

To perform a pudendal block, the patient is placed in the lithotomy position. The ischial spine is palpated vaginally. A 12- to 14-cm, 20 French gauge needle, attached to a 10-ml Luer-Lok syringe filled with local anesthetic solution, is guided to the ischial spine through the vaginal wall by the index and middle fingers. The needle is preferably introduced through a needle guide (Iowa Trumpet or Kobak instrument), which limits the penetration of the needle. When the needle is in the sacrospinous ligament, compression of the syringe with local anesthetic solution meets with considerable resistance. As the needle tip passes through the ligament, loss of resistance is felt, and the area should then be infiltrated with the 10 ml of local anesthetic solution. This procedure is then repeated on the other side.

Transperineal Pudendal Block

The transperineal route for pudendal block requires a skin wheal about 2 to 3 cm posteromedial to the ischial tuberosity. The 12 to 15-cm 20-gauge needle attached to a syringe as described above is guided to the ischial spine with the index finger usually placed in the vagina, or in the rectum if the fetal head is fully descended to the perineum.

Lidocaine (1%) with epinephrine (1:200,000) is the most commonly used drug. A total volume of 20 to 25 ml should be sufficient to produce the desired block, usually for 90 to 120 minutes. Chloroprocaine (1.5–2%) may also be used in similar volumes but will produce analgesia for a shorter period (60–90 min.). Pudendal block produces analgesia in the posterior two-thirds of the labia and part of the buttock. Analgesia of the anterior one-third of the labia requires local infiltration as described above. During the deposition of the local anesthetic drug in both of these blocks, it is mandatory that intravascular injection does not occur, and frequent aspirations of the syringe should be made.

The success rate of pudendal block is undoubtedly related to the clinician's experience in administering it. This block is often described as the "obstetricians' block." One study reported a bilateral success rate of 50 per cent in transvaginal blocks, and only 25 per cent in transperineal blocks, when they were performed by obstetric trainees.[195] Even when successful, the quality of analgesia is limited. In patients undergoing a mid-cavity or rotational forceps delivery, low subarachnoid or caudal analgesia is far more preferable and efficient. Finally, the danger of a systemic toxic local anesthetic reaction should not be underestimated. During a 6-month period in Glasgow, five episodes of major convulsions followed the use of 1-per-cent plain lidocaine for pudendal nerve block.[145] Pudendal block should only be performed by clinicians who are aware of the symptoms, signs, and treatment of toxicity (see Chap. 4).

PARACERVICAL BLOCK

First described by Gellert in Germany in 1926, paracervical block has been most popular in North America, Scandinavia and continental Europe, but

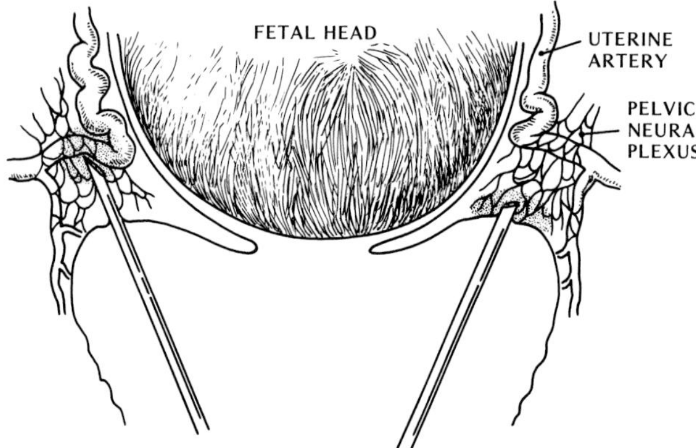

Fig. 18-7. Neurovascular anatomy associated with a paracervical block in obstetrics. The needle in the right fornix is short bevelled and shows distribution of the local anesthetic. (After Bloom)

not in the United Kingdom.[145] The differing enthusiasm for the technique originally reflected differences in obstetric management. In those countries where paracervical block is popular, the obstetrician is directly involved with management during labor, while in the United Kingdom, uncomplicated labor (including analgesia) has traditionally been managed by a midwife rather than a doctor.

The technique of paracervical block is simple. To avoid intravascular injection, a 12- to 14-cm French gauge needle is used with a guide (*e.g.*, Iowa Trumpet), so that the needle point can only protrude 5 to 7 mm. The guide, with the needle tip protected, is directed into the lateral fornix by the index and middle fingers, so that the tip of the guide does not depress the vaginal mucosa excessively. The technique as described by Bloom and colleagues,[12] in which only the bevel of the needle is placed through the vaginal mucosa, is recommended. In addition, a short beveled needle may be used, with the guide omitted (Fig. 18-7).

The success rate has ranged from 55 to 90 per cent in different case series. Apart from its relative simplicity, paracervical block results in no sympathetic efferent involvement compared to central neural blockade (although this is, in itself, of very dubious importance). The usefulness of the block is also limited because it relieves only uterine pain.

Paracervical block in obstetric analgesia is hindered by the brief duration of action of the local anesthetic drugs used. Lidocaine and mepivacaine (0.5–1.0%) have most frequently been administered; their effects last about 60 to 75 minutes. Bupivacaine (0.25%) has a somewhat longer action: 90 to 110 minutes.

The quality of pain relief with bupivacaine has been disappointing.[138] Etidocaine (0.125%, 25 mg) has also been used for paracervical block,[205] in an attempt to reduce dosage to a minimum, but the duration of analgesia was similar to that of lidocaine (100 mg). The addition of epinephrine (5 μg/ml) increases the duration of effect of lidocaine, but does not do so for bupivacaine or mepivacaine.[2] The use of continuous paracervical block has not gained acceptance, because it is difficult to maintain the correct position of the tip of the catheter. In addition, there may be extensive bleeding in the lateral fornix with the use of a catheter.

The major disadvantage of paracervical block in obstetrics is the incidence of fetal arrhythmia (particularly bradycardia), which has been described in almost every series. Furthermore, it is usually associated with fetal acidosis.[5,196] In studies in which continuous monitoring is used, the highest incidences of fetal bradycardia have been reported following paracervical block. Fetal death has occurred as a result of paracervical block, and there is an increased risk of fetal morbidity. Following paracervical block, the onset of fetal bradycardia occurs within 10 minutes, and the heart rate may fall as low as 60 beats per minute. Most studies show at least a 20-per-cent incidence with lidocaine and mepivacaine, although only a 6-per-cent incidence was found with chloroprocaine.[74,197,204] Fetal death has been reported following the use of mepivacaine and bupivacaine.[159,186] There also appears to be a high incidence of fetal bradycardia following paracervical block when the fetus is premature or had preexisting disease.

Whether the observed changes in fetal heart rate (FHR) represent a primary depressant effect of local anesthetics on the myocardium, or whether they are secondary to other factors following paracervical block remains controversial. Certainly absorption from the vascular paracervical area is rapid, with maximum maternal and fetal blood levels occurring within 10 minutes,[170] the period within which FHR changes begin to appear. Direct fetal myocardial depression by local anesthetics has accordingly been suggested as the basic mechanism,[1,5,203] with fetal acidosis as a secondary effect. In contrast, Liston and colleagues found that bradycardia commonly occurred even when fetal scalp blood concentrations of local anesthetics were low.[119] Furthermore, Freeman and colleagues, following direct injection of massive doses of mepivacaine (300 mg) into anencephalic fetuses, found that bradycardia did not occur until the terminal phase, even though there was evidence on the ECG of conduction depression (increased PR interval and widened QRS complex).[75] For these reasons, a direct local anesthetic action is unlikely.

A secondary increase in uterine tone following paracervical block has also been suggested as the principal mechanism leading to fetal acidosis. Although some investigators have reported a positive correlation between increased uterine tone and FHR changes,[76,213] others have not[30,140]; and, it seems that uterine tone is quite variable following paracervical block.

Recent reviews have reasoned that the high incidence of FHR changes is most likely to be due to fetal acidosis secondary to uterine vasoconstriction, with or without increase in myometrial tone.[30,81] Uterine vasoconstriction has been demonstrated in vitro with sufficiently high concentrations of local anesthetics,[77] and it is likely that such concentrations can be achieved following paracervical block. Other contributory factors may include mechanical distortion of uterine vessels and aortocaval compression owing to use of the supine position (which has commonly been ignored). Epinephrine has also been incriminated, but this explanation is unlikely, because a similar incidence of FHR changes is observed whether or not it is used.[196,203] Although the debate will probably continue, the most plausible primary mechanism of fetal bradycardia after paracervical block is a reduction in placental perfusion owing to uterine vasoconstriction.

Paracervical block is associated with a disturbingly high incidence of morbidity, and is inferior to properly conducted central neural blockade in terms of efficacy, flexibility, and safety. Prematurity, preexisting evidence of placental deficiency, and fetal acidosis should be absolute contraindications. Even in cases without these complications, it is difficult to recommend paracervical block in modern obstetrics.

LUMBAR EPIDURAL BLOCKADE

The application of local anesthetic agents into the epidural space has reached a pinnacle of success in the field of obstetrics. When properly managed, efficient analgesia is invariably assured, maternal satisfaction is high, and serious morbidity is very low. Careful documentation from several major world centers has successfully rebutted most of the misgivings and reticence which initially greeted this revolutionary source of pain relief for women in labor.

Furthermore, as new information accumulates, beneficial effects for the neonate are becoming apparent when epidural analgesia is used, as opposed to use of no analgesia or of other methods of pain relief.[89]

The flexibility and nuance provided by drugs that are introduced into the epidural space assures this method a permanent place in modern obstetrics and promises a further decade of progress. The epidural administration of narcotic drugs to women in labor has exciting potential. The absence of motor and sympathetic blockade (see Chap. 31) that such application suggests is particularly attractive.

Finally, the importance of ensuring high standards of practice and management must be stressed. Most, if not all, serious complications are avoidable when epidural analgesia is performed properly and managed by competent staff.

Technical Considerations

Technical considerations of epidural analgesia are discussed fully in Chapter 8 and in standard obstetric texts. There are certain difficulties that should be recognized in obstetric practice: The sitting position is uncomfortable when the patient is in strong labor, and the lateral position is therefore preferable; spinal flexion is limited and is more difficult to achieve; the patient may be very restless when experiencing strong contractions; and the epidural space may well have a positive pressure—especially during contractions—and a technique which relies on a negative pressure (*e.g.*, "hanging drop") is unsatisfactory. For these reasons, obstetric epidural practice is not suitable for a clinician who is a novice, and a good technique is essential if accidental dural puncture is to be prevented. Introduction of an epidural catheter allows subsequent doses to be administered with ease and can be tailored to each patient's needs.

Although reduced epidural local anesthetic requirements during pregnancy have been generally observed,[21] this is not a universal conclusion.[83] The importance of ensuring adequate hydration and avoiding aortocaval compression requires no further mention (see Chap. 8). Satisfactory rapport with the patient and an assurance that the patient is giving informed consent is most important.

Maintenance

Bupivacaine is currently the agent of choice for epidural analgesia during labor, although 2-chloroprocaine has been greeted favorably. Several "regimens" have been reported using various doses and concentrations ranging from 0.125- to 0.5-per-cent bupivacaine, with or without adrenaline. Reducing the concentration to 0.125 per cent reduces the

MANAGEMENT OF EPIDURAL ANALGESIA
INSTRUCTIONS

Patient's name .... Date ....

(1) Blood Pressure

B.P. should be taken every 5 mins for 20 mins after top-up

If B.P. falls below .... mmHg Systolic.

(i) turn patient on left side.

(ii) give i.v. infusion of....................

(iii) inform Dr...................

(2) Positioning

Always nurse on side. Use a wedge under the right buttock when patient is in the lithotomy position.

(3) Top-up doses.

* First dose through catheter given at ....(time) by

Dr....................... Agent ....Dose....ml.

*Anaesthetist in charge must be present for first dose through the catheter. Top-up doses may be given in the presence of a qualified midwife. The drug must be

(a) injected through the millipore filter

(b) double checked and

(c) any syringe with unlabelled contents must not be used.

DRUG (Block letters)	Strength	With or Without Adrenaline	Dose in ml	When necessary at intervals of

Signature of Anaesthetist....................

TOP-UP RECORD

TIME	DRUG	STRENGTH	DOSE GIVEN	GIVEN BY	CHECKED BY
1					
2					
3					
4					
5					
6					

Always inform the Anaesthetist if patient requires more analgesia sooner than prescribed for, or if concerned in any way.

Fig. 18-8. Epidural instruction sheet suitable for midwife management of top-up doses.

success rate,[201] In a double-blind trial this strength provided painless labor in only 30 per cent of patients,[120] although this rose to 50 per cent with the addition of epinephrine (1:200,000). The latter study also confirmed that increasing the concentration of bupivacaine to 0.5 per cent enhanced analgesia but increased the degree of motor block. The addition of epinephrine also increases motor blockade.[120] When an epidural catheter is inserted early in labor, then full advantage can be made of the flexibility of the technique by tailoring the strength of blockade according to each patient's needs. For example, 0.25-per-cent bupivacaine can provide acceptable analgesia during most labors, and many mothers prefer to remain aware of contractions and suffer the minimal motor blockade that this concentration allows. A more potent block can easily be provided with 0.5-per-cent bupivacaine if required.

In practice, top-up doses may be safely administered by a midwife trained in the management of epidural block (see Chap. 8), with instructions that have been ordered by the anesthesiologist (Fig. 18-8). However the anesthesiologist is solely responsible for these instructions, and it is imperative that a physician experienced in management of local anesthetics toxicity and extensive sympathetic blockade is readily available to the labor ward.

Although the above procedure is practical, simple, and safe, some hospitals have introduced refinements in order to reduce the local anesthetic dose or to provide more continuous analgesia by means of an infusion pump.[68,78] A segmental technique, aiming to block only T10 through T12 with small doses (4 ml of 0.5% bupivacaine) by way of a catheter has achieved favorable results for the first stage of labor only.[94] Other hospitals have avoided the use of catheters, and instead prefer to use a single-shot lumbar epidural during the first stage, and a single shot caudal (see Chap. 9) to provide perineal analgesia for delivery as necessary.

Indications

Apart from providing the most efficient method of pain relief in labor, it has become clear that there are several clinical conditions in which epidural analgesia provides additional benefits and can reduce morbidity and even mortality associated with childbirth.

Preeclampsia and Hypertension. Epidural analgesia results in valuable reductions in maternal blood pressure during labor[151] (by approximately 20%) and therefore reduces the cardiovascular and cerebral vascular complications of preeclampsia. The requirements for other medication (*e.g.*, narcotics, sedatives) in the prevention of eclampsia are also reduced, and consequently there is less potential for neonatal pharmacological depression. Although renal blood flow is unaltered following epidural analgesia,[103] recent evidence using the ^{133}Xe method* has demonstrated improvement in placental flow—especially in preeclampsia. Pain-free labor has other advantages for the fetus (see Fig. 18-5) and provides optimal conditions for delivery (*e.g.* prematurity).

Theoretical objections to epidural blockade on

* Personal communication, Joupilla and colleagues

the grounds that it aggravates hypovolemia have not been confirmed in fact, although naturally it is necessary to avoid aortocaval compression and provide adequate fluid replacement.[44] The clinician is faced with a dilemma when preeclampsia is associated with coagulopathy (see Chap. 8). The risk of epidural hematoma formation in the presence of mild coagulation defects is unknown, but it is reassuring that there have been no case reports suggesting a serious association. Patients with coagulation defects must be treated with caution. In practice, this degree of severity usually indicates cesarean section, in which general anesthesia would be the technique of choice.

High-Risk Fetus. A fetus is at high risk in a pregnancy that involves premature labor, maternal diabetes, preeclampsia, and conditions of intrauterine growth retardation. Avoiding use of narcotic agents and preventing progressive fetal acidosis (see Fig. 18-5),[168] which epidural analgesia may allow to develop, can only be beneficial. In one retrospective study, there was a significantly lower death rate in the first week of life in neonates weighing less than 2.5 kg, delivered with epidural analgesia, compared to those delivered with other methods of pain relief.[53] This study also noted a much higher rate of forceps use in the group receiving epidural analgesia, and it is probable that such a controlled and gentle expedition of the second stage is beneficial rather than harmful to the infant. A controlled trial is required to confirm the role of epidural analgesia in the high-risk fetus.

Breech Presentation. Formerly regarded as a contraindication to epidural analgesia, several studies have shown superior conditions for delivery and improved neonatal outcome in breech presentations. Initial fears that epidural analgesia would contribute to morbidity by increasing the breech extraction rate have not been substantiated. Retrospective studies of vaginal breech deliveries comparing epidural analgesia with "conventional" analgesia have found a small prolongation of labor but no increase in the incidence of operative intervention and a better neonatal condition in deliveries using epidural analgesia.[16,41,52,58] All of these studies recommended epidural analgesia. Recently, a prospective study concluded that epidural analgesia did not prolong labor, that breech extraction was reduced, and that the condition of the fetus (judged by fetal acid-base sampling) was better than when labor was conducted with other methods of analgesia.[20] There are several possible explanations for the favorable results observed when the breech is delivered vaginally with epidural analgesia. The mother is comfortable and cooperative, and the progress of labor can be determined by thorough vaginal examinations. The otherwise common urge to push before full dilatation is obtunded, and perineal relaxation provides optimal conditions for controlled delivery. For these reasons, epidural analgesia is strongly indicated whenever a vaginal breech delivery is proposed.

Multiple Pregnancy. Until recently, multiple pregnancy was regarded as a contraindication to epidural analgesia, on the grounds that a delay in the second stage of labor would lead to greater intervention and result in a contracted uterus that would jeopardize the second twin. It is universally agreed that mortality and morbidity is greater among second twins, and reflects contraction and even separation of the placental bed following delivery of the first infant. Multiple pregnancy is also commonly associated with premature labor and preeclampsia, which contribute further to a higher perinatal mortality. Obstetric intervention and the need for anesthesia are commonly indicated with urgency in order to expedite delivery of the second twin.

In the past few years, epidural analgesia for multiple births has been regarded favorably.[42,94,101,105,217] Although most of these studies reported a longer second stage of labor and increased operative intervention compared with other methods of analgesia, the neonatal outcome was similar. However, the facility with which obstetric intervention can be performed, without resource to the induction of urgent general anesthesia, has been favorably noted in all these studies to date. Even locked twins have been successfully and rapidly disimpacted under lumbar epidural blockade.[113]

Prolonged Labor and Trial of Labor. Prolonged labor is commonly associated with maternal fatigue and demoralization, apart from the unwanted physiological responses associated with pain summarised in Figure 18-5. A failure to progress due to incoordinate uterine action may well be causally related to these responses. Whatever the mechanisms, efficient analgesia in these circumstances is not only humane, but in the absence of disproportion may well allow labor to progress without resource to cesarean section. Uterine action usually improves under epidural analgesia in 70 per cent of cases, especially with the addition of intravenous oxytocin.[149] This has been confirmed by cardiotocography in one study, in which nine patients who were imminent candidates for cesarean section all safely delivered vaginally after epidural analgesia.[129]

Maternal Medical Complications. Cardiac disease

in women in labor is usually an indication for use of epidural analgesia. It is a useful adjunct in the prevention of heart failure. The physiological effects of pain (Fig. 18-5) are discussed elsewhere and the cardiovascular responses to a painful labor are particularly unwanted in patients with diminished cardiac reserve. Epidural analgesia not only reduces these effects but also lowers oxygen utilization during labor.[189] It is of interest that most maternal deaths involving cardiac complications have occurred in the second stage of labor or soon after delivery. The effects of pushing in the second stage of labor may be contributory. An elective forceps delivery is now usually advised. The risk of pulmonary edema is also lessened with epidural analgesia by virtue of dilation of the venous capacitance vessels, which are thus better able to accommodate the "autotransfusion" following delivery. Administration of ergometrine is dangerous in these cases. Despite theoretical objections to the reduction in peripheral resistance in the presence of Eisenmenger's syndrome, vaginal delivery conducted under epidural analgesia has been proposed as the best management for this serious condition.[47]

Epidural analgesia is indicated in patients with respiratory disease and previous cerebrovascular accident or brain surgery because of its superior homeostasis, minimal strain and lack of side-effects that are common to other methods of pain relief for labor. Maternal diabetes mellitus is also a relative indication for use of epidural analgesia in labor.[145]

Fetal Abnormality and Intrauterine Death. It seems both reasonable and humane to reduce pain as efficiently as possible in grief-stricken patients. Accordingly, epidural analgesia should be available, although caution is required in the patients with coagulopathy.

Cesarean Section. Following favorable reports in the past few years from several major medical centers, epidural analgesia has become increasingly popular as an alternative to general anesthesia for cesarean section. There are several advantages: blood loss is approximately halved compared with general anesthesia[143]; the risk of aspiration is reduced, and epidural analgesia can be continued into the postoperative period.[25] Many mothers, moreover, have a very strong desire to be aware of birth and to share this experience with their partner.[26] Close maternal-infant contact, including suckling, shortly after birth and in the immediate postoperative period is also facilitated by this method. This early mother-infant interaction may improve emotional "bonding,"[115] since the neonate is said to be in a heightened state of alertness in the first hour of life.[122] This alertness can encourage the mother's affectionate responses. Early suckling is certainly a significant factor in establishing successful breast feeding,[187] and this is much more likely with neural blockade than following general anesthesia.[26] An early return to normal diet is also facilitated with neural blockade, as opposed to narcotic analgesia, which delays gastric emptying.[160] For all of these reasons, highly motivated mothers will invariably express a preference for neural blockade both for a future cesarean section, and for other surgery when this is feasible.[26,146] Satisfied mothers also raise the consumer demand for cesarean section with epidural analgesia.

Cesarean section is a major test of epidural analgesia. Profound blockade of 17 segments is required (see Table 8-13), strong visceral stimulation is present, sudden cardiovascular changes can occur, and some discomfort is common.[25,128,141,146] Inadequate sacral nerve root blockade may be a source of discomfort during cesarean section with epidural analgesia,[146] and suggestions have been made to relieve this discomfort: a posture change alone,* to the added administration of a caudal or subarachnoid block.[25] It is necessary to ensure an adequate dose of local anesthetic. It should be injected in incremental doses and not as a bolus. The most commonly used agents are lidocaine (2%), bupivacaine (0.5–0.75%), and etidocaine (1.0–1.5%), with the addition of epinephrine (1:200,000) in volumes of 15 to 20 ml (see Chap. 8).

Providing careful management during surgery is performed as outlined in Chapter 8, with special attention to the prevention and treatment of hypotension, the immediate neonatal outcome following cesarean section under ideal epidural analgesia is similar to that under ideal general anesthesia.[8,63,73,95,102,128,164] However, a shorter time to sustained respiration usually occurs following the epidural technique. Recent studies suggest that the infant neurobehavioral outcome may be altered by anesthetic agents and technique. Thus, one study comparing epidural bupivacaine (0.75%) with subarachnoid tetracaine for cesarean section found no depression in neurobehavioral scores at 4 and 24 hours of age in either group.[126] (Subarachnoid analgesia can be discounted as having a direct depressive effect by virtue of the negligible blood levels attained.) Another study comparing epidural lidocaine with general anesthesia found a greater number of infants with weak sucking, rooting, and palmer grasp reflexes in the group delivered with

* Personal communication, Moir

epidural analgesia.[95] Of even greater interest in this study was the significant correlation observed between these weaker reflexes in the first 2 days and intraoperative hypotension; this suggests that the latter was the causative factor. Further comparative studies are awaited with interest. This study emphasizes the importance of avoiding hypotension during cesarean section.

Ultimate safety and success depends on cardiovascular stability, adequate placental perfusion, and supplementary oxygenation. Measures such as a prefluid load,[219] avoidance of aortocaval compression by tilting,[33,200] uterine displacement,[31] administration of atropine and ephedrine prophylactically[85] or therapeutically are therefore mandatory during cesarean section. Inflatable boots do not apparently contribute to the prevention or treatment of hypotension.[103] More detailed descriptions of management are described in standard texts.[1,14,21,145]

Contraindications

In practice there are remarkably few contraindications to the use of epidural analgesia in parturients. In fact, one leading authority proposes that there are no absolute contraindications, and that there are only three strong contraindications: patient disinclination, a blood clotting defect, and local or general sepsis. These and other relative contraindications are discussed in Chapter 8. Hypovolemia requires replacement before instituting epidural blockade. It should be stressed, however, that epidural analgesia, especially in patients with relative contraindications or in high-risk pregnancies, demands expertise and experience on behalf of all attending staff.

Obstetric emergencies that necessitate immediate delivery, such as placenta previa, a prolapsed cord, and acute fetal distress, are relative contraindications to regional blockade. All of these conditions require the swift intervention of the anesthesiologist, to provide adequate conditions for surgery and delivery of the infant. General anesthesia, therefore, is the optimum method for these procedures, unless a regional block has been administered in advance of the emergency.

Two relative contraindications are currently controversial. Epidural analgesia has been suspected to obscure the rupture of a uterine scar by masking the pain associated with impending rupture.[27,199] However, other investigators have argued that a painful scar is completely unreliable, and other signs are far more important in the diagnosis of uterine rupture.[137] In fact, the Oxford group commended the use of epidural (caudal) analgesia in these occasions: It allowed frequent palpations of the scar during labor. Furthermore, using relatively low doses of bupivacaine in labor, as is now common practice, it has been postulated that "pathological" pain is still appreciated by the patient.[44] The second controversial contraindication to epidural analgesia is placental abruption. Again, it has been suggested that a diagnosis may go unnoticed in the absence of pain. In a retrospective study, however, pain was associated with abruption in the majority of cases, and an increased risk in the presence of epidural analgesia was not demonstrated.[48]

Side-Effects and Complications

Detailed clinical analyses from several (Crawford, 1972(a): Crawford, 1972(b): Moore et al, 1974: Holdcroft and Morgan, 1976: Raabe and Belfrage, 1976: Hollmen et al., 1977, 174: Phillips et al., 1977: Doughty, 1975) major centers have made epidural analgesia in obstetrics one of the best documented areas of clinical anesthesia.[39,40,60,90,94,154,172,179]

Although when properly managed unwanted sequelae are invariably of little serious importance, there is a constant search for further improvement.

Nonobstetric complications of epidural analgesia (*e.g.*, dural puncture, total spinal, massive epidural, bladder dysfunction, backache, neurological damage, and epidural hematoma or abscess) are discussed fully in Chapters 7 and 8. The incidence of dural tap is related to operator experience.[40] The possible resultant severe headache is especially undesirable in a nursing mother. Fortunately, the therapy provided by postpartum epidural infusion or a blood patch is extremely effective. The incidence of bladder dysfunction is complicated because difficulty with micturition is a common consequence of labor. One study found no evidence of increased postpartum retention after epidural blockade had worn off in the puerperium.[210] Other prospective studies comparing upsets of micturition and backache after forceps delivery found that epidural block was comparable with those who received pudendal block.[112,148]

Neurological complications (excluding accidental dural tap) following epidural analgesia for labor in the case series cited above have been extremely rare and often unrelated to the technique. For example, patchy numbness on the outer aspect of the thigh occurred in three patients in one series of 2,000,[40] and in another series of 1,000 two complications (*i.e.*, one of lateral thigh numbness, and one of foot drop) were attributed to trauma following forceps delivery.[90] All three patients recovered completely within 6 weeks. It is conceivable, however, that the higher rate of forceps use and possibly a diminished "protective" muscle tone might have contributed to the incidence of temporary, epidural-associated neurological complications.

Case reports of prolonged block lasting 36 to 72 hours following epidural analgesia in women in labor have been described[50,165] even though technical difficulties were not always encountered. Bupivacaine with or without epinephrine was used on these occasions, and the total doses ranged from 10 to 36 ml. Neurological consultation is essential whenever delayed recovery occurs in order to exclude pathology (*e.g.*, epidural hematoma) requiring urgent intervention. These cases also stress the need for postpartum assessment—preferably by the anesthesiologist who administered the epidural block (see Chap. 8).

The most serious complications, such as toxicity, total spinal, and unexpected "high epidural" blockade (see Chap. 8), have been reported extremely rarely in obstetrics and are all either avoidable or readily treated with high standards of care and supervision. Nevertheless, their occurrence emphasizes the vital importance of having expert staff in the labor ward and close proximity of a physician experienced in resuscitation.

Failure of Analgesia. Satisfactory analgesia with epidural blockade has been reported to occur in 85 to 94 per cent of patients in labor.[39,40,60,90,94,145,154,179] Experience and attention to detail reduces the incidence of complete failure and allows corrective adjustments to be made in most cases in which pain relief is not complete. Doughty found that readjustments were required in 18.6 per cent of patients before satisfactory analgesia was achieved.[60] These adjustments included turning the patient to one side or into the sitting position while giving a further dose, withdrawal of the catheter, or reinsertion for persistent unilateral block. Other sources of dissatisfaction can include delay in providing adequate top-up doses. Perfection depends on frequent assessment, both during labor and after delivery, and the opportunity for critical reappraisal of current practices in the light of maternal opinions.

Unblocked segments are more frequently witnessed when epidural doses are administered through a catheter and occur in up to 7 per cent of cases,[65,90] of which a small number are persistent despite positioning and catheter withdrawal. The incidence of unblocked segments during labor does not appear to be influenced by a previous epidural or subarachnoid block.[18] Inadequate perineal analgesia for delivery is a more frequent nuisance,[93] although some authorities are convinced that a top-up dose in the sitting position is invaluable.[21,60] Patient faintness, pallor, and nausea may occur with this maneuver however. Some medical centers using low-dose segmental analgesia deliberately do not aim to achieve perineal analgesia.[112] When additional analgesia is required then a pudendal, caudal, or subarachnoid block can be considered.

Instrumental Delivery. One of the most contentious and difficult issues concerns the influence of epidural analgesia on the incidence of instrumental deliveries. Most large case series cited in this book have demonstrated an increased incidence of forceps deliveries in the patients given epidural block. However, this association is not as simple as it might appear. In most units, epidural analgesia is selected for patients in whom difficulties are anticipated (*e.g.*, trial of labor, malposition, placental insufficiency), and it is hardly surprising that instrumental delivery is more common. In cases of premature labor or maternal heart disease, epidural analgesia is specifically requested to aid an elective forceps delivery. On the other hand, when epidural analgesia is provided more extensively, then spontaneous delivery is more frequent—80%[59] or even higher[112] when low-dose regimes are used.

In addition, the indications for instrumental delivery have not always been stated, and yet they are needed, because obstetric practice is not uniform. For example, not all obstetricians agree on the signs of onset of the "second stage" (*e.g.*, full dilation of the cervix, or descent of the head). Some allow only a stipulated period of time to elapse in the "second stage," after which operative delivery is performed on the grounds of "delay in the second stage." Intervention may also be instituted for fetal distress following a period of active pushing in the supine position, when actually the patient may be better managed on her side, allowing spontaneous fetal descent in comfort.[127] Finally, there are, no doubt, occasions when it is convenient for the obstetrician to intervene! Individual obstetric practice is a significant factor in the rate of use of forceps: In one unit, visiting obstetricians have an interference rate ranging from 10 to 70 per cent.[61]

Despite these difficulties, in a recent prospective trial a five-fold increase in instrumental delivery and three-fold increase in malposition in the group given epidural analgesia was demonstrated compared with a control group.[98] Undoubtedly, the type of instrumental delivery is important in the current controversy. It is generally (although not universally[162]) accepted that an outlet forceps delivery is innocuous, whereas a rotational forceps application can be associated with traumatic morbidity. Clinical reports to date, however, have not distinguished whether rotational Kiellands forceps have been applied for deep transverse arrest or merely to rotate from a transverse position. The latter procedure is relatively innocuous when performed by skilled hands.[87]

Despite the reported increase in the forceps rate associated with epidural analgesia, there has been no reported increase in perinatal mortality. Indeed, the combination of epidural analgesia and forceps delivery may be advantageous for the premature infant.[53] Nevertheless, epidural analgesia obviously does modify the course of labor, especially in the second stage. Therefore, its use demands skilled obstetrics and midwifery.

In an attempt to increase the rate of normal delivery, some Scandinavian hospitals have successfully provided a very limited segmental block (T10–12) for the first stage of labor only.[94,112,130,132] This procedure maintains pelvic floor tone and the bearing-down reflex. The rate of normal deliveries (85–90%) and high degree of patient satisfaction in these studies is impressive and warrants similar studies in other hospitals. Perineal pain in the second stage of labor may not be as acceptable in other countries or cultures, but suitably informed patients may prefer to "trade off" some degree of pain for an increased likelihood of a normal delivery.

Perhaps anesthesiologists (usually male!) have naively and mistakenly assumed that patient satisfaction is identical with complete analgesia, and yet this is frequently not the case. Each patient has individual expectations and aspirations. When these are ascertained, it should be possible to tailor analgesia for each mother in labor by making full use of the flexibility that an epidural catheter provides. Another alternative approach, originally described in Cleland in 1952, provides for a second catheter introduced into the caudal space as a route for perineal analgesia. This double-catheter technique has been favoured recently using chloroprocaine (3%) administered by means of the caudal catheter for the second stage, once flexion and rotation of the head have been completed.[93]

"There is now an indisputable case for the safe practice of epidural analgesia: while it has been shown to give positive clinical benefits to both mother and baby, its most impressive effect is to bring tranquillity and humanity to the delivery suite as well as happiness and dignity to a woman on one of the most important occasions in her life."[61]

CAUDAL EPIDURAL ANALGESIA

The caudal approach to the epidural space has become less popular in obstetrics during the past decade. Earlier, large case series have reported high success rates with few complications.[57,67,136,153] The incidence of reported hypotension and accidental subarachnoid injection is similar with both routes.[144] Satisfactory cephalad spread sufficient to provide analgesia in the first stage of labor (*i.e.*, to T10) is more difficult to control and requires much larger early doses than those required with lumbar epidural analgesia. Toxicity is no less than and is probably greater than that produced by the lumbar approach. It is a common temptation in practice to inject local anesthetics during strong labor more rapidly than is prudent. Consequent rapid absorption or frank direct intravascular injection may occur.

Caudal analgesia is used as part of the two-catheter technique in some centers; and for the provision of perineal analgesia when delivery is imminent and time or conditions preclude a lumbar epidural block, or when an instrumental delivery is planned. Under the latter conditions, many anesthesiologists would prefer to use a low subarachnoid block instead.

SUBARACHNOID ANALGESIA

Subarachnoid blockade has been popular for many years in North America and has a most useful place in obstetrics. The rapid onset, profound degree of blockade, and lack of toxicity are particularly attractive properties for certain urgent obstetric maneuvers, whenever an epidural block is not already in effective use. These maneuvers include operative vaginal delivery, repair of third-degree tear or cervical laceration, and removal of the placenta. Low subarachnoid blockade is generally preferable to caudal block or peripheral nerve blocks on these occasions, and it is certainly preferable to the induction of general anesthesia.[45]

Either 0.5-per-cent tetracaine, 5.0-per-cent lidocaine, or 0.5-per-cent dibucaine are used in standard hyperbaric preparations—all in volumes of 0.75 to 1.5 ml (see Chap. 7). In the patients undergoing perineal or vaginal surgery, a sacral (saddle) block is quite adequate, but for a forceps delivery or placental removal, the patient should be so positioned to ensure a block to T10. In the patients with a hemorrhage, it is necessary, of course, to replenish blood volume before proceeding with subarachnoid block. Compared to epidural analgesia, the subarachnoid route has certain advantages for cesarean section also.[25] Complete sacral nerve root blockade can be assured, a quality which improves the patients' comfort during the procedure.[146] The standard hyperbaric preparations in volumes of 1.5 to 2.0 ml are required to ensure a block extending from T5 to S4. To provide bilateral blockade, the patient should be tilted to the opposite side immediately after subarachnoid injection and should not be placed in the supine position. No studies to date have compared epidural and subarachnoid analgesia on neonatal neurobehavior following cesarean section. However, one recent study[88] compared the effects of subarachnoid analgesia to those of two standard methods of general anesthesia on infant scores on the Neonatal Neurobehavioural Scale.[191] Subarachnoid analgesia was associated with the greatest percentage of high scores.

Management of cesarean section under subarachnoid block is exactly the same as that of epidural analgesia. Opinion differs as to whether hypotension is more frequent under subarachnoid analgesia,[146] but the same therapy is equally effective.[104]

A recent case series has confirmed a suspicion that obstetric patients are unfortunately more likely to experience headache (16.3%) after subarachnoid analgesia even following the use of a 25-gauge needle.[45] This high incidence probably reflects the early ambulation of mothers compared to other surgical series.

Part 2: Gynecological Procedures Suitable for Neural Blockade

DILATION AND CURETTAGE

Dilation and curettage has been performed for many years in the "day-surgery" setting when the indications are diagnostic or for therapeutic abortion up to 12 weeks' gestation. Paracervical block is a useful technique for a number of reasons. It is relatively easy to use and contributes significantly to patient safety as well as early recovery. In addition, it cuts the costs of medical care because only one physician is involved, and simplified medical facilities may be used. The dangers in this practice, however, should not be underestimated. In one report, toxic reactions led to the death of five women receiving paracervical block for termination of pregnancy.[82] Full facilities and the necessary resuscitative skills are essential requirements for any physician contemplating its use (see Chap. 4). As the procedure is short, 1-per-cent lidocaine with epinephrine can be used with a maximum volume of 40 ml (400 mg). Frequently, a smaller dose is sufficient. There would be little need to use the long-acting agents, such as bupivacaine, unless postoperative analgesia is required.

MAJOR VAGINAL SURGERY

Vaginal surgery can be conveniently separated into two groups, depending upon whether or not the ovarian pedicles are to be stretched or ligated as in vaginal hysterectomy. These structures have a sensory nerve supply from the T8 level, and therefore regional anesthesia to that level is necessary. Any one of the centrally acting blocks (caudal, lumbar epidural, subarachnoid) are suitable, provided there are no contraindications.

The local anesthetic drugs commonly used for lumbar epidural anesthesia are lidocaine (1.5–2%), 15 to 25 ml with epinephrine (1:200,000); or bupivacaine (0.5–0.75%), 15 to 20 ml. However, most major vaginal surgery does not involve the ovarian structures, and therefore, caudal analgesia is frequently suitable. Smaller doses of local anesthetic drug can be used and provide excellent analgesia for the procedure. Once again, lidocaine (1.5%) or bupivacaine (0.5%) may be used, depending on the duration of the procedure. Despite the adequacy of analgesia, many patients undergoing vaginal surgery require light sedation (*e.g.*, with low-dose intravenous infusion techniques).

INTRA-ABDOMINAL PELVIC SURGERY

Patients undergoing intra-abdominal pelvic surgery are eminently suited to regional block. The duration of the surgical procedure plays an important part, as some reconstructive surgery (tuboplasty, myomectomy) may be inordinately long. It is wise to ensure that the height of the block is sufficient: in these patients, to a level of T8. Of the three blocks mentioned above, the lumbar epidural is most frequently used. A relative contraindication to regional block is surgery in which huge uterine or ovarian tumors have to be excised. The supine hypotension syndrome may occur; however, the difficulty that the surgeon has in ligating the tumor is more important. The types and doses of drugs used for intra-abdominal pelvic surgery are similar to those used in major vaginal surgery, in which traction on the ovarian structures is to be anticipated. The important feature in this type of surgery is muscle relaxation, and bupivacaine (0.75%) is often used. Etidocaine (1%), which produces satisfactory motor blockade, may also be used. Even with blockade to T8, some patients experience pain owing to vagal afferent stimulation. Thus, light general anesthesia, administered by a face mask and inhalation agent, is often used to supplement epidural block (see Chap. 8).

There are two major advantages of regional anesthesia for pelvic surgery: There is a reduction in blood loss with an associated decrease in the surgical time; and, the time of recovery from the anesthetic technique is considerably shortened when compared with general anesthesia. Also, the patient has an earlier return of appetite and improved gut motility if epidural analgesia is continued after operation. It seems likely that the incidence of deep venous thrombosis may be reduced (see Chap. 8).

POSTPARTUM TUBAL LIGATION

In patients in whom continuous lumbar or caudal epidural block is already instituted, then it is a simple postpartum procedure to give more local anesthetic drug, to provide a suitable anesthetic level (T8) for tubal ligation. The incision is usually subumbilical (T10) and the procedure is short. However, it is important to ensure that cardiovascular stability is present before administering the dose of the local anesthetic.

Care should be taken to ensure adequate hydration, because frequently a significant loss of blood occurs during delivery. Should a regional block be instituted for the first time postpartum, it is necessary to assess maternal blood volume, because the potential for hypotension is high if epidural block is induced in the presence of unrecognised blood loss (see Fig. 8-17).

PELVIC LYMPH NODE DISSECTION

Major surgical procedures frequently benefit from the use of the continuous lumbar epidural technique. The reduction in blood loss and improved surgical access owing to a small gut makes for smoother surgery. However, the length of these procedures (4–6 hours) is often beyond the tolerance of most patients lying in just one position. Therefore, it is necessary on most occasions to supplement the regional block with a light general anesthetic with the patient intubated. This, therefore, ensures the airway and avoids hypoxia, which may occur from prolonged spontaneous respiration with intravenous sedation or inhalation anesthesia (see Chap. 8).

REFERENCES

1. Abouleish, E.: Pain control in obstetrics. pp. 268, 286, 342. Philadelphia, J.B. Lippincott, 1977.
2. Albright, G.A.: Anesthesia in Obstetrics. pp. 105, 157. California Addison-Wesley, 1978.
3. Ansari, I., Wallace, G., Clemetson, C.A.B., Mallikarjuneswara, V.R. and Clemetson, C.D.M.: Tilt caesarian section. J. Obstet. Gynaecol. Br. Commonw., *77*:713, 1970.
4. Arens, J.F., and Carrera, A.E.: Methemoglobin levels following peridural anesthesia with prilocaine for vaginal deliveries. Anesth. Analg. (Cleve.), *49*:219, 1970.
5. Asling, J.H., Shnider, S.M., Margolis, A.J., Wilkinson, G.L., and Way, E.L.: Paracervical block anesthesia in obstetrics. II: Etiology of fetal bradycardia following paracervical block anesthesia. Am. J. Obstet. Gynecol., *107*:626, 1970.
6. Assali, N.S., Brinkman, C.R., and Nuwayhid, B.: Uteroplacental circulation and respiratory gas exchange. *In* Gluck, (ed.): Modern perinatal medicine. p. 67. Year Book Medical Publishers, 1974.
7. Beard, R.W. and Simons, E.G.: Diagnosis of foetal asphyxia in labour. Br. J. Anaesth., *43*:874, 1971.
8. Belfrage, P., Irestedt, L., Raabe, N., and Arner, S.: General anaesthesia or lumbar epidural block for caesarean section? Effects on the foetal heart rate. Acta Anaesthesiol. Scand., *21*:67, 1977.
9. Belfrage, P., Raabe, N., Thalme, B., and Berlin, A.: Lumbar epidural analgesia with bupivacaine in labor. Determination of drug concentration and pH in fetal scalp blood, and continuous fetal heart rate monitoring. Am. J. Obstet. Gynecol., *121*:360, 1975.
10. Bevan, D.R., et al.: Closing volume and pregnancy. Br. Med. J., *1*:13, 1974.
11. Bieniarz, J., et al.: Aortocaval compression by the uterus in late human pregnancy. Am. J. Obstet. Gynecol., *100*:203, 1968.
12. Bloom, S.L., Horswill, C.W., and Curet, L.B.: Effects of paracervical blocks on the fetus during labor, a prospective study with the use of direct fetal monitoring. Am. J. Obstet. Gynecol., *114*:218, 1972.
13. Boehm, F.H., Wooddruff, L.F., Jr., and Growdon, J.H., Jr.: The effect of lumbar epidural anesthesia on fetal heart

rate baseline variability. Anesth. Analg. (Cleve.), *54*:779, 1975.
14. Bonica, J.J.: Principles and Practice of Obstetric Analgesia and Anesthesia pp. 531, 1338, 473. Philadelphia, F.A. Davis, 1967.
15. ______: Peripheral mechanisms and pathways of parturition pain. Br. J. Anaesth., *51*:3S, 1979.
16. Bowen-Simpkins, P., and Fergusson, I.L.: Lumbar epidural block and the breech presentation. Br. J. Anaesth., *46*:420, 1974.
17. Brackbill, Y., Kane, J., Manniello, R.L., and Abramson, D.: Obstetrical meperidine usage and assessment of neonatal status. Anesthesiology, *40*:116, 1974.
18. Bray, M.C., and Carrie, L.E.S.: Unblocked segments in obstetric epidural blocks. Anaesthesia, *33*:232, 1978.
19. Brazleton, T.B.: Neonatal behavioural assessment scale. Clinics in Developmental Medicine. No. 50. London, Spastics International Medical Publishers, 1973.
20. Breeson, A.J., Kovacs, G.T., Pickles, B.G., and Hill, J.G.: Extradural analgesia—the preferred method of analgesia for vaginal breech delivery. Br. J. Anaesth., *50*:1227, 1978.
21. Bromage, P.R.: Epidural Analgesia. pp. 523, 528, 564, 548. Philadelphia, W.B. Saunders, 1978.
22. Brown, W.U., Jr., Bell, G.C., and Alper, M.H.: Acidosis, local anesthetics and the newborn. Obstet. Gynecol., *48*:27, 1976.
23. Brown, W.U., et al.: Newborn blood levels of lidocaine and mepivacaine in the first postnatal day following maternal epidural anesthesia. Anesthesiology, *42*:698, 1975.
24. Brownridge, P.: Foetal hypoxia—an anaesthetists approach to classification and prevention. Anaesth. Intens. Care, *6*:5, 1978.
25. ______: Central neural blockade and caeserian section. Part 1: Review and case series. Anaesth. Intens. Care, *7*:33, 1979.
26. Brownridge, P., and Jefferson, J.: Central neural blockade and caesarian section. II: Patient assessment of the procedure. Anaesth. Intens. Care, *7*:163, 1979.
27. Brudenell, M., and Chakravarti, S.: Uterine rupture in labour. Br. Med. J., *2*:122, 1975.
28. Caldeyro-Barcia, R.: Effect of position changes on the intensity and frequency of uterine contractions during labor. Am. J. Obstet. Gynecol., *80*:284, 1960.
29. Casady, G.N., Moore, D.C., and Bridenbaugh, L.D.: Postpartum hypertension after use of vasoconstrictor and oxytocic drugs. J.A.M.A., *172*:1011, 1960.
30. Cibils, L.A., and Santonja-Lucas, J.J.: Clinical significance of fetal heart rate patterns during labor. III. Effect of paracervical block anesthesia. Am. J. Obstet. Gynecol., *130*:73, 1978.
31. Clark, R.B., Thompson, D.S., and Thompson, C.H.: Prevention of spinal hypotension associated with cesarean section. Anesthesiology, *45*:670, 1976.
32. Cleland, J.G.P.: Paravertebral anesthesia in obstetrics. Surg. Gynecol. Obstet., *57*:51, 1933.
33. Clemetson, C.A., Hassan, R., Mallikarjuneswara, V.R., and Wallace, G.: Tilt-bend cesarean section. Obstet. Gynecol., *42*:290, 1973.
34. Climie, C.R., et al.: Consumer satisfaction in the labour ward. Med. J. Aust., *2*:1081, 1973.
35. Cooper, L.V., Stephen, G.W., and Aggett, P.J.: Elimination of pethidine and bupivacaine in the newborn. Arch. Dis. Child., *52*:638, 1977.
36. Corke, B.C.: Neurobehavioural responses of the newborn. Anaesthesia, *32*:539, 1977.
37. Covino, B.G., and Vassallo, H.G.: Pharmacokinetic Aspects of Local Anesthetic Agents in Local Anesthetics: Mechanism of Action and Clinical Use. p. 103. New York, Grune & Stratton. 1976.
38. Craft, J.B., Jr., Epstein, B.S., and Coakley, C.S.: Effect of lidocaine with epinephrine versus lidocaine (plain) on induced labor. Anesth. Analg. (Cleve.), *51*:243, 1972.
39. Crawford, J.S.: Lumbar epidural block in labour: a clinical analysis. Br. J. Anaesth., *44*:66, 1972.
40. ______: The second thousand epidural blocks in an obstetric hospital practice. Br. J. Anaesth., *44*:1277, 1972.
41. ______: An appraisal of lumbar epidural blockade in patients with a singleton fetus presenting by the breech. J. Obstet. Gynaecol. Br. Commonw., *81*:867, 1974.
42. ______: An appraisal of lumbar epidural blockade in labour in patients with multiple pregnancy. Br. J. Obstet. Gynaecol., *82*:929, 1975.
43. ______: Epidural analgesia in pregnancy hypertension. Clin. Obstet. Gynaecol., *4*:735, 1977.
44. ______: Principles and Practice of Obstetric Anaesthesia. pp. 14, 182, 215, 267, 293. Oxford, Blackwell Scientific Publications, 1978.
45. ______: Experience with spinal analgesia in a British obstetric unit. Br. J. Anaesth., *51*:531, 1979.
46. Crawford, J.S.: Burton, M., and Davies, P.: Anaesthesia for section: further refinements of a technique. Br. J. Anaesth., *45*:726, 1973.
47. Crawford, J.S., Mills, W.G., and Pentecost, B.L.: A pregnant patient with Eisenmenger's syndrome. Case report. Br. J. Anaesth., *43*:1091, 1971.
48. Crawford, J.S., and Paterson, M.E.: Abruptio placentae and epidural block in labour. Anaesthesia, *33*:272, 1978.
49. Crawford, J.S., and Opit, L.J.: A survey of the anaesthetic services to obstetrics in the Birmingham region. Anaesthesia, *31*:56, 1976.
50. Cuerden, C., Buley, R., and Downing, J.W.: Delayed recovery after epidural block in labour. A report of four cases. Anaesthesia, *32*:773, 1977.
51. Cugell, D.W.: Pulmonary function in pregnancy; serial observations in normal women. Am. Rev. Tuberc., *67*:568, 1953.
52. Darby, S., Thorton, C.A., and Hunter, D.J.: Extradural analgesia in labour when the breech presents. Br. J. Obstet. Gynaecol., *83*:35, 1976.
53. David, H., and Rosen, M.: Perinatal mortality after epidural analgesia. Anaesthesia, *31*:1054, 1976.
54. Department of Health and Social Security. Report on Confidential Enquiries into Maternal Deaths in England and Wales, 1970–72. H.M.S.O., London, 1975.
55. Dick-Read, G.: Childbirth Without Fear. ed. 2. New York, Harper & Row, 1959.
56. Difazio, C.H.: Metabolism of local anaesthetics in the fetus, newborn and adult. Br. J. Anaesth., *51*:29S, 1979.
57. Dogu, T.S.: Continuous caudal analgesia and anesthesia for labor and vaginal delivery. A review of 4071 confinements. Obstet. Gynecol., *33*:92, 1969.
58. Donnai, P., and Nicholas, A.D.: Epidural analgesia. Fetal monitoring and the condition of the baby at birth with breech presentation. Br. J. Obstet. Gynaecol., *82*:360, 1975.
59. Doughty, A.: Selective epidural analgesia and the forceps rate. Br. J. Anaesth., *41*:1058, 1969.
60. ______: Lumbar epidural analgesia—the pursuit of perfection. With special reference to midwife participation. Anaesthesia, *30*:741, 1975.
61. ______: Epidural analgesia in labour: the past, the present and future. Proc. R. Soc. Med., *71*:879, 1978.

62. Downing, J.W., Coleman, A.J., Mahomedy, M.C., Jeal, D.E., and Mahomedy, Y.H.: Lateral table tilt for caesarian section. Anaesthesia, *29*:696, 1974.
63. Downing, J.W., Houlton, P.C., and Barclay, A.: Extradural analgesia for caesarian section: a comparison with general anaesthesia. Br. J. Anaesth., *51*:367, 1979.
64. Drummond, G.B., Scott, S.E.M., Lees, M.M., and Scott, D.B.: Effects of posture on limb blood flow in late pregnancy. Br. Med. J., *4*:587, 1974.
65. Ducrow, M.: The occurrence of unblocked segments during continuous lumbar epidural analgesia for pain relief in labour. Br. J. Anaesth., *43*:1172, 1971.
66. Eckstein, K.L., and Marx, G.F.: Aortocaval compression and uterine displacement. Anesthesiology, *40*:92, 1974.
67. Epstein, H.M., and Sherline, D.M.: Single-injection caudal anesthesia in obstetrics. Obstet. Gynecol., *33*:496, 1969.
68. Evans, K.R., and Carrie, L.E.S.: Continuous epidural infusion of bupivacaine in labour. Anaesthesia, *34*:310, 1979.
69. Finster, M., and Pedersen, H.: Placental transfer and fetal uptake of drugs. Br. J. Anaesth., *51*:25S, 1979.
70. Finster, M., et al.: Pharmacodynamics of 2-chloroprocaine. Fourth European Congress on Anesthesiology, Amsterdam. Exerpta Medica, *330*:189, 1974.
71. Finster, M., Poppers, P.J., Sinclair, J.C., Morishima, H.O., and Daniel, S.S.: Accidental intoxication of the fetus with local anesthetic drug during caudal anesthesia. Am. J. Obstet. Gynecol., *92*:922, 1965.
72. Fisher, A., and Prys-Roberts, C.: Maternal pulmonary gas exchange. Anaesthesia, *23*:350, 1968.
73. Fox, G.S., Smith, J.B., Namba, U., and Johnson, R.C.: Anesthesia for cesarean section: further studies. Am. J. Obstet. Gynecol., *133*:15, 1979.
74. Freeman, D.V., and Arnold, N.I.: Paracervical block with low doses of chloroprocaine—fetal and maternal effects. J.A.M.A., *231*:56, 1975.
75. Freeman, P.K., et al.: Fetal cardiac response to paracervical block anaesthesia. Am. J. Obstet. Gynecol., *113*:583, 1972.
76. Freeman, R.K., and Schifrin, B.S.: Whither paracervical block? *In* Advances in Fetal Monitoring and Obstetric Anesthesia. Int. Anesthesiol. Clin., *11, 2*:69, 1973.
77. Gibbs, C.P., and Noel, S.C.: Response of arterial segments from gravid human uterus to multiple concentrations of lignocaine. Br. J. Anaesth., *49*:409, 1977.
78. Glover, D.J.: Continuous epidural analgesia in the obstetric patient: a feasibility study using a mechanical infusion pump. Anaesthesia, *32*:499, 1977.
79. Goodlin, R.C.: Importance of the lateral position during labor. Obstet. Gynecol., *37*:698, 1971.
80. ———: Aortocaval compression during cesaran section. Obstet. Gynecol., *37*:702, 1971.
81. Greiss, F.C., Still, J.G., and Anderson, S.G.: Effects of local anesthetic agent on the uterine vasculature and myometrium. Am. J. Obstet. Gynecol., *124*:889, 1976.
82. Grimes, D.A., and Cates, W.: Deaths from paracervical anesthesia used in first trimester abortion 1972–1975. N. Engl. J. Med., *295*:1397, 1976.
83. Grundy, E.M., Zamora, A.M., and Winnie, A.P.: Comparison of spread of epidural anesthesia in pregnant and nonpregnant women. Anesth. Analg. (Cleve.), *57*:544, 1978.
84. Gullestad, S., and Sagen, N.: Epidural block in twin labour and delivery. Acta Anaesthesiol. Scand., *21*:504, 1977.
85. Gutsche, B.B.: Prophylactic ephedrine preceding spinal analgesia for cesarean section. Anesthesiology, *45*:462, 1976.
86. Hehre, F.W., Hook, R., and Hon, E.H.: Continuous lumbar peridural anesthesia in obstetrics. IV: The fetal effects of transplacental passage of local anesthetic agents. Anesth. Analg. (Cleve.), *48*:909, 1969.
87. Hibbard, B., et al.: Lumbar epidural analgesia in labour (letter). Br. Med. J., *1*:286, 1977.
88. Hodgkinson, R., Bhatt, M., Kim, S.S., Grewal, G., and Marx, G.F.: Neonatal neurobehavioural tests following cesarian section under general and spinal anesthesia. Am. J. Obstet. Gynecol., *132*:670, 1978.
89. Hodgkinson, R., Marx, G.F., Kim, S.S., et al.: Neonatal neurobehavioural tests following vaginal delivery under ketamine, thiopental and extradural anesthesia. Anesth. Analg. (Cleve.), *56*:548, 1977.
90. Holdcroft, A., and Morgan, N.: Maternal complications of obstetric epidural analgesia. Anaesth. Intens. Care, *4*:108, 1976.
91. Holdsworth, J.D.: Relationship between stomach contents and analgesia in labour. Br. J. Anaesth., *50*:1145, 1978.
92. Holland, R.: Special committee investigating deaths under anaesthesia: report on 745 classified cases, 1960–1968. Med. J. Aust., *1,* 573, 1970.
93. Hollmen, A.: Regional techniques of analgesia in labour. Br. J. Anaesth., *51*:17S, 1979.
94. Hollmen, A., Jouppila, R., Pihlajaniemi, R., Karvonen, P., and Sjostedt, E.: Selective lumbar epidural block in labour. A clinical analysis. Acta Anaesthesiol. Scand., *21*:174, 1977.
95. Hollmen, A., et al.: Neurologic activity of infants following anesthesia for cesarian section. Anesthesiology, *48*:350, 1978.
96. Holmes, F.: Spinal analgesia and caesarian section—maternal mortality. J. Obstet. Gynaecol. Br. Emp., *64*:229, 1957.
97. ———: Incidence of the supine hypotensive syndrome in late pregnancy. J. Obstet. Gynaecol. Br. Emp., *67*:254, 1960.
98. Hoult, I.J., Maclennan, A.H., and Carrie, L.E.S.: Lumbar epidural analgesia in labour: relation to fetal malposition and instrumental delivery. Br. Med. J., *1*:14, 1977.
99. Humphrey, M., Houslow, D., Morgan, S., and Wood, C.: The influence of maternal posture at birth on the foetus. J. Obstet. Gynaecol. Br. Commonw., *80*:1074, 1973.
100. Huovinen, K., Kivalo, I., and Teramo, K.: Factors influencing the incidence of fetal bradycardia after lumbar epidural block for vaginal labour. Abstracts of Proceedings of the 5th European Congress of Perinatal Medicine. Stockholm, Almqvist & Wiksell. 1976.
101. James, F.M., Crawford, J.S., Davies, P., and Naiem, H.: Lumbar epidural analgesia for labor and delivery of twins. Am. J. Obstet. Gynecol., *127*:176, 1976.
102. James, F.M. III, Crawford, J.S., Hopkinson, R., Davies, P., and Naiem, H.: A comparison of general anesthesia and lumbar epidural analgesia for elective cesarean section. Anesth. Analg. (Cleve.), *56*:228, 1977.
103. James, F.M. III, and Davies, P.: Maternal and fetal effects of lumbar epidural analgesia for labor and delivery in patients with gestational hypertension. Am. J. Obstet. Gynecol., *126*:195, 1976.
104. James, F.M., III, and Greiss, F.C., Jr.: The use of inflatable boots to prevent hypotension during spinal anesthesia for cesarean section. Anesth. Analg. (Cleve.), *52*:246, 1973.
105. Jaschevatzky, O.E., Shalit, A., Levy, Y., and Grunstein, S.: Epidural analgesia during labour in twin pregnancy. Br. J. Obstet. Gynaecol., *84*:327, 1977.
106. Johnstone, M.: The cardiovascular effects of oxytocic drugs. Br. J. Anaesth., *44*:826, 1972.
107. Jouppila, R., and Hollmen, A.: The effect of segmental epi-

dural analgesia on maternal and foetal acid-base balance, lactate, serum potassium and creatine phosphokinase during labour. Acta Anaesthesiol. Scand., *20*:259, 1976.

108. Jouppila, R., Hollmen, A., Jouppila, P., Kauppila, A., and Tuimala, R.: The effect of segmental epidural analgesia on maternal Acth, cortisol and tsh during labour. Ann. Clin. Res., *8*:378, 1976.
109. Jouppila, R., Jouppila, P., Hollmen, A., and Kuikka, J.: Effect of segmental extradural analgesia on placental blood flow during normal labour. Br. J. Anaesth., *50*:563, 1978.
110. Jouppila, P., Jouppila, R., Kaar, K., and Merila, M.: Fetal heart rate patterns and uterine activity after segmental epidural analgesia. Br. J. Obstet. Gynaecol., *84*:481, 1977.
111. Jouppila, R., Jouppila, P., Kuikka, J., and Hollmen, A.: Placental blood flow during caesarian section under lumbar extradural analgesia. Br. J. Anaesth., *50*:275, 1978.
112. Jouppila, R., Pihlajaniemi, R., Hollmen, A., and Jouppila, P.: Segmental epidural analgesia and post partum sequelae. Ann. Chir. Gynaecol. Fenn., *67*:85, 1978.
113. Kenney, A., Koh, L.S., and Pole, Y.L.: A case of locked twins managed under lumbar epidural analgesia. Anaesthesia, *33*:32, 1978.
114. Kerr, M.G., Scott, D.B., and Samuel, E.: Studies of the inferior vena cava in late pregnancy. Br. Med. J., *1*:532, 1964.
115. Klaus, M.H., and Kennell, J.H.: Maternal-Infant Bonding. St. Louis, C.V. Mosby, 1976.
116. Kobak, A.S., Evans, E.F., and Johnson, G.R.: Transvaginal pudendal block. Am. J. Obstet. Gynecol., *71*:981, 1956.
117. Lees, M.M., Scott, D.B., and Kerr, M.G.: Haemodynamic changes associated with labour. J. Obstet. Gynaecol. Br. Commonw., *77*:29, 1970.
118. Levinson, G., and Shnider, S.M.: Placental transfer of local anesthetics. Clinical implications. *In* Marx, G.F. (ed.): Parturition and Perinatology, pp. 173–185. Philadelphia, Williams & Wilkins, 1973.
119. Liston, W.A., Adjepon-Yamoah, K.K. and Scott, D.B.: Foetal and maternal lignocaine levels after paracervical block. Br. J. Anaesth., *45*:750, 1973.
120. Littlewood, D.G., Buckley, P., Covino, B.G., Scott, D.B., and Wilson, J.: Comparative study of various local anaesthetic solutions in extradural block in labour. Br. J. Anaesth., *51*:47S, 1979.
121. Lofstrom, B.: Aspects of the pharmacology of local anaesthetic agents. Br. J. Anaesth., *43*:194, 1970.
122. Lozoff, B., Brittenham, G.M., Trause, M.A., Kennell, J.H., and Klaus, M.H.: The mother-newborn relationship: limits of adaptability. J. Pediatr., *91*:1, 1977.
123. Lund, P.C., Cwik, J.C., Gannon, R.T., and Vassallo, H.G.: Etidocaine for caesarean section—effects on mother and baby. Br. J. Anaesth., *49*:457, 1977.
124. Lund, P.C., Cwik, J.C., and Pagdanganan, R.T.: Etidocaine (Duranest). A clinical and laboratory evaluation. Acta Anaesthesiol. Scand., *18*:176, 1974.
125. McDonald, J.S., Bjorkman, L.L., and Reed, E.C.: Epidural analgesia for obstetrics: a maternal, fetal and neonatal study. Am. J. Obstet. Gynecol., *120*:1055, 1974.
126. McGuinness, G.A., Merkow, A.J., Kennedy, R.L., and Erenberg, A.: Epidural anesthesia with bupivacaine for cesarian section: Neonatal blood levels and neurobehavioural responses. Anesthesiology, *49*:270, 1978.
127. McQueen, J., and Mylrea, L.: Lumbar epidural analgesia in labour (letter). Br. Med. J., *1*:640, 1977.
128. Magno, R.: Anesthesia for Cesarian Section [Thesis]. University of Goteborg, 1976.
129. Maltau, J.M., and Andersen, H.T.: Epidural anaesthesia as an alternative to caesarean section in the treatment of prolonged, exhaustive labour. Acta Anaesthesiol. Scand., *19*:349, 1975.
130. ———: Continuous epidural anaesthesia with a low frequency of instrumental deliveries. Acta Obstet. Gynecol. Scand., *54*:401, 1975.
131. Maltau, J.M., Andersen, H.T., and Skrede, S.: Obstetrical analgesia assessed by free fatty acid mobilisation. Acta Anaesthesiol. Scand., *19*:245, 1975.
132. Marx, G.F., and Greene, N.M.: Maternal lactate, pyruvate and excess lactate production during labour and delivery. Am. J. Obstet. Gynecol., *90*:786, 1964.
133. Matadial, L., and Cibils, L.A.: The effect of epidural anesthesia on uterine activity and blood pressure. Am. J. Obstet. Gynecol., *125*:846, 1976.
134. Mather, L.E., and Tucker, G.T.: Pharmacokinetics and biotransformation of local anesthetics. Int. Anesthesiol. Clin., *16*:4, 1978.
135. Matouskova, A., Dottori, O., Forssman, L., and Victorin, L.: An improved method of epidural analgesia with reduced instrumental delivery rate. Acta Obstet. Gynecol. Scand., *54*:231, 1975.
136. Meehan, F.P.: Continuous caudal analgesia in obstetrics. Proc. R. Soc. Med., *62*:185, 1969.
137. Meehan, F.P., Moolgaoker, A.S., and Stallworthy, J.: Vaginal delivery under caudal analgesia after caesarean section and other major uterine surgery. Br. Med. J., *2*:740, 1972.
138. Meis, P.J., Reisner, L.S., Payne, T.F., and Hobel, C.J.: Bupivacaine paracervical block: Effects on fetus and neonate. Obstet. Gynecol., *52*:545, 1978.
139. Mihaly, G.W., et al.: The pharmacokinetics of anilide-local anaesthetics in neonates. I: Lignocaine. Eur. J. Clin. Pharmacol., *13*:143, 1978.
140. Miller, F.C., Quesnel, G., Petrie, R.H., Paul, R.H., and Hon, E.H.: The effects of paracervical block on uterine activity and beat-to-beat variability of the fetal heart rate. Am. J. Obstet. Gynecol., *130*:284, 1978.
141. Milne, M.K., and Murray Lawson, J.I.: Epidural analgesia for caesarian section. Br. J. Anaesth., *45*:1206, 1973.
142. Mirkin, B.L.: Perinatal pharmacology, placental transfer, fetal localization and neonatal disposition of drugs. Anesthesiology, *43*:156, 1975.
143. Moir, D.D.: Anaesthesia for caesarian section: an evaluation of a method using low concentrations of halothane and 50 per cent oxygen. Br. J. Anaesth., *42*:136, 1970.
144. ———: Recent advances in pain relief in childbirth. II: Regional anaesthesia. Br. J. Anaesth., *43*:849, 1971.
145. ———: Obstetric Anaesthesia and Analgesia. pp. 56, 59, 171, 184, 193, 195, 216, 220. London, Bailliere Tindall, 1976.
146. ———: Extradural analgesia for caesarian section. Br. J. Anaesth., *51*:79, 1979.
147. Moir, D.D., and Amoa, A.B.: Ergometrine or oxytocin: Blood loss and side effects at spontaneous vertex delivery. Br. J. Anaesth., *51*:113, 1979.
148. Moir, D.D., and Davidson, S.: Postpartum complications of forceps delivery performed under epidural and pudenal nerve block. Br. J. Anaesth., *44*:1197, 1972.
149. Moir, D.D., and Willocks, J.: Management of inco-ordinate intrauterine action under continuous epidural analgesia. Br. Med. J., *3*:396, 1967.
150. ———: Epidural analgesia in British obstetrics. Br. J. Anaesth., *40*:129, 1968.

151. Moir, D.D., Victor-Rodrigues, L., and Willocks, J.: Epidural analgesia during labour in patients with pre-eclampsia. J. Obstet. Gynaecol. Br. Commonw., *79*:465, 1972.
152. Moodie, J.E., and Moir, D.D.: Ergometrine, oxytocin and extradural analgesia. Br. J. Anaesth., *48*:571, 1976.
153. Moore, D.C., Bridenbaugh, L.D., Bridenbaugh, P.O., and Tucker, G.T.: Caudal and epidural blocks with bupivacaine for childbirth. Report of 657 parturients. Obstet. Gynecol., *37*:667, 1971.
154. Moore, J., Murnaghan, G.A., and Lewis, M.A.: A clinical evaluation of the maternal effects of lumbar extradural analgesia for labour. Anaesthesia, *29*:537, 1974.
155. Morishima, H.O., et al.: Transmission of mepivacaine hydrochloride across the human placenta. Anesthesiology, *27*:147, 1966.
156. Morishima, H.O., et al.: Placental transfer and tissue distribution of etidocaine and lidocaine in guinea pigs. Abstracts of the Annual Meeting of the American Society of Anesthesiologists. pp. 83. Chicago, 1975.
157. Moya, F., Morishima, H.O., Shnider, S.M., and James, L.S.: Influence of maternal hyperventilation of the newborn infant. Am. J. Obstet. Gynecol., *91*:76, 1965.
158. Munson, E.S., and Embro, W.J.: Lidocaine, monoethylglycinexylidide, and isolated human uterine muscle. Anesthesiology, *48*:183, 1978.
159. Murphy, P.J., Wright, J.D., and Fitzgerald, T.B.: Assessment of paracervical nerve block anaesthesia during labour. Br. Med. J., *1*:526, 1970.
160. Nimmo, W.S., Littlewood, D.G., Scott, D.B., and Prescott, L.F.: Gastric emptying following hysterectomy with extradural analgesia. Br. J. Anaesth., *50*:559, 1978.
161. Nunn, J.F.: Hypoxia and oxygen transfer. *In* Gray and Nunn, (eds.): General Anaesthesia. ed. 3. vol. 1. p. 55. London, Butterworth, 1971.
162. O'Driscoll, K.: An obstetrician's view of pain. Br. J. Anaesth., *47*:1053, 1975.
163. Ostheimer, G.W.: Neurobehavioural effects of obstetric analgesia. Br. J. Anaesth., *51*:35S, 1979.
164. Palahniuk, R.J., Scatliff, J., Biehl, D., Wiebe, H., and Sankaran, K.: Maternal and neonatal effects of methoxyflurane, nitrous oxide and lumbar epidural anaesthesia for caesarean section. Can. Anaesth. Soc. J., *24*:586, 1977.
165. Pathy, G.V., and Rosen, M.: Prolonged block with recovery after extradural analgesia for labour. Br. J. Anaesth., *47*:520, 1975.
166. Pearson, J.F., and Davies, P.: The effect of continuous lumbar epidural analgesia on the acid-base status of maternal arterial blood during the first stage of labour. J. Obstet. Gynaecol. Br. Commonw., *80*:218, 1973.
167. ______: The effect of continuous lumbar epidural analgesia on maternal acid-base balance and arterial lactate concentration during the second stage of labour. J. Obstet. Gynaecol. Br. Commonw., *80*:225, 1973.
168. ______: The effect of continuous lumbar epidural analgesia upon fetal acid-base status during the first stage of labour. J. Obstet. Gynaecol. Br. Commonw., *81*:971, 1974.
169. ______: The effect of continuous lumbar epidural analgesia upon fetal acid-base status during the second stage of labour. J. Obstet. Gynaecol. Br. Commonw., *81*:975, 1974.
170. Pedersen, H., Morishima, H.O., and Finster, M.: Uptake and effect of local anesthetics in mother and fetus. Int. Anesthesiol. Clin., *16*:4, 1978.
171. Peskett, W.G.H.: Antacids before obstetric anaesthesia. A clinical evaluation of mist magnesium trisilicate, B.P.C. Anaesthesia, *28*:509, 1973.
172. Phillips, J.C., Hochberg, C.J., Petrakis, J.K., and Van Winkle, J.D.: Epidural analgesia and its effects on the "normal" progress of labor. Am. J. Obstet. Gynecol., *129*:316, 1977.
173. Poppers, P., Covino, B.G., and Boyes, R.N.: Epidural block with etidocaine for labour and delivery. Acta Anaesthesiol. Scand. (Suppl.), *60*:89, 1975.
174. Poppers, P.J.: Evaluation of local anaesthetic agents for regional anaesthesia in obstetrics. Br. J. Anaesth., *47*:322, 1975.
175. Poppers, P.J., and Finster, M.: Use of prilocaine hydrochloride for epidural analgesia in obstetrics. Anesthesiology, *29*:1134, 1968.
176. Power, G.G., and Longo, L.D.: Sluice flow in placenta: maternal vascular pressure effects on foetal circulation. Am. J. Physiol., *225*:1490, 1973.
177. Printz, J.L., and McMaster, R.H.: Continuous monitoring of fetal heart rate and uterine contractions in patients under epidural anesthesia. Anesth. Analg. (Cleve.), *51*:876, 1972.
178. Prowse, C.M., and Gaensler, E.A.: Respiratory and acid-base changes during pregnancy. Anesthesiology, *26*:381, 1965.
179. Raabe, N., and Belfrage, P.: Lumbar epidural analgesia in labour. A clinical analysis. Acta Obstet. Gynecol. Scand., *55*:125, 1976.
180. ______: Epidural analgesia in labour. IV: Influence on uterine activity and fetal heart rate. Acta Obstet. Gynecol. Scand., *55*:305, 1976.
181. Ralston, D.H., and Shnider, S.M.: The fetal and neonatal effects of regional anesthesia in obstetrics. Anesthesiology, *48*:34, 1978.
182. Ralston, D.H., Shnider, S.M., and De Lorimer, A.A.: Effects of equipotent ephedrine, metaraminol, mephentermine and methoxamine on uterine blood flow in the pregnant ewe. Anesthesiology, *40*:354, 1974.
183. Rekonen, A., Luotola, H., Pitkanen, M., Kuikka, J., and Pyorala, T.: Measurement of intervillous and myometrial blood flow by an intravenous 133xe method. Br. J. Obstet. Gynaecol., *83*:723, 1976.
184. Reynolds, F., Hargrove, R.I., and Wyman, J.B.: Maternal and foetal plasma concentrations of bupivacaine after epidural block. Br. J. Anaesth., *45*:1049, 1973.
185. Reynolds, F., and Taylor, G.: Plasma concentrations of bupivacaine during continuous epidural analgesia in labour: the effect of adrenaline. Br. J. Anaesth., *43*:436, 1971.
186. Rosefsky, J.B., and Petersiel, M.E.: Perinatal deaths associated with mepivacaine paracervical block anesthesia in labor. N. Engl. J. Med., *278*:530, 1968.
187. Salariya, E.M., Easton, P.M., and Cater, J.I.: Duration of breast feeding after early initiation of frequent feeding. Lancet, *2*:1141, 1978.
188. Saling, E., and Ligdas, P.: The effect on the foetus of maternal hyperventilation during labour. J. Obstet. Gynaecol. Br. Commonw., *76*:877, 1969.
189. Sangoul, F., Fox, G.S., and Houle, G.L.: Effect of regional analgesia on maternal oxygen consumption during the first stage of labor. Am. J. Obstet. Gynecol., *121*:1080, 1975.
190. Scanlon, J.W., and Alper, M.H.: Perinatal pharmacology and evaluation of the newborn. Int. Anesthesiol. Clin., *11*:163, 1973.
191. Scanlon, J.W., Brown, W.U., Weiss, J.B., and Alper, M.H.: Neurobehavioral responses of newborn infants after maternal epidural anesthesia. Anesthesiology, *40*:121, 1974.
192. Scanlon, J.W., et al.: Neurobehavioral responses and drug

concentrations in newborns after maternal epidural anesthesia with bupivacaine. Anesthesiology, *45*:400, 1976.

193. Schifrin, B.S.: Fetal heart rate patterns following epidural anaesthesia and oxytocin infusion during labour. J. Obstet. Gynaecol. Br. Commonw., *79*:332, 1972.
194. Scott, D.B., and Kerr, M.G.: Inferior vena caval pressure in late pregnancy. J. Obstet. Gynaecol. Br. Commonw., *70*:1044, 1963.
195. Scudamore, J.H., and Yates, M.J.: Pudendal block—a misnomer? Lancet, *1*:23, 1966.
196. Shnider, S.M., Asling, J.H., Hall, J.W., and Margolis, A.J.: Paracervical block anesthesia in obstetrics. I: Fetal complications and neonatal morbidity. Am. J. Obstet. Gynecol., *107*:619, 1970.
197. Shnider, S.M., and Gildea, J.: Paracervical block anesthesia in obstetrics. Am. J. Obstet. Gynecol., *116*:320, 1973.
198. Shnider, S.M., et al.: Vasopressors in obstetrics. I: Correction of fetal acidosis with ephedrine during spinal hypotension. Am. J. Obstet. Gynecol., *102*:911, 1968.
199. Smith, A.M.: Letter: Uterine rupture in labour. Br. Med. J., *2*:446, 1975.
200. Sprague, D.H.: Effects of position and uterine displacement of spinal anesthesia for cesarean section. Anesthesiology, *44*:164, 1976.
201. Stainthorp, S.F., Bradshaw, E.G., Challen, P.D., and Tobias, M.A.: 0.125% bupivacaine for obstetric analgesia? Anaesthesia, *33*:3, 1978.
202. Taylor, G., and Prys-Davies, J.: Prophylactic use of antacids in the prevention of the acid-pulmonary-aspiration syndrome. Lancet, *1*:288, 1966.
203. Teramo, K.: Effects of obstetrical paracervical blockade of the fetus. Acta Obstet. Gynecol. Scand. (Suppl.), *16*, 1971.
204. Teramo, K., and Widholm, Q.: Studies of the effect of anesthetics on the foetus. Part I: The effect of paracervical block with mepivacaine upon foetal acid-base values. Acta Obstet. Gynecol. Scand. (Suppl. 2), *46*:1, 1967.
205. Teramo, K., Kivalo, I., and Huovinen, K.: Obstetric paracervical blockade with etidocaine. Acta Anaesthesiol. Scand. (Suppl.), *60*:100, 1975.
206. Thalme, B., Belfrage, P., and Raabe, N.: Lumbar epidural analgesia in labour. I: Acid-base balance and clinical condition of mother, fetus and newborn child. Acta Obstet. Gynecol. Scand., *53*:27, 1974.
207. Tronick, E., et al.: Regional obstetric anesthesia and newborn behavior: Effect over the first ten days of life. Pediatrics, *58*:94, 1976.
208. Tucker, G.T.: Plasma binding and disposition of local anesthetics. Int. Anesthesiol. Clin., *13*:33, 1975.
209. Tucker, G.T., et al.: Binding of anilide-type local anesthetics in human plasma. II: Implications in vivo with special reference to transplacental distribution. Anesthesiology, *33*:304, 1970.
210. Tunstall, M.E., Donald, L.A., and Manson, H.G.: Proceedings: delivery-micturition intervals following spontaneous and forceps delivery. Anaesthesia, *30*:120, 1975.
211. Tyack, A.J., Parsons, R.J., Millar, D.R., and Nicholas, A.D.: Uterine activity and plasma bupivacaine levels after caudal epidural analgesia. J. Obstet. Gynaecol. Br. Commonw., *80*:896, 1973.
212. Ueland, K., Gills, R., and Hansen, J.M.: Maternal cardiovascular dynamics. I: Cesarian section under subarachnoid block anesthesia. Am. J. Obstet. Gynecol., *100*:42, 1968.
213. Vasicka, A., et al.: Fetal bradycardia after paracervical block. Obstet. Gynecol., *38*:500, 1971.
214. Warwick, R., and Williams, P.L. (eds.): Dorsal rami of the spinal nerves. *In* Grays Anatomy. p. 1032. ed. 35. Norwich, Longman, 1973.
215. Weaver, J.B., Pearson, J.F., and Rosen, M.: The effect of posture and epidural block upon limb blood flow and radial artery pressure in term pregnant women. Br. J. Obstet. Gynaecol., *82*:844, 1975.
216. ———: The implications of the valsalva manoeuvre on mother and foetus. Preliminary Communication, Obstetric Anaesthetists Association, Oxford.
217. Weekes, A.R., Cheridjian, V.E., and Mwanje, D.K.: Lumbar epidural analgesia in labour in twin pregnancy. Br. Med. J., *2*:730, 1977.
218. Weis, F.R., Markello, R., Mo, B., and Bochiechio, P.: Cardiovascular effects of oxytocin. Obstet. Gynecol., *46*:211, 1975.
219. Wollman, S.B., and Marx, G.F.: Acute hydration for prevention of hypotension of spinal anesthesia in parturients. Anesthesiology, *29*:374, 1968.
220. Zador, G., and Nilsson, B.A.: Low dose intermittent epidural anaesthesia in labour: influence on labour and fetal acid-base status. Acta Obstet. Gynecol. Scand. (Suppl.), *34*:17, 1974.
221. Zador, G., Lindmark, G., and Nilsson, B.A.: Pudendal block in normal vaginal deliveries: clinical efficacy, lidocaine concentrations in maternal and fetal blood, fetal and maternal acid-base values and influence on uterine activity. Acta Obstet. Gynecol. Scand. (Suppl.), *34*:51, 1974.
222. Zilianti, M., Salazar, J.R., Aller, J., and Aguero, O.: Fetal heart rate and ph of fetal capillary blood during epidural analgesia in labor. Obstet. Gynecol., *36*:881, 1970.

19 Neural Blockade for Plastic Surgery

Leo A. Keoshian

Plastic surgery is very frequently elective and performed for cosmetic reasons. It is especially desirable, then, to keep the risks incurred by the anesthesia as low as possible. Since most plastic surgery is in the head–neck region, the use of general anesthesia necessitates intubation and, often, muscle-relaxant techniques with a small but inevitable risk of airway obstruction, disconnection, and other complications of general anesthesia per se. In addition, many plastic surgeons require a bloodless field that may involve controlled hypotension if general anesthesia is employed.

The comparative simplicity and safety of neural blockade techniques are very appealing provided the anesthesiologist has a full knowledge of the physiology and pharmacology of local anesthetic agents and of the differential diagnosis of local anesthetic reactions and their treatment (see Chaps. 2–4, Table 4-8). Since quite large volumes of local anesthetic and vasocontrictor solutions are required for some plastic-surgery procedures, it is essential that the clinician carefully calculate the dose of both agents and ensures that they are within safe limits for the particular patient. In order to avoid fatalities in association with neural blockade procedures, it is essential to make adequate preparations, even for the peripheral nerve block and infiltration techniques described in this chapter. This entails adequate preoperative evaluation of the patient, premedication, and preparation of resuscitative equipment (see Chap. 6). It is wise routinely to start an intravenous infusion to ensure rapid access to the vascular system and it is essential to have the drugs and equipment for treatment of local anesthetic toxicity readily available (see Chap. 4). The intravenous infusion may also be useful for judicious injection of small doses of supplementary sedative, if they are required.

The neural blockade techniques described in this chapter represent a common range of practices for plastic surgery. Many of the techniques described elsewhere in this book have equal appeal for plastic surgery for reasons similar to those outlined above. Plastic surgeons should consult the appropriate section of the book for neural blockade techniques applicable to the region of the body for which plastic surgery is contemplated.

PREOPERATIVE AND OPERATIVE CONSIDERATIONS

Preoperative Evaluation and Consultation

The plastic surgeon who administers local anesthesia has a rather unique position in that he is responsible both for satisfactory anesthesia and for the surgery itself, which is usually considered his primary goal. These two factors are very closely related; in fact, superb results in plastic surgery are often dictated by the quality of anesthesia administered. The preoperative evaluation for anesthesia usually begins at the time of the initial consultation in the surgeon's office (see Chaps. 6 and 8). This evaluation is affected by such factors as the patient's experience with local anesthesia, what other people have told him of anesthesia, and what he has learned from nonprofessional journals and publications. In order to understand better the patient's position, often the surgeon must ascertain his response to previously administered local anesthetics. Thus, the surgeon has the opportunity to clarify many misconceptions and put the patient's mind at ease. Also, this preliminary period of consultation should provide information on the general state of health, history of allergy to medications, and medications regularly used. A complete history and physical examination as well as preoperative laboratory studies may be obtained at this time. The anesthetic consultation cannot be separated from the preoperative consultation since they are taking place simultaneously. If the patient is a poor anesthetic risk, surgery will not be considered. Establishing good rapport with the patient is just as important in administering the local anesthetic as it is in conducting the surgical procedure.

Premedication

Administering sedatives before the anesthetic is an established practice. The primary purpose of such premedication is to sedate a patient who experiences minimal discomfort or pain. In plastic surgery, since most patients do not arrive in the operating room in a painful state, the reason would be to render the patient tranquil.

"The basic concept of premedication," to quote Claude Bernard, "is mixed anesthesia." The selection of the particular agents is based on general medical status, psychological and emotional factors, the types of medication currently used by the patient, and finally, the extent of the surgical procedure anticipated. Sedation may be obtained by a wide range of central nervous system (CNS) depressant drugs; however, only minimal cardiorespiratory depression is desired. Because no single agent will give the optimal premedicative effects, a combination of drugs is necessary, generally consisting of a narcotic or a synthetic narcotic combined with barbituates, tranquilizers, or ataractics. A narcotic is used even when there is no preoperative pain in order to reduce anxiety and provide basal analgesia, both of which supplement the effect of the local anesthetic in abolishing pain. Thus, pain transmission is reduced, and the patient's response to pain is also altered; though he may experience minimal pain, he is oblivious to it. Although a certain measure of tranquility is obtained with low doses of narcotics, a moderate dose of a tranquilizer is more efficient. The end result is muscle relaxation, relief from anxiety, amnesia, and analgesia (see also Chap. 31).

Local Anesthetic Agents

Particularly in cosmetic surgery, a minimal volume of local anesthetic agent should be used so that there is minimal tissue distortion. This is quite important since many corrective procedures are measured or should be measured very accurately. This fact is one of the leading arguments presented by plastic surgeons using general anesthesia rather than local anesthesia on a regular basis. However, careful and judicious use of these local agents at precise sites minimizes the total quantity used, assuming that the administrator is quite aware of the normal anatomy and possible anomalies. Also, modern agents that have a long duration now minimize the need for reinjection in lengthy surgical procedures (see Chap. 4). An added benefit of the long-acting agents is that less analgesia is required in the postoperative period (see Chap. 25).

The selection of local anesthetic for the patient, or procedure, and duration of effect desired is discussed in Chapter 4 (see Fig. 4-1 and Tables 4-1–4) and also in Chapter 6. In general, 1 per cent lidocaine (or equivalent medium-duration agent) or 0.5 per cent bupivacaine (or equivalent long-acting agent) is adequate for the peripheral nerve blocks described in this chapter. Infiltration techniques are carried out with 0.5 per cent lidocaine (or equivalent) or 0.25 per cent bupivacaine. It should also be emphasized that the total volume required should first be estimated, then the minimal effective concentration of drug determined, and finally the administered dose calculated. If the dose is too high then consideration should be given to using a lower concentration of drug, if this is possible. For example, extensive infiltration requires 0.25 per cent lidocaine with epinephrine. Such large volumes are uncommonly required in plastic surgery; however, they may sometimes be useful in very aged patients (bearing in mind that onset of action may be much slower than with higher concentrations).

Vasoconstrictor Agents

Vasoconstrictor agents are added to local anesthetic agents in plastic surgery for a variety of reasons. First, there is less continuous bleeding during the surgical procedure. Second, since there is a slower release of the local anesthetic from the injection site, less anesthetic agent is necessary, and the total amount of local agent reaching the cardiovascular system and CNS is consequently reduced (see Table 3-6, Fig. 3-12, and Figs. 4-7 and 4-8). Also, the addition of epinephrine usually prolongs the duration of a given dose of local anesthetic (see Chaps. 3 and 4).

There is, however, a group of surgical patients who are particularly susceptible to the cardiovascular effects of the absorbed vasoconstrictor (see also Table 4-7 and Fig. 8-17). These patients are elderly, hypertensive, or hyperthyroid. The surgeon must be very careful to modify the dose in these patients or use a vasoconstrictor with minimal or no beta-adrenergic-stimulating properties.

Epinephrine is one of the most potent vasopressors known and perhaps the vasoconstrictor agent most commonly used in conjunction with the local anesthetics. There has been much debate about the proper concentration of epinephrine to be administered. In an experimental and clinical study, Siegel and colleagues demonstrated that effective hemostasis can be achieved by using less epinephrine with the local anesthetic than usual.[5] As little as 1:800,000 concentration of epinephrine appears to provide adequate cutaneous hemostasis in most plastic surgical procedures. In practice, 1:200,000 or 1:400,000 are effective solutions now available commercially. No patient should receive more than 0.25 mg (50 ml of 1:200,000 or 100 ml of 1:400,-000). Patients with cardiovascular disease or hyperthyroidism should be limited to half this dose or more appropriately, another vasoconstrictor without beta-adrenergic activity should be used.

At present the most promising vasoconstrictors, without direct cardiac activity, are derivatives of vasopressin: felypressin (Octapressin) and ornipressin (POR-8).[2] These are described in detail in Chapter 4. It should be remembered that significant vascular absorption of vasopressor may cause increased peripheral resistance and thus indirect cardiac effects, which include increased myocardial oxygen consumption and bradycardia. Thus dose should be carefully regulated (see Chap. 4).

Patient Monitoring

In this age of computerized patient-monitoring systems, it is alarming to discover the number of operative procedures performed without adequate provision for surveillance of vital signs during the procedure. Many times the vital signs are obtained only prior to premedicating the patient. However, not every operating room will have electronic equipment for continuous patient surveillance. Although continuous display of electrocardiogram and digital pulse waveform is extremely useful, it is not a substitute but merely a complement to regular measurements of blood pressure, pulse, and respiratory rate together with observations of level of consciousness, color, and capillary refill time (see Chap. 8). Thus, appropriate arrangements should be made for such observations since the plastic surgeon will not be able to make this evaluation objectively. Failure to allow for these observations may lead to a sudden and unexpected discovery of gross deterioration in the patient's condition. Anesthesiologists are all too familiar with this and would much prefer to be alerted at an earlier stage as a result of the detection of an early change in vital signs.

Also, it is well worthwhile to alert the anesthesiologist to potential difficulties beforehand, if at all possible. It is worth noting at this point the importance of draping with care to permit adequate access to the airway and also to permit routine administration of supplementary oxygen by way of nasal spectacles or oxygen mask. Patients who are sedated will benefit from an increased inspired oxygen concentration, which will provide some reserve if the patient's condition deteriorates and resuscitation is needed.

PLASTIC SURGERY PROCEDURES

Blepharoplasty, Meloplasty, and Mentoplasty

Local anesthesia with a vasoconstrictor is preferred to general anesthesia in combination with local anesthesia for procedures on the aging face because there is a significant reduction in bleeding.[7] In addition, this method facilitates the ease of positioning and draping and provides greater mobility of the head for surgical dissection. By combining local infiltration with nerve blocks, less agent is used and less tissue distention is noted. In meloplasty, 1 per cent lidocaine (Xylocaine) with epinephrine is used in the infraorbital, mandibular, and superior cervical plexus blocks. The major local infiltration (0.5%) is administered along the lines of the incision. Each case varies significantly, as does the distribution of the local infiltration and dissection. For example, more local anesthetic is used in the mastoid area and in the upper neck above the sternocleidomastoid muscle level since the skin is inherently associated with the overlying fascial tissue. Total quantity of local anesthetic used varies somewhat; however, usually not more than 500 mg of lidocaine with 1:400,000 epinephrine is used during the entire procedure, which may last up to 4 hours. The anesthetic is instilled into the area of dissection approximately 20 to 30 minutes prior to surgery.

Chlorpromazine (Thorazine), 2.5 to 50 mg, intramuscularly, is used for patients with a hypertensive tendency; dosage should be carefully tailored for age and the presence of other antihypertensive drugs.[1] It is important to control hypertension in order to minimize the risk of postoperative bleeding.[1]

Another benefit of nerve blocks plus infiltrative anesthesia is that the motor branches of the facial nerve can be stimulated and isolated for identification during the procedure itself, whereas during muscle-relaxant/general anesthesia techniques, responses of facial muscles may be abolished by the combined effects of neuromuscular blockade and general anesthesia.

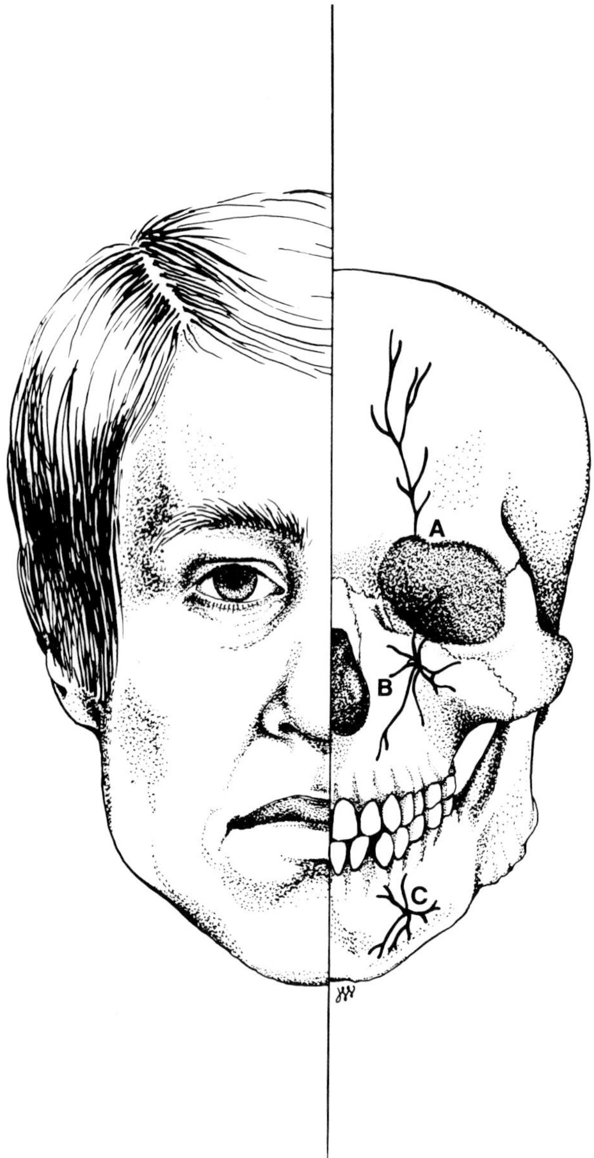

Fig. 19-1. Supraorbital (*A*), infraorbital (*B*), and mental nerves (*C*).

Techniques. As shown in Figure 19-1, the foramen of exit for the supraorbital, infraorbital, and mental nerves passes through a vertical line located just medial to the pupil in adults, but which bisects the pupil in children. (The sensory distribution for the following 3 blocks is shown in Fig. 19-3*B*; see also Fig. 15-10*B*.)

Infraorbital Block. The infraorbital foramen is located in line with the pupil, just below the bony margin (Fig. 19-2*A*). Approximately 2 ml of local agent are infiltrated in and around the infraorbital foramen.

Mandibular Block, by Way of the Mandibular Notch. The puncture site is below the zygomatic arch in the middle of the mandibular notch.

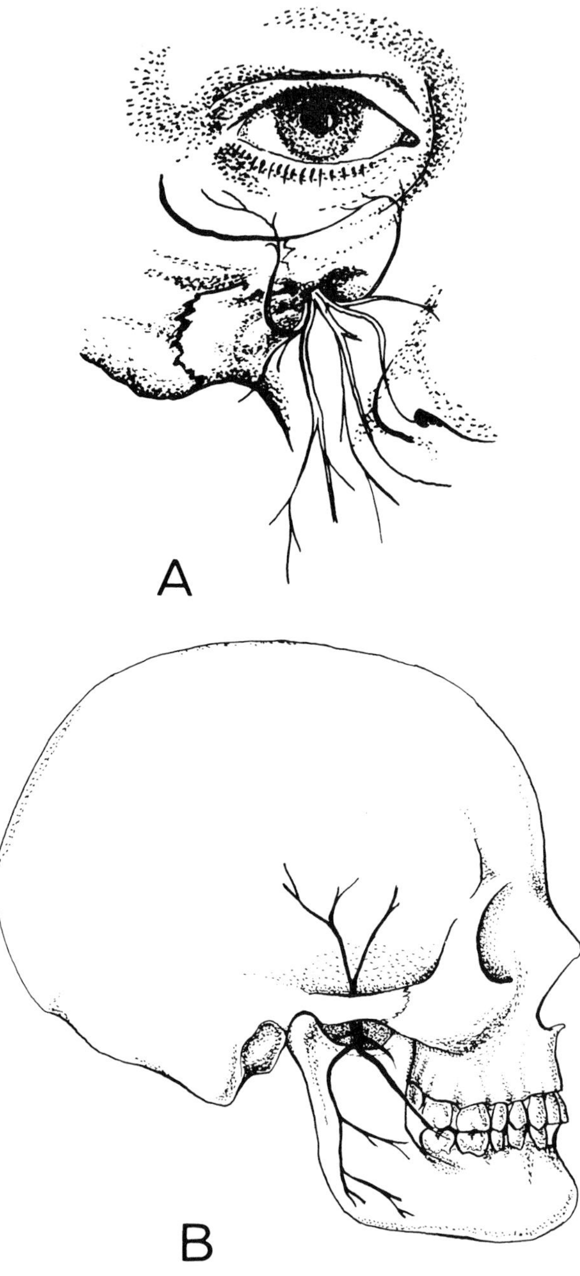

Fig. 19-2. (*A*) Infraorbital block. (*B*) Mandibular block by way of the mandibular notch.

The needle is directed perpendicular to the skin to a depth of about 4 cm. The mandibular nerve is found just posterior to the lateral pterygoid plate (Fig. 19-2*B*). Four ml of 1 per cent lidocaine is used. Chapter 15 should also be consulted for a more detailed account of the anatomy of this technique (see Fig. 15-6).

Superficial Cervical Plexus Block. Four ml of agent is instilled into the central area of the posterior margin of the sternocleidomastoid muscle (Fig. 19-3*A*). The distribution of the agent is both subcutaneous and subfascial.

Rhinoplasty

Technique. Ten to 20 minutes before surgery, cotton applicators moistened with 2 ml of 10% cocaine or 4% lidocaine are applied to the area of the nasociliary nerve and the sphenopalatine ganglion (Fig. 19-4*B*; see Chap. 15). While this topical anesthetic is taking effect, the local agent can be injected.[3] Approximately 6 to 10 ml of 2 per cent lidocaine with epinephrine, 1:200,000, is administered, using the least volume possible. The agent is injected slowly through a No. 27 hypodermic needle 4 cm in length. The rate of distention of the tissue appears to be directly related to the amount of pain incurred with the injection. Starting the injection in the glabellar area at the junction of the nose and forehead, the dorsum is infiltrated (Fig. 19-4*A*). Next, the infraorbital block is completed (see Chap. 15). Finally, the nasal spine is infiltrated for completion of the block. The cotton applicators are then replaced with 2.5 cm nasal packing that has been soaked in 1 to 2 ml of 4 per cent cocaine. The packing is used primarily to prevent blood from dripping into the nasopharyngeal area, but the local anesthetic effect is also important.

Mammoplasty (Augmentation)

Innervation of the Breast and Technique. Sir Astley Cooper's description in *Anatomy** is still appropriate. The innervation of the breast is from the lateral mammary rami of the anterior rami of the lateral cutaneous branches of the third to the sixth intercostal nerves and the medial mammary rami of the anterior branches of the third to the sixth intercostal nerves. In addition, the skin is supplied by the supraclavicular branch of the cervical plexus.

A field block in the subcutaneous tissue and in the retromammary space provides not only satisfactory anesthesia but also identification of that space for

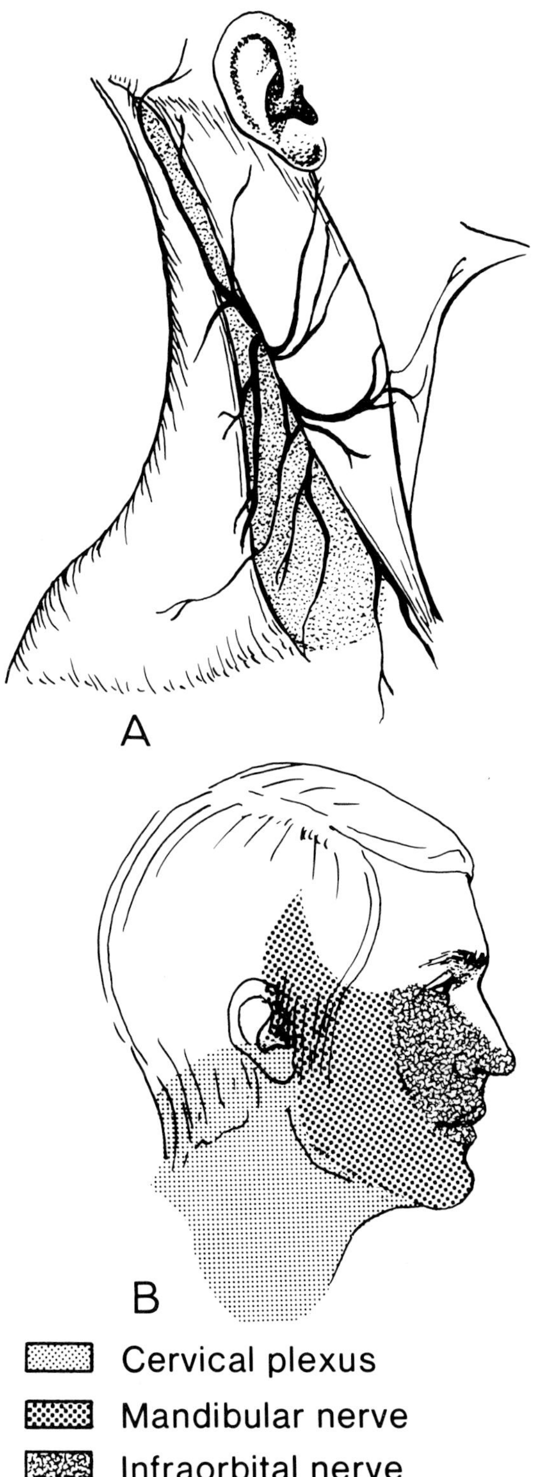

Fig. 19-3. (*A*) Superficial cervical plexus block. (*B*) Distribution of sensory loss after blockade of cervical plexus, mandibular nerve, and infraorbital nerves.

* London, Longman, 1840

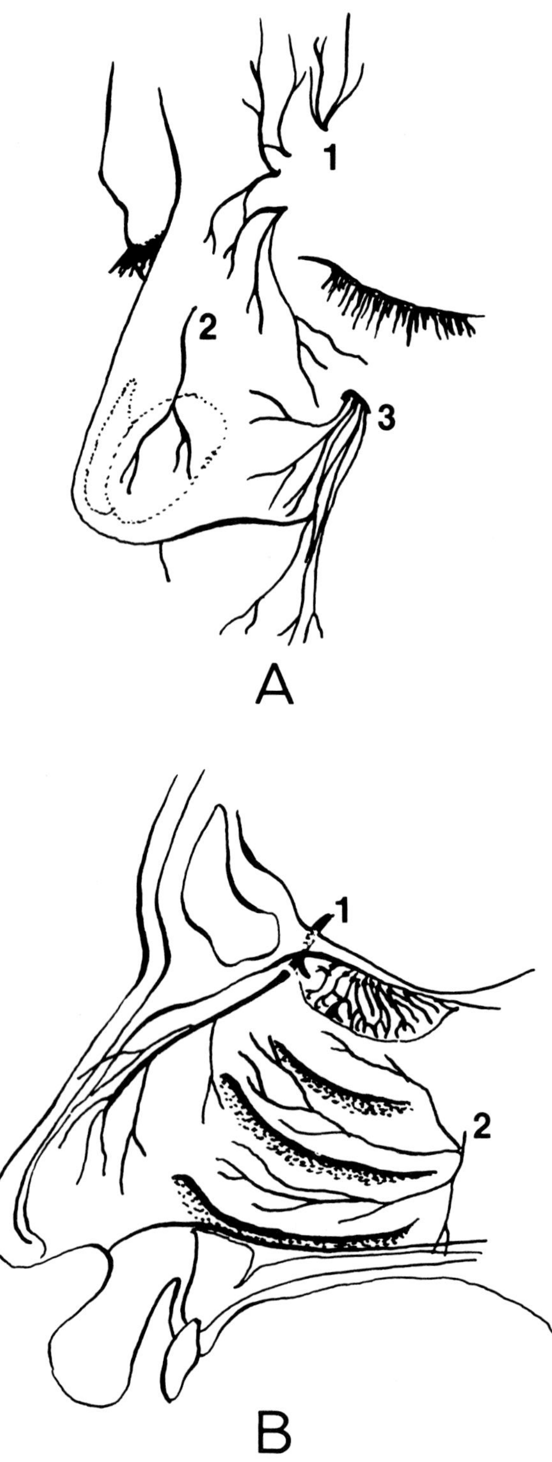

Fig. 19-4. Innervation of the nose as applied to rhinoplasty. (*A*) Nasal branches of the supraorbital nerve (*1*), external branch of the anterior ethmoid nerve (*2*), and nasal branches of the infraorbital nerve. (*B*) Anterior ethmoidal nerve (*1*) and sphenopalatine ganglion area (*2*).

insertion of the prosthesis. Also, dissection for insertion of the prosthesis has already been started by the administration of the local anesthetic. All of the volume (15–20 ml of 2% lidocaine with epinephrine, 1:200,000) can be inserted slowly through three or four injection sites using a No. 27 hypodermic needle 4 cm in length, since the size of the breast is generally quite small. Also, by placing the agent superficial to the pectoralis fascia, the risk of intravascular or intrathoracic injection is eliminated (Fig. 19-5).[6]

Although 1 per cent lidocaine with 1:200,000 epinephrine is quite adequate, the onset of blockade is much slower, and the 2 per cent solution is preferred unless bilateral mammoplasty is to be performed (the 1% solution is essential then to avoid overdose). If prolonged postoperative analgesia is desired, then 0.25 per cent bupivacaine with 1:200,000 epinephrine is an excellent choice.

Penile Block for Circumcision

Circumcision is generally performed for cosmetic reasons, usually as an elective procedure. Surprisingly, general anesthesia is very commonly used for this operation, whereas all that is required is 5 ml of local anesthetic. The size of the operative procedure and the relative risks of the two anesthetic techniques bring into question the routine use of general anesthesia for circumcision. Certainly the procedure has psychological overtones; however, adequate preoperative explanation and appropriate premedication can almost always alleviate such problems. Even if light general anesthesia is used in small children, the additional benefits of penile block are reduced reflex activity during the procedure and the possibility of prolonged postoperative pain relief. The alternative technique of single-shot caudal block is described in Chapter 9 for adults and Chapter 21 for pediatric patients.

Technique. The dorsal nerves of the penis may be blocked at the base of the penis by two separate injections of 1 ml of 1 per cent lidocaine by way of a 26-27 gauge needle inserted at the 10:30 o'clock and 1:30 o'clock positions on the penis; it is necessary for the needle to pierce the deep fascia, but great care should be taken that the needle does not lie in a blood vessel.

If the injection is made close to the pubic bone, the dorsal nerve is blocked before its posterior branches pass toward the undersurface of the penis. If the posterior branches are not blocked, the frenulum and undersurface of the penis will not be anesthetized, and a separate injection will be required along the lateral surface of the penis.

If postoperative analgesia is required, 0.25 to 0.5 per cent bupivacaine is employed. Circumferential infiltration at the base of the penis is avoided and vasoconstrictors are not used for fear of causing ischemia. Also, great care should be taken not to use large needles, which may cause hematomas.

Plastic Surgery of the Arm and Hand

Brachial Plexus Block. The axillary technique of brachial plexus block is well suited to plastic surgical operations on the arm or hand. This neural blockade technique is described in detail in Chapter 10. It should be stressed that it is a major plexus block requiring local anesthetic at doses close to toxic so that the knowledge, skill, and equipment to deal with local anesthetic toxicity is a prerequisite to its use (see Chap. 4).

Peripheral Nerve Blocks at the Elbow and Wrist. As described in Chapter 10, there is rarely any advantage in blocking the radial, median, and ulnar nerves at the elbow rather than at the wrist where blockade is easily accomplished by the plastic surgeon after draping and skin preparation. Sometimes it is desirable to produce sensory blockade without significant motor blockade so that movement can be evaluated during tendon-repair surgery. Experience has shown that motor block is very difficult to avoid if adequate sensory block is achieved by axillary brachial block. In this situation individual branches of peripheral nerves can be blocked at the wrist, leaving long flexors intact. If the duration of the operation is kept brief and the patient is adequately premedicated patients will tolerate the required arm tourniquet (see Chap. 10).

Digital Nerve Block is perhaps one of the most useful techniques for minor plastic surgery on the digits. The various approaches are described in Chapter 10.

Plastic Surgery on the Leg

Skin Graft With Infiltration or Nerve Block. Many skin grafting procedures are performed under general anesthesia in order to provide analgesia for the donor site on the thigh. Many years ago Hamilton Brailey described a very simple procedure for obtaining skin from the thigh under the cover of a circumscribed "fence" of local anesthesia. The area of thigh from which the graft is to be taken is marked as a rectangular area by an indelible marking pen or merely as an extra rectangle of preparation solution. This rectangular fence is then thoroughly infiltrated with 0.5 per cent lidocaine or 0.25 per cent bupivacaine. The latter is preferable because donor sites are often quite painful postoperatively. It is important that the area of infiltration is marked beforehand and that the graft be taken only from within this area. Alternatively, the technique of lateral femoral cutaneous nerve block extends the anesthetized area available for graft donation. This technique is described in Chapter 11.

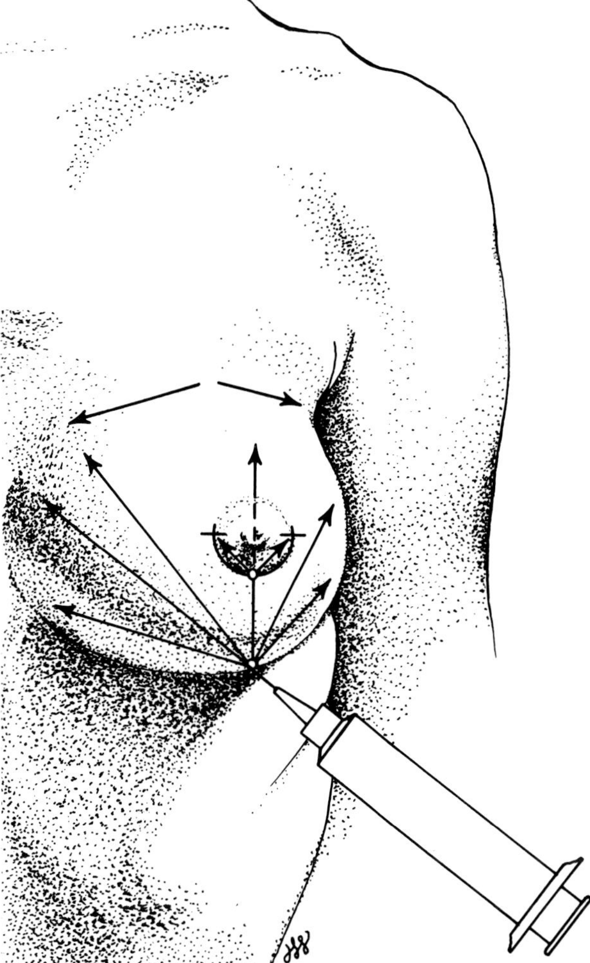

Fig. 19-5. Field block for augmentation mammoplasty.

Procedures on the Foot with Ankle Block. Neural blockade of the individual nerves at the ankle is an easy technique that provides excellent operating conditions for foot surgery and superb postoperative analgesia. These techniques are described in Chapter 11.

Acute Post-traumatic Procedures. A wide range of neural blockade techniques are applicable to repair of soft-tissue trauma in various regions of the body. Particular mention should be made of the following:

(1) For major lacerations of the scalp, circumferential infiltration above the level of the ears provides complete analgesia of the entire scalp (see Chap. 15).

(2) For superficial injuries in the region of the eye, a combination of topical and nerve block techniques is often useful (see Chap. 17).

(3) Repair of lacerations in the mouth, lips, and surrounding region lends itself to a considerable range of nerve block and infiltration techniques, which are common knowledge to dentists and oral surgeons but are too infrequently used by others.[4] These techniques are described in Chapter 16.

In particular inferior mental nerve block deserves more frequent use; block of this nerve with 5 ml of local anesthetic provides anesthesia of one-half of the lower jaw and its overlying mucous membrane including the lower lip (see Fig. 16-18).

REFERENCES

1. Berner, R.E., Morain, W.D., and Noe, J.M.: Postoperative hypertension as etiological factor in hematoma after rhytidectomy, prevention with chlorpromazine. Plast. Resconstr. Surg., *57*:314, 1976.
2. Clodius, L., and Smahel, J.: POR-8, A new vasoconstrictor substitute for adrenaline in plastic surgery. Br. J. Plast. Surg., *23*:73, 1970.
3. Kazanjian, V.H., and Converse, J.M.: The Surgical Treatment of Facial Injuries. ed. 2. pp. 649. Baltimore, Williams & Wilkins, 1959.
4. Macintosh, R., and Ostlere, M.: Local Analgesia, Head and Neck. ed. 2. Edinburgh, E. & S. Livingstone, 1967.
5. Siegel, J., Vistnes, L.M., and Iverson, R.E.: Effective hemostasis with less epinephrine, an experimental and clinical study. Plast. Resconstr. Surg., *51*:129, 1973.
6. Tabari, K.: Augmentation mammoplasty under local anesthesia. Plast. Resconstr. Surg., *43*:320, 1969.
7. Webster, G.V.: The ischemic face-lift. Plast. Resconstr. Surg., *50*:560, 1972.

20 Neural Blockade in the Outpatient Clinic, Emergency Room, and Private Office

F. R. Berry and J. A. Kirchoff

Compared to a fully equipped operating room, the outpatient clinic and private office are often rather primitive in both equipment and staff. The use of local analgesia is often the only choice in these circumstances, and in many places this is limited to a simple infiltration technique. Consequently, the use of a properly applied regional block—intravenous regional, peripheral nerve block, or simple field block—will have definite advantages.

The emergency room, while falling short of the fully equipped operating room in the range of anesthetic equipment and trained personnel, is usually well provided with resuscitation equipment and a "versatile" staff. The need for the use of local anesthetic methods in this acute environment is well-known and practiced; however, the extent of their potential is often not appreciated, particularly for acute pain relief.

The limiting factor in deciding whether a patient needs hospitalization for his operation need not be the requirements of anesthesia. Many operations can be performed very adequately under some kind of regional block if a few simple requirements in relation to equipment, the patient, and the surgeon are fulfilled.

ANESTHETIC REQUIREMENTS

Equipment

The simplicity of equipment necessary is an advantage of regional anesthesia. For the blocks, 2-, 5-, and 10-ml syringes and small-caliber 2.5-, 5-, and 10-cm needles will cover most of the needs that arise. To avoid possible contamination, disposable syringes and needles are preferred. The identification of the nerve to be blocked is generally not very difficult, provided sufficient care is taken in identifying the correct landmarks, but a nerve stimulator has proven to be of considerable help, especially with some of the more difficult blocks, such as the obturator nerve or the anterior approach to the sciatic nerve (see Chaps. 6 and 21).

Serious toxic reactions after properly administered regional blocks are very rare, but they must be treated immediately and correctly. Thus, no regional block should ever be attempted unless facilities to treat all complications are at hand.

The basic requirements for resuscitation equipment are a table that can be tipped to the head-down position and a means of providing a free airway and artificial ventilation with oxygen. A simple resuscitation kit that contains airways, masks, a self-inflating bag, and a manually operated suction apparatus is available. A vasopressor agent and an anticonvulsant should also be available (see p. 113).

The Patient

Cooperation and understanding by the patient are necessary if an operation is to be performed solely under local anesthesia. He must be willing to undergo surgery while awake, and he must submit to the slight discomfort of the application of the regional block. As compensation, he obtains the advantage of somewhat less rigid rules on fasting and probably less need for preoperative laboratory tests. In addition, he avoids the hazards of unconsciousness during general anesthesia and some of the sequelae of general anesthesia, such as nausea and vomiting.

Most patients will accept the decision to use local anesthesia, but a few are terrified by the thought of being awake during the procedure. It may be wise to reject these patients as candidates for regional blocks because, apart from upsetting the patient, it is highly likely that it will prove a failure.

How often this kind of patient is met will vary according to national and local tradition and, most important, local reputation. In countries where anesthesiology is not a specialty in its own right, local analgesia has been used extensively (and with great skill) to avoid the complications following poorly conducted general anesthesia. In some of the English-speaking countries, general anesthesia has been administered by specialists, only a few of whom bothered to learn regional blocks. To encourage a more extensive use of regional anesthesia, the public must be educated. Since patients learn quickly from the experience of others, the best way of introducing regional anesthesia as an accepted procedure is to make certain that no patient is forced to submit to a painful operation because of an insufficient regional block.

Small children cannot be expected to cooperate and should not be treated under local anesthesia alone. The age at which children can tolerate local anesthesia will vary individually and with the ability of the physician to gain the confidence of the child. In addition, some patients, such as the very obese, may produce technical difficulties in performing blocks.

The Physician

Skill and patience are the primary requirements of the physician. Skill can be acquired and maintained only if the physician is sufficiently interested in regional blocks to undergo a period of training that involves considerable practice. Even for an expert, a successful block will not be obtained in all cases, and a beginner certainly must expect a number of failures. Thus, it is recommended that the necessary experience be acquired by performing regional blocks as supplementary analgesia in patients for whom general anesthesia is part of the inpatient routine. The anatomy of landmarks can be learned from a textbook, but experience can be gained only by repeated administration.

Patience is mandatory because a block may take as long as 30 minutes to become completely effective. No surgery must ever be begun until the effect of the block has been tested.

SELECTION OF TECHNIQUE

Some of the techniques for regional block that are available to the physician are not as suitable in the outpatient setting because they require just as much preparation and patient supervision as general anesthesia requires; such is the case with spinal and epidural blocks. Also, sometimes special and prolonged attention may be needed postoperatively for unintended sequelae, such as pneumothorax. No amount of expertise will prevent the occasional pneumothorax following supraclavicular brachial plexus or intercostal nerve blocks, a complication for which symptoms may not develop for many hours and which is harmless only if diagnosed and treated correctly. Some would regard chest radiographs after a 3-hour observation period as essential with these blocks, but if the patient is warned to return should dyspnea occur, routine radiographs should not be necessary for experienced physicians.

For operations on the distal part of the extremities, the simplest technique is intravenous regional analgesia (see Chap. 12). It requires little skill to administer and usually produces sufficient muscle relaxation for reduction of fractures, and the tourniquet may be an advantage to the surgeon. However, this method does have limitations, and during training it is important to acquire experience with the more useful conduction block techniques, and to stay practiced in their use. If a regional block is chosen for an operation on an arm or a leg, a proximal block has certain advantages over a more distal block. The proximal block allows a tourniquet to be applied for a longer period; it overcomes the problem of variation in a peripheral nerve distribution; and in the upper limb, it does not require multiple needles. On the other hand, distal blocks are often all that are necessary and can be very useful, particularly in the Emergency Department, and patients who want to go home do not have to be managed for analgesia and paralysis of an entire arm or leg.

A study of anesthetic records of large numbers of surgical cases performed under regional block shows that the time to prepare and perform the block, plus the time until the effect of the block is complete, is, in most cases, longer than the duration of the operation itself. When the duration was recorded, the block was shown to last for an average of almost 2 hours after the end of the operation.* As a result, the timing of the sequence of events becomes important in exploiting the advantages of regional block over general anesthesia. It may be necessary to perform the regional block well in advance of the operation, preferably in an anteroom where the effect can be observed and supplementation, if necessary, can be administered.

The onset time varies with the particular block and depends mainly on how close the anesthetic solution has been placed to the nerve. Thus, the landmarks and how to use them are very important. A few nerves can be palpated directly under the skin; the ulnar nerve at the elbow and the peroneal nerve

* Kirchoff, J.A.: Unpublished data.

at the neck of the fibula represent their own landmarks. Other nerves, such as the femoral or the nerves of the brachial plexus, can be located by means of the large, easily palpable artery that runs in close proximity. The pulsation of the needle hub can be used as a sign that the tip lies close to the artery and is a fairly reliable indication that the block will eventually be effective. If the needle is disconnected from the syringe after the injection of a few milliliters, the solution will start to appear as a few drops from the hub of the needle, indicating that the injection has occurred in the right compartment, where it creates a slight overpressure.[4] When the patient feels a paresthesia in the area supplied by the nerve as the solution is being injected, a total block is almost certain to occur within a few minutes. The use of one or other of these signs to indicate proximity to the nerve avoids the possible hazards of damage that may ensue when paraesthesias are deliberately sought with the tip of the needle.

Other nerves, in particular the sciatic, can be located only by identifying bony landmarks, drawing lines on the skin, and calculating angles to the surface. This relatively coarse technique yields only an approximation to the nerve, and it is therefore necessary either to elicit paraesthesias or to use a nerve stimulator to place the needle into a position where the nerve can be blocked with a reasonable volume of local anesthetic agent.

USEFUL PROCEDURES IN THE EMERGENCY ROOM

Pain Relief

One of the most important aspects of the management of the patient presenting to the Emergency Department after injury is the relief of pain, for which there is a tendency to think only of parenteral analgesic agents. However, although use of nerve block is limited almost exclusively to the extremities, the appropriate nerve block can provide total analgesia of the affected limb and at the same time leave the remainder of the body unaltered for the observation of other signs and symptoms that have not been dulled by narcotic agents. Total pain relief is especially appreciated by patients who may have to wait some time for the completion of radiographs and transfer to hospital bed and operating room before definitive treatment is begun, even if a general anesthetic may subsequently prove to be necessary or desirable.

The introduction of a sympathetic block to the limb may also be advantageous in both short- and long-term management (see Chap. 13).

It is, of course, very important to assess neurovascular and tendon status before deliberately interrupting nerve supply.

In the upper limb, analgesia can be obtained by total brachial plexus block or by interruption of the brachial plexus branches farther down the arm. The approach to the brachial plexus depends on the physician's experience and the prevailing conditions, but a block from above the clavicle is usually most convenient because of difficulty in moving the injured limb to approach the axilla.

Major fractures of the lower limb frequently require nerve block analgesia because of the severity of the pain. A femoral nerve block yields almost total analgesia to the patient with a fractured shaft of the femur, and a sciatic and femoral nerve block combination provides total analgesia below the knee.[1] The anterior approach to the sciatic nerve would be advantageous if it were reliable; however, the patient can easily be rolled on his side for a classical approach, as long as the limb is adequately splinted.

Anesthesia for Surgery

The repair of wounds, the opening of abscesses, and the reduction of fractures and dislocations are procedures commonly performed in the Emergency Room, and topical, infiltration, field, and nerve block anesthesia are just as useful as in elective surgery. Most appropriate agents, concentrations, and doses are provided in Chapter 4. A well-planned procedure for the differential diagnosis and management of local anesthetic reactions should be well understood and the appropriate equipment should be available (see p. 113).

Topical Analgesia. The use of topical anesthetic solutions in the eye and mucous membrane, particularly of the nose and throat, is well-known and has considerable application, especially for the removal of foreign bodies. Another very rewarding use for topical local anesthetic is the application of the jelly as a temporary dressing on abrasions that are impregnated with road grit and other foreign material prior to their cleaning because this allows a thorough painless scrub.[5]

Infiltration anesthesia is commonly applied for the suture of wounds by either injection through the wound edges (which is relatively painless but risks contamination) or infiltration through the intact skin near the wound edge. These techniques, of course, are satisfactory for small clean wounds, but the

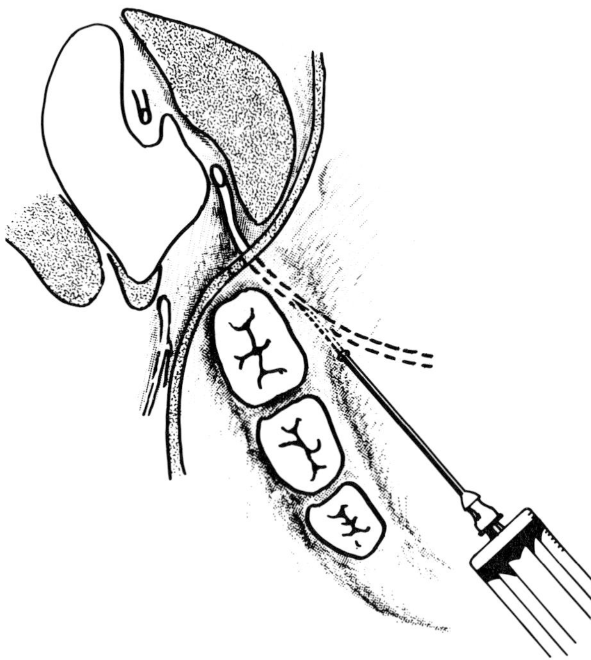

Fig. 20-1. Lingual nerve block. The lower right molar teeth are shown from above with the mandibular ramus cut in cross section. A 22 to 25 gauge needle is inserted below the last molar tooth at the reflection of the mucous membrane from the mandible.

wound and surrounding area must be cleaned and prepared prior to the injection of the local anesthetic, and this in itself is often a painful procedure. Injection of solution into or around dirty and macerated wounds, with the hazards of contamination and distortion and damage of tissue, should be avoided.

A small quantity of local anesthetic solution injected slowly into the dermis that overlies an abscess is highly satisfactory and is recommended over freezing with ethyl chloride or carbon dioxide.

Field Block. The procedure of depositing a wall of local anesthetic between the lesion and its nerve supply is a useful method of avoiding injections in and around the lesion but at the same time does not require a specific nerve block. This method of analgesia is obviously applicable only for subcutaneous infiltration and one must be aware not only from which direction the nerve supply is derived but where the nerves pierce the deep fascia. Analgesia of the scalp is probably the best described example of field blocking but it can be employed in many other parts of the body. It must be remembered that quite substantial volumes of solution may be necessary and also that analgesia does take some time to become effective (see Chap. 19).

Nerve Block. Areas of particular use follow.

Scalp and Ear. The supraorbital, supratrochlear, auriculotemporal, and greater occipital nerves supply the scalp on each side, and these can either be blocked individually or by field block (see Chap. 15). The auriculotemporal nerve can be conveniently blocked as it passes upward over the posterior root of the zygoma just behind the superficial temporal artery. The pinna and lobe of the ear can be repaired under block of the auriculotemporal nerve together with block of the great auricular and lesser occipital branches of the cervical plexus. These two nerves can easily be interrupted by field block with a subcutaneous wheal below the ear.

Lips. The whole lip structure of skin, vermillion, and mucous membrane is supplied by the infraorbital and mental nerves on each side with a contribution at the angle of the mouth from the long buccal nerve. Infraorbital and mental nerve blocks are extremely useful for the repair of lacerated lips and may be performed by the extraoral or intraoral approach (see Chaps. 15 and 16). However, the intraoral method, although normally easier and more reliable, is not always feasible because of the discomfort involved in everting the damaged lips.

Tongue. Lacerations to the tongue can be troublesome because this is a difficult, time-consuming, and painful area to infiltrate locally.

The lingual nerve, which supplies the anterior two-thirds of the tongue and the floor of the mouth, may be blocked with the inferior alveolar nerve by standard dental approach. However, it can be simply blocked on its own as it passes in direct relation to the mandible just below and behind the last molar tooth, where it can be palpated (Fig. 20-1; see Chap. 16). In performing a block at this site, it is important to deposit the solution just below the mucous membrane at its reflection from the mandible because too deep of an insertion may place it below the plane of the mylohyoid muscle.

Extremities. As has been stated, brachial plexus block and femoral and sciatic nerve blocks may be used for pain relief; the indications for the use of these and the more peripheral limb blocks are provided in Chapters 10 and 11. However, the physician should bear in mind a few specific blocks that are of considerable value in the Emergency Department for the repair of relatively minor or common injuries.

The interscalene approach to the brachial plexus is the method of choice for the reduction of dislocations or fractures of the shoulder (see Chap. 10).

The arm cannot be abducted to approach the axilla, and the "shrugged" position of the shoulder causes a routine supraclavicular approach to be much deeper, whereas position and landmarks for an interscalene block are not affected. Only blockade of the upper roots of the plexus is required so that only 10 to 15 ml of local anesthetic is necessary at the C5 or C6 level.

Colles' fractures are by far the most common skeletal injury in the upper limb requiring anesthesia for correction. An axillary block is preferred for this procedure because of its overall safety (see Chap. 10). One of the disadvantages of an axillary block is delay in onset; complete muscle relaxation and profound analgesia are rarely achieved under 20 minutes. No attempt should be made to reduce the fracture before this time has elapsed, even though other signs of autonomic, sensory, and motor block may have occurred.

For soft tissue repair as well as fracture and dislocation of the hands and fingers, the peripheral blocks, particularly at the wrist, are very useful (see Chap. 10).

In the lower limb, the sciatic and femoral combination is particularly valuable for fracture dislocations around the ankle (see Chap. 11). The use of regional anesthesia for surgery on the foot was reviewed and described by McCutcheon and more recently by Schurman, and the use of the posterior tibial nerve block for curettage of plantar warts was described by Laurie.[2,3,6] In warm climates, the barefooted sole of the foot is prone to cuts and foreign bodies, and like the palm, it is a very sensitive area but at the same time very tough and difficult to infiltrate. Posterior tibial block at the ankle is one of the most rewarding of all nerve conduction blocks, particularly in view of the alternatives, and it is very easy to perform. This nerve is blocked at about the point where it divides into medial and lateral plantar nerves behind the medial malleolus, and it can be approached either from a point directly over the nerve just behind the posterior tibial artery or, preferably, from a point at the medial border of the Achilles tendon at the level of the medial malleolus, with the needle then being directed anteriorly (Fig. 20-2). By this means, the fingers of the nonoperating hand can be used to palpate the posterior tibial artery and indirectly guide the tip of the needle to a site just posterolateral to the artery.

It is preferable to perform the posterior tibial block on patients in the prone position so that they cannot kick away from the needle when paraesthesias are elicited; also, the sural nerve can conveniently be blocked at the same time by a wheal from the lateral border of the Achilles tendon to the lateral malleolus. It is usually easier to perform surgery on the sole with the patient in the prone position.

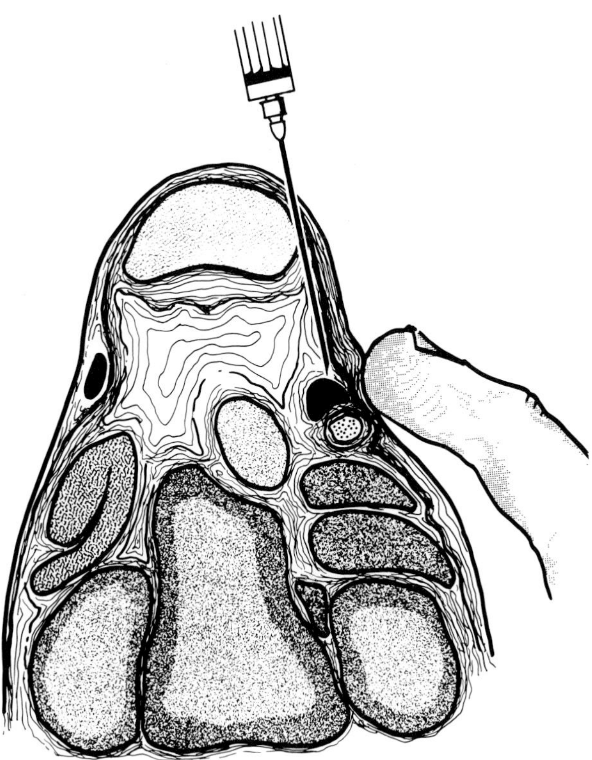

Fig. 20-2. Posterior tibial nerve block at the ankle. A horizontal section through the right ankle joint is shown from above. A 22 to 25 gauge needle is inserted at the medial edge of the Achilles tendon at the level of the medial malleolus and directed anteriorly. The posterior tibial artery is palpated as the needle is guided gently toward the nerve.

A midcalf tourniquet, if it is properly applied, is well tolerated by most patients for at least 30 minutes, and this is an essential for the removal of foreign bodies from the sole of the foot.

PREPARATION AND SUPERVISION OF THE PATIENT

A written record should be kept, which contains a short history with special attention given to previous experiences with local anesthetic agents. If a reaction to a local anesthetic agent has occurred, its nature must be explored.

Most patients are more nervous than they will admit, and the attitude of the medical personnel is of enormous psychological importance in relieving this anxiety. Some will benefit from a pharmacological sedative, however it must be remembered that this may lead to disorientation and lack of cooperation, particularly in the elderly. Heavy sedation will necessitate prolonged supervision, and any sedation at all leaves the patient unfit to go home unattended.

Patients scheduled in advance for minor surgery under neural blockade should be advised to have a light meal no later than 4 hours prior to the procedure and after that to have only sips of clear fluid.

All patients treated for emergencies are, on principle, assumed to have a full stomach, but if regional block can be used, there is no reason to subject them to the ordeal of manipulations with the stomach tube. Some of the patients who come to the Emergency Room will be under the influence of alcohol, which, in itself, is no contraindication to regional block. The decision for regional block is solely a matter of the patient's desire and ability to cooperate.

Ideally, all patients should have vital signs measured and recorded from the moment the block is started, but since local analgesics will normally not interfere with the physical or mental condition of the patient, it is necessary only to observe the following basic requirements: a patient must never be left alone; regular verbal contact with the patient must be maintained to ensure that he is conscious and comfortable; and pulse and blood pressure should be measured before starting and then as clinically indicated.

When the operation is completed, the block will still be effective, and, consequently, part of the patient's body will be anesthetic and so deprived of its normal protection against trauma. However, if the patient is properly instructed, he can be sent home during this period. The risk of a delayed toxic reaction after 30 minutes decreases rapidly and is very remote after 1 hour.

When the effect of the regional block wears off, the patient may need analgesics, which should be prescribed as part of instructions to the patient. It is well worth stressing that a very effective analgesic for operations on the extremities is provided by elevation and immobilization. If narcotics are demanded urgently by a patient in the immediate postoperative period, the possibility of a complication should be considered before they are administered because minor surgical operations will not normally be followed by severe pain. The masking of signs of surgical complications because of continuing nerve blockade is important, particularly in the patient who is not under direct medical supervision. Thus, the long-acting local anesthetic agents are usually best avoided for outpatients.

In institutions where procedures are performed on day patients under neural blockade, consideration should be given to providing the patients with a form that warns of possible sequelae, such as injury to a limb with residual analgesia, pneumothorax, hazards of driving; and other potential problems. It is also often useful to have a brief instruction sheet, which is given to patients at the time of booking for the operation. This may include advice about food or drink before the procedure, the need to be accompanied by someone, and other relevant information.

REFERENCES

1. Berry, F.R.: Analgesia in patients with fractured shaft of femur. Anaesthesia, *32*:576, 1977.
2. Laurie, W.G.R.M.: Plantar warts. Br. Med. J., *3*:116, 1972.
3. McCutcheon, R.: Regional anesthesia for the foot. Can. Anaesth. Soc. J., *12*:465, 1965.
4. Miranda, D.R.: Identification of the brachial plexus perivascular space. Br. J. Anaesth., *49*:721, 1977.
5. Mojares, E.C.: Xylocaine jelly for skin abrasions. JACEP, *6*:429, 1977.
6. Schurman, D.J.: Ankle block anesthesia for foot surgery. Anesthesiology, *44*:348, 1976.

21 Neural Blockade for Pediatric Surgery

Ottheinz Schulte-Steinberg

Although neural blockade techniques, such as spinal anesthesia, have been used in children as long ago as 1909[24] the only techniques commonly employed have been local infiltration for minor lacerations and topical techniques.

As with adults, there has been a recent increase in interest in the use of more significant neural blockade techniques in children. To some extent, this has been due to data obtained in adults relating to the pharmacokinetics, physiologic effects, and toxicity of local anesthetics; the physiologic effects of the major neural blockade techniques; and clarification of the anatomy of some block techniques and development of a "spectrum" of local anesthetics, including new long acting agents (see Chaps. 3 and 4).

At the present time, very little of the above has been duplicated in children. However, as in adults, if these factors are not taken into account for neural blockade, the potential advantages will be outweighed by considerable hazards. In particular, it is useful to remember that local anesthetics are relatively toxic drugs with a margin, in adults, between toxic blood level and maximum blood concentration after safe clinical doses of only 2. At present, it is assumed that this relationship also holds true in children. Thus, those who contemplate the use of neural blockade in children should first be familiar with the pharmacology, physiology, and anatomy in the adult. Considerable clinical experience with block techniques in adults is a wise prerequisite to pediatric neural blockade. A plan of preoperative assessment, preparation of resuscitative equipment, preventive measures, and management of toxicity should be a well-established part of the armentarium of the pediatric regional anesthesiologist (see p. 113).

GENERAL CONSIDERATIONS

There are known *anatomical* differences from the adult in the dura, spinal cord, spinal fluid, and epidural fat of children.[14,22,23,57,60] *Pharmacokinetic* differences from the adult are a higher rate of uptake from the respiratory tract and reduced metabolism of some amide local anesthetics.[13,17] Some differences in *physiologic* response may account for unproven claims that hypotension is less likely with epidural or spinal anesthesia in children.[5,20,29,35,45,54] There may be many more differences between adult and pediatric neural blockade, and additional objective data are needed. However, some very important practical aspects of management of neural blockade in children are well known.

The smaller the child, the smaller the neural "target" and the closer are other structures, such as blood vessels, pleura, and dura; thus, the likelihood of complications is increased. Most children do not like injections and are fearful of the theater environment so generally they should be unconscious during surgical procedures. This has led many to conclude that neural blockade has no place in pediatric anesthesia. However, this conclusion ignores the fact that the neural block technique may be carried out after the child is asleep. This spares the child any emotional trauma and still enables several benefits to be obtained.

First, a continuum of analgesia from the intra- to postoperative period can develop; thus, the dosage of inhalation agent can be reduced. The child awakens rapidly at the end of surgery but is comfortable and tranquil in the recovery room.

Second, use of neural blockade permits the suppression of undesirable autonomic reflexes such as laryngospasm during circumcision and perianal procedures.

Third, neural blockade allows the provision of excellent muscle relaxation without the use of muscle relaxant drugs or, sometimes, with minimal supplementary doses.

Fourth, a limb can be immobolized after delicate surgery such as nerve or tendon repair.

Fifth, use of neural blockade enables the possible modification of the "stress response,"[42] more rapid recovery, and a shorter hospital stay, which have been reported in adults.[7]

Modern general anesthesia with muscle relaxant,

Table 21-1. Local Anesthetic Agents and Doses in Children

	Topical Use		*Injection*	
Agent	*Concentration (%)*	*Dose (mg/kg)**	*Plain solution dose (mg/kg)**	*Dose With Epinephrine (mg/kg)**
Lidocaine	2–10	3†	5	7
Mepivacaine		5	5	7
Prilocaine			5–7 (Dose not to exceed 600 mg; single dose only)	7–9
Chloroprocaine and procaine			7	10
Bupivacaine			2	2
Etidocaine			3	3–4
Dibucaine	0.2–0.5	1	2 (Subarachnoid use only)	2
Cocaine	3–10	2		
Amethocaine (Tetracaine)	0.5–2	1	1.5 (Subarachnoid use only)	1.5

* These doses are the same on a milligram per kilogram basis as in adults and are based on measurements of plasma levels after safe clinical use, compared to toxic plasma levels (see Table 3-4).
† This low dose is preferable below the age of 3 years since plasma levels following topical use at this age are relatively higher than for older children.[17]

nitrous oxide techniques can usually provide excellent conditions for surgery and rapid awakening. However, it cannot, by itself, achieve the enumerated results indicated above. In particular, after very painful procedures children must either be treated with narcotic agents or be restless and crying with pain. If supplementary neural block techniques are used, the child may awake rapidly and in no pain and be able to resume normal oral fluid intake (if desirable). Effective neural blockade often reduces bleeding during surgery and lowers the risk of further bleeding and dislodgement of dressings in the recovery room if the child is pain-free and tranquil.

The benefits achieved with neural blockade techniques in adults can and should be extended to children. However, these techniques should be employed only if they offer a clear advantage to the child in question. There is no validity to the argument that neural blockade techniques in infants obviate the need for pediatric anesthetic equipment. On the contrary no anesthesia, be it regional or general, should be attempted in infants and children without adequate equipment to induce and maintain general anesthesia. Such equipment is one of the vital ingredients of effective treatment of local anesthetic toxicity, extensive sympathetic blockade, and other sequelae of neural blockade. It is worth repeating that neural blockade in children can be used effectively and safely only by application of the physiologic, pharmacologic, and anatomical knowledge outlined in Part I of this book and in the appropriate sections that deal with the various neural blockade techniques.

Dosage of Local Anesthetics in Children

At present, recommendations for safe maximum dose are based on adult data and a dose per weight calculation. It should be noted that this calculation is derived by dividing maximum adult doses by a theoretical 70 kg "lean" weight and is purely empirical. At present, data available show no relationship between body weight and blood concentration (see Chap. 3). However, until alternative data are available in children, determining doses on the weight basis seems most practical (Table 21-1). As in adults, the volume and concentration required for the block should be determined, and then the total dose should be checked. If the dose is too high, but volume is required, then the concentration may have to be reduced. For example, the maximum safe epidural dose of lidocaine without epinephrine in a 12-kg patient is 60 mg or 3 ml of 2-per-cent solution. If 4 ml is found to be required, the 2-per-cent solution would not be acceptable (an overdose of 80 mg); instead, 4 ml of a 1.5-per-cent solution would be employed (60 mg). Although higher doses of lidocaine than those in Table 21-1 have been reported to have been safely used, no blood level data were reported.[35] Dosage for patients younger than 3 years of age needs particularly careful control for tracheal use, as described below.[17]

Blood Concentrations and Toxicity

Factors that affect blood concentrations in children are probably similar to those discussed in Chapter 3 for adults, that is, *site of administration, speed of injection, dosage, use of vasoconstrictor, local anesthetic employed, and physiologic and pathologic factors*. Recent data suggest that children differ from adults in several ways. First, uptake from the respiratory tract is more rapid than in adults, particularly at ages below 3 years.[17] Second, lidocaine is less bound to plasma proteins than in adults; thus more free drug is available for tissue uptake with possibly an increase in toxic potential.[60] Third, in the newborn, enzyme systems responsible for a metabolism of mepivacaine are deficient; however, presumably these increase shortly after birth (see Chap. 3).[13]

The manifestations of local anesthetic toxicity and their management are discussed in Chapters 2 to 4. The blood levels at which toxicity occurs are presumed to be the same in adults and children, although precise data are lacking. Recent studies of blood levels in children following caudal, subcutaneous, and tracheal administration showed blood levels that in general were similar to those in adults.[17] However, after tracheal lidocaine administration, levels were significantly higher in children below 3 years of age than for older children given similar milligram per weight dosage (Fig. 21-1).[17] Despite venous plasma levels of up to 8 μg per ml in these lightly anesthetized patients, no signs of toxicity were observed. Following single-shot caudal block, blood levels were surprisingly low (1–2 μg/ml of lidocaine). For the present, it must be assumed that toxic blood levels and toxicity ratios of adults, as presented in Table 3-4, also apply to children. Thus, plasma concentrations of 5 to 6 μg per ml lidocaine and 1 to 1.6 μg per ml bupivacaine probably coincide with the onset of toxic symptoms

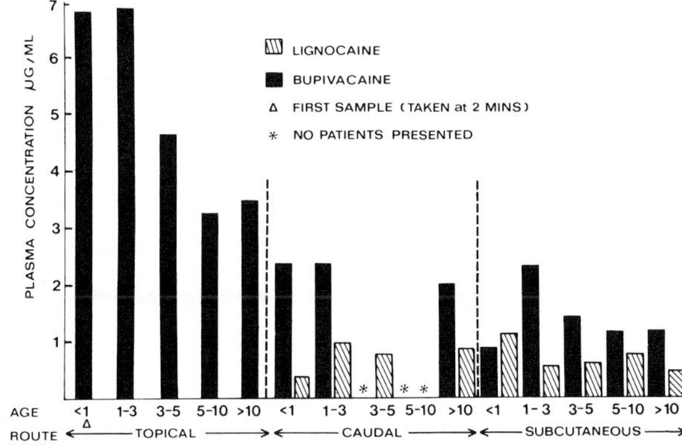

Fig. 21-1. Comparison of plasma concentrations for lidocaine (lignocaine), and bupivocaine administered topically, caudally, and subcutaneously to patients aged 1 to 10 years.

in unanesthetized patients,[61] whereas approximately double these concentrations are required for toxicity in anesthetized patients.[21]

The signs of toxicity in children are almost certainly the same as in adults (Fig. 4-14). Earliest signs in unanesthetized children are circumoral and tongue numbness and excitement and confusion leading to twitching and convulsions. Lidocaine may sometimes cause initial sedation at low blood concentrations. At very high blood concentrations, respiratory depression accompanies convulsions, and hypoxia combines with the local anesthetic to cause vasomotor depression.

The differential diagnosis of local anesthetic reaction is the same as in adults: direct intravascular injection; relative overdose or rapid absorption; reaction to vasoconstrictor; vasovagal reaction; and extensive sympathetic blockade due to the neural blockade technique per se (see Chap. 4).

Preparation for, prevention of, and management of toxicity are described in Chapter 4. Medical and nursing staff who care for children managed with neural blockade should be familiar with a simple procedure. The wisdom of having a secure intravenous route prior to neural blockade becomes even more evident in small children since access to veins during a convulsion would be compromised by the technical difficulties of small veins. Diazepam has been shown to raise the threshold for toxicity, and avoidance of acidosis reduces the rate of central nervous system (CNS) uptake of local anesthetic (see Chap. 2). General anesthesia markedly suppresses CNS toxicity from local anesthetics, as shown by Yoshikawa; five anesthetized patients developed muscle rigidity without convulsions fol-

Table 21-2. Premedication Guide for Infants and Children*

Age	Weight (kg)	Fentanyl plus Dehydrobenzperidol (combined in ml)	Fentanyl (mg)	Dehydrobenzperidol (mg)	Atropine (mg)
4 months	3–6				0.1
4–7 months	6–7				0.2
7–11 months	7–8	0.1	0.0025	0.125	0.2
11–18 months	8–9	0.2	0.0050	0.25	0.3
11–18 months	9–10	0.3	0.0075	0.375	0.3
18–24 months	11–13.5	0.4	0.01	0.5	0.3
3–5 years	13.5–15.5	0.5	0.0125	0.625	0.4
3–5 years	16–17.5	0.6	0.015	0.75	0.4
5–8 years	18–19.5	0.7	0.0175	0.875	0.6
5–8 years	20–25	0.8	0.02	1.0	0.6
10–12 years	25–35	1.0	0.025	1.25	0.6

* Alternatively, meperidine (1 mg/kg) and hyoscine (0.01 mg/kg) may be given.

lowing intercostal blocks with bupivacaine, which resulted in blood levels of 9 to 12 μg per ml.[64]

Considerable variation in toxic threshold should be expected among children. In addition, it has been shown in mice that toxic threshold varies widely with variation rhythm so that a toxic response may occur even though no such response was previously seen at a different time of day with the identical technique.[32]

Neural Blockade Without General Anesthesia

Some children, usually older than 7 years, may accept neural blockade alone if the technique is carefully explained and a tranquil environment is ensured in the anesthetic room and theater. This usually implies an operating team accustomed to working with an awake patient having a regional anesthesia. Neural blockade without general anesthesia may be useful in the following: as local infiltration or minor peripheral nerve block techniques for suturing minor lacerations; as topical analgesia for removal of foreign bodies; and in emergency procedures in a child with a full stomach when compromised vascular supply or other considerations preclude waiting the time recommended to reduce the risk from general anesthesia of inhalation of gastric contents (*e.g.*, supracondylar forearm fracture).

In all of these situations, highly apprehensive children should be excluded. Even in a cooperative, calm child, continued reassurance during the block is needed, and it is sometimes useful to employ 50 per cent nitrous oxide (self-administered) during the block if the child can tolerate the face mask; a clear plastic mask reduces the child's anxiety and gives a clear view of the mouth while *in situ*. A skilled assistant sympathetic to children is essential.

Generalized systemic disease may be an indication for use of neural blockade alone if the child is amenable, the operation is suitable, and the surgeon is accustomed to operating under regional analgesia. The following systemic diseases are some examples of possible indications:

- Family history of malignant hyperpyrexia
- Severely compromised respiratory function due to any cause (*e.g.*, severe scoliosis, chronic bronchitis, etc.)
- Severe integumental disease, such as epidermolysis bullosa
- Severe cardiovascular disease that requires cardiac catheterization
- Very difficult airway problems, such as those that accompany congenital craniofacial abnormalities or are due to tracheal stenosis, for example
- Other severe systemic disease, such as brittle diabetes mellitus

Neural Blockade with General Anesthesia

In most instances, neural blockade will be combined with light general anesthesia. As noted above, the addition of an appropriate neural blockade technique to the anesthetic regimen may be highly beneficial for many pediatric patients. It is important to choose the simplest block technique to achieve the desired aim for the proposed operation and for postoperative analgesia. Thus, for example, femoral nerve block may be a better choice for surgery of the front of the thigh than spinal anesthesia. Penile block may sometimes be preferable to caudal blockade for circumcision. In any case, a neural block technique should be added to the anesthetic regimen only if it offers clear advantages to the patient.

The same preoperative assessment, premedication, preparation of resuscitation equipment, and preventive measures used for adults should be carried out for children (see p. 113). Since blocks will usually be performed under general anesthesia, adequate premedication may be Omnopon (0.4 mg/kg), Scopolamine (0.006 mg/kg), or alternative regimen (*e.g.*, Table 21-2).

Adequate monitoring prior to neural blockade should include a precordial stethoscope, blood pressure and pulse measurements, electrocardiogram, and skin temperature (as for any pediatric anesthetic). Intravenous therapy is recommended to correct the effects of preoperative starvation and dehydration, particularly if central neural blockade (caudal and epidural or spinal) is employed.[48] The intravenous line also provides rapid access to the vascular system should local anesthetic toxicity occur. All drugs and equipment for neural blockade should be prepared prior to induction of general anesthesia. Once general anesthesia is induced and the patient's condition is stable, neural blockade is performed. A skilled assistant is required to maintain the airway. It is possible for the anesthesiologist to continue monitoring during the block by use of a monaural precordial stethoscope. The decision to intubate should be based on the usual criteria, such as a full stomach or upper abdominal surgery. The addition of a neural blockade does not reduce the requirements for airway control in such situations.

Lumbar, caudal and epidural, and spinal blockades are particularly suitable for use after induction of general anesthesia since their success does not depend on obtaining paresthesias. The lateral position is most convenient for carrying out these blocks; however, the assistant should be careful not to flex the head forward because airway obstruction occurs very easily in small children.

Peripheral nerve block procedures can be performed by using arterial pulsation (*e.g.*, axillary or femoral nerve block) or by using a peripheral nerve stimulator (*e.g.*, sciatic block; see Fig. 21-11).

Basal anesthesia may be accomplished by intravenous or inhalational methods or by intramuscular injection of 4 mg per kg of ketamine. After the block is completed only light general anesthesia is required (*i.e.*, nitrous oxide, oxygen, small increments of halothane [with avoidance of acidosis], ketamine [0.5–0.75 mg/kg IV], diazepam, etc.). Because of the danger from a full stomach, the procedure for basal anesthesia may be modified for an infant with an incarcerated hernia that is to be reduced only and to be operated at a later time. Here, caudal block alone may supply sufficient analgesia and relaxation for reduction of the hernia. If this is impractical, then intubation is necessary to protect the airway during general anesthesia.

Smith warned in his textbook that regional anesthesia was ill-advised in sick children with high fever and rapid pulse.[56] However, experience shows that in well-prepared children in whom the fluid, electrolyte, and acid-base balance has been corrected prior to surgery, the indications for regional anesthesia do not differ from those for the adult.

Regional blocks may offer a simple way to avoid postoperative vomiting, dehydration, and hyperthermia, which is sometimes seen after inhalation anesthesia in children in hot climates or in places without air-conditioning during the summer. Fortuna stresses this point from his experience in Brazil; he reported only 2 cases of vomiting out of 170 patients.[20] Berkowitz and Green report similar results with regional anesthesia in children in hot climates.[5]

NEURAL BLOCKADE APPROACHES IN CHILDREN

Any of the techniques described in this book may be performed in children, and the reader is advised to consult the appropriate section and acquire familiarity with the technique in adults before proceeding to its use in pediatric patients.

The following neural blockade techniques will be considered with respect to particular aspects of their use in children: central neural blockade, including spinal subarachnoid block, lumbar epidural block, and caudal epidural block; block of the extremities, including brachial plexus blockade and peripheral nerve blocks of the upper extremity, lumbar plexus blockade and peripheral nerve blocks of the lower extremity, and intravenous regional anesthesia; paravertebral and intercostal block; penile block; block for bronchography; and minor infiltration and topical techniques.

CENTRAL NEURAL BLOCKADE

Anatomy

It is important to realize that both the spinal cord and the dural sac extend farther down in small chil-

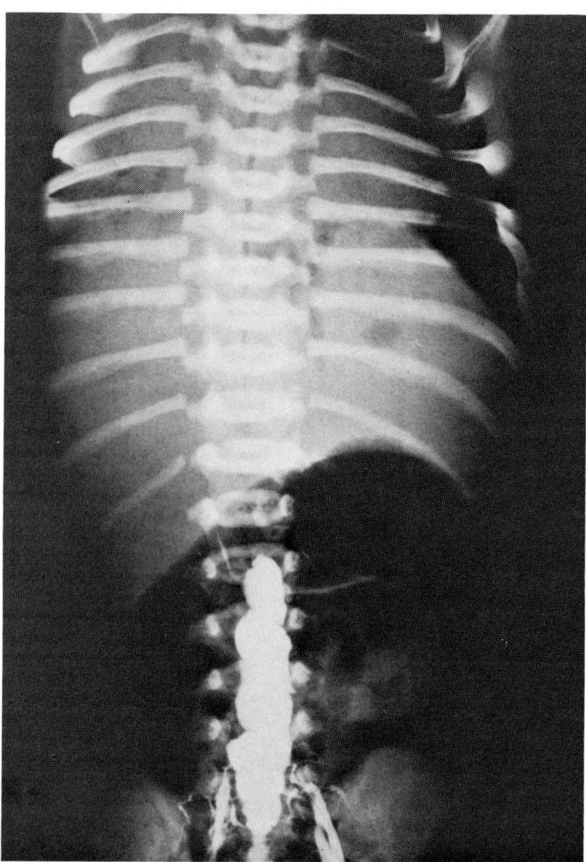

Fig. 21-2. This radiograph shows the spread of 2 ml radiopague material injected via the sacral hiatus of a stillborn baby. Note the spread to L1 and the escape from intervertebral foramina following the course of the nerves.

dren. According to Gray, the tip of the spinal cord at birth is at the level of L3.[23] At the age of 1 year, it has reached its permanent position at the L1 interspace. Ordinarily, the position of the lower end of the dural sac is independent of the tip of the spinal cord and it is found at the level of the S1–2 foramen. However, in one case the spinal cord reached down to the S1 foramen and the dural sac extended as far as the S4 foramen.[14] Spiegel even quotes the distance between the sacral hiatus and the dural sac in the newborn and infant as being as small as 1 cm.[57] This is said to be accentuated in Black children; however, precise documentation is lacking.

Infants and children who weigh less than 15 kg have a relatively higher total volume of spinal fluid (*i.e.*, 4 ml/kg, compared to 2 ml/kg for the adult). This is an important consideration in determining the volume of local anesthetic solution in infants and small children.[22]

There is yet another feature of the contents of the infantile neural canal that differs from that of the adult. The epidural fat of the newborn and the small child has a gelatinous, spongy appearance with distinct spaces between the individual fat lobules. This contrasts with the adult epidural fat where the lobules are more densely packed and interrupted by fibrous strands.[60] Thus, the juvenile epidural fat offers less of an obstacle to longitudinal spread of injected solutions.

Isakob and colleagues investigated the topographic anatomy of the thoracic epidural space and the features of distribution of injected colored solutions in corpses of children aged from 2 months to 15 years.[25] On opening the epidural space, they found that previously injected quantities of red dye had spread upward and downward within the epidural space. It also had emerged from the intervertebral foramina and colored the nerves and sympathetic ganglia. The epidural space of the children was easily identified, even in the thoracic section.

The patency of the sacral and intervertebral foramina is demonstrated in a radiograph of a baby who died 24 hours after birth. Two ml of Conray-60 injected through the sacral hiatus can be seen emerging from the spinal column and following the course of the nerves (Fig. 21-2).

For lumbar epidural block, Bromage has demon-

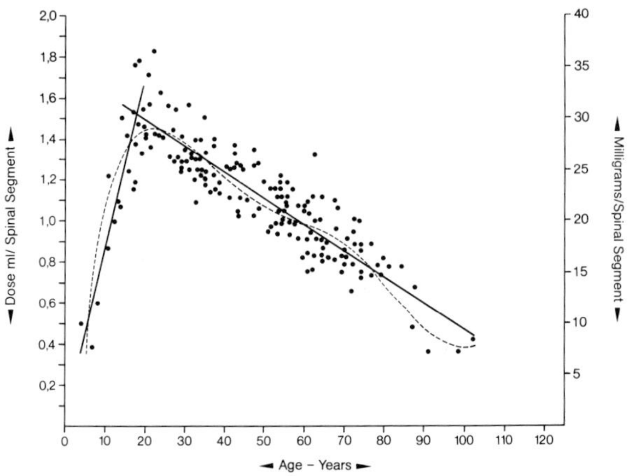

Fig. 21-3. Lumbar epidural block. Segmental dose requirements are related to age between 4 and 102 years. Computer-fitted linear (——) and curvilinear (---) lines have been drawn through the data points. Four children under the age of 12 years were included. Note the linear increase in dose requirements to age 20 and then linear decrease as age increases. (Bromage, P.R.: Ageing and epidural dose requirements: Segmental spread and predictability of epidural analgesia in youth and extreme age. Br. J. Anaesth., *41*:1016, 1969)

strated a relationship between dose requirements and age that is linear over a wide range of ages (Fig. 21-3).[6]

I have performed clinical studies of the distribution of local anesthetic solutions injected at the sacral hiatus in children.[50–52] The volumes of solution used and the number of dermatomes blocked at various ages were examined with multiple-regression techniques and the aid of a computer. It was found that in caudal anesthesia in children—contrary to the findings in adults (see Chap. 9)—there is a regular segmental spread related to age. This relationship holds reasonably well over the age range studied (2–140 months). However, it should be noted that there was as much as a twofold variation in dose to spinal segment requirement (Figs. 21-4–21-6).

In contrast, there is a poor correlation of dose and segmental spread in adults after caudal block (see Chap. 9). This may be due to transformation of the juvenile epidural fat into adult epidural fat tissue, which offers more resistance to longitudinal spread.

The cardiovascular effects of spinal and epidural block in children are reported to be less pronounced than in adults. This has been observed by a number of authors with extensive experience in these techniques.[5,20,29,35,38,39,44,45] Leigh and Belton refer to the pediatric patients' active sympathetic nervous system, which compensate rapidly for minor falls in blood pressure.[29] Ruston demonstrated in several patient records of infants the singular lack of the characteristic falls of blood pressure that are observed in adults following spinal or epidural blocks.[45] Melman and associates saw no instances

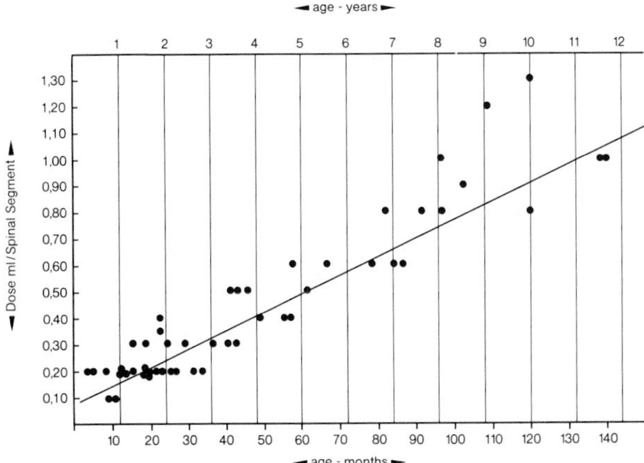

Fig. 21-5. Caudal epidural blockade in children. Segmental dose requirements of 1 per cent mepivacaine are related to age from birth to 11-½ years. Computer-fitted regression lines have been drawn through the data points. Note the high correlation between segmental spread and age; contrast this with the lack of correlation in adults (see Chap. 9).

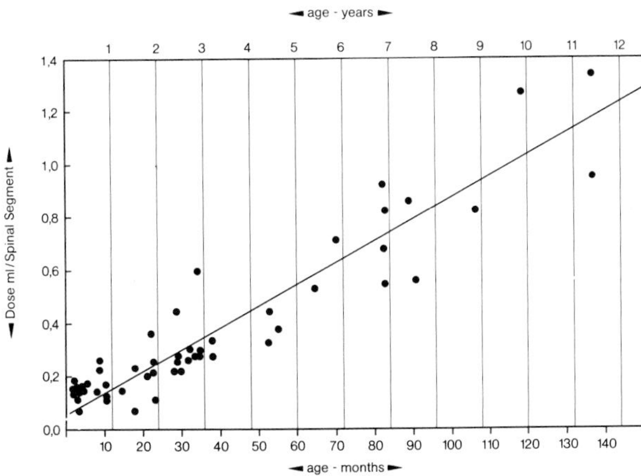

Fig. 21-4. Caudal epidural blockade in children. Segmental dose requirements of 1 per cent lidocaine are related to age from birth to 11-½ years. Computer-fitted regression lines have been drawn through the data points. Note the high correlation between segmental spread and age; contrast this with the lack of correlation in adults (see Chap. 9).

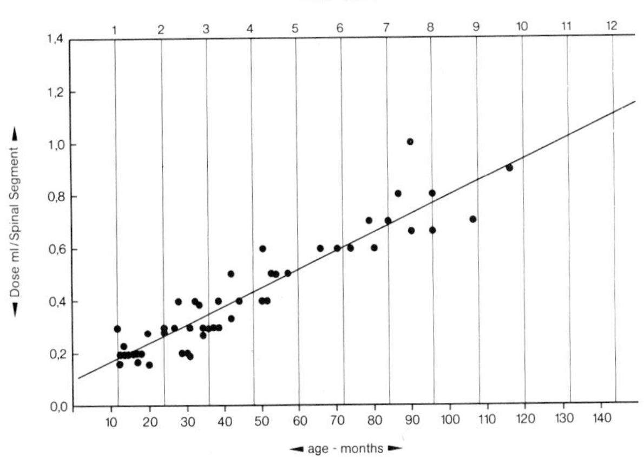

Fig. 21-6. Caudal epidural blockade in children. Segmental dose requirements of 0.25 per cent bupivacaine are related to age from birth to 11-½ years. Computer-fitted regression lines have been drawn through the data points. Note the high correlation between segmental spread and age; contrast this with the lack of correlation in adults (see Chap. 9).

of hypotension or alteration in either heart rate or respiratory rate in 200 cases of spinal, lumbar, and caudal epidural blocks.[35] Controlled data are not currently available.

The accentuated stress reaction of children is a common observation, although it is undocumented. Bromage found that stress reactions in adults during upper abdominal surgery could be modified by high epidural blocks.[7] Similar mechanisms may be expected in children. Clinical observations seem to support this opinion; however, further supporting investigations are necessary.

Advantages

Of the three major conduction blocks—spinal subarachnoid, lumbar epidural, and caudal—the first two have only very limited application because of modern inhalation-anesthesia techniques. Their use without general anesthesia is still indicated, particularly in very hot climate or high altitudes, which may interfere with the conduct of inhalation anesthesia. Some examples are surgical interventions in the presence of pulmonary complications and trauma of the lower extremities with simultaneous head injuries; the juvenile diabetic remains an excellent candidate for these techniques because there is less disturbance of the metabolism than with general anesthesia. Spinal subarachnoid block should be reserved for diabetics in whom profound relaxation is required. From the work of Parnes and Isakob, it appears that continuous epidural anesthesia can be useful for postoperative analgesia, which results in improved hemodynamics and respiration and has a favorable influence on the acid-base balance both in thoracic and upper abdominal procedures.[25,39]

Compared to the other two major conduction blocks, caudal anesthesia offers a number of distinct advantages. It is practically devoid of the hazard of dural puncture. Still, there is a highly predictable possibility of blocking higher dermatomes if so desired. Without the potential cardiopulmonary complications of general anesthesia, muscular relaxation can be obtained and the blood loss reduced.[36] The block is rapidly accomplished, usually in 1 minute. This is important if the operating schedule is busy. There is satisfactory pain relief in the immediate postoperative period, depending on the agent used and the duration of the operative procedure. The children are therefore quiet even after notoriously painful operations, such as circumcision and hypospadias.[27]

Caudal epidural anesthesia appears to be preferable to spinal and lumbar epidural block for all operations of the lower abdomen and lower extremities. Incarcerated hernias in infants can be reduced with ease or will reduce spontaneously, permitting an operation at a convenient time. It can also be used in outpatients.[10,27] If necessary, it can be performed without drapes with a no-touch technique (31).

Contraindications

Contraindications for all central neural blockade techniques are the following: spina bifida and other spinal defects, infected skin over the site of injection, bleeding disorders, uncorrected hypovolemia, and neurologic disease.

Spinal Subarachnoid Anesthesia

Spinal subarachnoid anesthesia in infants and children was developed by Gray as early as 1909.[24] There were a number of reports of its use in the 1930s and 1940s, particularly from Canada where it was even used for performing intrathoracic operations.[26,28,29,43,54] However, with the advent of better methods of general anesthesia, this blockade lost its advocates in the mid-1950s.*

The technique is easily and safely applied if the anatomic considerations noted above are heeded. Familiarity with lumbar puncture in children is an important prerequisite.

Choice of Agent. Both hypo- and hyperbaric solutions have been used, but the latter have enjoyed more popularity. The agents generally used are 5 per cent hyperbaric lidocaine and 1 per cent tetracaine with 10 per cent dextrose or 0.5 per cent dibucaine with 6 per cent glucose.

Five per cent hyperbaric lidocaine has been studied by Gouveia.[22] In this study, the duration of the blockade averaged 45 minutes with no further extension by the addition of vasoconstrictor agents. The dosage for children below 3 years of age and less than 15 kg body weight was found to be 2 mg per kg of lidocaine.

Older children required gradually decreasing doses down to the average adult dose of 1 mg per kg of body weight. The explanation for this discrepancy, according to Gouveia, rests with the fact that the relation between the amount of spinal fluid and body weight is 4 ml per kg in the younger age group, contrasted with 2 ml per kg in the adult.

One per cent tetracaine with 10 per cent dextrose will produce 45 to 90 minutes of anesthesia. Dosage

* Green, B.A.: Personal communication, 1975.

is calculated at 1 mg per year of age. With exceptionally small children it is better to gauge the dose of tetracaine by the calculation of 0.2 mg per kg body weight. The calculated dose of tetracaine is always matched by an equal amount of 0.2 ml of 10 per cent dextrose to ensure hyperbaricity. The increased dose requirements for children below 3 years of age follow the example set by lidocaine. At present, there are no such data available for tetracaine. Duration of blockade is extended 30 to 100 per cent if 1 per cent phenylephrine is added to the solution. Since it is difficult to measure small amounts of vasoconstrictor for younger children, Smith simplified the procedure by mixing 1 per cent phenylephrine in 10 per cent glucose prior to preparation of the anesthetic solution.[56] In adults, 2.5 to 5 mg of phenylephrine is used; a comparable amount for children may be obtained by mixing 4 mg of 1 per cent phenylephrine in 2 ml of 10 per cent glucose. A dosage schedule for lidocaine and tetracaine is outlined in Table 21-3. Cinchocaine, 0.5 per cent (dibucaine, Nupercaine), in glucose, 6 per cent, is a hyperbaric solution with a duration of action slightly longer than that of tetracaine.

Technique. Normal premedication is given. Since no paraesthesias are sought, the patient should receive basal anesthesia as described above. An intravenous infusion with Ringer's lactate is started. Spinal puncture is performed through the L3, L4, or L5 interspace with the patient lying on the side. For low analgesia, as required for operations confined to the area supplied by the lumbosacral nerves, the table is tilted steeply head up, basal anesthesia with ketamine is sometimes useful for this position since this agent has minimal cardiovascular depressant effect. After skin preparation, a wheal is raised, and local anesthetic is infiltrated subcutaneously through a 25-gauge hypodermic needle. Through a Sise introducer at the skin wheal, a 25-gauge short bevelled lumbar puncture needle 5 cm long is introduced. The small diameter obviates the complication of post-spinal-anesthetic headaches. With the "hanging drop" at the hub of the needle, the epidural space can be identified by the disappearance of the fluid. Subsequently, reappearance of the drop signals penetration of the dural sac. The correct position of the needle is reached once free flow of spinal fluid is seen to well from the hub. Injection is performed only if no muscle contraction has been observed, which would indicate direct contact of the needle with nerve structures. Otherwise, the needle is withdrawn 1 mm, still maintaining free flow of spinal fluid. The anesthetic solution should be administered at a rate not exceeding 1 cc per 5 seconds. Now the needle is removed swiftly, the patient turned on the back, and maintenance of supplementary anesthesia continued. The level of the cephalad spread of anesthesia can be gauged within the first few minutes by comparing the increase in skin temperature in the area to be blocked (due to almost immediate vasodilatation) and the unaltered segments above. This permits early recognition of an unsatisfactory cephalad spread. A well-controlled adjustment can be made by a 15° headward tilt of the table.

Table 21-3. *Recommended Dosages for Spinal Anesthesia in Children*

Agent	*Expected Duration of Anesthesia (min)*	*Dose*
Hyperbaric lidocaine, 5%	45	2 mg/kg (3 years of age), decreasing doses down to 1 mg/kg (3–10 years)
Tetracaine, 1%, plus 10% glucose	45–90	1 mg per year of age; below 3 years, 0.2 mg/kg
Dibucaine 0.5% in 6% glucose	100–160	0.2 mg/kg
Tetracaine, 1%, plus 10% glucose that contains 2 mg phenylephrine in 1 ml	100–200	0.2 mg/kg 1 mg per year of age; below 3 years, 0.2 mg/kg

(Data from Gouveia, M. A.: Raquinaestesia para pacientes pediatricos. Rev. Bras. Anest., *4*:503, 1970; and Berkowitz, S., and Green, B. A.: Spinal anesthesia in children: Report based on 350 patients under 13 years of age. Anesthesiology, *12*:376, 1951)

With excessive cephalad spread, timely anti-Trendelenburg positioning can be used long before somatic block has appeared. Of course, the fact that sympathetic blockade is always about 2 segments higher than the anticipated somatic block has to be taken into account. The final extent of block can be determined by noting pupil and blood pressure response to pinching with an Allis forceps.

The child is maintained on a mask or intubated and artifically ventilated with nitrous oxide and oxygen, depending on the site of the operation and the condition of the patient. Additional sedation, when required, may be provided by 0.5 per cent halothane and other inhalation agent or with small increments of 0.75 to 1.5 mg per kg ketamine or 0.3 mg per kg of diazepam.

Complications. In general, the complications of spinal subarachnoid block and their management are identical with those in adults. As has been mentioned, the cardiovascular system of children is surprisingly stable. This stability does not lessen the need to start an infusion with Ringer's lactate prior to the block to offset pooling. Hypovolemia is a contraindication to spinal anesthesia, as it is in the adult.

Particularly in very small children, it may be different to cannulate an upper limb vein securely; it is easier in the lower extremities. The onset of vasodilatation will facilitate the search for a vein after the block has been performed. Ephedrine, 1 mg per ml, or a solution of 5 per cent glucose in water with 5 to 10 mg of phenylephrine should be kept ready. Unexpected hypotension may be controlled by careful intravenous titration of either of these drugs; however, elevation of the legs and increased intravenous fluids usually suffice (see Chap. 7).

There is one complication during the subarachnoid block peculiar to infants and small children. Flexing the head on the chest may cause complete mechanical obstruction of the airway. This may occur even in the previously intubated child by kinking of the tube. Precordial (esophageal) stethoscopy with continuous monitoring of respiration and cardiac action will avert this type of complication.

Epidural Blockade

Epidural blockade in children was first reported in 1936 by Sievers and later by Schneider in 1951.[49,53] Ruston perfected the technique and introduced continuous methods.[45] Bromage evaluated dosage requirements for children in 1969.[6] However, epidural anesthesia in children did not receive general acceptance.

A new approach was described in 1971 by Russian authors: thoracic epidural anesthesia in children for postoperative analgesia after thoracic surgery.[25] They studied hemodynamic changes and effects on respiration in detail and obtained favorable results. An early publication on caudal epidural anesthesia in children appeared in 1933 by Campbell.[8] Spiegel reported on this technique in 1962.[57] Further reports appeared later by the same and other authors.[11,58] Analogously to Bromage's investigations in adults and children with lumbar epidural anesthesia, I studied segmental dose requirements for caudal anesthesia in children.[6,50–52]

The technical simplicity of caudal epidural blocks and the predictability of the spread of local anesthetic agents have recently made caudal epidural anesthesia more popular.[30] Lourey and McDonald recently reported 290 caudal blocks as a supplement to general anesthesia in children and observed excellent postoperative analgesia.[30]

In general, the caudal route to the epidural space is preferred in small children because of the increased difficulty in locating the narrow epidural space and the risk of spinal headache unless single-shot technique is employed with narrow-gauge needles. Total spinal analgesia is more likely to occur in children than in adults because of the small epidural space and the difficulty in determining that the dura has not been punctured.

Choice of Agent. Commonly employed drugs are 1- or 2-per-cent solutions of lidocaine or mepivacaine and 0.25 or 0.5 per cent bupivacaine. These solutions may be used with or without epinephrine, 1:200,000.

Dosage. Bromage applied computer techniques to find the best relationships between dose requirements and age for 2 per cent lidocaine in lumbar epidural blocks (see Fig. 21-3).[6] For children he found a linear increase of dose requirements from 4 to a maximum of 18-½ years—the general end point of growth. Although the number of children below 10 years of age in this study was small, they conformed well to this pattern. Later studies in a larger group of children with caudal epidural anesthesia confirmed Bromage's findings for equivalent solutions (Figs. 21-7 and 21-8).[50–52]

In the studies of caudal anesthesia, spread of analgesia was determined under basal narcosis with nitrous oxide and oxygen by means of the pinprick test. Segmental dose requirements of local anesthetic were examined by multiple-regression techniques with the aid of a computer for their correlation to the variables of age, weight, and height. There was strong correlation between dose and all three variables, but correlation was highest with age, with a correlation coefficient of 0.94. This applied to three local anesthetic agents examined (Fig. 21-7).[50–52]

Based on these two studies, the dose for lumbar or caudal epidural anesthesia in children can be calculated for 2 per cent lidocaine and mepivacaine and 0.5 per cent bupivacaine by the formula: 0.1 ml per 1 year of age per one spinal segment; for example, 0.3 ml per one segment for a child 3 years of age.

To avoid toxic levels, it is important to double-check dosage by calculating the volume on a milligram per kilogram of body weight basis as well. When maximum doses are reached, weaker solutions have to be used.

Follow-up doses in continuous techniques should be one-half of the initial dose, as in adults.

Isakob used volumes for thoracic epidural anesthesia in children similar to those obtained by the above formula for the lumbar approach.[25]

Lumbar and Thoracic Epidural Block

Technique. Normal premedication is given. Since no paresthesias are sought, the block is easily performed under anesthesia as described above. An intravenous infusion with balanced salt solution is started.

The patient is placed in lateral decubitus position with the lumbar spine extended. It is important to have an assistant secure the patient to avoid movement. After skin preparation, a wheal is raised over the site of the puncture at L3–4 or L4–5. The epidural puncture is performed in the same manner as in the adult. The epidural space may be identified with the hanging drop technique or with the loss of resistance test with normal saline or air. Care should be taken to inject as little saline as possible into the epidural space to avoid undue dilution of the calculated small quantities of local anesthetic. In thoracic epidural blocks, the preferred puncture sites are T5–7, as in the adult.

Single-shot techniques are best performed with a 22-gauge needle. Continuous techniques are performed with an 18-gauge Tuohy needle and polyvinyl or teflon catheters, the use of which has been described by Ruston for lumbar epidural blocks.[45–47] They are also used for prolonged thoracic epidural analgesia. In children, the catheter is advanced only approximately 3 cm beyond the point of the needle. Ruston described one case in which the catheter met a resistance on introduction and an epidural hematoma ensued.[45] After the anesthetic solution has been injected in single-shot procedures and once the catheter has been taped in continuous techniques, the patient is returned to his back. It is useful to immobilize small children, in particular, on a padded board and wrap them with flannel bandages. The child is maintained on a mask or intubated as described above, depending on the site of the operation and the condition of the patient.

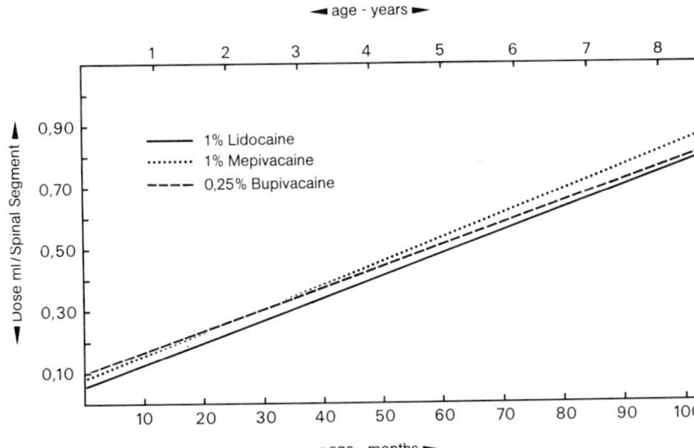

Fig. 21-7. Caudal epidural blockade in children. Segmental dose requirements of lidocaine, bupivacaine, and mepivacaine are related to age.

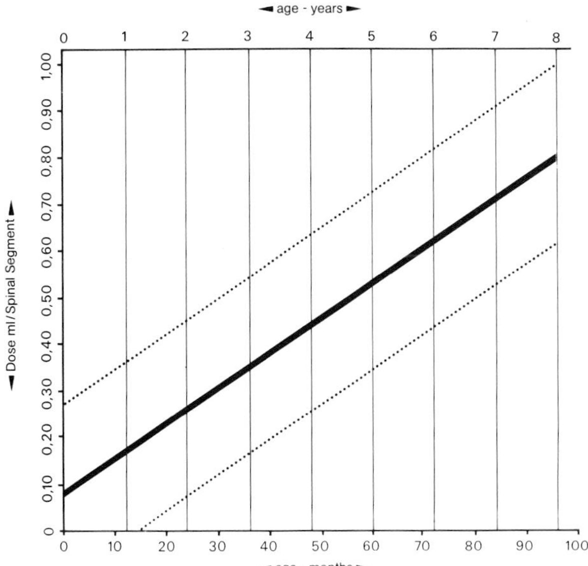

Fig. 21-8. Caudal epidural blockade in children. Segmental dose requirements are related to age for 1 per cent lidocaine, 1 per cent mepivacaine, and 0.25 per cent bupivacaine. Computer-fitted regression line with 95 per cent confidence limits.

Complications. The potential for unrecognized dural puncture is considerable in epidural block. The doses of local anesthetic employed for epidural block will rapidly produce total spinal analgesia if the dura is punctured, which requires rapid, effective treatment (see Chap. 7). Because failure to recognize this situation quickly may result in a catastrophe, epidural blockade in children should be employed only by those with considerable experi-

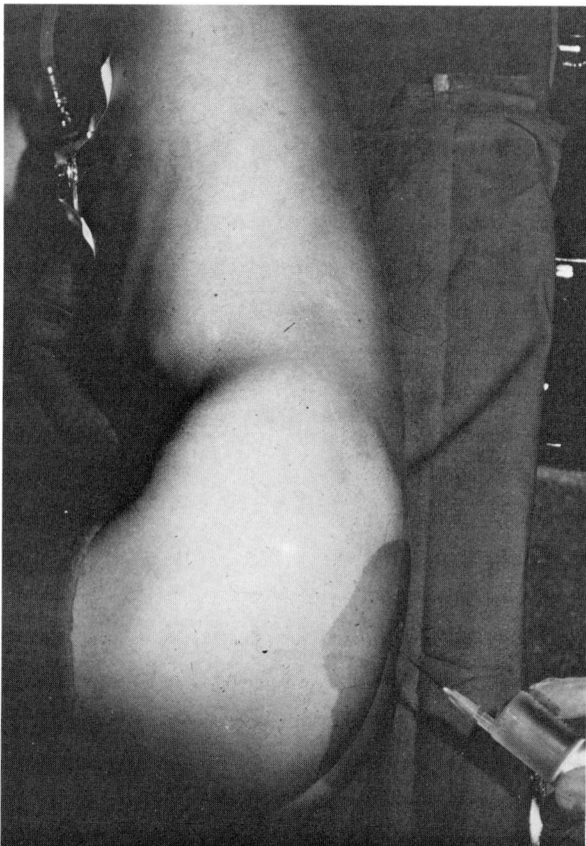

Fig. 21-9. Caudal epidural blockade in the child. This photograph shows technique for needle insertion with child in the lateral position using the "no-touch" approach; the drapes have been removed to aid orientation for the purposes of this illustration. Many prefer to steady the needle with a second hand, which is braced against the patients' buttock (see Chap. 9).

ence with the technique. There should be a clear advantage for the patient, and the anesthesiologist should consider whether alternative methods of providing neural blockade might be equally effective, and perhaps safer.

Caudal Epidural Blockade

In an increasing number of pediatric anesthesia units caudal epidural block is the neural technique most commonly employed as an adjunct to light general anesthesia. It has particular application for surgery below the umbilicus, especially for "sacral segment" procedures such as circumcision, hypospadeas repair, and perianal procedures. Many of these operations can be performed without endotracheal intubation, and caudal block greatly reduces the incidence of laryngeal spasm, which may otherwise occur under halothane anesthesia with a mask. Some pediatric anesthesiologists report that caudal block reduces bleeding, and it certainly prevents erection and provides excellent intra- and postoperative analgesia.* The analgesia often permits a tranquil postoperative period compared to the stormy scene that may follow general anesthesia alone.

Dosage. The linear increase in dose requirements related to age demonstrated by Bromage for lumbar epidural anesthesia was also found to be applicable for caudal blocks in children (Figs. 21-7 and 21-8).[6,50–52]

As noted above, the dosage for 1 per cent lidocaine, 1 per cent mepivacaine and 0.25 per cent bupivacaine is 0.1 ml per year per segment (±0.2 ml). For caudal block, in practice it is often easier to use 0.5 ml per kg of these solutions since autopsy studies with contrast media show that this volume, injected by way of the sacral hiatus, spreads consistently to L2–3 and sometimes to T10–11.† Higher levels of blockade may be obtained with 0.7 ml per kg; epinephrine, 1:200,000, is necessary with these higher doses. The total milligram per kilogram dosage should always be checked to ensure that it is below the recommended dose level.

Technique. The patient is placed in a lateral decubitus position as shown in Figure 21-9. After skin preparation, the sacral hiatus is palpated as a depression in the midline between the sacral cornu proximal to the sacrococcygeal joint.[59] A 21-gauge short-bevel needle is inserted slightly cephalad to this point in an upward direction at an angle of 65 to 70°, while the bevel is turned toward the feet. Figure 21-9 shows the direction of the needle with the drapes removed for better orientation. With a 21-gauge needle, a loss of resistance as the needle penetrates the sacrococcygeal membrane can be felt. Finer needles make this identification more difficult and also may puncture bone and lead to intraosseous injection.

If the needle strikes the posterior table of the bone, it is "walked" caudad until it pierces the sacrococcygeal ligament with a characteristic "give" and is arrested by the anterior table (Fig. 21-10). The caudal epidural space has now been entered.[59] Care is taken not to advance the needle up the sacral canal to avoid puncturing the dural sac, which may be very close to the hiatus in the infant. After aspiration to exclude bone marrow, dural puncture,

* Brown, T.C.K.: Personal communication.
† Brown, T.C.K.: Personal communication.

or venipuncture, a test dose of 1 ml of local anesthetic solution is injected; this should meet minimal resistance. The lack of resistance is another sign of correct positioning of the needle. Intravascular or subarachnoid injection may result in a rapid onset of hypotension. If the needle is posterior to the caudal canal, a subcutaneous swelling may be seen. The actual blocking procedure is accomplished in less than a minute. Even higher thoracic dermatomes may be anesthetized, depending on the dosage, since the condition of the infantile epidural fat permits longitudinal spread comparable to that with the lumbar epidural approach. Figures 21-7 and 21-8 show that spread of caudally injected solutions remains within the 95 per cent confidence limits up to the age of 12 years.

Complications. Dural puncture as a complication of caudal epidural block may occur owing to the dura's ending below S2. It is less likely to occur when the described technique is followed, and threading the needle into the caudal canal is carefully avoided. The sacral anomaly of failure of fusion of the lower sacral segments should be carefully sought prior to caudal block. This makes location of the caudal space more difficult but, more important, may lead to insertion of the needle at a higher than normal level with an increased chance of dural puncture.

If by chance spinal fluid is obtained on aspiration, the block should be abandoned. This will eliminate an accidental spinal anesthesia. In over 500 cases, no spinal fluid has been obtained on any occasion nor did any high spinal blockade occur using this technique. If the entire dose of local anesthetic for caudal block is injected into the subarachnoid space, a high spinal anesthetic may ensue with profound cardiorespiratory depression.

Intravascular Injection. Aspiration of blood is also an indication for abandonment of the procedure. However, I have observed two cases in which blood was neither found to appear from the detached needle nor could any be obtained on aspiration. Despite this, in both cases the children started to have convulsive movements, which disappeared in less than 30 seconds after controlled ventilation with oxygen by mask was started. It was believed that the convulsions were due to spillage of local anesthetic into a vessel that the needle passed through on its path to the anterior table of the sacrum. In this case, blood would not necessarily be obtained on aspiration. A needle's becoming plugged during introduction would also fail to show blood on the first aspiration. An effective epidural block ensued both times and appeared to exclude bone marrow

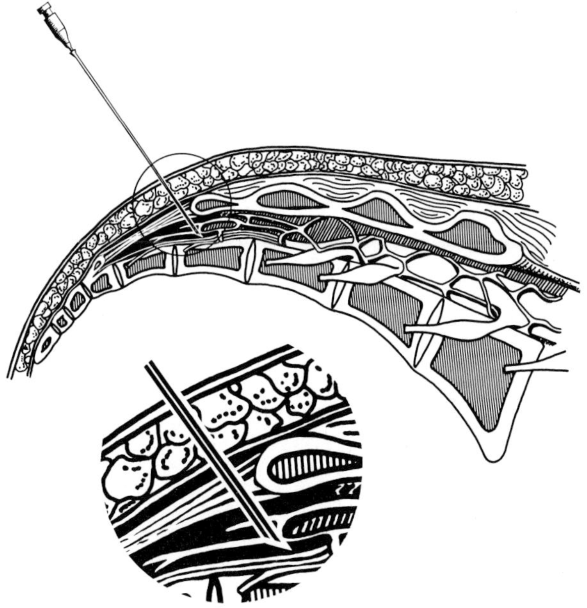

Fig. 21-10. Caudal epidural blockade in the child. Anatomical view of the needle path, which is directed at an angle of 65 to 70° and passes almost at a right angle through the sacrococcygeal ligament. The enlarged view (*inset*) shows the needle passing into the caudal epidural space, which offers no resistance to the advancing needle until it reaches the anterior table of the sacrum.

injections. Fortuna also saw this complication in 1.1 per cent of his cases.[20] Repeated aspirations during injection will help to avoid it, as will the use of short-bevel needles.

Intraosseous Injection is more likely with fine needles and may result in toxic blood levels.

Intrapelvic Injection may result from failure to recognize the shallowness of the sacral canal and insertion of the needle too deeply and into the pelvis. It is possible to aspirate fluid that, upon exposure to the nose, smells like feces; this indicates puncture of the rectum. Treatment is abandonment of caudal block, conservative measures with antibiotic therapy, and a low-residue diet.

Miscellaneous hazards include bleeding from punctured veins and hematoma formation, and rapid absorption of injected local anesthetic with subsequent onset of local anesthetic toxicity.

BLOCK OF EXTREMITIES

All peripheral nerve blocks used in adults can be performed in children as well. Children over 3 years

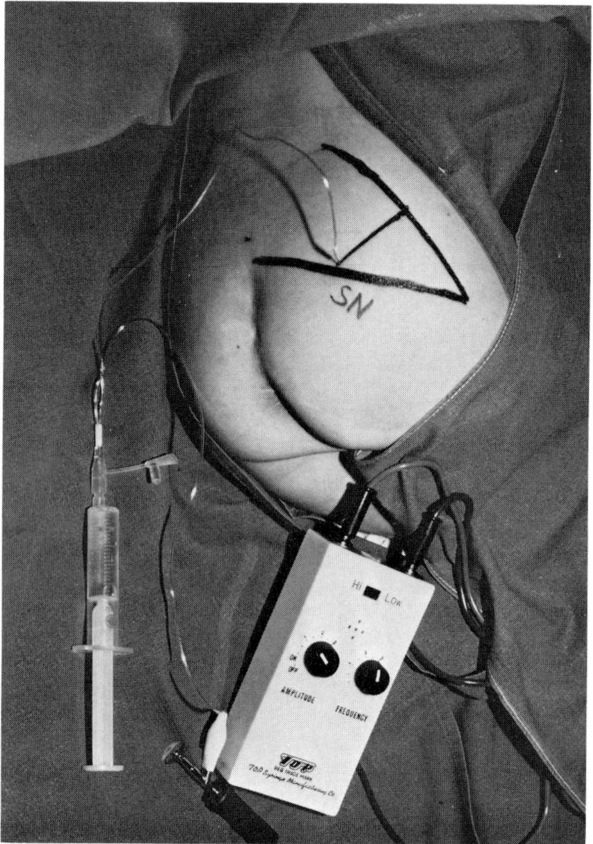

Fig. 21-11. Sciatic nerve block, using a peripheral nerve stimulator. The ground lead (right) is attached to the back of the thigh, while the stimulating lead (left) is attached to the fluid column of the injecting needle. Note the landmarks that best fit the location of the sciatic nerve, as identified with the stimulator. The upper line is drawn from the superior border of the greater trochanter to the posterior superior iliac spine. A second line is drawn from the greater trochanter to the uppermost end of the intergluteal fold where the sacral hiatus is usually palpable. A perpendicular line is drawn from the midpoint of the first line to cross the second line at the point of injection. The child is positioned as in the adult with the uppermost hip joint in 40° of flexion by ensuring that the lower leg is straight and the heel of the upper leg rests on the opposite knee.

of age are often surprisingly cooperative and will monitor paresthesias quite well. Contraction of the appropriate muscles will assist in recognizing a paresthesia. A warm sympathetic approach to a child is a prerequisite for gaining the child's cooperation.

But even when adequate cooperation cannot be obtained, peripheral nerve blocks are possible, including blocks of multiple nerves at different sites, following induction of light basal anesthesia with nitrous oxide and oxygen, ketamine, or barbiturates. Aizenberg described a very useful and dependable method of locating peripheral nerves in children—not requiring their cooperation.[2,3] He used an electric nerve stimulator to send intermittent currents of 0.3 to 1 ma down a sheathed injection needle with an uncovered metal tip (Fig. 21-11).

Once the probing needle is in direct contact with the nerve and electrical impulses are transmitted, contractions of corresponding muscle groups will occur. This indicates correct position of the needle and assures proper timing for the injection of the local anesthetic agent. This technique has been found very useful. Alternatively, perivascular techniques may be employed, as noted below.

Basal anesthesia may or may not be continued throughout the operative procedure. Postoperative supervision for the regional block itself does not need to be longer than 60 minutes past the application time. When there is no postoperative pain, the need for analgesics is drastically reduced, and early feeding is not threatened by the possibility of nausea and vomiting.

Upper Extremity

Brachial Plexus Blockade

Historical Review. Brachial plexus block in children was first described by Farr in 1920.[18] Since 1941, more reports have appeared.[31,33,41,55]

In 1948, DePablo mentioned as many as 3000 blocks, which, however, were not limited to children.[12] There were two fatal cases in this group. Only one of these could be explained—by an accidental intravascular injection. The axillary approach in children was described by Accardo and Adriani in 1949.[1] Previously, the supraclavicular method was generally employed. During the last 15 years, the axillary approach gained more favor in many institutions. Winnie introduced the interscalene brachial plexus technique.[62] Aizenberg was the first to use electrical stimulation to locate peripheral nerves for blocking in children.[2,3]

General Considerations. In children the axillary approach to the brachial plexus is preferable because of its safety and ease of performance. Technical details are the same as for the adult (see Chap. 10). Although the supraclavicular, subclavian perivascular, and interscalene techniques are equally applicable in children, they are probably most effective when axillary blockade is not possible because the arm cannot be abducted.

Axillary Brachial Plexus Block. *Choice of Agent.* The local anesthetics used are 1 per cent lidocaine, 1 per cent mepivacaine, 1 per cent prilocaine, 0.25 per cent bupivacaine with and without epinephrine, and other equipotent agents. Table 21-4 shows the volumes for axillary brachial plexus block with 1 per cent prilocaine and may be used as a guide for equipotent anesthetic solutions.[16]*

Technique. The arm is abducted and externally rotated, and the second and third fingers of one hand palpate and then compress the axillary artery against the humerus. The artery is easily palpated in children at the same level as in adults (*i.e.*, at the junction of pectoralis major and coracobrachialis). It should be remembered that the axillary vein overlies the axillary artery, and the vein should be compressed out of the way of the advancing needle. The fingers of the palpating hand should be kept firmly in position while the other hand grasps a short-bevel 23-gauge needle attached to the extension tubing of a syringe, which an assistant holds. The hand holding the needle should be braced against the patient for stability. The needle is advanced until paresthesias are obtained or arterial pulsation of the needle is seen. The plexus lies at an even more superficial level in children than in adults, and inappropriately deep injection is the commonest reason for failed block.

Eriksson has described some special considerations in axillary brachial plexus block in children.[16] He believes that it is better not to seek pulsation of the needle but to obtain paresthesias or muscle contraction in response to a nerve stimulator—the superficial location of the plexus makes paresthesias easy to obtain. Niesel, using a nerve stimulator, found a 60 per cent success rate when he sought paresthesias in children.[37] Either these were reported by the child or, when basal anesthesia was given, they were diagnosed by the observation of muscular contractions. When contractions or paresthesias occur, the needle is arrested and the entire calculated dose injected. Where no paresthesias can be provoked, the needle is advanced farther toward the artery, and pulsations are sought. The syringe is emptied at this site because it can be assumed that it now lies close to the artery and within the fascial space. Continued compression of this structure with a finger will keep the solution from running into the periphery along the nerves. Use of rubber tourniquet frequently leads to false positive signs of paresthesia.

* Niesel, H.C.: Personal communication, 1975.

Table 21-4. Axillary Brachial Plexus Block Volumes Equipotent to One Per Cent Prilocaine*

Age (years)	*Volume† (ml)*
1–3	6–9
4–6	9–11
7–9	14–20
10–12	21–25
13–15	28–35

* Alternatively, a volume of 0.6 to 0.7 ml per kg may be used as a guide.

† To avoid toxic levels, it is important also to calculate the dosage on a mg per kg basis and to reduce the volume accordingly. (Data from Eriksson, E.: Axillary brachial plexus anesthesia in children with Citanest. Acta Anaesthesiol. Scand., *16*:291, 1965; and Niesel, H.C., Rodrigues, P., and Wilsmann, I.: Regional Anaesthesie der oberen Extremitat bei Kindern. Anaesthetist, *23*:178, 1974)

As in adults, continued compression of the axillary artery and adduction of the arm aid spread of solution upward with an increased probability of blocking the musculocutaneous nerve, which has a high origin. A small skin wheal should be raised as the needle is withdrawn to block the intercostobrachial nerve if a tourniquet is to be used.

Interscalene Brachial Plexus Block. *Choice of Agent.* Local anesthetics used for interscalene brachial plexus block are lidocaine, mepivacaine, and bupivacaine with and without epinephrine. The concentrations and volumes may be taken from Table 21-5. As in other pediatric blocks, dosage in mg per kg should always be checked as a final safety measure.

Technique. Since paresthesias are required for this technique, no or light premedication is given when patient cooperation can be expected. When identification with a nerve stimulator is planned, heavy premedication may be administered. The landmarks and the actual blocking procedure are the same as for the adult and have been described in Chapter 10. When basal anesthesia is planned in a child, it is useful to identify the landmarks prior to induction. The fingers of one hand are inserted behind the sternomastoid at the level of the cricoid cartilage and rolled posteriorly until they sink into the groove between the anterior and posterior scalene muscles. At this point, the transverse process of C6 should be readily palpable only a few milli-

Table 21-5. Guide to Determination of Volume for Perivascular Anesthesia

	Male		*Female*			*Concentration*	
Age (years)	*Height (cm)*	*Volume (ml)*	*Height (cm)*	*Volume (ml)*	*Formula to Determine Volume (ml)*	*Lidocaine, Mepivacaine*	*Bupivacaine*
Birth	53	4	50	4			
1	76	6	76	6			
2	91	7	91	7	$\frac{\text{Height}}{12.5}$	0.7–0.8	0.1875
3	101	8	101	8			
4	109	9	109	9			
5	116	12	114	11			
6	124	12.5	121	12	$\frac{\text{Height}}{10.3}$	0.8–0.9	0.25
7	132	14	129	12.5			
8	137	14	134	13			
9	142	18.5	139	18			
10	147	19	146	19			
11	152	20	152	20			
12	157	21	160	21	$\frac{\text{Height}}{7.7}$	0.9–1	0.25
13	165	22	165	22			
14	172	23	167	22			
15	177	23	167	22			
16	180	25	167	22.5			

(Data from Winnie, A.P.: Interscalene brachial plexus block. Anesth. Analg. (Cleve.), *49*:455, 1970)

meters under the skin, in close proximity to the brachial plexus. The second hand inserts a 23-gauge short-bevel needle, as for axillary block, connected to extension tubing and remote syringe. It is very important to realize that the chance of entering the dural cuff or vertebral artery is much greater than in the adult because in the child the distances are short. Thus, the lateral aspect of the C6 transverse process should always be located with the palpating finger, and the needle should not be inserted to any great depth beyond this landmark. Paresthesias or muscle contraction in response to nerve stimulation should be obtained at a very superficial depth.

Complications. As in adults, injection into the vertebral artery may result in an immediate convulsion. Dural cuff injection results in total spinal anesthesia. Other complications such as phrenic nerve palsy are described in Chapter 10. Children who are to remain unsedated may become quite apprehensive as a result of unilateral phrenic nerve palsy or spread of solution to involve the recurrent laryngeal nerve. For these reasons, this technique is less appealing than axillary block unless analgesia and relaxation of shoulder muscles are required and light supplementary general anesthesia is to be used.

Supraclavicular Brachial Plexus Block, Short-Needle Technique. Because of the potential complication of pneumothorax, the supraclavicular technique is less commonly used than the axillary in children.

Choice of Agent. The local anesthetics used are 1 per cent lidocaine, 1 per cent mepivacaine, and 0.25 per cent bupivacaine, both with and without epinephrine. The volume of solution is calculated on the basis of 3 to 5 mg per kg for lidocaine and mepivacaine and 1.5 mg per kg for bupivacaine.

Technique. Since paresthesias are required for this technique, no or light premedication is given when patient cooperation can be expected. When identification with a nerve stimulator is planned, heavy premedication may be administered.

The landmarks and the actual blocking procedure are the same as for the adult and have been described in Chapter 10. When basal anesthesia is planned in a child, it is useful to identify the landmarks prior to induction. However, identification of landmarks is also possible when the patient is asleep and no cooperation is forthcoming.

For the supraclavicular approach to the brachial plexus, there are two main methods: the Kuhlenkampf method, in which the first rib is sought as a landmark and paresthesias are elicited, and the short-needle technique as described by Fortin.[19] The former is still popular but fraught with more complications. The short-needle technique avoids contacting the rib and thereby is not as prone to cause a pneumothorax as a primary complication. Therefore, and because it is particularly suitable for children, the short-needle technique is described in more detail here.

The success of the short-needle method depends on bringing the brachial plexus as close to the skin surface as possible. This is accomplished by placing the child on the table in supine position with a towel rolled lengthwise between the shoulders and along the upper thoracic spine. The shoulders are molded around the towel and backward until they touch the table. The head of the patient rests back on the table and is turned in the direction opposite to the side to be blocked. By these maneuvers, the first rib is elevated, carrying the brachial plexus and the subclavian artery close to the skin surface at the site of injection. As with other supraclavicular blocking techniques, the point of injection is 1 cm above the midpoint of the clavicle, just lateral to the subclavian artery. In the child, the pulsation of the artery can be palpated more easily than in the adult. Orientation in the child is further facilitated by a palpable first rib.

The anesthesiologist stands at the head of the table behind the shoulder to be blocked. The relatively thin layer of soft tissue separating the nerve structures from the surface of the skin permits almost exclusive use of 26-gauge needles not longer than 13 mm. Certainly, there is no need to use needles longer than 2.5 cm. The search for paresthesias by "walking" the small-gauge short needle in anterior-posterior direction can obviously proceed with little fear of piercing the pleura. Striking the first rib only indicates too deep a penetration past the intended nerve structures. The rib in this technique is considered only as a protective shield and not as a landmark for the block.

If the block is performed after induction of anesthesia, observation of the hand and forearm will reveal muscle twitching when parts of the plexus are touched by the needle. Often, the nurse holding the arm will first report these twitches. On the first paresthesia, the entire calculated amount of local anesthetic is injected without reorienting the needle since it has entered the subclavian perivascular space and the solution will inundate the entire nerve bundle.

When a nerve stimulator is to be used on a child under basal anesthesia, the procedure is duplicated. Again, the entire solution is injected when contractions of corresponding muscle groups are observed with the electrical stimulator.

Complications are identical with those that occur in the adult and require the same treatment. Phrenic nerve palsy may occur as in interscalene blockade with similar results. Pneumothorax should be avoided by ensuring that the needle is always lateral to the subclavian artery and by using the short-needle technique.

Subclavian Perivascular Technique

Subclavian perivascular technique is very similar to the short-needle approach and is described in detail in Chapter 10. The interscalene groove is identified and a finger run down the groove until it makes contact with the subclavian artery. A short needle is then inserted lateral to the artery so that its direction is in line with a line passing up immediately in front of the ear on the same side of the block. The needle should strike the middle trunk of the brachial plexus immediately lateral to the subclavian artery at a very superficial depth (see Chap. 10).

Peripheral Blocks

As in adults, there is little to be gained by blocking at the elbow, and the radial, ulnar, and median nerves can easily be blocked at the wrist with very small doses of 0.5 to 1 ml of local anesthetic, equivalent to 1 per cent lidocaine. In view of the minimal dosage, it is safe to employ fine-gauge (25 or 26) needles. Details are provided in Chapter 10.

Lower Extremity

Inguinal Paravascular

Inguinal paravascular block (three-in-one block) is block of the femoral nerve, obturator nerve, and lateral femoral cutaneous nerve.

The choice of agent, dosage, and volume employed are the same as described above for axillary brachial plexus block. A 22-gauge, short-bevel needle is inserted immediately lateral to the femoral artery, and the artery is compressed as local anesthetic is injected, employing the remote syringe as for brachial plexus block (see Chap. 10).[63] Blockade of L1–5 segments, but not sacral segments, follows.

Femoral Nerve Block

A simpler technique is to proceed as above but limit the volume injected and fan laterally beside the femoral artery. In a child, the femoral nerve is only 1–2 cms below the skin surface, and when the needle is in correct position it should pulsate from side to side as viewed from the foot of the bed. If it is inserted too deeply, pulsation will cease; whereas if it is on top of the artery, it will pulsate in and out.

Femoral nerve block is highly useful for pain relief in a child with a fractured femur since it will relieve muscle spasm and provide immediate analgesia. Because it is relatively safe, it may be employed as soon as the child is admitted to hospital (see also Chap. 11).

Paravertebral Lumbar Plexus Block

Paravertebral lumbar plexus block is a less attractive method of blocking lumbar segments in children but may sometimes be useful if a single-shot somatic block is required without sympathetic blockade (see Chapter 11).

Sciatic Nerve Block

Agents, dosages, and volumes for sciatic nerve block are similar to those used for interscalene brachial plexus block (see also Chap. 11).

Technique. Heavy premedication is given since this block is best performed under basal anesthesia. The patient is positioned along the lines described for the adult, that is, on the side opposite the one to be blocked with the uppermost hip joint in 40° of flexion. Aizenberg found with the aid of the nerve stimulator that, unlike those of the adult, the points of projection in the child are better described, as follows:[2] a line is drawn on the skin from the superior border of the greater trochanter to the posterior superior iliac spine. From the midpoint of this line, a perpendicular line is drawn in a downward direction. Where this line crosses another line drawn from the greater trochanter to the uppermost end of the intergluteal fold, the point of injection in the child can be found (see Fig. 21-11). Here, the sciatic nerve lies at a distance of 1.9 to 7.5 cm from the skin, depending on the age of the patient.[11] The injection of the local anesthetic agent is made at the moment when contractions of the muscles of the lower leg and foot are observed on electrical stimulation. The length of the sheathed needle should be 10 cm. The anterior approach, as described by Englesson, is also possible.[15]

Complications of the sciatic nerve block and their management are the same as in the adult.

Intravenous Regional Anesthesia

Smith mentioned intravenous regional anesthesia in pediatric patients in his book *Anesthesia for Infants and Children* in 1968.[56] Little has been published on this method in children, which suggests that it has not gained wide popularity.

Choice of Agent. The local anesthetic agents used are 0.5 per cent lidocaine and 0.5 per cent prilocaine without epinephrine. The dosage is calculated at 3 mg per kg for the upper extremity and 5 mg per kg for the lower. Prilocaine is safer than lidocaine because it is more rapidly metabolized.

Technique. The technique is similar to the one for adults (see Chap. 12). Since patient cooperation is not required, heavy sedation may be given prior to the procedure. Basal anesthesia may be used as well. The youngest children on record treated with this method were 3 years of age.

Tourniquet pressures used by Carrell and Eyring were 180 to 240 torr for the upper extremity and 350 to 500 torr for the lower. It is preferable to use small plastic cannulas to secure a safe intravenous access. The period of ischemia between inflation of the tourniquet and injection does not seem to influence the quality of anesthesia. After injection, the tourniquet should be kept inflated for 5 to 7 minutes. Then a second tourniquet is applied and inflated distal to the first, which is removed. Where an extremity is too painful for application of an Esmarch bandage for exsanguination, the procedure may be modified as in the adult. The limb is elevated merely for 3 minutes, and the arterial blood supply is occluded by digital compression prior to inflation of the tourniquet. Carrell and Eyring believe that manipulation of fractures under tourniquet ischemia may reduce bleeding during the procedure.[9] There is no evidence that intravenous injection of local anesthetics increases swelling at the fracture site.

PARAVERTEBRAL AND INTERCOSTAL BLOCK

Paravertebral blocks are rarely employed in children since their primary use in adults is in the diagnosis of pain syndromes, which are rare in children. Lumbar and thoracic paravertebral somatic and sympathetic blockade are described in Chapters 13 and 14.

Intercostal nerve blocks are very useful in providing somatic block of thorax and abdomen without accompanying sympathetic block. In addition, the use of long-acting agents such as bupivacaine permits analgesia that lasts in excess of 12 to 24 hours. This can be very useful in the management of chest trauma or following thoracic surgery. In the latter, the surgeon can inject the intercostal nerves under direct vision at the end of the operation; however, it is possible that local anesthetic remains in contact with intercostal nerve longer if the percutaneous technique is employed (see Chap. 14). It should be stressed that the rib must be carefully palpated and the needle inserted only 1 to 2 mm under the rib since the pleura is a very short distance from the skin in small children. The needle should not be inserted medial to the angle of the rib in children unless a chest drain is *in situ* (*e.g.*, after thoracic surgery) because there is no internal intercostal muscle at this part of the rib. Recent studies indicate excellent respiratory function restoration using intercostal block following thoracic surgery with minimal narcotic requirements.

PENILE BLOCK

Penile block is a useful alternative to caudal block for penile surgery, such as circumcision. It has the advantage that it can be performed after the patient is anesthetized but still in the supine position.

Agents and Dosages. Bupivacaine without epinephrine, 0.5 per cent, 1 to 4 ml, is employed, with adjustments made for age—1 ml in infancy and 4 ml at 12 years.[4] Epinephrine-containing solutions should not be employed because of the risk of ischemia of the penis.

Technique. The dorsal nerves of the penis enter from under the symphysis pubis and run below the deep fascia (Buck's) of the penis but superficial to the corpora cavernosa. The nerves then divide and supply branches to the entire circumference of the penis. The second and third fingers of one hand palpate the lower border of the symphysis pubis. A 25-gauge needle is then inserted at a right angle to the skin between these two fingers until bone is contacted. The needle is then directed to pass just inferior to the lower border of the symphysis but not deep to it; an aspiration test is then performed and local anesthetic injected.

Complications include direct intravascular injection with consequent local anesthetic toxicity or puncture of a blood vessel, causing a large hemotoma.

BRONCHOGRAPHY

Local anesthetic techniques may be employed in children for bronchography, as described for adults in Chapter 16. The tongue is initially anesthetized by giving the child viscous lidocaine solution to suck. Next, the superior laryngeal nerves are blocked either percutaneously or using 4-per-cent-cocaine-soaked pledgets, which are inserted into the piriform fossa. The epiglottis and larynx are anesthetized by instilling lidocaine, 2 to 4 per cent, by way of a catheter, which is inserted under direct vision through the cords into the trachea and then passed into the bronchus to be studied. Pelton and Conn have shown that maximum venous blood levels after 3 mg per kg of 10 per cent lidocaine tracheal spray were 3.2 μg per ml.[40] Thus, it would seem that a total dosage of lidocaine of 3 mg per kg would be safe. Great care should be taken to calculate the total dosage of local anesthetic (*i.e.*, cocaine and lidocaine), bearing in mind that the toxic potential is almost certainly additive.

MINOR INFILTRATION AND TOPICAL TECHNIQUES

Adequate prior sedation permits many minor procedures, such as suture of a small laceration, to be performed with local anesthesia. Attempts to carry out such procedures without adequate premedication are very likely to result in a highly distressed child who will then require general anesthesia.

REFERENCES

1. Accardo, N.J., and Adriani, J.: Brachial plexus block: A simplified technique using the axillary route. South. Med. J., *42*:920, 1949.
2. Aizenberg, VL.: The technique of regional anesthesia of the extremities in combination with nitrous oxide general anesthesia in children. Vestn. Khir., *108(5)*:88, 1972.
3. Aizenberg, V.L., and Moisenko, O.L.: Regional anesthesia of the upper extremity in combination with nitrous oxide analgesia in children. Khirurgiia (Mosk.), *48*:26, 1972.
4. Bacon, A.K.: An alternative block for post circumcision analgesia. Anaesth. Intensive Care, *5*:63, 1977.
5. Berkowitz, S., and Greene, B.A.: Spinal anesthesia in children: Report based on 350 patients under 13 years of age. Anesthesiology, *12*:376, 1951.

6. Bromage, P.R.: Ageing and epidural dose requirements: Segmental spread and predictability of epidural analgesia in youth and extreme age. Br. J. Anaesth., *41*:1016, 1969.
7. Bromage, P.R., Shibata, R.R., and Willoughby, H.W.: Influence of prolonged epidural blockade on blood sugar and cortisol responses to operations upon the upper part of the abdomen and thorax. Surg. Gynecol. Obstet., *132*:1057, 1971.
8. Campbell, M.F.: Caudal anesthesia in children. J. Urol., *30*:245, 1933.
9. Carrell, E.D., and Eyring, E.J.: Intravenous regional anesthesia for childhood fractures. J. Trauma, *11*:301, 1971.
10. Castanos, C.C., Rollano, J., and Beltran, J.J.: Anestesia peridural sacra em criancas. Rev. Bras. Anest., *20*:348, 1970.
11. Davenport, H.T.: Paediatric Anaesthesia. p. 97. London, Heinemann Medical Books, 1967.
12. De Pablo, J.S., and Diez–Mallo, J.: Experiences with 3000 cases of brachial plexus blocks: Its dangers: Report of a fatal case. Ann. Surg., *128*:956, 1948.
13. Eather, K.F.: Regional anesthesia for infants and children. Int. Anesthesiol. Clin., *13*:19, 1975.
14. Elze, C.: Centrales nervensystem. *In* Braus, H. (ed.): Anatomie des Menschen. Berlin, Springer-Verlag, 1932.
15. Engleson, S.: Anterior sciatic nerve blockade. *In* Erikson, E. (ed.): Atlas der Lokal-Anaesthesie. Stuttgart, Georg Thieme Verlag, 1970.
16. Eriksson, E.: Axillary brachial plexus anaesthesia in children with Citanest. Acta Anaesthesiol. Scand., *16*:291, 1965.
17. Eyres, R.L., Kidd, J., Oppenheim, R., and Brown, T.C.K.: Local anaesthetic plasma levels in children. Anaesth. Intensive Care, *6*:243, 1978.
18. Farr, R.E.: Local anesthesia in infancy and childhood. Arch Pediatr., *37*:381, 1920.
19. Fortin, G., and Tremblay, L.: the The short-needle technique in brachial plexus block. Can. Anaesth. Soc. J., *6*:32, 1959.
20. Fortuna, A.: Caudal analgesia: A simple and safe technique in paediatric surgery. Br. J. Anaesth., *39*:165, 1967.
21. Gianelly, R., von der Broeben, J.O., Spivack, A.P., and Harrison, D.C.: Effect of lidocaine on ventricular arrhythmias in patients with coronary heart disease. N. Engl. J. Med., *277*:1215, 1967.
22. Gouveia, M.A.: Raquianestesia para pacientes pediatricos. Rev. Bras. Anest., *4*:503, 1970.
23. Gray, H.: Anatomy of the Human Body. ed. 29, p. 792–802. Philadelphia, Lea & Febiger, 1973.
24. Gray, T.: Study of spinal anaesthesia in infants and children. Lancet, *25*:9; *10*:10, 1909; and *10*:6, 1910.
25. Isakob, Y.F., Geraskin, B.I., and Koshevnikov, V.A.: Long term peridural anesthesia after operations on the organs of the chest in children. Grudnaja Chirurija, *13*:104, 1971.
26. Junkin, C.I.: Spinal anesthesia in children. Can. Med. Assoc. J., *28*:51, 1953.
27. Kay, B.: Caudal block for post-operative pain relief in children. Anaesthesia, *29*:610, 1974.
28. Koster, H.: Spinal anesthesia in head and neck surgery. Am. J. Surg., *5*:554, 1928.
29. Leigh, M.D., and Belton, M.K.: Pediatric Anesthesia. ed. 2. New York, Macmillan, 1960.
30. Lourey, C.J., and McDonald, I.H.: Caudal anaesthesia in infants and children. Anaesth. Intensive Care, *1*:547, 1973.
31. Lundy, J.S., Tuphy, E.B., Adams, R.C., and Mousel, C.H.: Clinical use of local and intravenous anesthetic agents: General anesthesia from the standpoint of hepatic function. Proceedings of the Staff Meetings of the Mayo Clinic, *16*:73, 1941.
32. Lutsch, E.F., and Morris, R.W.: Circadian periodicity in susceptibility to lidocaine hydrochloride. Science, *156*:100, 1967.
33. Macintosh, R.R., and Mushin, W.W.: Local anaesthesia: Brachial Plexus. p. 1. Oxford, Blackwell, Scientific Publications, 1944.
34. Martelete, M., *et al.*: Anesthesia caudal em pediatra. Rev. Bras. Anest., *20*:512, 1970.
35. Melman, E., Pennelas, J., and Maruffo, J.: Regional anesthesia in children. Anesth. Analg. (Cleve.), *54*:387, 1975.
36. Moir, D.: Blood loss during major vaginal surgery: A statistical study of the influence of general anaesthesia and epidural analgesia. Br. J. Anaesth., *40*:233, 1968.
37. Niesel, H.C., Rodrigues, P., and Wilsmann, I.: Regional Anaesthesie der oberen Extremitat bei Kindern. Anaesthesist, *23*:178, 1974.
38. Parnes, D.I., and Gordeyev. V.I.: Some indices of external respiration in the conduct of postoperative peridural anesthesia in children. Vestn. Khir., *105*:66, 1970.
39. Parnes, D.I., *et al.*: Hemodynamics and respiration in the postoperative peridural blockade in children. Vestn. Khir., *106*:110, 1971.
40. Pelton, D.A., and Conn. A.W.: A bronchoscopic adapter for intermittent positive pressure breathing in children. Can. Anaesth. Soc. J., *15*:628, 1968.
41. Pitkin, G.P.: Conduction Anesthesia: Clinical Studies of George P. Pitkin. Southwerth, J.L., and Hingson, R. (eds.) p. 387. Philadelphia, J.B. Lippincott, 1946.
42. Reinauer, H., and Hollman, S.: Der Einfluss der Narkoseart auf den Gehalt an Adeninnucleotiden Lactat und Pyruvat in Herz, Leber und Milz der Ratte. Anaesthesist, *15*:327, 1966.
43. Robson, C.H.: Anesthesia in children. Am. J. Surg., *34*:468, 1936.
44. Rodrigues, I.A.: Anestesia peridural no pacienta pediatrico. Rev. Bras. Anest., *14*:116, 1964.
45. Ruston, F.G.: Epidural anaesthesia in infants and children. Can. Anaesth. Soc. J., *1*:37, 1954.
46. ______: Epidural anesthesia in pediatric surgery. Anesth. Analg. (Cleve.), *36*:76, 1957.
47. ______: Epidural anesthesia in paediatric surgery: Present status at the Hamilton General Hospital. Can. Anaesth. Soc. J., *11*:12, 1964.
48. Schettler, D.: Untersuchungen der Ventilation der Atemmechanik, der Blutgase und des Saeure-Basen-Haushaltes bei Saeuglingen mit Lippen-, Kiefer-, Gaumenspalten vor, waehrend und nach der Operation. Dusseldorf, Habil Schr, 1970.
49. Schneider Kinderklinik, Leipzig: Peridural Anaesthesie im Kindesalter. Z. Urol. Chir., *76*:704, 1951.
50. Schulte–Steinberg, O.: Die Caudalanaesthesie im Kindesalter unter besonderer Berucksichtigung der Frage der Ausbreitung und des Wirkungsortes von Lokalanaesthetika im Kindlichen Epiduralraum. Munich, Habil-Schr, 1976.
51. Schulte–Steinberg, O., and Rahlfs, V.W.: Caudal anaesthesia in children and spread of 1 per cent lignocaine: A statistical study. Br. J. Anaesth., *42*:1093, 1970.
52. ______: Caudal Anaesthesie bei Kindern und die Ausbreitung von 0.25%iger Bupivacaine Loesung. Anaesthesist, *21*:94, 1972.
53. Sievers, R.: Peridural Anaesthesue zur Cystoscopie beim Kind. Arch. Klin. Chir., *185*:359, 1936.
54. Slater, H.M., and Stephen, C.R.: Hypobaric pontocaine spinal anesthesia in children. Anesthesiology, *11*:709, 1950.
55. Small, G.A.: Brachial plexus block anesthesia in children. J.A.M.A., *147*:1648, 1951.

56. Smith, R.M.: Anesthesia for Infants and Children. ed. 3. St. Louis, C.V. Mosby, 1968.
57. Spiegel, P.: Caudal anesthesia in pediatric surgery: a preliminary report. Anesth. Analg. (Cleve.), *41*:218, 1962.
58. Spiegel, P.: Anestesia peridural sacra em pacientes pediatros. Panorama Atual Rev Bras Anest, *26*:566, 1976.
59. Touloukian, R.J., Wugmeister, M., Pickett, L.K., and Hehre, F.W.: Anesthesia for neonatal anoperineal and rectal operations. Anesth. Analg. (Cleve.), *50*:565, 1971.
60. Tretjakoff, D., and Mather, L.E.: Pharmacokinetics of local anaesthetic agents. Br. J. Anaesth., *47*:213, 1975.
61. Tucker, G.L.: Das Epidural Fettgewebe. Z. Anat., *79*:100, 1926.
62. Winnie, A.P.: Interscalene brachial plexus block. Anesth. Analg. (Cleve.), *49*:455, 1970.
63. Winnie, A.P., Ramamurthy, S.R., and Durrany, Z.: The inguinal perivascular technique of lumbar plexus anesthesia: The "3-in-1 block." Anesth. Analg. (Cleve.), *52*:989, 1973.
64. Yoshikawa, K., Mima, T., and Egawa, J.: Blood level of marcaine (LAC-43) in axillary plexus blocks, intercostal nerve blocks and epidural anaesthesia. Acta Anaesth. Scand., *12*:1, 1968.

PART TWO

Techniques of Neural Blockade

Section F: Complications of Neural Blockade

22 Complications of Local Anesthetic Neural Blockade

Mark Swerdlow

The various techniques of neural blockade may be followed by an intimidatingly large number of complications, and it is important that the anesthesiologist is aware of these hazards, the conditions under which they are most likely to occur, and the treatment that will be necessary should they, unfortunately, arise. The occurrence of accidental side-effects is sometimes the result of sheer "bad luck," but they are often due to errors in technique or management, and as such the incidence is related to the skill and experience of the anesthesiologist.

The injection of local anesthetics to produce neural blockade can result in exaggerated cardiovascular responses (due to vascular absorption or accidental intravascular injection or by causing sympathetic blockade) and systemic toxic reactions from relative or absolute overdose. Vasopressors added to local anesthetics will produce their own modification of cardiovascular function. These physiologic and pharmacologic responses to local anesthetic agents are discussed in Chapters 2 to 4. This chapter examines abnormal reactions, accidents, and complications that arise from aberrant placement or technique.

Neurologic sequelae can be avoided by careful selection of patients and preparation of equipment, an immaculate technique, and attentive observation during surgery. Before the block is administered, a detailed history should be taken and examination made to discover whether there is preexisting neurologic disease, marked blood deficiencies, major circulatory disturbance, and so forth (see Chap. 6). It is generally wise not to use regional anesthesia in patients with neurologic disease. Spinal or epidural analgesia should be avoided when surgery itself is liable to cause a spinal cord lesion either directly or by interfering with the blood supply to the cord. Finally, the anesthesiologist must have available the knowledge, agents, equipment, and facilities to institute effective treatment should complications ensue, and, when necessary, appropriate specialist colleagues should be consulted as soon as possible.

GENERAL COMPLICATIONS

The complications of local anesthetic neural blockade result from a number of different causes of which the following list makes note.

Complications due to introduction of a needle can result from

Breakage of a needle or catheter

Needle damage to tissue or nerves

Needle punctures of vessels, viscera, or special structures (*e.g.*, dura, pleura)

Complications due to neural blockade technique employed can result from

Overspill of anesthetic on unintended nerves (*e.g.*, phrenic block during supraclavicular brachial block)

Accidental injection into the dura or a dural cuff, viscera, vessels, and so forth (*e.g.*, total spinal anesthesia following interscalene block)

Accidental contamination with bacteria or irritating agents

Injected solution abnormally affecting nerves

Broken Needles and Catheters

A needle or catheter may break and the distal portion be retained within the body tissues, which is a potentially serious accident sometimes associated with regional nerve block. Needles are liable to break at the junction of the hub and shaft.[44] There is also a risk of breakage at the site of irregularity if a used needle is not completely straight. It is probably wiser to discard nondisposable, bent needles than try to straighten them. As Moore points out, needles "will rust when their polished surface has once been damaged, and this rusting results in a focal weak spot."[98] When bony landmarks are used in locating a nerve, the anesthesiologist should avoid forcing the needle against the bone. If the direction of the needle must be changed during performance of a block, the needle should be withdrawn until it is subcutaneous before it is re-

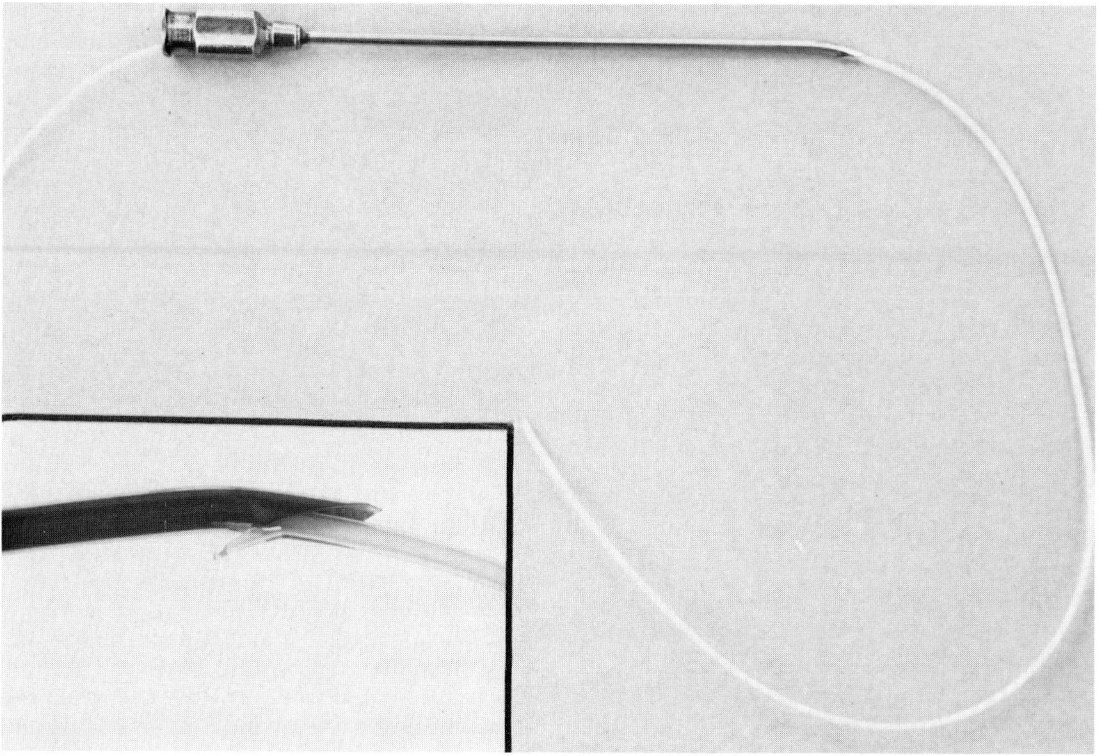

Fig. 22-1. This photograph shows a needle "shearing off" a catheter.

directed. The needle should never be inserted as far as the hub; if it breaks, it can easily be extracted as long as a piece of needle protrudes from the skin. Finally, a warning must be given against the use of needles of inadequate length and gauge for neural blockade procedures; Snow and colleagues described a case in which a disposable 25-gauge, 1.5-cm long needle broke off at the hub and could not be found at open exploration.[136]

Catheters used (especially in epidural analgesia) for continuous nerve blockade are liable to break either at the skin surface when a sharp pull is exerted or (as is or should be well known) at the needle bevel if the catheter is withdrawn after its tip has been pushed beyond the tip of the introducing needle. If for any reason it is necessary to withdraw a catheter that has been passed beyond the tip of the needle, then the needle must be withdrawn before or together with the catheter. "Shearing off" of the catheter by the needle has been reported by a number of authors (Fig. 22-1).[9,20,52] Chun and Karp described a case in which the beveled end of the needle had bent toward the lumen, forming a barb that cut through the catheter.[20] Elam advocated the use of Teflon, which he believed would not shear or fragment, even with repeated autoclaving.[43]

Breakage of an epidural needle or catheter is more common in caudal than in lumbar or thoracic epidural block, probably because caudal analgesia is predominantly used in obstetric procedures, during which considerable movement may occur. There have been a number of reports of the occurrence of this accident, although its precise incidence has not been determined. In Dawkins's analysis of published data, 12 cases of broken needles and six of broken catheters were reported.[31] Moore reported that in his practice, breakage of four needles and two catheters has required surgical intervention to recover retained portions.[98] I have had a patient for whom surgical exploration was necessary to retrieve a broken piece of epidural catheter. However, it is debatable whether the magnitude of intervention of a surgical laminectomy is warranted since many catheter tips have not been retrieved and there have been no ill effects.

It is well known that epidural catheters may curl or double back on themselves; this has been said to occur in about 50 per cent of cases.[104] An epidural catheter may also knot itself within the epidural space; in one such case the catheter was successfully removed by firm steady traction.[69,105] Elam wrote that if a knot were to form with Teflon, it would untie when external traction was applied.[43]

It is advisable to remove any portion of needle that has detached itself into the tissues. A broken piece of needle tends to "migrate" and may damage vessels, nerves, or viscera. If a plastic catheter breaks, it should be removed as long as this can be done without difficulty. However, plastic tubing may soften at body temperature and not be palpable, and, moreover, it may not be visible on radiograph. Because it seldom causes tissue reaction or injuries to organs and vessels, it has been suggested that the patient should be informed and allowed to join in making the decision whether or not to remove the tubing.[100] Dawkins reports a patient in whom a broken catheter was left *in situ* with no subsequent harm.[31]

Pain

Not infrequently, there is some residual pain and tenderness around the site of the needle puncture, but if pain persists for more than a few days after a nerve block, a cause other than local tissue trauma should be sought. Such causes include the accidental contamination with or mistaken injection of an antiseptic, neurolytic agent, or other irritant solution; infection; trauma to a nerve; and (in relevant block procedures) pneumothorax.

Epidural and spinal catheters have occasionally been the cause of irritation and infection at the site of introduction; an incidence of 10 per cent has been reported after prolonged epidural anesthesia.[138]

Backache

Backache, an annoying but relatively minor complaint, may follow spinal, epidural, or paravertebral block. However, backache may also follow surgery under general anesthesia, and one of the causes of such backache is flattening of the normal lumbar lordosis and stretching and straining of the joint capsules and ligaments of the spine during prolonged supine position on the operating table. Later, when analgesia (or general anesthesia) wears off, this stretching is felt as backache. Such an effect is exaggerated if the patient is "manipulated" during surgery (*e.g.*, lithotomy position).

In epidural and subarachnoid block, needle placement in the perivertebral tissues, possibly including accidental hemorrhage, may later result in pain in the back. There have also been some reports that suggested that accidental needle placement in an intervertebral disc during lumbar puncture may give rise to backache and, indeed, to a disc lesion.[2,38,45] The incidence of backache may be somewhat reduced by performing the block gently, by careful positioning of the patient while on the table, and by maintenance of the lumbar lordosis. Needless to say, the use of sharp needles and an aseptic technique are essential.

Ecchymosis and Hematoma Formation

Hemorrhage is not an uncommon complication of nerve block and is due to puncture or tearing of a blood vessel by the needle. Whether bleeding from a damaged vessel results in minor or serious consequences depends on the looseness and vascularity of the injected tissue, as well as on the nature of the agent injected and the patient's coagulation time. The tissues of the head, neck, and scrotum are particularly vulnerable. The risk of hemorrhage is accentuated in patients with blood dyscrasias and in those who are receiving anticoagulant therapy (large hematoma formation, in particular, has been reported[71,109]) following lumbar sympathetic block. It has been suggested that an additional cause is that local anesthetics with a vasodilator action may prevent retraction of the vessel and sealing of the puncture.[98] A hematoma rarely persists longer than a few weeks and usually disperses within a week or two. Hemorrhage in the intrathecal and epidural spaces and into the orbit is particularly dangerous and may be followed by serious neurologic sequelae, as will be seen below.

The incidence and degree of hemorrhage can be reduced by the use of fine, sharp-pointed needles, gentleness in technique, and the immediate and sustained application of pressure to the bleeding area, when this is possible. In addition, because of the hazard of hemorrhage, neural block should be avoided in patients on anticoagulant therapy or those with prolonged clotting time. Also, treatment should consist of application of cold packs to the hematoma and perhaps injection of hyaluronidase in saline into the surrounding area. When retroperitoneal or spinal hemorrhage has occurred, anticoagulants (if in use) should be reversed and a surgeon consulted.

Pneumothorax

Pneumothorax is due to puncture of the visceral pleura and may be encountered whenever a needle is introduced in close proximity to the thoracic cage.

In the neck
  Stellate ganglion block
  Brachial plexus block
  Cervical plexus block
In the chest
  Intercostal block
  Paravertebral block (sympathetic, somatic)

The risk of causing a pneumothorax is greater on the right side of the neck where the cupula of the pleura is normally higher and is also greater in tall, slim, long-necked people in whom the pleura reaches up higher into the neck. There is an added risk in patients who suffer from emphysema; puncture by the needle of an emphysematous bulla may lead to tension pneumothorax.

The reported incidence of pneumothorax following various nerve blocks is as follows:

Supraclavicular brachial plexus block (see Chap. 10)
  0.6–2%
Stellate ganglion block (see Chap. 13)
  Anterior approach
    0.25%
  Anterolateral approach
    0.5–8%
  Posterior approach
    3–13%
Thoracic paravertebral (somatic) block (see Chap. 14)
  0–6%
Thoracic paravertebral (sympathetic) block (see Chap. 13)
  1.4–7.9%

The signs and symptoms of pneumothorax are usually apparent within a short time of the pleural puncture, but they may not appear until as long as 12 hours later. The initial complaint is of pain in the chest, (accentuated by deep breathing), cough, or dyspnea. The degree of discomfort and distress will depend on the size of the pneumothorax, which can be ascertained by the physical signs in the chest and confirmed by radiograph (Fig. 22-2). Should the film be negative but symptoms persist and increase, a repeat film should be taken. With massive pneumothorax, of course, shift of the mediastinum can have severe respiratory and circulatory effects. (However, as Moore points out, if during nerve block in the neck there is coincidental block of the phrenic nerve, the chest movement on that side will be impaired even though there is no pneumothorax.)[98] Occasionally, there is also an escape of air into the subcutaneous and mediastinal tissues. I had a patient in whom emphysema occurred over a wide area of the lower neck and upper chest following stellate ganglion block. Hemopneumothorax, hemoptysis, and pleural effusion have also been reported following cervicothoracic sympathetic block or brachial plexus block.[87,98,110,159] One patient with "clicking" pneumothorax has been described following thoracic paravertebral block.[78] "Clicking," which may occur with a small pneumothorax on the left side, is thought to be due to the cardiac contractions moving a bubble of air, to cause forcible pleural separation.

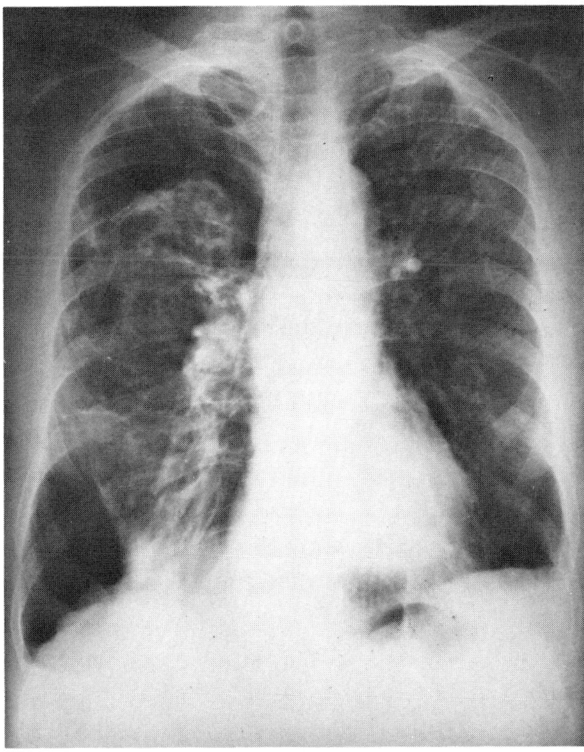

Fig. 22-2. Pneumothorax (right side) apex following stellate ganglion block.

A number of measures may be taken to reduce the incidence of pneumothorax. A gentle and careful technique is essential and the path of the needle should be kept as close to the bony landmark (rib or vertebra) as possible. The hand holding the needle should be braced against the patient at all times.[99] When blocks in the neck are performed, every effort should be made to remain cephalad to the cupula of the pleura. The patient should be adequately prepared and warned so that he does not move or jerk during performance of the block. It is wise not to perform nerve blocks listed above with the patient in a sitting position.[85] Bonica recommends that when thoracic paravertebral block is performed, the patient should be asked to empty the lungs as much as possible before the needle is advanced to the anterolateral aspect of the vertebral body.[7]

Bed rest and sedation will minimize the degree of pneumothorax after pleural puncture, while increased activity and respiration will accentuate the leakage of air from the lung. The treatment of pneumothorax depends upon its extent and the degree of upset that it causes. With a small pneumothorax, the patient should be kept under observation, reassured, and given a mild analgesic. With greater degrees of pneumothorax, he should be admitted to the ward and an underwater drain inserted.

Local Tissue Irritation

Swelling, cellulitis, abscess, gangrene, and sloughing may result from bacterial or chemical contamination of local anesthetic solutions or from inadequate sterilization of needles and syringes. Serious complications may also result from the accidental or unwitting introduction of particulate matter.[28] Gangrenous changes may also be due to vasoconstrictor agents added to solutions, especially for digital block. Furthermore, tissue irritation may result from the release of metallic ions by the action of local anesthetics on any metal-containing instruments employed or from synthetic rubber stoppers that contain excessive amounts of zinc oxide.[100] Finally, superficial sloughing may follow a large skin wheal made with a high concentration of vasoconstrictor.

Intraneural Injection

Direct accidental placement of needles in nerves or even intraneural injection of local anesthetic solution is unlikely to cause neurologic sequelae.[98] If neurologic effects should arise after nerve block, the possibility of other causes (*e.g.*, preexisting neurological deficiencies; contamination with preservatives, etc.[106] surgical trauma; postural nerve trauma during surgery) should be borne in mind. Damage is more likely to result from the needle if the nerve is composed of a single large funiculus than if it is composed of a number of small widely separated fiber bundles.[140] Selander and colleagues consider that damage is less likely if a 45°-bevel needle is used.[130] However, neurologic sequelae may follow intraneural injection of a peripheral nerve within 5 inches of the intervertebral foramen. Moore has shown that when the lumbar or cervical nerves of monkeys were injected intraneurally 3 to 4 cm from the intervertebral foramen, the solution spread centrally at once, reaching the parenchyma of the spinal cord in 2 to 5 minutes.[100] The solution took 10 to 15 minutes to pass through the pia or epineurium and approach the cerebrospinal fluid (CSF), and total spinal block resulted in 35 to 40 minutes. Moreover, Chen has shown that fluids injected under the perineural membrane of the peripheral nerves will travel centrally, and small quantities may reach the brain in this way; this is important in cranial nerve injections.[18]

Clinically, complete recovery of nerve function usually occurs after local anesthetic block, but signs of neuropathy have been reported, although it is not clear whether they were due to the needle or the anesthetic agent.[76,160] Löfström, Wennberg, and Widen recorded nerve action potentials in order to study nerve function during the weeks following ulnar nerve block with a variety of local anesthetic agents.[81] Three of their 21 subjects showed electroneurographic signs of nerve damage. All three had received local anesthetic after the nerve had been struck by the needle, and signs of neuropathy appeared 1 week or more after block, were maximal in about 3 weeks, and were diminishing after 2 to 3 months.

COMPLICATIONS DUE TO SPECIFIC TECHNIQUES

Spinal Anesthesia

The complications attributed to spinal anesthesia are bedeviled by its past reputation[144]—a reputation gained in the days of irritant solutions, nonaseptic techniques, unduly large needles, and imperfectly controlled methods. A number of studies of large series of spinal anesthetics performed under modern conditions have shown that this method is rarely the cause of serious complications. Thus, Sadove and colleagues published an analysis of 20,000 spinal anesthetics with 24 neurologic complications; Scarborough reported an incidence of complications of less than 0.16 per cent in 65,677 cases; and Noble and Murray recorded 78,000 spinal anesthetics with no major complications.[108,127,128] Lund summarized over 500,000 spinal anesthetics in a number of large series with no permanent neurologic sequelae (see Table 7-4). However, continuous spinal techniques may not be so relatively innocuous.[83]

It is important to realize that any neurologic abnormalities that follow spinal anesthesia and surgery are not necessarily due to the subarachnoid injection.[79,88] In fact, such abnormalities have been reported after surgery under general anesthesia.[21,57] The causes of such fortuitous post-spinal-anesthesia neurologic complications have admirably been analyzed by Noble and Murray.[108] Residual neurologic damage may also be due to preexisting neurologic disease or to exacerbation of it by the anesthetic.[38,98,148] In a study of 482 patients with neurologic complaints that appeared to be related to spinal anesthesia, Marinacci and Courville showed by electromyeography that in only four cases was spinal anesthesia actually the cause.[89]

Nevertheless, permanent and serious sequelae due to effects on the spinal cord and its coverings do occasionally follow spinal anesthesia. A legal case of great significance is Wooley and Roe, in which two patients who received spinal anesthesia on the same operating list subsequently developed permanent and painful paraplegia.[23] The cause was ascribed to seepage of the phenol solution used for storage through invisible cracks in the local anesthetic ampules. Sporadic cases due to various causes are still reported from time to time.[56,129] The occurrence of such cases, although fortunately rare, stresses the need for unremitting care and attention whenever lumbar puncture or spinal block is performed.

The importance of absolute sterility of solutions and equipment used in spinal anesthesia must be emphasized. The enzyme and antibody content of CSF is very low, and consequently the fluid is poorly equipped to combat any infection that might be introduced.[49] Moreover care should be taken to check not only the sterility but the precise identity and concentration of the solution to be used for subarachnoid injection. A case has been described in which gallamine triethiodide was mistakenly injected intrathecally instead of lidocaine—the results were somewhat alarming.[91] More recently, thiopentone was mistakenly injected epidurally instead of a local anesthetic.[50]

Headache. The commonest complication of spinal anesthesia is probably headache, which is thought usually to be due to leakage of CSF through the dural puncture. When spinal anesthesia is used for obstetric delivery, this leakage may be aggravated by the fact that after the birth of the infant the obstruction to the vena cava is removed and the vertebral venous plexus decongests, leaving more space for fluid to exude through the dural puncture.[40]

Headache after spinal anesthesia may, however, on occasion be due to infective or irritative conditions of the meninges. *Spinal headache* is brought on or aggravated by sitting or standing. It arises within an hour to a few days and is usually frontal or occipital. Although it is usually mild and disappears in a day or two, it may be severe and persist for a week or more and it may be accompanied by nausea, vomiting, and visual and auditory disturbances. Postoperative headache may, of course, be quite unrelated to spinal anesthesia, particularly in susceptible patients who react to the stress and anxiety of the preoperative and operative period. Such headache is not postural, is often not localized in one part of the head, and is usually not intense. The incidence of headache is variously reported to be from 1.4 to 12 per cent (see Chap. 7).[102] In less than 1 per cent of cases, headache is accompanied by temporary visual and auditory symptoms.[39,116,157]

Greene, Vandam and Dripps, and others have shown that the use of 24- or 26- gauge needles, perhaps employed with a Sise introducer, will reduce the incidence of post-spinal-anesthetic headaches.[61,149] The use of a pencil-point needle has been said, in addition, to reduce the incidence of headache.[15,67]

A number of methods have been advocated for the treatment of headache, including epidural injections of saline or Hartmann's solution, tight abdominal binders, the use of Trendelenburg tilt, intramuscular pituitary extract, inhalation of carbon dioxide, and the administration of fluids orally or, if necessary, parenterally (see Chap. 7).[94,121,134,137,154] It is of some historical interest that as long ago as 1930, Nelson advocated the use of a piece of catgut (passed through the lumbar puncture needle) to plug the dural hole; while this effectively reduced the incidence of headache, it frequently caused far more serious sequelae, such as cauda equina syndrome.[107] Use of tolazoline as a prophylactic against spinal-anesthetic headache has been suggested; the principle is that in the generalized vasodilatation produced by this drug, the passive dilatation of the subdural vessels may compensate for the CSF loss and subarachnoid hypotension associated with cephalalgia.[43] Another method of prevention is the injection of 2.5 ml of the patient's blood into the epidural space as the spinal needle is withdrawn through the dura. A fibrin patch forms and occludes the dural puncture.[36,59,150] However, although the method appears fundamentally to be effective and safe, Ostheimer and colleagues describe, following epidural blood patch, four cases of backache of 24 hours' duration and one patient who had symptoms of nerve root irritation that subsided within 10 days, and Walpole reports a case with temporary but severe pain in the back and legs.[111,150] Some doubt has also been expressed by Crawford on the wisdom of deliberately introducing blood into the epidural space, and clearly, conservative measures should be employed initially before blood patch is considered (see Chap. 7).[27]

Other Minor Complications. *Nausea and Vomiting.* The incidence of nausea and vomiting during spinal anesthesia has been greatly decreased by adequate premedication and suitable medication during surgery. Graves and colleagues have found atropine useful in treating nausea that accompanies spinal anesthesia.[60] Ratra and associates have found that the incidence of emesis after surgery under spinal analgesia was higher in patients whose systolic blood pressure fell below 80 torr and that chlorpromazine and oxygen inhalation both produced a lowering in the incidence of nausea and vomiting (see Chap. 7).[118]

Hypotension is a physiologic result of spinal sympathetic blockade. It must be remembered, however, that when certain agents, such as tranquilizers, and antihypertensive drugs are administered as premedication or in conjunction with spinal (or epidural) analgesia, they may disastrously aggravate hypotension or prevent response to or treatment of it. Hypotension from spinal anesthesia is commoner in pregnant than in nonpregnant patients, and Bonica believes it is commoner after spinal than after epidural anesthesia (see Chap. 8).[8,94] In Caesarian section under spinal anesthesia, the incidence of hypotension can greatly be reduced by prophylactic ephedrine and intravenous fluids.[90,103] The subarachnoid injection of vasoconstrictor drugs is probably quite safe in normal patients at appropriate concentration, as indicated by large series of patients who showed no sequelae (see Chap. 7).[83] Finch and Carter report a patient who, following spinal anesthesia administered at the L4–5 interspace with amethocaine and phenylephrine, developed paresis of the right quadriceps femoris muscle group without sensory deficit; recovery was complete 2 months later.[46]

Backache is commonly partly due to trauma caused by the needle in the supraspinous and interspinous ligaments and ligamentum flavum and occurs less frequently after the use of a 22-gauge or finer needle than when a larger needle is employed. Backache is unusual with modern atraumatic techniques; Wilkinson reports a 6 per cent incidence (see also Chap. 7, p. 172).[157]

Pain Across Shoulders. Abouleish states that pain across the shoulders and down the arms not uncommonly follows dural puncture and is usually accompanied by cephalalgia.[1] It normally takes 24 hours to develop but may occur immediately with dural puncture by a large epidural needle.

Neurologic Sequelae. Almost all of the following are also possible after diagnostic or therapeutic lumbar puncture. Thorsen classified neurologic lesions of the cord as follows[144]:

Nerve root trauma by the needle may temporarily produce pain, numbness, or paraesthesias in the corresponding dermatome.

Injection into a nerve root produces severe pain and paresis and sensory changes, which may be somewhat persistent.

Intramedullary injection causes sudden collapse, and, if the patient survives, signs of complete transverse myelitis are found. Thorsen discovered only seven such cases in the literature.

Toxic effect of the injected solution on nerve tissue may result in persistent and widespread paresis and sensory changes.

Toxic effect of the injected agent on the leptomeninges may result in proliferative arachnoiditis.

Available data indicate that uncontaminated local anesthetic solutions do not cause neurotoxicity or local tissue changes at clinical concentrations (see Chap. 4).

Temporary peripheral nerve palsy has been reported in 0.17 per cent and 0.3 per cent of patients after spinal anaesthesia.[102,116] Moore and colleagues also reported two patients in whom analgesia continuing longer than 12 hours occurred after spinal anesthesia with a local anesthetic.[102]

Temporary cranial nerve palsy sometimes occurs; paralysis of most of the cranial nerves has at one time or another been reported following spinal anesthesia. Most often affected is the abducens nerve, which is particularly vulnerable, probably because of its long course within the skull.[68] Diplopia is usually preceded by headache and may not appear until 2 or 3 weeks after administration of the anesthetic. The cause is thought to be low CSF pressure. Spontaneous recovery occurs in a large proportion of patients, and treatment should include covering the eye, muscle exercises, and fusion training. When no recovery has taken place after 2 years, surgical correction of the strabismus may be advised. Lund and Cwik wrote, "The incidence of cranial nerve palsies appears to vary directly with the extent of dural trauma, occurring more frequently following continuous spinal anesthesia conducted with large ureteral catheters."[83]

Chronic adhesive arachnoiditis is a most serious sequel of spinal anesthesia. It is a proliferative reaction of the arachnoid mater, which is followed by fibrosis and distortion of the arachnoid space. The pathologic changes are often most marked in the lumbosacral enlargement of the spinal cord and result in the *cauda equina syndrome*. Clinical symptoms and signs may not become apparent for weeks or even months after the anesthetic has been administered. In arachnoiditis, there is usually some weakness and numbness of the legs and impairment of bowel and bladder function. Gradually as the condition involves the spinal cord, there is increasing spasticity. Involvement of the posterior roots will result in a varying amount of pain. A wide variety of agents have been found responsible in reported cases of arachnoiditis, including nonpyrogen free distilled water, lysol, detergents, and pyrogen-contaminated dextrose.[56,72,120]

Payne and Bergentz and others suggest that one cause of arachnoiditis is a virus invasion of the nervous system, resistance of which has been lowered by spinal anesthesia; however, there is no evidence to support this.[113] Another possible source of danger has been cited by Brandus, who points out that a conventional 22-gauge spinal needle produces a core of epidermis in 75 per cent of cases.[12] The core is usually drawn into the syringe when CSF is being aspirated, but it may be reinjected into the CSF with the risk of septic or chemical contamination, which suggests the need for an introducer.

Direct damage to the cord is a possibility when the needle is introduced above the L2 interspace. Damage to the cord itself or to a nerve root usually produces an immediate disability in one region only, and the patient generally recovers from the paresis and sensory disturbance in a matter of months. On the other hand, the effects of arachnoiditis are somewhat delayed in onset and more widespread in distribution and chronic or progressive in character.[98] Rosenbaum and colleagues reported chronic adhesive arachnoiditis following saddle block analgesia.[124] It has been pointed out by Moore, however, that trauma to the cord may result in an aseptic meningeal reaction due to extravasated blood.[9] Neurologic damage, usually temporary, has also been reported to have been caused by injury to nerve roots and blood vessels by spinal catheters.[5] Elam considered that there is little danger to the cord and roots from an advancing catheter made of polyvinyl chloride, polyethylene, or Teflon.[43] As a means of avoiding damage to the cord from an advancing catheter, it has been suggested that injecting CSF through the catheter as it is advanced will "float" the tip away from any solid structures approached.[43]

Anterior spinal artery thrombosis is a rare complication of spinal anesthesia (and of epidural anesthesia[146]) although it would appear from anecdotal and medicolegal evidence that the incidence of this complication is greater than the sparse published reports might suggest. It may occur in patients who suffer from arteriosclerosis and results in necrosis of the central gray matter and degeneration of the periphery of the cord, leading to paraplegia and even death. The condition may be precipitated by a massive fall in blood pressure during spinal anesthesia. However, anterior spinal artery thrombosis has been attributed to acute flexion of the neck in patients with cervical spondylosis who have not received regional anesthesia. In one instance, permanent paraplegia immediately followed an unsuccessful attempt to introduce the needle within the vertebral canal for epidural puncture.* Figure 22-3 shows the abnormal myelogram of the cervical spine of another patient who was subsequently administered an intrathecal neurolytic injection; she had no symptoms or signs of compression of the cervical spinal cord. Had the neck been acutely flexed during the intrathecal injection, she might well have developed anterior spinal artery thrombosis (see also Fig. 8-13 and associated discussion).*

Subarachnoid hemorrhage is frequently symptomless; if the hemorrhage is heavy, the eventual organized clot may produce arachnoiditis and also thrombosis of the radicular arteries. The consequent neurologic symptoms may therefore not appear for days or weeks after performance of the lumbar puncture. A patient with a hemorrhagic diathesis or on anticoagulant therapy is liable to develop intrathecal hemorrhage if a vessel is accidentally damaged, and this may be followed by neurologic complications. Edelson and colleagues have cited four previously described cases of spinal subdural hematoma following lumbar puncture and reported eight patients with thrombocytopenia who developed subdural spinal hematoma following lumbar puncture. In three, the hematoma was associated with weakness and sensory loss in the lower extremities and with bladder dysfunction. One patient recovered spontaneously, but two remained paraplegic until their deaths several months later.

The source of subdural bleeding is not clear. The major intrathecal blood vessels usually enter the spinal canal above L3 but occasionally accompany the L4 or L5 nerve root (see Fig. 8-11). Lumbar puncture performed in the midline at the L4–5 interspace is unlikely to involve either subarachnoid or subdural vessels large enough to cause important bleeding because such vessels are laterally too distant. However, lumbar puncture should not be undertaken in patients who receive anticoagulants.[92]

* Swerdlow, M.: Unpublished data.

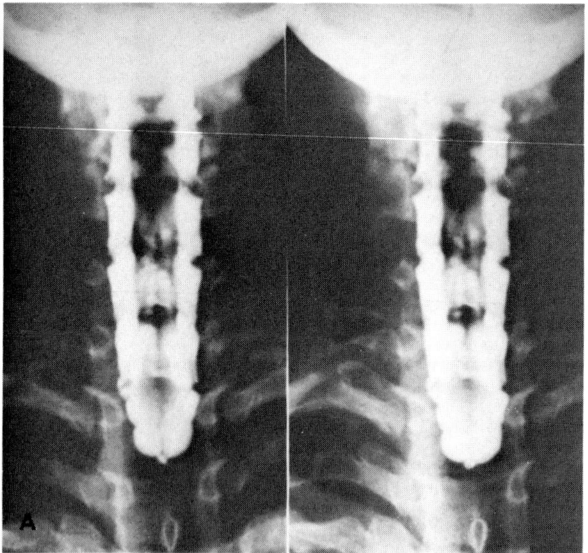

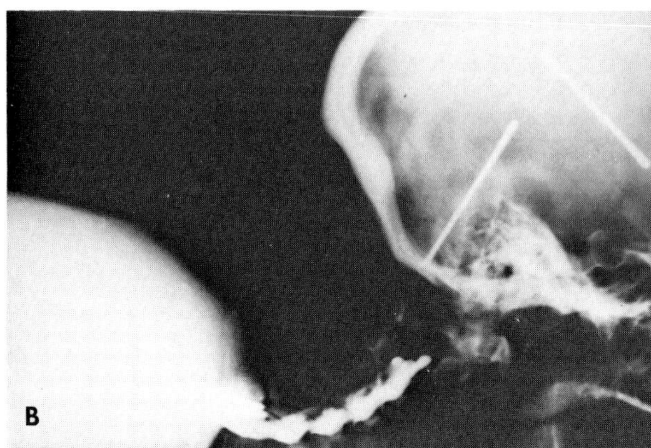

Fig. 22-3. Myelogram of cervical spine.

Edelson and his colleagues consider that lumbar puncture is potentially dangerous in patients with thrombocytopenia and that the lower the platelet count the greater the risk of hematoma.[41] Moreover, the more difficult the puncture and the more punctures made, the greater is the risk. After lumbar puncture, if pain or neurologic signs develop, the patient should be given a platelet transfusion. Bender and Christoff advocate the medical treatment of subdural hematoma (corticosteroids and intravenous hyperosmolar solutions), resorting to surgery only if the patient is comatose or if there is progressive worsening of the condition.[3] A number of cases of vertebral osteomyelitis have also been reported after lumbar puncture.[119]

Cardiac Arrest. Finally, cardiac arrest is, fortunately, an extremely unlikely hazard, but two cases have been recorded after sinus bradycardia following high spinal anesthesia.[55] Sadove and colleagues have reported four cases of cardiac arrest (3 of whom died) under spinal anesthesia.[127] It should be possible to prevent this complication by close observation of the level of block and early treatment of cardiovascular depression (see Chap. 7).

Epidural Analgesia

Epidural analgesia has been regarded as being responsible for fewer and mostly less serious complications than spinal analgesia.[82] In a review of the complications of 32,718 reported epidural blocks, Dawkins found the following incidence of sequelae: backache—2%; retention of urine—1%; dural puncture—1.2%; accidental spinal injection—0.2%; intravascular injection causing convulsions—0.2%; and central nervous system lesions, transient—0.1% and permanent—0.02%.

Most of the complications are due to errors in technique; overdose is the commonest fault attributable to the anesthetic agent itself. Systemic reactions from absorption or from accidental intravascular injection are considerably more likely after epidural than after spinal anesthesia because of the much larger volume of local anesthetic administered and the large plexus of extradural veins. An additional danger exists in obstetric analgesia in which, according to Eckenhoff, if the patient is improperly positioned or if she has a contraction during or immediately after the injection, there may be a rapid absorption of local anesthetic through the engorged vertebral venous plexus.[40] A more recent large survey by Usubiaga indicated that, in light of the complete range of expertise, the incidence of neurologic complications of epidural block was about 1 in 10,000 (see Chap. 8).

Backache not uncommonly results following epidural blockade and according to Foldes and associates is the one complication commoner after epidural than after spinal analgesia.[48] The incidence of backache rises markedly if very blunt needles are used to avoid piercing the dura.[19] It is usually of short duration and is attributed by some to superficial tissue injury at the site of the injection.[24]

Urinary retention has been reported by a number of workers to occur no more frequently after delivery under epidural analgesia than under pudendal nerve block or under natural spontaneous delivery.[63,95] Also, the incidence has been found to be considerably lower than in similar patients whose operations were performed with spinal anesthesia (see Chap. 25).[48]

Headache is unusual after epidural block, and its occurrence should suggest accidental dural puncture. Moore and his colleagues report spinal type headache in 0.069 per cent of 3,312 epidural anesthesias.[102] Grove found that the incidence of headache in women who deliver under epidural analgesia was not dissimilar from that in women in the same hospital who delivered without regional analgesia.[63] Episodes of dizziness and of "ear popping" have also been reported during the first 2 or 3 days after delivery under epidural analgesia.[27]

The spread of analgesia after epidural injection of local anesthetic solution is highly variable.[141]

Massive extradural is a rare and as yet unexplained complication; according to Dawkins only 28 cases have so far been reported.[31] Twenty to 30 minutes after the institution of epidural anesthesia, the respirations disappear; the patient loses consciousness, the pupils dilate, but the blood pressure remains satisfactory. If artificial ventilation is applied, the patient recovers consciousness and full activity within 1 to 2 hours. A few cases have also been reported of delayed and exaggerated spread of epidural anesthesia in elderly patients with arteriosclerosis.[34]

Transient Neurologic Defects. Numbness and weakness has been reported to persist 24 hours after epidural block with bupivacaine, 0.25 per cent, with epinephrine, 1:200,000, and 60 hours after 0.5 per cent bupivacaine, without epinephrine.[37,112] In another report, an area of paresthesia was found to have persisted for 3 weeks.[139] Crawford has reported two patients with residual patches of numbness that lasted 6 weeks after obstetric epidural anesthesia.[26] It is difficult to know whether such sequelae are due to the effects of the injected solution; to trauma on nerve roots, perhaps, by the needle or catheter; or to pressure on peripheral nerves when a patient who has analgesia and some degree of muscle relaxation is incorrectly positioned.

Dural puncture is relatively common and is an accident not too serious as long as it is recognized in time and nothing is injected. Failure to realize that the needle is subarachnoid, with subsequent injection of an epidural dose of local anesthetic, would result in total spinal anesthesia—a condition that requires cardiovascular and ventilatory support. According to Dawkins, dural puncture occurs in 2.9 per cent of cases of epidural anesthesia, in which the loss-of-resistance method is used to locate the epidural space, and in 1.6 per cent of cases in which a visual indicator is employed. Accidental subdural injection of anesthetic has also been reported.[10]

An epidural catheter is considered by some to be a safety precaution against accidental subarachnoid injection, but cases have been reported in which the dura was punctured by the catheter during its introduction and also at the time of subsequent "top-up" doses.[26,48,58,96,115] The use of an extradural catheter can lead to additional complications, such as kinking or breaking of the catheter, and the catheter may impinge on the spinal cord and cause damage. Radiculitis following epidural analgesia with a stiff catheter has been reported.[30] When extradural catheter techniques are used to provide postoperative analgesia, the main problems are reported to be drug overdose and tachyphylaxis, hypotension, and the effects of bacterial contamination.[132,138]

Extradural Hematoma. Hemorrhage and hematoma formation are a serious hazard of epidural anesthesia. The extradural venous plexus is large, and the veins are thin-walled and vulnerable to needle puncture. Over 100 cases of spinal epidural hematoma have been reported, about one-third being associated with anticoagulant therapy. It appears that the hematoma usually lies dorsal to the dural sac and extends over several vertebral segments.[14] Epidural hematoma may produce a compression syndrome, just as an extradural abscess or tumor would; the differential diagnosis is shown in Table 22-1.[31] In the sacral space, a hematoma may produce little in the way of symptoms, whereas in the lower thoracic or upper lumbar areas, compression will produce marked neurologic signs because the epidural space is so restricted (Fig. 22-4). A case of paraparesis due to an epidural abscess following thoracic epidural analgesia has been reported.[126]

It must be pointed out that extradural hemorrhage may occur spontaneously or be precipitated by minor trauma and can progress to paraplegia within hours or days.[32]

Paraplegia is a rare sequel of epidural block; Usubiaga reported that a thorough search of the world literature revealed a total of 54 cases of paraplegia following epidural analgesia; of these, 9 recovered almost completely (see Chap. 8).[147] The cause is not always established, but anterior spinal artery

Table 22-1. Differential Diagnosis of Epidural Abscess, Epidural Hemorrhage, and Anterior Spinal Artery Syndrome

	Epidural Abscess	*Epidural Hemorrhage*	*Anterior Spinal Artery Syndrome*
Age of patient	Any age	50% over 50 years	Any age
Previous history	Infection*	Efforts–anticoagulants	Arteriosclerosis
Onset	1–3 days	Sudden	Sudden
Generalized symptoms		None during epidural block; sharp transient pain otherwise	None
Sensory involvement	None or paresthesias		
Motor involvement	Flaccid paralysis, later spastic	Flaccid paralysis	Flaccid paralysis
Segmental reflexes	Exacerbated*–later obtunded	Abolished	Abolished
Queckenstedt's sign and myelogram	Signs of extradural compression	Signs of extradural compression	Normal
Cerebrospinal fluid	Increased cell count	Normal	Normal
Blood data	Rise in red cell sedimentation rate	Prolonged coagulation time*	Normal

* Infrequent findings (Usubiaga, J. E.: Neurological complications of spinal and epidural analgesia. *In* Saidman, L. J., and Moya, F. (eds.): Complications of Anesthesis, Springfield, Charles C Thomas, 1970).

thrombosis is a possibility.[146] Such thrombosis produces a degree of necrosis of the anterior two-thirds of the cord, causing motor signs without great sensory changes; symptoms may occur within the first few postoperative days.[11] Davies and colleagues have described a case of paraplegia due to anterior spinal artery syndrome following epidural anesthesia, in which there was no actual thrombosis.[30] The occlusion, although temporary, was sufficient to cause permanent changes in the anterior part of the cord due to ischemia. They considered that it was due either to hypotension or to the vasospastic action of the epinephrine injected with the local anesthetic.[16,66] A case of paraplegia of 16 months duration occurred owing probably to contamination with benzyl alcohol preservative.[25] Permanent bilateral paresis of the quadriceps muscles has also been reported after epidural anesthesia.[102]

Miscellaneous Sequelae. Moore and associates have reported a patient who developed cardiac arrest after a precipitous fall in blood pressure 20 minutes after epidural block and before surgery started; resuscitation was successful.[102] Rapid epidural injection of 30 ml of local anesthetic solution has been

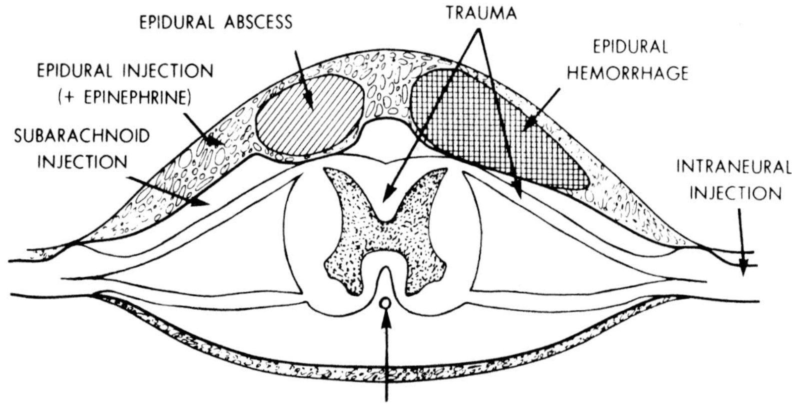

Fig. 22-4. Illustration of the site of epidural abscess, epidural hemorrhage, and anterior spinal thrombosis.

reported to produce intraocular hemorrhage, perhaps owing to the rise in CSF pressure, causing subhyaloid bleeding.[22]

Meningitis has developed in two patients after epidural injection and was attributed to contamination of the syringe with antiseptic; both recovered within 7 days.[29] Epidural abscess has also occurred 16 days after obstetric epidural analgesia as a result of blood-borne spread of infection to an epidural hematoma.[27] It is suggested that patients with evidence of systemic infection should be treated with antibiotics when extradural block is to be administered. Extradural hematoma may, of course, occur spontaneously (see also Chap. 8, pp. 257–261).[27]

Caudal Block

The possibility of puncture of the dura and of intravascular injection must always be borne in mind and avoided by taking proper precautions. A further hazard that has recently been pointed out is that of intraosseous injection.[35,84] The sacral cortex is sometimes very thin, and intraosseous injection of a large volume of local anesthetic may, through rapid absorption, give rise to toxic effects. In obstetric caudal block, misdirection of the needle with injection of local anesthetic into the fetal cranial cavity may result in serious consequences.[47]

Finally, it must be asserted that despite this rather frightening list of possible complications, epidural analgesia is basically an eminently safe procedure when it is carefully and expertly practiced. The vast majority of the serious sequelae that have been reported were due to faults in technique or equipment.[70,84]

Paracervical Block

A number of cases of fetal acidosis have been reported following paracervical block with mepivacaine and bupivacaine whereas paracervical injection of placebo produces no such changes.[133,142,143] Cases of fetal and neonatal death have also been reported after paracervical block (see also Chap. 18).[123]

Infiltration of the uterovaginal plexus (especially if it is supplemented with pudenal block to anesthetize the vulva) may involve a large total quantity of anesthetic producing fetal distress (especially bradycardia) and maternal disorientation, tachycardia, hypertension, and even death.[4,62] The fetal liver has insufficient amidase to metabolize the amide group of local anesthetics. Paracervical block itself may result in injection into the placenta or even the fetus.[17] The use of continuous paracervical block technique has been reported, on occasion, to cause maternal hamorrhage and fetal depression. Wenger and Gitchell report two cases and quote six previously recorded cases of infection following pudendal or paracervical anesthesia.[155] The infection that begins in the paracervical or paravaginal areas, spreads behind the hip joint, into the gluteal musculature or into the retropsoas space.

Paravertebral Block

The complications that follow paravertebral nerve block could, to a large extent, be predicted from the topography of the site of the injection and, to some extent, can be prevented by due care and forethought. In somatic nerve block, there is a possibility of encountering the dura or a dural cuff and of producing spinal or epidural block.[73] This complication, although less likely, is also possible after paravertebral sympathetic block. Gay and Evans have reported two cases of total spinal anesthesia following paravertebral lumbar sympathetic block with local anesthetic.[54] They have pointed out that when the needle is perfectly situated near the sympathetic chain, injection of more than 10 ml of solution can cause a spread backward along the sympathetic rami to the epidural space. If the needle is not directed anteriorly enough, subarachnoid puncture may occur in the dural sleeve, or, possibly, some solution may diffuse through the dura.[53]

White has indicated that during paravertebral thoracic block, the risk of accidental intrathecal injection is greatest if the needle is passed over the upper border of the rib in a cephalad direction.[156] In sympathetic nerve block, the needle will be sited very close to the aorta or vena cava, and intravascular injection must be avoided. In both somatic and sympathetic block, the needle passes through a large bulk of muscle, and hemorrhage from vessels in the muscle is a hazard. Spread of local anesthetic solution within the psoas muscle sheath may lead to involvement of neighboring somatic nerves and yield temporary paresis and analgesia in the lower limb.

Finally, with paravertebral block in the L1 or thoracic segments, pneumothorax is a serious hazard. There has been a report of one death due to pneumothorax in an elderly patient with massive pulmonary metastatic disease and essentially no pulmonary reserve, even though the pneumothorax was promptly recognized and treated.[33]

The importance of absolute sterility must again be stressed. Wright reported a patient who, following a series of local anesthetic paravertebral somatic blocks, developed osteomyelitis of the spine with associated extradural abscess and spinal cord compression.[161]

Intercostal Nerve Block

In expert hands, intercostal nerve block is a remarkably effective and safe procedure. The most important (and most feared) hazard is pneumothorax, the incidence of which ranges from as little as 0.092 per cent to as high as 19 per cent, depending on the skill of the operator.[101]

Brachial Plexus Block

The brachial plexus bears a close relationship to the subclavian artery and vein, to the cupula of the pleura and to sundry small vessels and nerves. To the danger of inadvertently involving one of these structures must be added the risks from deliberate or accidental needle puncture of the trunks of the plexus during performance of the block. Burkhardt has reported neuritis and paresthesias in 16 patients following 1,054 supraclavicular brachial plexus blocks; in 14 patients, symptoms disappeared within 3 weeks, in two additional patients, recovery took 5 and 8 weeks, respectively.[13] The spinal cord is not inaccessible, and high epidural anesthesia and total spinal block have both been reported following brachial plexus block.[77,125] It is not surprising, therefore, that a number of different approaches are advocated, at least partly in the hopes of reducing the incidence of complications.

Supraclavicular Block. Harley and Gjessing found the following complications in 41 patients with supraclavicular brachial plexus block[65]: eight patients with Horner's syndrome, four patients with phrenic nerve block, 13 with arterial puncture, and two with pneumothorax.

The incidence of pneumothorax after supraclavicular brachial plexus block is stated to be 0.5 to 6 per cent; hemopneumothorax has also been reported by Hamelburg and Jacoby.[64,100] This method has also been reported to cause transient neurologic sequelae in about 5.7 per cent of patients.[93]

Axillary Block. In the axilla, the nerves from the plexus are enclosed in a sheath within which the solution is deposited. There is no hazard of pleural puncture or of phrenic nerve block, and direct needle placement in neural tissues is not required to locate the plexus. With axillary brachial plexus block, hematomas from inadvertent puncture of the artery are not uncommon but do not seem to produce sequelae.* Kirchoff reports two cases of paresthesias, one in the radial, the other in the ulnar nerve, lasting 3 and 6 weeks, respectively.*

The interscalene route has recently been advocated for brachial plexus block. The level at which interscalene brachial plexus block is performed renders pneumothorax an unlikely complication, and Winnie reported that the interscalene approach has not caused subarachnoid block, epidural block, vertebral artery injection, or phrenic nerve block "in many hundreds of cases"[158] However, Ward has encountered the following complications in 33 patients after interscalene brachial plexus block: one patient with hematoma, one patient with block of recurrent laryngeal nerve, two patients with unilateral phrenic nerve block, one with pneumothorax, and one with arterial puncture.[152] Hoarseness and Horner's syndrome have also been reported.[131]

Siler and colleagues have reported a patient in whom, following interscalene brachial plexus block, a carotid bruit developed and lasted for about 2.5 hours.[135] It has been suggested that narrowing of the carotid artery was caused by distension of the perineural sheath, of the brachial plexus, of the carotid, or of the wall of the carotid artery. It has been pointed out that such compression of the carotid artery might be dangerous in the elderly and those with arteriosclerosis.

Infraclavicular Block. It is said that the dangers of pneumothorax, phrenic nerve block, sympathetic block, epidural and subarachnoid block, and intravascular injection may be avoided by using the infraclavicular route to the brachial plexus, in which the needle is directed in a lateral direction under the midpoint of the clavicle.[117]

Block in the Head and Neck

The head and neck are liberally endowed with blood vessels and nerves, and nerve blocks in this part of the body must be performed with particular care and attention.

Inadvertent injection of local anesthetic into the cerebral subarachnoid space may occur during injection of cranial nerves, especially during gasserian ganglion block. Sudden loss of consciousness and respiratory paralysis may ensue. Two cases of abducens palsy have been reported; in the first it was considered that some of the anesthetic injected into the sphenopalatine fossa could have reached the abducens nerve by way of the inferior orbital fissure. Abducens nerve palsy has been recorded following local anesthetic block of the posterior branch of the second cervical nerve. It was thought that either the needle accidentally penetrated the dural sleeve of the second cervical nerve or the an-

* Kirchoff, J.: Personal communication, 1974.

esthetic solution infiltrated through the sleeve to produce the abducens palsy.[75]

The phrenic nerve may accidentally be involved in cervical blocks. While unilateral phrenic block is relatively innocuous in a healthy patient, bilateral phrenic paralysis may produce severe hypoxia in the presence of pulmonary pathology. Moore has reported two such cases in patients with pneumothorax in whom continuous oxygen was required for the duration of the block.[98] With phrenic nerve block itself there is the possibility of coincidental block of the vagus nerve, the sympathetic chain, and the recurrent laryngeal nerve.[42]

Another risk in cervical nerve blocks is puncture of the esophagus, which leads to dysphagia with tenderness at the site of the puncture and pyrexia and requires treatment with antibiotics.

Stellate Ganglion Block

The commonest complications of stellate ganglion block are accidental intravascular injection, recurrent laryngeal nerve block, brachial plexus block, and pneumothorax. Puncture of the dura sometimes occurs and should be avoided by keeping the trajectory of the needle toward the (palpated) tip of the transverse process. CSF pressure in the dural cuff is low within the intravertebral foramen so that there may be no flow of CSF to warn that the dura has been punctured. Hematoma formation is a nuisance but is not a hazard and requires no specific treatment. Partial brachial plexus block may occur after block with local anesthetic and is not serious—however, the patient should be reassured that the arm weakness is purely transient. If the needle is inclined too far medially, Horner's syndrome may appear on the opposite side, especially if a large volume of solution is injected.[153]

A not uncommon complication is pneumothorax due to puncture of the cupula of the pleura; it is especially liable to occur if the patient is emphysematous or if the needle is inserted in too caudad a direction. This hazard can be diminished by inserting the needle at C_6 (see Chap. 13).

Peng and colleagues have reported convulsions during stellate ganglion block, owing to inadvertent injection of lidocaine into the vertebral artery.[114] Moore has recommended the injection of a preliminary test dose (1–2 ml) of local anesthetic, which, if it was introduced into the vertebral or carotid artery, would cause dizziness, faintness, and nausea since the agent reaches the brain directly without the mixing that follows injection into a peripheral artery.[97]

Accidental subarachnoid injection in a patient with a traumatic cervical meningocele has been reported; the injection was followed by collapse, which responded to resuscitative measures.[74]

Accidental subarachnoid puncture has also been reported during stellate ganglion block with the anterior approach; Magora stresses the importance of the patient's keeping still during the injection.[51,86]

Dental Analgesia

Facial nerve palsy, immediate or delayed, is a complication of inferior dental nerve block and is thought to be due either to action of the local anesthetic on the facial nerve within the parotid gland or to a reflex spasm of the vessels that supply the nerve in the stylomastoid foramen region—recovery is always complete.[80] A case of hemifacial palsy has been reported after inferior dental nerve block.[145] The palsy was thought to be due to a sympathetic vascular reflex that resulted in ischemic paralysis.

Walsh reported two patients in whom blindness followed maxillary infiltration block with an oily solution of procaine; oily emboli reached the central retinal vessels.[151] Transient blindness has been reported following local anesthetic block of the inferior dental nerve and also of the superior dental nerve. The suggested mechanism was accidental intra-arterial injection in a patient with an anomalous vascular anastomosis between the external and internal carotid systems.[6]

Leopard has reported diplopia following local anesthetic block of the posterior superior alveolar nerve.[80] Three possible explanations were offered. First, diplopia might have resulted from block of the abducens nerve intra-orbitally—the needle having entered the inferior orbital fissure. Second, there might have been injection into the neighboring pterygoid venous plexus or, third, injection into the posterior superior alveolar artery.

Rood has reported temporary ptosis and diplopia following inferior dental nerve block; it is suggested this, too, might be due to accidental intravascular injection with retrograde flow to the orbital vessels.[122]

REFERENCES

1. Abouleish, E.: The inadvertent continuous spinal continued. Br. J. Anaesth., *46*:628, 1974.
2. Baker, A.H.: Lesion of the intervertebral disc caused by lumbar puncture. Br. J. Surg., *34*:385, 1947.
3. Bender, M.B., and Christoff, N.: Neurosurgical treatment of subdural haematomas. Arch. Neurol., *31*:73, 1974.
4. Berger, G., Tyler, C., and Harrod, E.: Maternal deaths as-

sociated with paracervical block anesthesia. Am. J. Obstet. Gynecol., *118*:1142, 1974.
5. Bizzarri, D.: Continual spinal anesthesia using a special needle and catheter. Anesth. Analg. (Cleve.), *43*:393, 1964.
6. Blaxter, P.L., and Britten, M.J.A.: Transient amaurosis after mandibular nerve block. Br. Med. J., *1*:681, 1967.
7. Bonica, J.J.: The Management of Pain. Philadelphia, Lea & Febiger, 1953.
8. ———: Principles and Practice of Obstetric Analgesia and Anesthesia. Philadelphia, F.A. Davis, 1967.
9. Bonica, J.J., *et al.*: Peridural block: Analysis of 3,637 cases and a review. Anesthesiology, *18*:723, 1957.
10. Boys, J.E., and Norman, P.F.: Accidental subdural analgesia: A case report possible clinical implications and relevance to "massive extradurals." Br. J. Anaesth., *47*:1111, 1975.
11. Braham, J., and Saia, A.: Neurological complications of epidural anaesthesia. Br. Med. J., *2*:657, 1958.
12. Brandus, V.: The spinal needle as a carrier of foreign material. Can. Anaesth. Soc. J., *15*:197, 1968.
13. Burkhardt, V.: The place of brachial plexus analgesia in modern anesthetic practice. *In* Recent Progress in Anesthesiology and Resuscitation. p.57. Amsterdam, Excerpta Medica, 1975.
14. Butler, A.B., and Green, C.D.: Haematoma following epidural anaesthesia. Can. Anaesth. Soc. J., *17*:635, 1970.
15. Cappe, B.E., and Deutsch, E.V.: A maleable core-tip needle for fractional spinal. Anesthesiology, *14*:398, 1953.
16. Catterburg, J., and Insausti, T.: Paraplejias consecutivas a anestesia peridural (estudio clinico y experimental). Revista de la Associacion Medica Argentina, *78*:1, 1964.
17. Chastain, G.M.: Acute blood levels of lidocaine following paracervical block. J. Med. Assoc. Ga., *58*:426, 1969.
18. Chen, C.J.: The perineural space of the peripheral nerve. MSc. Thesis, Magill University, 1945.
19. Cheng, P.A.: The anatomical and clinical aspects of epidural anesthesia. Anesth. Analg. (Cleve.), *42*:398, 1963.
20. Chun, L., and Karp, M.: Unusual complications from placement of catheters in caudal canal in obstetrical anesthesia. Anesthesiology, *27*:96, 1966.
21. Ciliberti, B.J.: Paraplegia following inhalation anaesthesia for subtotal gastrectomy. Anesthesiology, *9*:439, 1948.
22. Clarke, C.J., and Whitwell, J.: Intradural haemorrhage after epidural injection. Br. Med. J., *2*:1612, 1961.
23. Cope, R.W.: The Wooley and Roe case. Anaesthesia, *9*:249, 1954.
24. Cotev, S., Robin, G.C., and Davidson, J.T.: Back pain after epidural analgesia. Anesth. Analg. (Cleve.), *46*:259, 1967.
25. Craig, D.B., and Habib, G.G.: Flaccid paraparesis following obstetrical epidural anesthesia: Possible role of benzyl alcohol. Anesth. Analg. (Cleve.), *56*:219, 1977.
26. Crawford, J.S.: The second thousand epidural blocks in an obstetric hospital practice. Br. J. Anaesth., *44*:1277, 1972.
27. ———: Pathology in the epidural space. Br. J. Anaesth., *47*:412, 1975.
28. Crawford, J.S., Williams, M.E., and Veales, S.: Particulate matter in the extradural space. Br. J. Anaesth., *47*:807, 1975.
29. Cyriax, J.H.: Lumbar disc lesions. Acta Orthop. Belg., *27*:442, 1961.
30. Davies, A., Solomon, B., and Levene, A.: Paraplegia following epidural anaesthesia. Br. Med. J., *2*:654, 1958.
31. Dawkins, C.J.M.: An analysis of the complications of extradural and caudal block. Anaesthesia, *24*:554, 1969.
32. Dawson, B.H.: Paraplegia due to spinal epidural haematoma. J. Neurol. Neurosurg. Psychiatry, *26*:171, 1963.
33. de Krey, J.A., Schroeder, C.F., and Buechal, D.R.: Selective chemical sympathectomy. Anesth. Analg. (Cleve.), *47*:1968.
34. Defalque, R.J.: Exaggerated spread of epidural block. Anesthesiology, *28*:229, 1967.
35. DiGiovanni, A.J.: Inadvertent intraosseous injection—A hazard of caudal anesthesia. Anesthesiology, *34*:92, 1971.
36. DiGiovanni, A.J., and Dunbar, B.S.: Epidural injections of autologous blood for post lumbar puncture headache. Anesth. Analg. (Cleve.), *49*:268, 1970.
37. Downing, J.W.: Bupivacaine: A clinical assessment in lumbar extradural block. Br. J. Anaesth., *41*:427, 1969.
38. Dripps, R.D., and Vandam, L.D.: Hazards of lumbar puncture. J.A.M.A., *147*:1118, 1951.
39. ———: Long term follow up of patients who received 10,098 spinal anesthetics. J.A.M.A., *156*:1486, 1954.
40. Eckenhoff, J.E.: The vertebral venous plexus. Can. Anaesth. Soc. J., *18*:487, 1971.
41. Edelson, R.N., Chernick, N.L., and Posner, J.B.: Spinal subdural haematomas complicating lumbar puncture: Occurrence in thrombocytopenic patients. Arch. Neurol., *31*:134, 1974.
42. Eisele, J.H., Noble, M.I.M., Katz, J., *et al.*: Bilateral phrenic-nerve block in man. Technical problems and respiratory effects. Anesthesiology, *38*:393, 1973.
43. Elam, J.O.: Catheter subarachnoid block for labor and delivery: A differential segmental technic employing hyperbaric lidocaine. Anesth. Analg. (Cleve.), *49*:1007, 1970.
44. Eng, M., and Zorotovich, R.A.: Broken-needle complication with a disposable spinal introducer. Anesthesiology, *46*:147, 1977.
45. Epps, P.G.: A case of degeneration of the intervertebral disc following lumbar puncture. Proc. R. Soc. Med., *35*:220, 1942.
46. Finch, J.S., and Carter, S.H.: Isolated neurologic deficit following spinal anesthesia. Anesthesiology, *28*:785, 1967.
47. Finster, M., *et al.*: Accidental intoxication of the fetus with local anesthetic during caudal anesthesia. Am. J. Obstet. Gynecol., *92*:922, 1965.
48. Foldes, F.F., Colavincenzo, J.W., and Birch, J.H.: Epidural anesthesia: A re-appraisal. Anesth. Analg. (Cleve.), *35*:89, 1956.
49. Foldes, F.F., and Swerdlow, M.: The use and abuse of anaesthetic drugs. Pa. Med. J. *57*:1160, 1954.
50. Forestner, J.E., and Raj, P.P.: Inadvertent epidural injection of thiopental: A case report. Anesth. Analg. (Cleve.), *54*:406, 1975.
51. Forrest, J.B.: An unusual complication after stellate ganglion block by the paratracheal approach. A case report. Can. Anaesth. Soc. J., *23*:435, 1976.
52. Frumin, M.J., and Schwartz, H.: Continuous lumbar peridural anesthesia. Anesthesiology, *13*:488, 1962.
53. Frumin, M.J., Schwartz, H., and Burns, J.J.: The appearance of procaine in the spinal fluid during peridural block in man. J. Pharmacol. Exp. Ther., *100*:102, 1953.
54. Gay, G.R., and Evans, J.A.: Total spinal anesthesia following lumbar paravertebral block: A potentially lethal complication. Anesth. Analg. (Cleve.), *50*:344, 1971.
55. Gerbershagen, H.V., and Kennedy, W.F.: Herzstillstand nach hoher Spinalanaesthesie. Anaesthetist, *20*:192, 1971.
56. Gibbons, R.B.: Chemical meningitis following spinal anesthesia. J.A.M.A., *210*:900, 1969.
57. Gilbert, R.G.: Neurological complications of spinal anaesthesia. Can. Anaesth. Soc. J., *2(2)*:116, 1955.
58. Gillies, I.D.S., and Morgan, M.: Accidental total spinal analgesia with bupivacaine. Anaesthesia, *28*:441, 1973.
59. Gormley, J.B.: Treatment of post spinal headache. Anesthesiology, *21(5)*:565, 1960.
60. Graves, C.L., Underwood, P.S., Klein, R.L., and Ki, Y.I.:

Intravenous fluid administration as therapy for hypertension secondary to spinal anesthesia. Anesth. Analg. (Cleve.), *47*:548, 1968.

61. Greene, B.A.: A 26-gauge lumbar puncture needle—Its value in prophylaxis of headache following spinal anesthesia for vaginal delivery. Anesthesiology, *11*:464, 1950.
62. Grimes, D.A., and Cates, W.: Deaths from paracervical anesthesia used for first trimester abortion. N. Engl. J. Med., *295*:1397, 1976.
63. Grove, L.H.: Backache, headache and bladder dysfunction after delivery. Br. J. Anaesth., *45*:1147, 1973.
64. Hammelburg, W., and Jacoby, J.J.: Pneumothorax following brachial plexus. Anesth. Analg. (Cleve.), *38*:251, 1959.
65. Harley, N., and Gjessing, J.: A critical assessment of supraclavicular brachial plexus block. Anaesthesia, *24*:564, 1969.
66. Harrison, P.D.: Paraplegia following epidural analgesia. Anaesthesia, *30*:778, 1975.
67. Hart, J.R., and Whitacre, R.J.: Pencil point needle in prevention of post-spinal headache. J.A.M.A., *147*:657, 1951.
68. Hayman, I.R., and Wood, P.M.: Abducens nerve paralysis following spinal anaesthesia. Ann. Surg., *115*:864, 1942.
69. Hehre, F.W., and Muechler, H.C.: Complications associated with use of extradural catheter in obstetric anesthesia. Anesth. Anal. (Cleve.), *44*:245, 1965.
70. Hingson, R.A.: Continuous caudal anesthesia and analgesia in obstetrics. Int. Anesthesiol. Clin., *1(3)*:575, 1963.
71. Hohf, R.P., Dye, W.S., and Julian, O.C.: Danger of lumbar sympathetic blocks during anticoagulant therapy. J.A.M.A., *152*:399, 1953.
72. Joseph, S.J., and Denson, J.S.: Spinal anesthesia, arachnoiditis and paraplegia. J.A.M.A., *168(10)*:1330, 1958.
73. Joshi, S.M., and Hehre, F.W.: Peridural block complicating lumbar sympathetic block. Anesth. Analg. (Cleve.), *56*:873, 1977.
74. Keim, H.A.: Cord paralysis following injection into traumatic cervical meningocele. Complication of stellate ganglion block. N. Y. State J. Med., *70*:2115, 1970.
75. Kepes, E.R., and Foldes, F.F.: Transient abducens paralysis following therapeutic nerve blocks of head and neck. Anesthesiology, *38*:393, 1973.
76. Killian, H.: Lokalanasthesie und Lokalanasthetika. Stuttgart, Georg Thieme Verlag, 1959.
77. Kumar, A., Battit, G.E., and Froese, A.B.: Bilateral cervical and thoracic epidural blockade complicating interscalene brachial plexus block. Report of 2 cases. Anesthesiology, *35*:650, 1971.
78. Lall, N.G., and Sharma, S.R.: Clicking pneumothorax following thoracic paravertebral block. Br. J. Anaesth., *43*:415, 1971.
79. Leatherdale, R.A.L.: Spinal analgesia and unrelated paraplegia. Anaesthesia, *14*:274, 1959.
80. Leopard, P.J.: Diplopia following injection of a local anaesthetic. Dental Practitioner, *22*:92, 1971.
81. Löfström, B., Wennberg, A., and Widen, L.: Late disturbances in nerve function after block with local anaesthetic agents. Acta Anaesthesiol. Scand., *10*:111, 1966.
82. Lund, P.C.: Peridural Analgesia and Anesthesia. Springfield, Charles C Thomas, 1966.
83. Lund, P.C., and Cwik, J.C.: Modern trends in spinal anaesthesia. Can. Anaesth. Soc. J. *15*:118, 1968.
84. McGown, R.G.: Accidental marrow sampling during caudal anaesthesia. Br. J. Anaesth., *44*:613, 1972.
85. Macintosh, R.R., and Mushin, W.W.: Local Anaesthesia, Brachial Plexus. Oxford, Blackwell Scientific Publications, 1944.
86. Magora, F.: An unusual complication after stellate ganglion block. A case report. Br. J. Anaesth., *36*:379, 1964.
87. Mandl, F.: Paravertebral Block in Diagnosis, Prognosis and Therapy. New York, Grune & Stratton, 1947.
88. Marinacci, A.A.: Neurological aspects of complications of spinal anesthesia. Bull. Los Angeles Neurol. Soc., *24*:170, 1960.
89. Marinacci, A.A., and Courville, C.B.: Electromyogram in evaluation of neurological complications of spinal anesthesia. J.A.M.A., *168*:1337, 1958.
90. Marx, G.F., Cosmi, E.V., and Wollman, S.B.: Biochemical status and clinical condition of mother and infant at caesarean section. Anesth. Analg. (Cleve.), *48*:986, 1969.
91. Mersy, S., and Baradaran, J.: Accidental intrathecal injection of gallamine triethiodide. Anaesthesia, *29*:301, 1974.
92. Messer, H.D., Forshan, V.R., Brust, J.C., and Hughes, J.E.O.: Transient paraplegia from haematoma after lumbar puncture. A consequence of anticoagulant therapy. J.A.M.A., *235*:529, 1976.
93. Moberg, E., and Dhuner, K.: Brachial plexus block analgesia with xylocaine. J. Bone Joint Surg., *33A*:884, 1951.
94. Moir, D.D.: Recent advances in pain relief in childbirth: Regional anaesthesia. Br. J. Anaesth., *43*:849, 1971.
95. Moir, D.D., and Davidson, S.: Postpartum complications of forceps delivery performed under epidural and pudendal nerve block. Br. J. Anaesth., *44*:1197, 1972.
96. Moir, D.D., and Hesson, W.R.: Dural puncture by an epidural catheter. Anaesthesia, *20*:373, 1965.
97. Moore, D.C.: Stellate Ganglion Block. Springfield, Charles C Thomas, 1954.
98. ______: Complications of Regional Anaesthesia. Oxford, Blackwell Scientific Publications, 1955.
99. ______: Regional Block. ed. 4. Springfield, Charles C Thomas, 1965.
100. ______: In anestheriques locaux en anesthesie reanimation. Paris, Arnette, 1974.
101. Moore, D.C., and Bridenbaugh, L.D.: Intercostal nerve block in 4,333 patients: Indications, technique and complications. Anesth. Analg. (Cleve.), *41*:1962.
102. Moore, D.C., Bridenbaugh, L.D., Bagdi, P.A., Bridenbaugh, P.O., and Stander, H.: The present status of spinal (subarachnoid) and epidural (peridural) block. Anesth. Analg. (Cleve.), *47*:40, 1968.
103. Moya, R., and Smith, B.E.: Resuscitation of depressed newborns. Some clinical considerations. J. Med. Soc. N. J., *63*:552, 1967.
104. Muneyuki, M., Shirai, K., and Inamoto, A.: Roentgenographic analysis of the positions of catheters in the epidural space. Anesthesiology, *33*:19, 1970.
105. Nash, T.G., and Openshaw, D.J.: Unusual complication of epidural anaesthesia. Br. Med. J., *2*:700, 1968.
106. Nathan, P.W., and Sears, T.A.: Action of methyl hydroxybenzoate on nervous conduction. Nature, *192*:668, 1961.
107. Nelson, M.O.: Postpuncture headaches: A clinical and experimental study of the cause and prevention. Arch. Dermatol. *21*:615, 1930.
108. Noble, A.B., and Murray, J.G.: A review of the complications of spinal anaesthesia with experiences in Canadian teaching hospitals from 1959–1969. Can. Anaesth. Soc. J., *18*:5, 1971.
109. O'Connor, W.R., Preston, F.W., and Theis, F.V.: Retroperitoneal haemorrhage following lumbar sympathetic block during treatment with dicourmarol. Report of fatality. Ann. Surg., *131*:575, 1950.
110. Orkin, L.R., Papper, E.M., and Rovenstine, E.A.: The complications of stellate and thoracic sympathetic nerve blocks. J. Thorac. Surg., *20*:911, 1950.
111. Ostheimer, G.W., Palahniuk, R.J., and Shnider, S.M.: Epidural blood patch for post lumbar headache. Anesthesiology, *41*:307, 1974.

112. Pathy, G.V., and Rosen, M.: Prolonged block with recovery after extradural analgesia for labour. Br. J. Anaesth., *47*:520, 1975.
113. Payne, J.P., and Bergentz, S.E.: Paraplegia following spinal anaesthesia. Lancet, *1*:666, 1956.
114. Peng, A.T.C., Bufalo, J., and Blancato, L.S.: Rare complication during stellate ganglion block: A case report. Can. Anaesth. Soc. J., *17*:640, 1970.
115. Philip, J.H., and Brown, W.V.: Total spinal anesthesia late in the course of obstetric bupivacaine epidural block. Anesthesiology, *44*:451, 1976.
116. Phillips, O.C., Ebner, H., Nelson, T.A., and Black, M.H.: Neurologic complications following spinal anesthesia with lidocaine. A prospective review of 10,440 cases. Anesthesiology, *30*:284, 1969.
117. Raj, P.P., *et al.*: Infraclavicular brachial plexus block: A new approach. Anesth. Analg. (Cleve.), *52*:897, 1973.
118. Ratra, C.K., Badola, R.P., and Bhargava, K.P.: A study of factors concerned in emesis during spinal anaesthesia. Br. J. Anaesth., *44*:1208, 1972.
119. Redo, S.F.: Spinal complications following lumbar puncture. Surgery, *33*:690, 1953.
120. Rendell, C.M.: Chemical meningitis due to syringes stored in lysol. Anaesthesia, *9*:281, 1954.
121. Rice, G.G., and Dabbs, H.C.: The use of peridural and subarachnoid injection of saline solution in the treatment of severe post-spinal headaches. Anesthesiology, *11*:17, 1950.
122. Rood, J.P.: Ocular complication of inferior dental nerve block. Br. Dent. J., *132*:23, 1972.
123. Rosefsky, J.B., and Petersiel, M.E.: Perinatal deaths associated with mepivacaine paracervical block anesthesia in labour. N. Engl. J. Med., *278*:530, 1968.
124. Rosenbaum, H.E., Long, F.B., Hinchey, T.R., *et al.*: Paralysis with saddle block anesthesia in obstetrics. Arch. Neurol. Psychiat., *68*:783, 1952.
125. Ross, S., and Scarborough, C.D.: Total spinal anesthesia following brachial plexus block. Anesthesiology, *39*:458, 1973.
126. Saady, A.: Epidural abscess complicating thoracic epidural analgesia. Anesthesiology, *44*:244, 1976.
127. Sadove, M.S., Levin, M.J., and Rant–Sejdinaj, I.: Neurological complications of spinal anesthesia. Can. Anaesth. Soc. J., *8*:4, 1961.
128. Scarborough, R.A.: Spinal anesthesia from the surgeon's standpoint, J.A.M.A., *168*:1324, 1959.
129. Seigne, T.D.: Aseptic meningitis following spinal analgesia. Anaesthesia, *25*:402, 1970.
130. Selander, D., Dhuner, K.G., and Lundbörg, G.: Peripheral nerve injury due to injection needles used for regional anesthesia. Acta Anaesthiol. Scand., *21*:182, 1977.
131. Selzer, J.L.: Hoarseness and Horner's syndrome after interscalene brachial plexus block. Anesth. Analg. (Cleve.), *56*:585, 1977.
132. Shanks, C.: Epidural analgesia for post-operative pain. Med. J. Aust., *56*:399, 1969.
133. Shnider, S.M., Asling, J.H., Margolis, A.J., *et al.*: High fetal blood levels of mepivacaine and fetal bradycardia. N. Engl. J. Med., *279*:947, 1968.
134. Sikh, S.S., and Agarwal, G.: Postspinal headache: A preliminary report on the effect of inhaled carbon dioxide. Anesthesiology, *29*:297, 1974.
135. Siler, J.N., Lief, P.L., and Davis, J.: A new complication of interscalene brachial plexus block. Anesthesiology, *38*:590, 1973.
136. Snow, J.C., Kripke, B.J., Sakellarides, H., *et al.*: Broken disposable needle during an axillary approach to block the brachial plexus, Anesth. Analg. (Cleve.), *53*:89, 1974.
137. Solomon, H.C.: Raising cerebrospinal fluid pressure with especial regard to the effect on lumbar puncture headache. J.A.M.A., *82*:1512, 1924.
138. Spoerel, W.E., Thomas, A., and Gerula, G.R.: Continuous epidural analgesia. Experience with mechanical injection devices. Can. Anaesth. Soc. J., *17*:37, 1970.
139. Steel, G.C., and Massey–Dawkins, C.J.: Extradural lumbar block with bupivacaine (MarcaineLAC-43): A clinical trial in lower abdominal and perineal surgery. Anaesthesia, *23*:4, 1968.
140. Sunderland, S.: Nerves and Nerve Injuries. Edinburgh, Churchill Livingstone, 1978.
141. Swerdlow, M., and Brown, J.: The effects of extradural injection of dilute local anaesthetics. Br. J. Anaesth., *33*:642, 1961.
142. Teramo, K.: Foetal acid base balance and heart rate during labour with bupivacaine paracervical block anaesthesia. Journal of Obstetrics and Gynaecology of British Commonwealth, *76*:81, 1969.
143. Teramo, K., and Widholm, G.: Studies of the effects of anaesthetics on the foetus I: The effect of paracervical block with mepivacaine upon foetal acid-base values. Acta Obstet. Gynecol. Scand. (suppl.) *46*:23, 1967.
144. Thorsen, G.: Neurological complications after spinal anaesthesia and results from 2,493 follow-up cases. Acta Chir. Scand., *95*:21, 1947.
145. Tiwari, I.B., and Keane, T.: Hemifacial palsy after inferior dental block for dental treatment. Br. Med. J., *1*:798, 1970.
146. Urquhart–Hay, D.: Paraplegia following epidural analgesia. Anaesthesia, *24*:461, 1969.
147. Usubiaga, J.E., and Usubiaga, L.B.: Classificacao das sindromes—Neurologicas pos-anestesia raquidea e peridural. Rev. Bras. Anestesiol., *19*:518, 1969.
148. Vandam, L.D., and Dripps, R.D.: Exacerbation of pre-existing neurological disease after spinal anesthesia. N. Engl. J. Med., *255*:843, 1956.
149. ———: Long term follow-up of patients who received 10,098 spinal anesthetics. J.A.M.A., *161*:586, 1956.
150. Walpole, J.B.: Blood patch for spinal headache. A recurrence and a complication. Anaesthesia, *30*:783, 1975.
151. Walsh, F.B.: Clinical Neuro-ophthalmology. Baltimore, Williams & Wilkins, ed. 2. p.1202.
152. Ward, M.E.: The interscalene approach to the brachial plexus. Anaesthesia, *29*:147, 1974.
153. Warwick, J.W.: Stellate ganglion block in treatment of Meniere's disease and in the symptomatic relief of tinnitus. Br. J. Anaesth., *41*:699, 1969.
154. Weintraub, F., Antine, W., and Raphael, A.J.: Postpartum headache after low spinal anesthesia in vaginal delivery and its treatment. Am. J. Obstet. Gynecol., *54*:682, 1947.
155. Wenger, D.R., and Gitchell, R.G.: Severe infections following pudendal block anesthesia: Need for orthopaedic awareness. J. Bone Joint Surg., *55*:202, 1973.
156. White, J.C.: Technique of paravertebral alcohol injection. Surg. Gynecol. Obstet., *71*:334, 1940.
157. Wilkinson, W.M.: Two thousand spinal anaesthetics. Br. J. Anaesth., *35*:711, 1963.
158. Winnie, A.P.: Interscalene brachial plexus block. Anesth. Analg. (Cleve.), *49*:455, 1970.
159. Wishart, H.Y.: Pneumothorax complicating brachial plexus block. Br. J. Anaesth., *26*:120, 1954.
160. Wooley, E.J., and Vandam, L.D.: Neurological sequelae of brachial plexus nerve block. Ann. Surg., *149*:53, 1959.
161. Wright, R.L.: Septic complications of neurosurgical spinal procedures. Springfield, Charles C Thomas, 1970.

23 Complications of Neurolytic Neural Blockade

Mark Swerdlow

GENERAL CONSIDERATIONS

The performance of neurolytic neural blockade entails the general hazards described in Chapter 22, but, in addition, the introduction of irritating sclerosing substances involves risks that are generally longer-lasting and more serious than those caused by local anesthetics. This is especially so if the neurolytic agent inadvertently overspills the intended site or is unknowingly injected into an unseen hazard (*e.g.*, dural cuff).

Because the dose of neurolytic agent injected is much smaller than in the corresponding local anesthetic block, complications that result from overflow or spread of a relatively large volume of anesthetic are less likely. If the neurolytic solution, however, impinges upon a neighboring structure, the effects will be more long-lasting and destructive; thus, for example, overflow onto the brachial plexus while chemical stellate block is being performed may yield protracted sensory and motor loss in the arm. The prolonged duration of action of the agents must particularly be borne in mind when chemical nerve block is contemplated in patients with existing physical disabilities, especially neurologic or respiratory. In such patients, an unexpected complication caused by injection of local anesthetic might result in temporary difficulties and embarrassment, but the same accident produced by a neurolytic drug could prove serious. Thus, in a case reported by Peyton and his colleagues, paresis due to a spinal cord lesion was precipitated into complete paralysis by a subarachnoid injection of alcohol.[51] Similarly, inadvertent chemical phrenic nerve block could be dangerous in a patient with respiratory difficulty.

With regard to the effect on nerve tissue itself, Sunderland has stated that the neural damage sustained by injection of sclerosing substances varies in severity from rapidly reversible changes that cause only transient loss of function to permanent constrictive scarring in and about the nerve, sufficient to prevent recovery in the affected fibers.[62] The extent and severity of damage are influenced by such factors as the internal structure of the nerve at the site of injection, the amount of material injected, and its sclerosing properties. A further important risk is vascular damage caused by the neurolytic agent, especially damage to the vascular supply of the central nervous system (CNS).[63] Phenol has been stated to have an even greater affinity for vascular tissue than for brain (see also Chap. 5).[47]

In light of the dangers of chemical neurolysis, it is clear that with peripheral nerve blocks a preliminary injection of a test dose (1–2 ml) of local anesthetic is usually advisable, especially when there is doubt about which nerve is involved and whether blocking it will provide effective pain relief. Such prognostic blocking has the added advantage that it may provide the patient with a chance to evaluate possible side-effects. This is not always the case because the path taken by the needle in a subsequent neurolytic injection might not be identical, and a blood vessel, dural cuff, or pleura involved on the first occasion would not necessarily be involved during the subsequent neurolytic injection and, of course, *vice versa*.

Following neurolytic block, a day or two should be allowed to elapse before the degree of depletion of nerve function that has resulted is determined. After phenol, this depletion may not be as serious as appeared at first, perhaps because of the biphasic effect of the agent.[45] Thus, for example, phenol injected into the cisterna has been reported to have produced quadriplegia that "lasted for 30 minutes in full intensity, then gradually cleared."[75]

If a neurolytic solution does cause persistent unwanted nerve block, the nerve will regenerate in time (except for the optic nerve), and treatment should be aimed at relieving pain, preventing disuse atrophy, and reassuring the patient. To reduce the anxiety that the occurrence of a complication may cause the patient (and the anesthesiologist!) and to

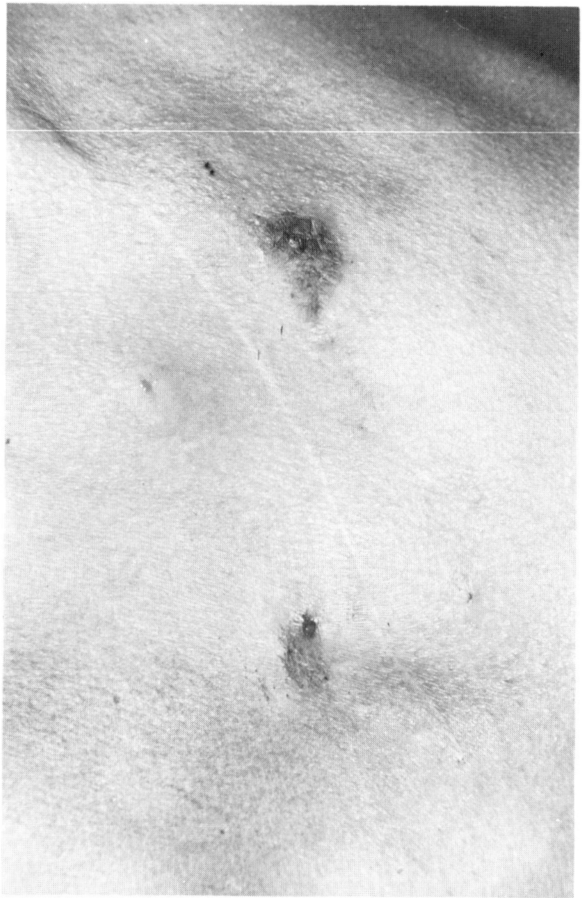

Fig. 23-1. Sloughing of a small area of skin over the chest after intercostal phenol block.

avoid legal action, it is well to explain the procedure and likely complications to the patient and to have a "consent" form signed *before* commencing treatment. Needless to say, if complications do occur, appropriate specialists should be consulted so that recovery and rehabilitation are as complete and expeditious as possible.

Injection of neurolytic solutions is sometimes followed by pain at the site of injection that lasts a few days and is presumably due to local tissue irritation. Persistence of the pain suggests the possibility of some complication such as a slough or sterile abscess formation. Chemical neurolysis may also be followed by a troublesome neuritis, especially after alcohol. If this is of moderate degree, it should be treated with appropriate analgesics; in more severe cases of neuritis, a somatic nerve block plus sympathetic block may be indicated, and occasionally the help of a neurosurgeon may be required.

Swelling, cellulitis, and sloughing of tissues have all been reported in perineural tissues, and May found that alcohol caused severe adhesions as well as neurolysis.[35] When the needle is being withdrawn following neurolytic block, there is a risk that some of the chemical will be left in the track of the needle with troublesome sequelae. It is advisable, therefore, to inject a little saline or local anesthetic as the needle is being removed. There is a special risk when a chemical is being injected at a superficial site (*e.g.*, intercostal block, neurolytic block for coccydinia); the dose at such sites should be minimal, and the needle should be flushed out with the saline during withdrawal. I had one patient with sloughing of a small area of skin over the coccyx after injection of 1 ml of 10 per cent phenol and a similar complication after intercostal phenol block (Fig. 23-1). Complete healing occurred eventually in both patients.

Intravascular injection should be avoided by aspirating repeatedly during injection of alcohol, phenol, or other neurolytic agents. Intravascular injection of 10 per cent phenol causes "severe tinnitus and flushing within a few seconds but recovery is rapid and complete."[53] Phenol stimulates the CNS causing muscle tremors and eventually convulsions.[14] However, absorption of large amounts of phenol will depress consciousness and blood pressure and cause renal damage.[16] Accidental intravascular injection of absolute alcohol results in effects that are "entirely pleasurable and will require no specific therapy."[7] However, intravenous alcohol may sometimes cause thrombosis of the vessel.

Neurolytic chemical agents are used for a more restricted and defined range of nerve blocks than local anesthetics, and this reflects, in part, the risks involved. Because of these risks, thermogangliolysis or neurosurgery rather than chemical neurolysis may be advised for specific nerves (*e.g.*, trigeminal ganglion, thoracic sympathetic ganglia).

SUBARACHNOID CHEMICAL BLOCK

Intrathecal neurolysis is undoubtedly a most valuable means of providing relief for intractable pain. However, the accessibility of the spinal nerve roots within the theca to injected fluids is a mixed blessing because unintended motor, sensory, and autonomic nerves may inadvertently be involved by the injected chemical (see Chap. 5). The complications that result are usually only temporary, but, as will be seen below, they sometimes persist and give rise to difficulties in patient management.

Table 23-1. Analysis of Agent Injected in Swerdlow's Series of 300 Patients Given Intrathecal Injections

Drugs Administered	*Number of Patients*
Phenol, 5% or 7% in glycerine	145
Chlorocresol, 1:50 or 1:40 in glycerine	138
Phenol and chlorocresol	17
Total	300

It is difficult to make any valid comparison among reported differences in incidence of the various complications because of the great individual variation in the patients treated. The majority of patients who undergo intrathecal neurolysis are suffering from pain due to malignant disease, and a number of factors may affect the incidence of complications. There are considerable between-patient differences in the size and position of the primary or secondary tumor that causes the pain and also in whether or not the patient has had radiotherapy. Furthermore, many of the patients already have some degree of sensory, motor, or autonomic impairment in the painful region of the body before the injection is given.[64] It is therefore difficult to conduct a comparative study of the complication potentiality of different intrathecal neurolytic agents other than to encompass a very large number of patients in the hope, thereby, of eliminating these variables. A further difficulty in assessing reported results is that the degree and duration of the complications are not always described.

The incidence of complications depends to a great extent on which part of the cord is being blocked and how many nerve roots are involved. Thus, paresis will be in evidence only when the cervicothoracic or lumbar cord is blocked, and bladder or rectal sequelae are very unlikely after subarachnoid blocks solely at the thoracic level. However, I had one patient who developed bladder paralysis after phenol block at T11 following three previous uncomplicated blocks at lower spinal levels and a second patient who developed bladder paresis after phenol block at T7.[65] The second patient had previously received extensive radiotherapy to the lower thoracic spine. On the other hand, Tank, Dohn, and Gardner, who administered 37 intrathecal alcohol blocks for intractable sacral plexus pain, report that half their patients suffered transient loss of bladder control and three had permanent loss, and Papo and Visca noted five permanent and 10 temporary interruptions of bladder function after phenol saddle block in 39 patients.[49,67] Finally, injection in the cervical part of the subarachnoid space entails the risk of respiratory arrest.[63]

The incidence of complications must, of course, be considered in relation to the quality of results obtained. A new agent or method that gave rise to an increased incidence of complications might be acceptable if it provided longer and more complete pain relief—it would certainly not be welcomed if it did not! These facts should be remembered in considering the following incidence of reported complications.

I have analyzed the complications that occurred in 300 patients who had received a total of 453 intrathecal injections at the Regional Pain Relief Centre, Hope Hospital (University of Manchester School of Medicine). All the cases, as detailed in Table 23-1, had been followed for at least 3 months or until death (if this occurred earlier).

Table 23-2. Complications That Lasted 72 Hours or Less

Drugs Administered	*Number of Patients*							
	Bladder Paresis	*Bowel Paresis*	*Muscle Paresis*	*Headache*	*Paresthesia*	*Numbness*	*Hyperesthesia*	*Others*
Phenol	7			5		7		Nausea
Chlorocresol	4		7	4	1	13	2	Backache, nausea (2)
Phenol and chlorocresol	2	2			1	2		Backache Involuntary movements of contralateral leg
Total	13	2	7	9	2	22	2	6

Table 23-3. Complications That Lasted Longer than 7 Days

Drugs Administered	Number of Patients					
	Bladder Paresis	Bowel Paresis	Muscle Paresis	Headache	Paresthesia	Numbness
Phenol	8	1	3		1	4
Chlorocresol	11	1	7	1	1	5
Phenol and chlorocresol	3	1		1		1
Total	22	3	10	2	2	10

Table 23-2 lists the complications that lasted for not more than 3 days. Of the total 300 patients:

48 had one or more complications that persisted more than 3 days; 21 of these patients had received more than one intrathecal injection

28 had one or more complications that persisted more than 1 week

19 had one or more complications that persisted more than 2 weeks

10 had one or more complications that persisted more than 1 month

Table 23-3 cites patients who had one or more complications that persisted for more than a week.

Nathan reported a 12 per cent incidence of sphincter disorder following intrathecal phenol.[44] Bonica found that vesical paralysis, rectal dysfunction, or limb paralysis occurred in 25 per cent of patients after subarachnoid neurolytic injection.[5] It has been claimed that phenol in isophendylate (Pantopaque) has a less injurious effect on bladder innervation, but Pantopaque may introduce complications of its own.[22,67] Interference with bladder function will necessitate the use of an indwelling catheter, while timely doses of carbachol may be both prognostic and therapeutic. The data provided by other publications on phenol are summarized in Table 23-4.[34,36,49,61,73]

With regard to the sequelae of alcohol injection, Derrick performed 685 intrathecal alcohol blocks in 322 patients, 18 of whom developed muscle weakness or bladder disturbance, two with permanent paralysis of both legs.[11] Wilber reports 485 subarachnoid alcohol blocks in 322 patients; the incidence of complications was 5.2 per cent (see also Table 27-4).[74]

Hand has reported the use of subarachnoid ammonium sulphate in 50 patients.[19] Transient complications were nausea, retching, and headache while paresthesias or a burning sensation occurred in 30.4 per cent of patients, especially when 500 mg was given, and lasted 2 to 14 days.

In view of the pain-riddled state of many of the patients who receive intrathecal neurolytics and the new sensations that the patient experiences immediately following the procedure, it is somewhat problematic whether subarachnoid alcohol some-

Table 23-4. Reported Complications of Intrathecal Phenol

Authors	Total Number Patients	Number of Patients					
		Bladder Paralysis	Bowel Paralysis	Headache	Paresis	Dysesthesia	Loss of Proprioception
Papo and Visca (1974)[49]	270	15			24		
Stovner and Endresen (1972)[61]	151	6	2	14	10	3	
Mark and colleagues (1962)[34]	30				4	4	4
White and Sweet (1969)[73]	26	2			6	2	
Mehta (1973; phenol or chlorocresol)[36]	55	8		2	10	27	

times causes alcohol neuritis. In one such possible case, Katz has suggested that the neuritis may have been caused by spilling of alcohol into the epidural space during the intrathecal injection.[27]

Meningismus is a rare complication of subarachnoid alcohol block.[4] Three to 4 days after the injection, the patient exhibits headache, neck rigidity, and pain over the vertebral column; the CSF pressure is found to be raised. Treatment consists of bed rest, removal of CSF and administration of appropriate analgesics. It has been suggested that the relatively scanty subarachnoid space in the cervical part of the spine could predispose a patient to a meningeal reaction there.[57]

Cauda equina lesion may, on occasion, be a sequel of intrathecal injection of alcohol, although the reported cases date from before the introduction of the autoclave.[56,70] Finally, posterior spinal artery thrombosis has been reported following intrathecal injection of phenol; the syndrome appeared on the second day and had practically cleared up a week later.[23]

Subarachnoid Hypertonic Saline

A number and variety of complications have been reported following intrathecal administration of hypertonic saline. Lucas and his colleagues have reviewed the adverse reactions encountered by a number of workers in a total of 2105 patients.[30] Complications of some degree occurred in 10.59 per cent of the patients; in 1.03 per cent there was "significant morbidity." Two patients treated by this method died as a result of myocardial infarction. It has been shown that during saline injection, sinus tachycardia or ventricular ectopic beats may be exhibited and that when the injection is administered intracisternally, sinus bradycardia may occur.[31] Hammermeister and Reichenbach suggested that intrathecal saline may excite a sympathetic discharge that could cause myocardial damage.[18] It would, therefore, appear inadvisable to employ this method in patients who suffer from cardiovascular or hypertensive disease.

Ventafridda and Spreafico have reported localized paresis lasting for many hours and paresthesias that sometimes persisted for weeks.[71] Transient hemiplegia has also been reported to follow subarachnoid hypertonic saline injection, and Thompson recorded a patient who developed pulmonary edema that responded to treatment with diuretics.[48,68] Hitchcock has stated that after cisternal injection of hypertonic saline, one patient developed pain in the ear and vestibular disturbances that persisted for some weeks.[20] Finally, persisting loss of sphincter control with sacral anesthesia has occurred in two patients who had "presumptive evidence of gross arteriosclerosis in the blood supply to the roots of the cauda equina."[6]

EXTRADURAL ANALGESIA

In theory, the extradural route should have advantages for the production of chemical neurolysis but there are relatively few reports of the results of this procedure or of its drawbacks.[9,65]

Epidural injection of alcohol may be followed by distressing neuritis, and there is a risk of inadvertent motor involvement. Impaired bladder function has also been reported following extradural administration of alcohol.

BLOCKS OF THE HEAD AND NECK

Trigeminal Nerve

Gasserian Ganglion Block. Because of the anatomical situation of the ganglion, gasserian chemical block is liable to be followed by a number of different complications, many of which are of serious import; indeed, Stender reports an 0.9 per cent fatality rate after alcohol blocks for trigeminal neuralgia.[60] The risks of diffusion of alcohol can be so serious that boiling water has been suggested as a safer means of destroying the ganglion cells, although new radiofrequency techniques now appear the best choice (see Chap. 15).[24]

Puncture of veins in the subtemporal region can cause hemorrhage, which spreads in the temporal fossa and cheek and should be controlled by firm pressure. Care, gentleness, experience, and a careful study of the anatomy all help, to some extent, to decrease the incidence of complications, as, it is hoped, will some more recent techniques.[46] In particular, in performing gasserian ganglion block the greatest care should be taken that there is no accidental movement of the needle tip once accurate placement has been assured; the dosage must be precisely checked, and the injection should be slow and controlled.

Some patients find the resulting anesthesia of the face a great disability, but they can be reassured that some sensation will return. A number of side-effects, which are usually neither grave nor lasting, are liable to follow shortly after the injection of alcohol. Thus, block of the paratrigeminal sympathetic fibers produces Horner's syndrome, which gradually diminishes, while involvement of the motor fibers of the trigeminal nerve will interfere with mastication.[8] The parasympathetic fibers of the third cranial nerve may be affected, giving rise to mydriasis with an irregular oval pupil that does not react to light. Block of the oculomotor nerve itself causes strabismus and diplopia, which usually fades in a few days. The abducens nerve is not uncommonly affected, and Ruge and colleagues have reported two patients with permanent lateral rectus palsy.[55] It has been suggested that the patient should be requested to move the eyes during the injection and that if signs of incipient muscle weakness become apparent, the injection should be discontinued.[46]

Involvement of other nearby nerves may be more serious. Thus, diffusion of solution to the eighth nerve causes loss of hearing, while involvement of the cochlear-vestibular nerve results in dizziness (aggravated by postural changes), nausea, vomiting, and nystagmus; the vestibular effects are usually short-lasting. Spread of alcohol may also occur in the space around the posterior root of the facial nerve; the facial muscles on the blocked side are paralyzed and the eye will not close; the prolonged inability to close the eyelid may result in corneal ulcer or keratitis. The facial weakness may prove to be temporary or permanent.[43,55] Corneal ulcers or keratitis may follow gasserian ganglion block because the nerve to the cornea travels through the ganglion. The corneal reflex is obtunded, which exposes the eye to trauma. If the ganglion has been blocked with chemical; therefore, long-term protection must be provided for the eye. In one reported series, keratitis occurred in 28 of 64 patients.[52] Cervical sympathectomy has been advocated in the treatment of keratitis.[12]

The later results of destruction of the ganglion can, according to Thurel, be divided into trophic disturbances and anesthesia dolorosa, and herpes simplex of the lips and delayed facial paralysis.[69] Trophic disturbances include mucous erosions in the mouth, nasal ulceration, keratitis, and facial "algae." These may result from trauma in an anesthetic area in the presence of diminished tissue resistance from neuromotor disturbances. Bactericidal ointments and the wearing of gloves at night are useful therapeutic measures. Anesthesia dolorosa and paresthesia in the numb area may follow gasserian ganglion alcohol injection; Sperling and Stender reported that 10 of 85 patients given ganglion block suffered later from burning pain in the blocked area, and Ramb had similar complications in four of 46 patients.[52,59] The use of a "drop-by-drop" method with positioning of the patient's head during injection has produced a diminution in the incidence of these complications. Jefferson's method of injecting the ganglion with 5 per cent phenol in glycerine (with the patient in a sitting position) appears to control even better the spread of the neurotoxic agent; of 50 patients reported by Jefferson, none developed either corneal ulceration or anesthesia dolorosa.[25]

Overflow onto the optic nerve may occur if the needle is directed incorrectly during gasserian ganglion block or supra- or infra-orbital nerve block. Chemical block of the optic nerve yields partial or total blindness, which may persist.[40,52] Overflow onto the glossopharyngeal nerve may also occur, resulting in dysphagia. Another complication that has been reported after gasserian ganglion block is osteomyelitis of the mandible.[55]

According to Labat, alcohol frequently causes an inflammatory reaction, which produces adhesions in the tissues around the ganglion—this may later render surgery difficult.[29] Labat considered that neurolytic agents should never be used in the retrobulbar area (*e.g.*, ophthalmic nerve, ethmoidal nerve block) because of the proximity of the optic, trochlear, and oculomotor nerves.[29]

Supraorbital Nerve Block. The dose of neurolytic solution injected should not exceed 0.5 ml because of the risk of diffusion into the orbit. If injected too superficially, it may cause sloughing of superficial tissues and skin overlying the nerve.

Maxillary Division Trigeminal Nerve. Neurolytic solutions must be used with caution when they are given extraorally. Not more than 1 ml of solution should be injected because excess may pass through the inferior orbital fissure into the orbit and damage the optic and oculomotor nerves, producing visual difficulties and even blindness. Alcohol block (or indeed surgical section) of the maxillary nerve at the foramen rotundum or of the infraorbital nerve can be followed by ulceration and sloughing of the cheek and ala of the nose or of the soft or hard palate (Fig. 23-2). I had one patient in whom a small area of ulceration occurred on the cheek following infraorbital block with 10 per cent aqueous phenol. Such damage usually occurs in the area innervated by the infraorbital nerve but Moore reports a patient in whom sloughing occurred in the posterior part of the superior ridge of the maxilla.[32,40,50] With ulceration of the cheek, stellate ganglion block may be helpful by improving the circulation.

Mandibular Nerve Block. As it emerges from the foramen ovale, the mandibular nerve contains motor as well as sensory fibers. Consequently, neurolytic block may result in paresis or paralysis of the muscles of mastication on the affected side, and the mandible may deviate from the midline. If a neurolytic solution is used, not more than 1 to 2 ml should be injected lest some solution pass upward and affect the gasserian ganglion. White and Sweet report one patient who developed permanent anesthesia dolorosa following alcohol block of the third division of the trigeminal nerve at the foramen ovale.[73] When trigeminal branch block is being performed by way of the mandibular notch, the facial nerve may also be involved. Finally, a fatality due to injury to the carotid artery in the cavernous sinus has been reported.[21]

Facial Nerve. Neurolytic agents should be used with the greatest caution in the facial nerve because they may cause permanent paralysis of facial muscles.

Glossopharyngeal nerve may be blocked near the stylomastoid process, but the vagus accessory and hypoglossal nerves are in close proximity and are at risk if neurolytic agents are injected. Montgomery and Cousins have recommended that glossopharyngeal nerve block should always be carried out under radiographic control.[39] Glossopharyngeal block causes dysphagia from paralysis of pharyngeal muscles, and it is recommended that unilateral block only should be performed.[1] Furthermore, neurolytic solutions may cause sloughing and fibrosis in surrounding tissues, and, in particular, the carotid artery and internal jugular vein may be involved with erosion or thrombosis. Facial nerve block may also follow chemical glossopharyngeal block distal to the jugular foramen.[54] Despite these hazards, surgery of the nerve is often not preferable to neurolytic block since patients who are candidates for this procedure are terminal or have severe systemic contraindication to surgery.

Cervical Nerve. Block of the cervical nerves should be performed with the greatest of care to avoid the risk of accidental intrathecal or intravascular injection. In addition, introducing the needle too deeply into the neck may result in involvement of the esophagus or of the spinal accessory nerve, causing paresis of the trapezius. Overflow onto the cervical sympathetic nerve will lead to Horner's syndrome; the patient may complain of ptosis or of nasal congestion.

Brachial Plexus. The use of neurolytic agents is not advised for the brachial plexus because of the risk of paresis or paralysis of muscles of the upper limb and because of the danger of erosion or thrombosis of blood vessels.

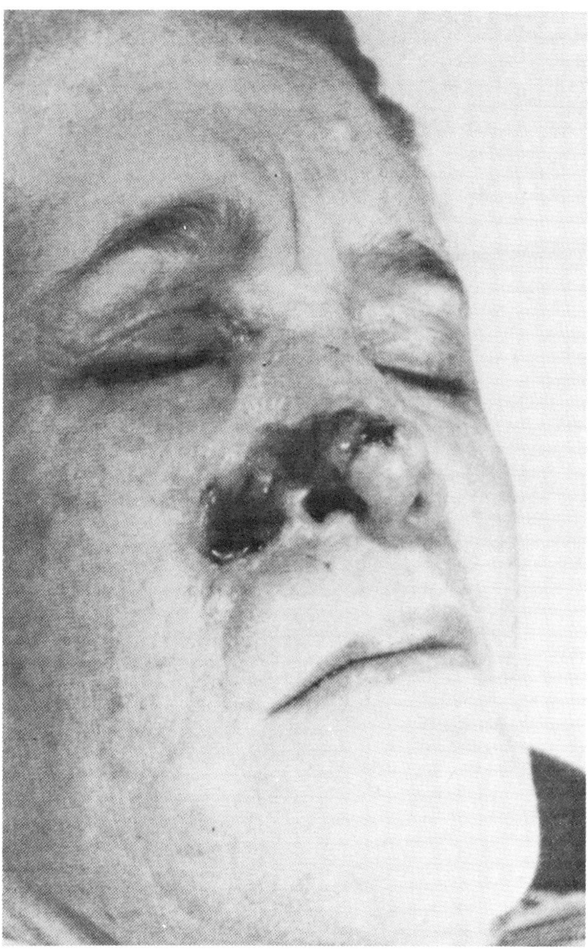

Fig. 23-2. Ulceration and sloughing of the cheek and ala of the nose after alcohol block of the maxillary nerve. (Macomber, D.W.: Plas. Reconstr. Surg., *11*:337, 1953)

Stellate Ganglion. Chemical block of the stellate ganglion carries the risks of prolonged Horner's syndrome and of possible involvement of the brachial plexus or of the recurrent laryngeal nerve. Recurrent laryngeal nerve block causes hoarseness and some difficulty in swallowing, but both are temporary and require no more than the reassurance of the patient. In addition to these risks, the solution may spread paravertebrally, which, in a case reported by Superville-Sovak and colleagues, gave rise to extensive extraspinal lesions and spinal cord infarction.[63]

Parastellate injections may reach the subarachnoid space, especially in the presence of enlarged or damaged dural root sleeves.[28] Intrathecal extension of a stellate injection is often heralded by severe headache and may cause respiratory arrest.[2]

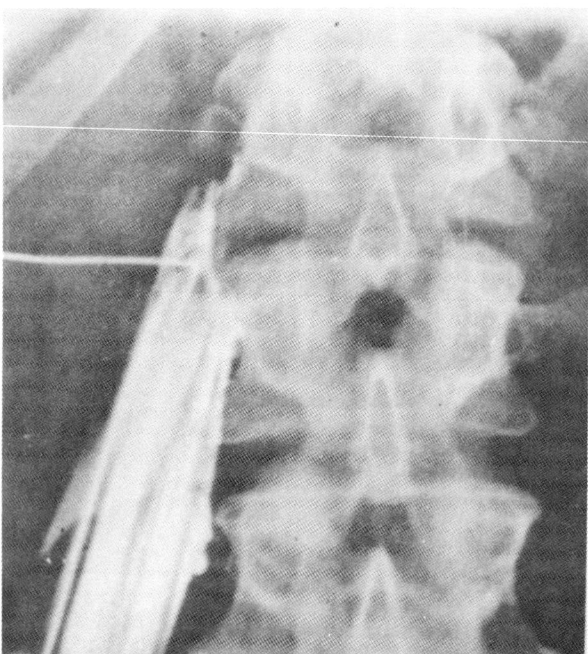

Fig. 23-3. Spread of phenol in the psoas sheath. (Feldman, S.A., Yeung, M.L.: Treatment of intermittent claudication. Lumbar paravertebral somatic block with phenol. Anaesthesia, *30*:174, 1975)

CHEMICAL ABLATION OF THE PITUITARY

The destruction of the pituitary by alcohol injected from needles inserted by the nasal transphenoidal route commonly results in diabetes insipidus, hypothyroidism, hypoadrenalism, and diminished libido.[42] In addition to these physiologic sequelae, Moricca has reported a number of complications, namely signs of meningeal irritation, rhinorrhea, ptosis, hemianopia, and diplopia, all of which he said are of short duration.[42] Headache and nasal hemorrhage may also be troublesome.*

INTERCOSTAL NEUROLYSIS

Injection of neurolytic agents onto intercostal nerves can be follwed by distressing neuritis, especially if alcohol is used. Another danger is of subcutaneous and cutaneous tissue sloughing.

If solutions of local anesthetic in oil or glycol are used, particularly in generous quantity, there is a risk of pleural irritation and effusion and nerve damage.[41]

PARAVERTEBRAL SYMPATHETIC BLOCK

Because of the anatomical position of the sympathetic chain, there is a genuine risk of the needle's entering the aorta, the vena cava, or the theca. Subarachnoid injection is a very serious hazard; the first complaint may be dyspnea or paralysis of the arms, and there is also a sharp fall in blood pressure.[7] It is important to remember that the dural cuff extends out of the intervertebral foramen, and it may accidentally (and perhaps unwittingly) be punctured while paravertebral nerve block is being performed; if a neurolytic solution is being injected, troublesome neurologic sequelae may well result. This emphasizes the added safety provided by radiographic confirmation of needle position.

Backache is a common sequel of lumbar paravertebral block and usually clears up in 24 to 48 hours. Less common and more troublesome is spillover of neurolytic agent onto intercostal nerves or onto paravertebral somatic nerves, in particular the genitofemoral and lumboinguinal nerves; this may cause motor or sensory loss.

Figure 23-3 shows how phenol spreads in the psoas sheath. Paravertebral spillover is usually the result of not having the needle point advanced far enough, but it may also be caused by drug spilling as the needle is withdrawn past the nerve. Because of the risk of adventitious neuritis, many workers and I prefer to use phenol rather than alcohol.[10,33] Reid and colleagues reported the complications encountered in 1666 injections of 6.7 per cent aqueous phenol onto the lumbar sympathetic chain. They found that 9 per cent of injections produced neuritis in the groin or the medial aspect of the thigh and occasionally the outer side of the thigh. Pain may be accompanied by hyperesthesia or numbness; the numbness may outlast the pain, which rarely persists more than 6 to 8 weeks although Miles and Rothman had one patient in whom neuritic pains in the thighs lasted over 4 months.[37]

Encroachment of the needle and injection into the abdomen are occasionally the cause of troublesome complications. Feldman and Yeung have reported one patient who developed transient abdominal pain and slight tenderness, due possibly to extraperitoneal spread of phenol.[13] Puncture of the kidney sometimes occurs and is recognized by a pendulum swing of the needle or by the escape of urine

* Lipton, S.: Personal communication, 1976

through the needle. Injury of the kidney may produce hematuria, renal colic, or dysuria, but in most cases the symptoms are transient and full recovery results. The ureter has also been involved following lumbar paravertebral block with 10 per cent phenol with subsequent sloughing and development of a urinary fistula in the loin.* Bilateral lumbar sympathetic block causes loss of ejaculation; impotence does not occur and the patient may not be sterile.

Pneumothorax is a not infrequent complication of upper thoracic block and has also been reported after high lumbar sympathetic block. Hemoptysis has occurred on a few occasions without sequelae.[53] Following paravertebral block of the highest sympathetic ganglia with alcohol, White has reported a patient with severe pleuritic pain that he considered to be due to alcohol leaking into the pleural cavity.[72] Molitch and Wilson reported a case of temporary Brown-Sequard paralysis following paravertebral injection of alcohol beneath the first rib for anginal pain.[38] The chemical may reach the spinal cord by way of an extended dural cuff of the perineural space or because of a misdirected needle. Intercostal neuritis, perhaps with hyperesthesia of the chest wall and medial aspects of the arm, is a not uncommon complication of paravertebral sympathetic block in the thoracic segments; it usually clears in a month or two.

Beddard has advised against the performance of lumbar sympathetic block in patients who receive anticoagulant treatment because this may "spread the necrosive action of the phenol"; he has reported a patient in whom "the greater part of the psoas muscle was found gangrenous at autopsy."[3]

CELIAC PLEXUS BLOCK

The anatomical position of the celiac plexus renders it susceptible to many hazards from nerve block.[66] Accidental subarachnoid or intravascular injection and pneumothorax are ever-present possibilities, as is the risk of hemorrhage. The dangers are accentuated by the relatively large volume of alcohol commonly injected. Spinal or paraspinal pain at the level of injection is not uncommon; it may be severe and last 24 to 48 hours and may be due to spilling of alcohol in the track of the needle. Spill of alcohol onto the first lumbar (somatic) nerve can give rise to neuritis.[26,33]

Hypotension commonly follows celiac plexus block and is usually well-compensated in younger patients. In the older and arteriosclerotic, however, postural hypotension may require bed rest and the use of an abdominal binder and elastic stockings for a few days. It has been suggested that preliminary local anesthetic block should be performed, and if an exaggerated hypotensive response results, alcohol block should not be given.[17]

Two cases of paraplegia have been reported following celiac plexus block with 6 per cent aqueous phenol. In one, vascular ischemia of the cord was thought to be the cause, although the possibility of injection of phenol into a dural cuff in the paravertebral region was not ruled out.[15] In the other, some of the phenol was thought to have entered the subarachnoid space.[58] Loss of ejaculation and also pleural effusion has been reported by at least one group (see Table 27-7). The use of radiologic control during the performance of this procedure will diminish the risk of some of these complications.

* Rose, S.S.: Personal communication, 1975

REFERENCES

1. Adriani, J.: Regional Anesthesia. Labat. ed. 3. Philadelphia, W.B. Saunders, 1967.
2. Adriani, J., Parmley, J., and Ochsner, A.: Fatalities and complications after attempts at stellate ganglion block. Surgery, *32*:615, 1952.
3. Beddard, J.R.J.: Twenty years' of clinical nerve blocking. Br. J. Anaesth., *30*:367, 1958.
4. Bonica, J.J.: Management of Pain. Philadelphia, Lea & Febiger, 1953.
5. ———: Diagnostic and therapeutic blocks: A reappraisal based on 15 years' experience. Anesth. Analg. (Cleve.), *37*:58, 1958.
6. Booth, A.E.: Intrathecal hypertonic saline. Proc. R. Soc. Med., *67*:772, 1974.
7. Challenger, J.: Sympathetic nervous system blocking. *In* Swerdlow, M. (ed.): In relief of Intractable Pain. Amsterdam, Excerpta Medica, 1974.
8. Crimeni, R.: Clinical experience with mepivacaine and alcohol in neuralgia of the trigeminal nerve. Acta Anaesthesiol. Scand. *24*[*Suppl.*]:173, 1966.
9. Debeule, F., and Schotte, A.: Nouvelle etapes dans la lutte contre la douleur. Alcoolisation paravertebrale et epidurale. Alcoolisation du plexus solaire. Rev. Belge. Sci. Med., *6*:357, 1934.
10. Dekrey, J.A., Schroeder, C.F., and Buechel, D.R.: Selective chemical sympathectomy. Anesth. Analg. (Cleve.), *47*:633, 1968.
11. Derrick, W.S.: Subarachnoid alcohol block for the control of intractable pain. Acta Anaesthesiol. Scand. *24*[*Suppl.*]:167, 1966.
12. Dott, N.H.: Facial pain. Proc. R. Soc. Med., *44*:1034, 1951.
13. Feldman, S.A., and Yeung, M.L.: Treatment of intermittent claudication. Lumbar paravertebral somatic block with phenol. Anaesthesia, *30*:174, 1975.
14. Felsenthal, G.: Pharmacology of phenol in peripheral nerve blocks; A review. Arch. Phys. Med. Rehabil., *55*:1, 1974.
15. Galizia, E.J., and Lahiri, S.K.: Paraplegia following coeliac plexus block with phenol. Br. J. Anaesth., *46*:539, 1974.

16. Goodman, L.S., and Gilman, A.: A Pharmacological Basis of Therapeutics. ed. 4. London, Macmillan, 1970.
17. Gorbitz, C., and Leavens, M.E.: Alcohol block of the celiac plexus for control of upper abdominal pain caused by cancer and pancreatitis. J. Neurosurg., *34*:575, 1971.
18. Hammermeister, K.E., and Reichenbach, D.D.: QRS changes, pulmonary edema, and myocardial necrosis associated with subarachnoid hemorrhage. Am. Heart J., *78*:94, 1969.
19. Hand, L.V.: Subarachnoid ammonium sulfate therapy for intractable pain. Anesthesiology, *5*:354, 1944.
20. Hitchcock, E.: Osmotic neurolysis for intractable facial pain. Lancet, *1*:434, 1969.
21. Horowitz, N.H., and Rizzoli, H.V.: Postoperative Complications in Neurosurgical Practice. P. 666. Baltimore, Williams and Wilkins, 1967.
22. Howland, W.J., Curry, J.L., and Butler, A.K.: Pantopaque arachnoiditis; Experimental study of blood as a potentiating agent. Radiology, *80*:489, 1963.
23. Hughes, J.T.: Thrombosis of the posterior spinal arteries. Neurology (Minneap.), *20*:659, 1970.
24. Jaeger, R.: The results of injecting hot water into the gasserian ganglion for the relief of tic douloureux. J. Neurosurg., *16*:656, 1957.
25. Jefferson, A.: Trigeminal neuralgia: Trigeminal root and ganglion injections using phenol in glycerin. *In* Knighton, R.S., and Dumke, P.R. (eds.): Pain. P. 365. Boston, 1966.
26. Jones, R.R.: Technic for injection of splanchnic nerves with alcohol. Anesth. Analg. (Cleve.), *36*:75, 1957.
27. Katz, J.: Pain theory and management. *In* Scurr, C.B., and Feldman, S. (eds.): Scientific Foundations of Anaesthesia. P. 226. London, Heinmann, 1970.
28. Keim, H.A.: Cord paralysis following injection into traumatic cervical meningocele. Complication of stellate ganglion block. N. Y. State J. Med., *70*:2115, 1970.
29. Labat, G.: Regional anesthesia technique and clinical applications. ed. 3. Adriani, J. (ed.): Philadelphia, 1967.
30. Lucas, J.T., Ducker, T.B., and Perot, P.L.: Adverse reactions to intrathecal saline injection for control of pain. J. Neurosurg., *42*:557, 1975.
31. McKean, M.C., and Hitchcock, E.: Electro-cardiographic changes after intrathecal hypertonic saline solution. Lancet, *2*:1083, 1968.
32. Macomber, D.W.: Necrosis of the nose and cheek, secondary to treatment of trigeminal neuralgia. Plast. Reconstr. Surg., *11*:337, 1953.
33. Mandl, F.: Aqueous solution of phenol as substitute for alcohol in sympathetic block. J. Int. Coll. Surg., *13*:566, 1950.
34. Mark, V.H., White, J.C., Zervas, N.T., Ervin, F.R., and Richardson, F.P.: Intrathecal use of phenol for the relief of chronic severe pain. N. Engl. J. Med., *267*:589, 1962.
35. May, O.: The functional and histological effects of intraneural and intraganglionic injections of alcohol. Br. Med. J., *2*:465, 1912.
36. Mehta, M.: Intractable Pain. London, W.B. Saunders, 1973.
37. Miles, E., and Rothman, J.S.: Experiences with the use of 10% aqueous phenol for chemical sympathectomy. Preliminary report. Am. J. Surg., *87*:830, 1954.
38. Molitch, M., and Wilson, G.: Brown-Sequard paralysis following a paravertebral alcohol injection for angina pectoris. J.A.M.A., *97*:247, 1931.
39. Montgomery, W., and Cousins, M.J.: Aspects of management of chronic pain illustrated by ninth nerve block. Br. J. Anaesth., *44*:383, 1972.
40. Moore, D.C.: Epidural anaesthesia. *In* Complications of Regional Anaesthesia. Springfield, Charles C Thomas, 1965.
41. Moore, D.C., and Bridenbagh, L.D.: Intercostal nerve block in 4,333 patients: Indications, technique and complications. Anesth. Analg. (Cleve.), *41*:1, 1962.
42. Moricca, G.: Chemical hypophysectomy for cancer pain. Adv. Neurol., *4*:707, 1974.
43. Mousel, L.H.:Treatment of intractable pain of the head and neck. Anesth. Analg. (Cleve.), *46*:705, 1967.
44. Nathan, P.W.: Control of pain. Ann. R. Coll. Surg. Engl., *41*:82, 1967.
45. Nathan, P.W., and Sears, T.A.: Effects of phenol on nervous conduction. J. Physiol., *150*:565, 1960.
46. Northfield, D.W.C.: The Surgery of the Central Nervous System. Oxford, Blackwell, 1973.
47. Nour–Eldin, F.: Preliminary report: Uptake of phenol by vascular and brain tissue. Microvasc. Res., *2*:224, 1970.
48. O'Higgins, J.W., Padfield, A., and Clapp, H.: Possible complication of hypothermic-saline subarachnoid injection. Lancet, *1*:567, 1970.
49. Papo, I., and Visca, A.: Phenol rhizotomy in the treatment of cancer pain. Anesth. Analg. (Cleve.), *53*:99, 1974.
50. Peet, M.M.: Major trigeminal neuralgia post-op. complications. Lewis's Practice of Surgery. *12*:48, 1954.
51. Peyton, W.T., Semansky, E.J., and Baker, A.B.: Subarachnoid injection of alcohol for relief of intractable pain with discussion of cord changes found at autopsy. Am. J. Cancer, *30*:709, 1937.
52. Ramb, H.: Die Alkoholinjektion ins Ganglion Gasseri bei der Trigeminusneuralgie. Dtsch. Med. Wochenschr., *74*:826, 1949.
53. Reid, W., Watt, J.K., and Gray, T.G.: Phenol injection of sympathetic chain. Br. J. Surg., *47*:45, 1970.
54. Rovenstine, E.A., and Papper, E.M.: Glossopharyngeal nerve block. Am. J. Surg., *75*:713, 1948.
55. Ruge, D., Brochner, R., and Davis, L.: A study of the treatment of 637 patients with trigeminal neuralgia. J. Neurosurg., *15*:528, 1958.
56. Sloane, P.: Syndrome referrable to the cauda equina following the intraspinal injection of alcohol for the relief of pain. Arch. Neurol. Psychiatr., *34*:1120, 1935.
57. Smith, M.C.: Histological findings following intrathecal injections of phenol solutions for relief of pain. Br. J. Anaesth., *36*:387, 1964.
58. Smith, R.C., Davidson, N.McD., and Ruckley, C.V.: Hazard of chemical sympathectomy. Br. Med. J., *1*:552, 1978.
59. Sperling, E., and Stender, A.: Tic Douloureux und Gesichtsschmerz (Therapeutische und Pathogenetische Betrachtungen) Dtsch. Zahn. Mund. Kieferheilkd., *173*:161, 1955.
60. Stender, A.: Excerpta Medica International Congress Series. Washington D.C., *36*, 1961.
61. Stovner, J., and Endresen, R.: Intrathecal phenol for cancer pain. Acta Anaesthesiol. Scand., *16*:17, 1972.
62. Sunderland, S.: Nerves and Nerve Injuries. Edinburgh, E. & S. Livingstone, 1978.
63. Superville–Sovak, B., Rasminsky, M., and Finlayson, M.H.: Complications of phenol neurolysis. Arch. Neurol., *32*:226, 1975.
64. Swerdlow, M.: 4 year's pain clinic experience. Anaesthesia, *22*:568, 1967.
65. ———: Intrathecal and Extradural Block. *In* Relief of Intractable Pain. 2nd ed. Amsterdam, Excerpta Medica, 1978.
66. ———: Peripheral nerve blocking in the relief of pain. *In* Lipton, S. (ed.): Persistent Pain. London, Academic Press, 1977.
67. Tank, T.M., Dohn, D.F., and Gardner, W.J.: Intrathecal injections of alcohol or phenol for relief of intractable pain. Cleve. Clin. Q., *30*:111, 1963.
68. Thompson, G.E.: Pulmonary edema complicating intrathe-

cal hypertonic saline injection for intractable pain. Anesthesiology, *35*:425, 1971.

69. Thurel, R.: Alcoolisation du ganglion de gasser. Complications tardives troubles trophiques et sympathalgies. Rev. Neurol., *104*:334, 1961.
70. Tureen. L.L., and Gitt, J.J.: Cauda equina syndrome following subarachnoid injection of alcohol. J.A.M.A. *106*:18, 1936.
71. Ventafridda, V., and Spreafico, R.: Subarachnoid saline perfusion. Adv. Neurol., *4*:477, 1974.
72. White, J.C.: Technique of paravertebral alcohol injection. Surg. Gynecol. Obstet., *71*:334, 1940.
73. White, J.C., and Sweet, W.H.: Pain and the Neurosurgeon. Springfield, Charles C Thomas, 1969.
74. Wilber, S.A. A discussion in L.H. Mousel. Anesth. Analg. (Cleve.), *46*:710, 1967.
75. Wilkinson, H.A., Mark, V.H., and White, J.C.: Further experiences with intrathecal phenol for the relief of pain. J. Chronic Dis., *17*:1055, 1964.

PART THREE

Neural Blockade in the Management of Pain

24 Neurologic Mechanisms of Pain: Modifications by Neural Blockade

Peter R. Wilson

Pain has most recently been defined as "an unpleasant sensory and emotional experience associated with acutal or potential tissue damage, or described in terms of such damage." [128]

The following is further noted:

> Pain is always subjective. Each individual learns the application of the word through experiences related to injury in early life. Biologists recognize that those stimuli which cause pain are liable to damage tissue. Accordingly, pain is that experience which we associate with actual or potential tissue damage. It is unquestionably a sensation in a part or parts of the body, but it is also always unpleasant and therefore also an emotional experience. Experiences which resemble pain, *e.g.* pricking, but are not unpleasant, should not be called pain. Unpleasant abnormal experiences (dysesthesia) may also be pain but are not necessarily so because, subjectively, they may not have the usual sensory qualities of pain.
>
> Many people report pain in the absence of tissue damage or any likely pathophysiological cause; usually this happens for psychological reasons. There is no way to distinguish their experience from that due to tissue damage if we take the subjective report. If they regard their experience as pain, and if they report it in the same ways as pain caused by tissue damage, it should be accepted as pain. This definition avoids tying pain to the stimulus. Activity induced in the nociceptor and nociceptive pathways by a noxious stimulus is not pain, which is always a psychological state, even though we may well appreciate that pain most often has a proximate physical cause.

This chapter deals primarily with the structure and function of nociceptive pathways, and the means by which activity in those pathways can be modulated. Where possible, reference is made to clinical experience. Most fundamental research has involved nociceptive systems of animals. It must be kept in mind that such research usually involves acute noxious stimuli in unphysiological settings and may not have direct application to chronic pain in humans. Similarly, questions of neuroantomy answered by animal models (including subhuman primates) may not necessarily apply to clinical cases. Despite these problems, animal models have contributed greatly to understanding human pain and continue to be needed to gain further knowledge.

Questions of human anguish and suffering receive less emphasis in this chapter, although these are important considerations in management of chronic pain syndromes (see Chap. 28).

Part 1: Anatomy and Physiology

It is necessary to determine the structure and function of nociceptive pathways in order to provide a framework for rational pain therapy. The discussion below begins with peripheral receptors and proceeds centrally to demonstrate the importance of different components of the nociceptive loop.

PERIPHERAL SENSORY RECEPTORS

There is some justification for classifying peripheral sensory receptors on structural grounds.[130] Some correlation between structure and function can be made for some of these receptors (*e.g.*, Pacinian corpuscles, Golgi-Mazzoni receptors, hair follicle receptors, Meissner corpuscles, Merkel "touch spots," and Ruffini endings). These are presumed to be simple, encapsulated nerve endings, which could possibly perform mechanoreceptor function. There are also more complex structures in skin, and also nerve endings that are apparently bare. However, there are no anatomic structures defined for most cutaneous sensory functions.[302] Mechanisms of transduction are not understood for

Table 24-1. Human Peripheral Receptors*

Receptor Type	*Best Stimulus*	*Signal*	*Conduction Velocity (m/sec)*
Cutaneous mechanoreceptors			
Type I	Indentation of skin (dome receptors)	Displacement & velocity	≃60
Type II	Skin deformation	Displacement & velocity	≃45
Meissner corpuscle	Skin indentation	Velocity	≃55
Pacinian corpuscle	Pressure changes	Vibration	≃50
Warm	Increased temp.	Warming	≃ 0.5
Cutaneous nociceptors			
C Polymodal)	(Noxious heat	Threat or damage	≃ 1†
)	(Mechanical damage		
C Mechanical)	(Algesic chemicals		
C Cold)	(Extreme cold		
Aδ mechanical)	(Noxious heat	Threat or damage	≃17†
Aδ heat)	(Mechanical damage		
Aδ cold)	(Algesic chemicals		

* The following nociceptors are described in various animals, and may be assumed to be present in humans: muscle nociceptors—Group III and IV; joint nociceptors—?Aδ and C; visceral nociceptors—?Aδ and C
† Data from Dyck and colleagues[84]; and Torebjörk[270]
(Price, D. D., and Dubner, R.: Neurons that observe the sensory discriminative aspects of pain. Pain, *3*: 307, 1977; Willis, W. D., Coggeshall, R. E.: Sensory Mechanisms of the Spinal Cord. New York, Plenum Press, 1978)

any somatosensory receptor, although Pacinian corpuscles may function by a lamellar-axon interaction.[245]

Classification of cutaneous receptors on functional grounds is more useful. Cutaneous mechanoreceptors in human skin (and presumably mechanoreceptors elsewhere) are supplied by large myelinated fibers, with conduction velocities of 30 to 60 m per second. Primate cutaneous receptors with afferent fiber conduction velocities less than 30 m per second have been grouped according to their optimal peripheral stimulus. Data for human receptors appear above (Table 24-1).[226,302]

Cutaneous nociceptors are supplied by fine myelinated (Aδ) and unmyelinated (C) fibers. A comprehensive study cannot be made in man, but animal studies suggest that nociceptors have two distinguishing features:[225] high threshold to all natural stimuli compared with other receptors in the same tissue; and progressively augmenting response to repeated or increasingly noxious stimuli (sensitization).

Recordings have been made from human nerves during skin stimulation by electric shocks, heat[272,273] and chemicals applied to blister bases.[65] In all cases, pain was experienced when activity in Aδ and C fibers reached a certain level. Sensitization has been produced by a number of chemicals: bradykinin (or other polypeptides), a prostaglandin, histamine, and serotonin. This sensitization (and nociceptor firing rate) could be reduced by antiinflammatory drugs such as indomethacin and aspirin.[140,160] Sensitization of receptors by heating to mechanical stimulation has been demonstrated in human skin also.[274]

There is a profusion of naturally-occurring toxins that can produce pain: This subject has been comprehensively reviewed by Chahl and Kirk.[44] Despite this large number, they can be grouped by about 10 major classifications. The possibility that a single cutaneous receptor may exist was indirectly suggested by the report of Janscó and colleagues.[135] They observed that capsaicin applied to the skin produced burning pain. However, repeated applications were painless. Other mechanical sensations were apparently unimpaired. It has been shown recently that this treatment depletes fine cutaneous nerve endings of substance P, an 11-amino acid peptide.[63] It is tempting to speculate that noxious cutaneous thermal and chemical transduction involves release of substance P. Additional evidence has also been presented that substance P is present in tooth

Table 24-2. Types of Peripheral Neuropathies

Peripheral Neuropathy	*Pathologic Anatomy*	*Pathological Physiology*	*Clinical Example*
I	Selective decrease in large myelinated fibers	Loss of touch—pressure; 2-point discrimination	Friedreich's ataxia
II	Selective decrease in unmyelinated and small myelinated fibers	Loss of pain, warm and cold, autonomics	Dominantly inherited amyloidosis
III	All fibers lost	Loss of touch—pressure, 2-point discrimination, pain, warm and cold	Hereditary sensory radicular neuropathy
NIL (CNS disease)	Normal fibers	Loss of touch—pressure, 2-point discrimination, pain, warm and cold	Tabes dorsalis

pulp, and is released by painful electrical stimulation to the pulp.

It is clear that mechanisms of cutaneous nociception are poorly understood. Much more information is needed before techniques for specific blockade of nociceptive information at the periphery become available. Also, surprisingly, little is known about anatomical pathways and mechanisms of visceral pain.

There has been a controversy about "specificity" within the somatosensory system.[200] The "specificity theory" assigned a particular psychophysical response to the activity of a particular receptor and its specific neural pathway. On the other hand, the "pattern theory" proposed that temporal and spatial patterns of afferent impulses signaled peripheral events. Neither of these theories can account for all described phenomena. For example, Perl described increasing sensitivity of certain peripheral receptors to repeated thermal stimuli:[225] Heat sensitization was incompatible with either theory.

Wall has reevaluated the concept of specificity in the light of such data.[290] He stated that there are two completely different uses of the word "specificity": diagnostic and prognostic. The diagnostic use is appropriate when discussing responses of individual receptors and nerve fibers. It can be shown that under defined conditions, there is a fixed and specific relationship between stimulus and response. The prognostic use purports to be able to predict the psychophysical consequences of activity in a particular nerve. There is not necessarily a fixed relationship between the electrical activity in a nerve fiber and perceived sensation.[270,271] Single-fiber studies in humans indicated that sensation of touch is dependent on activity in thick myelinated nerve fibers.[22,81,109] Cold and pricking pain depends on Aδ fibers, and heat and delayed pain on C fibers. Pressure on peripheral nerves blocked activity in large fibers first, with early impairment of tactile and vibratory stimuli. Differential nerve blocks showed that small-diameter fibers were more susceptible than large fibers. Perception of pain was decreased before all other modalities except temperature. This is of obvious significance in neural blockade (see Table 24-2).

It is clear that there are a number of peripheral receptors that are capable of signaling stimulation of skin by noxious mechanical, thermal, or chemical events. Peripheral receptors may have certain specificity, but nociceptors are often polymodal, responding to more than one form of noxious stimulus. Mechanisms of transduction are unknown, but substance P and noradrenaline are likely to be involved. Nociceptive information is transmitted in peripheral nerves by way of the fine myelinated Aδ fibers and unmyelinated C fibers. Structure, function and connections of muscle, joint, and visceral nociceptors are yet to be determined.

PERIPHERAL NERVES

Compound action potentials of peripheral nerves were first described by Gasser and Erlanger in 1927. It was recognized that nerve fibers had differential sensitivity to cocaine and other local anesthetics, related to their size.

Dyck and colleagues measured sensation by quantitative methods and attempted to correlate these findings with histological appearance of nerve fibers.[84] Conduction and morphometric studies in a number of patients with various neurologic diseases led to a revision of the classical view of peripheral neural function. Dyck and colleagues described three types of sensory loss in disorders affecting primary afferent neurons: Types I, II and III peripheral neuropathies (see Table 24-2). They concluded from their studies that pain and temperature fibers in cutaneous nerves of man were contained in the $A\delta$ and C groups, while the high sensitivity fibers for touch-pressure and two-point discrimination were in the $A\alpha$ group.

These studies have shown that "pain" messages are transmitted by $A\delta$ and C fibers. These fibers have widely different conduction velocities. Human sural nerve has been shown to have $A\delta$-fiber conduction velocities of 10 to 27 m per second (mean = 17) and C-fiber velocities of 1.0 to 1.8 m per second (mean = 1.4).[84] Both fiber groups transmit nociceptive information: C-fiber activity would be appreciated as much as 1.5 seconds later than $A\delta$ activity. It can be argued from this that the terms "first" and "second" pain have physiological justification.[230]

The question of whether sensation other than pain can be transmitted by C fibers in humans has been addressed in a recent review by Mumford and Bowsher.[210] They reported that nonpainful sensations were able to be elicited from tooth pulp, cornea, and skin in its early stages of repair. Electrical stimulation of teeth in human subjects caused pain. Threshold stimulation caused other sensations such as coldness, heat, pins and needles, and tingling. They also defended the use of the term "protopathic" for the ill-defined sensory experiences evoked by the activation of small primary afferent fibers in the absence of large fiber activity. There can be no justification for the use of this term in its original context, with "epicritic," to describe two divisions of the peripheral nervous system.[302] LaMotte and Campbell have also shown that C fibers transmit thermal information, as well as nociception.[171] C-fiber firing frequency may encode intensity of stimulation.

Correlations between nerve lesions and presence (or absence) of pain are not simple. Pain occurs in various peripheral neuropathies[82,83,268] but causes are usually not known. There are also apparent paradoxes. Pain in Fabry disease has been reported to be associated with selective decrease in small myelinated and unmyelinated peripheral nerve fibers.[220] Pain in other neuropathies has been shown to be associated with acute breakdown of myelinated fibers.[85] It is clear that mechanisms involved in producing pain have yet to be determined.

Coding in Peripheral Nerves

Concepts of information transmission in the nervous system constitute a problem that is also not solved. A stimulus has four dimensions: position in space, temporal behavior, amplitude, and modality.[260] This information has to be transmitted to the CNS for processing. Peripheral axons transmit binary digital information from specific anatomical locations. Activity in peripheral axons usually defines whether a stimulus is perceived or not ("signal" or "noise"). The question of amplitude discrimination has been unanswered since 1846, when Weber described the logarithmic relationship between stimulus amplitude and perception response. Coding of information about the stimulus occurs at the site of transduction in the periphery. Demodulation-decoding must begin to occur at the first relay (*e.g.,* in spinal cord dorsal horn).[286] There is a limit to the number of bits of information able to be carried along a nerve by a succession of action potentials.[260] This information must be coded as a frequency-modulated signal (action potential amplitudes and duration are identical, and an unstimulated receptor is silent). Problems related to somatic sensation have been discussed by Kenton and colleagues, who have shown temperature dependence of some mechanoreceptors.[143] This work showed that certain receptors changed their firing rate in response to a certain pressure if test probe temperature was altered. It raises difficult questions about the encoding process. There are similar problems of transduction, encoding, and decoding in other sensory systems, and these are similarly unresolved.

Animal Models of Chronic Pain

There is no entirely satisfactory animal model of chronic pain.[293] Usefulness of such a model is obvious, but there are ethical objections to such research. Wall stated that it was unacceptable "to perform experiments where the animal was unable to indicate or arrest the onset of suffering."[288] Criteria proposed by Sternbach were as follows: "i) the pain stimuli must be above threshold, but below tolerance, as judged by ii) the animals ability initially to continue such usual activities as eating, sleeping, grooming and sexual behaviours. . . ."

There have been a number of attempts to induce chronic pain in animals. Applications of toxins (*e.g.*, tetanus toxin, strychnine) and chemicals (*e.g.*, KCl, penicillin, and ouabain) in agar (for prolonged release) to spinal cord led to severe self-mutilation by the animal[166] and would fall outside the above guidelines. Other models of experimental central chronic pain have included intraspinal alumina injections,[181] generation of localized trigeminal epileptic foci,[23] and dorsal rhizotomy.[183] Peripheral origin of chronic pain has been induced by adjuvant arthritis.[57]

Amplitude is a difficult concept to bring to a discussion of the physiology of pain. In animal experiments, motor responses (avoidance, withdrawal, or vocalization) have to be used to determine the threshold of stimulus (*e.g.*, heat, cold, pressure) that is presumably "painful": that magnitude of stimulus sufficient to evoke escape behavior on a certain percentage of occasions.

Experimental Pain in Humans

Signal detection theory (sensory decision theory) has been applied to studies of pain threshold in humans. Its place in clinical and laboratory pain research, having its proponents[46] and detractors,[243] is undetermined. It describes the ability of a subject to discriminate between painful and nonpainful stimuli, to determine whether a painful stimulus has occurred. It is also said to allow an estimate of the magnitude of a painful stimulus. It is not applicable to animal studies, which rely on observable behavioral responses (reflex or learned) to a particular stimulus. Such responses may be highly reproducible (*e.g.*, hot plate and tail flick tests[322]), which is not the case in humans, whose verbal and behavioral responses may be altered by numerous psychological factors.

Estimation of pain threshold and tolerance in humans is difficult and unreliable, and results may depend on the nature of the test and site tested. Lynn and Perl used pinprick, pinch, and heat and cold on the neck, abdomen, and thigh.[185] They found that the neck was most sensitive to cold, the abdomen to heat, and the thigh least sensitive to all tests. They also found a barely statistically significant tendency for subjects relatively sensitive on one test to be also relatively sensitive on other tests. Correlation coefficients between any two tests in the same subject ranged from an r of 0.10 (pinch vs. cold) to an r of 0.56 (pinprick vs. cold). For all four tests at the three sites, the average correlation was 0.25, not significantly different from zero.

There are major problems in assessing response to neural blockade and other therapies in acute and chronic pain and also that to clinical and experimental pain. Attempts to achieve reliable quantification have included questionnaires,[62,195] verbal rating scales,[3,12] and visual analogue scales.[219,240,247] Questionnaires and verbal scales rely on a high fluency in English (there are 78 adjectives in the McGill Questionnaire, 87 in another.[175] Using such semantics, it has been suggested that pain has three dimensions:[198] *quality*—sensory qualities of temporal, spatial, nature of perceived stimulus; *quantity*—evaluative qualities that describe the subjective overall intensity of the pain experience; *emotion*—affective properties related to the fear, tension, autonomic effects, and punitive aspects.

Despite these problems, such questionnaires have been shown to have good reliability.[77] In psychophysical testing using hand-grip strength, Gracely and colleagues showed that ratio scales of sensory and affective verbal pain descriptors were valid, reliable, and objective.[102] They also showed that their verbal scales were reliable for description of electrical stimulation of skin. In an important subsequent experiment, they showed that intravenous diazepam (5 mg) significantly lowered affective descriptor responses without altering sensory descriptor or handgrip responses.[103] However, they make the cautionary point that their subjects were balanced for sex, age, and education, all of which may alter responses and attitudes to pain. Socioeconomic status and ethnic origin may also affect responses, as may anxiety,[283] depression, family dynamics and marital adjustment.[207]

In view of these often insurmountable problems, there is a requirement for objective measurement of pain. There is initial evidence that endorphin levels in human cerebrospinal fluid (CSF) may contribute to pain threshold and tolerance.[6,284] Patients with chronic somatogenic pain had levels of "endorphin" that tended to be lower than those of patients with predominantly psychogenic pain. Evidence of biochemical changes induced by pain is contained in a report that nonesterified fatty acids in serum increased by about 40 per cent in patients undergoing trigeminal ganglion destruction.[163]

Electrophysiological events related to sensory stimulation are also under investigation. Somatosensory evoked potentials recorded from scalp have been shown to be related to peripheral events.[47,60] There are overall similarities of wave form, latency, and amplitude. In a systematic study of scalp potentials evoked by electrical dental stimulation, Chen and colleagues demonstrated a relationship between subjective painfulness and amplitudes of the second negative-positive wave (N175 − P260 m/sec, r = 0.63) and following positive-negative wave (P260 − N340 m/sec, r = 0.65).[47] These later waves possibly represent psychological evaluation processes.

Unfortunately, other tests of pain threshold and tolerance do not measure or predict responses to pain with great accuracy.[105,208,223] It has been shown that present measures and tests of clinical and experimental pain are not highly reliable. Electrophysiological and biochemical measures are also crude and nonspecific at present. There is a need for continuing research in these fields before pain responses can be adequately quantitated for accurate assessment of experimental and therapeutic maneuvers.

Central Mechanisms

Dorsal Root Ganglion. Cell bodies of primary afferent fibers are contained in dorsal root ganglia and trigeminal sensory ganglia. Several types of cell (cyton) are described and reviewed by Willis and Coggeshall.[302] Large cytons give rise to large myelinated fibers, and small cytons supply small myelinated and unmyelinated fibers. There is not a clear division into these two groups. An extensive morphometric analysis of human dorsal root ganglia (first sacral[221]) has defined their composition. Each contained some 60,000 cytons, 15 to 110 μm in diameter with a nonstandard distribution. Most were 35 to 40 μm in diameter.

Dorsal root ganglia cytons may be divided into two groups using immunohistochemical criteria. Substance P has been shown in small cells of dorsal root ganglia.[121,122] It was also shown in peripheral and central branches of these primary afferent transmitters. This suggests that there are at least two functional classes of dorsal root ganglia cells.

Dorsal root ganglion cell bodies usually do not initiate primary afferent transmission de novo. Activity begins in peripheral processes, and action potentials travel centrally. These travel past dorsal root ganglion cells, which they may depolarize[176] before entering dorsal horn layers. Sensory axons may branch within dorsal roots.[173] Dorsal root ganglion cells are not normally sources of afferent impulses.[181] Under certain experimental conditions (*e.g.*, scarring with alumina), they may become mechanosensitive and as sources of additional sensory input.

Spinal Nerve Roots

Dorsal Root. Axons from peripheral somatic nerves enter the spinal cord by way of dorsal roots. There is known to be dermatomal distribution of dorsal roots.[69] Such dermatomes are not fixed in size. Overlapping of primary afferent fibers occurs within dorsal horn.[17,115] Axons in any particular dorsal root may extend over five (or more) spinal cord segments. This implies that any point on the body is innervated by fibers from five dorsal roots. This is only evident if neighboring dorsal roots are sectioned, if Lissauer's tract is sectioned, or if strychnine is given.[69] In clinical practice, an area of skin is supplied by two adjoining dorsal roots (see Chap. 27).

There may be some segregation of large and small fibers as they enter the dorsal horn. Large fibers enter dorsal columns, with collaterals also to dorsal horn. Lissauer reported that fine fibers entered separately to form a longitudinal tract that now bears his name.[179] Lissauer's tract (dorsolateral fasciculus) contains a majority of fine primary afferent fibers[49,152] and fibers from substantia gelatinosa.[202] Comparative studies have shown some species differences, with no segregation of fine fibers in cats, but some in monkeys.[255] A similar conclusion was reached by Carlstedt,[40] who described C fibers (their ventrolateral aspects in particular) being redistributed to the periphery of dorsal rootlets. Such redistribution was thought to be of possible significance for surgical control of pain. Ranson and Billingsley suggested that cutting the lateral part of dorsal roots abolished nociceptive reflexes.[238] However, any changes of this type are likely to be a result of damage to the cord[253] caused by damage to nutritive vessels running in the lateral aspect of dorsal roots (see Chap. 8).

Ventral Root. Ventral roots contain efferent (motor) fibers as well as "recurrent" fibers.[251] Myelinated sensory fibers had been detected in ventral roots.[74] Unmyelinated fibers (below the resolution of the light microscopes) were demonstrated by Coggeshall and colleagues.[53,54] These fibers arose from dorsal root ganglion cells.[8] Physiological recordings showed them to be sensory nerves.[50,51,55] This evidence shows that 15 to 30 per cent of axons in ventral roots are sensory and enter by way of ventral roots.[193] This is a partial explanation for failure of dorsal rhizotomy to relieve pain.[52] More anatomical and physiological data are required before functions can be assigned to these ventral root afferents.

Dorsal Horn Structure. Spinal cord is known to be

comprised of a central butterfly-shaped "grey" zone, surrounded by "white" matter.[302] Gray matter can be divided into ten groups based on cell morphology.[241] This is not an ideal classification,[101] because the spinal cord is not a laminar structure. Cell groups I to VI are involved in sensory transmission and comprise dorsal horn. Figure 24-1 shows the general arrangement.

Lamina I: Marginal Zone. Lamina I, marginal zone of Waldeyer, forms a thin dorsal cap on the dorsal horn. It contains cells of all sizes, including large marginal cells of Waldeyer.[285] These large, flattened cells[236] have long dendrites[246] and contribute to contralateral spinothalamic tracts,[275,278] as well as forming local connections.[36,41] Excitatory input to marginal cells is from primary afferents ending on distal dendrites. Inhibition is probably from substantia gelatinosa axon terminals on the soma.[153,211]

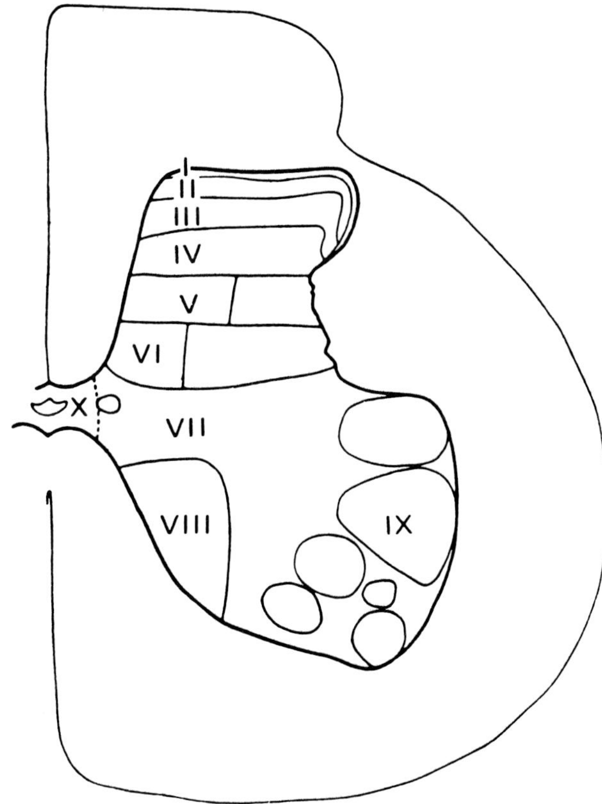

Fig. 24-1. Lamination of the spinal cord. Lamina I: marginal zone; II, III: substantia gelatinosa; IV, V, VI; nucleus proprius; VII, VIII, IX, X: motor areas. (Adapted from Rexed, B.: The cytoarchitectonic organization of the spinal cord in the cat. J. Comp. Neurol., *96*:415, 1952)

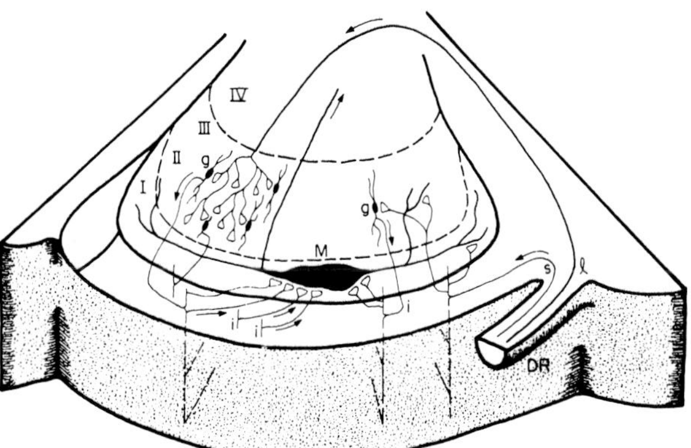

Fig. 24-2. Afferent input to marginal cells and substantia gelatinosa. Small primary afferents (*s*) from dorsal root (*DR*) bifurcate in the medial aspect of the tract of Lissauer and contact distal dendrites of marginal neurons (*M*) and gelatinosa neurones (*g*). Gelatinosa axons terminate from the intrinsic fibres (*i*) of the tract of Lissauer, synapse with and inhibit the soma and proximal dendrites of marginal cells. (Kerr, F.N.L.: Pain: a central inhibitory balance theory. Mayo Clin. Proc., *50*:685, 1975)

Marginal cells respond to peripheral stimulation of three types:[169] noxious mechanical stimulation only, noxious mechanical or thermal stimulation, and innocuous thermal change as well as polymodal nociception.[35,42] Identified high threshold afferents have been shown to end in lamina I.[176]

Laminae II and III: Substantia Gelatinosa. It is convenient to consider laminae II and III together as substantia gelatinosa.[246] Significant differences may exist between layers.[302] Ramon y Cajal described very small cells in these layers with extensive dendrites.[236] These dendritic arborizations are closely related to terminal arborizations of primary afferent fibers. There is general radial arrangement of these terminals.[262]

Cells of substantia gelatinosa are of four main types according to their projections: short axon cells, with axons that do not leave dorsal horn; cells with axons that enter tract of Lissauer or propriospinal pathways[98,187]; cells with two axons[100]; and spinothalamic neurons.[303]

A possible wiring diagram has been suggested by Kerr[153] and appears as Figure 24-2.

Primary afferent input to substantia gelatinosa occurs partly by means of collaterals of large primary afferents.[152] These have been demonstrated by a number of workers with injection of horseradish peroxidase.[16,32] Fine primary afferents and their collaterals also enter substantia gelatinosa.[49,170]

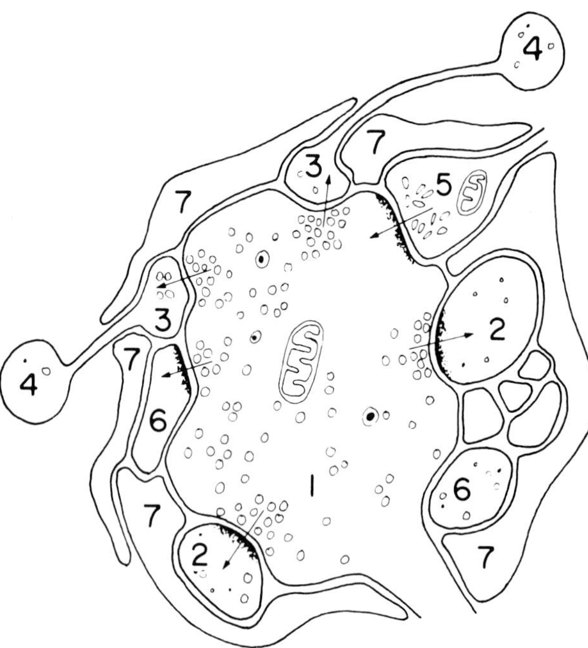

Fig. 24-3. Primary afferent glomerulus in substantia gelatinosa. (*1*) Primary afferent terminal. (*2*) Secondary dendrite of lamina IV cell. (*3*) Spine heads of gelatinosa dendrite. (*4*) Gelatinosa dendrite. (*5*) Bouton with flattened vesicle: origin unknown, function presumably inhibitory. (*6*) Gelatinosa dendrite. (*7*) Glial lamella. (Kerr, F.W.L.: Pain: a central inhibitory balance theory. Mayo Clin. Proc., *50*:685, 1975)

Glomeruli are present in this region. These are complex synaptic arrays[148,152,235] contained in glial lamellae (Fig. 24-3). Primary afferents provide central endings, which are presynaptic to dendrites of lamina IV and V neurons and to spines of gelatinosa dendrites.[99] They are postsynaptic to boutons with flattened vesicles. Some evidence suggests that GABA is an inhibitory transmitter.[13] Axodendritic, axoaxonal, dendrodendritic, and dendroaxonal synapses are probably all present within these structures, whose integrative functions[276] must be assumed from their structure.

Cells of substantia gelatinosa are too small for usual physiological recording. Perl illustrated responses of a gelatinosa neuron to heating,[225] with firing only when C-fiber activity was present, and expanded this finding subsequently.[168] Other workers were also able to record from substantia gelatinosa.[43,321] Further investigations have shown that substantia gelatinosa has inhibitory effects transmitted by way of Lissauer's tract, possibly mediated by an opiate-like mechanism.[202]

Laminae IV, V, and VI: Nucleus Proprius. Laminae IV, V, and VI are considered together, although there are differences between them. Lamina VI is only present in the cervical and lumbosacral enlargements. Cells in these layers are variable in size. Extensive cone-shaped dendritic fields radiate in all directions.[246] The apex of the cone is directed ventrally, and dorsal arborizations are extensive.

Cells in these layers have different functional characteristics. Cutaneous stimulation produces responses in all layers. Lamina IV receives convergent input from mechanoreceptors and tactile receptors (narrow dynamic range). Some cells respond to pressure and pinching in addition (wide dynamic range). Lamina V cells have larger receptive fields, and Lamina VI cells are the only ones which respond to joint movement.[287] There are also cells that respond to noxious stimuli.[165,201] Somatic and visceral input converges onto certain of these neurons.[111]

Attempts have been made to classify dorsal horn interneurons.[302] These classifications are based on responses of cells to electrical and/or natural stimulation. No scheme is entirely satisfactory. Definition of cell response requires knowledge of stimulus specificity and intensity, bandwidth (narrow—or wide—dynamic range), axonal projection, and mechanisms of inhibition (see Table 24-3).

Somatotopic arrangement may be present in these laminae,[34] with lateral cells having proximal receptive fields.[71]

Axons from cells in laminae IV to VI project in three ways: contralateral thalamus; ipsilateral lateral cervical nucleus; and propriospinal fibers to other spinal segments.[152,302]

Spinothalamic cells have been identified in these

Table 24-3. Classification of Dorsal Horn Interneurons

Lamina	*Afferent Fibers*	*Stimuli*
I	Mainly Aδ and C	Innocuous, mechanical, thermal, polymodal noxious
IV	Aαβ, Aδ and C	Innocuous, mechanical, wide dynamic range
V	A, C cutaneous, Group III muscle	Intense, mechanical, wide dynamic range
VI	A, C, Group I muscle	Proprioceptive, wide dynamic range

(Willis, W.D., and Coggeshall, R.E.: Sensory Mechanisms of the Spinal Cord, New York, Plenum Press, 1978) layers by retrograde transport of horseradish peroxidase.[277,279] They have also been identified by antidromic stimulation from thalamus.[152,304]

Ascending Sensory Pathways

Structure and function of ascending sensory pathways have been reviewed by Dennis and Melzack,[68] Kerr and Wilson,[157] and Willis and Coggeshall.[302] Nociceptive information is transmitted by a number of classical systems which include neospinothalamic tract, from laminae I, IV to VI directly to contralateral thalamus; paleospinothalamic tract to midline-intrathalamic regions; spinoreticular system, from cord to regions: brainstem reticular formation; dorsal columns, from cord to ipsilateral dorsal column nuclei; and spinocervical tract, to lateral cervical nucleus. There are also diffuse, polysynaptic connections that relay nociceptive information within the cord.[16]

Spinothalamic tracts are the most important in nociception in humans. Figure 24-4 illustrates ascending projections.

Spinothalamic Tracts. Axons from second-order neurons in laminae I, IV, V, and VI cross the midline to ascend in anterolateral quadrants as lateral and ventral spinothalamic tracts.[154] They terminate mainly in posterior thalamic nuclei and ventroposterolateral nuclei. These tracts are the main pathway for second-order nociceptive afferents in humans.[152,191] Electrical stimulation of lateral spinothalamic tract produced sensations of tingle, warmth, or cooling. Higher current intensities caused usually burning pain, but aching, cramping, and sharp pain were also reported.

Spinothalamic tracts convey tactile information in addition to nociception. Noordenbos and Wall reported a patient who had her cord transected completely and cleanly at T3 apart from part of one anterolateral quadrant.[216] She had the expected preservation of temperature and pinprick identification on the contralateral side below the lesion. There were additional unexpected findings below the lesion. Localization of touch and pressure was present on both sides. Pain could be evoked on both sides. Light touch (Von Frey hairs) could be detected on both sides, with threshold decreasing during repeated stimulation. Passive movement could be detected on the ipsilateral side. This observation adds weight to animal studies,[68] that specific ascending systems do not transmit information of a single modality. No unmyelinated fibers have been found in crossed ascending systems.[177] Input of information by unmyelinated fibers must be relayed by myelinated fibers. Some relay could occur by intrinsic unmyelinated fibers. Anterolateral cordotomy is effective in producing relief from intractable pain in some cases.[190] Species differences in ascending systems have been reviewed by Kerr.[152] It should be noted that he did not use the classical terms "neo- and paleospinothalamic" tracts. Lateral and ventral spinothalamic tracts[154] in macaque monkeys were described as dividing into lateral and medial "currents." The lateral component projected to ventroposterolateral nucleus of thalamus. This is similar to a "neospinothalamic" projection. Medial components projected (inter alii) to periaqueductal gray, nucleus cuneiformis, and bilaterally to paralamina nuclei of thalamus (similar to "paleospinothalamic" projections). He suggested that medial components of spinothalamic tracts were concerned mainly with affective and motivational aspects of nociception. Lateral components were thought to be concerned with discriminatory functions. Lateral and ventral spinothalamic tracts have different connections in brain stem and a different course through pons.[156] Evidence that ventral spinothalamic tracts are involved in nociception is only indirect, and confirmation requires further research (Fig. 24-5).

Other Tracts. Postsynaptic fibers reponding to noxious stimuli were described in dorsal columns of cats.[7,295] There is no evidence that the dorsal column-medial lemniscus system has a direct role in nociception.[302] Spinocervical tracts are well developed in cats, rudimentary in subhuman primates, and probably absent in humans.[152] Propriospinal (intraspinal) and spinoreticular tracts may be important in transmission and modulation of nociceptive information. They may be involved in local inhibitory mechanisms and may be necessary to evoke descending inhibition.[157]

It is apparent that extremely complex connections involve diverse areas of the nervous system, in contrast to earlier concepts of a dedicated spinothalamic "pain" system.

Descending Control of Spinal Cord Function

Concepts of descending control of sensory input have been long recognized.[31] Physiological support for such hypotheses was supplied by Hagbarth and Kerr.[108] They showed that primary afferent volleys in spinal cord could be markedly depressed by stimulation of brain stem reticular formation and certain higher brain areas. The potential behavioral power of descending control was not recognized until later. Reynolds stimulated brain stem of rats and produced enough analgesia to perform laparotomies.[242] Bowsher,[27] Wall,[289] Mayer and Price,[190] Fields and Basbaum,[88] and Fields and Anderson[87] have reviewed brain stem and midbrain contributions to nociception and analgesia.

Electrical stimulation of periaqueductal gray and brain stem raphe and reticular formations produces naloxone-reversible analgesia.[78,189,192,222] The anatomic routes for these inhibitions are not clear,[302] but are probably within dorsolateral fasciculus.[18] Some project by way of ventrolateral and ventral funiculi.[19] Cortical and pyramidal stimulation also depress the activity of spinothalamic neurons,[58] by an unknown mechanism.

Brain Stem Reticular Formation

Anatomically, the brain stem is a complicated area. It transmits all ascending and descending information, and contains numerous nuclear groups.[263] Responses of brain stem units and their projections have been described.[94,95] Ascending connections were with medial, posterior, and ventral thalamus, cerebral cortex, intralaminar nuclei, and a number of other areas not usually regarded nociceptive. Descending connections were shown to suppress spinal unit activity. Bowsher reported that reticular formation cells were excited most strongly by peripheral Aδ activity.[27] They had variable receptive fields, and did not exhibit strict somatotopic arrangements.

The raphe nuclei are particularly important as the origin of descending inhibition. Their arrangement and projections (in cat) are described by Bobillier and colleagues.[24]

Thalamus. Thalamic nuclei are relays for nociceptive information.[26,75] Pain sensations are due to widespread activity in thalamic nuclei, and a gating mechanism that allows information to reach cortical areas. Recordings of thalamic activity correlated with pain have been made in conscious humans.[93] Despite the complexity of thalamic connections, both stimulation and ablation have been attempted in pain control with unpredictable success.[184]

Cerebral Cortex. Early attempts to correlate painful stimuli with cortical evoked potentials have not been successful. Recent evidence indicated that electrical potentials recorded from scalp in humans have a strong linear correlation with painful dental stimulation.[47] This technique may allow quantitation of cortical responses to peripheral stimuli and may aid in assessing neural blockade.

Trigeminal System. The trigeminal nerve is the cranial nerve analogue of a spinal nerve.[205] It comprises a motor nucleus and motor division to supply muscles of mastication. Three sensory branches supply skin of face, as well as cornea, part of oral and nasal mucosae, and pulps of all teeth. Proprioceptive information is also transmitted.

Peripheral receptors within trigeminal distribution have similar characteristics to skin elsewhere.[205] There are important modifications. Face skin is very sensitive to gentle mechanical stimuli. Cornea is innervated by fine, beaded nerve terminals only. Sensations from cornea include touch, warm, and cold, as well as pain. Tooth receptors, unmyelinated nerve endings, are also able to signal touch and temperature in addition to pain.[210] Vibrissal receptors, important in many animals, are not found in humans and are probably not found in subhuman primates.[158]

Arrangement of trigeminal sensory nuclei has some similarities to spinal nerve organization, but there are many important differences.[69,101,147,157] All projection to mesencephalic nuclei is ipsilateral.[144] Bilateral axonal degeneration patterns have been reported after unilateral tooth pulp removal in cats.[301] Mesencephalic nucleus of trigeminal has primary afferent cell bodies and receives proprioceptive information. There is somatotopic organization of nucleus caudalis similar to that of the sensory root, demonstrated by anatomical[145] and physiological[157] methods.

In both sites, ophthalmic fibers are most ventral, maxillary fibers intermediate, and mandibular fibers most dorsal. Nucleus caudalis (spinal nucleus) is arranged in a similar way to spinal cord, with marginal zone,[92] substantia gelatinosa[148] with glomeruli, and a deeper laminar structure. This nuclear complex extends from pons to upper cervical segments of spinal cord. It contains neurons from cranial nerves, five, seven, nine and ten and spinal nerves C1, C2 and C3.[145–147,151]

There may be some functional organization in the mediolateral axis.[157] Touch and pressure units tend to be more lateral than glabrous skin and oral cavity units. Nociceptive units have been described in marginal zone and magnocellular layer.[76,92,156] Nucleus caudalis cells project to contralateral thalamic nuclei, and presumably transmit all nociception from that area.[35,76]

The trigeminal system has many features analogous with spinal systems. Somatic sensation and nociception are represented in a similar way, and marginal neurons of nucleus caudalis are equivalent to spinal cord spinothalamic neurons.

Fig. 24-4. Ascending pathways of the spinal cord in humans. (*1*) Ventral spinothalamic tract. (*2*) Lateral spinothalamic tract. (*3*) Lissauer's tract: dorsal root entry zone. (*4*) Substantia gelatinosa. (*5*) Laminae IV, V, VI.

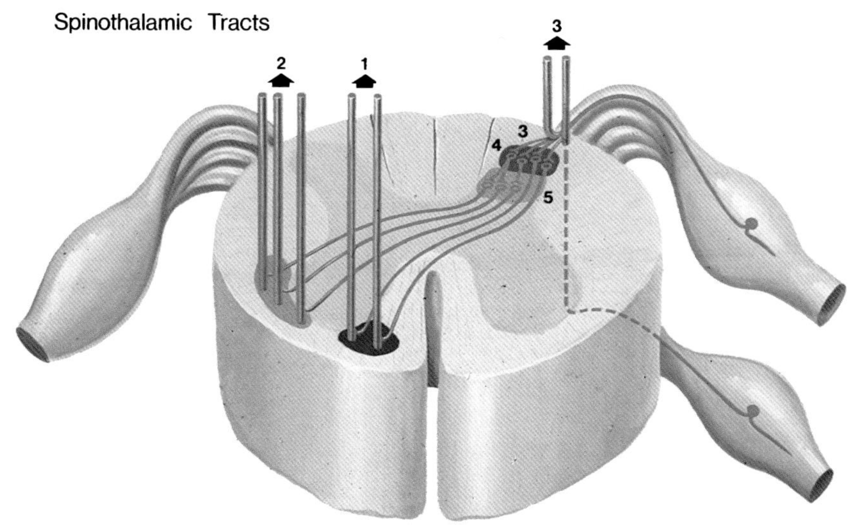

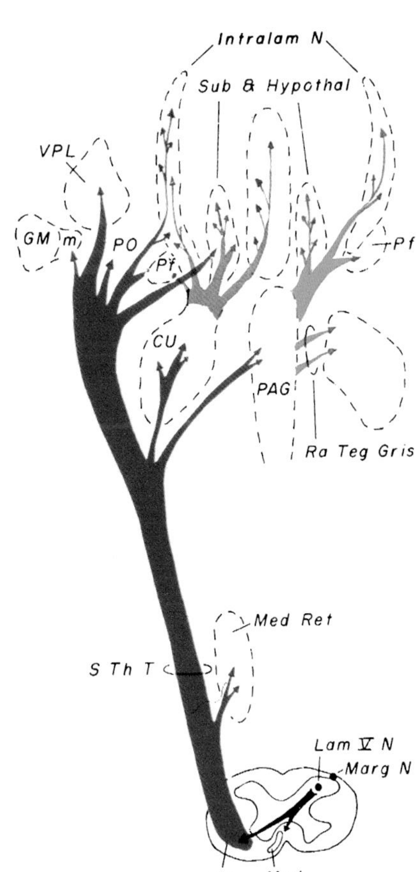

Fig. 24-5. Spinothalamic projections. Nociceptive input excites marginal (*Marz*) and lamina V (*Lam V*) neurons. These project to medial (*Med*) and lateral (*Lat*) spinothalamic tracts (*STLT*). These tracts ascend to thalamus with collaterals to medial reticular formation (*Med Ret*), periaqueductal gray (*PAG*), nucleus cuneiformis (*CU*), and thalamic nuclei and sub- and hypothalamus.

Part 2: Pharmacology of Pain and Analgesia

Significant advances in concepts of somatosensory function and pain (and nociception) occurred when Hagbarth and Kerr demonstrated descending modulation of incoming information at spinal cord level.[108] Melzack and Wall proposed a gate control theory of pain incorporating this observation.[199] This theory stimulated resurgence of interest and research into pain mechanisms and pain management. Although it was unable to explain all phenomena and was based on the admittedly incomplete physiological knowledge of the time, it has become a standard reference on this subject. A general restatement of the gate control theory has been made recently by Wall:[290]

1. Information about the presence of injury is transmitted to the central nervous system by peripheral nerves. Certain small diameter fibres (Aδ and C) respond only to injury, while others with lower thresholds increase their discharge frequency if the stimulus reaches noxious levels.
2. Cells in the spinal cord or fifth nerve nucleus which are excited by these injury signals are also facilitated or inhibited by other peripheral nerve fibres which carry information about innocuous events.
3. Descending control systems originating in the brain modulate the excitability of the cells which transmit information about injury.

This theory emphasizes that perception depends upon the actual content or characteristics of physiologically defined peripheral stimuli and also upon modulatory processes occurring within spinal cord and brain stem. Thus, nociception must be considered in terms of both afferent and efferent limbs. Nociception is only a part of perception of pain. Pain can be perceived in the absence of noxious stimulation, and a noxious stimulus does not necessarily cause pain.

Classically, pain control has depended upon the blockade of afferent pathways, by interruption with local anesthetics,[66] chemical agents,[308] or surgical lesions.[261] However, such methods are neither specific for pain nor reliable in the long term. Neurosurgical intervention has attempted to interrupt an essential link in ascending pathways that carry nociceptive information. This approach is basic to the assumption that there is an anatomical separation between those systems carrying nociceptive information and those carrying other somatosensory modalities. Unfortunately, this assumption is invalid. Nociceptive information is not the only information carried by the fine Aδ and C fibers. It also ascends by way of a number of ascending pathways.[68,152,159] Surgery also causes interruption of descending pathways in the area, intrinsic connections with the cord necessary for modulation.

Selectivity of local anesthetic blockade depends on physical properties of myelinated versus unmyelinated fibers.[257] Because of the difficulties in achieving and maintaining a stable local anesthetic concentration (along with anatomical problems mentioned above), it is virtually impossible to maintain a stable, prolonged block of pain—specific nerves, even if such nerves do exist.[84] Local anesthetic blocks for pain are therefore usually complicated by some degree of autonomic, motor and general sensory blockade. It is clear that these classical approaches to pain therapy are handicapped by their lack of specificity.

In recent years, there have been considerable advances in understanding pharmacology of systems within brain and spinal cord which mediate transmission and modulation of nociceptive information. These advances have occurred most rapidly in two fundamental areas: structure and activity of brain and spinal cord systems underlying the analgetic* actions of opiates; and pharmacology of primary afferent systems.

New findings in these areas now suggest that selective pharmacological interventions may permit specific modifications of transmission within the nociceptive system. The discussion below therefore deals broadly with four topics: mechanisms of opiate analgesia; pharmacology of primary afferent transmission and afferent modulation; experimental and therapeutic applications; and speculation on possible future applications to anesthesia and pain management.

MECHANISMS OF OPIATE ANALGESIA

Brain Sites

Although opium has been known for centuries to possess analgetic properties, it is only recently that sites of action of opiates have been defined.[319] Briefly, microinjections of morphine into certain brain sites of primates produced behavioral analge-

* Oxford English Dictionary: anaesthesia/anaesthetic; hence, analgesia/analgetic.

sia.[227] The most active sites were in periaqueductal gray matter in the midbrain. A most important observation in rats was that periaqueductal morphine blocked the tail-flick, *a spinal reflex!* This could only have occurred by descending inhibition of the spinal cord itself. Behavioral changes observed after periaqueductal gray injections of morphine could have been explained on the basis of blockade at the midbrain level.

It became apparent with subsequent anatomical, physiological, and pharmacological studies in a number of laboratories that this spinal analgetic effect was mediated by means of a descending serotonergic and/or adrenergic link.[4,88,203,234,312] This analgetic effect of intracerebral microinjections of morphine was shown to be similar to that of systemically administered morphine.[133] Narcotic agonists were also shown to have a direct spinal action, producing local effects,[79,162] as well as behavioral analgesia.[318] These effects fulfilled the criteria for opiate receptor activation; dose dependency, stereospecificity, naloxone reversibility, and existence of a well-defined structure-activity series of narcotic agonists.

Spinal Cord Sites

Initial demonstration of a spinal serotonin link in antinociception was provided by Wang[298] and confirmed by Yaksh and Wilson.[322] Behavioral experiments used lumbar intrathecal administration of serotonin in rats. Manipulations of a spinal serotonin system were able to influence analgesia produced by intrathecal injection of serotonin. Resulting analgesia was antagonized by methysergide and cyproheptadine and increased by pretreatment with monoamine oxidase inhibitors or serotonin uptake blockers. However, it was not affected by naloxone, implying that there was no opiate link in this direct spinal effect. These effects were demonstrated in rats, cats, and rabbits and, subsequently, in primates. Yaksh has shown that lumbar intrathecal administration of methysergide (serotonin antagonist) was able to block inhibition of a spinal reflex (tail flick in intact rats) produced by microinjections of morphine into periaqueductal gray matter.[310]

This suggests that serotonin terminals in spinal cord are mediators for inhibition caused by periaqueductal morphine. Additional corroborative evidence was demonstration of spinal serotonin release after periaqueductal morphine microinjection.[320] Other behavioral evidence showed noradrenaline to be involved in morphine activity.[254] Noradrenaline selectively reduced firing of nociceptive units in cat spinal cord.[114]

Baclofen (β-[*p*-chlorophenyl] GABA) produced a dose-dependent stereospecific analgetic effect when injected into the lumbar intrathecal space of rats and cats.[307] This effect was not antagonized by naloxone. Yaksh reported that morphine, serotonin, and baclofen had synergistic analgetic effects in this preparation.[307] These findings suggest that these three compounds do not act through a final common pathway.

Concurrent investigations had shown the presence of opiate-specific binding sites in the CNS.[9,10,167] This provided additional corroboration for specific opiate action. Isolation of endogenous opiate-like peptides (enkephalins, β-endorphin[256]) suggested the possibility that the system could be a tonic homeostatic (feedback) mechanism. Evidence for this is equivocal so far. These (and other) peptides have been shown to produce analgesia when administered intrathecally.[313] Dose-response curves and dose ratio plots have been described for morphine, methionine enkephalin, methionine enkephaline amide, and D-alanine-enkephaline amide. These suggest a common locus of action.

It must be pointed out that tolerance develops during narcotic agonist administration. This reduction in efficacy occurs not only with different routes of administration, but also between different agonists (cross tolerance).[117,315]

Morphine and other narcotic analgetics have been shown to exert both a direct and indirect (via serotonin) inhibition of nociceptive transmission at the spinal level.

PRIMARY AFFERENT TRANSMISSION

A question that has frustrated workers in nociception and pain research is whether pain is a specific sensation.[224] It is clear that nociceptive information is carried in some (but not all) Aδ and C fibers (conduction Aδ, 10–20 m/sec; C, 1–2 m/sec[84]) in peripheral nerves. Some larger fibers with faster conduction velocities (to 45 m/sec) also conduct this information.[129] Certain cells in dorsal horn respond preferentially or exclusively to nociceptive input (marginal cells, lamina I[48]; polymodal nociceptors[42,231]). Wall addressed the issue of specificity and pointed out that the term is acceptable in a diagnostic sense, in that under defined conditions there is a "fixed and specific relation between stimulus and response."[290] However, the term is invalid if used in a "predictive prognostic" sense.

This implies that if an impulse is detected in a particular nerve, it is not possible to predict the sensation experienced as a result. It is clear that a nerve fiber, dorsal horn cell, or, indeed, any single cell can not "feel" pain: Perception of pain is the hallmark of the intact organism. There are, however, certain relatively simple reflex circuits that detect nociception and initiate simple motor response (*e.g.*, spinal withdrawal reflex or trigeminal jaw-opening reflex). Single-fiber and single-cell studies are invaluable in elucidating fundamental mechanisms, but behavior of intact animals must be used as the criterion of perception of pain (for discussion of the problems involved in the study of pain in animals and humans see Wall and Sternbach[293]; Procacci and colleagues[233]).

Substance P and Nociception

Anatomical organization of the spinal cord is not yet clear.[152,159,302] It is also not surprising that neurochemistry of primary afferent transmission is still unclear. There is accumulating evidence that substance P, an undecapeptide, may be involved in primary afferent transmission in dorsal horn of spinal cord. Substance P-like immunoreactivity has been described in a number of brain sites. Highest levels have been seen in trigeminal nucleus and superficial layers of dorsal horn of spinal cord.[14,64,121–123,264] Substance P is also found within axons and cell bodies of primary afferents in dorsal root ganglia.[120] On the basis of size and relative numbers, it was suggested that these may have been type B cells—small cells with unmyelinated processes. Rhizotomy causes an almost total loss of dorsal horn immunoreactivity[122] (and also fluoride-resistant acid phosphatase[136,164]). Substance P has been shown to be stored by some trigeminal ganglion neurones and possibly released at axon terminals in medulla and sensory terminals in skin.[63] Substance P is constantly absent from dorsal column nuclei,[142] suggesting that it is not associated with terminals of large primary afferents.

Substance P has been shown to cause depolarization of a number of CNS neurones.[265] Henry has shown that iontophoresis of substance P onto spinal neurons with a wide dynamic range potentiates responses of those cells to heat, but not to innocuous stimuli.[116] Substance P has also been shown to be released from slices of trigeminal nucleus and spinal cord in vitro.[137] This potassium-evoked release was inhibited by an enkephalin. Significant release has also been measured in vivo from rat and cat spinal cord after electrical stimulation of sciatic nerves at Aδ/C intensities.[311]

Capsaicin, an extract of red peppers, has been shown to produce pain when administered to humans or animals.[135] Curiously, subsequent doses did not cause pain. Jessell and colleagues have shown that capsaicin caused depletion of substance P in primary sensory neurones.[138] Evidence from intact rats suggested that substance P is released into cerebrospinal fluid by capsaicin applied to lumbar intrathecal space and that cord levels of substance P are depleted.[311] Seventy per cent of these rats demonstrated prolonged (to 20 weeks) insensitivity to noxious thermal (hot plate, tail flick) and chemical (formalin) stimuli, with other modalities (perhaps except bladder control) intact. This evidence provides some persuasive corroboration that substance P is a candidate as a primary afferent transmitter for noxious thermal and chemical stimuli.

It is known that stimulation of the large rapidly conducting myelinated primary afferents is able to modify the transmission of small-fiber information. Anatomical and biochemical substances by which this inhibition occurs are not known. One hypothesis has been proposed by Kerr.[153] Large afferent fibers (which comprise the dorsal column-medial lemniscus system) supply collaterals to substantia gelatinosa through deeper layers. They synapse onto small, inhibitory gelatinosa neurons. Axons of these neurons travel for 50 to 100 μm in the lateral part of the tract of Lissauer and reenter dorsal horn to mediate inhibition.[296] There is some question of whether the inhibitory transmitter in this case is GABA, glycine,[96] cyclic GMP,[56] or an opiate link.[80] It is clear that significant inhibition is mediated by means of a substantia gelatinosa link carried in the lateral part of the tract of Lissauer.[70] There are unpublished data* suggesting that substantia gelatinosa cell firing correlates with dorsal horn nociceptor cell inhibition. Wall and Yaksh have shown that microstimulation of the tract of Lissauer causes localized inhibition.[296] There is obviously much still to be learned about this critical anatomical area where the first modulation can occur.

It now seems possible that substantia gelatinosa receives collaterals of nociceptive (thermal and chemical) information and that inhibition of this transmission occurs at the spinal cord level in substantia gelatinosa. It is likely that several systems

* Personal communication, P.D. Wall

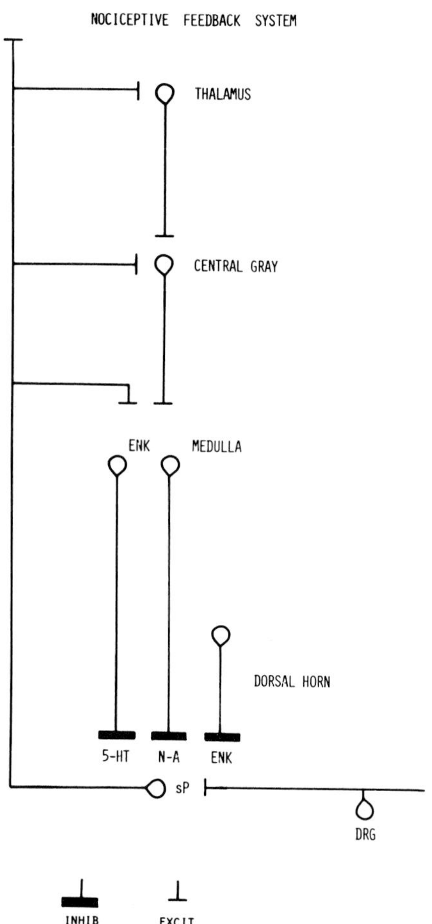

Fig. 24-6. Theoretical model of nociceptive system: dorsal root ganglion (*DRG*). substance P (*SP*). serotonin (*5-HT*). noradrenaline (*N-A*). enkephalin (*ENK*). Primary afferent nociceptive impulses are conducted by way of DRG to spinothalamic neurons in the dorsal horn with substance P as transmitter. Collaterals supply medulla and central gray matter. Descending pathways are activated. Enkephalin (or other morphine-like transmitters) activates descending serotonergic and noradrenergic pathways that inhibit primary afferent transmission. Within dorsal horn there are local enkephalin (opiate) inhibitory systems.

may be involved: opiates (endogenous and exogenous) by a dual action (descending via 5HT and direct local effects); serotonin; noradrenaline; GABA system.

Taking into account evidence presented here, it is possible to construct a theoretical model of the nociceptive system (Fig. 24-6). It must be remembered that this model is derived from information presently available and will doubtless be modified or corrected as knowledge of this system expands. For example, cholecystokinin-octapeptide-like immunoreactivity has been shown to be in maximum density in the periaqueductal gray matter,[131] vasoactive intestinal peptide may be functional in the spinal cord,[311] and neurotensin has been shown to excite lamina I to III neurons.[206]

Experimental and Therapeutic Applications

Having restated the concept of a nociceptive circuit with afferent and efferent limbs, it is possible to review sites at which electrical or pharmacological stimulation might be expected to alter the transmission of information in the system (or systems).

Electrical Stimulation

An obvious prediction of the gate control theory of pain was that stimulation of large-diameter peripheral nerve fibers should effect some blockade of nociceptive information transmission in dorsal horn. Consequently, transcutaneous electrical stimulation (TCS) was introduced.[294] This has subsequently been shown to have a certain place in management of chronic pain of peripheral origin.[184] This assertion must be qualified, because the only double-blind cross-over trial of TCS has shown that a placebo effect is also present.[269] Transcutaneous stimulation is now an established therapeutic modality in acute (*e.g.*, postoperative[228,244] or obstetrical[11]) and chronic pain.

Using the same rationale, pain control has been attempted using dorsal column electrical stimulation with transcutaneous[281] or implanted electrodes.[215] However, the success of this method has not resulted in widespread utilization. Similarly, stimulation of other areas of brain has not been shown to be highly effective in controlling pain.[184]

Stimulation of brain sites in a putative nociceptive loop has been attempted. Reynolds showed that stimulation of periaqueductal gray could produce profound analgesia in animals.[242] This observation was applied to clinical cases by Hosobuchi and his colleagues.[126] Evidence was presented that analgesia resulting from stimulation of electrodes implanted in brain stem of patients was reversed by naloxone.[2] This implicated an opioid link. Further evidence for this has been the demonstration of enkephalin-like material in cerebrospinal fluid (CSF) of patients who had analgesia resulting from focal brain stimulation.[5] This observation has not yet been confirmed by other workers, although Terenius has shown an increase in enkephalin-like material after acupuncture analgesia.[267]

The place of such heroic intervention in pain management has been questioned in an international forum.[106] Gybels commented on difficulties involved in such studies. He warned that proper evaluation of these techniques would involve careful selection of patients, unequivocal quantification of results, and collection of anatomic data supplemented with appropriate animal models. It is apparent that there is much more work to be done before the place of regional brain stimulation is defined in clinical practice.

PHARMACOLOGICAL MANIPULATION OF THE NOCICEPTIVE LOOP

Systemic Narcotic Analgetics

Narcotic analgetics have been used from time immemorial to impair perception of pain, leaving the perception of other modalities intact. There has only been desultory investigation of this phenomenon until the last decade, in which time research has burgeoned. Yaksh and Rudy have presented an overview of the development of understanding of narcotic analgesia.[319] They discussed the evidence that narcotics produce analgesia by supraspinal actions and also by direct effects on spinal cord function. The relative contribution of the spinal and supraspinal effects is to be determined. They addressed this question and suggested that opiate analgesia was not just a simple addition of function of these two components. They present a more attractive hypothesis that a complex interaction with multiplicative and additive components is present. They also point out that analgesia produced by systemic administration of narcotics depends both on passive (at primary afferent terminals in dorsal horn) and active actions (excitation of descending pathways from brain stem and medulla). The concept of a nociceptive feedback loop makes it possible to conceive manipulations that are likely to have clinical relevance.

Intrathecal Narcotics

Yaksh and Pert showed that administration of very small quantities of narcotics directly into spinal subarachnoid space of animals produced a dose-dependent, stereospecific naloxone-reversible analgesia.[316,317] This was "pure" analgesia as measured by spinal reflex and complex behavioral responses to noxious stimuli. Blockade of the nociceptive responses occurred, without detectable motor or sensory alterations other than analgesia. Wang conducted a double-blind clinical trial of intrathecal morphine in patients with severe intractable pain from pelvic cancer.[299] They found that 0.5 to 1.0 mg morphine by this route was able to produce 12 to 24 hours of pain relief. A similar result was described for cervical intrathecal injections of 0.5 mg morphine.[282] It is clear that this alternative route of narcotic administration is highly effective. Little is known about its pharmacodynamics. Kaiko and colleagues have reported initial studies of blood and CSF narcotic levels after therapeutic systemic doses.[141] As narcotics presumably act by means of cerebrospinal fluid, it would be reasonable to expect endorphins, enkephalins, and their analogues to act in the same way. Beta-endorphin has been reported to produce analgesia in humans when so used.[91,125]

These animal and human studies show that intrathecal administration is the most effective and specific route. There is potential for respiratory depression if narcotic should spread to respiratory centers of brain stem.[90] The full potential of this method has yet to be determined.[323] Its place in the diagnosis and management of acute and chronic pain is also unknown.

Intrathecal administration has intrinsic problems (*e.g.*, infection, spinal, headache, cord damage, discomfort caused by repeated punctures), and it was rational to attempt the epidural route. Initial animal studies suggested that analgesia produced by epidural narcotics was less potent and of shorter duration than that by intrathecal administration.[305] A preliminary communication of ten clinical cases was made independently of this laboratory.[20] Epidural morphine (2 mg) was given 1 to 3 times per day for 1 to 4 days, with partial to complete pain relief. In a contemporaneous clinical study, Cousins and colleagues showed that epidural meperidine produced high levels of CSF merperidine. Onset of analgesia occurred when CSF meperidine concentration reached analgetic concentrations predicted from blood pharmacodynamic studies (0.5 mg/L). Blood concentrations did not reach this level. In this series also, duration of analgesia was widely variable (4.5–20 hours) and without detectable effects on sensory, motor, or sympathetic systems. This is another technique that must be investigated fully to determine its place in clinical practice (see also Figs. 31-1 to 31-3).

Enkephalins and Endorphins

Enkephalins and endorphins have been shown to produce analgesia when applied to spinal cord of animals.[313,314] These substances are rapidly hydrolyzed, and active analogues that resist such degradation have been tested for analgetic properties.[45] These agents have been administered by intrathecal, intravenous,[91,125] and oral routes. Once again, it is too early to comment on the final place of this group of compounds in clinical practice.

Other Antinociceptive Systems

It has been shown that a number of putative neurotransmitters are involved in the nociceptive loop. Opioid peptides, serotonin,[298,322] noradrenaline,[114] GABA and glycine,[96] cyclic-GMP,[56] glutamic acid,[139] neurotensin,[280] and somatostatin[15,237] are included. It is possible that modification of one or more of these systems could affect responses to extrinsic (or intrinsic) analgetics. There is some evidence that such is the case. Yaksh and Wilson showed that the analgesia produced by intrathecal serotonin was augmented by blockade of serotonin uptake, or monoamine oxidase inhibition, and antagonized by serotonin antagonists.[322] Naloxone had no effect. Manipulations of the noradrenaline system had similar effects; analgesia was produced by agents mimicing or prolonging the action of noradrenaline. Baclofen (chlorophenyl-GABA) has been shown to produce dose-dependent stereo-specific analgesia when applied to spinal cord of animals.[307] The significance of this is not yet known. Again, it is clear that much more research is required to elucidate the types of drug interactions that are operative at spinal cord level. An indication of the probable complexity of this subject has been given by Yaksh.[309] He showed that subanalgetic doses of morphine, serotonin and baclofen, administered intrathecally, produced a higher degree of analgesia than could be explained by simple additive effects. It is also interesting to note that lanthanum is able to produce an analgesia with cross-tolerance with morphine.[113] Intraventricular calcitonin is also able to produce analgesia.[28]

There are a number of sites in the nociceptive loop at which physiological or pharmacological manipulation could be carried out. There is obviously a need for continued research into the detailed physiology and pharmacology of primary afferent transmission, in order to determine which, if any, manipulations have clinical relevance.

Pituitary Ablation

A special case must be made of pituitary ablation in management of chronic pain. Hypophysectomy has been established in management of metastatic breast cancer.[239] The technique of chemical hypophysectomy (with alcohol) for intractable pain was proposed by Morrica.[209] There have been a number of studies of this phenomenon, which is reported to have a satisfactory analgetic effect in a majority of patients.[178] Any hypophysectomy has an obligate morbitity (hormonal dysfunction: ADH, ACTH, TSH). A low incidental and unexpected morbidity (cranial nerve damage, rhinorrhea) and low mortality was reported in Lipton's series (155 injections in 106 patients; four deaths in the first week after injection).

Other methods have been used for pituitary ablation: radioactive Yttrium implants (*e.g.,* Juret, cited by Gye and colleagues[107]), and local freezing.[107] Mechanisms of analgesia are not known. It is tempting to speculate that endorphins (or ACTH) contained in the pituitary have a role. (For example, is this analgesia naloxone-reversible?)

Opiate Tolerance

The nemesis of opiate analgesia is the ability of the opiate receptors to become tolerant, or to suffer a decrease in sensitivity with repeated exposure to any narcotic agonist. (It is not the purpose of this review to discuss in detail receptor tolerance, physical dependence and opiate withdrawal.[182] There is evidence that tolerance develops after single intracerebral (PAG, 5 μg) microinjection or single intraperitoneal (20 mg/kg) injection of morphine in rats.[61] This was suggested by the observation that a second dose of morphine 6 to 24 hours after the first produced less analgesia than the first. A central mechanism was implicated. Physical dependence has also been demonstrated after a single injection of opiates.[29] This phenomenon was elicited by the induction by naloxone of behavioral withdrawal symptoms ("jumping responses"). Withdrawal signs have also been observed in single cells (myenteric neurons).[217] On the other hand, there has been a report that rats with chronic pain may fail to develop tolerance to narcotic analgesia.[57] The authors of this present review have observed this phenomenon in two patients* with chronic pain treated with daily meperidine (800–1200 mg/day). In each case, the analgetic blood level remained at 0.5 mg/L when tested before and after 3 months of this self-administered narcotic dosage.

New evidence has been produced that physical dependence on morphine (measured by naloxone-precipitated withdrawal) could be prevented, without altering the analgetic potency.[297] Profound implications can be made based on this observation.

* Unreported data, Pain Clinic, Flinders Medical Center

It should be pointed out that with pure narcotic agonists and antagonists available, there can be no argument for the use of drugs with mixed agonist-antagonist activities. There is no evidence that equianalgetic doses are less likely to produce tolerance or dependence than are pure agonists. The greatest hope is for the discovery of different morphine receptors (M[analgesia], M[euphoria] M[respiratory depression]). Preliminary data suggest this might be so.[132,300]

Speculations

The intrathecal route is now established with certain clinical indications. However, many questions remain. What is the place of this technique in management of acute pain (*e.g.*, operative, obstetrical)?[323] What is the optimal dose? (At which dosage are receptors fully occupied?[124] How rapidly does significant tolerance develop?[315] Is a reservoir system and continuous infusion feasible?[91] Are there "better" opiates? Is the epidural route more applicable than the intrathecal?[59] Is it possible to utilize the nonnarcotic analgetic systems for clinical analgesia? What is the place of the intrathecal route in the differential diagnosis of peripheral versus central pain? (If the intrathecal narcotic does not produce a naloxone-reversible analgesia, does the pain arise from a structure central to the spinal cord?)

Part 3: Clinical Aspects of Pain

Concepts of nociception and its modulation by means of a feedback loop were discussed earlier in this chapter. This section deals in two parts with certain clinical syndromes with respect to these concepts: pain syndromes with predominantly peripheral and somatic components (somatogenic), and pain syndromes with predominantly psychological components (psychogenic).

PERIPHERAL SOMATIC PAIN SYNDROMES (SOMATOGENIC)

Pain associated with peripheral nerve injuries and lesions has received considerable attention (*e.g.*, in the definitive monograph of Sunderland[261]).

In the context of the nociceptive system, it is possible for "pain" to arise from a number of sites in the periphery. Wall has suggested a list of possible sources of altered neural activity following peripheral nerve injury which could be interpreted as pain (see next column).[291]

One or more of these mechanisms is likely to contribute to symptoms or syndromes discussed below. Precise roles of each remain speculative.

This scheme is useful in devising a rational sequence of diagnostic, prognostic, and therapeutic nerve blocks. Such blocks should begin as close to the periphery as possible. Each successive block should be at the next logical step towards the spinal cord. Using such a sequence, symptoms arising in the periphery may be controlled in the most parsimonious way.

Sources of Altered Neural Activity Following Peripheral Nerve Injury

Peripheral end organs
Axon terminals
Collateral sprouting (of intact neighbor)
Sprouting of damaged axons[72,292]
Sympathetic fibers in location of damage[25]
Changes in axons proximal to the damage
Changes in dorsal root ganglion cells[127]
Differential regeneration/maturation of sprouts[218,268]
Reaction of Schwann cells[268]
Changes in central terminals of damaged axons
Changes in central terminals of intact neighbouring axons
Changes in spinal cord cells that have lost part of normal input[73]

Trigeminal Neuralgia

Trigeminal neuralgia (tic doloreaux) has certain characteristic clinical features:[149,150]

Pain is limited to some part of the distribution of the trigeminal nerve (rarely glossopharyngeal or nervus intermedius).

Pain is paroxysmal, unilateral, superficial, brief and intense, sudden in onset and termination, with pain-free intervals.

Frequency and severity of episodes tends to increase with age.

No neurological deficit is detectable (or minimal sensory loss).

Trigger points for nonnociceptive stimuli are present at some time, commonly perioral.

Fewer than 5 per cent start in the ophthalmic division; 3 per cent are ultimately bilateral.

Onset usually occurs after age 40, and it is more common in women.

Mechanical factors involving root or ganglion may produce a similar syndrome.

Sensory rhizotomy produces relief (at least temporary).

Decompression or compression procedures on trigeminal ganglion produces relief.

Trigeminal-evoked averaged cortical potentials may be abnormal in patients with trigeminal neuralgia.[21]

These features provide some evidence to support a peripheral etiology. Two additional theories emphasize a peripheral origin. Exaggerated trigeminal dorsal root reflexes or additional action potentials arising at sites of altered myelination may contribute to, or cause trigeminal neuralgia.[39,104]

Compression of the trigeminal ganglion or nerves by adjacent arteries has also been proposed.[112,134] A recent study of normal anatomy in 50 patients without trigeminal neuralgia demonstrated that superior or anterior inferior cerebellar arteries made contact with 29 nerves or ganglia. A conclusion could be drawn that such neurovascular contacts were coincidental.

Management of tic doloreaux has been reviewed by Loeser.[180] Medical therapy relies on carbamazepin and phenytoin. These anticonvulsants produce significant improvement in symptoms (of 70% and 20%, respectively).

There may be some improvement with mephenesin or chlorphenesin. Mechanisms of action are unknown. It is tempting to suggest that they might act by suppressing a central reverberation (seizure) in the trigeminal system.

Surgical therapy may be needed if medical management does not control the symptoms. Coagulation of part of trigeminal ganglion (percutaneous radiofrequency trigeminal neurolysis) is a safe and effective method. Improvement has been reported as 80 per cent at 1 year.[180] It should be carried out with intermittent general anesthesia to avoid corneal anesthesia. The patient is allowed to wake between each incremental application of radiofrequency heating to report changes in sensation. Patients considering this operation should first have local anesthetic block of the trigeminal nerve, both for diagnosis and to allow them to experience facial anesthesia.

Suboccipital craniectomy and release of putative pressure on trigeminal ganglion has an indeterminate place in management of tic doloreaux. Trigeminal tractotomy is also a major surgical endeavour, whose place is unknown.

Anesthesia dolorosa is pain in the distribution of an interrupted nerve. It occurs in a small number of patients who have undergone gangliolysis. It has some of the features of phantom limb pain and also of causalgia. Its cause is not known and treatment is unrewarding at present.

Facial Neuralgia

Nonparoxysmal facial neuralgia, atypical facial pain, is an obscure syndrome of chronic, continuous deep-seated pain of moderate intensity. It usually involves more than one trigeminal branch and has no trigger points. There are no apparent underlying causes.[38,155] It may represent a central pain syndrome (*i.e.*, a disorder of the nociceptive feedback loop). Psychiatric abnormalities are common. Nonmedical treatment (psychotherapy, hypnotherapy) should be used in conjunction with drug therapy.[97] Postherpetic neuralgia is also a difficult disease of unknown etiology requiring multiple therapies.[213,266]

Causalgia: Reflex Sympathetic Dystrophy (Dysfunction)

Reflex sympathetic dystrophy[25,232] is a term that includes a spectrum of clinical conditions: causalgia, post-traumatic pain syndrome, shoulder-hand syndrome, Sudeck's atrophy, post-traumatic vasomotor disorder. These syndromes appear to have a similar pathophysiological etiology, clinical presentation, and response to therapy.[259]

Causalgia is the extreme case of this syndrome. It has been extensively studied and reviewed by Sunderland.[261] There are specific characteristics of the pain of causalgia:

Characteristics of the Pain of Causalgia

Follows injury to a nerve
Severe, spontaneous and persistent
Burning in nature, but also crushing or tearing
Present in hand or foot
Accompanied by hyperalgesia or hyperesthesia
Accompanied by vasomotor and sudomotor changes
Accompanied by edema and muscular dysfunction
Aggravated by environmental and/or emotional factors
Leads to disuse of limb and osteoporosis ("Sudeck's atrophy")

In later stages, there may develop progressive trophic changes in the skin and its appendages, weakness and atrophy of muscles, bones and joints. Causalgia develops in the first few weeks after injury, in the distribution of the injured nerve. Brachial plexus, median, or sciatic nerves are involved in the majority of cases. Once the pain is established, it may be greatly exacerbated by increased activity of the limb, or by trivial somatosensory input to the causalgia area. Sunderland considered three mechanisms of pain and sympathetic dysfunction:[261]

Some pain impulses undoubtedly arise from the region of the damaged nerve (neuroma).[292] These are not sufficient to cause all the vasomotor effects.

Damaged nerves possibly change in composition and act as a source of aberrant impulses. Causalgia may be particularly severe after spinal root avulsion when no recovery of nerves is possible. Peripheral factors may exacerbate or perpetuate causalgia, but are unlikely to cause it. A more likely explanation is to be found below.

Turbulence hypothesis: This hypothesis proposes disorderly neural activity in spinal cord somatic and autonomic interneurons. Indirect evidence for this has been presented by Torebjörk and Hallin.[273] Patients with causalgia relieved by sympathectomy had hyperalgesia induced in previously causalgic skin by local application of noradrenaline.[110]

Treatment of causalgia must be initiated early in the course of the syndrome (see Chaps. 13 and 31). Sympathectomy by some method is fundamental in management. It can be carried out with regional intravenous guanethidine, local anaesthetic blockade of sympathetic outflow (see Chap. 13), chemical sympathectomy (with phenol), or by surgical sympathectomy. Unfortunately, little is known about the role of the autonomic nervous system in pain states, so this therapy must be regarded as empirical.

Causalgia has also been treated successfully with transcutaneous stimulation and hypnosis. Interesting preliminary data were reported by Finer and colleagues.[89] Subjects under hypnosis were able to imagine "hyperalgesia." This was accompanied by increased sympathetic efferent activity in skin nerves. Conversely, imagined "hypoalgesia" was accompanied by a decrease in sympathetic outflow. This work suggests the intriguing possibility that voluntary control of causalgia may be feasible.

Sunderland lists a number of surgical ablative procedures used to attempt to control the pain of causalgia.[261] He concludes "at whatever level pain is attacked, the whole nervous system seems to make a co-ordinated and determined effort to re-establish the pathway by developing some alternative route."

Phantom Limb Pain

Amputation of a limb causes almost all patients to experience sensory illusions that the limb is still present. This phantom limb is a natural and almost invariable sequela of amputation.[261] Phantom sensations may also occur in paraplegia.[196] Phantom limb phenomena are usually transient. The phantom is said to gradually fade or "telescope" in about half the cases. Persistent phantom limb phenomena have certain characteristics: they are more common with upper than with lower limbs; limbs are usually perceived as distorted or incomplete; movement can be perceived; and, sensation can be perceived, particularly if the stump is stimulated.[194,261]

Origins of phantom limbs are unknown. Peripheral nerves are severed during amputation. Neuroma formation occurs as part of healing. Such neuromas may be the source of spontaneous activity.[292] Central mechanisms are also important.[30,261] Pain occurs in phantom limbs in 5 to 37 per cent of cases.[261] Phantom limb pain has a number of characteristics:

It may be felt in the phantom limb or stump. It may be intermittent or continuous. It may commence without warning.

Peripheral stimuli and psychological factors may be related to the onset of pain. Pain may last for seconds to days; pain-free intervals may last for years.

Pain is bizarre and often described as burning, cramping, aching, stabbing, or as having causalgic features.

Pain usually fades and disappears, but recovery may be punctuated by acute exacerbations.[306] Rarely, it persists in a severe, intractable, and incapacitating form.

Phantom limb pain is more likely if the limb was painful prior to amputation, and if amputation was delayed for a long period after the injury (see Chap. 13).

Phantom limb pain is difficult to treat because of its unknown etiology. Sunderland emphasized that any operation for phantom limb pain is more likely to fail than to succeed. Conservative measures should be used aggressively and directed at peripheral and central components. Preventative measures include early amputation and prevention of pain in the limb (see Chap. 13). Sympathectomy may be necessary to aid demarcation in obliterative vascular disease.

Nerve block, within the stump, at segmental level or extradural-intrathecal blockade may produce temporary or long lasting improvement. Such blocks may be repeated when necessary. Transcutaneous and dorsal column stimulation have been used successfully in management of phantom limb pain.[184,204] Phantom pain associated with spinal cord damage is resistant to any treatment.[196,204,212]

Good relief of pain has been claimed for psychological methods.[250] Relaxation training helped 14 of 16 amputees, by breaking a putative "pain-anxiety" cycle. Hypnosis may also have a place in management.[118,119]

Backache

Back pain is a major social and economic problem with interrelated mechanical and psychological factors.[37]

Mechanical factors play a large part in the genesis of low back pain,[86] and they must be considered in the differential diagnosis.[249] Extraskeletal and skeletal factors were considered in detail by Selecki and colleagues.[249] Mechanical factors that cause pain are often related to overload of tissues.[86] Axial compression and torsional overloads injure bony and soft-tissue structures and may lead to pain. Other causes may include chemical radiculitis from disc material,[188] nerve root compression or traction, and joint stresses.[161] Diagnosis of spinal disease is difficult, and the source of opposing views between orthopaedists and neurosurgeons.[249] Cervical pain is likely to be caused by nerve compression or traction within foramina. Back pain is more likely to be caused by disc-protrusion or annular disruption. Posture is an important consideration at both levels. There is a place for neural blockade in management of back pain. Individual blockade of particular nerve roots, facets, or other joints may aid in localizing sources of pain. Provocation of back or leg pain by discography, and subsequent relief by local anesthetic may also localize abnormalities. Differential spinal and epidural local anesthetic blockade may also be useful in determining the fine-fiber contribution to the pain. It will be necessary to assess intrathecal narcotics as a diagnostic tool. It might be expected that intrathecal narcotics would block pain arising from spinal or more peripheral lesions. It might not block pain arising from structures rostral to spinal cord. In this way, it might be possible to distinguish pain of "somatic" origin (see Chap. 31).

Just as diagnosis of the mechanisms of back pain is difficult, so is diagnosis of significant personality factors (see Chap. 31).[37,174,175,186]

Management of back pain is a contentious subject.[249] Multidisciplinary approaches are difficult[214] because of the lack of unanimity among specialities. Within a conservative framework, there are places for epidural and intrathecal local anesthetic and steroid injections.[1,33]

Myofascial Syndromes

Myofascial syndrome is a term used to describe ill-defined pain in muscles, tendons, or fascial planes. Such pain is not necessarily related to a specific incident of tissue damage. The syndrome is characterized by intermittent pain of variable intensity and radiation. A "trigger point" is present. Pressure on such a point reproduces pain in its usual distribution. A self-perpetuating cycle is suggested as the cause: A focus of local pain (trigger point) causes reflex muscle spasm in its region. Such muscle spasm becomes painful (*e.g.*, tourniquet test), and this pain perpetuates the cycle. This hypothesis receives indirect corroboration from the observation that cervical epidural block is able to relieve acute wry-neck (torticollis) by relieving the pain-spasm-pain cycle.* Stimulation of trigger points (by acupuncture, dry needling, intense cold, or electrically), or blockade with local anesthetic may paradoxically diminish or abolish the pains for days, weeks, or sometimes permanently.[200] Causes of the myofascial syndromes are unknown, and treatment is therefore empirical. Melzack and colleagues attempt to correlate trigger points with acupuncture points in a large number of myofascial syndromes.[197] The investigators studied maps of trigger points and acupuncture points prepared by other workers. Close correlation was found. No evidence was presented for the existence of either type of point. Conclusions cannot be drawn. However, the review is useful as it contains lists of clinical syndromes of myofascial origin and a discussion of principles of referred pain.

Myofascial syndromes have no clear pathophysiology. The occurrence of these syndromes is undoubted, but any treatment must be empirical. A particular type of myofascial syndrome is thought to cause headache.[252] Occipital neuralgia causes a "tension" headache that may be relieved by blockade of the occipital nerves at the occiput. It is not known how these syndromes relate to other forms

* Personal communication, Wang

of headache. The reader is referred to the monograph on that subject by Lance.[172]

Referred Pain

Referred pain is well known as a clinical entity, but little is known about its etiology. Convergence of visceral and somatic input onto single dorsal horn neurons has been described,[111] and this might be the best explanation.

PSYCHOGENIC PAIN

Pain, by definition, is an experience that is expressed in terms of tissue damage. Some pain has clearly defined somatic cause. Other pain is better described and understood in psychological language.[258] "Psychogenic" is a descriptor of causative relationship. Sternbach's use of "psychogenic pain" refers to "pain which is better understood in psychological than in physical language." Patients are designated as experiencing psychogenic pain when no adequate somatic (nociceptive) cause for such symptoms can be found. It is a diagnosis of exclusion.

Pain is a symptom associated with a number of mental states (see below). Not all patients with these conditions have pain.

In 250 patients with orofacial pain of unknown origin, multiple problems were present, but a majority had obvious psychiatric illness.[97] Depression was present in 39 per cent, anxiety neurosis in 31 per cent, and hysterical conversion reaction in 11 per cent.

In a different type of study, complaints of pain were elicited in 38 per cent of 227 consecutive psychiatric hospital admissions.[67] Pain was relatively often associated with anxiety, depression, personality disorders (hysterical, antisocial, inadequate, passive-aggressive), and alcoholism. It was less frequently associated with schizophrenia, mania, mental retardation, organic brain syndrome, and transient situational disturbances. Pain is often associated with abnormal illness behavior[229] in health professionals.*

Mechanisms of pain in such cases are unknown. The concept of "nocebo" has been proposed.[248] Subjects were told that a (nonexistent) electric current would be passed through their heads. More than two-thirds reported headaches. A different study demonstrated that high anxiety was related to decreased pain tolerance.[283] These experiments suggest that central mechanisms may "set" pain threshold and tolerance.

Other indirect evidence relates to endorphins.[6] Patients classified as having "organic" pain had lower lumbar CSF levels of endorphin-like material than those with "psychogenic" pain. (Depressed patients in both groups had higher levels than non-depressed patients.) In another study, pain-sensitive patients were found to have lower levels of endorphin than pain-insensitive patients.[284]

* Unpublished observations, Pain Management Unit, Flinders Medical Center

REFERENCES

1. Abram, S.E.: Subarachnoid corticosteroid injection following inadequate response to epidural steroids for sciatica. Anesth. Analg. (Cleve.), *57*:313, 1978.
2. Adams, J.E.: Naloxone reversal of analgesia produced by brain stimulation in the human. Pain, *2*:161, 1976.
3. Agnew, D.C., and Merskey, H.: Words of chronic pain. Pain, *2*:73, 1976.
4. Akil, H., and Liebeskind, J.C.: Monoaminergic mechanisms of stimulation-produced analgesia. Brain Res., *94*:279, 1975.
5. Akil, H., Richardson, D.E., Hughes, J., and Barchas, J.D.: Enkephalin-like material elevated in ventricular cerebrospinal fluid of pain patients after analgetic focal stimulation. Science, *201*:463, 1978.
6. Almay, B.G.L., Johansson, F., Von Knorring, L., Terenius, L., and Wahlstrom, A.: Endorphins in chronic pain. I: Differences in CSF endorphin levels between organic and psychogenic pain syndromes. Pain, *5*:153, 1978.
7. Angaut-Petit, D.: The dorsal column system: 1. Existence of long ascending post-synaptic fibres in the cat's fasciculus gracilis. Exp. Brain Res., *22*:257, 1975.
8. Applebaum, M.L., et al.: Unmyelinated fibres in the sacral 3 and caudal 1 ventral roots of the cat. J. Physiol., *256*:557, 1976.
9. Atweh, S.F., and Kuhar, M.J.: Autoradiographic localization of opiate receptors in rat brain. I: Spinal cord and lower medulla. Brain Res., *123*:53, 1977.
10. ———: Autoradiographic localization of opiate receptors in rat brain. II: The brain stem. Brain Res., *129*:1, 1977.
11. Augustinsson, L.-E., et al.: Pain relief during delivery by transcutaneous electrical nerve stimulation. Pain, *4*:59, 1977.
12. Bailey, C.A., and Davidson, P.O.: The language of pain: intensity. Pain, *2*:319, 1976.
13. Barber, R.P., Vaughn, J.E., Saito, K., McLaughlin, B.J., and Roberts, E.: Gaba ergic terminals are presynaptic to primary afferent terminals in the substantia gelatinosa of the rat spinal cord. Brain Res., *141*:35, 1978.
14. Barber, R.P., et al.: The origin, distribution and synaptic relationships of substance P axons in rat spinal cord. J. Comp. Neurol., *184*:331, 1979.
15. Barchas, J.D., Akil, H., Elliott, G.R., Hollman, R.B., and Watson, S.J.: Behavioral neurochemistry: neuroregulators and behavioral state. Science, *200*:964, 1978.
16. Basbaum, A.I.: Conduction of the effects of noxious stimulation by short-fiber multisynaptic systems of the spinal cord in the rat. Exp. Neurol., *40*:699, 1973.

17. Basbaum, A.I., Clanton, C.H., and Fields, H.L.: Three bulbospinal pathways from the rostral medulla of the cat: an autoradiographic study of pain modulating systems. J. Comp. Neurol., *178*:209, 1978.
18. Basbaum, A.I., and Fields, H.L.: The dorsolateral funiculus of the spinal cord: a major route for descending brain stem control. Soc. Neurosci. Abstr., *3*:499, 1977.
19. Basbaum, A.I., and Wall, P.D.: Chronic changes in the response of cells in adult cat dorsal horn following partial deafferentation: the appearance of responding cells in a previously non-responsive region. Brain Res., *116*:181, 1976.
20. Behar, M., Magora, F., Olshwang, D., and Davidson, J.T.: Epidural morphine in treatment of pain. Lancet, *1*:527, 1979.
21. Bennett, M.H., and Jannetta, P.J.: Evoked potentials in trigeminal neuralgia. Pain Abstr., *1*:66, 1978.
22. Bessou, P., and Perl, E.R.: Responses of cutaneous sensory units with unmyelinated fibres to noxious stimuli. J. Neurophysiol., *32*:1025, 1969.
23. Black, R.G.: A laboratory model for trigeminal neuralgia. Adv. Neurol., *4*:651, 1974.
24. Bobillier, P., et al.: The raphe nuclei of the cat brain stem: a topographical atlas of their efferent projections as revealed by autoradiography. Brain Res., *113*:449, 1976.
25. Bonica, J.J.: Causalgia and other reflex sympathetic dystrophies. Pain Abstr., *1*:11, 1978.
26. Bowsher, D.: Thalamic convergence and divergence of information generated by noxious stimulation. Adv. Neurol., *4*:223, 1974.
27. ———: Role of reticular formation in responses to noxious stimulation. Pain, *2*:361, 1976.
28. Braga, P., Ferri, S., Santagostino, A., Olgiati, V.R., and Pecile, A.: Lack of opiate receptor involvement in centrally induced calcitonin analgesia. Life Sci., *22*:971, 1978.
29. Brands, B., Hirst, M., Gowdey, C.W., and Baskerville, J.C.: Analgesia duration and physical dependence in mice after a single injection of three heroin salts and morphine sulphate in various vehicles. Arch. Int. Pharmacodyn. Ther., *231*:285, 1978.
30. Bromage, P.R., and Melzack, R.: Phantom limbs and the body schema. Can. Anaesth. Soc. J., *21*:267, 1974.
31. Brouwer, B.: Centrifugal influence on centripetal systems in the brain. J. Nerv. Mental Dis., *77*:621, 1933.
32. Brown, A.G., Rose, P.K., and Snow, P.J.: The morphology of hair follicle afferent fibre collaterals in the spinal cord of the cat. J. Physiol. (Lond.), *272*:779, 1977.
33. Brown, F.W.: Management of diskogenic pain using epidural and intrathecal steroids. Clin. Orthop., *129*:72, 1977.
34. Brown, P.B., and Fuchs, J.L.: Somatotopic representation of hindlimb skin in cat dorsal horn. J. Neurophysiol., *38*:1, 1975.
35. Burton, H., Craig, A.D., Jr., Poulos, D.A., and Molt, J.T.: Efferent projections from temperature sensitive recording loci within the marginal zone of the nucleus caudalis of the spinal trigeminal complex in the cat. J. Comp. Neurol., *183*:753, 1979.
36. Burton, H., and Loewy, A.D.: Descending projections from the marginal cell layer and other regions of the monkey spinal cord. Brain Res., *116*:485, 1976.
37. Caldwell, A.B., and Chase, C.: Diagnosis and treatment of personality factors in chronic low back pain. Clin. Orthop., *129*:141, 1977.
38. Calvin, W.H.: Facial neuralgias: What do normal and pathophysiological mechanisms suggest? Pain Abstr., *1*:88, 1978.
39. Calvin, W.H., Loeser, J.D., and Howe, J.F.: A neurophysiological theory for the pain mechanism of tic douloureux. Pain, *3*:147, 1977.
40. Carlstedt, T.: Observations on the morphology at the transition between the peripheral and the central nervous system in the cat. IV: Unmyelinated fibres in S1 dorsal rootlets. Acta Physiol. Scand., (Suppl. 446): 61, 1977.
41. Cervero, F., Iggo, A., and Molony, V.: Ascending projections of nociceptor-driven lamina I neurones in the cat. Exp. Brain Res., *35*:135, 1979.
42. Cervero, F., Iggo, A., and Ogawa, H.: Nociceptor driven dorsal horn neurones in the lumbar spinal cord of the cat. Pain, *2*:5, 1976.
43. Cervero, F., Moloney, V., and Iggo, A.: Extracellular and intracellular recordings from neurones in the substantia gelatinosa rolandi. Brain Res., *136*:565, 1977.
44. Chahl, L.A., and Kirk, E.J.: Toxins which produce pain. Pain, *1*:3, 1975.
45. Chang, J.K., Fong, B.T.W., Pert, A., and Pert, C.B.: Opiate receptor affinities and behavioral effects of enkephalin: structure-activity relationship of ten synthetic peptide analogues. Life Sci., *18*:1473, 1976.
46. Chapman, C.R.: Sensory decision theory methods in pain research: a reply to Rollman. Pain, *3*:295, 1977.
47. Chen, A.C.N., Chapman, C.R., and Harkins, S.W.: Brain evoked potentials are functional correlates of induced pain in man. Pain, *6*:365, 1979.
48. Christensen, B.M., and Perl, E.R.: Spinal neurons specifically excited by noxious or thermal stimuli: marginal zone of the dorsal horn. J. Neurophysiol., *33*:293, 1970.
49. Chung, K., Langford, L.A., Applebaum, A.E., and Coggeshall, R. E.: Primary afferent fibres in the tract of Lissauer in the rat. J. Comp. Neurol., *184*:587, 1979.
50. Clifton, G.L., Coggeshall, R.E., Vance, W.H., and Willis, W.D.: Receptive fields of unmyelinated ventral root afferent fibres in the cat. J. Physiol. (Lond.), *256*:573, 1976.
51. Clifton, G.L., Vance, W.H., Applebaum, M.L., Coggeshall, R.E., and Willis, W.D.: Responses of unmyelinated afferents in the mammalian ventral root. Brain Res., *82*:163, 1974.
52. Coggeshall, R.E., Applebaum, M.L., Fazen, M., Stubbs, T.B., III, and Sykes, M.T.: Unmyelinated axons in human ventral roots, a possible explanation for the failure of dorsal rhizotomy to relieve pain. Brain, *98*:157, 1975.
53. Coggeshall, R.E., Coulter, J.D., and Willis, W.D., Jr.: Unmyelinated fibers in the ventral root. Brain Res., *57*:229, 1973.
54. ———: Unmyelinated axons in the ventral roots of the cat lumbosacral enlargement. J. Comp. Neurol., *153*:39, 1974.
55. Coggeshall, R.E., and Ito, H.: Sensory fibres in ventral roots L7 and S1 in the cat. J. Physiol. (Lond.), *267*:215, 1977.
56. Cohn, M.L., Cohn, M., and Taylor, F.H.: Guanosine 3′, 5′-monophosphate: a central nervous system regulator of analgesia. Science, *199*:319, 1978.
57. Colpaert, F.C.: Long-term suppression of pain by narcotic drugs in the absence of tolerance development. Arch. Int. Pharmacodyn. Ther., *236*:293, 1978.
58. Coulter, J.D., Maunz, R.A., and Willis, W.D.: Effects of stimulation of sensorimotor cortex on primate spinothalamic neurons. Brain Res., *65*:351, 1974.
59. Cousins, M.J., Mather, L.E., Glynn, C.J., Wilson, P.R., and Graham, J.R.: Selective spinal analgesia. Lancet, *1*:1141, 1979.
60. Cracco, R.Q., and Cracco, J.B.: Somatosensory evoked

potential in man: far field potentials. Electroenceph. Clin. Neurophysiol., *41*:460, 1976.

61. Criswell, H.E., Dahlberg, S.T., and Cwiertniewicz, J.S.: Delayed onset of single dose tolerance to morphine analgesia. Life Sci., *21*:1735, 1977.
62. Crockett, D.J., Prkachin, K.M., and Craig, K.D.: Factors of the language of pain in patient and volunteer groups. Pain, *4*:175, 1977.
63. Cuello, A.C., Delfiacco, M.D., and Paxinos, G.: The central and peripheral ends of the substance P-containing sensory neurones in the rat trigeminal system. Brain Res., *152*:499, 1978.
64. Cuello, A.C., Polak, J.M., and Pearse, A.G.E.: Substance P: a naturally-occurring transmitter in human spinal cord. Lancet, *2*:1054, 1976.
65. Dash, M.S., and Deshpande, S.S.: Human skin nociceptors and their chemical response. *In* Bonica, J.J., and Albe-Fessard, D.G. (eds.): Advances in Pain Research and Therapy. vol. 1. pp. 47–51. New York, Raven Press, 1976.
66. De Jong, R.H.: Neural blockade by local anesthetics. Life Sci., *20*:915, 1977.
67. Delaplaine, R., Ifabumuyi, O.I., Merskey, H., and Zarfas, J.: Significance of pain in psychiatric hospital patients. Pain, *4*:361, 1978.
68. Dennis, S.G., and Melzack, R.: Pain-signalling systems in the dorsal and ventral spinal cord. Pain, *4*:97, 1977.
69. Denny-Brown, D., Kirk, E.J., and Yanagisawa, N.: The tract of Lissauer in relation to sensory transmission in the dorsal horn of spinal cord in the macaque monkey. J. Comp. Neurol., *151*:175, 1973.
70. Denny-Brown, D., and Yanagisawa, N.: The function of the descending root of the fifth nerve. Brain, *96*:783, 1973.
71. Devor, M., and Wall, P.D.: Dorsal horn cells with proximal cutaneous receptive fields. Brain Res., *118*:325, 1976.
72. ______: Type of sensory nerve fibre sprouting to form a neuroma. Nature, *262*:705, 1976.
73. ______: Reorganization of spinal cord sensory map after peripheral nerve injury. Nature, *275*:75, 1978.
74. Dimsdale, J.A., and Kemp, J.M.: Afferent fibres in ventral roots in the rat. J. Physiol. (Lond.), *187*:25P, 1966.
75. Dong, W.K., Ryu, H., and Wagman, I.H.: Nociceptive responses of neurons in the posterior group of nuclei and medial thalamus. Fed. Proc., *37*:2228, 1978.
76. Dubner, R., Gobel, S., and Price, D.D.: Peripheral and central trigeminal "pain" pathways. *In*, Bonica, J.J., and Albe-Fessard, D.G. (eds.): Advances in Pain Research and Therapy. vol. 1. pp. 137–148. New York, Raven Press, 1976.
77. Dubuisson, D., and Melzack, R.: Classification of clinical pain descriptions by multiple group discriminant analysis. Exp. Neurol., *51*:480, 1976.
78. Duggan, A.W., and Griersmith, B.T.: Inhibition of the spinal transmission of nociceptive information by supraspinal stimulation in the cat. Pain, *6*:149, 1979.
79. Duggan, A.W., Hall, J.G., and Headley, P.M.: Morphine, enkephalin and the substantia gelatinosa. Nature, *264*:456, 1976.
80. ______: Suppression of transmission of nociceptive impulses by morphine: selective effects of morphine administered in the region of the substantia gelatinosa. Br. J. Pharmacol., *61*:65, 1977.
81. Dyck, P.J.: Pathologic alterations of the peripheral nervous system of man. *In*, Dyck, P.J., Thomas, P.K., and Lambert, E.H. (eds.): Peripheral Neuropathy. pp. 296–336. Philadelphia, W.B. Saunders, 1975.
82. ______: Peripheral neuropathy. *In*, Tower, D.B. (ed.): The Nervous System. vol. 2. pp. 307–321. The Clinical Neurosciences. New York, Raven Press, 1975.
83. Dyck, P.J., and Kiely, J.M.: Differential diagnosis of neuropathy associated with cancer. Adv. Neurol., *15*:149, 1976.
84. Dyck, P.J., Lambert, E.H., and Nichols, P.C.: Quantitative measurements of sensation related to compound action potential and number and sizes of myelinated and unmyelinated fibres of sural nerve in health, Friedreich's ataxia, hereditary sensory neuropathy and tabes dorsalis. *In* Remond, A. (ed.): Handbook of Electroencephalography and Clinical Neurophysiology. vol. 9. pp. 83–118. Amsterdam, Elsevier, 1971.
85. Dyck, P.J., Lambert, E.H., and Obrien, P.C.: Pain in peripheral neuropathy related to rate and kind of fiber degeneration. Neurology (Minneap.), *26*:466, 1976.
86. Farfan, H.F.: Mechanical factors in the genesis of low back pain. Pain Abstr., *1*:216, 1978.
87. Fields, H.L., and Anderson, S.D.: Evidence that raphe-spinal neurons mediate opiate and midbrain stimulation-produced analgesias. Pain, *5*:333, 1978.
88. Fields, H.L., and Basbaum, A.I.: Brainstem control of spinal pain transmission neurons. Annu. Rev. Physiol., *40*:193, 1978.
89. Finer, B.L., Hallin, R.G., and Torebjork, H.E.: Sympathetic outflow in human skin nerves during hypnosis. Pain Abstr., *1*:33, 1978.
90. Florez, J., and Mediavilla, A.: Respiratory and cardiovascular effects of met-enkephalin applied to the ventral surface of the brainstem. Brain Res., *138*:585, 1977.
91. Foley, K.M., Kaiko, R.F., Inturrisi, C.E., Posner, J.B., and Li, C.H.: Intravenous and intraventricular administration of beta-endorphin in man. Pain Abstr., *1*:17, 1978.
92. Fukushima, T., Grabow, J.D., and Kerr, F.W.L.: The organization of trigemino-thalamic neurons as determined by horseradish peroxidase retrograde labelling. Soc. Neurosci. Abstr., *3*:481, 1977.
93. Fukushima, T., Mayanagi, Y., and Bouchard, G.: Thalamic evoked potentials to somatosensory stimulation in man. Electroenceph. Clin. Neurophysiol., *40*:481, 1976.
94. Fuller, J.H.: Brain stem reticular units: some properties of the course and origin of the ascending trajectory. Brain Res., *83*:349, 1975.
95. ______: Brain stem reticular units: synaptic responses to stimulation within the ascending reticular pathways. Brain Res., *112*:229, 1976.
96. Game, C.J.A., and Lodge, D.: The pharmacology of the inhibition of dorsal horn neurones by impulses in myelinated cutaneous afferents in the cat. Exp. Brain Res., *23*:75, 1975.
97. Gerschman, J.A., Burrows, G.D., and Reade, P.C.: Chronic oro-facial pain. Pain Abstr., *1*:279, 1978.
98. Giesler, G.J., Cannon, J.T., Urca, G., and Liebeskind, J.C.: Long ascending projections from substantia gelatinosa rolandi and the subjacent dorsal horn in the rat. Science, *202*:984, 1978.
99. Gobel, S.: Synaptic organization of the substantia gelatinosa glomeruli in the spinal trigeminal nucleus of the adult cat. J. Neurocytol., *3*:219, 1974.
100. ______: Neurons with two axons in the substantia gelatinosa layer of the spinal trigeminal nucleus of the adult cat. Brain Res., *88*:333, 1975.
101. ______: Principles of organization in the substantia gelatinosa layer of the spinal trigeminal nucleus. *In* Bonica, J.J., and Albe-Fessard, D.G. (eds.): Advances in Pain Research

and Therapy. vol. 1. pp. 165–170. New York, Raven Press, 1976.

102. Gracely, R.H., McGrath, P., and Dubner, R.: Ratio scales of sensory and affective verbal pain descriptors. Pain, *5*:5, 1978.
103. ______: Validity and sensitivity of ratio scales of sensory and affective verbal pain descriptors: maniuplation of affect by diazepam. Pain, *5*:19, 1978.
104. Gregg, J.M., Banerjee, T., Ghia, J.N., and Campbell, R.: Radiofrequency thermoneurolysis of peripheral nerves for control of trigeminal neuralgia. Pain, *5*:231, 1978.
105. Grieve, N., et al.: An analysis of tourniquet induced ischaemic pain in relation to the McGill pain questionnaire and the Cornell Medical Index. Biobehav. Rev. [In Press].
106. Gybels, J.: Electrical stimulation of the central gray for pain relief in humans: a critical review. Pain Abstr., *1*:170, 1978.
107. Gye, R.S., Stanworth, P.A., Stewart, J.A., and Adams, C.B.T.: Cryohypophysectomy for bone pain of metastatic breast cancer. Pain, *6*:201, 1979.
108. Hagbarth, K.-E., and Kerr, D.I.B.: Central influences of spinal afferent conduction. J. Neurophysiol., *17*:295, 1957.
109. Hallin, R.G., and Torebjork, H.E.: Studies on cutaneous A and C fibre afferents, skin nerve blocks and perception. *In* Zotterman, Y. (ed.): Sensory Functions of the Skin in Primates with Special Reference to Man. pp. 137–149. Oxford, Pergamon Press, 1976.
110. ______: Observations on hyperalgesia in the causalgic pain syndrome. Pain Abstr., *1*:48, 1978.
111. Hancock, M.B., Foreman, R.D., and Willis, W.D.: Convergence of visceral and cutaneous input onto spinothalamic tract cells in the thoracic spinal cord of the cat. Exp. Neurol., *47*:240, 1975.
112. Hardy, D.G., and Rhoton, A.L., Jr.: Microsurgical relationships of the superior cerebellar artery and the trigeminal nerve. J. Neurosurg., *49*:669, 1978.
113. Harris, R.A., Iwamoto, E.T., Loh, H.H., and Way, E.L.: Analgetic effects of lanthanum: cross-tolerance with morphine. Brain Res., *100*:221, 1975.
114. Headley, P.M., Duggan, A.W., and Griersmith, B.T.: Selective reduction by noradrenaline and 5-hydroxytryptamine of nociceptive responses of cat dorsal horn neurones. Brain Res., *145*:185, 1978.
115. Heimer, L., and Wall, P.D.: The dorsal root distribution to the substantia gelatinosa of the rat with a note on the distribution in the cat. Exp. Brain Res., *6*:89, 1968.
116. Henry, J.L.: Effects of substance P on functionally identified units in cat spinal cord. Brain Res., *114*:439, 1976.
117. Herz, A., and Teschemacher, H.: Development of tolerance to the antinociceptive effect of morphine after intraventricular injection. Experientia, *64*:64, 1973.
118. Hilgard, E.R.: The alleviation of pain by hypnosis. Pain, *1*:213, 1975.
119. Hilgard, E.R., and Hilgard, J.R.: Hypnosis in the relief of pain. Kaufmann, Los Altos, 1975.
120. Hokfelt, T., et al.: Immunohistochemical evidence for separate populations of somatostatin-containing and substance P-containing primary afferent neurons in the rat. Neuroscience, *1*:131, 1976.
121. Hokfelt, T., Kellerth, J.O., Nilsson, C., and Pernow, B.: Substance P: localization in the central nervous system and in some primary sensory neurons. Science, *190*:889, 1975.
122. ______: Experimental immunohistochemical studies on the localization and distribution of substance P in cat primary sensory neurons. Brain Res., *100*:235, 1975.
123. Hokfelt, T., Ljungdahl, A., Terenius, L., Elde, R., and Nilsson, G.: Immunohistochemical analysis of peptide pathways possibly related to pain and analgesia: enkephalin and substance P. Proc. Natl. Acad. Sci. U.S.A., *74*:3081, 1977.
124. Hollt, V.: The in vivo occupation of opiate receptors. *In* Adler, M.W., Manara, L., and Samanin, R. (eds.): Factors Affecting the Action of Narcotics. pp. 207–220. New York, Raven Press, 1978.
125. Hosobuchi, Y., and Li, C.H.: A demonstration of the analgesic activity of human beta-endorphin in six patients. Pain Abstr., *1*:18, 1978.
126. Hosobuchi, Y., Adams, J.E., and Linchitz, R.: Pain relief by electrical stimulation of central gray matter in humans and its reversal by naloxone. Science, *197*:183, 1977.
127. Howe, J.F., Calvin, W.H., and Loeser, J.D.: Impulses reflected from dorsal root ganglia and from focal nerve injuries. Brain Res., *116*:139, 1976.
128. Iasp Subcommittee on Taxonomy. Pain Terms: A List with Definitions and Notes on Usage. Pain, *6*:249, 1979.
129. Iggo, A. Peripheral and spinal "pain" mechanisms and their modulation. *In* Bonica, J.J., and Albe-Fessard, D.B. (eds.): Advances in Pain Research and Therapy. vol. 1. pp. 381–394. New York, Raven Press, 1976.
130. ______: Is the physiology of cutaneous receptors determined by morphology? Prog. Brain Res., *43*:15, 1976.
131. Innis, R.B., Correa, F.M.A., Uhl, G.R., Schneider, B., and Snyder, S.H.: Cholecystokinin octapeptide-like immunoreactivity: histochemical localization in rat brain. Proc. Natl. Acad. Sci. U.S.A., *76*:521, 1979.
132. Jacquet, Y.F., Klee, W.A., Rice, K.C., Iijima, I., and Minamikawa, J.: Stereospecific and nonstereospecific effects of ( )- and (−)-morphine: evidence for a new class of receptors? Science, *198*:842, 1977.
133. Jacquet, Y.F., and Lajtha, A.: The periaqueductal gray: site of morphine analgesia and tolerance as shown by 2-way cross-tolerance between systemic and intracerebral injections. Brain Res., *103:* 501, 1976.
134. Jannetta, P.J.: Arterial compression of the trigeminal nerve at the pons in patients with trigeminal neuralgia. J. Neurosurg., *26*:159, 1967.
135. Jansco, N., Jansco-Gabor, A., and Szolcsanyi, J.: The role of sensory nerve endings in neurogenic inflammation induced in human skin and in the eye and paw of the rat. Br. J. Pharmacol., *33*:32, 1968.
136. Jansco, G., and Knyihar, E.: Functional linkage between nociception and fluoride-resistant acid phosphatase activity in the rolando substance. Neurobiology, *5*:42, 1975.
137. Jessell, T.M., and Iversen, L.L.: Opiate analgesics inhibit substance P release in rat trigeminal nucleus. Nature, *268*:549, 1977.
138. Jessell, T.M., Iversen, L.L., and Cuello, A.C.: Capsaicin-induced depletion of substance P from primary sensory neurones. Brain Res., *152*:183, 1978.
139. Johnson, J.L.: Glutamic acid as a synaptic transmitter candidate in the dorsal sensory neuron: reconsiderations. Life Sci., *20*:1637, 1977.
140. Juan, H.: Prostaglandins as modulators of pain. J. Gen. Pharmacol., *9*:403, 1978.
141. Kaiko, R.F., Foley, K.M., Houde, R.W., and Inturrisi, C.E.: Analgesic drug levels in cerebral spinal fluid and plasma in cancer patients. Pain Abstr., *1*:200, 1978.
142. Kanazawa, I., and Jessell, T.M.: Post-mortem changes and regional distribution of substance P in the rat and mouse nervous system. Brain Res., *117*:362, 1976.

143. Kenton, B., Crue, B.L., and Carregal, E.J.A.: The role of cutaneous mechanoreceptors in thermal sensation and pain. Pain, *2*:119, 1976.
144. Kerr, D.I.B., Haugen, F.P., and Melzack, R.: Responses evoked in the brain stem by tooth stimulation. Am. J. Physiol., *183*:253, 1955.
145. Kerr, F.W.L.: Structural relation of the trigeminal spinal tract to upper cervical roots and the solitary nucleus in the cat. Exp. Neurol., *4*:134, 1961.
146. ______: Facial, vagal and glossopharyngeal nerves in the cat. Arch. Neurol., *6*:264, 1962.
147. ______: The divisional organization of afferent fibres of the trigeminal nerve. Brain, *86*:721, 1963.
148. ______: The ultrastructure of the spinal tract of the trigeminal nerve and the substantia gelatinosa. Exp. Neurol., *16*:359, 1966.
149. ______: Correlated light and electronmicroscopic observations on the normal trigeminal ganglion and sensory root in man. J. Neurosurg., *26*:132, 1967.
150. ______: Evidence for a peripheral etiology of trigeminal neuralgia. J. Neurosurg., *26*:168, 1967.
151. ______: Central relationships of trigeminal and cervical primary afferents in the spinal cord and medulla. Brain Res., *43*:561, 1972.
152. ______: Neuroanatomical substrates of nociception in the spinal cord. Pain, *1*:325, 1975.
153. ______: Pain: a central inhibitory balance theory. Mayo Clin. Proc., *50*:685, 1975.
154. ______: The ventral spinothalamic tract and other ascending systems of the ventral funiculus of the spinal cord. J. Comp. Neurol., *159*:335, 1975.
155. ______: Facial neuralgias: mechanisms, diagnosis and treatment. Pain Abstr., *1*:87, 1978.
156. Kerr, F.W.L., and Fukushima, T.: A new concept of the organization of the spinothalamic system. Pain Abstr., *1*:193, 1978.
157. Kerr, F.W.L., Kruger, L., Schwassmann, H.O., and Stern, R.: Somatotopic organization of mechanoreceptor units in the trigeminal nuclear complex of the macaque. J. Comp. Neurol., *134*:127, 1968.
158. Kerr, F.W.L., and Lysack, W.R.: Somatotopic organization of trigeminal ganglion neurons. Arch. Neurol., *11*:593, 1964.
159. Kerr, F.W.L., and Wilson, P.R.: Pain. Annu. Rev. Neurosci., *1*:83, 1978.
160. King, J.S., Gallant, P., Myerson, V., and Perl, E.R.: The effects of anti-inflammatory agents on the responses and the sensitization of unmyelinated (C) fiber polymodal nociceptors. *In* Zotterman, Y. (ed.): Sensory Functions of the Skin in Primates with Special Reference to Man. pp. 441–461. Oxford, Pergamon Press, 1976.
161. Kirkaldy-Willis, W.H.: Five common back disorders: how to diagnose and treat them. Geriatrics, *33*:32, 1978.
162. Kitahata, L.M., Kosaka, Y., Taub, A., Bonikos, K., and Hoffert, M.: Lamina-specific suppression of dorsal-horn unit activity by morphine sulfate. Anesthesiology, *41*:39, 1974.
163. Knitza, R., Clasen, R., and Fischer, F.: Pain-induced alterations in the individual non-esterified fatty acids in serum. Pain, *6*:91, 1979.
164. Knyihar, E., and Csillik, B.: Regional distribution of acid phosphatase-positive axonal systems in the rat spinal cord and medulla, representing central terminals of cutaneous and visceral nociceptive neurons. J. Neural Transmission, *40*:227, 1977.
165. Kolmodin, G.M., and Skoglund, C.R.: Analysis of spinal interneurons activated by tactile and nociceptive stimulation. Acta Physiol. Scand., *50*:337, 1960.
166. Kryzhanovsky, G.N.: Experimental central pain and itch syndromes: modeling and general theory. *In* Bonica, J.J., and Albe-Fessard, D.G. (eds.): Advances in Pain Research and Therapy. vol. 1. pp. 225–230. New York, Raven Press, 1976.
167. Kuhar, M.J., Pert, C.B., and Snyder, S.H.: Regional distribution of opiate receptor binding in monkey and human brain. Nature, *245*:447, 1973.
168. Kumazawa, T., and Perl, E.R.: Differential excitation of dorsal horn and substantia gelatinosa marginal neurons by primary afferent units with fine (A-delta and C) fibers. *In* Zotterman, Y. (ed.): Sensory Functions of the Skin in Primates with Special Reference to Man. pp. 67–89. Oxford, Pergamon Press, 1976.
169. ______: Excitation of marginal and substantia gelatinosa neurons in the primate spinal cord: indications of their place in dorsal horn functional organization. J. Comp. Neurol., *177*:417, 1978.
170. La Motte, C.: Distribution of the tract of Lissauer and the dorsal root fibers in the primate spinal cord. J. Comp. Neurol., *172*:529, 1977.
171. Lamotte, R.H., and Campbell, J.N.: Comparison of responses of warm and nociceptive C-fiber afferents in monkey with human judgements of thermal pain. J. Neurophysiol., *41*:509, 1978.
172. Lance, J.W.: Mechanisms and Management of Headache. London, Butterworths, ed. 3., 1978.
173. Langford, L.A., and Coggeshall, R.E.: Branching of sensory axons in the dorsal root and evidence for the absence of dorsal root efferent fibers. J. Comp. Neurol., *184*:193, 1979.
174. Leavitt, F., Garron, D.C., D'Angelo, C.M., and McNeill, T.W.: Low back pain in patients with and without demonstrable organic disease. Pain, *6*:191, 1979.
175. Leavitt, F., Garron, D.C., Whisler, W.W., and Sheinkop, M.B.: Affective and sensory dimensions of back pain. Pain, *4*:273, 1978.
176. Light, A.R., and Perl, E.R.: Central termination of identified cutaneous afferent units with fine myelinated fibers. Soc. Neurosci. Abstr., *3*:486, 1977.
177. Lippman, H.H., and Kerr, F.W.L.: Light and electron microscopic study of crossed ascending pathways in the anterolateral funiculus in monkey. Brain Res., *40*:496, 1972.
178. Lipton, S., Miles, J., Williams, N., and Bark-Jones, N.: Pituitary injection of alcohol for widespread cancer pain. Pain, *5*:73, 1978.
179. Lissauer, H.: Beitrag zum faserverlauf im hinterhorn des menschlichen ruckenmarkes und verhalten desselben bei tabes dorsalis. Arch. Psychiat. Nervenkrankh., *17*:377, 1886.
180. Loeser, J.D.: The management of tic douloureux. Pain. *3*:155, 1977.
181. Loeser, J.D., and Peirce, K.R.: Intraspinal alumina injection: the relationship between epileptiform focus, root scarring and chronic pain. Pain, *5*:245, 1978.
182. Loh, H.H., Tseng, L.F., Holaday, J.W., and Wei, E.: Endogenous peptides and opiate actions. *In* Adler, M.L., Manara, L., and Samanin, R. (eds.): Factors Affecting the Action of Narcotics. pp. 387–402. New York, Raven Press, 1978.
183. Lombard, M.-C., Nashold, B.S., Jr., Albe-Fessard, D., Salman, N., and Sakr, C.: Deafferentation hypersensitivity

in the rat after dorsal rhizotomy: a possible animal model of chronic pain. Pain, *6*:163, 1979.

184. Long, D.M., and Hagfors, N.: Electrical stimulation in the nervous system: the current status of electrical stimulation of the nervous system for the relief of pain. Pain, *1*:109, 1975.
185. Lynn, B., and Perl, E.R.: A comparison of four tests for assessing the pain sensitivity of different subjects and test areas. Pain, *3*:352, 1977.
186. McCreary, C., Turner, J., and Dawson, E.: Differences between functional versus organic low back pain patients. Pain, *4*:73, 1977.
187. Mannen, H., and Sugiura, Y.: Construction of neurons of dorsal horn proper using golgi-stained serial sections. J. Comp. Neurol., *168*:303, 1976.
188. Marshall, L.L., Trethewie, E.R., and Curtain, C.C.: Chemical radiculitis. A clinical, physiological and immunological study. Clin. Orthop., *129*:61, 1977.
189. Mayer, D.J., and Liebeskind, J.C.: Pain reduction by focal electrical stimulation of the brain: an anatomical and behavioral analysis. Brain Res., *68*:73, 1974.
190. Mayer, D.J., and Price, D.D.: Central nervous system mechanisms of analgesia. Pain, *2*:379, 1976.
191. Mayer, D.J., Price, D.D., and Becker, D.P.: Neurophysiological characterization of the anterolateral spinal cord neurons contributing to pain perception in man. Pain, *1*:51, 1975.
192. Mayer, D.J., Wolfle, T.L., Akil, H., Carder, B., and Liebeskind, J.C.: Analgesia from electrical stimulation in the brainstem of the rat. Science, *174*:1351, 1971.
193. Maynard, C.W., Leonard, R.B., Coulter, J.D., and Coggeshall, R.E.: Central connections of ventral root afferents as demonstrated by the hrp method. J. Comp. Neurol., *172*:601, 1977.
194. Melzack, R.: Central neural mechanisms in phantom limb pain. Adv. Neurol., *4*:319, 1974.
195. ———: The McGill pain questionnaire: major properties and scoring methods. Pain, *1*:277, 1975.
196. Melzack, R., and Loeser, J.D.: Phantom body pain in paraplegics: evidence for a central "pattern generating mechanism" for pain. Pain, *4*:195, 1978.
197. Melzack, R., Stillwell, D.M., and Fox, E.J.: Trigger points and acupuncture points for pain: correlations and implications. Pain, *3*:3, 1977.
198. Melzack, R., and Torgerson, W.S.: On the language of pain. Anesthesiology, *34*:50, 1971.
199. Melzack, R., and Wall, P.D.: Pain mechanisms: a new theory. Science, *150*:971, 1965.
200. ———: On the nature of cutaneous sensory mechanisms. Brain, *85*:331, 1962.
201. Menetrey, D., Giesler, G.J., and Besson, J.M.: An analysis of response properties of spinal cord dorsal horn neurones to nonnoxious and noxious stimuli in the spinal rat. Exp. Brain Res., *27*:15, 1977.
202. Merrill, E.G., Wall, P.D., and Yaksh, T.L.: Properties of two unmyelinated fibre tracts of the central nervous system: lateral Lissauer tract, and parallel fibres of the cerebellum. J. Physiol. (Lond.), *284*:127, 1978.
203. Messing, R.B., and Lytle, L.D.: Serotonin-containing neurons: their possible role in pain and analgesia. Pain, *4*:1, 1977.
204. Miles, J., and Lipton, S.: Phantom limb pain treated by electrical stimulation. Pain, *5*:373, 1978.
205. Miles, T.S.: Features peculiar to the trigeminal innervation. Can. J. Neurol. Sci., *6*:95, 1979.
206. Miletic, V., and Randic, M.: Neurotensin excites cat spinal neurones located in laminae I–III. Brain Res., *169*:600, 1979.
207. Mohamed, S.N., Weisz, G. M., and Waring, E.M.: The relationship of chronic pain to depression, marital adjustment and family dynamics. Pain, *5*:285, 1978.
208. Moore, P.A., Duncan, G.H., Scott, D.S., Gregg, J.M., and Ghia, J.N.: The submaximal effort tourniquet test: its use in evaluating experimental and chronic pain. Pain, *6*:375, 1979.
209. Morrica, G.: Chemical hypophysectomy for cancer pain. Adv. Neurol., *4*:707, 1974.
210. Mumford, J.M., and Bowsher, D.: Pain and protopathic sensibility. A review with particular reference to the teeth. Pain, *2*:223, 1976.
211. Narotzky, R.A., and Kerr, F.W.L.: Marginal neurons of the spinal cord: types, afferent synaptology and functional considerations. Brain Res., *139*:1, 1978.
212. Nashold, B.S., Zorub, D.S., Urban, B., and Wilfong, R.F.: Focal coagulation of the spinal substantia gelatinosa for relief of phantom arm pain. Pain Abstr., *1*:295, 1978.
213. Nathan, P.W.: Chlorprothixene (taractan) in post-herpetic neuralgia and other severe chronic pains. Pain, *5*:367, 1978.
214. Newman, R.I., Seres, J.L., Yospe, L.P., and Garlington, B.: Multidisciplinary treatment of chronic pain: long-term follow-up of low-back pain patients. Pain, *4*:283, 1978.
215. Nielson, K.D., Adams, J.E., and Hosobuchi, Y.: Phantom limb pain. Treatment with dorsal column stimulation. J. Neurosurg., *42*:301, 1976.
216. Noordenbos, W., and Wall, P.D.: Diverse sensory functions with an almost totally divided spinal cord. A case of spinal cord transection with preservation of part of one anterolateral quadrant. Pain, *2*:185, 1976.
217. North, R.A., and Zieglgansberger, W.: Opiate withdrawal signs in single myenteric neurones. Brain Res., *144*:208, 1978.
218. Ochoa, J., and Noordenbos, W.: Pathology and disordered sensation in local nerve lesions: an attempt at correlation. Pain Abstr., *1*:8, 1978.
219. Ohnhaus, E.E., and Adler, R.: Methodological problems in the measurement of pain: a comparison between the verbal rating scale and the visual analogue scale. Pain, *1*:379, 1975.
220. Ohnishi, A., and Dyck, P.J.: Loss of small peripheral sensory neurons in Fabry disease—histologic and morphologic evaluation of cutaneous nerves, spinal ganglia and posterior columns. Arch. Neurol., *30*:120, 1974.
221. Ohta, M., Offord, K., and Dyck, P.J.: Morphometric evaluation of first sacral ganglia of man. J. Neurol. Sci., *22*:73, 1974.
222. Oliveras, J.L., Redjemi, G., Guilbaud, G., and Besson, J.M.: Analgesia induced by electrical stimulation of the inferior centralis nucleus of the raphe in the cat. Pain, *1*:139, 1975.
223. Peck, C.L., and Nayman, J.: The submaximal effort tourniquet test as a predictor of post operative clinical pain. Pain Abstr., *1*:210, 1978.
224. Perl, E.R.: Is pain a specific sensation? J. Psychiatr. Res., *8*:273, 1971.
225. ———: Sensitization of nociceptors and its relation to sensation. *In* Bonica, J.J., and Albe-Fessard, D.G. (eds.): Advances in Pain Research and Therapy. vol. 1. pp. 17–28. New York, Raven Press, 1976.
226. Perl, E.R., Kumazawa, T., Lynn, B., and Kenins, P.: Sensitization of high threshold receptors with unmyelinated (C) afferent fibers. Prog. Brain Res., *43*:263, 1976.
227. Pert, A., and Yaksh, T.L.: Sites of morphine induced anal-

gesia in the primate brain: relation to pain pathways. Brain Res., *80*:135, 1974.
228. Pike, P.M.H.: Transcutaneous electrical stimulation. Its use in the management of postoperative pain. Anaesthesia, *33*:165, 1978.
229. Pilowsky, I., and Spence, N.D.: Illness behaviour syndromes associated with intractable pain. Pain, *2*:61, 1976.
230. Price, D.D.: Modulation of first and second pain by peripheral stimulation and by psychological set. *In* Bonica, J.J., and Albe-Fessard, D.G. (eds.): Advances in Pain Research and Therapy. vol. 1. pp. 427–431. New York, Raven Press, 1976.
231. Price, D.D., and Dubner, R.: Neurons that subserve the sensory-discriminative aspects of pain. Pain, *3*:307, 1977.
232. Procacci, P., Francini, F., Zoppi, M., Maresca, M., and Giovannini, L.: Role of sympathetic system in reflex dystrophies. *In* Bonica, J.J., and Albe-Fessard, D.G., (eds.): Advances in Pain Research and Therapy. vol. 1. pp. 953–57. New York, Raven Press, 1976.
233. Procacci, P., Zoppi, M., and Maresca, M.: Experimental pain in man. Pain, *6*:123, 1979.
234. Proudfit, H.K., and Anderson, E.G.: Morphine analgesia: blockade by raphe magnus lesions. Brain Res., *98*:612, 1975.
235. Ralston, H.J.: Organization of the substantia gelatinosa rolandi in the cat lumbosacral cord. Z. Zellforsch., *67*:1, 1965.
236. Ramon, Y., and Cajal, S.: Histologie du systeme nerveux de l'homme et des vertebres. Madrid, Inst. Cajal, [Reprint] 1952.
237. Randic, M., and Miletic, V.: Depressant actions of methionine-enkephalin and somatostatin in cat dorsal horn neurones activated by noxious stimuli. Brain Res., *152*:196, 1978.
238. Ranson, S.W., and Billingsley, P.R.: The conduction of painful afferent impulses in the spinal nerves. Am. J. Physiol., *40*:571, 1916.
239. Reed, P.I., and Pizey, N.C.D.: Trans-sphenoidal hypophysectomy in the treatment of advanced breast cancer. Br. J. Surg., *54*:369, 1967.
240. Revill, S.I., Robinson, J.O., Rosen, M., and Hogg, M.I.J.: The reliability of a linear analogue for evaluating pain. Anaesthesia, *31*:1191, 1976.
241. Rexed, B.: The cytoarchitectonic organization of the spinal cord in the cat. J. Comp. Neurol., *96*:415, 1952.
242. Reynolds, D.V.: Surgery in the rat during electrical analgesia induced by focal brain stimulation. Science, *164*:444, 1969.
243. Rollman, G.B.: Signal detection theory measurement of pain. A review and critique. Pain, *3*:187, 1977.
244. Rosenberg, M., Curtis, L., and Bourke, D.L.: Transcutaneous electrical nerve stimulation for the relief of postoperative pain. Pain, *5*:129, 1978.
245. Santini, M.: The "receptripse": the desmosome-like lamellar-axonal junction subserving mechano-electric transduction and effecting the sympathetic actions on the pacinian sensor. *In* Zotterman, Y. (ed.): Sensory Functions of the Skin in Primates with Special Reference to Man. pp. 37–42. Oxford, Pergamon Press, 1976.
246. Scheibel, M.E., and Scheibel, A.B.: Terminal axonal patterns in cat spinal cord. II. The dorsal horn. Brain Res., *9*:32, 1968.
247. Scott, J., and Huskisson, E.C.: Graphic representation of pain. Pain, *2*:175, 1976.
248. Schweiger, A., and Parducci, A.: Nocebo. The psychological induction of pain in the absence of either noxious stimulation or hypnotic suggestion. Pain Abstr., *1*:35, 1978.
249. Selecki, B.R., Ness, T.D., and Williams, H.B.L.: Low back pain: aetiology, differential diagnosis and pathogenesis. *In* Selecki, B.R. (ed.): Low Back Disability. Neurosurgical Orthopaedic and Radiological Symposium. pp. 1–11. Glebe, Australasian Medical Publishing, 1978.
250. Sherman, R.A., Gall, N., and Gormly, J.: Treatment of phantom limb pain with muscular relaxation training to disrupt the pain-anxiety-tension cycle. Pain, *6*:47, 1979.
251. Sherrington, C.S.: On the anatomical constitution of nerves of skeletal muscles; with remarks on recurrent fibers in the ventral spinal nerve root. J. Physiol. (Lond.), *17*:211, 1894.
252. Sicuteri, F.: Headache as the most common disease of the antinociceptive system. Pain Abstr., *1*:95, 1978.
253. Sindou, M., Quoex, C., and Baleydier, C.: Fiber organization at the posterior spinal cord-rootlet junction in man. J. Comp. Neurol., *153*:15, 1974.
254. Slater, P., and Blundell, C.: The effects of a permanent and selective depletion of brain catecholamines on the antinociceptive action of morphine. Arch. Pharmacol., *305*:227, 1978.
255. Snyder, R.: The organization of the dorsal root entry zone in cats and monkeys. J. Comp. Neurol., *174*:47, 1977.
256. Snyder, S.H., and Childers, S.R.: Opiate receptors and opioid peptides. Annu. Rev. Neurosci., *2*:35, 1979.
257. Staiman, A., and Seeman, P.: The impulse-blocking concentrations of anesthetics, alcohols anticonvulsants, barbiturates and narcotics on phrenic and sciatic nerves. Can. J. Physiol. Pharmacol., *52*:535, 1974.
258. Sternbach, R.A.: Pain Patients. Traits and Treatments. New York, Academic Press, 1974.
259. Sternschein, M.J., Myers, S.J., Frewin, D.B., and Downey, J.A.: Causalgia. Arch. Phys. Med. Rehab., *56*:58, 1975.
260. Stubbs, D.F.: Frequency and the Brain. Life Sci., *18*:1, 1976.
261. Sunderland, S.: Nerves and Nerve Injuries. ed. 2. p. 1046. Edinburgh, Churchill-Livingstone, 1978.
262. Szentagothai, J.: Neuronal and synaptic arrangement in the substantia gelatinosa rolandi. J. Comp. Neurol., *122*:219, 1964.
263. Taber, E.: The cytoarchitecture of the brainstem of the cat. I: Brainstem nuclei of cat. J. Comp. Neurol., *116*:27, 1961.
264. Takahashi, T., Konishi, S., Powell, D., Leeman, S.E., and Otsuka, M.: Identification of the motoneuron-depolarizing peptide in bovine dorsal root as hypothalamic substance P. Brain Res., *73*:59, 1974.
265. Takahashi, T., and Otsuka, M.: Regional distribution of substance P in the spinal cord and nerve roots of the cat and the effect of dorsal root section. Brain Res., *87*:1, 1975.
266. Taub, A.: Relief of postherpetic neuralgia with psychotropic drugs. J. Neurosurg., *39*:235, 1973.
267. Terenius, L.: Endogenous peptides and analgesia. Annu. Rev. Pharmacol., *18*:189, 1978.
268. Thomas, P.K.: Painful neuropathies. Pain Abstr., *1*:9, 1978.
269. Thorsteinsson, G., Stonnington, H.H., Stillwell, G.K., and Elveback, L.R.: The placebo effect of transcutaneous electrical stimulation. Pain, *5*:31, 1978.
270. Torebjork, H.E.: Afferent C units responding to mechanical, thermal and chemical stimuli in human non-glabrous skin. Acta Physiol. Scand., *92*:374, 1974.
271. Torebjork, H.E., and Hallin, R.G.: Perceptual changes accompanying controlled perferential blocking of A and C fibre responses in intact human skin nerves. Exp. Brain Res., *16*:321, 1973.
272. ———: A new method for classification of C-unit activity in intact human skin nerves. *In* Bonica, J.J., and Albe-Fes-

sard, D.G. (eds.): Advances in Pain Research and Therapy. vol. 1. pp. 29–34. New York, Raven Press, 1976.

273. ______: Hyperalgesia related to abnormal reactivity in peripheral nerve endings with A-delta and C fibres. Pain Abstr., *1*:5, 1978.
274. ______: Hyperalgesia accompanying sensitization of nociceptors in human skin. Pain Abstr., *1*:236, 1978.
275. Trevino, D.L.: The origin and projections of a spinal nociceptive and thermoreceptive pathway. *In* Zotterman, Y. (ed.): Sensory Functions of the Skin in Primates, with Special Reference to Man. pp. 367–376. Oxford, Pergamon Press, 1976.
276. ______: Integration of sensory input in laminae I, II, and III of the cat's spinal cord. Fed. Proc., *37*:2234, 1978.
277. Trevino, D.L., and Carstens, E.: Confirmation of the location of spinothalmic neurons in the cat and monkey by the retrograde transport of horseradish peroxidase. Brain Res., *98*:177, 1975.
278. Trevino, D.L., Coulter, J.D., and Willis, W.D.: Location of cells of origin of spinothalamic tract in lumbar enlargement of the monkey. J. Neurophysiol., *36*:750, 1973.
279. Trevino, D.L., Maunz, R.A., Bryan, R.M., and Willis, W.D.: Location of cells of origin in the spinothalamic tract in the lumbar enlargement of cat. Exp. Neurol., *34*:64, 1972.
280. Uhl, G.R., and Snyder, S.H.: Regional and subcellular distributions of brain neurotensin. Life Sci., *19*:1827, 1976.
281. Urban, B.J., and Nashold, B.S., Jr.: Percutaneous epidural stimulation of the spinal cord for relief of pain. Long-term results. J. Neurosurg., *48*:323, 1978.
282. Ventafridda, V.: Cervical subarachnoidal morphine infusion. Pain Abstr., *1*:199, 1978.
283. Von Graffenried, B., Adler, R., Abt, K., Nuesch, E., and Spiegel, R.: The influence of anxiety and pain sensitivity on experimental pain in man. Pain, *4*:253, 1978.
284. Von Knorring, L., Almay, B.G.L., Johansson, F., and Terenius, L.: Pain perception and endorphin levels in cerebrospinal fluid. Pain, *5*:359, 1978.
285. Waldeyer, H.: Das gorilla-ruckenmark. Akad. Wissensch. Berlin, pp. 1–147, 1888.
286. Wall, P.D.: Presynaptic control of impulses at the first central synapse in the cutaneous pathway. Prog. Brain Res., *12*:92, 1964.
287. ______: The laminar organization of dorsal horn and effects of descending impulses. J. Physiol. (Lond.), *188*:403, 1967.
288. ______: Editorial. Pain, *1*:1, 1975.
289. ______: Modification of pain by non-painful events. *In* Bonica, J.J., and Albe-Fessard, D.G. (eds.): Advances in Pain Research and Therapy. vol. 1. pp. 1–16. New York, Raven Press, 1976.
290. ______: The gate control theory of pain mechanisms. A re-examination and restatement. Brain, *101*:1, 1978.
291. ______: Sensory physiology after various types of peripheral nerve injury. Pain Abstr., *1*:10, 1978.
292. Wall, P.D., and Gutnick, M.: Ongoing activity in peripheral nerves: the physiology and pharmacology of impulses originating from a neuroma. Exp. Neurol., *43*:580, 1974.
293. Wall, P.D., and Sternbach, R.A.: The need for an animal model of chronic pain. Pain, *2*:1, 1976.
294. Wall, P.D., and Sweet, W.H.: Temporary abolition of pain in man. Science, *155*:108, 1967.
295. Wall, P.D., and Werman, R.: The physiology and anatomy of long ranging afferent fibres within the spinal cord. J. Physiol. (Lond.), *255*:321, 1976.
296. Wall, P.D., and Yaksh, T. L.: Effect of Lissauer tract stimulation on activity in dorsal roots and in ventral roots. Exp. Neurol., *60*:570, 1978.
297. Walter, R., Ritzmann, R.F., Bhargava, H.N., and Flexner, L.B.: Prolyl-leucyl-glycinamide, cyclo (leucylglycine), and derivatives block development of physical dependence on morphine in mice. Proc. Natl. Acad. Sci. U.S.A., *76*:518, 1979.
298. Wang, J.K.: Antinociceptive effect of intrathecally administered serotonin. Anesthesiology, *47*:269, 1977.
299. Wang, J.K., Nauss, L.A., and Thomas, J.E.: Pain relief by intrathecally applied morphine in man. Anesthesiology, *50*:149, 1979.
300. Watson, S.J., Akil, H., Richard, C.W., III, and Barchas, J.D.: Evidence for two separate opiate peptide neuronal systems. Nature, *275*:226, 1978.
301. Westrum, L.E., Canfield, R.C., and Black, R.G.: Axonal degeneration patterns in the cat brainstem spinal trigeminal nucleus after tooth pulp removal. *In* Bonica, J.J., and Albe-Fessard, D.G. (eds.): Advances in Pain Research and Therapy. vol. 1. pp. 161–164. New York, Raven Press, 1976.
302. Willis, W.D., and Coggeshall, R.E.: Sensory Mechanisms of the Spinal Cord. New York, Plenum Press, 1978.
303. Willis, W.D., Leonard, R.B., and Kenshalo, D.R.: Spinothalamic tract neurons in the substantia gelatinosa. Science, *202*:986, 1978.
304. Willis, W.D., Trevino, D.L., Coulter, J.D., and Maunz, R.A.: Responses of primate spinothalamic tract neurons to natural stimulation of hindlimb. J. Neurophysiol., *37*:358, 1974.
305. Wilson, P.R., Person, J.R., Su, D.W., and Wang, J.K.: Herpes zoster reactivation of phantom limb pain. Mayo Clin. Proc., *53*:336, 1978.
306. Wilson, P.R., and Power, G.A.: Actions of Narcotics in the Epidural Space in Animals. Scientific Meeting of Australasian Chapter of the International Association for the Study of Pain. Surfers Paradise, Australia, 1979.
307. Wilson, P.R., and Yaksh, T.L.: Baclofen is antinociceptive in the spinal intrathecal space of animals. Eur. J. Pharmacol., *51*:323, 1978.
308. Wood, K.M.: The use of phenol as a neurolytic agent: a review. Pain, *5*:205, 1978.
309. Yaksh, T.L.: The synergistic interaction of three pharmacologically distinct spinal systems mediating antinociception: the intrathecal action of morphine serotonin and baclofen. Soc. Neurosci. Abstr., *4*:437, 1978.
310. ______: Direct evidence that spinal serotonin and noradrenaline terminals mediate the spinal antinociceptive effects of morphine in the periaqueductal gray. Brain Res., *160*:180, 1979.
311. ______: Pain and Analgesia—Pharmacology of the Nociceptive Feedback Loop. Scientific Meeting of Australasian Chapter of the International Association for the Study of Pain. Surfers Paradise, Australia, 1979.
312. Yaksh, T.L., Du Chateau, J., and Rudy, T.L.: Antagonism by methysergide and cinanserin of the antinociceptive action of morphine administered into the periaqueductal gray. Brain Res., *104*:367, 1976.
313. Yaksh, T.L., Frederickson, R.C.A., Huang, S.P., and Rudy, T.A.: In vivo comparison of the receptor populations acted upon in the spinal cord by morphine and pentapeptides in the production of analgesia. Brain Res., *148*:516, 1978.
314. Yaksh, T.L., Huang, S.P., and Rudy, T.A.: The direct and specific opiate-like effect of met-5-enkephalin and analogues on the spinal cord. Neuroscience, *2*:593, 1977.

315. Yaksh, T.L., Kohl, R.L., and Rudy, T.A.: Tolerance and withdrawal in rats receiving morphine in the spinal subarachnoid space. Eur. J. Pharmacol., *42*:275, 1977.
316. Yaksh, T.L., and Pert, A.: Chronic catheterization of the spinal subarachnoid space. Physiol. Behav., *17*:1031, 1976.
317. ______: Analgesia mediated by a direct spinal action of narcotics. Science, *192*:1357, 1976.
318. Yaksh, T.L., and Rudy, T.A.: Narcotic analgesia produced by a direct action on the spinal cord. Science. *192*:1357, 1976.
319. ______: Narcotic analgetics: CNS sites and mechanisms of action as revealed by intracerebral injection techniques. Pain, *4*:299, 1978.
320. Yaksh, T.L., and Tyce, G.M.: Microinjection of morphine into the periaqueductal gray evokes the release of serotonin from spinal cord. Brain Res. [In Press].
321. Yaksh, T.L., Wall, P.D., and Merrill, E.G.: Response properties of substantia gelatinosa neurones in the cat. Soc. Neurosci. Abstr., *3*:495, 1977.
322. Yaksh, T.L., and Wilson, P.R.: Spinal serotonin terminal system mediates antinoception. J. Pharmacol. Exp. Ther., *208*:446, 1979.
323. Yaksh, T.L., Wilson, P.R., Kaiko, R.F., and Inturrisi, C.E.: Analgesia produced by a spinal action of morphine and effects upon parturition in the rat. Anesthesiology. [In Press].

25 Acute Traumatic and Postoperative Pain Management

F. Peter Buckley and B. Roy Simpson

Pain has a teleological function in warning the patient that something is amiss and a protective function of protecting him from further insult (*e.g.*, by tightening of the abdominal musculature after abdominal surgery). Postoperatively, these functions are to some extent unnecessary because the etiology of the pain is known and the patient can, to a large extent, be protected from further harm. It is also possible that some of the protective functions may exert deleterious effects on body functions (*e.g.*, respiration) and that pain may hinder early mobilization and recovery.[27,81] Therefore, adequate pain relief may not only be indicated on humanitarian grounds but may also ameliorate some of the harmful effects.

Centrally acting narcotic analgesics have certain limitations, for while they often relieve pain at rest, they will not relieve the pain associated with moving and coughing. Efforts to provide improved analgesia by increasing the dosage of such drugs frequently results in an unacceptable incidence of central nervous system (CNS) depressive side-effects. Despite widespread efforts in the synthesis and investigation of new narcotic analgesics, there has not been a material advance in the quality of the analgesia provided nor a decrease in the incidence of undesirable side-effects associated with the use of these drugs.

For some time it has been believed that regional analgesia can provide a superior quality of pain relief and avoid many of the side-effects of a conventional narcotic analgesic. But despite this, regional analgesia has not been widely used postoperatively, for several reasons. It is much simpler and less time-consuming to permit the nursing staff to administer doses of narcotic agents intramuscularly at their convenience than for a medical specialist to perform repeated intercostal blocks or to maintain a prolonged epidural block. Until recent years, the local anesthetic drugs available were of a limited duration of action, and there were fears of the possible complications as a result of cumulative toxicity. However, with newer longer-acting drugs and careful documentation of the sequelae of neural blockade, many of these limitations have been shown to be specious.

Some carefully executed and reported studies of regional analgesia are supporting the belief that neural blockade may provide superior analgesia to narcotics. It would also appear that the patients receiving regional blocks may recover from surgery more rapidly than those receiving narcotics.[18,72] If this last contention is correct, one of the major barriers to the wider use of regional blocks—namely, that they are time-consuming and expensive—may be removed. If the patients can be discharged from the hospital earlier, the financial savings may more than justify the expense and effort of making neural blockade readily available for postoperative and post-traumatic pain.

With any analgesic technique, there is always the price to be paid of a certain incidence of complications, and the benefits that result from the technique must be measured against this incidence. Regional analgesia has suffered rather badly in this respect, inasmuch as the complications of regional blocks are usually obvious and localized (*e.g.*, a pneumothorax with an intercostal block or hypotension with an epidural block), whereas the complications of using narcotics are much less easily highlighted. It is far more difficult to assess the role of pain or of a narcotic analgesic in the patient's development of a deep vein thrombosis or pneumonia than it is to assess the role of an epidural block in producing hypotension. As a result of careful studies, it would appear that the incidence of the complications specific to regional blocks may be at a level far below that previously feared, particularly if they are routinely employed and medical and nursing staffs are familiar with their physiologic effects and develop a management routine.

SITES AND TECHNIQUES

The sites at which it is possible to inject a local anesthetic to produce analgesia can be divided into three major categories: infiltration and peripheral neural blockade, paravertebral blockade (somatic and autonomic), and central neural blockade (extradural and subarachnoid).

Although in theory any of these sites may be used, in practice the range is restricted to what technique is practical and what is least likely to lead to undue complications. A continuous subarachnoid technique, with the risk of infection and headache, and a thoracic paravertebral technique, which may carry an unacceptable incidence of pneumothorax, are thus rarely used. Moreover, just as satisfactory results can be achieved by using other techniques (*e.g.*, peripheral nerve or epidural blockade) without the aforementioned complications. In selecting the appropriate technique, it is necessary to be aware of which part of the peripheral nervous system carries the pain impulses. For instance, only partial success may result in the use of only intercostal blockade of somatic afferents during an attempt to relieve the postoperative pain of pancreatectomy, in which some of the afferent impulses are also carried by the visceral fibers by way of the celiac plexus.

INFILTRATION AND PERIPHERAL NEURAL BLOCKADE

Infiltration and peripheral blockade were among the earliest regional techniques to be used to relieve postoperative pain. While the efficacy of these techniques in producing analgesia was appreciated by the early investigators, these researchers were restricted by the properties of the drugs at their disposal, all of which had a limited duration of action. Efforts to circumvent this problem were directed in two ways: first, to find and use substances that had a prolonged duration of action and thus would require only a single administration or, second, to devise techniques that would permit repeated injection of available drugs through tubes placed in or near wounds.

In the former group a variety of substances, many of which would not be regarded as local anesthetics by today's definition, were used. These substances included qunidine and urea, local anesthetics dissolved in oil, and a number of other substances.[27,31,33,54,96,98] The use of these substances was found to produce a number of problems—patchy analgesia, an occurrence of wound sloughs, and the destruction of nerves by neurolytic substances present in the injected mixtures—and so their use has not been sustained.[13,39] Today, of course, these problems have been overcome with the availability of bupivacaine and etidocaine.

The second approach to wound infiltration was to leave hollow needles or catheters in the wound, and, through these, local anesthetic was periodically injected.[26,48,79] While such techniques apparently produced satisfactory analgesia and a low incidence of side-effects, their use has not been widespread nor have they been investigated thoroughly. If, on critical appraisal, they do provide adequate analgesia and a low incidence of side-effects, such techniques would appear to have a certain promise. They are simple; repeated "top- ups" can easily and safely be given by the nursing staff; and, with the advent of relatively inert plastic catheters and of bacterial filters, the likelihood of wound sloughs and infections would be minimized. In addition, the availability of safe long-acting agents would reduce the volume and frequency of injection.

INTERCOSTAL BLOCKS

Intercostal blocks have been used widely and have distinct advantages. They can be performed with a minimum of equipment in a body area that has a constant anatomy. They can, however, be used only when the pain is produced in thoracic or upper abdominal regions and does not involve visceral afferents.

For thoracotomy wounds, only unilateral blocks are necessary, but it is imperative that the injection be as proximal as possible in the nerve's course (*i.e.*, at the angle of the rib) in order to include the posterior division of the nerve into whose distribution the incision may extend. The nerves of the intercostal space through which the incision is made, plus the nerves of the two or three adjacent spaces, should be blocked, as should the nerves that supply the area through which the chest drains, if any emerge. It should be noted that dissection toward the apex of the lung may cause postoperative pain that involves the lower roots of the brachial plexus. This may be relieved by interscalene or other technique of brachial block. This fact was well known to surgeons who performed thoracoplasty under regional anesthesia and quickly realized that complete

(*Text continues on p. 590.*)

Table 25-1. Use of Local Anesthetics in Intercostal Block

Study	*Technique*	*Operation*	*Drug/Concentration*	*Dose/Nerve (ml)*	*Duration (hrs)*	*How Duration Assessed*
Moore and Bridenbaugh (1962)[86]	Percutaneous	Abdominal and thoracic	Tetracaine, 0.1–0.25%, + epinephrine	4–5	5–9	Not stated
Telivuo (1966)[88]	Percutaneous	Thoracic	Bupivacaine, 0.5%, + epinephrine	4	16.3	C.A.
			Bupivacaine, 0.5%	4	13.6	C.A.
Bergh and colleagues (1966)[10]	Percutaneous	Thoracic	Bupivacaine, 0.25%, + epinephrine	3–4	10–14	C.A.
Yoshikawa and colleagues (1968)[97]	Percutaneous	Abdominal, bilateral	Bupivacaine, 0.5%, + epinephrine		5–7	S.A.
Moore (1971)[69]	Percutaneous	Abdominal	Bupivacaine, 0.25%, + epinephrine		8.5	Onset regression C.A.
					11	Complete regression
Bridenbaugh (1975)[18]	Percutaneous	Abdominal	Etidocaine, 0.5%		5	
			Etidocaine, 0.5%, + epinephrine		6	
			Etidocaine, 0.5%, + epinephrine		5.5	Onset regression C.A.
			Bupivacaine, 0.25%, + epinephrine		6	
Delikan (1973)[36]	Intrathoracic	Thoracic	Bupivacaine, 0.5%, + epinephrine	4	8.5	S.A.

Dhuner (1975)[37]	Percutaneous	Abdominal, unilateral	Etidocaine, 0.5%	3	5	
			Etidocaine, 0.5%, + epinephrine		7.5	Onset regression
		Abdominal, bilateral	Bupivacaine, 0.5%, + epinephrine		7	C.A.
			Etidocaine, 0.5%, + epinephrine		7.5	
Engberg (1975)[41]	Percutaneous	Abdominal, unilateral	Etidocaine, 1.0%, + epinephrine	3	10	S.A.
		Abdominal	Etidocaine, 1.0%, + epinephrine	3	6	
Willdeck-Lund and Edstrom (1975)[95]	Intrathoracic	Thoracotomy	Etidocaine, 1%, + epinephrine		6 11	S.A. C.A.
			Bupivacaine, 0.5%, + epinephrine	2	5 11	S.A. C.A.
Galway and colleagues (1975)[47]	Intrathoracic	Thoracotomy	Bupivacaine, 0.5%, + epinephrine	5	Little useful analgesia	S.A.
			Lidocaine, 2%, + epinephrine			
Cronin and Davies (1976)[34]	Percutaneous	Abdominal, unilateral and bilateral	Bupivacaine, 0.5%, + epinephrine	3	6–18	S.A.

Key: C.A., Cutaneous analgesia;
S.A., Subjective analgesia

pain relief required both intercostal and brachial plexus blockade.

For abdominal incisions, it is not necessary to block the nerves as far posteriorly as for chest incisions, but the site of blockade should be no farther anteriorly than the posterior axillary line in order to anesthetize the lateral division of the nerve. For a subcostal incision, a unilateral block may suffice, but for paramedian or midline incisions, bilateral blocks are necessary. The nerves that supply the dermatomes through which the incision passes, plus the nerve above and below, should be blocked; thus if the incision passes through dermatomes at the level of T5–10 the nerves blocked should be T4–11.

When the block is performed will depend upon whether the block is to be a part of the anesthetic technique or is accomplished purely for postoperative analgesia. In abdominal surgery, it is feasible to use the block in company with light general anesthesia; and thus the block may be administered prior to surgery. In thoracic surgery, blocks are most useful for postoperative analgesia. In order to obtain maximum duration of postoperative analgesia, it is probably best to perform the blocks at the conclusion of the operation.

The position of the patient when the block is instituted is largely a matter of personal preference and convenience. For posterior bilateral blocks, it is easiest to have the patient prone with arms hanging loose over the sides of the table in order to rotate the scapuli out of the way and afford easy access to both sides. For posterior unilateral blocks, the lateral position with the upper arm extended forward over the chest may be acceptable. For bilateral blocks for abdominal surgery, the patient may be left supine but tilted from side to side and still afford adequate access to the posterior axillary line. A further alternative is to have the patient sitting. This is, however, practical only if the patient is not heavily sedated and an assistant is available to hold the patient.

The volume of solution used to block an individual nerve should be 4 to 5 ml and, naturally, should be accurately placed. Studies have shown that while inaccurate placement and the use of smaller volumes produce a transiently satisfactory block, the duration of action tends to be much shorter than with an accurately placed block with a larger volume of solution.[88]

Choice of Drug and Concentration

The history of the development of intercostal blocks parallels that of infiltration blocks to the degree that when the blocks were first used, the only available drugs were of a limited duration of action, so investigators turned to long-acting "anesthetic mixtures" or, alternatively, to catheter techniques. The long-acting anesthetic mixtures were plagued by complications of patchy analgesia.[8,54,87,98] Techniques were also developed in which catheters were placed along the intercostal nerves either with an open chest post-thoracotomy or, with the chest closed, with intravenous cannuli.[2,12]

The development of intercostal blocks for postoperative pain relief has proceeded with the use of conventional long-acting local anesthetics. The ideal drug for use in repeated intercostal blocks has, in clinically useful concentrations and doses, a prolonged duration of action without producing excessively high blood levels that would result in systemic side-effects. Irrespective of which drug is used, it is probably mandatory that epinephrine be included in the injected solution, for even with the long-acting drugs (bupivacaine and etidocaine), inclusion of epinephrine will tend to lower peak blood levels of the drug.[67] This is of particular importance with intercostal blocks, because for a given dose they are associated with the highest blood levels of all techniques.[16,67,97]

The inclusion of epinephrine is not without its own problems, because adverse cardiovascular effects can occur in some patients. In certain instances (*e.g.*, patients with cardiac disease, severe hypertension, or thyrotoxicosis or on monoamine oxidase inhibitors), the inclusion of epinephrine may actually be contraindicated.

In the development of long-acting drugs, attention was first focused upon tetracaine and more recently upon the long-acting local anesthetics bupivacaine and etidocaine (Table 25-1).[18,34,36,37,41,43,47,67,68,69]

The majority of studies have been concerned with single intercostal blocks, with bupivacaine initiated for surgical anesthesia with a residuum of analgesia postoperatively. As can be seen from Table 25-1, the mode of assessment of the duration of the drug's effect varies, some investigators using cutaneous analgesia and others using the patient's assessment of pain. In general, cutaneous analgesia lasts rather longer than subjective analgesia, and unilateral blocks for thoracic or upper abdominal surgery provide a longer period of patient comfort than bilateral blocks for surgery through midline or paramedian incisions. For abdominal surgery, it has been reported that blocks repeated every 8 to 12 hours provide satisfactory relief.[34,67] Concentrations of bupivacaine of 0.25 per cent and 0.5 per cent are used most frequently and while a longer duration of effect might be expected from increasing the mass of drug (*i.e.*, with 0.5% solution), this has not been studied. The addition of epinephrine would appear to prolong the duration of effect, but whether this extension is statistically significant is in doubt. One of the major fears associated with the use of bupivacaine for bilateral intercostal blocks is that in order to block all necessary nerves with 0.5-per-cent solution, the recommended maximum dose may be exceeded. For example, six nerves blocked on each side with 5 ml of 0.5 per cent bupivacaine (25 mg) consumes a total dose of 300 mg and with that comes the risk of systemic toxic effects. With frequently repeated doses, it should be anticipated that accumulation of the drug will occur. However, this is unlikely if the blocks are 6 to 9 hours apart (see Chap. 3). To date, blood levels after such repeated doses have not been measured, but clinical studies of repeated blocks using up to 200 mg every 12 hours have not reported evidence of toxicity.[34]

The use of etidocaine in intercostal blocks has also been reported at concentrations of 0.5 per cent and 1 per cent.[18,37,41,95] The addition of epinephrine appears to prolong the duration of action.[37] As with the data for bupivacaine, there is considerable variation in methods of assessing duration of analgesia. In general, in both abdominal and thoracic procedures, etidocaine, 0.5 per cent, produces about 6 hours of analgesia. As yet, its use for repeated blocks in the postoperative period has not been reported. With doses up to 360 mg (3 ml of 1% etidocaine on each of 12 intercostal nerves), no systemic complications were noted.[41]

It would seem that the choice of drug is between etidocaine, 0.5 per cent, and bupivacaine, 0.5 per cent, both with epinephrine. Both drugs produce longer durations of action than tetracaine.[18] In order to compare the toxicity of the two drugs on a dose for dose basis, it is necessary to know that etidocaine produces lower blood levels than bupivacaine, but bupivacaine may be effective in lower concentrations. However, etidocaine is more rapidly metabolized and has a greater volume of distribution (see Chap. 3).

As can be seen from Table 25-1, the duration of effect of the long-acting drugs is about 8 to 12 hours. Thus, to provide analgesia for a patient who has undergone thoracic or abdominal surgery, the anesthesiologist will have to repeat the block three or even four times in order to provide continuous postoperative analgesia. In order to avoid such repeated blocks, a search for a drug that will have a very long duration of action (24–48 hours) has been undertaken. In this search, workers have mixed dextrans with local anesthetics.[28,55,60] When local anesthetic/dextran mixtures are assessed objectively for peripheral nerve block, they do not show an appreciably longer duration of action than local anesthetics alone.[28] Nevertheless, the researchers do report increases in the duration of subjective analgesia (Table 25-2). It should be stressed that while these are subjective reports of prolonged analgesia, more studies with objective data will be necessary before the efficacy of dextran in prolonging local anesthesia can be advocated.

Quality of Analgesia

Those who use the technique widely are in virtual agreement that the analgesia provided by intercostal blocks is superior to that provided by narcotics. However, in most studies, the methods of measuring the quality of the analgesia have been indirect—patient reference; time to patient's request for, or nurse's assessment of the need for further analgesia; asking the patient if he was in pain; or abdominal palpation.[18,34] Quality of analgesia has been evaluated objectively in a small series of patients, which has shown that intercostal blocks are better than narcotics.[55] However, a larger series in which the quality of analgesia in patients who had had thoracotomies was scored by an independent observer differed markedly.[47] Obviously, there is a need for further studies by unbiased observers of quality of analgesia in a series of comparable patients, one group receiving their analgesia by blocks and the other by narcotics.

Cardiovascular Effects

There are no available studies of the cardiovascular effects of intercostal blocks alone or of the cardiovascular changes produced when pain is relieved by a block. The block alone would be expected to produce very minor changes in cardiovascular variables, the extent depending upon the drug and dose used and the presence of epinephrine, because all have been shown to produce changes in cardiovascular function.[57] When these blocks are used in the postoperative period, their cardiovascular effects would be a part of a composite picture with the cardiovascular effects of pain and pain relief.

Respiratory Effects

The effects upon respiratory function of intercostal blocks alone have not been studied. The physicians who first used intercostal blockade for analge-

Table 25.2. Nerve Block With Local Anesthetic/Dextran Mixtures

Study	*Technique*	*Operation*	*Drug/Concentration*	*Dose/Nerve (ml)*	*Duration (hrs.)*	*Duration Assessment*
Loder (1962)[60]	Intrathoracic	Thoracotomy	Lidocaine, 1% + epinephrine ± 10% dextran	5	No block, 1.75 Block, 5.75	S.A.
Chinn and Wirjoatmadja (1967)[28]	Ulnar nerve		Tetracaine, 0.15%, + epinephrine	1	5.5	Regression C.A.
			Tetracaine, 0.15%, + epinephrine + dextran	1	6.5	
	Various	Various	Tetracaine, 0.15%, + epinephrine		Up to 10	C.A.
			+ dextran, 5%		Up to 17	S.A.
Kaplan and colleagues (1975)[55]	Intrathoracic	Thoracic	Bupivacaine, 0.375%	3	More than 12	C.A.
			Bupivacaine, 0.375%, + dextran		36	S.A.

Key: C.A., Cutaneous Analgesia
S.A., Subjective Analgesia

sia expected that the superior analgesia and lack of primary respiratory side-effects would result in a lower incidence of postoperative respiratory complications.[31] It is clear that certain factors (*e.g.*, abdominal and chest surgery, advancing age, and a history of respiratory disease) all predispose patients to an increase in the incidence and severity of both hypoxemia and pulmonary infection. However, the role of the pathophysiologic changes (*e.g.*, decreased functional residual capacity [FRC], abdominal distension, and hypoventilation) has not been determined. It is also not clear which respiratory function studies are the best indices for assessing these problems. The effects of intercostal blocks on some dynamic indices of respiratory function and blood gases have been studied (Table 25-3). Unfortunately, studies to date have concerned fit patients rather than those expected to derive the most benefit from intercostal blocks (*e.g.*, the elderly and those with marked respiratory disease).

Studies that report the respiratory effects of intercostal blocks in thoracic surgery have utilized blocks performed once at the end of surgery, with either bupivacaine or etidocaine, and compared them with similar groups of patients who received narcotics. Following thoracic operations, patients consistently show marked reductions in effort-dependent tests of respiratory function (*e.g.*, PEF and FVC). Compared with patients receiving narcotics, the intercostal block group of patients consistently showed significantly less impairment of these indices. This implies that the patients who have had blocks are able to cough more effectively and to participate in respiratory therapy procedures.

While effort-dependent tests yield an estimate of the mechanical aspects of respiratory function, they do not necessarily correlate with the changes in blood gas values seen after thoracic surgery. Investigations on Pco_2 changes with intercostal blocks generally show that patients with and without blocks have similar Pco_2 levels, usually within the normal range. The effects of intercostal blocks on postoperative hypoxemia are not as consistent; some authors have found little or no alleviation of hypoxemia, whereas others have found significant reduction in postoperative hypoxemia.[36,43,55] Also, in patients who receive a single intercostal block the respiratory sparing effects produced persisted 12 to 16 hours, which is beyond the period of time that effective analgesia from the blocks would be expected to last.[10,55]

In abdominal surgery, a difference in respiratory effects of intercostal blocks has been reported between patients having subcostal incisions and those having midline incisions. Patients having subcostal incisions, who received single-injection intercostal blocks, had significantly less impairment of PEF, FVC, and Pao_2 than patients who received narcotics.[41] These differences persisted well beyond the expected duration of the block. In the same study, patients who received midline incisions showed changes in PEF and FVC similar to those of the patients receiving narcotics. Although single-dose intercostal blocks may alleviate some of the respiratory problems, there is also evidence that if analgesia is provided by a series of blocks or a combination of blocks plus limited narcotics, there will be less impairment of Pao_2 during the immediate postoperative period than with narcotics alone. Also, the blood gases return to normal values earlier.[19]

Thus, there appears to be increasing evidence that patients who receive intercostal blocks show better respiratory posture in the postoperative period. In practical terms, the fact that a single block may provide beneficial effects of long duration renders the technique worthwhile, especially in patients with chronic lung disease or in whom the use of narcotic analgesics would be hazardous.

Prevention of Respiratory Complications

As mentioned previously, one of the rationales for intercostal blocks is to produce a reduction in the incidence of postoperative respiratory infections. However, while studies of this have been performed, they are plagued by the difficulties in defining chest infection using such variable indices as pyrexia, purulence, and sputum and radiologic changes (Table 25-4). As can be seen, the results are equivocal, but the evidence suggests a lesser incidence of infection in patients treated with blocks. As with respiratory effects of blocks, more detailed studies of the incidence of chest infection after blocks, with more precise criteria, are necessary.

Early Ambulation and Discharge

Even if regional analgesia by intercostal blocks does not confer benefits in other respects, its use may be attractive if patients fare better in general and can be discharged from the hospital earlier than those who receive narcotics. There is some evidence that this may be the case, but as yet the numbers involved are too small to draw firm con-

(*Text continues on p. 596.*)

*Table 25-3. **Postoperative Respiratory Effects of Intercostal Blocks***

Study	Operations and Technique	Time of Test	Type of Test	Effects
Bergh and colleagues (1966)[10]	Thoracotomy; percutaneous single shot	1st postoperative day, 2 hours post-block	Bupivacaine vs. narcotics	PEFR improved by block and significantly better than narcotic group on 2nd and 3rd post-operative days Blood gas changes similar
Bridenbaugh and colleagues (1973)[19]	Cholecystectomy; per-cutaneous repeated	Postoperative Days 1, 2, and 3	Tetracaine more than 4 blocks 1 and 2 blocks ± narcotics 3 Tetracaine less than 4 blocks + narcotics N Narcotics	Patients in Groups 1 and 2, lesser falls in Pao_2, patients in 1, 2, and 3 tended to have lower $Paco_2$
Delikan and colleagues, (1973)[36]	Thoracotomy; intrathoracic single shot	Postoperative 4 hours after block	Bupivacaine vs. narcotics	Lesser falls in PERF and Pao_2 in blocked group
Engberg (1975)[41]	Upper abdominal; single shot unilateral incision	Postoperative 1 and 4 hours and 1 and 2 days	Etidocaine, 1%, + epinephrine vs. narcotics	PEFR and FVC significantly less reduced in blocked group; minimal falls in Pao_2 Effects persisted into 1st postoperative day
	Midline incision			PEFR and FVC and Pao_2 and reductions all similar (both groups)
Faust and Nauss (1975)[43]	Thoracotomy; percutaneous day of surgery	Day of operation	Bupivacaine, 0.5%, vs. narcotics	Lesser falls in FVC; lesser falls in MNV; blood gases similar
Galway and colleagues (1975)[47]	Thoracotomy; intrathoracic single shot	Postoperative 1, 2, 24 hours after block	Bupivacaine and lidocaine vs. narcotics	No differences in PEFR, FVC, and $Paco_2$ between groups
Kaplan and colleagues (1975)[55]	Thoracotomy; intrathoracic single shot	Postoperative 4 hours 1, 2, and 3 days	Bupivacaine, 0.375%, + Dextran Bupivacaine, 0.375% Dextran only	PEFR and FVC and Pao_2 falls less in blocked groups
Willdeck-Lund and Edstrom (1975)[95]	Thoracotomy; intrathoracic single shot	Postoperative .5 to 1.5 and 1.5 to 2 hours	Bupivacaine, 0.5%, vs. Etidocaine, 1%	PEFR and blood gas changes similar

*Table 25-4. **Influence of Intercostal Block on Postoperative Respiratory Complications***

Study	*Operation*	*Number of Blocks*	*Diagnostic Criteria*	*Incidence*	
				Narcotics	*Blocks*
Delikan and colleagues (1975)[36]	Thoracic	Single	Radiology	3/20	1/20
Bridenbaugh (1973)[19]	Cholecystectomy	Repeated	Radiology and leukocytosis	1/15	1/11 (Pneumo)
Engberg (1975)[41]	Upper abdomen	Single	Clinical symptoms	7/118	2/112 (1 Pneumo 1 Asthma)
Faust and Nauss (1976)[43]	Thoracic	Single	Radiology	2/14	Not stated

clusions.[19] If these findings are confirmed, the extra effort entailed in performing these blocks in the postoperative period may be warranted by the savings in use of hospital beds and associated expenses.

Complications

With any technique, however efficacious and reliable, complications do occur and, when the practicability and risk-to-benefit ratio are evaluated, these must be taken into consideration. With intercostal block, pneumothorax is the complication that has aroused most anxiety, the quoted incidence varying from 19 per cent in one series to 0.073 per cent in another.[34,67] It would appear that the incidence of pneumothorax with experienced anesthesiologists is relatively low. The danger of pneumothorax is primarily found in patients who have undergone abdominal surgery and is virtually lacking in patients who have undergone thoracic procedures, because the blocks will be performed only on the operative side and the patient will either not have a lung to puncture (as in the case of a pneumonectomy) or will have chest drains *in situ* (as in the case of a lobectomy, pleurectomy, or mitral valvotomy).

As has been mentioned , the peak blood levels of local anesthetic produced by intercostal blocks are high in comparison with other techniques, and thus there is a potential for a toxic reaction from the absorbed drug. The toxic reaction, however, appears to be relatively rare. Intrathoracic blocks are also performed under direct vision at the time of surgery. The unusual complication of a total spinal anesthetic has been reported from this technique. The explanation of this may be an inadvertent subarachnoid puncture or, alternatively, a spread or direct injection of the drug through the dural cuff of the nerve root and then to the subarachnoid space.[9]

PARAVERTEBRAL BLOCKADE

With paravertebral blockade, local anesthetic is placed close to the nerves shortly after they leave the vertebral column and prior to their division into somatic and visceral divisions, with resultant blockade of both somatic and autonomic afferents. Such a technique was advocated for the provision of postoperative analgesia.[52] It is, however, a relatively difficult technique to perform, requiring multiple punctures, and has a distinct incidence of complications, such as hypotension due to the associated sympathetic block. These problems, allied with availability of extradural or intercostal analgesia, have caused the technique to fall into disuse.

EXTRADURAL BLOCKADE

Extradural blockade has been used extensively to provide postoperative analgesia. Initially, its use was restricted to upper abdominal operations and chest wall trauma, which caused the most pain and the greatest degree of physiologic derangement. Recently, its use has been extended to procedures in which pain is not as severe, such as hip surgery and urologic and gynecologic surgery. A block of the desired extent can be achieved by introducing a catheter by way of the commonly used caudal or lumbar routes and then injecting an appropriate dose of drug. While this method of initiating and maintaining the block is feasible, it involves large doses of drug and also unnecessarily blocks areas that may not be a source of pain. For example, a low lumbar approach to block at the level of T5–T10 for upper abdominal incisional pain, will also block the segments L1 to S5 and thus produce leg weakness and urinary retention. These problems can be circumvented by putting the catheter in the extradural space at, or near, the middle of dermatomes to be blocked and injecting a limited amount of drug to produce "segmental analgesia."

When segmental extradural blocks were first used, methods of passing catheters into the thoracic and lumbar extradural space were unavailable. Stiff catheters with stylets were introduced by way of the caudal hiatus and passed cephalad to the desired level.[30] Today, techniques and equipment are available to enable the extradural space to be catheterized at virtually any level.

When an extradural catheter is introduced for analgesia, it is best to place a short length (3–4 cm) of the catheter within the extradural space at, or near, the middle of the segments to be blocked. Thus, for an upper abdominal incision to extend through dermatomes at the level of T6 to T10, the catheter should be introduced at T7–8 or T8–9 or for a lower abdominal incision to extend through dermatomes at T10–L1, atT12–L1 or T11–12. Attempts to pass catheters to a level remote from the puncture site may be unsuccessful because it has been fairly conclusively shown that, once placed in the extradural space, such catheters may loop, travel in the wrong direction, and even pass out of the extradural space by way of the intervertebral foramina.[17,80] While it is quite feasible to block thoracic dermatomes by using a lumbar catheter, this will entail the disadvantages mentioned earlier—high dosage and excessive block.

Techniques of catheter placement are fully discussed in Chapter 8. Avoidance of infection during prolonged epidural analgesia requires meticulous attention to sterile technique with each refill. This may be aided by adding a bacterial filter of the kind used for hyperalimentation lines to the catheter injection site. It is possible for the filter membranes to rupture, and it is prudent practice to replace the filter at 24-hour intervals.

Techniques and Drugs

In order to maintain an analgesic concentration of local anesthetic within the desired area of the extradural space, one of two techniques is used. The original method, here termed the *"top-up" technique,* was to administer the drug through the catheter at intervals. Alternatively, a constant infusion of drug, here termed *infusion technique,* could be used. Each technique and its result are discussed separately and then respective advantages and deficiencies noted.

The "Top-up" Technique. With the "top-up" technique, a dose of drug is administered either when the patient complains of returning pain or at predetermined intervals appropriate to the effective duration of action of the drug being used. The second method was used in order to spare the patient intervals of pain that might occur between doses. In using such a technique, it is important to bear in mind that the speed of regression of analgesia is much faster than seen with conventional narcotic analgesia. Thus, when the patient complains of returning pain, little time should be lost in providing a reinforcing dose, both in order to spare the patient discomfort and to reduce any tachyphylaxis that might occur.[22]

For the administration of the top-up injection, the patient is usually placed supine, and control measurements of pulse and blood pressure are taken. The appropriate dose of drug is administered, with appropriate sterility precautions (Table 25-5). The patient should be left supine for about 30 minutes in order to permit the maximum sympathetic block effects, to be observed by pulse and blood pressure readings repeated at 5-minute intervals. If, after this time, the cardiovascular measurements are satisfactory, the patient may be placed in any desired position. If changes in position result in a significant change or blood pressure, he should be returned to the supine position and have an increased rate of intravenous infusion (see Chap. 8).

Drugs. In theory, it is possible to use any local anesthetic agent for continuous extradural analgesia. However, when the properties of some of the available drugs are considered, the range is substantially narrowed. Procaine, with its unreliable action and short duration of action, is not suitable, nor is prilocaine because doses of 600 mg, which lead to the production of methemoglobinemia, are likely to be exceeded.

Early workers reported satisfactory results using dilute solutions of 0.15 per cent to 0.25 per cent tetracaine.[13,30] Later studies used lidocaine in concentrations of 1 per cent and 1.5 per cent.[20,25,64,81] As seen in Table 25-5, the duration of action of lidocaine is from 60 to 90 minutes. Mepivacaine has not been widely used, but it has been reported satisfactory and of duration similar to lidocaine.[85]

The advent of the newer longer-acting drugs, bupivacaine and etidocaine, has made them the current drugs of choice. Bupivacaine has been used in concentrations of 0.25 per cent and 0.5 per cent and etidocaine in solutions between 0.5 per cent and 1 per cent. These drugs appear to produce effective durations of analgesia between 1.5 and 3 hours, depending upon the circumstances and concentration and dose used.

It is readily apparent from Table 25-5 that the quoted durations of action of the various local anesthetic drugs, for analgesia in segmental extradural block are considerably shorter than when the same drugs are used to provide extradural anesthesia for surgical operations or when they are used for peripheral nerve blocks. These differences are reflections of differences in technique and clinical circumstances. In using an extradural block for surgical purposes, a large dose of drug is used to provide a wide area of blockade, whereas for analgesic purposes a small dose is used to provide blockade of a circumscribed area. In the latter case, absorption and disposition of drug occur more quickly, and thus the block does not last as long.

The addition of epinephrine to solutions used in extradural block for analgesia does not appear to produce the prolongation of action that is seen when the drugs are used in other circumstances. This applies to both the short-acting drugs and the longer-acting drugs.[1,40,78,81]

Concentration. The choice of concentration will depend upon the anatomic segments to be blocked. Some segments (*e.g.*, L5–S1) are more resistant to blockade, a finding that has been correlated with the size of nerve roots.[46] These segments will thus require a higher concentration of drug. There do, however, appear to be concentrations below which

Table 25-5. Prolonged Segmental Epidural Block—"Top-up" Technique

Study	Operation	Catheter Site	Drug/Concentration	Volume (ml)	Duration of Action (min.)	Total Dose mg/hr (Calculation from Available Data)	Plasma Concentrations (ug/ml)
Cleland (1949)[30]	Abdomen	Caudal Lumbar	Tetracaine, 0.15% Epinephrine, 1:200,000 Dibucaine, 0.2% Epinephrine, 1:100,000	6–15	Not given		
Bonica (1953)[13]	Various	Various	Tetracaine, 0.05–0.1%				
Bromage (1954)[20]	Upper abdomen	Not known	Lidocaine, 0.8%				
Simpson and colleagues (1961)[81]	Upper abdomen	Thoracic	Lidocaine, 1.5%	Mean 9 S.D. 0.7	80–95 Epinephrine did not extend the duration	Approximately 90	
Burn (1964)[25]	Upper and lower abdomen	Thoracic	Lidocaine, 1.5% + epinephrine	5–9	Approximately 120	35–65	
Ellis and colleagues (1968)[40]	Upper abdomen	Thoracic	Lidocaine, 1.5% Prilocaine, 1.5% Bupivacaine, 0.375%	5–7 3–6 5–6	(60 Epinephrine (67 did not extend (125 duration		
Renck (1969)[74]	Prostatectomy	Lumbar	Bupivacaine, 0.5%, + epinephrine	8–12	Approximately 240	25	
Stanton-Hicks (1971)[86]	Hip	Lumbar	Bupivacaine, 0.5%, + epinephrine	64	180–360	10–15	
Spence and Smith (1971)[84]	Upper abdomen	Thoracic	Bupivacaine, 0.5%, + epinephrine	5–7	Approximately 120	12.5–17.5	
Abel, Salem, and Scott (1975)[1]	Hysterectomy	Lumbar	Bupivacaine, 0.5% Etidocaine, 1.0%	10 10	160 SEM ± 9 149 SEM ± 9 Addition of epinephrine had little effect	20	
Griffiths and colleagues (1975)[51]	Thoracic	Thoracic	Bupivacaine, 0.5%, + epinephrine	5.7 ISD 0.7	163 S.D. 51	12	
Buckley and Simpson (1975)[24]	Upper abdomen	Thoracic	Bupivacaine, 0.5% Bupivacaine, 0.375% Etidocaine, 0.5%	5–9	100–150 85–130 85–110		
Renck (1976)[76]	Upper abdomen	Thoracic	Etidocaine, 1.0%	4–5	No stated doses given at 300-minute intervals		0.5–1
Miller and colleagues (1976)[64]	Upper abdomen	Thoracic	Lidocaine, 1–2%		No stated doses at 1- to 2-hour intervals	(Mean of 40)	

satisfactory analgesia cannot be produced. For lidocaine, this is in the region of 0.8 per cent and 1 per cent; for bupivacaine, 0.25 per cent; and for etidocaine, 0.5 per cent. While the lower quoted concentrations may be effective, they produce a short duration of action. Workers have therefore used higher concentrations—lidocaine, 1 per cent to 1.5 per cent; bupivacaine, 0.375 per cent to 0.5 per cent; and etidocaine, up to 1 per cent. There are no data on the maximum concentration of drug that can be used in these circumstances, but it should be kept in mind that higher concentrations increase total dose and with it the likelihood of toxic reactions.

Dosages. Once the appropriate concentration to be used has been selected, it is then necessary to decide the volume of solution required to produce analgesia of the relevant segments. As with concentration, this is governed by site; the sacral region needing larger volumes than the lumbar region, which in turn requires more than the thoracic region. Age and body weight also influence the size of dose, the young needing more than the old and the obese less than the average-sized (Table 25-5). It should be stressed that these quoted doses are only guidelines. The volume and concentration of drug used to obtain desired analgesia should be determined for each patient. In general, small doses of drug (4–5 ml) can be initiated and increased from there as necessary. This is especially applicable for the elderly and in thoracic extradural blockade.

Repeated doses for continuous postoperative analgesia may result in tachyphylaxis. That is, the extent, intensity and duration of the block tend to diminish with successive doses. It has been suggested that tachyphylaxis can be avoided by repeating doses empirically rather than allow the block to wear off between doses.[22]

Toxicity. Amide-type local anesthetics are metabolized by the liver. As the amount of drug reaching the circulation exceeds the metabolic rate, accumulation of the drug in the circulation will occur. This can be seen to occur with intermittent injections, the blood levels peaking some 15 to 20 minutes after each "top-up" and then falling away, only to rise again with a successive injection, producing a graph with a "saw-toothed" pattern. This rise in the peak blood levels has been shown to occur with lidocaine, but with etidocaine this rise in peak levels is slow (see Chap. 3). In contrast, the predicted quantity of drug remaining at the site of injection is greater with etidocaine than with lidocaine.[91] Bupivacaine pharmacokinetics has not been studied in postoperative analgesia, but from work in obstetrics the rise in peak plasma concentration levels would also appear to be slow.[77,89] Thus, it would seem that the likelihood of producing plasma concentrations that would lead to a toxic reaction is greater with the short-acting drugs, a problem that may be compounded by the fact that tachyphylaxis is more likely to occur with these agents, with their need for larger doses at more frequent intervals.

The addition of epinephrine to local anesthetic mixtures is a time-honored method of reducing peak blood levels of local anesthetic agents. This has not been studied following repeated injections for postoperative analgesia. Research in obstetrics, however, would suggest that while this lowering is significant in the case of lidocaine, it is less significant with bupivacaine.[89] It may prove to be so with the larger dosage used in postoperative analgesia, however.[78] Other factors that may influence the rise in blood levels of the drug are the inability of the liver to metabolize the drugs, for instance, in hepatic failure or when there is a low cardiac output with low hepatic perfusion rates (see Chap. 3).[90]

Infusion Technique. The second method of maintaining continuous extradural analgesia is by a continuous infusion of local anesthetic into the extradural space, at a rate that equals that at which the drug is removed by the extradural vessels. This technique was developed to avoid the occasional periods of pain between tardy "top-ups" and, in fact, the need for "top-ups" at all.[50,62] The infusion has been maintained by either a *gravity-feed drip* or by a variety of infusion-pumping devices.[72,85]

Drugs. Details of the drugs used and the infusion rates are provided in Table 25-6. The most widely used drug for this technique has been lidocaine. Originally, 1 per cent lidocaine was used, but following an accidental overdose, workers turned to 0.5-per-cent or 0.4-per-cent solutions. Another advantage of the reduced concentration is the possibility that a faster flow rate could be used and would minimize the blockage rate of the fine extradural catheter. The effects of prolonged diluted infusion on physiologic parameters (cardiorespiratory), with apparently satisfactory results, have been reported.[65,82] Other workers found they could achieve better results using either 1-per-cent or 1.5-per-cent solutions of lidocaine.[85] Bupivacaine (0.1%–1%) has also been used in this technique.[51,72,75,76]

Dosages. Thoracic blocks with lidocaine after abdominal operations required a wide variation in dosage from 5 to 150 mg per hour to 3.2 mg per kg per hour (224 mg/hour for a 70-kg man).[63,82,85] Whether the use of a dilute solution is associated with a reduced dose requirement is not clear, although some

Table 25-6. Prolonged Epidural Block —Infusion Technique

Study	*Operation*	*Catheter Site*	*Drug/Concentrations*	*Duration of Study*	*Dose (mg/hour)*	*Peak Blood Levels ($\mu g/ml$ + sample time)*
Greene and Dawkins (1966)[50]	Upper and lower abdomen	Thoracic and lumbar	Lidocaine, 0.5%–1%, + epinephrine		163 S.D. 73	4.8–6.9 $\mu g/ml$
Spoerel (1971)[85]	Abdomen	T11–L2	Lidocaine, 0.5%, + epinephrine	10–15 hours	50–120	
	Abdomen	L3–4–T9–10	Lidocaine, 1.2%, ± epinephrine	Mean 49 hours	50–150	
Sjögren and Wright (1972)[82]		Lumbar			4.5 ± 0.3 mg/kg/hr (315 mg/hr for 70-kg man)	Mean 4.81 (3–5.1)
	Cholecystectomy		Lidocaine, 0.4%	2 days		
		Thoracic			3.2 ± 0.1 mg/kg/hr (224 mg/hr for 70-kg man)	Mean 4.18 (2.2–7.5) at 38 hours
Modig and Holmdahl (1975)[65]			Lidocaine, 0.4%			4.25 ± SEM 0.2
	Hip	Lumbar	Lidocaine, 0.4%, + epinephrine	3 days	Not given	4.0 ± SEM 0.5 2nd day
Griffiths and colleagues (1975)[51]	Thoracic	Thoracic	Bupivacaine, 0.25%	48 hours	22	0.95–3.76 48 hours
			Bupivacaine, 0.125%		16	2.24–2.36 48 hours
Renck (1975)[75]		Thoracic	Bupivacaine, 0.1%	30 hours	15–20	3 $\mu g/ml$ (approximate)
			Bupivacaine, 1%	50 hours	7–18	1.2 $\mu g/ml$ (approximate)
Pflug and colleagues (1974)[72]	Upper abdomen and hip	T10–11 abdominal;	Bupivacaine, 0.25–0.5%	72 hours		0.73 (0.29–0.95), 24 hours
		T2–3, hip	Concentration decreasing with time			1.49 (0.85–2.34), 48 hours
						1.39 (0.62–2.85), 72 hours
Renck (1976)[76]	Upper abdomen	Thoracic	Bupivacaine, 1%	24–48 hours	Initial, 7	
					24 hours, 11	0.65, 24 hours
					48 hours, 18	1.25, 43 hours

work suggests that this might be so. For example, in one study 0.5 per cent lidocaine had to be given as 50 to 150 mg per hour, as did lidocaine, 1.2 per cent.[85] Studies with bupivacaine reported conflicting date, a higher dosage and a lower one with dilute solutions.[51,76] With the shorter-acting drugs, the addition of epinephrine did not appear to decrease the dose requirement.[65]

Toxicity. As with the "top-up" technique, the prolonged administration of a local anesthetic at a rate faster than it is metabolized will lead to a gradual accumulation of the drug in the body, as reflected by a gradual rise in blood levels. In contrast to that of the "top-up" technique, this rise is likely to be fairly smooth. At some point, it is likely that a state of equilibrium between infusion and metabolism could be reached, being reflected by steady blood levels of the drug. This time would appear to be at, or around, 40 to 48 hours after the start of the infusion for both the short-acting and for the long-acting drugs.[65,76,82] Other than the incidents that might result from an inadvertent overdose of the drugs, there is no evidence that such a technique produces toxicity. The blood level data that have been reported are below the levels that are thought to produce serious toxic effects. Peak levels apparently are unaffected by the addition of epinephrine. Some workers have reported what they interpreted as subjective signs of toxicity (*i.e.*, drowsiness, with blood levels of greater than 1.5 ug/ml of bupivacaine), whereas other workers found no signs of toxicity with higher blood levels (up to 2.8 ug/ml).[51,72,76]

Quality of Analgesia

When extradural analgesia has proceeded smoothly, there is little doubt that the quality of analgesia is excellent. In a small number of cases, failure to provide satisfactory analgesia will result from problems of catheter placement or displacement, kinking or blocking.[81,85] If there are no technical problems, what is the quality of analgesia that can be expected (Table 25-7)? As with intercostal blocks, it is difficult to reach clear-cut conclusions because of the varying criteria of analgesia used by different authors, and because of the paucity of controlled data that compare patients who receive blocks with patients who receive conventional narcotic analgesia.

With the "top-up" technique, early workers were enthusiastic but did not provide data on efficacy and duration.[13,21,30] Simpson and colleagues were the first to provide such data.[81] In their series of 57 patients, analgesia was classified as excellent (complete freedom from pain even when coughing and moving) in all but three, in whom the failure was associated with catheter extrusion. Stanton–Hicks, using 0.5 per cent bupivacaine with epinephrine, had three failures associated with catheter problems in his series of patients following hip surgery.[86] While he did not classify the analgesia directly, he noted that none of the patients required any analgesics. Addisson and colleagues used a linear analogue scale to compare analgesia in a group of patients receiving a thoracic epidural block with 0.5 per cent bupivacaine against a series of patients receiving narcotics following cholecystectomy. Their findings were that on Day 1, 60 per cent of the blocked patients had more than 70 per cent of pain relief, and on Day 2, 56 per cent had more than 70 per cent pain relief, figures that were superior to the narcotic-treated group. In using the same drug post-thoracotomy, Griffiths, and associates found that no patient suffered more than slight pain and four out of seven suffered no pain at all.[51] However, they did not use a control group receiving narcotics. When the continuous infusion mode of administration is used, the results are general. In a more recent series of patients following upper abdominal operations and using small volumes of 1 per cent bupivacaine, Renck reported only moderate pain relief.

Thus, the notion that the continuous mode of analgesia provides a smoother course than the "top-up" mode appears not to be supported by the available data. In addition, there is the potential problem of catheter movement into a blood vessel or subarachnoid space while infusion continues. The "top-up" technique offers the opportunity for careful aspiration prior to injection and close surveillance during the following 30 minutes when maximum plasma concentrations and sympathetic blockade will occur. The availability of long-acting drugs further supports the "top-up" approach as being quite practical, as well as potentially safer.

Cardiovascular Effects

Extradural block can influence the patient's cardiovascular status in a number of ways: extent of vasomotor blockade; blocking of the cardiac sympathetic fibers; pharmacologic effects of absorbed local anesthetic on the cardiovascular system, systemic effects of vasoactive substance injected with the local anesthetic, elevation of cerebrospinal fluid (CSF) pressure, and the condition of the patient—

(*Text continues on p. 604.*)

Table 25-7. Prolonged Epidural Block—Overall Assessment of Analgesia

Study	*Operation*	*Number of Patients*	*Catheter Site*	*Drug/ Concentration*	*Duration of Study*	*Success*	*Mode of Assessment*
"Top-up" technique							
Simpson and colleagues (1961)[81]	Upper abdomen	57	Thoracic	Lidocaine, 1.5%	48 hours	93%, Excellent 7% Failure due to catheter problems	Assessed by author Excellent = free from pain or coughing or movement
Stanton-Hicks (1971)[86]	Hip	22	Lumbar	Bupivacaine, 0.5%, + epinephrine	3 days	17, Good 3 Failures due to catheter problems	Good = no narcotics required
Addison and colleagues (1974)[3]	Cholecystectomy	25	Thoracic	Bupivacaine, 0.5%	2 days	Day 1, 60% > 70% relief Day 2, 56% > 70% relief	By visual analogue scale
Griffiths and colleagues (1975)[51]	Thoracic	7	Thoracic	Bupivacaine, 0.25%, + epinephrine	48 hours	4/7, No pain 3/7, Slight pain	Assessed by patient 10 days postoperatively
Infusion techniques							
Green and Dawkins (1966)[50]	Upper abdomen	42	T5–6	Lidocaine, 0.4%	Average 71 hours	83%, No narcotic 9%, 1 dose narcotic 8%, 1 dose narcotic	By ward nursing staff
		91	T9–10	Lidocaine, 1%, + epinephrine		65%, No narcotic 35%, 1 or more narcotic	
		22		Lidocaine, 0.5%, + epinephrine		71%, No narcotic 28%, 1 or more narcotic	

Spoerel and colleagues (1971)[85]	Abdomen pancreatic, and vascular disease	95	T9–10 or L3–4 Mechanical Intermittent	Lidocaine or Mepivacaine, 1–2%, + epinephrine	Average 70 hours	76% (73), Good 16% (16), Fair 7% (6), Poor	Good = not more than 100 mg pethidine/day
		31	Mechanical Continuous		Average 76 hours	77% (24), Good 13% (7), Fair	Fair = some relief but more than 100 mg pethidine /day
Griffiths and colleagues (1971)[51]	Thoracic	8	Thoracic	Bupivacaine, 0.25 or 0.125%	48 hours	Amount of pain None, 3 Slight, 2 Moderate, 2 Severe, 1	Recall by patient 10 days post-operatively
Pflug (1974)[72]	Upper abdomen Hip	10 10	T10–11 L2–3	Bupivacaine, 0.5–0.25%	72 hours	Excellent	Not stated
Renck (1976)[26]	Upper abdomen	16	Not stated	Bupivacaine, 1%	48 hours	Mean pain, Score approximately 2	Scale 1 Pain free on coughing 2 Moderate pain on coughing 3 Severe pain on coughing

vasomotor tone, blood volume, efficiency of homeostatis mechanisms.[14] In general, the effects are mild provided hypovolemia is avoided (see Chap. 8).

Most studies of cardiovascular function following epidural block have had young and healthy volunteers, and it may well be invalid to extend that data to postoperative patients, in whom a number of other factors may influence the cardiovascular response: concurrent medication—especially CNS-depressant drugs that reduce CNS sensitivity or peripheral and central cardiovascular responses, blood volume deficits either as a result of blood or fluid loss or fluid deprivation (patients with blood loss tolerate epidural block poorly[15], and age and any significant medical condition such as severe cardiovascular disease).

Only a few studies have addressed themselves to these factors. Renck, studying elderly patients receiving either morphine or epidural block analgesia (bupivacaine, 0.5%, plus epinephrine), found that both groups had a hyperdynamic circulation with raised cardiac output, but this was significantly greater following epidural block.[74] Similar results were found in patients undergoing hip surgery treated with 0.4 per cent lidocaine infusion or pentazocine.[65] In a much larger series of patients undergoing chloecystectomy and treated with 0.4 per cent lidocaine infusion, similar evidence of a hyperkinetic circulation indicated that cardiac output was increased by 43 per cent over the preoperative value and total peripheral resistance and mean arterial pressure decreased. Although heart rate and stroke volume were raised, cardiac-work indices were not affected.[82] In these patients, when the block was stopped and pain experienced, further rises in cardiac output and mean arterial pressure were seen, but at a penalty of a rising cardiac work.

Thus, the clinical picture of a patient who received a continuous epidural block in the postoperative period shows vasodilatation with a dynamic circulation and a mean arterial pressure lower than the preoperative value. This picture will be affected, however, by such variables as level of block, the inclusion of epinephrine, blood levels of circulating local anesthetic, and the blood-volume status of the patient. Although detailed investigations do not indicate significant change in mean arterial pressure, many papers have reported episodes of hypotension in patients receiving epidural block. These are potential sources of serious complications for those unfamiliar with the technique (Table 25-8). It is worth noting that no consistent definition of hypotension is followed. While episodes of hypotension undoubtedly occur, this may best be avoided by a restriction of the extent of the sympathetic blockade, careful patient monitoring, and the provision of adequate intravenous fluids. If blockade has extended into the upper thoracic segments and bradycardia and persistent hypotension are present, then atropine, 0.6 mg, intravenously may be beneficial. More rarely, ephedrine or alternative vasopressor therapy may be used.

Respiratory Effects

As with the provision of postoperative analgesia by intercostal blocks, early workers enthusiastically advocated extradural analgesia, believing that the superior analgesia permitted a better respiratory posture postoperatively and reduced the incidence of postoperative chest infections. Detailed investigation of these claims has tempered the initial enthusiasm with objective findings.

The effects of extradural block alone, without intervening surgery, upon a variety of respiratory parameters have been studied and are small (see Chap. 8).[24,61,66,76,82,92,94] The most consistent finding is a clinically insignificant fall in effort-dependent tests (forced vital capacity [FVC], forced expiratory volume in 1 second [FEV_1], and peak expiratory flow rate [PEFR]). An early finding that an extensive motor block (T2) reduced expiratory reserve volume would suggest that perhaps a fall in functional residual capacity (FRC) could be predicted, but direct studies of FRC following blockade of the extent useful for postoperative analgesia have not shown any significant reduction in FRC.[45,61,93] All these studies relate to the effects of a single injection of the drug; the effect of a prolonged block upon respiratory parameters has not been studied.

Many surgical operations, particularly those on the upper abdomen, are attended by significant incidence of chest infections, the pathogenesis of which is poorly understood. Early users of extradural blocks believed that relief of pain would enable patients to deep breathe and cough better and thus reduce this incidence of infection (Table 25-9). Published results differ owing to a variety of criteria for the definition of chest infection. However, the results of series of extradural blocks show a lesser incidence of pulmonary infection than do series with narcotics. It should be pointed out that the studies have not involved high-risk patients, that is, those with a history of chest problems and the elderly. Controlled studies with these patients may well resolve the question.

(*Text continues on p. 608.*)

Table 25-8. Incidence of Hypotension

Study	*Operations*	*Block and Site*	*Drug/Concentration*	*Number of Patients*	*Incidence*	*Criterion*
Simpson and colleagues (1961)[81]	Upper abdomen	Thoracic	Lidocaine, 1.5%	40	6% of injection	Systolic blood pressure less than 80 torr on sitting up (in all cases returned to normal when returned to lying position)
Burn (1964)[25]	Lower abdomen and upper abdomen	Lumbar	Lidocaine, 1.5% Lidocaine, 1.5%	40	Frequent Rarely	Not Stated
Green and Dawkins (1971)[50]	Upper abdomen	T5–6	Lidocaine, 0.4–1%	42	25% of patients	1 dose vasopressor, more than 1 dose vasopressor (but all patients routinely received 1 dose vasopressor at operation)
	Lower abdomen	T9–10		113	34% of patients 11% of patients	1 dose vasopressor, more than 1 dose vasopressor (40% of these had blood pressure less than 99 torr at some time postoperative)
Spoerel and colleagues (1970)[85]	Various abdomen		Lidocaine, 1–2%, mepivacaine, + 2%	135	17 patients had	Not stated
Addison and colleagues (1974)[3]	Cholecystectomy	Thoracic	Bupivacaine, 0.5%	25	1 patient	Not stated
Griffiths and colleagues (1975)[51]	Thoracic	Thoracic	Bupivacaine, 0.5%, + epinephrine	10	3 patients	Not stated
			Bupivacaine, 0.125–0.25%, infusion	10	2 patients	
Renck (1976)[76]	Upper abdomen	Thoracic	Bupivacaine, 1%, infusion	14	2–1 due to excessive dosage	Systolic blood pressure 80–85 torr

Table 25-9. Incidence of Postoperative Chest Complication

Study	*Operation*	*Number of Patients*	*Incidence*	*Definition of Complication*
Simpson and colleagues (1961)[81]	Mainly upper abdomen	60	1	Not stated
Green and Dawkins (1966)[50]	Upper abdomen	42	Halved	Opinion of ward sister
	Lower abdomen	113	None	
Spence and Smith (1971)[84]	Gastric	11, Epidural block	2/11	Pyrexia + clinical changes and film changes or pyrexia + purulent sputum
		10, Morphine	7/10	
Addison (1974)[3]	Cholecystectomy	25, Epidural block	5%	Not stated
		25, Meperidine	20%	
Pflug and colleagues (1975)[72]	Upper abdomen	13, Epidural block	6/13	Purulent sputum, clinical signs, film changes
		11, Morphine	9/11	
	Hips	11, Epidural block	1/7	
		11, Morphine	3/7	
Miller and colleagues (1976)[64]	Upper abdomen	10, Epidural block	1/10 (pulmonary embolism)	Not stated
		10, Meperidine	1/10 (atelectasis)	

Table 25-10. Postoperative Vital Capacities During Extradural Block

Study	Operation	Number of Patients	Drug/Concentration	Time of Study	FVC as % of Preoperative FVC
Bromage (1955)[20]	Upper abdomen	18, Extradural block	Lidocaine, 0.8%	Postoperatively	86 (range, 75–100)
Simpson and colleagues (1961)[81]	Upper abdomen	54, Extradural block	Lidocaine, 1.5%	24 hours postoperatively	Mean, 69
					Mean, 83
	Lower abdomen	6, Extradural block	Lidocaine, 1.5%		Mean, 84.8
					Mean, 94.7
Ellis and colleagues (1968)[40]	Upper abdomen	3 } Extradural block	Lidocaine, 1.5%	Postoperatively	60–71
		3 } Extradural block	Prilocaine, 1.5%		56–73
		3 } Extradural block	Bupivacaine, 0.375%		52–76
Spence and Smith (1971)[84]	Gastric	10, Morphine	Bupivacaine, 0.5%, + epinephrine	Postoperative Day 1	Morphine, 32
		11, Extradural block (morphine by night)			Extradural block, 27
				Postoperative Day 2	Morphine, 42
					Extradural block, 52
Sjögren and Wright (1972)[82]	Cholecystectomy	24, Extradural block	Lidocaine, 0.4%	Postoperative Day 1	Thoracic, 52
					Lumbar, 46
Pflug (1975)[72]	Upper abdomen	13, Extradural block	Bupivacaine, 0.25%–0.5%	Postoperative Day 1	Extradural block, 74
		11, Morphine			Morphine, 54
				Postoperative Day 3	Extradural block, 85
					Morphine, 71
Miller and colleagues (1976)[64]	Upper abdomen	10, Extradural block	Lidocaine, 1–2% + epinephrine	3–4 hours postoperatively	Extradural block, 49.9
		10, Morphine			Meperidine, 36.5
				24 hours postoperatively	Extradural block, 45.6
					Meperidine, 42.1

Postoperative changes in lung volume (*e.g.*, FVC) have been known to occur for a long time. Early workers suggested that extradural analgesia might reduce such changes to some degree (Table 25-10). In patients who are already having pain postoperatively, the institution of a peridural block can dramatically improve FVC to a much greater extent than can narcotics.[20] Early workers found values of FVC of 70 per cent of the preoperative values in patients following upper abdominal operations (usual values in such patients are 25–50% of the preoperative value).[81] Subsequent investigations that compared patients receiving extradural block or narcotics have not reported such dramatic results but, in general, have tended to confirm the contention that patients who receive epidural blockade do suffer less postoperative impairment of FVC. Although FVC tends to be preserved by extradural block in the postoperative period following upper abdominal operations, these effects have not been studied after thoracic operations.

FRC is known to decrease after upper abdominal operations, and this may contribute to postoperative hypoxia with FRC falling within closing volume (CV) and producing atelectasis. In patients who had undergone abdominal operations under general anesthesia and who developed postoperative pain, the institution of an extradural block did not improve FRC[38,93] Extending intraoperative extradural analgesia into the postoperative period—with a regime of extradural block by day, morphine and extradural block by night—did not preserve FRC to any greater extent than in a control group of patients receiving morphine alone.[83]

As noted previously, hypoxia frequently occurs after upper abdominal surgery. The ability of extradural analgesia to reduce this hypoxia has been studied in various circumstances (Table 25-11). Patients who have pain and then receive analgesia with either narcotics or extradural block generally show a fall in Pa_{O_2}, whereas those receiving extradural blockade show a stable or an increased Pa_{O_2}.[38,53,70,71] The institution or regression of an extradural block does little to alter the P_{CO_2} values.

The aforementioned studies all dealt with intermittent blockade, and the use of a sustained block in the postoperative period cannot be extrapolated from their data. With a sustained block after upper abdominal operations, it has been found that the block did not prevent the development of some degree of hypoxia, which was not compared to other forms of analgesia.[82] Studies of patients postgastrectomy who received either morphine analgesia as necessary or extradural block by day and morphine at night showed that the group who had had blocks had significantly less fall in both $A\text{-}a_{DO_2}$ and Pa_{O_2} than the group treated with narcotics, which the researchers attributed to the undesirable respiratory effects of the narcotic.[84] However, subsequent work showed that much larger doses of narcotics could be used without producing respiratory impairment, and perhaps the poor performance of the earlier group treated with narcotics was a consequence of too little analgesia rather than too much.[4] This theory was tested in a further trial, one group of patients receiving, as before, extradural block by day and morphine by night, and the other group receiving higher doses of morphine (10 mg), every 4 hours.[83] With these regimes, they found the differences were not significant.

Studies on patients who undergo elective hip surgery compared the effects of a continuous extradural block with liberal doses of pentazocine.[65] They showed that although the group with blocks had only minimal changes from preoperative Pa_{O_2} over the 3 days of the study, the group treated with pentazocine showed a significant decrease. A similar study could not confirm these findings.[72] In fact, the group treated with morphine showed lesser falls in Pa_{O_2}, although the group with blocks tended to return toward normal earlier.

As with the studies of the influence of extradural blocks upon the incidence of postoperative chest infections, the data on the effect of such blocks upon the magnitude of postoperative hypoxema, although suggestive of a possible protective effect, do not constitute definitive evidence. It is evident that more detailed studies must be performed to identify the technique that produces the best results, in light of a particular patient's age and sex, the kind of surgery, and medical history.

Renal Function

Because renal function is affected by changes in cardiovascular function and by changes in the endocrine system (*e.g.*, ADH secretion), which are believed to be mediated by pain, it would not be surprising to find that an extradural block had some influence on renal function after surgery.

In fit volunteers, lidocaine without epinephrine caused a small fall in effective renal plasma flow (ERPF), probably as a result of a slightly lowered mean arterial pressure (MAP) and a slight rise in renal vascular resistance (RVR) and similar small falls in glomerular filtration rate (GFR).[56] Almost identical changes in GFR were seen in patients who had lidocaine plus epinephrine, despite greater falls in MAP, RVR, and ERPF, thus implying that the kidney is capable of compensating for changes in cardiovascular function by renal autoregulation. The effects of the local anesthetic drug upon the renal vasculature were not studied, but because the changes produced were similar to those produced by spinal anesthetic, this would suggest that the effects of the drug, if any, are small (see Chap. 8).

Although many researchers have commented on satisfactory urinary excretion, there is only one detailed study of the effect of prolonged blockade upon renal function.[11] This examined epidural analgesia for patients following gastric operations. Epidural block from T4–12 was achieved with 0.5 per cent bupivacaine plus epinephrine—other patients received narcotics—and all were subjected to a varying fluid and electrolyte load. Postoperatively, the patients with blocks did not retain sodium to the same extent as the patients who were given narcotics. They did, however, retain water to the same extent. This was interpreted to mean that the block of the renal sympathetic nerves prevented afferent renal vascular constriction, thereby preventing renin angiotensin secretion, and permitting a greater blood flow to the renal cortex with a consequent natriuresis. It should be pointed out, however, that the fluid loads in the patients were very conservative by today's standards, some patients only receiving 1500 ml of fluid in the first 24 hours.

Hepatic Effect

Concern with hepatic function during prolonged extradural block is not purely academic for, as the liver is responsible for metabolism of amide-type local anesthetics, any impairment of hepatic function will lead to decreased metabolism of the drug and a consequent rise in blood drug levels.

Unfortunately, there are no studies of the effect of prolonged extradural block on hepatic function in the postoperative period. However, studies of the effects of single-shot extradural blocks are available (see Chap. 8).

Metabolism

Trauma causes an increase in basal metabolic rate (BMR), which is reflected by an increase in oxygen consumption (VO_2). This rise in VO_2 may be of the order of 10 to 15 per cent in an elective abdominal operation. In patients who are in pain, the institution of analgesia with either narcotics or regional block can be shown to produce a fall in VO_2.[70,82] In comparing patients who received either narcotics or prolonged extradural block for postoperative analgesia, inconsistent results have been found, some studies showing patients with blocks having less rise in VO_2; others show little or no differences between the two groups.[65,74,84]

The effect of regional block upon some aspects of postoperative metabolism—namely, the rise in blood glucose, impairment of glucose tolerance, and the associated hormonal responses—has been studied fairly widely. A rise in blood glucose is commonly seen postoperatively and is directly related to the magnitude of stress.[29,35] This may be due to catecholamine secretion or sympathetic activity, causing hepatic glycogenolysis and should account for other aspects of postoperative metabolism, (*e.g.*, the suppression of insulin release).[6,73] Because it is extremely difficult to measure serum catecholamines and to assess the level of sympathetic activity in the postoperative period, the validity of this has not been assessed. Regional block may help to mitigate these changes either by reducing the patient's pain or by block of the sympathetic nerves that supply the splanchnic bed and the renal medulla. However, levels of other hormones that may raise blood glucose and impair glucose tolerance are also changed in the postoperative period (*e.g.*, glucagon, human growth hormone, and cortisol).

It has been known for a long time that high spinal or extradural blocks may attenuate the rise in blood glucose during surgery.[5] As soon as the block wears off, however, the blood glucose picture is indistinguishable from that in patients who receive a general anesthetic.[58] Without regard to surgical site, if the blockade is sustained into the postoperative period, the rise in blood glucose can be attenuated or abolished.[23,42]* Low blockade (*e.g.*, T8) in patients undergoing gynecologic operations markedly attenuates the rise in blood glucose, but raising the blocks to the T4 level completely abolishes the hyperglycemic response.

Following trauma, glucose intolerance and a fall in insulin response to glucose challenge is also known to occur, but it is not clear whether these are due to stress and catecholamine release or other hormone secretion.[5] Prolonged extradural blockade, plus light general anesthesia in patients who are undergoing lower abdominal surgery, while markedly attenuating the rise in blood glucose,

(*Text continues on p. 612.*)

* Buckley, F.P., Arthur, R.G., Scott, D.B., Kehlett, H., and Cameron, E. A.: Effect of epidural block upon the reduced glucose tolerance and suppression of insulin release postop. Unpublished data, 1978.

Table 25-11. Postoperative Arterial Oxygenation Changes —Extradural Block and Narcotics

Study	Operation	Kind of Study	Number of Patients	Age	Time of Study	Significant Differences
Pain vs. analgesia studies						
Maneyuki and colleagues (1968)[70]	Cholecystectomy	Pain vs. analgesia	11, Narcotic	49	90 minutes postoperatively	No changes with analgesia
		Meperidine, IV,	13, Epidural	48		
		Mepivacaine epidural block	6, Narcotic	29	4 hours postoperatively	No changes with analgesia
			6, Epidural	46		Narcotic,
			6, Narcotic	29	15 hours postoperatively	Pa_{O_2} ↓ (93.3 → 88.3)*
			6, Epidural	46		Pa_{O_2} ↓ (103 → 98)
						Epidural block,
						Pa_{O_2} ↑ (83 → 87)*
						Pa_{O_2} ↑ (100 → 104)
Hollmen and Saukkonen (1972)[53]	Cholecystectomy	Pain vs. analgesia	10, Narcotic	46	2 hours postoperatively	Narcotic, Pa_{O_2} ↓ (83 → 78)
		Opiate or bupivacaine epidural block	10, Epidural	40		Epidural block, Pa_{O_2} stable
Sjögren and Wright (1972)[82]	Cholecystectomy	Epidural block allowed to wear off	20		1st day postoperatively	No changes with onset of pain
Muneyuki and colleagues (1972)[70]	Upper abdomen	Pain vs. analgesia	6, Narcotic	67	6 hours postoperative	No difference
		Mepivacaine or epidural block	7, Epidural	63	17 hours postoperative	
Drummond and Littlewood (1972)[38]	Lower abdomen	Preop. vs. pain vs. epidural analgesia	14	37	Preoperative 24 hours postoperative	No change with analgesia

						Morphine		Epidural Block	
						PaO_2	A-aDO_2	PaO_2	A-aO_2
Prolonged blocks									
Spence and Smith (1971)[84]	Gastric	Morphine vs. epidural block by day and morphine by night	10, Narcotic	37	Preoperative	93	8	95	7
			11, Epidural	42	Postoperative Day 1	69	33*	83	19*
					Day 2	68	30*	82	22*
					Day 5	83	25*	92	7*
Spence and Logan (1975)[83]	Gastric	Morphine every 4 hours vs. epidural block by day and morphine by night			Preoperative	86	14	90	13
					Postoperative Day 1	63	35	74	29
					Day 3	64	34	77	27
					Day 5	85	18	88	17
Pflug and colleagues (1972)[72]	Upper abdomen	Morphine vs. epidural block	11, Narcotic	43	Preoperative	76	31	77	36
			13, Epidural	47	Postoperative Day 1	67*	41	73*	41
					Day 3	78	33	83	30
	Hip fracture surgery		9, Narcotic	62	Preoperative	69	43	65	44
			7, Epidural	59	Postoperative Day 1	65	48	59	55
					Day 3	70	42	72	41
Modig and Holmdahl (1975)[65]	Elective hip surgery	Pentazocine vs. epidural block	10, Narcotic	52	Preoperative	Extradural patients PO_2 stable			
			19, Epidural	72	Postoperative Day 1, 2, and 3	Pentazocine patients ↓ PO_2			
Miller and colleagues (1976)[64]	Upper abdomen	Meperidine vs. epidural block	10, Narcotic	55	Immediately postoperative	156	FIO_2 28%	128	
			10, Epidural	49	3–4 hours postoperative	137		133	
					24 hours postoperative	63*	Air	80.7	

* Significant intergroup difference at that time

showed only slight attenuation of glucose intolerance and slight suppression of insulin release to glucose challenge.[25]*

Cortisol levels are also known to rise with surgery. However, cortisol responses after extradural blockade are similar to those in patients receiving a general anesthetic for the same operation.[23,42] Extending the block to T4 and maintaining it at that level not only abolish the rise in blood glucose but also abolish the cortisol response.

A comprehensive study of the effects of prolonged extradural block (T8) in patients undergoing lower abdominal operations indicated that although the extradural block markedly attenuated the hyperglycemic response, this could not be uniformly correlated with changes in plasma insulin, glucagon, growth hormone, or prolactin. It is not yet clear whether these effects of regional block upon postoperative metabolism are of practical or therapeutic use.

REGIONAL BLOCK IN THE MANAGEMENT OF CHEST INJURIES

Patients who suffer chest trauma may present with a wide variety of injuries from the most severe hemopneumothorax, severe lung contusion, and chest wall instability to the most mild, with a few fractured ribs and chest wall bruising. The patients in the former group are likely to suffer life-threatening respiratory failure from the time of injury and may need prompt endotracheal intubation and prolonged artificial ventilation. The mild injury group may need no therapy other than simple analgesia. Within these two extremes, there exists a group of patients who may develop respiratory failure with atelectasis, as a consequence of their painful inability to take deep breaths and cough adequately. If the chest wall pain can be relieved, respiratory failure can be halted or contained and the necessity for more invasive modes of therapy avoided. Analgesia by narcotic drug may fail to provide adequate analgesia or depress respiration. Moreover, narcotics may be contraindicated in patients who have suffered a head injury as well as a chest injury. In such patients, regional blockade can provide a superior quality of analgesia and circumvent the problems of CNS depression. A pneumothorax is not necessarily a contraindication to regional blockade, provided that once it has been properly treated the patient does not have residual respiratory difficulty. Patients with a relatively stable chest wall and who suffer a mild degree of respiratory distress are the prime candidates for regional blockade. Patients with fractures of the ribs are also greatly benefited. Once a regime of regional analgesia has been selected, it should be followed closely with special regard to the patient's condition. The patient should be carefully reviewed clinically and radiologically and with blood gas determinations. Should deterioration in his respiratory status become apparent, further appropriate measures such as bronchoscopy, suction, endotracheal intubation, and artificial ventilation should be instituted.

Techniques

Thoracic extradural analgesia is probably the most commonly used technique for chest injuries. Although the block may be extended to all thoracic segments, the policy of those who have used this technique widely is to restrict the degree of spread to the area of rib fractures.[49,59] Occasionally, the block is not extended to upper rib fractures because they are usually not as painful, and the block of a wide area may be unwise in patients who have a potential circulating volume deficit. There are reports of severe falls in blood pressure and even circulatory arrest following institution of such a block in these circumstances. It is therefore, essential that, if indicated, the patient's volume be adequately replenished prior to the inception of the block.

Intercostal blocks have also been used but suffer from the disadvantage of having to be repeated at intervals over a period of several days. Their reported use has been restricted to rib fractures.[49] The agents and dosage used will, to a large extent, parallel those used to provide postoperative analgesia. As with postoperative patients, it is probably both wise and kind to treat patients with a mild sedative to ensure a good night's sleep.

Complications

The complications of using a prolonged extradural block to provide postoperative analgesia are primarily the complications associated with the use of an extradural block in any circumstances.

A persistent fear with continuous extradural blocks over a prolonged period is that infections may occur in the extradural space. Although there have been reports of extradural abscesses occurring

* Buckley, F.P., Arthur, R.G., Scott, D.B., Kehlett, H., and Cameron, E.A.: Effect of epidural block upon the reduced glucose tolerance and suppression of insulin release postop. Unpublished data, 1978.

Table 25-12. Incidence of Urinary Retention

Study	Operation	Catheter Site	Drug/Concentration	Technique	Incidence
Simpson (1961)[81]	Upper and lower abdomen	Thoracic	Lidocaine, 1.5%	"Top-up"	0
Burn (1964)[25]	Upper and lower abdomen	Thoracic	Lidocaine, 1.5%	"Top-up"	0
Green and Dawkins (1966)[50]	Upper and lower abdomen	Thoracic	Lidocaine, 1%–0.5%	Infusion	0
Sjögren and Wright (1972)[82]	Cholecystectomy	Thoracic Lumbar	Lidocaine, 0.4%	Infusion	50% 90%
Addison (1974)[3]	Cholecystectomy	Thoracic	Bupivacaine, 0.5%	"Top-up"	1/25
Griffiths (1975)[51]	Thoracic	Thoracic	Bupivacaine, 0.5%, + epinephrine	"Top-up"	3/8
			Bupivacaine, 0.25% or 1.25%	Infusion	9/9
Renck (1975)[75]	Thoracic	Thoracic	Etidocaine, 1%	"Top-up"	10–20%
			Bupivacaine, 1%	Infusion	67%

spontaneously or following lumbar punctures, there have been only two cases reported following prolonged blocks.[32,44]

Urinary Retention

When an extradural block is used to provide analgesia for an incision in certain dermatomes, it may impair functions of the organs supplied by the nerves of those blocked dermatomes. If a caudal block is used to provide analgesia for a perineal operation, urinary retention may well occur, or similarly, if a lumbar block is used to provide analgesia for an abdominal operation, urinary retention and leg weakness may occur. However, there is evidence that even if a segmental thoracic block is used and the extent of sensory spread does not encroach upon sacral segments, urinary retention may occur (Table 25-12).

REFERENCES

1. Abdel-Salem, A., and Scott, D.B.: Bupivacaine and etidocaine in epidural block for postoperative relief of pain. Acta Anaesthesiol. Scand., *60*[*Suppl.*]:80, 1975.
2. Ablondi, M.A., Ryan, J.F., O'Connell, C.T., and Haley, R.W.: Continuous intercostal nerve blocks for postoperative pain relief. Anaesth. Analg., *45*:185, 1966.
3. Addison, N.V., Brear, F.A., Budd, K., and Whittacker, M.: Epidural analgesia following cholecystectomy. Br. J. Surg., *61*:850, 1974.
4. Alexander, J.I., Parikh, R.K., and Spence, A.A.: Postoperative analgesia and lung function. Br. J. Anaesth., *45*:346, 1973.
5. Alison, S.P., Prowse, K., and Chamberlain, M.J.: Failure of insulin response to glucose load during operation and after myocardial infarction. Lancet, *478*:1, 1967.
6. Annamunthodo, H., Keating, V., and Patrick, S.: Liver glycogen alterations in anaesthesia and surgery. Anaesthesia, *13*(4):429, 1958.
7. Bartlett, R.W.: Bilateral intercostal blocks for upper abdominal surgery. Surg. Gynecol. Obstet., *71*:194, 1940.
8. Bartlett, R.W., and Eastwood, P.W.: Long acting bilateral intercostal blocks for upper abdominal surgery. Surgery, *32*:956, 1952.
9. Benumof, J.L., and Semenza, J.: Total spinal anesthesia following intrathoracic intercostal nerve blocks. Anesthesiology, *43*:124, 1975.
10. Bergh, W.P., Dottori, O., Axisonhof, B., Simonsson, B.G., and Ygge, H.: Effect of intercostal block on lung function after thoracotomy. Acta Anaesthesiol. Scand., *24*[*Suppl.*]: 85, 1966.
11. Bevan, D.R.: Modification of metabolic response to trauma under extradural analgesia. Anaesthesia, *26*:188, 1971.
12. Blades, B., and Ford, W.A.: A method for the control of postoperative pain. Surg. Gynecol. Obstet., *91*:524, 1950.
13. Bonica, J.J.: The Management of Pain. London, Henry Kimpton, 1953.
14. Bonica, J.J., Akamatsu, T.J., Berges, P.U., Morikawa, K., and Kennedy, W.F., Jr.: Circulatory effects of peridural block: II. Effects of epinephrine. Anesthesiology, *34*:514, 1971.
15. Bonica, J.J., Kennedy, W.F., Jr., Akamatsu, T.J., and Gerbershagen, M.U.: Circulatory effects of epidural block: III. The effects of acute blood loss. Anesthesiology, *36*:219, 1972.
16. Braid, D.P., and Scott, D.B.: The systemic absorption of local analgesic drugs. Br. J. Anaesth., *37*:394, 1965.
17. Bridenbaugh, L.D., Moore, D.C., Bagdi, P., and Bridenbaugh, P.O.: The position of plastic tubing in continuous block techniques. An x-ray study of 552 patients. Anesthesiology, *29*:1047, 1968.
18. Bridenbaugh, P.O.: Intercostal nerve blockade for the evalu-

ation of local anaesthetic agents. Br. J. Anaesth., *47*:306, 1975.

19. Bridenbaugh, P.O., DuPen, S.L., Moore, D.C., Bridenbaugh, L.D., and Thompson, G.E.: Postoperative intercostal nerve block analgesia versus narcotic analgesia. Anaesth. Analg., *52*:81, 1973.
20. Bromage, P.R.: Spirometry in the assessment of analgesia after abdominal surgery. Br. Med. J., *2*:589, 1955.
21. ———: Extradural analgesia for pain relief. Br. J. Anaesth., *29*:721, 1967.
22. Bromage, P.R., Pettigrew, R.T., and Crowell, D.E.: Tachyphylaxis in epidural analgesia. 1. Augmentation and decay of local analgesia. J. Clin. Pharmacol., *9*:30, 1969.
23. Bromage, P.R., Shibata, H.R., and Willoughby, H.W.: The influence of prolonged epidural blockade on blood sugar and cortisol responses to operations in the upper abdomen and thorax. Surg. Gynecol. Obstet., *132*:1051, 1971.
24. Buckley, F.P., and Simpson, B.R.: Relief of pain following upper abdominal surgery by thoracic epidural block with etidocaine. Acta. Anaesthesiol. Scand., *60*[*Suppl.*]:76, 1975.
25. Burn, J.M.B.: Prolonged epidural analgesia. Anaesth. Analg., *43*:568, 1963.
26. Cappelle, W.: Die Dedeutang des Wundschmerzes und sied Ausschaltung für den Ablauf der Atmung bei Laparotomeirten. Deutsche Z. Chir., *246*:466, 1935–36.
27. Cherney, L.S.: Tetracaine hydroiodide: A long lasting local anesthetic for the relief of postoperative pain. Anesth. Analg., *42*:477, 1963.
28. Chinn, M.A., and Wirjoatmadja, K.: Prolonging local anaesthesia. Lancet, *2*:835, 1967.
29. Clarke, R.S.J.: The hyperglycaemic response to different types of surgery and anaesthesia. Br. J. Anaesth., *42*:45, 1970.
30. Cleland, J.G.P.: Continuous peridural and caudal analgesia in surgery and early ambulation. Northwest Med., *48*:26, 1949.
31. Collins, M.L.: Eucupin infiltration in abdominal surgery. J. Kans. Med. Soc., *42*:106, 1941.
32. Crawford, J.S.: Particulate matter in the extradural space. Br. J. Anaesth., *47*:807, 1975.
33. Crile, G.: Local Anaesthesia. *In* Bickham: Operative Surgery. Philadelphia, W.B. Saunders, 1944.
34. Cronin, K.D., and Davies, M.J.: Intercostal block for postoperative pain relief. Anaesth. Intensive Care, *4*:259, 1976.
35. Cullingford, D.W.J.: The blood sugar response to anaesthesia and surgery in southern Indians. Br. J. Anaesth., *463*:38, 1966.
36. Delilkan, A.E., Lee, C.K., Young, W.K., Ong, S.C., and Gannendran, A.I.: Post-operative local analgesia for thoracotomy with direct bupivacaine intercostal blocks. Anaesthesia, *28*:561, 1973.
37. Dhuner, K.G., and Lund, N.: Intercostal nerve blocks with etidocaine. Acta Anaesthesiol. Scand., *60*[*Suppl.*]:39, 1975.
38. Drummond, G.B., and Littlewood, D.G.: Respiratory effects of extradural analgesia after lower abdominal surgery. Br. J. Anaesth., *49*:999, 1977.
39. Duncan, D., and Jarvis, W.H.: A comparison of the action on nerve fibres of certain anesthetic mixtures and substances dissolved in oil. Anesthesiology, *4*:465, 1943.
40. Ellis, R.H., Hillman, G., and Simpson, B.R.: The duration of action of local analgesic drugs in the extradural space. *In* Simpson, B.R. *et al.:* Progress in Anaesthesiology. Amsterdam, Excerpta Medica, 1241, 1961.
41. Engberg, G.: Single dose intercostal nerve block for pain relief after upper abdominal surgery. Acta Anaesthesiol. Scand., *60*[*Suppl.*]:43, 1975.
42. Engquist, A., Brandt, M.R., Fernandes, A., and Kehlet, M.: The blocking effect of epidural anaesthesia on the adrenal hyperglycaemic responses to surgery. Acta. Anaesthesiol. Scand., *21*:330, 1977.
43. Faust, R.J., and Nauss, L.A.: Post-thoracotomy intercostal block: comparison of its effects on pulmonary function with those of intramuscular meperidine. Anesth. Analg., *55*:542, 1976.
44. Ferguson, J.F., and Kirsch, W.: Epidural empyema following thoracic extradural block. J. Neurosurg., *41*:762, 1974.
45. Freund, F.G., Bonica, J.J., Akamatsu, T.J., and Kennedy, W.F., Jr.: Ventilatory reserve and the level of motor block during high spinal and epidural anaesthesia. Anaesthesiology, *28*:834, 1967.
46. Galindo, A., Hernandez, J., Benavides, O., Ortegon de Munoz, S., and Bonica, J.J.: Quality of spinal extradural analgesia. The influence of spinal root diameter. Br. J. Anesth., *47*:41, 1975.
47. Galway, J.E., Caves, P.K., and Dundee, J.W.: Effect of intercostal nerve blockade during operation on lung function and relief of pain following thoracotomy. Br. J. Anaesth., *47*:730, 1975.
48. Gerwig, W.J., Jr., Thompson, C.W., and Blades, B.: Pain control following upper abdominal operations. Arch. Surg., *62*:678, 1952.
49. Gibbons, J., James, O., and Quail, A.: Relief of pain in chest injury. Br. J. Anaesth., *45*:1136, 1973.
50. Green, R., and Dawkins, C.J.M.: Postoperative analgesia: The use of a continuous drip epidural block. Anaesthesia, *21*:372, 1966.
51. Griffiths, D.P.G., Diamond, A.W., and Cameron, J.D.: Postoperative extradural analgesia following thoracic surgery. A feasibility study. Br. J. Anaesth., *47*:48, 1975.
52. Guis, J.A.: Paravertebral procaine block in the treatment of postoperative atelectasis: A preliminary report. Surgery, *8*:832, 1940.
53. Hollmen, A., and Saukonen, J.: The effects of postoperative epidural analgesia versus centrally acting opiate on physiological shunt after upper abdominal operation. Acta Anaesth. Scand., *16*:147, 1972.
54. Jason, A.M., and Shaffel, M.E.: The problem of postoperative pain. Am. J. Surg., *83*:549, 1952.
55. Kaplan, J.A., Miller, E.D., and Gallagher, E.G.: Postoperative analgesia for thoracotomy patients. Anaesth. Analg. (Cleve.), *54*:773, 1975.
56. Kennedy, W.F., Jr., Everett, C.B., Cobb, L.A., and Allen, G.D.: Simultaneous systemic and hepatic haemodynamic measurements during high peridural anaesthesia in normal man. Anaesth. Analg., *50*:1069, 1971.
57. Kennedy, W.F., Jr., *et al.:* Cardiorespiratory effects of epinephrine when used in regional analgesia. Acta Anaesth. Scand., *23*[*Suppl.*]:320, 1966.
58. Lindseth, R.G.: Postoperative glucose metabolism in diabetic and nondiabetic patients. Arch. Surg., *741*:105, 1972.
59. Lloyd, J.W., and Rucklidge, M.A.: The management of closed chest injuries. Br. J. Surg., *56*:721, 1969.
60. Loder, R.E.: A long acting local anaesthetic solution for the relief of pain after thoracotomy. Thorax, *17*:375, 1962.
61. McCarthy, G.S.: The effect of thoracic extradural analgesia on pulmonary gas distribution functional residual capacity and airway closure. Br. J. Anaesth., *48*:243, 1976.
62. Massey–Dawkins, C.J.: Analysis of the complications of extradural and caudal block. Anaesthesia, *24*:554, 1969.
63. Massey–Dawkins, C.J., and Steel, G.C.: Thoracic extradural block for upper abdominal surgery. Anaesthesia, *26*:41, 1971.

64. Miller, J.L., Gertel, M., Fox, G.S., and Maclean, P.D.: A comparison of the effect of narcotic and epidural analgesia on postoperative respiratory function. Am. J. Surg., *131*:291, 1976.
65. Modig, J., and Holmdahl, M.H.: The role of regional block versus parenteral analgesics in patients management with special emphasis on the treatment of postoperative pain. Br. J. Anaesth., *47*:264, 1975.
66. Moir, D.: Ventilatory function during epidural anaesthesia. Br. J. Anaesth., *35*:568, 1963.
67. Moore, D.C.: Intercostal nerve block for postoperative somatic pain following surgery of the thorax and upper abdomen. Br. J. Anaesth., *47*:284, 1975.
68. Moore, D.C., and Bridenbaugh, L.D.: Intercostal nerve block in 4333 patients: Indications, technique and complications. Anaesth. Anal., *41*:1, 1962.
69. Moore, D.C., Bridenbaugh, P.O., Bridenbaugh, L.D., and Thompson, G.E.: Bupivacaine hydrochloride, a summary of investigational use in 3274 cases. Anaesth. Anal., *50*:856, 1971.
70. Muneyuki, M., Ueda, Y., Urabe, N., Takeshita, H., and Inamoto, A.: Postoperative pain relief and respiratory function in man: comparison between intermittent intravenous injections of meperidine and continuous lumbar epidural analgesia. Anesthesiology, *29*:304, 1968.
71. Muneyuki M, *et al.:* Oxygen breathing and Q_s/Q_t during postoperative pain relief in man. Can. Anaesth. Soc. J., *19*:230, 1972.
72. Pflug, A.E., Murphy, T.M., Butler, S.H., and Tucker, G.T.: The effects of postoperative peridural analgesia on pulmonary therapy and pulmonary complications. Anesthesiology, *41*:8, 1974.
73. Porte, D., Jr., and Robertson, P.R.: Control of insulin secretion by catecholamines stress and sympathetic nervous system. Fed. Proc., *32*:1792, 1973.
74. Renck, H.: The elderly patient after anaesthesia and surgery with special regard to certain respiratory, circulatory, metabolic and muscular functions. Acta Anaesth. Scand., *1*[*Suppl.*], 1969.
75. Renck, H.: Discussion on the use of long acting local anaesthetics. Acta Anaesth. Scand., *60*[*Suppl.*]:124, 1975.
76. Renck, H., Edstrom, H., Kinneberger, B., and Brandt, G.: Thoracic epidural analgesia. II. Prolongation in the early postop. period by continuous injection of 1.0% Bupivacaine. Acta Anaesth. Scand., *20*:476, 1976.
77. Reynolds, F., and Taylor, G.: Maternal and neonatal blood concentrations of bupivacaine in comparison with lignocaine during continuous epidural analgesia. Anaesthesia, *24*:14, 1970.
78. ______: Plasma concentrations of bupivacaine during continuous epidural analgesia in labour: The effect of adrenaline. Br. J. Anaesth., *43*:436, 1971.
79. Samarji, W.N.: Rectus sheath analgesia in the control of postoperative abdominal pain and its influence in pulmonary function and pulmonary complications. Proc. Vth World Congress of Anaesthesiology at Kyoto, Amsterdam, Excerpta Medicine, 1972.
80. Sanchez, R., Amna, L., and Rocha, F.: An analysis of the radiological visualisation of catheters placed in the extradural space. Br. J. Anaesth., *39*:485, 1967.
81. Simpson, B.R.J., Parkhouse, J., Marshall, R., and Lambrechts, W.: Extradural analgesia and the prevention of respiratory complications. Br. J. Anaesth., *33*:628, 1961.
82. Sjögren, S., and Wright, B.: Circulation, respiration and lidocaine concentration during continuous epidural blockade. Acta Anaesth. Scand., [*Suppl.*]*46* 16:5, 1972.
83. Spence, A.A., and Logan, D.A.: Respiratory effects of extradural nerve block in the postoperative period. Br. J. Anaesth., *47*:281, 1975.
84. Spence, A.A., and Smith G.: Postoperative analgesia and lung function: a comparison of morphine with extradural block. Br. J. Anaesth., *43*:144, 1971.
85. Spoerel, W.E., Thomas, A., and Gerula, G.R.: Continuous epidural analgesia: Experience with mechanical injection devices. Can. Anaes. Soc. J., *17*:37, 1970.
86. Stanton-Hicks, M.D.A.: A study using bupivacaine for continuous epidural analgesia in patients undergoing surgery of the hip. Acta Anaesth. Scand., *15*:97, 1971.
87. Starr, A., and Gilman, S.: The effect of postoperative intercostal block on pulmonary ventilation. N. Engl. J. Med., *227*:102, 1942.
88. Telivuo, L., and Perttala, Y.: Use of x-ray contrast medium to control intercostal nerve blocks. Ann. Chir. Gynaecol. Fenn., *55*:185, 1966.
89. Thomas, C.J., Climie, C.R., and Mather, L.E.: The maternal plasma levels and placental transfer of bupivacaine following epidural anaesthesia. Br. J. Anaesth., *41*:1035, 1969.
90. Thompson, P.D., *et al.:* Lignocaine pharmacokinetics in advance of heart failure, liver disease and renal failure in humans. Ann. Intern. Med., *78*:499, 1973.
91. Tucker, G.T., *et al.:* Observed and predicted accumulation of local anaesthetic agents during continuous extradural analgesia. Br. J. Anaesth., *49*:237, 1977.
92. Wahba, W.M., Craig, D.B., Don, H.F., and Becklake, M.R.: The cardiorespiratory effects of thoracic epidural anaesthesia. Can. Anaesth. Soc. J., *19*:5, 1972.
93. Wahba, W.M., Don, H.F., and Craig, D.B.: Postoperative epidural analgesia: Effects on lung volumes. Can. Anaesth. Soc. J., *22*:519, 1975.
94. Ward, R.J., *et al.:* Epidural and subarachnoid anaesthesia: Cardiovascular and respiratory effects. J.A.M.A., *191*:275, 1965.
95. Willdeck-Lund, G., and Edstrom, H.: Etidocaine in intercostal nerve block for pain relief after thoracotomy. Acta Anaesth. Scand. *60*[*Suppl.*]:33, 1975.
96. Yoemans, F., Gorsh, R.V., and Mattesheimer, J.L.: Benacol in the treatment of pruritis. Am. Med. J., *127*:19, 1928.
97. Yoshikawa, K., Mima, T., and Egawa, J.: Blood levels of marcaine (LAC-43) in axillary plexus blocks, intercostal blocks, and epidural anesthesia. Acta Anaesth. Scand., *12*:1, 1968.
98. Zollinger, G.: Observations on use of prolonged anaesthetic agents in upper abdominal incisions. Surgery, *42*:106, 1941.

26 Chronic Pain and Local Anesthetic Neural Blockade

Ronald D. Miller, William L. Munger, and Patrick E. Powell

APPROACH TO THE PATIENT WITH CHRONIC PAIN

Local anesthetic nerve blocks can have an important role in the diagnosis and therapy of chronic pain. This chapter emphasizes the pre- and postblock evaluation of the patient because interpretation of the results of the block, in our experience, is far more difficult than the mechanical performance of the block. To this end, the success of several pain clinics and units in the treatment of various pain problems is presented. However, because pain frequently does not correspond to expected anatomic sites and frequently is associated with dramatic and confusing psychological dimension, standard criteria for diagnosis and the evaluation of therapy are lacking. For these reasons, we often caution against rigidly comparing the results of one pain clinic with those of another. Nevertheless, guidelines can be established and are offered below.

Interview

The overall objective of an interview is to determine whether a nerve block or other pain-removing procedure will be helpful with the diagnosis or treatment of the patient's pain, according to his or her description of it. Obviously, the specific nerve block selected depends on the location and kind of pain.

Although the interview should be a free-flowing conversation, answers to the following questions should be sought.

What has been the duration of the pain?

Is the pain constant or intermittent?

What precipitates or exacerbates the pain? (*i.e.*, certain movements, temperature, etc.). Is sleep disturbed by pain?

How does the family react to the patient's pain behavior? How has the pain affected behavior?

What kind of work does the patient do? How have fellow workers responded to the patient's pain behavior?

If the patient is unemployed, from what source is income obtained?

What is the patient's history of pain medication?

Is there litigation or some form of financial compensation involved that may be lost if the pain were to be removed?

How would the patient's life change if the pain were to be removed?

From the answers to these questions can be learned not only what precipitates or exacerbates the pain but also the rewards or consequences of the pain. Almost every patient who has chronic pain will lose something in the process of readjustment if the pain is removed. Will the patient lose family, sympathy, and attention? If litigation is involved, the patient may subconsciously not be willing to risk this loss of income by getting better. If the patient is taking narcotic analgesics, perhaps addiction is more of a problem than chronic pain. Treatment by nerve block, then, consists not only of removing the noxious neural traffic responsible for the pain but also of altering the maladaptive behaviors created by chronic pain.

The physician should explain that nerve blocks rarely remove the organic cause of the pain (*i.e.*, pancreatic cancer or protruding lumbar disc) but rather block perception of the pain.

These answers will also allow the physician to determine how satisfied and happy a patient would be were the noxious stimulation removed. Our experience is that patients with the following characteristics tend to respond better to removal of pain.

Happily married with adequate family support

Continuing his occupation even if the position has been made less demanding

Has tried prescribed analgesics but found them unsatisfactory and stopped taking them

Has had pain for months (rather than years)

In contrast, patients who are unemployed and on welfare and drug addicts or alcoholics will respond poorly even if the neural traffic responsible for the pain is removed. Thus, it becomes evident that interpretation of results of nerve blocks is far more difficult than the technical administration of the block. For example, differences from clinic to clinic in success rates for a given block are related to the source of the pain and the patient's personality type, and multiple other variables (socioeconomic class, ethnic background, personality of the physician, etc.).

Psychological Tests

Many clinics perform psychological screening tests of some kind prior to administration of any diagnostic or therapeutic nerve block. Probably the most commonly used test is the "Minnesota Multiphasic Personality Inventory."[91,94] Four profiles most commonly encountered in patients with chronic pain are the following: hypochondriasis, reactive depression, somatization, and manipulative reaction.

With hypochondriasis there is a preoccupation with a large number and variety of bodily complaints. Most of these complaints are unrelated to any underlying pathologic process. A reactive depressive patient insists that his depression is in response to living with pain. In contrast, the patient with a somatization profile usually focuses on physical symptoms to repress awareness of latent depression. This patient will indicate that his life is fine except for pain and insist that the doctor eliminate the pain. A patient who is manipulative attempts to persuade surgeons to perform unnecessary surgery, anesthesiologists to perform unnecessary nerve blocks, and doctors in general to write narcotic orders or sign disability claims.[91,99] Sternbach and colleagues found manipulative profiles in patients with chronic low back pain who had litigation pending.[91] If the personnel at a pain clinic wish an impressive record of success, they might select for treatment patients whose profiles show either reactive depressions or somatization reactions. Patients who are hypochondriacal or manipulative will need not only physical therapy of the pain state itself but also help with social integration and self-control.

Physicians who are inexperienced in treating patients who have chronic pain frequently label many of them "crocks." These physicians frequently forget that chronic pain leads to despair, demoralization, worry, and, sometimes, hostility. Neurotic behavior is a natural response to chronic pain.[111] Physicians should be tolerant of such neurotic behavior because it frequently disappears with removal of the pain.[95] Obviously, patients should not be excluded from treatment because of their personality profiles. Psychotic patients are entitled to the same pain relief as "normal" patients. The interview and personality testing are intended to determine not only whether or not to perform a block or surgery but if additional forms of therapy are necessary. As we said, patients with hypochondriacal or manipulative profiles may also require behavior modification[4] or operant conditioning.[38]

Measurement of Pain

Although several methods of measuring pain have been proposed, the *pain estimate* and *tourniquet ratio* are sometimes useful and practical.[23,26] With the pain estimate, the patients merely assign a number to the intensity of their pain. Patients are asked to rank their pain on a scale of 0 to 100, where "0" refers to no pain and "100" refers to pain so severe that suicide would be considered. Several numbers may be assigned each day; for example, one number might be the average pain per day and another might be the worst pain. Patients can record these numbers before and after nerve block to assess the magnitude and duration of pain relief.

The pain estimate may be influenced by psychological and cultural factors that lead, for example, to differences in verbal description of pain. "Gnawing" pain may not be the same pain to different patients.[90] Producing a painful physical stimulus against which patients may match their clinical pain level is helpful. The submaximum effort tourniquet technique is commonly used.[87] Blood is drained from the nondominant arm by means of a tight rubber bandage, which is removed after a blood pressure cuff is inflated above systolic blood pressure. Then the patient squeezes a hand exerciser 20 times slowly, and a stopwatch is started. The patient matches the intensity of his usual clinical pain with the experimentally induced ischemic pain (in seconds of ischemia), and the maximum experimentally induced pain that can be tolerated is also noted. These two times (clinical pain level and maximum pain tolerance) are recorded. The tourniquet pain ratio is computed by dividing the time required to reach the clinical pain level by the pain tolerance, and multiplying the result by 100.

The pain estimate and tourniquet ratio score both may be used to measure the magnitude and duration of pain relief. If the pain estimate is much higher than the tourniquet ratio score, these results may confirm a preliminary diagnosis of hypochondriasis or manipulativeness. Recent studies indicate that patients with chronic pain have a respiratory alkalosis so that blood gases may be a useful objective test (see Chap. 31).

Physical Examination

The physical examination should follow the usual patterns of inspection, palpation, percussion, and auscultation and include a thorough neurologic examination. When patients with chronic pain are examined, the following areas should receive particular attention:

The Painful Region Should be Mapped Out as Accurately as Possible. If the area is not too tender, we outline the painful area with a felt-tip pen. This can be recorded freehand or on a standard dermatome chart. Perhaps better documentation might be provided by a photograph of the patient after the painful areas have been localized. If possible, the painful area should be identified according to peripheral nerve or dermatome areas.

The skin often provides clues to sympathetic dysfunction. Red, warm, dry, smooth skin with coarse hair is evidence of vasodilatation. Nails are ridged and usually long because the patient avoids trimming them. Vasoconstricted skin is blanched, clammy, cool, thin and glistening with thin to sparse hair, and the nails are fragile.

Muscle and Joint. Evidence of guarding, wasting, deformity, swelling and temperature changes (telethermometry) should be noted.

Maneuvers that Relieve Pain. Reduced movements and warmth are used by some patients to relieve their pain.

Maneuvers that cause pain may include pressure (particularly on a trigger point) or movement in general. Neck movement is particularly useful to elicit cervical root irritation, and straight leg-raising, to elicit lumbar root irritation.

Characterizing the pain is helpful in determining the diagnosis. An attempt should be made to differentiate between somatic and visceral pain. In contrast to somatic pain, visceral pain is poorly localized. Except in patients with colic, visceral pains are usually dull rather than sharp because viscera are sensitive only to chemical and tension changes rather than crushing, burning, or cutting.

DIAGNOSTIC NERVE BLOCKS IN PATIENTS WITH CHRONIC PAIN

Indications

Diagnostic nerve blocks with local anesthetics may be performed for one of several reasons:[13] to localize anatomically the pain pathway, to differentiate pharmacologically the size of fibers that mediate the pain, to differentiate central pain from peripheral pain, or to determine whether a neurolytic block or surgical resection of the nerve should be performed. Techniques of nerve block and the pharmacology of local anesthetics have been discussed in preceding chapters.

Because pain can arise by way of many pathways, nerve blocks with local anesthetics may help determine whether the pain is transmitted by specific nerves. If the source of pain can be localized to specific neural pathways, a neurolytic nerve block might be considered. Diagnostic nerve blocks allow the patient to undergo a "trial run" without permanent change. When, on occasion, the numbness or motor weakness is too unpleasant for the patient to withstand, a neurolytic block may be unwise.

To some extent, nerve blocks can differentiate the size of nerve fibers mediating the pain. Low concentrations of local anesthetic (*i.e.*, 0.5% lidocaine) will block small-diameter sympathetic fibers but not the larger somatic fibers. If relief of pain is not obtained from the sympathetic nerve block, the larger somatic fibers may be involved in the production of the pain. Likewise, if peripheral nerve blocks relieve the pain, then a central origin can be excluded. As simple and logical as this approach may appear, relief of pain by peripheral nerve block may not exclude a central source of pain. By acutely changing the pattern of peripheral input into the central nervous system (CNS), central pain may be abolished temporarily. However, the CNS apparently adapts to this change in sensory input, and the centrally induced pain will reappear. Therefore, relief of pain from repeated nerve blocks is required to confidently exclude a central source of pain.

Similarly, continuous epidural anesthesia may be used to detect drug addiction. If a patient with chronic pain still requires his normal dosage of analgesic drugs during administration a continuous epidural anesthetic that lasts for several hours, addiction or severe drug dependency should be suspected. (These issues are considered in detail when specific pain syndromes are discussed.)

Placebo Injection

Placebo injection is the administration of a solution without known pharmacologic action that relieves pain. A placebo effect is associated with any procedure or drug that alleviates pain. Postoperatively, Beecher found that one-third of patients received marked analgesia from injection of inactive agents.[9] Taub has suggested that the placebo effect is statistical and may not occur in every instance.[95] For example, a placebo may relieve pain only 30 to 40 per cent of the time in any one patient. Therefore, nerve blocks should be repeated. The inactive (placebo) and active drugs should be randomized.

Taub has also advised that the administrator of the block should not be the evaluator although the use of a double-blind technique is uncommon in busy pain or block clinics. While this technique requires more personnel and time, it does enhance the objectivity of the evaluation of pain. However, problems with interpretation remain. For example, success of a placebo agent in relieving pain may depend on how convincing the person is who administers it.

Anticipation of analgesia is a well-known placebo effect.[62] Also, if a patient does not experience expected secondary effects of the block, he may suspect a placebo. If a patient has had two stellate ganglion blocks, the lack of a warm feeling with the third injection may clue the patient that a placebo has been given. To avoid this problem, the placebo must be given frequently before the patient would experience the secondary effects of the nerve block. Last, it must be determined that the "inactive" drug genuinely is inactive. For example, normal saline in multiple-dose containers frequently contains benzyl alcohol as a preservative; benzyl alcohol is a local anesthetic!

The placebo response often is normal and should not be used to classify a patient as a "crock." Many authors have expressed concern over the professional disdain for the placebo effect that has apparently become widespread.[11] As indicated above, the patient's psychological state is important in regard not only to a placebo but also to how the patient responds to an active drug. If analgesia from the placebo is as effective as that from medication, is it bad medical practice to use it?

Differential Nerve Blocks

Because fiber size is the primary factor that governs sensitivity to local anesthetics, differential nerve blocks can be used to distinguish placebo effect and sympathetic and somatic sensory fibers as mediators of nociception. The graduated spinal block technique recommended by Ahlgren and associates and Winnie and associates sometimes can accomplish this distinction.[2,107] After a lumbar puncture, the following solutions are injected at 10-minute intervals. (In the lateral position, it is important to use isotonic solutions to ensure a bilateral effect.)

7 ml of "artificial CSF" with no preservatives (placebo)*
7 ml of 0.2% procaine (sympathetic block)
7 ml of 0.5% procaine (sensory block)
7 ml of 1% procaine (motor block)

* Hypotonic solutions injected into the CSF, result in blockade of pain conduction (see p. 124). Thus, slow withdrawal of CSF and then reinjection 5 minutes later is a preferable technique. Alternatively, a solution isotonic with CSF may be composed. The new technique, **selective spinal analgesia,** is discussed in Chapter 31.

If relief occurs with the placebo, the pain probably is psychogenic. If 0.2 per cent procaine provides relief, a sympathetic pathway of transmission should be considered.

Similarly, sympathetic pain can be differentiated from pain of somatic sensory origin. If pain persists after 1 per cent procaine has been administered, then pain of more central origin or psychogenic pain should be considered. For accurate interpretation, sympathetic (skin temperature, oscillometry, liquid-crystal thermography, pulse monitor, or psychogalvanic response),[10,32] sensory (pinprick), or motor (mobility) function should be monitored identically after each injection. Methods for monitoring these functions are discussed in other chapters.

Unfortunately, a patient cannot move during differential spinal anesthesia (unless a catheter technique is used) and perform the maneuvers that elicit pain. A differential epidural anesthetic by catheter technique may offer an advantage in this respect.

With the differential spinal anesthetic, it is assumed that 0.2 per cent procaine will not block small sensory fibers. If there is any question whether a pure sympathetic block occurred with a spinal injection, the following approach can be used for the lower extremity:

Needles should be inserted as if to perform a paravertebral lumbar sympathetic block at L2 or L3: however, instead of injecting a local anesthetic, 10 ml of saline is administered (placebo).

If pain persists, then 10 ml of 0.5% lidocaine is injected.

If pain persists after 15 to 30 minutes of a well documented sympathetic block, then a sciatic, femoral, or epidural block should be performed to obtain a somatic block.

At many clinics a diagnostic paravertebral sympathetic block is used initially. If pain is not relieved, a differential spinal or epidural block is performed. Again, if pain persists in spite of a complete block, a central or psychogenic basis for pain must be considered.

Upper extremity pain can be evaluated by the following general approach:

A needle is inserted into the area of the stellate ganglion, after which 10 ml of normal saline (without preservative) is injected (placebo). If relief is obtained, psychogenic pain should be suspected.

If relief does not occur within 10 minutes, then 10 to 15 ml of 0.5% lidocaine is injected to achieve a sympathetic block.

If relief does not occur with objective evidence of a sympathetic block, a brachial plexus block to achieve a somatic block is performed with 1 to 1.5% lidocaine or mepivacaine (see Chap. 13).

DIAGNOSTIC SPINAL USE OF NARCOTICS (see Chap. 31)

THERAPEUTIC LOCAL ANESTHETIC NERVE BLOCKS

Local anesthetic nerve blocks can be therapeutic in patients with chronic pain in five situations: interruption of reflex sympathetic response that secondarily contribute to noxious stimulation; temporary neural blockade to allow physical therapy; reduction of inflammatory response, usually with steroid injection; occasional instances when one or more local anesthetic nerve blocks lead to prolonged or permanent relief of pain; or to improve vascular supply in "acute on chronic" ischemia in patients with vascular disease (see Chap. 13).

MANAGEMENT OF SPECIFIC PAIN SYNDROMES WITH LOCAL ANESTHETIC BLOCK

CAUSALGIA AND REFLEX SYMPATHETIC DYSTROPHIES

Clinical Features

Causalgia is characterized by chronic, severe, burning pain; autonomic dysfunction; and atrophic changes.[91,92,99,111] The pain has been described as burning, aching, intense, or agonizing. Generally, pain spreads to other areas of the same limb or even to the trunk, head, or contralateral limb. Anything that increases activity in the limb or CNS may exacerbate the pain of causalgia. These activities include mechanical stimulation, movement, and application of heat or cold. Many patients find some relief in keeping the limb moist with cool water or wet dressings. Some actually keep the limb continually wet and avoid touching dry objects with it.

Central nervous system factors that may exacerbate the pain include somatosensory experiences (visual and auditory stimuli) and emotional factors (looking down from heights, arguments, noise, excitement). These emotional factors further complicate diagnosis and treatment because, at the very least, they cause irritation and withdrawal.

Initially, vascular changes, probably resulting from altered sympathetic nervous system activity lead to a red, warm, dry, swollen extremity. Later, the extremity will become cool, clammy with pallor, and possibly cyanotic. The late consequence of causalgia is atrophy of the skin and underlying muscle and decreased density of bones. The trophic changes may be due to disuse or altered sympathetic activity. The radiographic findings consist of trabecular, subchondral, intracortical, and endosteal bone resorption. Cortical thickness and bone mineral content decrease 30 to 40 per cent.[42] These kinds of changes have been called *shoulder-hand syndrome, Sudeck's atrophy,* and *post-traumatic osteoporosis.* Presently, the most commonly accepted term is *reflex sympathetic dystrophy syndrome.*[42]

Causalgia has been divided into "major" and "minor" types. The division is based on severity of injury and, to some extent, symptoms, although atrophy and bone changes can occur with both kinds.[48,103]

Mechanism

Although several theories have been advanced, three have emerged as the most popular explanation of pain from causalgia. These are the "gate control" theory, the "vicious cycle of reflexes" theory, and the "artificial synapse" theory. The gate control theory of Melzack and Wall has attracted most recent attention (see Chap. 24).[66]

According to the gate control theory, certain cells in the substantia gelatinosa of the dorsal horn act as "gates," either allowing or preventing peripheral impulses from entering the CNS. When the gate is open, the rapid firing of the next order neurons, the so-called action system, is interpreted in higher centers as pain. Impulses arriving at the dorsal horn by way of large-fiber afferents have an inhibitory effect upon transmission of impulses arriving by way of the smaller afferent fibers. On the other hand, tonic small-fiber input tends to facilitate transmission to the action system. Higher centers in the nervous system can influence inhibition at the spinal gate.

Causalgia is explained as an abnormal state in which the spinal gate remains open, allowing normal sensory stimuli to be interpreted as pain. Consistent with this theory, large-fiber stimulation has provided relief of pain from causalgia during physical therapy.[67] (See also Chap. 24.)

According to the "vicious cycle of reflexes theory," a chronic irritative lesion in a peripheral nerve causes the spinal cord to be bombarded with afferent impulses.[42] In addition to causing pain, this excites internuncial pools of neurons in the lateral and anterior horns. These pools of neurons excite sympathetic efferent fibers, which, in turn, cause vasomotor changes in the extremity, secondarily causing additional stimulation of the irritative lesion.

The internuncial pool activity becomes self-sustaining and thus contributes to the chronicity of the pain. Eventually, according to this theory, the internuncial pool activity is so well established that it can continue even when the sympathetic efferent fibers are severed, as by sympathectomy. This theory attempts to unite several different pain states under one mechanism (*i.e.*, post-traumatic reflex sympathetic dystrophy, or minor causalgia, and major causalgia). However, the almost invariably successful result of sympathectomy in major causalgia lends credit to the argument that causalgia is, in fact, a unique syndrome, which probably does have a different mechanism.

The most credible of the proposals for this mechanism is the "artificial synapse" theory, which states that when a nerve lesion destroys the electrical insulation between different fibers or alters the anatomy in some way, efferent sympathetic fibers, which are tonically active, stimulate somatic afferent fibers.[34] Afferent fiber depolarization occurs both orthodromically and antidromically. Constant orthodromic bombardment is interpreted by the CNS as pain. Antidromic depolarization, in addition, sensitizes the peripheral nerve endings, perhaps through the release of neurokinin. As a result of the peripheral sensitization, either the damaged neurons themselves or their neighboring normal neurons hyperreact to stimulation. This also results in transmission of impulses that are interpreted by the CNS as pain (Fig. 26-1).

Although experimental confirmation of interaction between sympathetic efferent and somatic afferent fibers is lacking, motoneurons can stimulate somatic afferent fibers in regions of nerve damage. This theory is supported by the fact that a humoral factor is secreted at the peripheral nerve endings, which, when injected elsewhere, causes pain.[24] This may explain why a local anesthetic block of a peripheral nerve distal to the lesion sometimes relieves pain.[55]

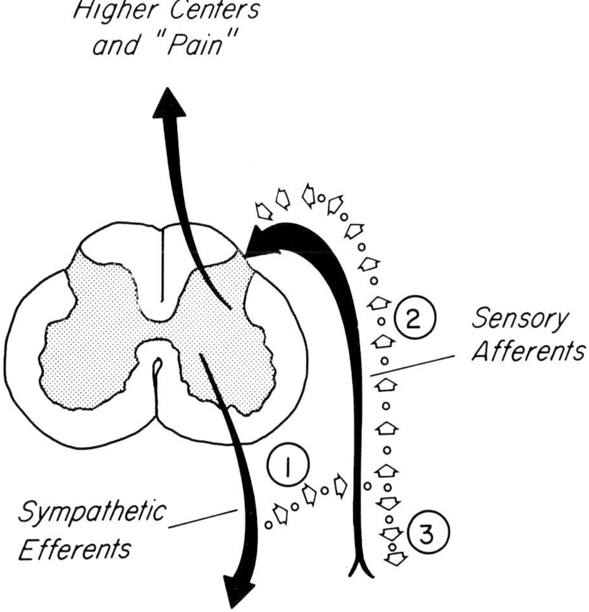

Fig. 26-1. A description of the "artificial synapse" theory. (*1*) Artificial synapse between sympathetic efferent and somatic sensory nerves; (*2*) orthodromic impulses that cause increased sensory activity; (*3*) antidromic impulses cause release of substances which decrease sensory nerve thresholds. (Adapted from Sternschein, M.J., *et al.:* Causalgia. Arch. Phys. Med. Rehabil., *56*:58, 1975)

One serious problem with this theory is that it does not explain the occasional patient with causalgia who has had complete transection of the peripheral nerve. Such a patient may form artificial synapses in the proximal stump but could not have the antidromic stimulation of primary afferent neurons.

Additional circumstantial evidence for the artificial synapse theory comes from the specific nerves usually involved with causalgia. Injuries to the median nerve, the tibial division of the sciatic nerve, and the inferior trunk of the brachial plexus most often result in causalgia.[76] These nerves carry sensory neurons, whose ultimate destination is in the hand or the foot, and provide the majority of sympathetic innervation to the entire extremity. Many of the sympathetic fibers are given off in the upper portion of the extremity, however, especially to the elbow and knee. Thus, the inferior trunk of the bra-

Table 26-1. Results of Various Treatments for Causalgia

Study	Total Cases	*Markedly Improved or Cured With* Physical Therapy	Perineural Infiltration	Stellate or Lumbar Sympathetic Block	Surgical Sympathectomy	No or Little Relief
Omer and Thomas (1974)[72]	41	9	5	10	9	8
Kleinert and associates (1973)[58]	323	147	*	*	*	176
Kleinert and associates (1973)[58]	183	*	*	121	23	39
Thompson and associates (1975)[98]	113	6		56	47	4
Wirth and associates (1970)[110]	32	*	*	4	24	3
Baker and associates (1969)[8]	28	*	*	3	23	2
Omer and Thomas (1971)[71]	70	14	14	16	15	6 (5)†

* This therapy not used
† 5 patients received other therapeutic procedures not listed

chial plexus, the median nerve, and tibial division of the sciatic nerve have an unusually high proportion of sympathetic fibers to sensory fibers, compared with other nerves in the body. Perhaps the lower incidence of "true" causalgia that occurs with damage to the median and tibial nerves below the elbow or knee is due to the lower proportion of sympathetic fibers at these levels and therefore less likelihood of development of artificial synapses.

In any event, according to the artificial synapse theory, sympathectomy or sympathetic block stops the pain of causalgia by interfering with the tonic efferent activity in sympathetic fibers. Additional evidence for this hypothesis is that stimulation of the cervical sympathetic chain causes pain only in patients with causalgia. These effects are now said to be due, at least in part, to increased or decreased activity in sympathetic fibers, which are in evidence near sensory receptors (see Chap. 13).

TREATMENT

Although Carron states that pain usually does not recur after five stellate ganglion blocks in patients with sympathetic dystrophy, other authors take exception to this.[8,22,58,71,72,98,110] There have been voluminous descriptions of various treatments. We have reviewed the recent reports, however, and have summarized them in Table 26-1. Differences among reports probably reflect different criteria for diagnosis of causalgia, variations in skill, and the personalities performing the therapeutic maneuvers. In general, if the pain cannot at least temporarily be relieved with a local anesthetic sympathetic block, the diagnosis of causalgia should be suspect. When the diagnosis of causalgia is confirmed by the signs and symptoms described previously and pain relief is provided by a stellate ganglion block (or lumbar sympathetic block with the lower extremity), the following approach is recommended.

Physiotherapy

Physiotherapy may be sufficient for milder forms of causalgia and has been described by Baker and colleagues.[8] (See also Chap. 31, p. 710.)

Periodic Perineural Infiltration

If a specific trigger area or zone can be identified by deep pressure, a catheter is inserted through a needle along the nerve proximal to the trigger area for 3 to 5 cm.[8,71] A test-dose of 0.5 ml of 1.5 per cent lidocaine is administered. If pain is relieved, the catheter is taped in place, and the patient is taught to administer 0.5 ml repeated as often as necessary for as long as 2 weeks. This permits resumption of physiotherapy and active use of the extremity.

Stellate Ganglion or Lumbar Sympathetic Block

Up to five to seven stellate ganglion or lumbar sympathetic blocks can be performed on alternate days, and one of the following results may occur (see Chap. 13 for technique[8]):

(1) Permanent adequate relief with one block would negate, of course, the necessity of performing repeated blocks.
(2) The postblock pain may be significantly less than the preblock pain.
(3) The duration of pain relief may exceed the expected duration of the local anesthetic used. Furthermore, subsequent blocks may provide progressively longer pain-free intervals.
(4) The duration of pain relief may exceed the expected duration of the local anesthetic, but, unfortunately, the duration of pain relief from subsequent blocks is progressively shorter.
(5) Pain relief may last only for the duration expected from the local anesthetic.
(6) There might be no pain relief.

For results (4), (5), (6), the benefits to be obtained from repeated stellate ganglion or lumbar sympathetic blocks are probably minimal. With results (4) and (5), it may be useful to proceed with an intravenous sympathetic blockade (described below) or, for lower limb pain, neurolytic or, rarely, surgical sympathectomy. Caution is recommended with patients in group (4) because there is a strong likelihood of a placebo effect. Patients who fall into categories (2) or (3) will benefit from repeated stellate ganglion or lumbar sympathetic block or intravenous sympathetic block because lasting pain relief is possible (see Table 26-1).

Intravenous Regional Sympathetic Blockade

A sympathetic blockade can be performed by infusing a sympatholytic drug intravenously into an extremity isolated from the general circulation by a tourniquet. This prevents general spread of the sympatholytic agent until it has been fixed to the tissues. The results of this technique are not listed on Table 26-1 because its use has been limited. Hannington-Kiff has reported dramatic relief of pain and increase in skin temperature in several patients, although the duration of relief was not well defined.[46] Subsequent studies have indicated the effectiveness of the technique in blocking sympathetic activity and relieving causalgia pain (see Chap. 13).

Technique. The procedure should be performed only when full resuscitation facilities are available, including an established intravenous infusion and a tilting table that allows the patient to be placed in a head-down position in case of hypotension upon release of the tourniquet.

After insertion of an indwelling intravenous catheter into the extremity to be blocked, the limb is elevated to drain it of venous blood, and the tourniquet is inflated to 50 to 100 torr above systolic blood pressure. Guanethidine, 10 to 20 mg, or if this is not available, reserpine, 1 to 2 mg in 20 to 25 ml of normal saline, is injected through the indwelling needle into the extremity. The extremity is isolated from the circulation for 10 minutes to allow binding of guanethidine or reserpine to the tissues; then the tourniquet is slowly released. Sympathetic function of the blocked limb should be monitored as previously described. In the presence of severe ischemia, slow intra-arterial injection into brachial or femoral artery achieves the same end result, although duration of the block is reduced (see Chap. 13).

The intravenous regional sympathetic block technique appears to be useful in a patient who shows signs of returning sympathetic tone despite apparently adequate surgical excision of the sympathetic ganglia. This procedure is also useful in patients taking anticoagulants, for which it provides an attractive alternative to neurolytic or surgical sympathectomy. Most patients with upper limb syndromes tolerate the procedure better than a series of stellate ganglion sympathetic blocks with local anesthetic.

Surgical or Neurolytic Sympathectomy

In patients who receive unquestioned, but unfortunately not prolonged, relief from pain with a local anesthetic sympathetic block, surgical or neurolytic sympathectomy usually provides the prolonged relief, even in patients with causalgias of several years' duration (see Table 26-1; Chap. 13). Poor results occur when technical difficulties make complete sympathectomy difficult or when the diagnosis is incorrect. For this reason, a diagnostic local anesthetic sympathetic block is valuable. Lack of pain relief from such a block is reason to question the diagnosis and the decision to operate.

If "permanent" sympathectomy is so successful, why waste time with physiotherapy, perineural infiltration, or multiple stellate ganglion or lumbar sympathetic blocks? A diagnostic local anesthetic sympathetic block and subsequent neurolytic block or surgical sympathectomy would save days (weeks?) of hospitalization or outpatient visits and protracted pain. The merits of this view must be weighed against the risk of surgery and anesthesia; surgical sympathectomy and complications of neurolytic techniques should be compared to the chance of relieving pain with less dramatic forms of therapy. Unfortunately, these risks are impossible to measure because objective data are nonexistent. Thus, the final decision is subjective. It seems reasonable to reserve "permanent" sympathectomy until the other forms of therapy fail, but often such a prolonged approach is not possible (see Chap. 13).

Transcutaneous Stimulation

Transcutaneous stimulation is used in some clinics to assist with pain relief during physiotherapy.

Prognosis and Less Popular Forms of Therapy

Whatever form of sympathetic blockade is chosen, relief of pain should be coupled with physical therapy to maintain function and prevent atrophy. Some physicians believe prophylactic sympathetic blocks should be performed in all patients with peripheral nerve injuries in order to prevent the development of causalgia. They recommend that a series of sympathetic blocks be performed at the first indication of causalgia. The blocks should be continued until no pain is present. One problem with this approach is that even if the sympathetic block removes the causalgic pain, the underlying deficits from peripheral nerve injury, such as paresthesias and dysesthesias, will persist.

Oral administration of propranolol has been recommended for treatment of causalgia on the basis of its successful use in two patients.[86] This approach deserves further consideration. In patients unable to tolerate 10 minutes of tourniquet time, an alternate is the intra-arterial administration of guanethidine; this has been employed in vascular disease (see Chap. 13). If the regional intravenous guanethidine technique is effective, then, in theory, intra-arterial guanethidine may be even more effective because of better access to constricted capillaries.

SPECIFIC PAIN SYNDROMES

Raynaud's Disease and Raynaud's Phenomenon

Raynaud's disease is characterized by episodic constrictions of small arterioles in extremities in response to cold or emotional stimuli; it occurs most frequently in young women. The minimum criteria for diagnosis are intermittent attacks of pallor, cyanosis, or rubor in one or more extremities; lack of arterial occlusion (*i.e.*, thrombus); symmetric or bilateral distribution; and trophic changes limited to the skin and never consisting of gross gangrene. Secondary criteria are the exclusion of primary diseases that can give rise to vasospastic symptoms. If vasospastic attacks occur in association with a systemic disease such as rheumatoid arthritis, cervical rib syndrome, thromboangitis obliterans, scleroderma, or periarteritis nodosa, the condition is properly termed Raynaud's *phenomenon,* not Raynaud's *disease*. In both conditions, attacks are usually limited to the arms and only occasionally involve the feet and toes.

As the process progresses to severe attacks, patients become significantly incapacitated by the almost constant presence of cold, numb, tingling fingers. Later, they may develop painful ulcers on the tips of the fingers, an occurrence more likely in Raynaud's phenomenon than in the disease.

Mild forms of the condition are managed by careful avoidance of exposure to cold whenever possible. Treatment for the more symptomatic patient has been based on numerous medications, with varying results reported. These medications include oral administration of reserpine, triiodothyronine, androgens, griseofulvin, methyldopa, phenoxybenzamine, guanethidine, topical nitroglycerine paste, and intra-arterial injections of guanethidine; hypnosis and operant conditioning have also been utilized. The number of therapies advocated is probably indicative of their lack of effectiveness.

The role of local anesthetic sympathetic block in Raynaud's disease and phenomena is controversial, and objective data are lacking.[7,52] Since stellate ganglion or lumbar sympathetic blocks may alleviate numbness and tingling and are associated with little risk, it is reasonable to perform a diagnostic block to evaluate the likely benefit for each patient. If Raynaud's disease has progressed to digital ulceration, stellate ganglion blocks (alternating the sides) every other day may facilitate healing. The interval between attacks may be lengthened by stellate ganglion blocks if these are performed early in the course of disease and during the cold months when the symptoms are most severe. Surgical sympathectomy may be performed when severe disability occurs. (Of course, a diagnostic local anesthetic sympathetic block should precede the operation.) Unfortunately, although immediate relief of pain frequently occurs, relapse is common, and surgery is not recommended by many physicians. Consequently, therapy for Raynaud's disease, or phenomenon, is a difficult long-term problem; however, patients may be helped over an "acute on chronic" attack by judicious use of sympathetic blockade.

Arterial Insufficiency of Lower Extremities

Arteriosclerosis obliterans refers to chronic peripheral vascular occlusion due to atherosclerotic plaque. The disease usually occurs in people over 60 years of age but occurs at a younger age in diabetics and patients with hyperlipidemias. Common signs and symptoms include intermittent claudication, rest pain, cyanosis, swelling, and occasionally gangrene.

To date, local anesthetic sympathetic blocks have been of limited diagnostic value in predicting the results of surgical or neurolytic lumbar sympathectomy. The role of lumbar sympathectomy has been debated for years. In order to assess its rational use, it is important to differentiate rest pain from intermittent claudication. The latter is due to inadequate blood supply to muscles during exerise. Although skeletal muscle has sympathetic vasoconstrictor fibers, no evidence exists that the increasing blood flow in response to exercise is a result of decreased sympathetic tone.[52] Therefore, sympathectomy usually does not relieve intermittent claudication. Those who claim improvement with chemical or surgical sympathectomy report results similar to those observed in patients who take placebos.[52,78] However, there is some evidence that the level of arterial obstruction may influence the effect of sympathectomy on claudication (see Chap. 13).

In contrast to intermittent claudication, a diagnostic local anesthetic sympathetic block may be useful to determine if rest pain is relieved. If so, lumbar sympathectomy should be considered. Also, there are those who maintain that even if intermittent claudication is not relieved, sympathectomy should still be performed to improve circulation to the skin of the extremity and to prevent ischemic changes.[88,93] In one series, over a 5- to 10-year period, only 8 per cent of the patients with intermittent claudication treated by sympathectomy developed severe ischemia that required amputation. A large number of pharmacologic and other treatments, apart from arterial reconstruction, have been used in the treatment of the pain of claudication.

Kim and associates performed lumbar sympathectomies on 61 patients who had end-stage occlusive vascular disease manifested by gangrene on less than 50 per cent of the foot, ulcerating ischemic lesions, rest pain or rapidly progressive, markedly limiting intermittent claudication.[56] The immediate postoperative mortality was 6.5 per cent, yet only 40 per cent had to have an amputation. The implication was that all the patients would have required amputation without sympathectomy. In spite of these encouraging results, Kim and associates still concluded that the effect of lumbar sympathectomy is unpredictable.[56] Obviously, patients with arterial insufficiency who have been treated with sympathectomy and patients who have not must be followed to resolve this question. Also, the accuracy of diagnostic lumbar sympathetic block in predicting long relief from surgical sympathectomy is not yet known. (See Chap. 13.)

Even if a diagnostic block suggests the possibility of improvement, it is necessary to be concerned about denervation hypersensitivity or rapid deterioration of the sympathectomized limb, or what surgeons refer to as *paradoxical reaction,* which has been reviewed by Richards and Shaw.[77,82] This has led some to advocate continuous catheter techniques for prolonged assessment with local anesthetics (see Chap. 13).

Buerger's disease (thromboangiitis obliterans) is a disease of peripheral vessels, usually of the lower limbs, usually in men, and usually occurring in patients before the age of 30 years. Both smaller arteries and veins suffer progressive obliteration resulting in ischemia and ultimately gangrene of the toes (possibly fingers). The etiology is unknown, but episodic inflammation of the arterial and venous walls causes thickening and thrombus formation. Treatment includes cessation of smoking and avoidance of cold. The role of sympathetic block and surgical sympathectomy is again controversial. Even optimistic reports indicate improvement that is undefined in only 30 to 70 per cent of the patients, which is only slightly better than a placebo response.[50,69,83] In these patients, it is reasonable to perform diagnostic, placebo, and local anesthetic sympathetic blocks. If dramatic improvement occurs with repeated block, then neurolytic block or surgical sympathectomy may be undertaken.

Vascular Facial Pain

Although many pain syndromes may be categorized as *vascular facial pain,* it is necessary here to consider only migraine and temporal arteritis. Migraine headaches probably are caused by periodic dilatation of parts of the extracranial vasculature, resulting in throbbing, usually unilateral, headaches associated with vertigo, nausea, and photophobia. However, since the pain of migraine is due to vascular dilatation (stretching of vessels causes the pain), stellate ganglion block would be expected to have no effect. Some patients, however, have their migraine triggered by suboccipital muscle spasm; this mechanism can sometimes be modified for quite long periods by a series of suboccipital nerve blocks.

On the other hand, the pain of temporal arteritis, which affects elderly patients, is characterized by severe, throbbing pain in the temple, ear, or face, and may be relieved by infiltration of local anesthetic around the superficial temporal artery.

Angina Pectoris

Nerve pathways from the heart traverse the upper four thoracic sympathetic ganglia. Emotional stress resulting in sympathetic augmentation can cause angina pectoris. Blockade of the sympathetic innervation of the heart has been advocated for many years for treatment of angina pectoris. The paravertebral approach to the upper thoracic sympathetic ganglia has been used successfully, but we discourage it because of the unacceptable risk of pneumothorax in these seriously ill patients.[15] Although stellate ganglion block does reduce post-exercise ST depression and the severity of angina, patients with severe angina can withstand the more specific surgical vascularizing procedure.[105] Surgery plus various drug therapies probably eliminates the need for stellate ganglion block in patients with angina pectoris.

Although not widely recognized as a discrete entity or as causalgia itself, *cardiac causalgia* is characterized by chronic precordial chest discomfort, which varies in intensity and distribution. It frequently follows the onset of angina pectoris, but, in contrast, it is burning, constant, and unrelated to exertion. Movement of the body or stimulation of trigger areas on the anterior chest wall may increase the pain. Hyperesthesia of the skin overlying the painful area is commonly present. Although administration of nitroglycerin does not relieve the pain, steroid administration has been partly successful. Because cardiac causalgia resembles causalgia of the limbs, the sympathetic nervous system may play a significant role in its pathogenesis, although this possibility has not been evaluated with sympathetic blockade.[20]

Abdominal Visceral Pain

The splanchnic nerves contain all the sympathetic and visceral afferent pain fibers in the upper abdominal viscera. Blocking these nerves will relieve pain caused by disorders of these viscera. Therefore, splanchnic plexus (celiac plexus) block can allow the differentiation of abdominal pain arising from the body wall from that arising from abdominal viscera.

Sustained hypotension from celiac plexus block is rare if patients are rendered normovolemic, so that this procedure earns a valuable place in the diagnosis of abdominal pain. If the pain is relieved by a diagnostic block, then an alcohol block should follow.[3,19] (The details of this are in Chaps. 14 and 27.)

Another cause of pain is "pinching" of the thoracic and upper lumbar nerves as they emerge from the rectus sheath. The pain is chiefly abdominal but may radiate to the back. A tentative diagnosis can be made by having the patient (usually a woman) tense her abdominal wall. The physician then presses the outer side of the rectus muscle with a blunt probe, which intensifies the pain. The diagnosis can be confirmed by an injection of local anesthetic on the nerve as it exits the sheath.[31] Longer relief can be obtained with injection of steroids. Some advocate injection of neurolytic agents. However, this may not be consistently effective and may result in a neuralgia.

Acute Vasospastic Disorders

With *thrombophlebitis,* perivenous lymphangitis is precipitated by some stimulus to produce an inflammatory process in the venous wall; the clot is secondary to this process. The clot is a white or mixed thrombus that is firmly attached to the wall of the vein and rarely becomes detached. The signs and symptoms are pain, fever, decreased peripheral pulse, and a white, swollen extremity.

With *phlebothrombosis* the clot is not attached to the venous wall because there is no inflammation of the venous wall. The clinical picture is not well defined but usually consists of tenderness in the calf or plantar aspect of the foot. There is obviously a life-threatening hazard of pulmonary emboli.

A sympathetic block does not appear to offer any advantage in treatment of phlebothrombosis because of the possibility of dislodging the clot. On the other hand, sympathetic block has been recommended for diagnosis and treatment of thrombophlebitis.[70,74] The radiographic evidence of venospasm associated with thrombophlebitis can be alleviated with sympathetic block.[74] Therefore, sympathetic block can be used as a diagnostic test to determine whether venospasm is present. Ochsner reports dramatic relief of pain, fever, and edema following sympathetic blockade.[70] In contrast, Snyder and colleagues found that sympathetic denervation actually accentuated the clinical course of thrombophlebitis by increasing venous congestion.[89] In view of these contrasting opinions, it is wise to perform a diagnostic lumbar sympathetic block only upon the recommendation of a specialist in peripheral vascular disease.

Frostbite constitutes another form of vasospastic disease and is characterized by arteriolar constriction and increased capillary permeability. This results in edema, stasis, and loss of tissue viability. Sympathectomy promotes resolution of edema, relieves the pain, hastens demarcation of viable tissue, and heals ulcerated areas and amputation stumps.[40] A sympathectomy of long duration is required, and therefore neurolytic block or surgical sympathectomy is preferred. Continuous paravertebral sympathetic block with plastic catheters and periodic injection of local anesthetic can be used when neurolytic agents or a surgical sympathectomy are not advisable.[61,104]

Phantom Limb Pain

Most patients report phantom limb sensations almost immediately after surgical amputation. At first the phantom limb feels normal in size and shape, but in time it usually becomes smaller and may telescope into the stump. Tingling is the dominant sensation although various types of pain have been reported; eventually these sensations will usually disappear. However, pain occasionally persists and is described as "cramping," "shooting," "burning," or "crushing" sensations. Melzack has characterized the following major properties in phantom limb pain[63]:

The pain remains for months or years after tissues heal.

More comonly, the pain will develop in patients who have suffered pain in the limb for some time prior to amputation.

Trigger zones may spread to healthy areas on the same or opposite sides. For example, pressure on the opposite limb may trigger pains in the phantom limb.

The pain may be dramatically attenuated or eliminated by decreases or increases in somatic input.

These observations have led to several explanations for phantom limb pain, which have been reviewed by Melzack.[63] These explanations have been the basis for many therapeutic maneuvers, none of which is completely effective, suggesting that the complete mechanism still is not known.

Before a therapeutic maneuver is attempted, phantom limb pain must be distinguished from stump pain. Stump pain takes several days or weeks to develop and usually is thought to be caused by physical irritation of cut nerves, accompanied by pressure between adjacent bone and a poorly fitting prosthesis, or by pressure on a terminal bulbous neuroma, which may have formed after amputation. Collagen deposition and perineural cell proliferation at the operative site during healing conducts regenerating nerve fibers away from the nerve stump; the development of neuroma follows about 1 month later. The neuroma will enlarge and adhere to fascia of adjacent tissues while axons grow extensively in all directions. Wall has reported the generation of abnormal impulses in neuromas (see Chap. 24). This may result in a locally painful stump. Sometimes, local stump pain can be alleviated for some time by pounding directly over the sensitive neuroma with a firm object such as a wooden applicator with crutch rubber on one end. Infiltration of the painful stump with local anesthesia may provide prolonged relief in some cases for reasons not understood. If relief lasts only as long as the duration of the local anesthetic, then surgical resection of the neuroma may be considered. However, unfortunately, new neuromas form after surgical resection. Of prime importance, is fashioning the amputation stump with plenty of fatty tissue between the end of the bone and skin to improve the fit of the prosthesis.

Since no single therapeutic maneuver will universally relieve phantom limb pain, several approaches can be attempted, and many involve local anesthetics. Injection of local anesthetic into the stump tissues may relieve the pain for days or weeks. Sometimes, successive injections may produce increasingly longer periods of relief. Occasionally, injections of hypertonic saline into the stump may provide pain relief. Injection of either hypertonic saline or local anesthetic into interspinous tissue initially may cause pain, which radiates into the phantom limb, but eventually provides relief of phantom limb pain for days or weeks.[63] Even temporary relief of pain by local anesthetic blocks will allow increased use of the stump prothesis, which increases activity of the remaining musculature and

Table 26-2. The Effect of Epidural Injections on Relief of Chronic Back Pain

Study	Patients Injected	Number Cured or Improved	Per cent Cured or Improved	Steroid Injected	Volume Injected (ml)	Local Anesthetic Injected	Number Treated After Surgery	Control or Placebo Group
Warr (1972)[101]	500	315	63	yes	40	yes	?	none
Swerdlow (1970)[94,*]	208	98	47	no	50	yes	?	none
Swerdlow (1970)[94,*]	117	76	65	yes	5	no	?	none
Cho (1970)[25]	16	14	88	yes	20–30	yes	3	none
Coomes (1961)[28]	20	12	60	no	50	yes	none	5/20‖
Kelman (1944)[54,*]	116	94	81	no	50–100	yes	none	none
Goebert (1961)[43]	113	82	73	yes	30	yes	44	none
Ito (1971)[51]	142	89	63	yes	2	no	?	none
Ito (1971)[51]	136	98	72	yes	10	yes	?	none
Brevik (1976)[16,*]	16	9	56	yes	20	yes	4	none
Brevik (1976)[16,*]	19§	5	26	no§	100	yes	7	none
Winnie (1972)[108,†]	20	19	95	yes	2	no	7	none
Davidson (1961)[29]	28	16	57	no	72‡	no	3	none
Arnhoff (1977)[5]	140	54	39	yes	10	yes	?	none
Dilke (1973)[33]	35	21	60	yes	10	no	none	11/36‖

* Caudal block
† 10 with epidural and 10 with subarachnoid block
‡ Saline alone
§ Of the 14 patients who did not receive relief, 11 did get relief with the steroid.
‖ Number of patients who received significant relief of the total who were in control group or received placebo

often exerts an inhibiting influence on phantom limb pain. Unfortunately, spinal anesthesia or injection of local anesthesic into the stump provides unpredictable results and occasionally may increase the pain, which presumably is related to sensory deprivation.

At times, signs of sympathetic hyperactivity (vasoconstriction and sweating) occur in the stump. These discomforts may be relieved by a sympathetic blockade if it is performed early. However, sympathetic blockade is invariably successful only after digital amputation because sympathetic blockade rarely relieves postamputation pain above the wrist or ankle. Prophylaxis also involves early operation and possibly the use of a transcutaneous stimulator (see Chap. 24).

NEURALGIAS

Chronic Back Pain

Chronic back pain represents a significant health problem. Various conservative and surgical treatments frequently are ineffective. The result is chronic pain, loss of productivity, and occasionally disability. Mechanical factors such as a protruding disc or degenerative changes such as osteophytes may exert pressure on spinal nerve roots; however, inflammatory or circulatory changes such as interosseous hypertension may be the cause.[6,80] Epidural injection of local anesthetic or steroid for chronic back pain is by far the most commonly administered block at many pain relief centers. This is one of many kinds of therapy used for treatment of chronic back pain.[36,41]

Although Arnhoff and colleagues have stated that reports of successful therapy for low back pain with epidural injections of steroids alone or in combination with local anesthetic solutions vary considerably, a careful analysis of the literature indicates the contrary.[5] Arnhoff and colleagues have indicated the lowest incidence of pain relief of any of the accounts evaluated (Table 26-2). Of the 10 groups who have reported treating more than 25 patients, a mean of 62 ± 3.9 (SE); (range 39–81) per cent of the patients received complete or significant relief of pain (Table 26-2). In light of the differing techniques, drugs, criteria for diagnosis, and success of treatment, these results are amazingly consistent and considerably above the anticipated 30 per cent placebo effect. Only two studies utilized a control group. Coomes reported a group of 20 patients who were treated by bed rest alone, and five of these patients experienced significant relief of pain.[28] Dilke and colleagues found that 11 of 36 patients experienced relief when 1 ml of saline was injected into the epidural space.[33] The groups who received epidural injection of steroid or larger volume of local anesthetics had a greater incidence of pain relief than the control group (Table 26-2). Acupuncture resulted in an incidence of relief similar to the control groups and less than that from epidural steroids or local anesthetics.[49] We are unable to explain the low success rate reported by Arnhoff and associates except that they may have followed more rigid criteria for defining "significant relief of pain."[5] It would seem important in future studies to use objective criteria of the result of successful placement of local anesthetic in the epidural space (*e.g.*, increased skin temperature in the lower limbs).

If epidural injection of local anesthetics or steroids is assumed to be effective for many cases of low back pain, the following questions arise: What is the effect produced by the volume of solution injected (*i.e.*, would a large volume of saline be as effective as a large volume of local anesthetic). Does the local anesthetic have a beneficial effect? Do the steroids enhance the incidence of pain relief?

Davidson and Robin reported a 57 per cent incidence of pain relief when a mean of 72 ml (range 35–120 ml) of saline was injected into the epidural space.[29] This suggests that volume and not the presence of local anesthetic is important. In fact, those who used large volumes of local anesthetic (without steroid) reported 47, 60, 81, and 26 per cent incidence of pain relief (Table 26-2). These varying results suggest that large volumes of local anesthetic are no more effective than large volumes of saline.

Steroids appear to reduce pain by an effect that is independent of volume effect.[81] Even small volumes of steroids (less than 6 ml) appear to provide significant relief of pain (Table 26-2). Two studies that compared epidural injections with and without steroids report a higher incidence of relief with steroids.[94] In fact, of 14 patients who did not receive relief with 100 ml of local epidural anesthetic, 11 received relief with 20 ml of local anesthetic and steroid.[16] Green has reported a 50 to 60 per cent incidence of significant pain relief after a series of intramuscular dexamethasone injections.[44] Perhaps, the steroid effect is systemic and need not be injected epidurally. Epidurally injected methyl prednisolone (80–160 mg) has been shown to exert a systemic effect, reflected by depression of plasma cortisol levels.[21]

In spite of Green's report, it is reasonable to conclude that the epidural injection of steroids is therapeutically beneficial and to adopt the following routine.[44] After careful diagnostic evaluation (including consultation with a neurosurgeon or orthopaedic surgeon), the patient should be advised of possible complications and benefits of epidural steroid injection and the possibility of no relief from these injections; in fact, the anesthesiologist should probably inform patients that their pain might get worse. All information given and received at this time should be recorded in the patient's chart.

During the block, the patient is placed in the lateral position so the affected side is dependent. Then a test-dose of local anesthetic (8–12 ml of 1% lidocaine [other local anesthetics could be used]) is injected. The local anesthetic is injected to provide temporary pain relief and confirm that the tip of the needle is in the epidural space. The use of a skin temperature probe aids further.

Methylprednisolone (Depo-Medrol), 80 to 160 mg, is injected. The patient is asked to remain in the lateral position for 15 minutes. As Winnie has pointed out, methylprednisolone is a suspension, not a solution, and should be vigorously shaken prior to injection.[108] Since it is rather heavy, it is important that the patient lie on the affected side.

We tend to be liberal with our indications for the epidural injection of steroids for chronic back pain although the acute cases tend to respond more favorably. This liberal attitude should not preclude a careful examination so that infection or a space-occupying lesion are not missed or masked.[12,79] Although we usually perform all our injections epidurally, intrathecal steroids may be indicated for pantopaque arachnoiditis.[80,108] The anesthesiologist should be careful to use steroids without neurolytic preservatives intrathecally. Most multiple-dose vials contain some kind of preservative. (See Chap. 22.)

Trigeminal Neuralgia

Trigeminal neuralgia is characterized by recurrent paroxysmal, usually intense, sharp pain and usually is unilateral in the face and oral cavity (see also Chaps. 15 and 27). Pain is usually provoked by touching a specific area of face or mouth or by movement of the head, face, tongue, or jaw. It is stabbing, explosive, and so severe that it frequently immobilizes the patient while it lasts, for a few seconds to a few minutes. A series of pains often persists for weeks, disappears for months, and then recurs. Women are affected more often than men, and the right side of the face is affected more often than the left. The diagnosis depends entirely on the history and observation of the patient during an attack because neurologic examination is normal except for hyperesthesia during an attack. Diagnostic local anesthetic blocks of the ganglion or mandibular or maxillary divisions, become useful in these cases (see Chap. 15).

Occasionally, trigeminal neuralgia (tic douloureux) is associated with multiple sclerosis or a small neoplasm. Accordingly, neurologic examination and skull radiography should be performed in all cases and other special examinations, when indicated.

The vast majority of patients are treated successfully with carbamazepine (Tegretol) or diphenylhydantoin (Dilantin) although controlled studies have not been performed to demonstrate the efficacy of either drug. Nevertheless, they are most useful initially for controlling the frequency and severity of attacks, but increasing doses are required with time. During high-dose therapy, undesirable neurologic (vertigo, ataxia) and systemic (bone-marrow depression) side-effects occur.[49] Failure of drug therapy necessitates attempts to block the nerve directly by nerve block, radiofrequency coagulation, or surgery.[78]

Local anesthetics compared to other treatments. Local anesthetic block of the division of the affected trigeminal nerve or the gasserian ganglion itself may be used to differentiate facial pain of trigeminal origin from that due to other causes (for technique, see Chap. 15). These blocks are also helpful in predicting the outcome of surgical operation and allowing the patient to experience temporary anesthesia or paresthesia in the affected area prior to a more permanent lesion of the nerve.[45] For example, facial anesthesia is poorly tolerated by as many as 20 per cent of those who undergo surgical destructive procedures.[102]

Surgical denervation and alcohol block of the gasserian ganglion are fairly successful in relieving the pain; however, there are problems with both procedures. Surgical division of the preganglionic rootlets between the brain stem and ganglion results in facial anesthesia and, in some cases, facial paralysis, corneal keratitis or ulceration, extraocular palsy, and hemiparesis and aphasia.[102] Although alcohol block is not associated with as many complications, the pain does tend to recur in months or years. Some surgeons feel the alcohol produces scar tissue, which makes subsequent surgery technically difficult.

Many of the problems associated with surgery and alcohol block have been reduced by the recent introduction of percutaneous thermocoagulation of the gasserian ganglion or its preganglionic rootlets. For a time radiofrequency current heats the carefully positioned probe to a temperature sufficient to coagulate small, poorly myelinated pain fibers, resulting in loss of pain perception, but sparing larger myelinated fibers and thereby preserving touch and proprioceptive sensation over the affected zone.[73] As attractive as this technique appears, it still results in occasional complications such as corneal keratitis, ulceration, and anesthesia of the face but to a lesser extent than does surgical excision.[78]

Carbamazepine, alcohol block, or thermocoagulation are the most frequently used methods for treating trigeminal neuralgia. Recently, other forms of therapy have been described, which include beta-adrenergic blockers, a different technique of the alcohol blockade, and repeated bupivacaine blocks.[1,35,59] Kranzl and Kranzl have suggested a significant sympathetic and parasympathetic component in trigeminal neuralgia because the trigeminal nerve is accompanied by both sympathetic and parasympathetic fibers, particularly in the first two divisions.[59] This hypothesis is further supported by abnormal glucose tolerance or increased cholesterol levels in 28 of 30 patients with trigeminal neuralgia. These researchers have used beta-blockers and atropine in 230 patients. Less than half responded well.[30] A positive response was defined as a patient who was asymptomatic for protracted periods of time after propranalol, atropine, and only a few infiltrations; *infiltrations* was not defined. Although beta-blockers and atropine may deserve a trial, the results reported by Kranzl and Kranzl are within the range expected from placebo, particularly when associated with *infiltrations,* which can be assumed to mean infiltrations with local anesthetics.[59]

Ecker has renewed some enthusiasm for alcohol gasserian ganglion injections.[35] In a study of 42 patients, miniscule quantities (0.05 ml) of absolute alcohol were injected with meticulous radiographic and neurosensory controls; 39 patients had complete relief from pain. Ecker believes that this technique produces relief for a longer period of time than does thermocoagulation although thermocoagulation has not been used for as many years as is needed for thorough evaluation.

Adler utilized bupivacaine gasserian ganglion blocks in five patients in whom medical therapy had failed.[1] Under fluoroscopic control, 0.6 to 1.5 ml of 0.5 per cent bupivacaine were injected into the ganglion. In two patients, with the cannula secured in place, a second injection was given 3 to 5 hours later. It was not explained why the second injection was performed at that particular time. Although sensory function returned within 24 to 72 hours, pain relief lasted for 7 months to 4 years. Although Adler's series is too small for objective conclusions, this approach may be useful before attempting procedures associated with more complications, such as alcohol block, surgery, or thermocoagulation.

Glossopharyngeal Neuralgia

Compared with trigeminal neuralgia, glossopharyngeal neuralgia is relatively rare. It is characterized by severe pain in the posterior third of the tongue, palatal tonsil, and lateral wall of the oropharynx spreading to the middle ear. The pain frequently is spontaneous but may be precipitated by swallowing, coughing, or talking. A cotton applicator applied to the base of the tongue or in the external auditory meatus may provoke an attack. These areas are called *trigger zones*. The course of therapy is much the same as for trigeminal neuralgia, and most patients can be treated with carbamazepine or diphenylhydantoin. With resistant cases, an alcohol block may be considered but has potential complications because of the close approximation of the ninth and 11th cranial nerves, internal carotid artery, and internal jugular vein. Thus, glossopharyngeal nerve block with local anesthetic should be used for diagnostic purposes and to determine whether the patient can tolerate the effects of no glossopharyngeal function, which would result from surgery.[97] Repeated local anesthetic blocks with long-acting local anesthetics have not been attempted. Aoki and Tokunaga reported successful treatment of this neuralgia by local anesthetic blockade of the great auricular nerve in two patients.[3] This approach has not been evaluated by others.

Brena and Bonica have recommended a combined medication and nerve block.[18] They use diphenylhydantoin and carbamazepine in conjunction with repeated local anesthetic nerve blocks. The blocks are thought to reduce the amount of sensory input from facial structures and thereby decrease abnormal excitatory states in the central neurons of the trigeminal and glossopharyngeal innervated muscles. They have found that the dose of anticonvulsant medication can be reduced, thereby eliminating many toxic side-effects of the drugs. This therapy has not been evaluated in an objective, controlled manner.

Other Facial Pain

A variety of painful syndromes can occur when chronic irritative lesions develop at various tendon or ligament attachments to bone and articular joints. This kind of pain is accentuated by exercise and is alleviated by rest.[17,39,75] The most common occurrence of this pain is in the temporomandibular joint. It is characterized by an aching, poorly localized, unilateral pain. An important diagnostic clue may be a worsening of the pain associated with chewing or other movement of the jaw.[75] Treatment consists primarily of instructing the patient about proper movements of the jaw.[75] Brena has recommended infiltrations of local anesthetics into sensitive areas to relieve muscle spasms and decrease undesirable stimulation from the temporomandibular joint.[17]

Atypical facial neuralgia refers to a peculiar kind of facial pain of unknown origin. The characteristics of the pain are almost similar to the more classic neuralgias, but the paroxysms are often more prolonged and less severe and occur frequently in bizarre facial distribution. Neurologic examinations usually fail to detect any abnormality. Attacks are almost always unilateral, and trigger zones usually are not found. Since it is difficult to ascribe such pain to organic factors, many patients with this complaint are labeled as *psychoneurotics*. Although some neurotic element is commonly present, lack of correlation between distribution of pain and known anatomic distribution of nerves should not detract from the fact that many patients respond satisfactorily to the drug therapy outlined for trigeminal neuralgia. If drug therapy is not effective, then a diagnostic stellate ganglion block may be performed; if pain is relieved, then repeated blocks may provide prolonged relief.

Intercostal Neuralgia and Post-thoracotomy Pain

Intercostal neuralgia following thoracotomy or fracture of ribs or vertebrae is characterized by paresthesia and pain in response to touch or movement of the thorax. The pain usually subsides within 2 weeks but occasionally persists for several months or years and requires active treatment. In most cases, destructive nerve blocks with alcohol or phenol and surgical removal of neuroma or rhizotomy offer little help. Alcohol or phenol injections are succeeded by 10 to 50 per cent incidence of postblock neuritis.[68] Surgical remedies not only have irrevocable effects but frequently provide only temporary relief. One approach is to perform local anesthetic intercostal or paravertebral blocks. During the pain-free time, physical therapy can be performed, which may be helpful. Repeated efforts of this kind occasionally will result in prolonged periods pf pain relief. In severe cases, 10 per cent ammonium sulfate has been used, and, while this is not effective in all cases, it is reported not to be associated with any complications such as postblock neuritis.[68]

In the initial postoperative days following thoracotomy, patients frequently are treated with narcotics for incisional and shoulder pain. Numerous studies have shown that ventilation is improved if postoperative pain is treated by intercostal nerve blocks rather than narcotics, and this may reduce the incidence of persistent neuralgic pain. The availability of long-acting local anesthetics such as etidocaine or bupivacaine makes this approach practical.

Postherpetic Neuralgia

Herpes zoster usually occurs in older people probably, because the varicella-zoster virus, which had been dormant in the posterior root ganglia, begins to multiply and invades the corresponding sensory nerves. The virus usually attacks only one to three nerves because renewed immunity develops as it multiplies. The cutaneous lesions gradually disappear in 2 to 4 weeks, after which the pain usually subsides; however, sometimes the pain and scarring persist. Local anesthetic, alcohol, or phenol intercostal nerve blocks are not effective in relieving this pain. Early cases (less than 3 months) can be treated by sympathetic nerve blocks with local anesthetic. Colding believes that repetitive sympathetic blocks can reduce the incidence of postherpetic neuralgia although this has not been documented.[27]

The intralesional injection of local anesthetic and steroids has been advocated by Moya and Epstein.[37,*] We have prepared a solution of 2 mg of triamcinolone per ml of 0.25 per cent bupivacaine. We have injected up to 25 to 30 ml per kg subcutaneously under the painful skin. Although Moya and Epstein are enthusiastic about this approach, we have not had sufficient experience for objective conclusions.[37,*] It is possible that the concomitant administration of prolixin and a tricyclic antidepressant (amitriptyline) are more responsible for the pain relief than are steroids and local anesthetic.

* Moya, F.: Personal communication.

Lateral Femoral Cutaneous Neuralgia (Meralgia Paresthetica)

Lateral femoral cutaneous neuralgia is characterized by burning pain, numbness, and tingling in the anterolateral aspect of the thigh and frequently is associated with obesity and prolonged pressure from belts. Although it is possibly associated with anatomical entrapment (such as passage of the lateral femoral cutaneous nerve through, rather than deep, to the inguinal ligament), a specific cause frequently is not identified. A simple valuable test to aid in the diagnosis of meralgia paresthetica is injection of local anesthetic into the lateral femoral cutaneous nerve at a point adjacent to the anterior superior iliac spine.[53] Relief of pain confirms the diagnosis although placebo injections should also be attempted. A word of caution is in order; lack of pain relief does not exclude the diagnosis of meralgia paresthetica. Intrapelvic lesions, such as carcinoma of the uterus or prostate, may cause this same pain syndrome because the lateral femoral cutaneous nerve has a long intrapelvic course and lies just under the parietal peritoneum. If the lesion were intrapelvic rather than near the inguinal ligament, a diagnostic block performed near the anterior superior iliac spine would fail to relieve pain despite the involvement of that nerve.

Usually, the pain disappears spontaneously with weight reduction or loosening of the belt.[100] Repeated infiltration with a long-acting local anesthetic and, in resistant cases, 2 ml of methylprednisolone (Depo-Medrol) will result in sustained relief.[53] Although alcohol blocks occasionally have been recommended, we believe they probably are not indicated because thay may result in painful neuritis, which could be worse than the original pain.[47,57] Teng has reported great success with surgery.[96] Block of the lateral femoral cutaneous nerve with local anesthetic and possibly steroids seems to be a more reasonable initial approach, reserving surgery for treatment failures.

MYOFASCIAL PAIN SYNDROME

Many chronic pain states of obscure origin depend on feedback cycles from myofascial trigger points. Travell has defined a *trigger point* in skeletal muscle as a localized area of tenderness in a palpably firm band of muscle with a positive *jump sign*, which is a visible shortening of the part of the muscle that contains the band when it is stimulated at the point of maximum tenderness.[100] When the jump sign is elicited by palpation of such a band, a transient burst of motor unit action potentials can be detected.[84] These trigger points will elicit pain in a fairly predictable anatomical distribution. The constancy of the myofascial pain patterns allows easier location of trigger points associated with the pain.[100,109] Melzack and colleagues have found a close correlation between trigger point areas and acupuncture points for pain.[64]

The trigger point concept has been difficult for many physicians to accept because the precise neuroanatomic connections between the trigger point and the pain are not understood. Motor unit action potentials will appear when trigger points are palpated.[84] Furthermore, histologic examination of trigger points obtained by biopsy reveals waxy degeneration and destruction of muscle fibers, an increase in number and agglomeration of nuclei of muscle fibers, and fatty infiltration.[60] These findings provide objective evidence for the existence of trigger points as anatomical and physiologic entities. Their function is yet unknown. Myofascial pain syndromes have been reviewed thoroughly by Simons.[85]

Brief intense stimulation of trigger points by dry needling, intense cold, injection of normal saline, and transcutaneous electrical stimulation may diminish or abolish myofascial pain for days or weeks.[64] More sustained relief has been obtained by injecting muscular trigger points with 10 ml of 0.25 per cent bupivacaine or other local anesthetic. These techniques have been amply described by several authors.[60] For trigger points at bones, ligaments, or fascial areas, the addition of 2 per cent methylprednisolone seems to be effective.

CANCER PAIN

Cancer can cause pain by one or a combination of the following mechanisms.[17]

Compression of nerve roots, trunks, or plexuses
Infiltration of nerves and blood vessels by malignant cells
Obstruction or distension of a viscus
Occlusion of blood vessels resulting in venous engorgement or local ischemia
Inflammation, swelling, or necrosis of invaded tissues

Local anesthetic blocks have little or no role in therapy of cancer pain. Sustained relief of pain can be obtained only with neurolytic blocks or surgery. The role of local anesthetic blocks then is diagnostic, to help predict the outcome of neurolytic block or surgery. Also, the possibility of the block producing results (*i.e.*, numbness) more undesirable than the pain may be assessed. Neurolytic blocks are described in Chapter 27.

EVALUATION OF NERVE BLOCK

Evaluation of a patient's physiologic and psychological response to a nerve block often is more difficult than the technical procedure required to produce the block. Diagnostic and therapeutic blocks require different criteria for evaluation of results because of different goals. The goal of a diagnostic nerve block is either to identify anatomical features of pain transmission or to predict the results of nerve ablation. However, the use of local anesthetic blocks to predict the success of a neurolytic block or surgical resection of a nerve is difficult. Too often a naive anesthesiologist or surgeon will say, "If the diagnostic block relieves the pain, then a neurolytic block or surgical resection certainly will be successful." Diagnostic local anesthetic blocks allow the patient to experience briefly the numbness and other side-effects that are likely to be permanent from nerve ablation techniques; nevertheless, they are not always accurate predictors of long-term pain relief. Diagnostic blocks provide little help in evaluation of the influence of pain relief on psychological factors such as family interactions, litigation (financial gain), or narcotic use. For a variety of reasons, therefore, local anesthetic diagnostic blocks have limited prognostic value for neurolytic block or surgery other than to help isolate the anatomical source of the pain.[14]

Evaluation of results from a therapeutic nerve block requires more thorough questioning than "Is your pain gone?" The patients should record daily as much information as possible, using the guidelines of Arnhoff and Brena and Bonica (see next page).[5,18]

These recorded lists should be analyzed for changes that may reflect important consequences of the block. If the patient states that the pain has been relieved and yet his recorded activities have not changed, then the conclusion about the effectiveness of the block should be guarded.

(1) List frequency and intensity of pain daily
(2) Record number of hours in bed and number of hours spent standing or reclining daily
(3) Estimate ability to walk, bend, and work
(4) Evaluate whether each item on a checklist of 13 to 20 activities (such as making beds, washing car, tying shoes, etc.) can be performed before and after nerve block
(5) Briefly describe recreational and social activities before pain; describe how the pain has altered these activities and whether the block has helped the return to the preblock level of activity
(6) List the medication taken daily

Objective criteria for determining the long-term success of neural blockade are lacking. For example, most studies measured the success of nerve blocks by asking patients simply whether their pain was relieved, with no evaluation by more extensive criteria of the responses. Because of such superficial evaluation of the results of blocks reported by the majority of authors, objective assessment of many of the results reported in this chapter is very difficult.

Arnhoff and colleagues have suggested that appropriate experimental designs and statistical methods for evaluation of nerve block effects remain generally unapplied.[5] Indeed, the complex nature of most chronic pain problems makes evaluation of the results of nerve blocks difficult. However, Arnhoff and colleagues have emphasized that the complexities of total treatment and isolation of the effect of a single factor are not unique to nerve block therapy.[5] They have pointed out that techniques available to isolate direct treatment effects are widely used in other areas of medicine. Until applied to nerve block therapy, chapters and conclusions such as ours will continue to be based on "art" rather than "science."

REFERENCES

1. Adler, P.: The use of bupivacaine for blocking the gasserian ganglion in major trigeminal neuralgia. Int. J. Oral Surg., *4*:251, 1975.
2. Ahlgren, E.W., *et al.:* Diagnosis of pain with a graduated spinal block technique. J.A.M.A., *195*:813, 1966.
3. Aoki, H., and Tokunaga, Y.: A new approach to the treatment of glossopharyngeal neuralgia, using the great auricular nerve. Folia Psychiatr. Neurol. Jpn., *19*:346, 1965.
4. Arkin, A.M., *et al.:* Behaviour modification. N.Y. State J. Med., *76*:190, 1976.
5. Arnhoff, F.N., Triplett, H.B., and Pokorney, B.: Follow-up status of patients treated with nerve blocks for low back pain. Anesthesiology, *46*:170, 1977.
6. Arnoldi, C.C.: Intraosseous hypertension. Clin. Orthop., *115*:30, 1976.
7. Atkinson, L.: The management of intractable pain. Med. J. Aust., *1*:786, 1976.
8. Baker, A.G., and Winnegarner, F.G.: Causalgia. Am. J. Surg., *117*:690, 1969.
9. Beecher, H.K.: The powerful placebo. J.A.M.A., *159*:1602, 1955.
10. Beene, T.K., and Eggers, G.W.N., Jr.: Use of the pulse monitor for determining sympathetic block of the arm. Anesthesiology, *40*:412, 1974.
11. Benson, H., and Epstein, M.D.: The placebo effect. A neglected asset in the care of patients. J.A.M.A., *232*:1225, 1975.
12. Bernard, W.N., Presbitero, J.V., and Dolorico, V.N.: Subarachnoid methylprednisolone for relief of sciatic pain secondary to space-occupying lesion: A case report. Anesth. Analg. (Cleve.), *53*:744, 1974.
13. Black, R.G.: The management of pain with nerve blocks. Minn. Med., *57*:189, 1974.
14. Black, R.G., and Bonica, J.J.: Diagnostic and therapeutic blocks in pain therapy. Compr. Ther., *1*:32, 1975.
15. Braun, K.: Paravertebral block and the electrocardiogram in angina pectoris. Br. Heart J., *8*:47, 1946.
16. Breivik, H., *et al.:* Treatment of low back pain and sciatica: Comparison of caudal epidural injections of bupivacaine and methylprednisolone with bupivacaine followed by saline. *In* Bonica, J.J., and Albe–Fessard, D. (eds.): Advances in Pain Research and Therapy, vol 1. pp. 927–932. New York, Raven Press, 1976.
17. Brena, S.: Current status of regional anesthesia for diagnosis and therapy. *In* Bonica, J.J. (ed.): Regional Anesthesia: Recent Advances and Current Status. pp. 168–191. 1971.
18. Brena, S., and Bonica, J.J.: Nerve blocks for managing pain in the elderly. Postgrad. Med., *47*:215, 1970.
19. Bridenbaugh, L.D., Moore, D.C., and Campbell, D.D.: Management of upper abdominal cancer pain. J.A.M.A., *190*:877, 1964.
20. Burch, G.E., and Giles, T.D.: Cardiac causalgia. Arch. Int. Med., *125*:809, 1970.
21. Burn, J.M.B., and Langdon, L.: Duration of action of epidural methylprednisolone. Am. J. Phys. Med., *53*:29, 1974.
22. Carron, H.: Management of common pain problems. Reg. Ref. Courses in Anesthesiology, *3*:51, 1975.
23. Chapman, C.R., Murphy, J.M., and Butler, S.H.: Analgetic strength of 33 percent nitrous oxide: A signal detection theory evaluation. Science, *179*:1246, 1973.
24. Chapman, L.F., *et al.:* Neurohumoral features of afferent fibers in man. Arch. Neurol., *4*:49, 1961.
25. Cho, K.O.: Therapeutic epidural block with a combination of a weak local anesthetic and steroids in management of complicated low back pain. Am. Surg., *36*:303, 1970.
26. Clark, W.C.: Pain sensitivity and the report of pain. Anesthesiology, *40*:272, 1974.
27. Colding, A.: The effect of regional sympathetic blocks in the treatment of herpes zoster. Acta Anaesthesiol. Scand., *13*:113, 1969.
28. Coomes, E.N.: A comparison between epidural anaesthesia and bed rest in sciatica. Br. Med. J., *1*:20, 1961.
29. Davidson, J.T., and Robin, G.C.: Epidural injections in the lumbosciatic syndrome. Br. J. Anaesth., *33*:595, 1961.
30. Delilkan, A.E., *et al.:* Post-operative local analgesia for thoracotomy with direct bupivacaine intercostal blocks. Anaesthesia, *282*:561, 1973.

31. Devalera, E., and Raftery, H.: Lower abdominal and pelvic pain in women. *In* Bonica, J.J., and Albe–Fessard, D. (eds.): Advances in Pain Research and Therapy. pp. 935–937. New York, Raven Press, 1976.
32. Diaz, P.M.: Use of liquid-crystal thermography to evaluate sympathetic blocks. Anesthesiology, *44*:443, 1976.
33. Dilke, T.F.W., Burry, H.C., and Grahame, R.: Extradural nerve root compression. Br. Med. J., *2*:635, 1973.
34. Doupe, J., Cullen, C.H., and Chance, G.Q.: Post-traumatic pain and causalgia syndrome. J. Neurol. Psychiatry, *7*:33, 1944.
35. Ecker, A.: Tic douloureux. N.Y. State J. Med., *74*:1586, 1974.
36. Edelist, G., Gross, A.E., and Langer, F.: Treatment of low back pain with acupuncture. Can. Anaesth. Soc. J., *23*:303, 1976.
37. Epstein, E.: Intralesional triamcinolone therapy in herpes zoster and postzoster neuralgia. Eye Nose Throat, *52*:61, 1973.
38. Fordyce, W.E., *et al.:* Operant conditioning in the treatment of chronic pain. Arch. Phys. Med. Rehabil., *54*:399, 1973.
39. Foster, J.B.: Facial pain. Br. Med. J., *4*:667, 1969.
40. Galati, S.M., Kapur, B.M.L., and Talwar, J.R.: Sympathectomy in management of frostbite: An experimental study. Indian J. Med. Res., *58*:343, 1970.
41. Gardner, W.J., Goebert, H.W., and Sehgal, A.D.: Intraspinal corticosteroids in the treatment of sciatica. Trans. Am. Neurol. Assoc., *86*:214, 1961.
42. Genant, H.K., *et al.:* The reflex sympathetic dystrophy syndrome. Radiology, *117*:21, 1975.
43. Goebert, H.W., *et al.:* Painful radiculopathy treated with epidural injections of procaine and hydrocortisone acetate. Anesth. Analg. (Cleve.), *40*:130, 1961.
44. Green, L.N.: Dexamethasone in the management of symptoms due to herniated lumbar disc. J. Neurol. Neurosurg. Psychiatry, *38*:1211, 1975.
45. Greenberg, C., and Papper, E.M.: The indications for gasserian ganglion block for trigeminal neuralgia. Anesthesiology, *31*:566, 1969.
46. Hannington-Kiff, J.G.: Intravenous regional sympathetic block with guanethidine. Lancet, *1*:1019, 1974.
47. ______: Spinal and limb pain. *In* Pain Relief. Pp. 111–112. London, Heinemann Medical Books, 1974.
48. Hardy, W.G., *et al.:* The problem of minor and major causalgias. Am. J. Surg., *95*:545, 1958.
49. Henderson, W.R.: Trigeminal neuralgia: The pain and its treatment. Br. Med. J., *1*:7, 1967.
50. Hill, G.L.: A rational basis for management of patients with the Buerger's syndrome. Br. J. Surg., *61*:476, 1974.
51. Ito, R.: The treatment of low back pain and sciatica with epidural corticosteroids injection and its pathophysiological basis. Nippon Seikeigeka Gakkai Zasshi, *45*:67, 1971.
52. Jacobson, A.M., *et al.:* Raynaud's phenomenon. J.A.M.A., *225*:739, 1973.
53. Jones, R.K.: Meralgia paresthetica as a cause of leg discomfort. Can. Med. Assoc. J., *111*:541, 1974.
54. Kelman, H.: Epidural injection therapy for sciatic pain. Am. J. Surg., *64*:183, 1944.
55. Kibler, R.F., and Nathan, P.W.: Relief of pain and paraesthesiae by nerve block distal to a lesion. J. Neurol. Neurosurg. Psychiatry, *23*:91, 1960.
56. Kim, G.E., Ibrahim, I.M., and Imparato, A.M.: Lumbar sympathectomy in end stage arterial occlusive disease. Ann. Surg., *183*:157, 1976.
57. Kitchen, C., and Simpson, J.: Meralgia paresthetica—A review of 67 patients. Acta Neurol. Scand., *48*:547, 1972.
58. Kleinert, H.E., *et al.:* Post-traumatic sympathetic dystrophy. Orthop. Clin. North Am., *4*:917, 1973.
59. Kranzl, B., and Kranzl, C.: The role of the autonomic nervous system in trigeminal neuralgia. J. Neural Transm., *38*:77, 1976.
60. Kraus, H.: Trigger points. N. Y. State J. Med., *73*:1310, 1973.
61. Kyosola, K.: Clinical experiences in the management of cold injuries: A study of 110 cases. J. Trauma, *14*:32, 1974.
62. Laska, E., and Sunshine, A.: Anticipation of analgesia—A placebo effect. Headache, *13*:1, 1973.
63. Melzack, R.: Phantom limb pain. Anesthesiology, *35*:409. 1971.
64. Melzack, R., Stillwell, D.M., and Fox, E.J.: Trigger points and acupuncture points for pain: Correlations and implications. Pain, *3*:3, 1977.
65. Melzack, R., and Torgerson, W.S.: On the language of pain. Anesthesiology, *34*:50, 1971.
66. Melzack, R., and Wall, P.D.: Pain mechanisms: New theory. Science, *150*:971, 1965.
67. Meyer, G.A., and Fields, H.L.: Causalgia treated by selective large fibre stimulation of peripheral nerve. Brain, *95*:163, 1972.
68. Miller, R.D., Johnston, R.R., and Hosobuchi, Y.: Treatment of intercostal neuralgia with 10 percent ammonium sulfate. J. Thorac. Cardiovasc. Surg., *69*:476, 1975.
69. Nakata, Y., *et al.:* Effects of lumbar sympathectomy in thromboangiitis obliterans. J. Cardiovasc. Surg., *16*:415, 1975.
70. Ochsner, A.: Venous thrombosis. Postgrad. Med., *31*:539, 1962.
71. Omer, G., and Thomas, S.: Treatment of causalgia. Tex. Med., *67*:93, 1971.
72. ______: The management of chronic pain syndromes in the upper extremity. Clin. Orthop., *104*:37, 1974.
73. Onofrio, B.: Radiofrequency percutaneous gasserian ganglion lesions. Results in 140 patients with trigeminal pain. J. Neurosurg., *42*:132, 1975.
74. Papper, E.M., and Imler, A.E.: The use of phlebography and lumbar sympathetic block in the diagnosis of venospasm of the lower extremities. Surgery, *15*:402, 1944.
75. Poser, C.M.: Facial pain: Diagnostic dilemma and therapeutic challenge. Geriatrics, *30*:110, 1975.
76. Richards, R.L.: Causalgia. Arch. Neurol., *16*:339, 1967.
77. ______: Lumbar sympathectomy for chronic occlusive arterial disease. Am. Heart J., *81*:735, 1971.
78. Rish, B.L.: Cerebrovascular accident after percutaneous thermocoagulation of the trigeminal ganglion. J. Neurosurg., *44*:376, 1976.
79. Roberts, M., Sheppard, G.L., and McCormick, R.C.: Tuberculous meningitis after intrathecally administered methylprednisolone acetate. J.A.M.A., *200*:190, 1967.
80. Sehgal, A.D., Gardner, W.J., and Dohn, D.F.: Pantopaque "arachnoiditis." Cleve. Clin. Q., *29*:177, 1962.
81. Sehgal, A.D., Tweed, D.C., and Foote, M.K.: Laboratory studies after intrathecal corticosteroids. Arch. Neurol., *9*:74, 1963.
82. Shaw, R.S., Austen, W.G., and Stipa, S.: A ten year study of the effect of lumbar sympathectomy on the peripheral circulation of patients with arteriosclerotic occlusive disease. Surg. Gynecol. Obstet., *119*:486, 1964.
83. Shionoya, S., *et al.:* Diagnosis, pathology and treatment of Buerger's disease. Surgery, *75*:695, 1974.
84. Simons, D.G.: Electrogenic nature of palpable bands and "jump sign" associated with myofascial trigger points. *In* Bonica, J.J., and Albe–Fessard, D. (eds.): Advances in

Pain Research and Therapy. Pp. 913–918. New York, Raven Press, 1976.

85. ______: Muscle pain syndromes. Am. J. Phys. Med., *55*:15, 1976.
86. Simson, G.: Propranolol for causalgia and Sudek atrophy. J.A.M.A., *227*:327, 1974.
87. Smith, G.M., *et al.:* Experimental pain produced by the submaximal effort tourniquet technique: Further evidence of validity. J. Pharmacol. Exp. Ther., *163*:468, 1968.
88. Smithwick, R.H.: Lumbar sympathectomy in treatment of obliterative vascular disease of the lower extremities. Surgery, *42*:415, 1957.
89. Snyder, M.A., Adams, J.T., and Schwartz, S.I.: Sympathectomy in iliofemoral venous thrombosis. Surg. Gynecol. Obstet., *124*:49, 1967.
90. Spiro, H.M.: Pain and perfection—The physician and the "pain patient." N. Engl. J. Med., *294*:829, 1976.
91. Sternback, R.A., *et al.:* Traits of pain patients: The low-back "loser." Psychosomatics, *14*:226, 1973.
92. Sternschein, M.J., *et al.:* Causalgia. Arch. Phys. Med. Rehabil., *56*:58, 1975.
93. Strand, L.: Lumbar sympathectomy in the treatment of peripheral obliterative arterial disease. Acta Chir. Scand., *135*:597, 1969.
94. Swerdlow, M., and Sayle-Creer, W.: A study of extradural medication in the relief of lumbosciatic syndrome. Anaesthesia, *25*:341, 1970.
95. Taub, A.: Factors in the diagnosis and treatment of chronic pain. J. Autism Child. Schizophr., *5*:1, 1975.
96. Teng, P.: Meralgia paresthetica. Bull. Los Angeles Neurol. Soc., *37*:75, 1972.
97. Thompson, G.E., and Robb, J.V.: Glossopharyngeal neuralgia—Implications for the anesthesiologist. Anesthesiology, *37*:660, 1972.
98. Thompson, J.E., Patman, D.R., and Persson, A.V.: Management of post-traumatic syndromes (causalgia). Am. Surg., *41*:599, 1975.
99. Timmermans, G., and Sternback, R.A.: Factors of human chronic pain: An analysis of personality and pain reaction variables. Science, *184*:806, 1974.
100. Travell, J.: Myofascial trigger points: Clinical view. *In* Bonica, J.J., and Albe-Fessard, D. (eds.): Advances in Pain Research and Therapy. Pp. 919–926. New York, Raven Press, 1976.
101. Warr, A.C., *et al.:* Chronic lumbosciatic syndrome treated by epidural injection and manipulation. Practitioner, *209*:53, 1972.
102. Wepsic, J.G.: Tic douloureux: Etiology, refined treatment. N. Engl. J. Med., *288*:680, 1973.
103. White, J.C.: 'Minor' causalgia. Arch. Surg., *100*:743, 1970.
104. Whitelaw, G.P., and Smithwick, R.H.: Some secondary effects of sympathectomy with particular reference to disturbance of sexual function. N. Engl. J. Med., *245*:121, 1951.
105. Wiener, L., and Cox, W.J.: Influence of stellate ganglion block on angina pectoris and the post-exercise electrocardiogram. Am. J. Med. Sci., *252*:69, 1966.
106. Willdeck-Lund, G., and Edstrom, H.: Etidocaine in intercostal nerve block for pain relief after thoractomy: A comparison with bupivacaine. Acta Anaesthesiol. Scand., *60*:33, 1975.
107. Winnie, A.P., and Collins, V.J.: Differential neural blockade in pain syndromes of questionable etiology. Med. Clin. North Am., *52*:123, 1968.
108. Winnie, A.P., *et al.:* Pain clinic II: Intradural and extradural corticosteroids for sciatica. Anesth. Analg. (Cleve.), *51*:990, 1972.
109. Winter, A.A., and Yavelow, I.: Oral considerations of the myofascial pain dysfunction syndrome. Oral Surg., *40*:720, 1975.
110. Wirth, F.P., Jr., and Rutherford, R.B.: A civilian experience with causalgia. Arch. Surg., *100*:633, 1970.
111. Woodforde, J.M., and Merskey, H.: Personality traits of patients with chronic pain. J. Psychosom. Res., *16*:167, 1972.

27 Chronic Pain and Neurolytic Neural Blockade

Brian Dwyer and David Gibb

GENERAL CONSIDERATIONS

Neurolytic blockade offers a great potential for pain relief in patients with severe, advanced pain, mostly due to cancer but also due to other noncurable conditions such as occlusive vascular disease. The techniques of subarachnoid, celiac plexus, and lumbar sympathetic block are capable of a very high degree of success with an acceptable level of side-effects in the patient who has not obtained satisfactory pain relief by other methods. It should be stressed that neurolytic blockade is generally not suitable for young patients with undiagnosed medical problems or for patients (apart from occlusive vascular disease) who are likely to live for a long period of time.

Neurolytic block should be regarded as only one aspect of the overall management of patients with intractable pain. The general care of these patients is best undertaken in a Pain Relief Clinic in which a multidisciplinary approach simplifies their management and considerably improves the results of treatment.[6,9,17,32] Consultations among specialists in the fields of anesthesiology, neurology, neurosurgery, psychiatry, radiotherapy, and social work within the structure of the Pain Relief Clinic have proved invaluable. Assistance from dentists and orthopedic or general surgeons is essential in specific instances.

At the first interview, a detailed history should be taken with emphasis on the features of the pain; the preceding pathology and its treatment; and the personal, social, and domestic situation of the patient. A physical examination is then performed, concentrating primarily on the painful condition.

Psychological support by means of personal interest, reassurance, and encouragement is an integral part of the management. Depression is a common accompaniment of chronic pain and requires appropriate treatment, usually with a tricyclic antidepressant (*e.g.*, imipramine, amitriptyline, or nortriptyline). A suggested regime is amitriptyline, 25 mg, three times a day, and 75 mg, at night, gradually increased over a period of 2 weeks. Slow increase and adequate evening dosage reduces the unpleasant anticholinergic, hypotensive, and sedative effects of the drug. It is important to inform the patient that no subjective improvement in his mood will occur for 2 to 3 weeks. When anxiety, agitation, and muscle spasm are present, diazepam, 5 mg, two to four times daily, should be added to the drug regime. Barbiturates are avoided because they tend to be antanalgesic, and long-term therapy frequently induces depression. Combination analgesic-barbiturate drugs (*e.g.*, sodium pentobarbitone and codeine) are particularly unsuitable for these reasons. Phenothiazines are prescribed by some clinicians, but, again, they may aggravate depression and are best reserved for the treatment of insomnia or, in terminal cases, to keep the patient totally unaware of his environment.[41]

Patients with chronic pain have invariably been treated with analgesic drugs for a considerable time. It is usually failure of the powerful narcotic analgesics to relieve pain, or the fear of producing addiction, that motivates the medical practitioner to seek advice on alternative forms of therapy. The best time to refer a patient for assessment is when the moderately strong, oral analgesics (*e.g.*, codeine phosphate) have ceased to be effective. This may be due to an increase in the intensity of the pain, the development of tolerance to the analgesic, or the appearance of such distressing side-effects as loss of appetite, gastric irritation, or constipation. Once a patient has become physically dependent on a powerful narcotic analgesic, it may be exceedingly difficult to assess the efficacy of a nerve block or plan a satisfactory sequential analgesic regime. It should be remembered that even when a neurolytic block has been a technical success, supplementary analgesics may be required because the disease has spread beyond the anatomical limits of the block or the patient has developed drug dependence. In malignant disease a primary objective of a neurolytic block is to keep the patient ambulant and on oral medication during the advanced stages of his illness. Regular injections of morphine or meperidine (pethidine) may be required, but the patient can usually be maintained on oral codeine, pentazocine, or methadone, three to four times daily.

Techniques. Precise unilateral segmental blocks can be produced at any spinal level from the cervical region to the perineum, by the *subarachnoid injection* of a neurolytic agent. *Epidural injection* can achieve similar results, but the anesthesia is bilateral and may not be as profound. Because the pain-carrying fibers of a spinal nerve cannot be selectively destroyed, neurologic complications are unavoidable in a percentage of patients; they are uncommon in the midthoracic region but are more common in the sacral area.

Celiac plexus block will denervate upper abdominal organs and relieve pain due to disease in these viscera and in the abdominal aorta. The latter may occur together with lower limb pain and necessitate lumbar sympathetic block as well. *Lumbar sympathetic block* alone will relieve lower limb pain when it has an autonomic component.

Peripheral nerves may effectively be blocked with a neurolytic agent by simple modification of the standard techniques used with local analgesics. In the sensory branches of the cranial nerves, the effect of these blocks in relieving pain from head and neck cancer has been most encouraging. With peripheral sensory nerves, however, experience has been less rewarding, owing to the relatively high incidence of neuritis, tissue necrosis, and, more rarely, transverse myelitis and motor paresis. In some clinics, intercostal block has been an exception to these problems (see Chap. 26).[28]

When a destructive procedure is contemplated, careful consideration should be given to the most effective method available. For example, evidence is now accumulating that *thermogangliolysis* is an excellent alternative to surgical section of the trigeminal ganglion.[48] It seems clear that *surgery* or thermogangliolysis are the treatments of choice for trigeminal neuralgia, which is unresponsive to carbamazepine, since the results of these two approaches are more predictable than alcohol injection. As a general rule, surgery, or gangliolysis, may be preferred in the young, fit patient, while the elderly, frail patient with a short life expectancy may be better treated with gangliolysis or, more rarely, by alcohol block. More recently *cryoanalgesia* has been used to control pain of both benign and malignant origin.[2,30] While the technique appears useful for postoperative pain, its role in the treatment of chronic pain requires further evaluation.

The results of permanent nerve block are disappointing in patients with widespread or poorly localized pain, when drug addiction or dependence are established, in midline lower back pain, in the ambulant patient with minimal pain, and, in subarachnoid block, in the presence of vertebral metastases.[28]

Before any permanent nerve block is performed, the implications must be discussed with the patient or his relatives and the advantages and possible complications of the procedure fully understood by all. It is most unwise to attempt such procedures in unwilling or uncooperative patients. Workers at many pain clinics believe that it is essential to employ an initial diagnostic block with reversible local anesthetic agent as part of the workup to assess the suitability of the patient for a permanent block. Sometimes the use of placebo agents is also favored in assessment.

Assessment of Results. Considerable objective improvement in drug requirements, sleep pattern, appetite, general activity, and mood can be observed after a technically successful nerve block. Subjectively, however, patients may deny any significant relief. This response may be due to the unmasking of other pains, preoccupations with side-effects of the block, depressions, narcotic addiction, or other causes. Assessment of the results of a block is, therefore, difficult, and, while it is not suggested that the patient's opinion be disregarded, other factors should also be considered.[22,28,32,50] In contrast, success may be obscured by withdrawal symptoms following too rapid cessation of analgesic therapy; it is thus extremely important to reduce analgesic therapy slowly. Finally, the opinions of relatives, friends, and nursing staff are invaluable in the final assessment.

SUBARACHNOID BLOCK

The subarachnoid injection of a neurolytic agent is an effective method of pain control and is restricted, ideally, to patients with advanced malignancy in whom the pain is unilateral and limited in extent to a few spinal segments. It should be used with great caution when the pain is bilateral or widespread and when it is due to neurologic or undiagnosed disease.[31,50]

Particular care must be taken to avoid increasing the patient's disability through motor weakness, sphincteric incompetence, and loss of positional sense, unless it can be justified by the degree of pain relief that is achieved. The aim is to produce a chemical posterior rhizotomy and interrupt the pain pathways from the affected area. Alcohol, phenol, chlorocresol, cold saline, and ammonium salts have been used in the manner described below.

Subarachnoid Absolute Alcohol

The use of alcohol was first described by Dogliotti in 1931.[16] To produce a precise block of profound intensity and adequate duration, the patient must be positioned carefully in order that the maximum concentration of the hypobaric alcohol solution reaches the posterior nerve roots. This means that the patient is placed in the lateral oblique position with the painful side uppermost. Alcohol may be injected where the affected nerve leaves the spinal cord or where it leaves the vertebral canal through the intervertebral foramen. Hay and Swerdlow state that the injection should be at cord level because alcohol exerts its maximal effect on the fine rootlets leaving the spinal cord.[22,50] On the other hand, the alcohol concentration is probably greater where the posterior root enters the dura, and, for this reason, injection at the vertebral level may be preferred. The controversy relates only to the lumbosacral and lower thoracic spinal nerves because, at higher levels, the nerves pass horizontally from the cord to their point of exit at intervertebral foramina (Fig. 27-1). The principal pathologic effects produced by alcohol are demyelination and degeneration of the dorsal root with some chromatolysis and swelling of the dorsal root with secondary degeneration of the posterior columns (see Chap. 5).[22,23]

Technique has been well described.[7,22,28,31,50] The patient is placed on an operating table with the affected side upward, in the oblique lateral position with the body about 45° to the horizontal (Fig. 27-2–27-4). Breaking the table at the proposed injection site assists in maintaining the posterior roots in the uppermost position. The free-flow of cerebrospinal fluid (CSF) through a fine needle may be minimal, owing to low intrathecal pressure, but it may be improved through rotation of the spinal needle or aspiration with a syringe.

To limit the spread of alcohol in the subarachnoid space to the affected segments, the volume of solution injected should be small and the rate of injection slow. If the area involved is relatively extensive, multiple segmental injections of a small volume are preferable to a single larger injection. If the pain is confined to one or two spinal segments, a single injection of 0.5 to 1.0 ml may be injected at each alternate interspace up to a total dose of 1.5 ml and the injection time should be more than 2 minutes at each site. The patient may experience a burning pain or unpleasant paresthesia for a few seconds, but this rapidly subsides as complete analgesia supervenes. However, it can be a valuable guide that the correct segments are being blocked.

Matsuki, Kato, and Ichiyanagi demonstrated that when the dose does not exceed 1 ml, the alcohol concentration in the CSF falls rapidly and allows the patient to be repositioned in the supine posture in 15 to 20 minutes without any fear of an unwanted extension of the block.[39] The supine position will reduce the incidence of spinal headache, particularly when a dural tap has been performed at several levels.

Bilateral Pain. Two techniques have been described to treat bilateral pain. The patient may be placed in the prone position with the affected segments uppermost over the break in the operating table. The injected alcohol will then spread to both posterior roots. Alternatively, each side may be blocked on separate occasions, 2 to 3 days apart, when the effect of the initial injection can be assessed before the second procedure is attempted.

An extradural block may also be used, particularly when a previous diagnostic block with a local analgesic has produced satisfactory pain relief and, preferably, in the thoracic and lumbar regions. A volume of 2 to 4 ml absolute alcohol per segment is recommended (see Chap. 8). In the opinion of these authors, this is much inferior to the subarachnoid technique. Finally, a new technique, *subdural block,* has been described.[26] Its role has yet to be defined (see Chap. 8).

Results. The difficulty of assessing results has already been mentioned, but within the limitations imposed by the subjective nature of the patient's response, various authors have claimed that approximately 50 per cent of the results are good, 30 per cent fair, and 20 per cent poor (Table 27-1).[8] The duration of effect varies from weeks to a year or more but can be expected to average 3 to 4 months.

Subarachnoid Phenol

Phenol has been recommended as a neurolytic agent on the basis that its action is differential, sparing the large myelinated fibers while destroying the small unmyelinated C fibers.[35,38,44] However, Bonica and Lund do not regard this differential effect as significant clinically, and there is now a wealth of experimental evidence to support this view (see Chap. 5).[7,31] The block produced by phenol tends to be less profound and of shorter duration than that of alcohol, but it can be used to advantage when the risk of motor paresis or loss of bladder and bowel control is high since the incidence of bladder paresis

Table 27-1. Results of Subarachnoid Block With Alcohol

Author	Number of Cases	Percentage Results		
		Good	Fair	Poor
Dogliotti (1931)[16]	150	59	25	16
Stern (1934)	50	63	27	10
Greenhill and Schmitz (1935)	25	80	12	8
Abbot (1936)	25	84	8	8
Adson (1937)	36	44	25	31
Peyton, Semansky, and Baker (1937)	33	34	27	39
Greenhill (1947)	>100	60	10	30
Bonica (1958)[8]	Unstated	50	30	20
Hay (1962)[22]	252	46	32	22
Tank, Dohn, and Gardner (1963)	13	54	15	31
Kuzucu, Derrick, and Wilber (1966)[28]	322	58.2	26.1	15.7

(Data from Kuzucu, E.Y., Derrick, W.S., and Wilbur, S.A.: Control of intractable pain with subarachnoid alcohol block. J.A.M.A., *195*:541, 1966; and Swerdlow, M. (ed.): Relief of Intractable Pain. Amsterdam, Excerpta Medica, 1974)

is reported to be lower than with alcohol (Table 27-2; see also Tables 27-1 and 27-4).

Phenol has been used as a 5-per-cent to 6-per-cent solution in glycerine (with or without silver nitrate, 0.6 mg/ml) or as a 7.5-per-cent to 10-per-cent solution in iophendylate.[1,31,35,38,44,50] Silver nitrate as an additive has largely been abandoned because of the meningeal irritation it can produce.[44] Phenol in glycerine is more effective than phenol in iophendylate because the glycerine diffuses more rapidly from the solvent to produce a higher neurolytic concentration.[38,44] Unlike absolute alcohol, all these phenol solutions are hyperbaric and viscous and deteriorate during storage, although this has been overemphasized since deterioration takes at least 1 year.[37] Glycerine delays release of the active constituent phenol and thus facilitates the use of gravity to direct the neurolytic solution downward past structures not to be blocked and onto nerve roots delineated for blockade (Fig. 27-5).

Technique. Segmental subarachnoid blocking with phenol requires that the patient lie on the painful side in a semilateral/supine position so that the posterior nerve roots are dependent (Figs. 27-2, 27-3, and 27-5). This may be quite distressing for some patients. In other respects, the technique is similar to that previously described for alcohol. Swerdlow states that phenol acts on the nerve root just before it pierces the dura, and, therefore, the injection should be made at the vertebral level that corresponds to the spinal cord segments involved.[50]

The phenol solution should have been prepared

Table 27-2. Results of Subarachnoid Block With Phenol

Author	Number of Cases	Percentage Results		
		Good	Fair	Poor
Mark and colleagues (1962)	57	26	24	50
	(phenol in iophendylate)			
	30	30	40	30
	(phenol in glycerine)			
Stovner and Endresen (1962)	151	77		23
Tank, Dohn, and Gardner (1963)	23	48	18	34
Wilkinson, Mark, and White (1963)	30	70		30
Ball, Pearce, and Davies (1964)	51	41	33	26
Maher (1972)	433	62	6	32
Brown (1972)	114	68	5	27

(Data from Swerdlow, M. (ed.): Relief of Intractable Pain. Amsterdam, Excerpta Medica, 1974) within the past 6 to 12 months or within an expiration date determined by the pharmacy. It may be warmed to reduce viscosity, but a moderately wide-bore spinal needle is still required for the injection (although the use of a 1-ml tuberculin syringe obviates this). Swerdlow places emphasis on choosing the most favorable interspace in relation to the segments required to be blocked but injects up to 1 ml at this single site with subsequent posturing of the patient to assist with the spread of solution to adjacent segments.[49]

In addition to its neurolytic effect, phenol has an initial local anesthetic action, producing warmth and a tingling, or prickling, sensation over the distribution of the affected nerve. Ichiyanagi and colleagues considered that if this local anesthetic effect does not develop within 2 to 3 minutes, the concentration of phenol is insufficient to produce an effective neurolytic block.[24] They stated that rapid dilution and diffusion of the phenol in the CSF prevents extension of the block even if the patient is repositioned. Like alcohol, the concentration of phenol in the CSF falls below that required for neurolysis within 15 minutes, and the patient need be specially positioned only for that period.[24]

Because phenol is hyperbaric, it has a particular advantage when it is used to produce saddle block anesthesia in patients with midline pain due to pelvic cancer. With the patient in the sitting position, 1 to 2 ml of 6 per cent phenol in glycerine injected at L4–5 or L5–S1 provides excellent pain relief with minimal or transient motor weakness or sphincteric disturbance (Fig. 27-6). Swerdlow, however, prefers unilateral blocks on both sides and reserves the saddle block for the terminal or advanced cases and when unilateral block fails.[50]

Results. The results, as reported in Table 27-2, are slightly inferior to the figures for subarachnoid alcohol block and the effects are of shorter duration.

Subarachnoid Chlorocresol

Maher and Swerdlow have reported the use of intrathecal cholorocresol and claimed that the agent was more effective than phenol, although Swerdlow recorded an increased incidence of complications (in particular, paresis and numbness; Table 27-3).[36,50] The solution used, 1:50 or 1:40 chlorocresol in glycerine, is hyperbaric. The technique was similar to that described for phenol. Chlorocresol does not produce any sensation on injection, and the anesthesiologist must wait for the disappearance of pain or onset of numbness to confirm the correct positioning of the needle. Swerdlow uses the repeated injection of 0.1-ml increments of chlorocresol at a single site and tilts the operating table to produce the desired effect. Five-tenths to 0.7 ml is recommended in the sacral region, 0.5 to 0.8 ml in the lumbar region, and 0.6 to 1.0 ml in the thoracic region.

Table 27-3. Comparison of Neurolytic Effects of Phenol and Chlorocresol

Agent	*Number of Cases*	*Percentage Results*		
		Good	*Fair*	*Poor*
Phenol	46	41	26	33
Chlorocresol	42	48	33	19

(Data from Swerdlow, M.: Intrathecal chlorocresol. A comparison with phenol in the treatment of intractable pain. Anaesthesia, *28*:297, 1973)

Subarachnoid Cold Saline

The intrathecal injection of cold 0.9 per cent saline (2°–4°C), is claimed to have a specific action on the pain-carrying C fibers, sparing the larger fibers that subserve other sensory, motor, and autonomic functions.[31] Cerebrospinal fluid is withdrawn, and the cold saline is then injected rapidly. Ten ml is the recommended dose, although up to 60 ml has been given. The procedure is quite distressing to the patient, and heavy sedation or even general anesthesia is recommended. The incidence of complications with subarachnoid cold saline is low but significant, and the pain relief is usually only short-lived (see Chap. 23).

Subarachnoid Ammonium Salts

In 1943, Bates described the intrathecal use of an extract of the insectivorous pitcher plant, *Sarracenia purpurea,* for the treatment of intractable pain.[3] The active ingredient was ammonium sulphate, which appeared to exert a specific action on the pain-carrying C fibers.

Prolonged pain relief was reported but Hand, Bonica, and Lund were disappointed with the results.[7,21,31] Complications such as nausea and vomiting, headache, paresthesia, and spinal cord damage have been documented.[20,21]

COMPLICATIONS

The complications encountered are usually of two kinds. First, there are those seen with any in-

Table 27-4. Complications That Result from Intrathecal Neurolytic Block

		Percentage Recorded				
Author	*Agent*	*Paresis*	*Rectal and Urinary Dysfunction*	*Sensory Loss*	*Paraesthesia Neuritis*	*Other*
Maher (1955)	Phenol (± silver nitrate)	8	13			Headache, vomiting
Nathan and Scott (1958)	Phenol (± silver nitrate)	14	12			Meningitis
Bonica (1958)	Alcohol	25				
Hay (1962)	Alcohol	1	0.7	1		
Mark and colleagues (1962)	Phenol	8	2.3	2.3	3.4	
McEwen and colleagues (1965)	Alcohol	5	10	10		
Kuzucu and colleagues (1966)	Alcohol	4.6	3.4	3.7	0.3	Tremor, headache
Swerdlow (1973)	Phenol		24	8.7	4	Headache
	Chlorocresol	12	26	21	2.4	Headache

trathecal injection—the self-limiting spinal headache—or the very rare problems of mechanical neural damage, infection, and arachnoiditis.[31]

Second, there are complications that result from the action of neurolytic substances on nerve fibers not concerned in the mediation of pain. These include motor paresis, loss of sphincteric function, impairment of touch and proprioception, and troublesome dysesthesias (see Chap. 23).

Complication rates reported by various authors are shown in Table 27-4 (see also Tables 23-1–23-4). Fortunately, complications are usually transient, although fatal meningitis, paraplegia, and permanent impairment of urinary function have been recorded.[22,28] The reported case of fatal meningitis was believed to have arisen as a result of meningeal irritation from silver nitrate incorporated in the neurolytic solution. The patients with postblock paraplegia were subsequently found to have vertebral metastases.

FAILURE

Finally, the block may fail for reasons that are often difficult to explain anatomically or physiologically. However, it is known that previous radiation therapy, inflammation in the region of the nerve roots, widespread disease, or narcotic addiction will reduce the efficacy of the procedure.[28,50]

TRIGEMINAL NERVE BLOCK

Neurolytic block of the trigeminal nerve and its branches has been used very effectively in the management of chronic pain. Maxillary and mandibular nerve blocks are particularly useful in controlling pain of malignant origin that arises from structures that the nerves supply. In the past, injection of the gasserian ganglion with alcohol was used widely in the treatment of trigeminal neuralgia, but, as indicated earlier, other methods, such as surgical rhizotomy and thermogangliolysis, have largely superseded this technique. Gasserian ganglion blockade is a difficult procedure, and, of the many methods described, Härtel's approach has proved most popular. This technique has been well described and illustrated in Chapter 15 and requires no further description here.[7]

Maxillary Nerve Block

The maxillary nerve supplies the maxilla, the maxillary antrum, the teeth of the upper jaw, the lower part of the nose, the nasopharynx, the roof of the mouth, part of the tonsillar fossa, and the skin over the middle third of the face. Maxillary nerve block is used to treat intractable pain in this area that commonly results from malignant disease and also trigeminal neuralgia, or post-traumatic neuralgia. Because tumors, which initially arise in the structures supplied by the maxillary nerve, may spread locally to areas innervated by other cranial nerves or metastasize to glands in the neck, additional blockade of the appropriate nerves is often necessary.

Technique. Maxillary nerve block can be performed by lateral percutaneous, oral, or transorbital routes (see Chaps. 15 and 16). The lateral percutaneous method described by Macintosh and Ostlere is preferred because it is simple and predictable.[33] The skin landmark lies over the anterior border of the masseter where a vertical line from the lateral orbital margin crosses a horizontal line through the middle of the upper lip. With the patient supine, the needle is passed into the pterygopalatine fossa to a depth of 4 cm by following a line in the direction of the pupil, 30° to the horizontal and immediately posterior to the tuberosity of the maxilla. The injection should be free from any resistance, and there should be no distension of the lower eyelid, which indicates diffusion of the solution into the periorbital tissues through the inferior orbital fissure. Accurate positioning of the needle is essential because it is possible to advance the needle to too great a depth and thereby come into close proximity to the optic nerve. A test dose of 2 ml of 2 per cent lidocaine with epinephrine is desirable to confirm the siting of the needle and to reduce the pain of injection of the neurolytic agent. Larger volumes of local anesthetic should be avoided because they will dilute the alcohol, which would reduce the effectiveness and duration of the neurolytic block and increase the risk of alcohol neuritis.

Because the injection is very painful, heavy sedation or general anesthesia is recommended. Intravenous meperidine, 50 mg (or fentanyl, 50 μg) promethazine, 25 mg; and, when required, diazepam, 5 to 10 mg, will generally produce adequate sedation. Once the patient is satisfactorily prepared, 1 to 2 ml of absolute alcohol is injected. The needle, cleared with 1 ml air, is then repositioned, and the procedure is repeated, yielding a total volume of 2 to 4 ml of alcohol.

In maxillary carcinoma, preliminary tomography of the base of the skull is recommended to exclude direct spread of the disease because once the tumor has invaded the skull, the results of maxillary blockade are likely to be disappointing.

A diagnostic block with 2 ml of local anesthetic should be performed 1 to 2 days prior to the alcohol injection to indicate the probable extent of the proposed neurolytic block. An alternative technique is described in Chapter 15 for both local anesthetic and neurolytic maxillary nerve block.

Results. The patient is reviewed on the following day when the effect of the heavy sedation has worn off. If the pain relief is incomplete, consideration is given to a further block after 2 to 3 weeks.

The results have been similar to those described by McEwen and colleagues (70% of patients with good or fair relief and 30% with little or no relief).[36] Pain alleviation may last from a few weeks to more than a year. Nerve block can be repeated, but as the tumor spreads it becomes increasingly difficult to produce a satisfactory result. Once the base of the skull has become infiltrated, the patient is best managed on potent oral analgesics such as pentazocine, 50 mg; dextromoramide, 10 mg, or methadone, 10 mg, every 4 to 6 hours.

Mandibular Nerve Block

The mandibular nerve carries sensory fibers from the lower jaw, the anterior two-thirds of the tongue, the external auditory meatus, the temporal region and anterior part of the ear, the temporomandibular joint, and the lower part of the face.

Intractable pain due to malignancy and other lesions in this area may be effectively treated by mandibular nerve block.[7,8,14,18,32] The distribution of pain varies. It may be confined to the site of the lesion or may spread widely over the entire area supplied by the mandibular nerve. The pain may be aggravated by the associated trismus, difficulty in swallowing and speaking, facial swelling, foul breath, anorexia, and malnutrition.

Metastatic spread to the cervical glands or postoperative neuromas of the cervical plexus can produce a constant or a triggered pain into and behind the ear, around the angle of the jaw, and into the neck or shoulder. Local or metastatic spread can, therefore, involve branches of the facial, glossopharyngeal, and vagus nerves, and the cervical plexus. Partial failure of a mandibular nerve block may be due to involvement of these other nerves.

Technique. Mandibular nerve block may be performed intraorally or extraorally. Two extraoral methods have been described; a lateral approach in which the needle is passed perpendicular to the skin through the mandibular notch and an anterolateral approach similar to that used to block the gasserian ganglion.[7,32] Radiographic localization has been recommended, but if the lateral extraoral method is used, the landmarks (mandibular notch, lateral pterygoid plate) are sufficient to allow accurate placement without radiography. A diagnostic block with 2 to 5 ml of 2 per cent lidocaine with epinephrine may be used to indicate the probable extent of the proposed neurolytic block.

Table 27-5. Nerve Blocks to Control Pain due to Carcinoma of Tongue and Floor of Mouth

Blocks Performed	*Number of Patients*	*Number of Treatments*
Mandibular nerve block	27	35
Intrathecal cervical plexus block	15	25
Mandibular nerve block and cervical plexus block	5	5
Mandibular glosso-pharyngeal, and vagus nerve block	5	5
Total	52	70

Absolute alcohol is used for the therapeutic block. Again, heavy sedation is necessary because the injection of absolute alcohol is extremely painful. The pain of the injection may also be modified by an injection of 2 ml of 2 per cent lidocaine with epinephrine immediately prior to the alcohol block. One to 2 ml of absolute alcohol is injected initially, the needle is repositioned, and the procedure repeated, using a total of 2 to 4 ml of alcohol (see also Chaps. 15 and 16).

Results. When the patient is reviewed on the following day, if pain relief is incomplete, the area of anesthesia produced is determined, and a decision is made whether to repeat the mandibular block or to extend the area of anesthesia by performing a glossopharyngeal, vagus, or intrathecal cervical plexus block. Table 27-5 records the combination of blocks used by Dwyer in 52 patients with carcinoma of the tongue and floor of the mouth.[18] Eighty per cent of these patients received significant relief from the injection. The pain of the remaining 20 per cent was unrelieved, and potent oral analgesics (pentazocine, 50 mg; dextromoramide, 10 mg; or methadone, 10 mg, every 4 to 6 hours), were required.

As with the maxillary block, pain relief may last from a few weeks to more than a year, and the block may be repeated if necessary. In malignancy, failure may be due to faulty technique but usually indicates spread of the disease to the skull and middle-cranial fossa.

Glossopharyngeal and Vagus Nerve Blocks

Glossopharyngeal and vagus nerve blocks are used in the treatment of intractable pain that arises from the pharynx, larynx, and related structures. They may be used singly when the lesion is discrete and confined to the area supplied by the nerves or, more frequently, in combination with other blocks (*e.g.*, mandibular or maxillary).[7,8,14,18]

The glossopharyngeal nerve supplies the pharyngeal wall, the palatine tonsils, and the posterior one-third of the tongue. The vagus through the internal branch of its superior laryngeal division supplies sensory fibers to the base of the tongue, the epiglottis, the larynx above the vocal cords, and the immediately adjacent pharynx. Both nerves leave the skull through the jugular foramen where they are anatomically related to the internal jugular vein, the internal carotid artery, the accessory nerve, the hypoglossal nerve, and the cervical sympathetic trunk.

The glossopharyngeal and vagus nerves are blocked at the base of the skull, at their exit through the jugular foramen (see Chap. 15). Invariably, the accessory and hypoglossal nerves are affected at the same time, causing weakness of the trapezius muscle and partial paralysis of the tongue. A Horner's syndrome due to sympathetic block also occurs. For these reasons, together with the effects of the laryngeal paralysis and persistent tachycardia that occurs when both vagus nerves are blocked, bilateral injections should not be attempted. McEwen and associates recorded a death due to respiratory obstruction following a vagal block in a patient with postcricoid carcinoma.[32]

Technique. The method used to block the glossopharyngeal and vagus nerves at the base of the skull has been described by Macintosh and Ostlere.[33] The patient lies flat on the operating table facing straight upward, and the needle is inserted just anterior to the tip of the mastoid process. It is directed forward at a right angle to the body axis and at an angle of 50° to the horizontal, to a depth of 4 cm, having passed just in front of and beyond the tip of the transverse process of C1. Two to 3 ml of absolute alcohol is then injected after careful aspiration to eliminate the greater than usual risk of an intravascular injection (see also Chap. 15).

In order to block the glossopharyngeal nerve and spare the vagus, Bonica recommends inserting the needle perpendicular to the skin, midway between the tip of the mastoid and the angle of the jaw, and injecting just anterior and medial to the styloid process.[7] Montgomery and Cousins report that accurate placement at the jugular foramen is aided by radiographic control.[42] Bonica further suggests as an alternative to a complete vagal block with its attendant risks that the internal laryngeal branch of the superior laryngeal nerve may be injected separately.[7] This is of particular advantage when the lesion extends across the midline, and the pain is bilateral. The nerve is approached as it enters the thyrohyoid membrane just anterior to the superior cornu of the thyroid cartilage deep to the posterior border of the thyrohyoid (see Chap. 15). The block can be performed by a midline or a lateral approach. Accurate placement of 2 to 3 ml of absolute alcohol is necessary to produce an effective block. The patient is instructed not to speak, swallow, or cough during the procedure.

Careful premedication and follow-up, as previously described, are essential.

Results. Glossopharyngeal and vagal nerve blocks are used infrequently, and it is difficult to assess their success. However, the results appear comparable to those achieved with other neurolytic blocks.

SYMPATHETIC BLOCKS

CELIAC PLEXUS AND LUMBAR SYMPATHETIC BLOCK

Celiac plexus block has been employed in the management of a large number of disorders, but its use is now primarily restricted to the treatment of pain due to malignancy of the upper abdominal viscera and chronic pancreatitis (for further information on sympathetic blocks, see Chap. 13).[4–6,8,11–13,15,19,20,29,45–47] In combination with lumbar sympathetic block, the procedure is used to treat ischemic or painful disorders of the abdomen and lower limb due to peripheral vascular disease, phantom limb pain, and causalgia (see also Chap. 13).[40] The following is a list of uses of celiac plexus block.

In malignancy and peripheral vascular disease, alcohol has been used because the effect is profound and long-lasting. Neurolytic block is preferable to surgical splanchnicectomy because the patients are frequently old, frail, and suffer from a terminal illness. Satisfactory surgical results have, however, been reported in patients with chronic pancreatitis.[52] When the origin of the pain is obscure—as in causalgia, phantom limb pain, and the dysesthesias—a local anesthetic is employed to block the sensory afferent pathway. This may achieve a permanent break in the cycle of nervous activity, which is thought to be responsible for the appreciation of pain.

Technique

Celiac plexus and lumbar sympathetic block has been performed by a posterior approach and anterior approach and under direct vision following a laparotomy (see also Chap. 14).[10,27,51] The anterior approach proved dangerous and inaccurate, and the results following laparotomy were not superior to those of the posterior approach, which has survived as the most practical.

Several methods of performing these blocks have been described. The patient may be placed in the prone, sitting, or lateral positions.[5,11,13,15,19,27,34,45–47] Some authors strongly advocate radiographic location of the needle tip to ensure injection.[13,19,25,26] Gorbitz and Leavens recommend the radiographic placement of a teflon cannula, which is used initially for a diagnostic block and subsequently for the destructive block.[19] Other authors consider that these methods are unnecessarily time-consuming and technically complex and fail to guarantee accurate placement of the needle.[5,11]

Historical Indications for Celiac Plexus Block

Abdominal malignancy	Gastrointestinal dysfunction	Postcholecystectomy syndrome
Achalasia	Herpes zoster	Postoperative visceral pain
Acrocyanosis	Hiccough (persistent)	Post-traumatic edema
Acute arterial occlusion	Hirschsprung's disease	Postphlebitic sequelae
"Angina abdominis"	Hyperhidrosis	Pylorospasm
Aortic pain	Hypertension	Raynaud's disease
Arthritis	Immersion foot	Raynaud's phenomenon
Cardiospasm	Ischemic ulceration	Shock
Causalgia	Mesenteric artery occlusion	Sympathalgia
Charcot's joint	Pancreatitis	Tabetic crisis
Cold injury	Paralytic ileus	Thromboangiitis obliterans
Cystalgia	Peptic ulceration	Thrombophlebitis
Delayed union of fractures	Peripheral vascular disease	Traumatic vasospasm
Dysmenorrhea	Phantom limb	Trench foot
Fibrocystic disease	Phlegmasia alba dolens	Ureteric colic
Frostbite	Poliomyelitis deformities	Urinary retention

Because the celiac plexus is a diffuse bilateral structure that spans the posterior abdominal wall at T12–L1, the best results are obtained when a bilateral block is performed with a large volume of local anesthetic or neurolytic agent.

During the preoperative visit, the patient is assessed and the procedure explained. Bridenbaugh, Moore, and Campbell recommend the suspension of ganglion blocking agents that are likely to enhance the hypotensive effect of the block and anticoagulants that may produce excessive bleeding.[11] Some authors do not premedicate the patient nor give narcotic analgesics for some hours preoperatively in order that the immediate effect of the block on the pain can be better judged. While premedication may be unnecessary for a diagnostic block, sedation, as previously described for maxillary nerve block, will not interfere with the performance of a destructive block and should contribute significantly to the patient's comfort.

Although many methods have been described, the following technique and that described in Chap. 14 are recommended. The patient is placed in the lateral position with the side to be injected uppermost. This is reasonably comfortable and more convenient than the sitting position, particularly because hypotension may occur. The spine is flexed and the needle is inserted below the 12th rib, four finger-breadths (7–8 cm) from the midline. This site of entry is at T12 or L1. The needle is passed forward and angled slightly toward the midline to make an angle of 30° with the sagittal plane and about 60° with the skin surface. As the needle is advanced, it will encounter either the transverse process of L1 or L2 superficially or the body of L1 more deeply. A deliberate effort is made to locate the transverse process, identified by the smooth, hard surface, prior to redirecting the needle to the deeper vertebral body with its soft, pitting surface. This assures the anesthesiologist that he is at the correct depth. Once the vertebral body has been located, the needle is withdrawn and reinserted at an increasing angle to the skin surface until the tip of the needle slips off the side of the vertebral body into the retroperitoneal space (Fig. 27-7). During this manipulation, local anesthetic (0.5% lidocaine with epinephrine) is continually infiltrated along the needle track. At the point where the needle just slips off the vertebral body, the depth of insertion is marked, and the needle is then advanced 1 to 2 cm into the retroperitoneal space. The distance from the skin to the tip of the needle will vary considerably, but it may be considered to be 7 to 10 cm in the average patient. When the needle is correctly positioned in the loose areolar tissue around the celiac plexus, there should be a negative aspiration test, and the injection of the solution should meet with minimal resistance. In this way, inadvertent penetration of major vessels, viscera, or muscle is immediately detected.

With the technique described here, the block is invariably performed bilaterally, and repositioning of the patient is necessary after the initial injection. Many favor the alternative use of the prone position so that both sides can be blocked at the same time (see Chap. 14). For diagnostic blocks, 20 ml of 1 per cent lidocaine with 1:200,000 epinephrine is used on each side. For destructive blocks, 10 to 20 ml of absolute alcohol is used on each side, preceded by about 5 ml of 2 per cent lidocaine with epinephrine, which reduces the unpleasant sensation of a "kick in the stomach," that the patient commonly experiences with a successful block. By repositioning the needle twice on each side, the spreading of alcohol can be improved to produce a more extensive block. Some pain relief is usually apparent immediately after the block, but relief may take some days to be complete.

Spread of the alcohol over the upper roots of the lumbar plexus may result in numbness and paresthesias over the lower abdominal wall and upper thigh and is a source of temporary discomfort. Injection of a small volume of air or saline through the needle at the termination of the block may assist in preventing contamination of the lumbar plexus with alcohol as the needle is withdrawn through the psoas major.

Lumbar Sympathetic Block

In cases of peripheral vascular disease, causalgia, and phantom limb pain in the lower limb, a lumbar sympathetic block may be indicated (see Chap. 13). With the same basic technique as for a celiac block, 5 ml of absolute alcohol is deposited at the L2 level and a further 5 ml at the L3 level.* A successful sympathetic denervation is indicated by change in color and temperature and venous filling occurring within 30 minutes.[5] This is accompanied by a gradual improvement in pain over 24 hours with full benefit of the block not necessarily apparent for some days.

The patient should be nursed in the supine position with a 10° head-down tilt for the first hour following the injection. Hypotension may occur and is best treated by intravenous fluid therapy. The pa-

* Alternatively, if a solution of 10 per cent phenol in Conray-420 dye is injected under image-intensifier control, as little as 1 ml of solution at each level may be seen to provide coverage of the sympathetic chain (see also Chap. 13).

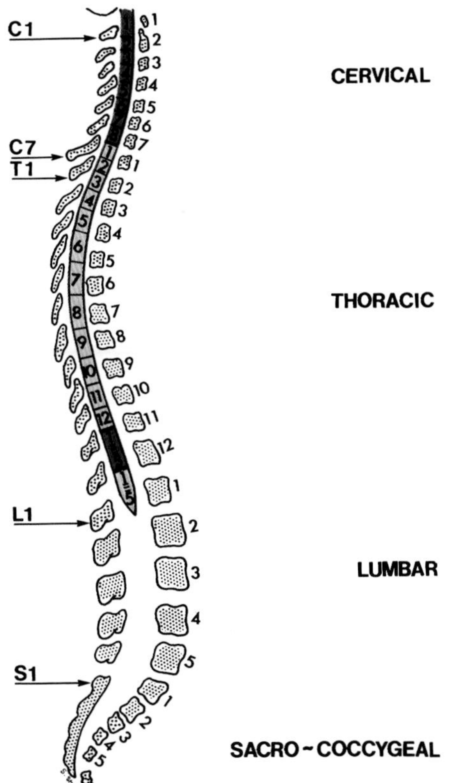

Fig. 27-1. This drawing of the vertebral column and spinal cord indicates their segmental relationships. Significant difference between the vertebral and cord levels occurs only in the lower thoracic and lumbosacral regions.

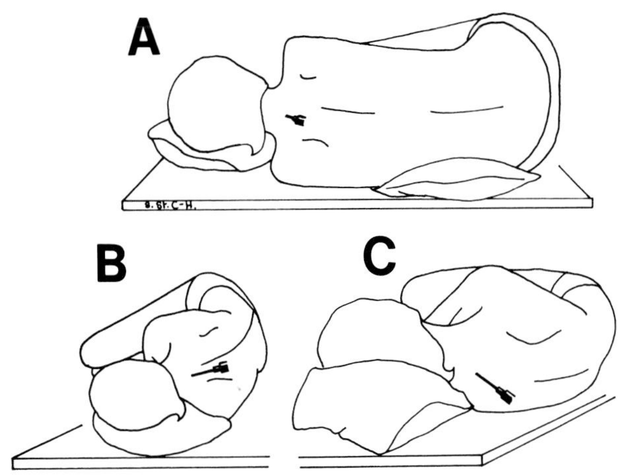

Fig. 27-3. Positioning for the patient for subarachnoid injection in the thoracolumbar region. (*A*) Posterior view. (*B*) Lateral-prone position used for the injection of absolute alcohol. (*C*) Lateral-supine position used for the injection of hyperbaric solutions.

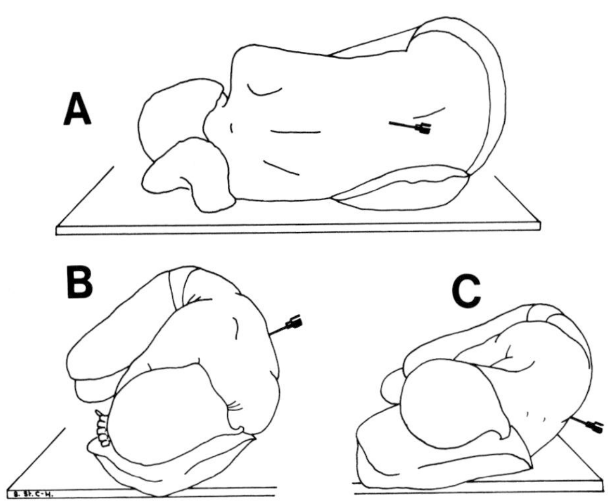

Fig. 27-2. Positioning of the patient for a cervical subarachnoid injection. (*A*) Posterior view. (*B*) Lateral-prone position used for the injection of absolute alcohol. (*C*) Lateral-supine position used for the injection of hyperbaric solutions.

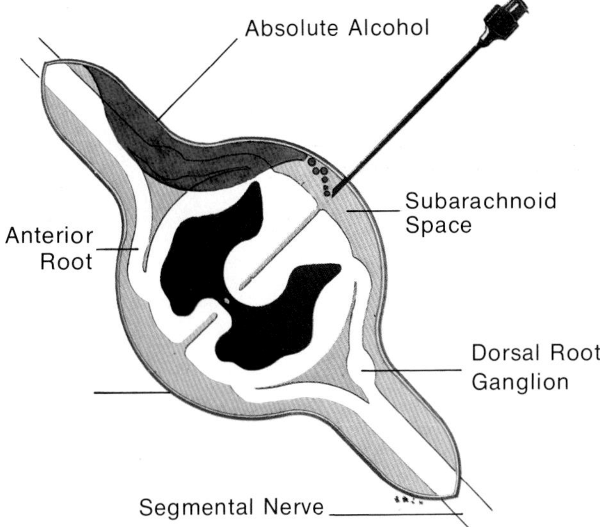

Fig. 27-4. The lateral-prone position used for the injection of absolute alcohol places the posterior nerve roots uppermost.

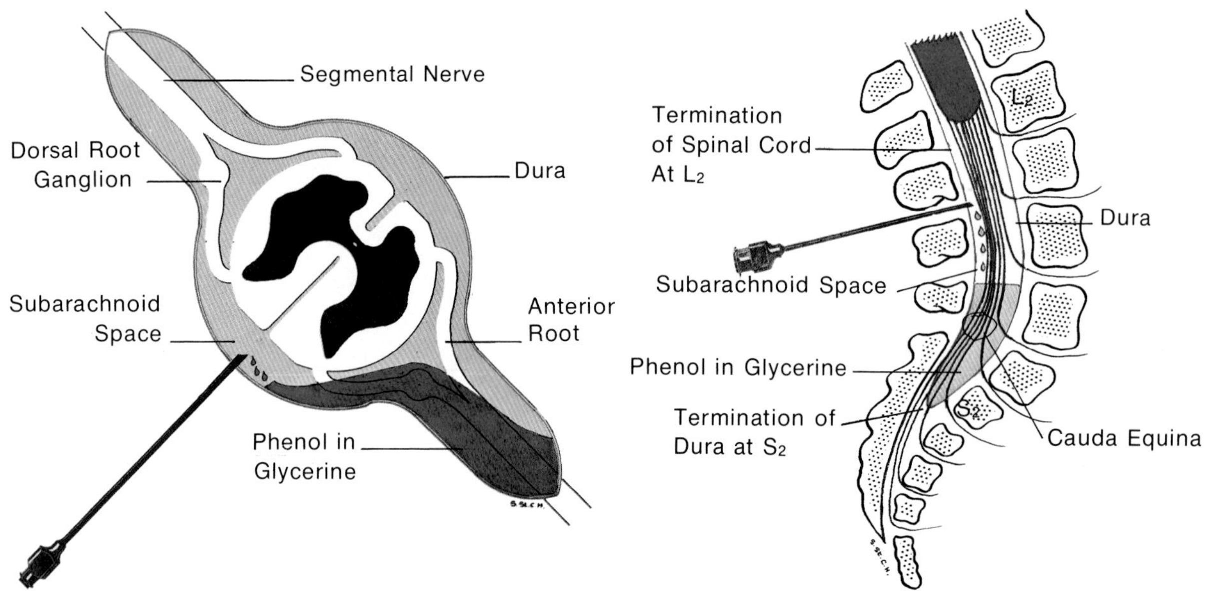

Fig. 27-5. The lateral-supine position used for the injection of phenol and other hyperbaric solutions ensures that the posterior nerve roots are dependent.

Fig. 27-6. Saddle block with phenol and other hyperbaric solutions is used in the treatment of midline perineal pain of malignant origin.

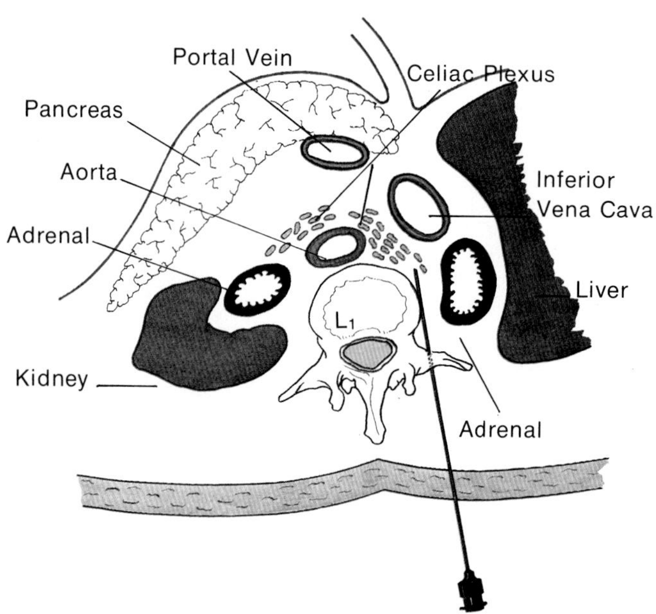

Fig. 27-7. Cross section of the body at the level of L1 indicates the placement of the needle in celiac plexus block.

Table 27-6. Results of Celiac Plexus and Lumbar Sympathetic Block With Alcohol

Author	Indication	Number of Cases	Percentage Results		
			Good	Fair	Poor
Bridenbaugh and colleagues (1964)	Upper abdominal cancer	41	73	24.5	2.5
Gorbitz and Leavens* (1971)	Upper abdominal cancer	11 (9)	56	17.5	26.5
Black and Dwyer (1973)	Carcinoma of pancreas	20	70	30	0
	Other abdominal malignancy	37	70	17	13
	Chronic pancreatitis	21	62	5	33
	Peripheral vascular disease	21	38	29	33
	Other	14	15	28	57

* Represents results for nine of 11 patients

tient should remain hospitalized at least 24 hours to allow stabilization of blood pressure, observation of the effect of the block, and recognition of any complications.

Results. Satisfactory relief of pain is obtained with upper abdominal malignancy, especially carcinoma of the pancreas, provided the posterior abdominal wall has not been extensively invaded (Table 27-6). The relief usually lasts for a period of 1 month to 1 year and frequently persists until the time of death.[5,11]

In chronic pancreatitis, 60 to 70 per cent of the patients are relieved for variable periods that are usually in excess of 1 month. In these patients the block may be repeated at appropriate intervals over a number of years. In peripheral vascular disease, there is a similar incidence of symptomatic relief. However, in causalgia, phantom limb pain, and musculoskeletal conditions, the results are disappointing.

COMPLICATIONS

Back pain around the injection site and postural hypotension in elderly patients are the most commonly recorded complications.[5,11,19] Both usually resolve within 48 hours. Involvement of the lumbar somatic nerves is not uncommon, and hyperalgesia from this cause may persist for 1 to 2 months.

Table 27-7 indicates the incidence of persistent complications recorded by Black and Dwyer in 104 patients treated over a 10-year period.[5]

Table 27-7. Complications That Occurred in 104 Celiac Plexus Blocks

Complication	Incidence (%)
Weakness or numbness T10–L2 distribution	8
Lower chest pain	3
Failure of ejaculation	2
Postural hypotension	2
Warmth and fullness of leg	1
Urinary difficulty	1

(Data from Black, A., and Dwyer, B.: Coeliac plexus block. Anaesth. Intensive Care, *1*:315, 1973)

NEUROLYTIC SOMATIC NERVE BLOCKADE

Although considerable benefit can be obtained in various pain states with local anesthetic somatic nerve blockade, neurolytic blockade has not enjoyed great popularity. The primary reasons for this are that it is generally held that the incidence of neuritis is high and that the often accompanying motor blockade poses the risk of a useless limb. The former problem may be partially related to technical difficulties since somatic neurolytic block must be performed with a smaller dose than the equivalent local anesthetic block, and, thus, needle placement must be very precise. It is possible that some cases of neuritis are due to imprecise needle placement and incomplete neurolysis. If larger volumes of neurolytic solution are used, necrosis of surrounding tissues may occur.

Despite the dictum by some authors that, apart from cranial nerve block, somatic nerve block should never be performed with a neurolytic agent, there may be occasions when the appropriate agent and sufficient technical skill, sometimes aided by a peripheral nerve stimulator, can greatly benefit the patient. Examples are intercostal block, infraorbital block, and obturator nerve block.*

* Bridenbaugh, P.O.: Unpublished data

Intercostal Block

In intercostal nerve block, a maximum of 1 ml of neurolytic solution should be employed for each intercostal nerve (see Chap. 14). Because of dermatomal overlap, it is also necessary to block the adjacent segments. In view of the high incidence of neuralgia with absolute alcohol, 6 to 7 per cent aqueous phenol or 10 per cent ammonium sulphate has been used. Cryoanalgesia shows great promise although its duration of effect is often as little as 10 days.[2,30] At most clinics the subarachnoid approach is preferred because of its greater predictability and avoidance of the problem of neuritis, although of course it may pose more serious complications.

Infraorbital Nerve Block

A maximum dose of neurolytic agent of 1 ml is employed in infraorbital nerve block and care must be taken to avoid direct periosteal injection (see Chap. 15 for technical details).

Some patients with trigeminal neuralgia have pain localized to infraorbital distribution and obtain complete relief with infraorbital block rather than the more extensive maxillary block. The advent of carefully controlled thermogangliolysis has probably substantially reduced the indications for infraorbital block. However, more recent cryoanalgesia has been used with considerable success.[2]

Obturator Block

Pain due to osteoarthritis of the hip may be relieved by obturator block and blockade of the nerve to quadratus femorus (for technique, see Chap. 11). The use of 0.25 per cent bupivacaine often yields weeks of pain relief so that the indications for the use of neurolytic solutions are minimal. It is essential to employ radiographic control (and often a peripheral nerve stimulator) if a neurolytic agent is to be used since needle placement is difficult.

On occasion the neurolytic technique can be used to assist nursing patients with paraplegia and adductor spasm although percutaneous adductor tenotomy is very simple and effective.

Cervical Plexus

Individual cervical nerve blockade is performed by a technique that is identical to the description of interscalene blockade except that the cervical nerve is injected separately (see Chap. 10). In general, chronic pain that involves the cervical and brachial plexus is best treated by the cervical subarachnoid technique described above. Some patients for whom the use of the subarachnoid approach presents problems may benefit from blockade of one or more cervical nerves. Initial block with 1 to 2 ml 0.25 per cent bupivacaine should be tried since it will often yield several weeks of pain relief. More rare, 1 ml of 6 to 10 per cent phenol in water or 10 per cent phenol in Conray-420 dye (with radiographic control) may be required at each level.

Other Peripheral Neurolytic Techniques

Coccidynia. Neurolytic solutions have been used in the treatment of coccidynia. Either 10 per cent phenol or 10 per cent ammonium sulphate is injected onto the last sacral and coccygeal nerve. Superficial slough is a hazard, and at many clinics more conservative measures are preferred since these patients usually have a long life expectancy and are otherwise healthy.

Nerve Entrapment. In general, diagnostic local anesthetic blocks are used for nerve entrapment, and, if successful, the patient may be best managed by surgical lysis or sometimes by local anesthetic blocks with steroid included in the solution (see Chap. 20). The same applies to the syndrome in which a thoracic cutaneous nerve is trapped in the posterior wall of the rectus sheath. However, on occasion, if surgery is not feasible, injection of 5 to 7 per cent aqueous phenol into the lateral part of the rectus compartment may be considered.

Neurolytic Stellate Ganglion Block

Neurolytic stellate ganglion block is extremely difficult and potentially hazardous. At many clinics it is believed that the complications of dural puncture, and extensive paresis and other serious sequelae, are too severe to warrant exposing a patient to potentially more disability than prior to the block. However, there may be a small number of instances, such as severe upper limb or mediastinal pain, in which this technique can be used with benefit.[50] The neurolytic block should always be performed at the C7 level to minimize the risk of permanent Horner's syndrome, and a diagnostic local anesthetic block should always be performed initially. A small volume (1–3 ml) of 0.25 per cent bupivacaine is appropriate. If the patient has satisfactory pain relief and no side-effects with this dose, then neurolytic block with 10 per cent phenol in Conray-420 may be performed under radiographic control. A dose of 1 ml of solution should not be exceeded. Neff performed over 12 neurolytic stellate blocks, using the above technique, for severe pain following frostbite; when the dose was kept to 1 ml, no serious side-effects ensued.* Today the safety of this procedure may be increased by employing a dye-containing neurolytic agent and injecting under radiograph. It should be noted that some patients obtain satisfactory results with a single or a series of local anesthetic stellate blocks.

Alcohol Injection of the Pituitary

A new technique, *pituitary neuroadenolysis*, has been reported to be useful for pain relief in disseminated cancer. Moricca has now treated over 1,000 patients by injecting 0.6 to 1.0 ml of absolute alcohol into the pituitary fossa with a needle inserted by way of the nostril.[43] Control with an image-intensifier is essential. The mechanism of pain relief is not certain since even tumors thought not to be hormone-dependent appear to respond. It is possible that alcohol spreads retrograde to the hypothalamus and thereby interferes with central pain transmission (see Chap. 24).

REFERENCES

1. Ball, H.C., Pearce, D.J., and Davies, J.A.: Experience with therapeutic nerve blocks. Anaesthesia, *19*:250, 1964.
2. Barnard, J.D.W., Lloyd, J.W., and Glynn, C.J.: Cryosurgery: In the management of intractable facial pain. Br. J. Oral Surg., Vol. 16, no. 2, 135–142, 1978.
3. Bates, W.: Control of somatic pain. Am. J. Surg., *59*:83, 1943.
4. Bentley, F.H.: Observations of visceral pain: Visceral tenderness. Ann. Surg., *128*:881, 1948.
5. Black, A., and Dwyer, B.: Coeliac plexus block. Anaesth. Intensive Care, *1*:315, 1973.
6. Bleasel, K.: The pain clinic at St. Vincent's Hospital, Sydney. Mod. Med. Aust., *17*:5, 1974.
7. Bonica, J.J.: The Management of Pain. Philadelphia, Lea & Febiger, 1953.
8. ______: Diagnostic and therapeutic blocks. A reappraisal based on 15 years experience. Anesth. Analg. (Cleve.), *37*:58, 1958.
9. Bonica, J.J., and Black, R.G.: Organisation and function of a pain clinic. *In* Swerdlow, M. (ed.): Relief of Intractable Pain. Amsterdam, Excerpta Medica, 1974.
10. Braun, H.: Ein Hilfsinstrument zur Ausfuehrung der Splanchnicusänasthesie. Zentralbl. Chir., *48*:1544, 1921.
11. Bridenbaugh, L.D., Moore, D.C., and Campbell, D.D.: Management of upper abdominal cancer pain. Treatment with celiac plexus block with alcohol. J.A.M.A., *190*:877, 1964.
12. Challenger, J.H.: Sympathetic nervous system blocking and pain relief. *In* Swerdlow, M. (ed.): Relief of Intractable Pain. Amsterdam, Excerpta Medica, 1974.
13. Dale, W.A.: Splanchnic block in the treatment of acute pancreatitis. Surgery, *32*:605, 1952.
14. Dam, W., and Larsen, J.J.V.: Peripheral nerve blocks in relief of intractable pain. *In* Swerdlow, M. (ed.): Relief of Intractable Pain. Amsterdam, Excerpta Medica, 1974.
15. De Takats, G.: Splanchnic anaesthesia: Critical review of theory and practice of this method. Surg. Gynecol. Obstet., *44*:501, 1927.
16. Dogliotti, A.M.: Traitement des syndromes douloureux de la peripherie par l'alcoolisation sub-arachnoidienne des racines postérieurs à leur émergencede la moelle épinière. Presse Med., *39*:1249, 1931.
17. Dwyer, B.: Le traitement de la douleur en australie. Cah. d'Anesthesiologie, *17*:633, 1969.
18. ______: Treatment of pain of carcinoma of the tongue and floor of the mouth. Anaesth. Intensive Care, *1*:59, 1972.
19. Gorbitz, C., and Leavens, M.E.: Alcohol block of the celiac plexus for control of the upper abdominal pain caused by cancer and pancreatitis. J. Neurosurg., *34*:575, 1971.
20. Guttman, S.A., and Pardee, I.: Spinal cord level syndrome following intrathecal ammonium sulphate and procaine hydrochloride. A case report with autopsy findings. Anesthesiology, *5*:347, 1944.
21. Hand, L.V.: Subarachnoid ammonium sulphate therapy for intractable pain. Anesthesiology, *5*:354, 1944.
22. Hay, R.C.: Subarachnoid alcohol block in the control of intractable pain: Report of results in 252 patients. Anesth. Analg. (Cleve.), *41*:12, 1962.
23. Hay, R.C., Yonezawa, T., and Derrick, W.S.: Control of intractable pain in advanced cancer by subarachnoid alcohol block. J.A.M.A., *169*:1315, 1959.
24. Ichiyanagi, K., Matsuki, M., Kinefuchi, S., and Kato, Y.: Progressive changes in the concentration of phenol and glycerine in the human subarachnoid space. Anesthesiology, *42*:622, 1975.
25. Jackson, S.H., Jacobs, J.B., and Epstein, R.A.: A radiographic approach to celiac plexus block. Anesthesiology, *31*:373, 1969.
26. Jacobs, J., Jackson, S., and Doppman, J.: A radiographic approach to celiac ganglion block. Radiology, *92*:1372, 1969.
27. Kappis, M.: Erfahrungen mit Localanästhesie bei Bauchoperationen. Verh. Dtsch. Ges. Chir., *43*:1. teil 87, 1914.
28. Kuzucu, E.Y., Derrick, W.S., and Wilber, S.A.: Control of intractable pain with subarachnoid alcohol block. J.A.M.A., *195*:541, 1966.
29. Lassner, J.: l'Analbesie prolongee par l'alcoolisation du ganglion coeliaque. Traitement palliatif des tumeurs abdominales hautes inoperables. Anesth. Anal. (Paris), *25*:335, 1968.
30. Lloyd, J.W., Barnard, J.D.W., and Glynn, C.J.: Cryoanalgesia: A new approach to pain relief. Lancet, *2*:932, 1976.
31. Lund, P.C.: Principles and Practice of Spinal Anesthesia. Springfield, Charles C Thomas, 1971.
32. McEwen, B.W., *et al.*: The pain clinic: A clinic for the management of intractable pain. Med. J. Aust., *1*:676, 1965.
33. Macintosh, R., and Ostlere, M.: Local Analgesia: Head and Neck, ed. 2. Edinburgh, E. & S. Livingstone, 1967.
34. Macintosh, R.R., and Bryce Smith, R.: Local Analgesia: Abdominal Surgery. Edinburgh, E. & S. Livingstone, 1953.
35. Maher, R.M.: Relief of pain in incurable cancer. Lancet, *1*:18, 1955.
36. ______: Intrathecal chloroscresol in the treatment of pain in cancer. Lancet, *1*:965, 1963.
37. Maher, R.M., and Mehta, M.: Spinal (intrathecal) and extradural analgesia. *In* Lipton, S. (ed.): Persistent Pain: Modern Methods of Treatment. New York, Grune & Stratton, 1977.
38. Mark, V.H., White, J.C., Zervas, N.T., Ervin, F.R., and Richardson, E.P.: Intrathecal use of phenol for the relief of chronic severe pain. N. Engl. J. Med., *267*:589, 1962.

* Neff, W: Personal communication

39. Matsuki, M., Kato, Y., and Ichiyanagi, K.: Progressive changes in the concentration of ethyl alcohol in the human and canine subarachnoid spaces. Anesthesiology, *36*:617, 1972.
40. Melzack, R.: Phantom limb pain: Implications for treatment of pathologic pain. Anesthesiology, *35*:409, 1971.
41. Merskey, H.: Psychological aspects of pain relief: Hypnotherapy; psychotropic drugs. *In* Swerdlow, M. (ed.): Relief of Intractable Pain. Amsterdam, Excerpta Medica, 1974.
42. Montgomery, W., and Cousins, M.J.: Aspects of the management of chronic pain illustrated by ninth nerve block. Br. J. Anaesth., *44*:383, 1972.
43. Moricca, G.: Pituitary neuroadenolysis in the treatment of intractable pain from cancer. Lipton, S. (ed.): Persistent Pain: Modern Methods of Treatment. New York, Grune & Stratton, 1977.
44. Nathan, P.W., and Scott, T.G.: Intrathecal phenol for intractable pain: Safety and dangers of the method. Lancet, *1*:76, 1958.
45. Ochsner, A.: Indications for sympathetic nervous system block. Anesth. Analg. (Cleve.): *30*:61, 1951.
46. Pereira, A., and A. de Sousa: Blocking of the splanchnic nerves and the first lumbar sympathetic ganglion: technic, accidents and clinical indications. Arch. Surg., *53*:37, 1946.
47. Quimby, C.W.: Intercostal-celiac block for abdominal surgery in the poor risk patient. J. Arkansas Med. Soc., *68*:266, 1972.
48. Sweet, W.H., and Wepsic, J.G.: Controlled thermocoagulation of the trigeminal ganglion and rootlets for differential destruction of pain fibres. Part 1. Trigeminal neuralgia. J. Neurosurg., *39*:143, 1974.
49. Swerdlow, M.: Intrathecal chlorocresol. A comparison with phenol in the treatment of intractable pain. Anaesthesia, *28*:297, 1973.
50. Swerdlow, M. (ed.): Relief of Intractable Pain. Amsterdam, Excerpta Medica, 1974.
51. Wendling, H.: Ausschaltung der Nervi Splanchnici durch Leitungsanästhesie bei Magenoperationen und andern Eingriffen in der oberen bauchhöhle ein Beitrag zur Kenntnis der Sensibilität der Bauchhöhle. Beitr. Z. Klin. Chir., *110*:517, 1918.
52. White, T.T., *et al.*: Treatment of pancreatitis by left splanchnicectomy and celiac ganglionectomy. Am. J. Surg., *112*:195, 1966.

28 Chronic Pain: Alternatives to Neural Blockade

David E. Bresler and Ronald L. Katz

THE NATURE OF CHRONIC PAIN

Chronic pain has become the nation's most expensive, debilitating, yet common disorder. It has been estimated that 8 to 10 per cent of the population of most Western countries suffer from some form of migraine, and there are at least 50 million Americans with arthritis, 20 million of whom require medical care.[5,185] Each year, arthritis claims 600,000 new victims, and its cost to the national economy is estimated to nearly $13 billion.[5]

According to the National Center for Health Statistics, low back pain has disabled 7 million Americans and generates nearly 19 million visits to physicians annually. Add to these the victims of chronic facial and dental pain, neuralgia and neuritis, cancer, and other problems, and it becomes evident why chronic pain is estimated to cost the nation's economy nearly $50 billion annually. Its cost in terms of human suffering is incalculable.

Few would argue that we live in a time of medical miracles. With the development of immunizations, antibiotics, and improved health conditions, we have witnessed the virtual elimination of infectious diseases that once decimated entire civilizations. Infant mortality has dropped significantly, and, almost daily, we read of astounding medical advances that would have been unthinkable only a few years ago.

Yet in an age in which the energy of the atom has been harnessed and man has walked on the moon, there is still no single form of therapy that is completely safe and effective for treatment of pain. Many of the more successful therapies were in fact discovered by ancient civilizations, not modern man, and they remain fundamentally unchanged over thousands of years. For example, opium was used extensively by the early Egyptians, and the Incas chewed on the leaves of the coca plant. Over 5,000 years ago, the Chinese employed acupuncture, herbs, and physical therapy (heat, cold, and massage) for management of pain. Transcutaneous electrical stimulation was first utilized by a Greek surgeon who applied a torpedo fish as a source of electricity.

Acute vs. Chronic Pain

By refining and expanding the insights of ancient civilizations, we have created an almost endless variety of pharmaceutical products, many of which are available over the counter. In the management of acute or self-limiting pain, these agents are usually highly effective, for they provide temporary relief while the body heals itself. With the development of neural blockade and other modern anesthetic techniques, patients who undergo operative procedures are generally spared even the slightest degree of surgical discomfort.

Yet the sophisticated approaches that have proven so successful in the management of acute pain are often unsatisfactory for treatment of chronic or long-term pain. Whereas acute pain improves by itself as the body heals, chronic pain often becomes worse with time. Patients with chronic pain are referred endlessly from physician to physician, for even if temporary relief is obtained, the pain frequently returns with time.

Most pain therapists now recognize the importance of a multidisciplinary approach to the problem of chronic pain. Although new drugs and surgical techniques continue to be introduced, pain researchers have begun to take a second look at alternative procedures that appear to mobilize the body's intrinsic pain-relieving abilities. Many of these new approaches focus on the unique psychophysiologic nature of the chronic pain experience, and they include techniques such as acupuncture, hypnosis, biofeedback, and guided imagery. This chapter provides a brief overview of the many alternatives available for control and management of chronic pain.

The Pain Experience

A painful *sensation* (mental awareness of a noxious stimulus) can be distinguished from the pain *experience* (the total subjective experience of suffering due to pain). Beecher made a similar distinction between the primary and secondary components of pain.[15] The primary component includes the sensation, perception, discrimination, and recognition of the noxious stimulus, whereas the secondary component involves the suffering and reactive aspects, including anxiety and other emotional responses to pain.

It is important to recognize that there is not necessarily any direct relationship between the sensation and experience of pain. For example, Beecher found that soldiers seriously wounded in battle reported only mild discomfort for they were elated to learn that they were to be sent home for the duration of the war.[15] In contrast, phantom limb pain often produces agonizing discomfort even when the entire stump is anesthetized.[161]

Pain is well known to be influenced by learning and early developmental predispositions. For example, animals raised in a pain-free environment show insensitivity to noxious stimuli in later life.[162,179] Social, cultural, and ethnic differences in the experience of pain are also well documented.[74,221,248] A vivid example is the initiation rituals of many primitive tribes, which would be considered nothing short of torture if practiced by members of Western cultures.

Aristotle was the first to suggest that "pain is an emotion," as pervasive as anger, terror, or joy. For the early philosophers, the answer to the question "what is pain?" was that "it is the opposite of pleasure." The emotional component of pain is inexorably bound to other aspects of the pain experience, for anxiety and agitation are the natural consequence of a painful sensation that tells higher cognitive centers that "something is wrong." If the "something" can be clearly identified and appropriate corrective action taken, the (acute) pain experience is terminated.

However, for most patients with chronic pain, the "something" is vague, and fear of continued pain in an unknown future produces even greater anxiety. On a physiologic level, sympathetic hyperactivity develops, as manifested by increased cardiac rate, blood pressure, respiration and palmar sweating, and muscle tension.[223] In patients with musculoskeletal pain, this increased muscle tension can often augment the sensation of pain, which further increases anxiety, which, in turn, produces even greater muscular tension. The relationship between pain and anxiety is well known to clinicians, for treatment of one frequently provides relief for the other as well.[74,221,223,248]

With time, exhaustion of sympathetic hyperactivity is inevitable, and more vegetative signs and symptoms soon emerge. These are characterized by feelings of helplessness, hopelessness, and despair with subjective reports of sleep and appetite disturbances, irritability, decreased interests and libido, and erosion of personal relationships with family and friends, as well as increased somatization of complaints.[223] Thus, acute pain and anxiety become chronic pain and depression. It is well known that the most notable emotional change in patients with chronic somatic and visceral pain is the development of reactive depression.[103,166,223] This may be overt or masked to both patient and health-care practitioner alike. As with acute pain and anxiety, chronic pain is often relieved by treating the associated depression.[166]

It is important to emphasize the psychophysiology of chronic pain. Pain is a complex subjective experience that involves physical, perceptual, cognitive, and emotional factors. When a patient with discogenic disease reports "my back hurts," his or her pain experience could also involve anxiety or depression (producing insomnia, loss of appetite, and decreased sexual desire); drug dependence or addiction; numerous secondary gains; separation from work, family, and friends; masochistic behavior; and a host of other problems. These may remain indelibly associated with the experience of back pain, even after the entire back has been anesthetized.

Clearly, a modern approach to control of chronic pain must involve both physical and psychological orientations to the problem. From this perspective, it seems nonsensical to wonder if the patient with chronic pain has "real" *versus* "unreal" (imaginary) pain, "physiologic" *versus* "psychological" pain, or "legitimate" *versus* "illegitimate pain."

Evaluation of the Patient With Chronic Pain

The most important aspect of evaluating a patient with chronic pain is to establish close rapport. Because pain is a totally subjective experience with few reliable objective indices of discomfort, a proper evaluation of its etiology, present status, and response to therapy must depend upon the patient's ability and willingness to relate honestly to the pain therapist. At the U.C.L.A. Pain Control Unit, each patient is assigned a "patient manager" who reviews all medical records, conducts a comprehensive workup, and develops a treatment program. Although a patient may be referred to other specialists for therapy (*e.g.*, nerve blocks, acupuncture, biofeedback training, etc.). it is the patient manager who also conducts periodic re-evaluations of the patient's progress.

As previously discussed, a careful evaluation of the patient with chronic pain must include not only the physical components of the problem but also the emotional, motivational, and cognitive components as well. The most common error made by clinicians is to evaluate and treat only the physical aspect of pain, for they assume that the objective of therapy is to treat the pain. In reality, however, the objective of therapy is to treat the patient-in-pain.

Since the pain experience involves a complex interaction of physical, emotional, motivational, and cognitive influences, the patient manager should freely utilize the services of consultants who can evaluate areas of involvement beyond his expertise. Such consultants may include psychiatrists, psychologists, anesthesiologists, neurologists, nutritionists, and marital, family, and vocational counselors. Only through a comprehensive or *holistic* understanding of each patient's situation can an appropriate total treatment plan be developed.

The Ideal Analgesic

Because of the complexity of the chronic pain experience, it is easy to understand why no single form of therapy has been found to be safe and effective for the treatment of all pain problems. Although medical scientists continue the search for the "penicillin of pain," a few pioneering clinicians have begun to explore the variety of unconventional therapeutic alternatives. The long-term effectiveness and safety of these approaches has yet to be determined, but preliminary evidence suggests that they can provide dramatic relief for many pain patients who have not responded to standard therapy.

One of the greatest difficulties in determining the effectiveness and safety of new analgesic procedures lies in the numerous problems inherent in clinical research. It is difficult, if not impossible, to obtain the cooperation of large numbers of patients for a long-term study so that appropriate follow-up observations can be made. Patients vary widely in the types and amounts of medications they take and in their activity levels, both of which may affect the outcome of a particular therapy. The private physicians who manage these patients may differ in their treatment philosophy, and the host of psychological differences among patients can never be adequately assessed.

For ethical reasons, it is sometimes impossible to employ appropriate controls—in order not to deprive a patient who is in pain of an effective therapy—just to create a "no treatment" control group. In most studies, the number of patients observed is usually too small to provide adequate data, and a comparison of various techniques is often difficult because many investigators do not describe their methods or present their data in sufficient detail. In addition, the most important clinical data on the efficacy of these techniques are with private practitioners, and, at present, there are no agencies available to unify, compile, analyze, and integrate this massive amount of information.

Critical research studies that provide a sufficiently large number of patients, uniformity in the management of matched subjects, comprehensive psychological information for each patient, and sufficient incentives to ensure long-term patient cooperation are needed. Because it is unlikely that adequate funding will be available to support such studies, pain therapists will continue to be faced with the difficult decision of which analgesic technique will be appropriate for a particular pain patient. To approach this question optimistically, it is possible to consider the criteria that an ideal analgesic therapeutic technique should meet.[28]

It should be highly efficient and reliable in its ability to alleviate pain. Not only should it eliminate pain, it should also be effective every time it is used.

Its analgesic effects should be immediate and long-lasting.

It should be safe to administer and should not make the patient more ill, even acutely.

It should be simple to administer with a minimum of expensive equipment. If a therapy is beyond the financial reach of a patient, it is useless to him.

It should not adversely affect the patient's personality or cognitive ability.

It should be nonaddicting.

It should not destroy normal neural tissue or interfere with normal physiologic functioning. The discovery of endogenous analgesic substances within the nervous system indicates that neural tissue may be involved in initiating pain as well as in terminating it.

It should not produce other long-term adverse effects, which might range from the possibility of chronic infection to emotional dependence on the therapist.

Although no single form of therapy can meet all of these criteria, these provide useful guidelines for

Table 28-1. Commonly Used Analgesic Drugs

Class of Drugs	*Analgesic Potency*	*Side-Effects*	*Abuse Liability*
Nonnarcotic agents			
Acetylsalicylic acid (aspirin)	Mild	Mild–Moderate	Low–Moderate
Para-aminophen (phenacetin)	Mild	Moderate–Severe	Low
Pyrazoles (Butazolidin)	Selective	Moderate–Severe	Low
Diphenylhydantoin (Dilantin)	Selective	Mild–Moderate	Low
Carbamazepine (Tegretol)	Selective	Moderate–Severe	Low
Weak narcotic agents			
Codeine	Moderate	Moderate–Severe	Moderate
Propoxyphene (Darvon)	Mild–Moderate	Mild–Moderate	Moderate
Pentazocine (Talwin)	Mild	Moderate–Severe	Moderate
Potent narcotic agents			
Meperidine (Demerol)	Strong	Severe	High
Morphine and other derivatives	Strong	Severe	High

the establishment of a comprehensive therapeutic program. *Such a program should begin with the safest and simplest techniques and progress to more invasive approaches only as needed.*

PHARMACOLOGIC THERAPIES

Analgesics

Technological developments in pharmacology over the past 30 years have made analgesic medications the most commonly utilized tool for controlling pain. While usually effective for acute pain, they fare poorly with chronic pain.

Analgesics act in unknown ways on the central nervous system (CNS) to reduce the sensation or experience of pain without producing unconsciousness. When they are properly used, they have the advantage of simplicity of administration and low cost. These same two factors can also lead to improper application owing to incorrect dosage or overuse by abuse-prone patients.

Some of the most commonly used analgesics are listed in Table 28-l along with their relative analgesic potencies, side-effects, and abuse liabilities. For purposes of simplicity, analgesic potency is divided into mild, moderate, strong, and selective (for agents that lack general analgesic effects); side-effects into mild, moderate and severe; and abuse liability into low, moderate, and high.

As is evident from Table 28-1, the most effective analgesics also produce the most severe side-effects and carry the highest liability for abuse potential. For example, some of the desirable and undesirable effects of morphine are shown in the following list.[93]

Effects of Morphine and Its Surrogates

Desirable effects
- Effective analgesia
- Relief of anxiety
- Euphoria*
- Sedation*

Undesirable effects
- Psychological dependence
- Tolerance
- Physical dependence
- Mental clouding
- Dysphoria
- Nausea, vomiting
- Spasmogenic effects
- Euphoria*
- Sedation*
- Constipation*
- Respiratory depression*
- Suppression of cough reflex*

* May be desirable or undesirable depending on circumstances

In addition, tolerance to narcotic analgesics develops quite rapidly, and their effectiveness usually decreases with time. Thus, patients often rapidly increase their dosage with the hope of obtaining continued pain relief. Typically, this produces significantly increased side-effects, profound dependence, and, yet, only a minimal degree of comfort. When patients tolerant of high doses of narcotics attempt to reduce their medication levels, the associated withdrawal symptoms only exacerbate the degree of discomfort.

The repeated use of narcotics should therefore be deferred until non-narcotic drugs and other kinds of therapy no longer provide adequate pain relief. Even for patients with inoperable or recurring malignancies, chronic administration of narcotics should be prescribed only as a last resort, for their use is often incompatible with a productive life. Drowsiness or sleepiness associated with chronic narcotic administration is a prevalent side-effect, and, as a result, the patient is left only a small amount of time in which he is neither sleepy nor drowsy yet pain-free. In addition, because a particular life expectancy is often difficult to estimate, premature introduction of opiates may lead to early tolerance so that the patient may not derive sufficient relief even with massive doses in the later stages of the disease.

The one notable exception to these several observations is methadone. We have utilized oral methadone for cancer patients and have been able to keep them comfortable and able to function relatively naturally in society. The duration of beneficial effects has been for as long as 4 or more years.

While their exact mechanism remains unknown, narcotic analgesics may act by binding to specific receptor sites located in "analgesia centers" within the medial brain stem, thereby mimicking the effects of an endogenous analgesic substance (*enkephalin*).[128] Preliminary evidence also suggests that the therapeutic effectiveness of certain nonpharmacologic therapies, such as acupuncture, may be due to their ability to activate enkephalin release.[190] Clinically, patients who are chronically medicated with narcotic analgesics often respond less favorably to acupuncture, guided imagery, and other modalities. Perhaps, the analgesic receptor sites of these patients have become desensitized to endogenous enkephalin release following prolonged administration of exogenous opiates.[115] This notion is consistent with clinical experience, which indicates that patients with chronic benign pain show greater improvement following detoxification from long-term narcotic dependence.

Chronic administration of non-narcotic analgesics is also known to produce unacceptable risks for many patients in pain. Acetylsalicylic acid for example, is perhaps the most widely used analgesic for treatment of musculoskeletal pain, and its anti-inflammatory actions are also of therapeutic value in the management of rheumatoid arthritis. Yet, a single dose can produce severe gastrointestinal (GI) hemorrhage in susceptible patients, and its prolonged administration is known to affect hemostasis.[80] Phenacetin can cause methemoglobinemia and sulfhemoglobinemia, and less frequently, hemolytic anemia following prolonged administration.[79]

For all of these reasons, the continued administration of systemic analgesics may be less satisfactory therapy than other approaches that provide significantly fewer risks.

Psychotropic Medication

Promising recent reports suggest that pain tolerance may be enhanced by the judicious use of major and minor tranquilizers or antidepressants.[114,125] Major tranquilizers such as chlorpromazine hydrochloride are thought to increase analgesia by decreasing the overall activation of the CNS. This approach is particularly helpful in patients with chronic pain who have uncontrollable psychotic ideation, but it should not be routinely prescribed since chronic use can strongly exacerbate depression.

Minor tranquilizers of the benzodiazepine class (*e.g.*, diazepam) are thought to produce muscular relaxation by a central mechanism and are therefore widely used in the management of musculoskeletal disorders in which anxiety, agitation, and muscle spasm are prominent. However, their dosage should be carefully controlled for they are also known to produce depression when they are administered in large doses over a long period of time. In our opinion, the carbamates (*e.g.*, meprobamate) should not be prescribed for chronic pain since they are strongly addictive with occurrences of insomnia, vomiting, tremors, anorexia, ataxia, and even epilepsy reported on withdrawal.[80]

Tricyclic antidepressants have been used successfully not only for psychoneurotic complaints but also to alleviate pain caused by a variety of pathologic conditions including terminal carcinoma and rheumatoid arthritis.[71,202] Unfortunately, symptomatic relief of depression or pain is usually delayed 2 to 3 weeks following introduction of tricyclics, and patient compliance with a recommended dosage regime is therefore often quite poor. Even when careful instructions and a thorough explanation of the delay is provided, many patients with chronic pain will quickly stop taking a medication that produces no immediate effects. Perhaps, this problem can be overcome as additional trials utilizing tricyclics in combination with other drugs are conducted.[57,114]

Amino Acid Precursors

A considerable amount of scientific and clinical evidence indicates that the sensation or experience of pain may be modulated by the brain monoamine serotonin.[187,224] The administration of L-tryptophan, its amino acid precursor, is known to increase the synthesis or levels of serotonin in the brain, and when it is given with a pyrrolase inhibitor such as nicotinamide, L-tryptophan is reported to be beneficial in the treatment of depression.[8,65] In some studies, L-tryptophan has been shown to be comparable in effectiveness to the tricyclic antidepressants and even superior to unilateral electroconvulsive shock therapy in unipolar depression.[84,105,141]

L-tryptophan is also reported to be an effective hypnotic agent for it reduces sleep latency in rats, in normal humans, and in patients with mild insomnia. Most important, its use does not generate the distortions of sleep physiology characteristic of other hypnotics, even with long-term administration or after withdrawal.[82,83]

For the past several years, Bresler has recommended the supplemental use of L-tryptophan in moderate doses (500 mg, at bedtime) with vitamin B_6 (100 mg) and niacinamide (100 mg) for pain patients with agitated depression and sleep difficulties. While controlled clinical data are not yet available, more than half of these patients have reported strikingly positive results. Although the possibility that these results represent nothing more than a placebo effect remains to be explored, the use of L-tryptophan is one of the safest pharmacologic therapies available since 1 to 2 g are ingested daily in the normal diet.

While the administration of an amino acid in pure form may produce effects different from those of the same amount taken in a mixture of amino acids and other nutritional substances, there are no reports to our knowledge of allergy or other complications in the clinical literature.[65]

One study with rats has suggested that direct implantation of crystals of certain tryptophan metabolites into the bladder may be carcinogenic, and the clinical implications of this finding should certainly be investigated further.[33] However, Coppen has reported that doses as high as 6 to 9 g per day have been taken by several thousand patients in England over a period of many months with very few side-effects and no serious complications.[83]

Placebos

The placebo effect is one of the most neglected yet powerful aspects of patient care. Shapiro has defined the placebo as ". . . any therapeutic procedure (or that component of any therapeutic procedure) which is given deliberately to have an effect, or unknowingly has an effect on a patient, symptom, syndrome or disease, but which is objectively without *specific* activity for the condition being treated. The therapeutic procedure may be given with or without conscious knowledge that the procedure is a placebo, may be an active (non-inert) or non-active (inert) procedure, and includes, therefore, all medical procedures no matter how specific—oral and parenteral medication, topical preparations, inhalants, and mechanical, surgical and psychotherapeutic procedures."[206] Numerous studies have indicated that placebos can provide relief for a variety of pain-related disorders including angina, rheumatoid and degenerative arthritis, peptic ulcer, duodenal ulcer, and other chronic pain problems.[4,7,14,58,59,227,237] One controlled study that compared the effectiveness of analgesic drugs reported that although 82 to 87 per cent of patients with chronic headache responded to active analgesics, 60 per cent responded to placebo medications.[104]

Another study found that 72 per cent of patients with postoperative pain responded to morphine injections, but 40 per cent of these same patients responded equally well to placebo injections.[123] In addition, approximately 70 per cent of patients with herniated lumbar discs who were given a general anesthetic and injected with a placebo obtained pain relief.[150]

Nearly 30 per cent of cancer patients who undergo controlled trials of oral analgesics reported 50 per cent or greater pain relief from placebo formulations.[172] Those who showed a change with placebos had a greater rate of response to active drugs but also a higher incidence of CNS side-effects to placebo medications. In this study, patients responsive to placebo included those with a high educational level, farmers, professionals, women working outside the home, and patients who were widowed, separated, or divorced. Those resistant to placebo included patients with a low level of education, unskilled workers, housewives, married women without children, and smokers.

Compared to nonresponders, those who responded to placebos were typically more dependent, anxious, self-centered, and emotionally unstable. They were less self-confident and dominant in personal relationships but more socially extroverted. Placebo responders tended to have a greater awareness of bodily functions, more stress-related symtoms, and greater dependence on analgesics, sedatives, and cathartics.[106,123]

Although it is commonly assumed that the placebo effect is a form of suggestion, most studies have found no significant relationship between suggestibility and the placebo response.[58] Perhaps the best working hypothesis is that the administration of a placebo produces a reduction of chronic anxiety, which in turn is accompanied by a decrease in pain perception.[221]

Evans has summarized the pharmacologic characteristics of placebo analgesia as follows:[58]

Placebo medication tends to be more effective in relieving severe pain, although its effectiveness may decrease with continued treatment.

The pharmacologic properties of the placebo closely mimic the pharmacologic properties of the active agent with which it is being compared.

The effects of placebo and other active medications tend to interact.

As with most active drugs, higher medication dosages are clinically more effective. For example, two placebo capsules typically produce a substantially stronger clinical effect than one capsule.

A placebo injection is usually more effective than oral administration.

The placebo effect is substantially more potent if given under double-blind conditions than if it is given nonblind.

It is also more potent if patients are told a powerfully effective drug has been given, compared to being told an experimental drug with unknown effects has been given.

The placebo effect is stronger when the placebo is administered by physicians who are more likely to prescribe medications than it is by physicians who tend to use medication as a last resort.

Because of their clinical effectiveness and minimal side-effects, placebos are an important part of the pain therapist's armamentarium. We have found the judicious use of placebos to be extremely helpful in detoxifying patients from opiates and other addicting medications, for the drug-giving ritual often provides initial assurance, security, and confidence in the therapist. It is subsequently easier to wean drug-dependent patients from a "new medication" (placebo) than from one identified with long-term use.

Placebos may be used as an adjunct to psychotherapy but never as a substitute.[207] Nor should placebos be prescribed simply to save time and trouble and "to see what happens." A placebo therapy should be administered with the same deliberate concern for indications as a more specific therapy, and only if the therapist himself believes that it may help.

NERVE BLOCKS

Diagnostic and Prognostic Blocks

The injection of chemical agents to block neuronal activity for the alleviation of pain dates back over a century. The wide variety of techniques and agents employed and their indications and contraindications are reviewed extensively elsewhere in this volume (see Chaps. 26 and 27).

Diagnostic nerve blocks can often be used effectively to identify the neuronal components related to the pain sensation. For example, the complete elimination of burning pain following sympathetic nerve block is one of the most reliable diagnostic indices of sympathetic reflex dystrophy. In addition, the effectiveness of anesthetic *versus* placebo blocks and the relative contributions of somatic *versus* psychological factors to the pain experience can often be distinguished. Diagnostic blocks may also be helpful in allowing the therapist to evaluate how the patient's overall level of discomfort is influenced by the lack of the pain sensation.

Prognostic nerve blocks permit patients to experience the sensation, temporarily, of long-term interruption of nerve pathways following neurosurgery or injection of neurolytic agents. By experiencing the numbness and other side-effects that often follow neurosurgical or neurolytic destruction, patients can determine in advance whether or not such procedures will be truly worthwhile.

Therapeutic Blocks With Local Anesthetic Agents

Local anesthetics injected around nervous tissue or into epidural or subarachnoid spaces often provide immediate pain relief, but, unfortunately, their effects usually last for only a few hours. Thus, because of the impracticality of regularly repeated injections, therapeutic blocks with such agents are not a satisfactory long-term treatment for the majority of patients with chronic pain.

Occasionally, however, a single therapeutic block will provide improvement that far exceeds the duration of the anesthetic—perhaps because of the way it can change a patient's attitude. Patients with chronic pain are typically characterized by feelings of helplessness, hopelessness, and depression, but these can be significantly ameliorated by a dramatic demonstration that pain relief is possible (at least temporarily). Nerve blocks can greatly reduce anxiety and fear of future pain because a patient whose pain is successfully blocked knows that if his discomfort becomes truly unbearable, relief is available. Thus, blocks can affect not only the pain sensation but the pain experience as well.

For patients with certain musculoskeletal pain problems, repeated nerve blocks can occasionally produce longer and longer periods of pain alleviation. Thus, while the first block may alleviate discomfort for 2 to 3 hours, subsequent blocks may provide days, weeks, months, or even years of pain relief.

Neurolytic Blocks

The longer-acting therapeutic blocks often require the destruction of nerve fibers with neurolytic agents. When they are injected for neural destruction either into the subarachnoid space or directly around the nerve itself, phenol and alcohol can cause complications much greater than the original pain problem. A postinjection neuritis can result from using these agents, producing pain that can be far more severe than the original complaint. Occasionally, the nerves blocked with these agents have motor fibers in them, thus resulting in a semipermanent or permanent paralysis of the area supplied by that motor nerve. (For example, following subarachnoid blocks with these agents, transient motor paralysis of the legs can occur with an indefinite motor paralysis of the bladder and rectum.) In addition, an inflammatory response may produce an adhesive arachnoiditis and a secondary pain syndrome. Thus, neurolytic blocks are generally reserved for patients with terminal cancer or for the treatment of patients with severe intractable pain who are not candidates for surgery (see Chap. 23).

NEUROSURGICAL PROCEDURES

Neuroablative Techniques

A wide variety of neuroablative techniques have been developed for the treatment of intractable pain, many of which are listed below (see Chap. 29).

Neuroablative Techniques for Treatment of Pain

Peripheral neurectomy
Sympathectomy
Rhizotomy
Surgical chordotomy
Percutaneous chordotomy
Commissural myelotomy
Medullary tractotomy
Mesencephalic tractotomy
Thalamotomy
Leukotomy
Postcentral gyrectomy
Cingulotomy
Frontal lobotomy

Although these techniques have been used to provide pain relief when all other therapeutic attempts have failed, they are all associated with some degree of mortality and morbidity. For example, the reported mortality following unilateral chordotomy ranges from 4 per cent to 10 per cent and increases up to 30 per cent following bilateral cervical chordotomy.[68] Varying kinds and degrees of complications have been reported in the literature, including motor paralysis, development of palsies, mental aberrations, sensory loss, dysesthesias, impotence, bladder dysfunction, and so forth.

In addition to these considerations, many ablative procedures are not indicated for debilitated patients owing to the risks attendant upon surgery in general. Even the less traumatic percutaneous techniques (*e.g.*, percutaneous chordotomy) are contraindicated in patients with certain illnesses (*e.g.*, asthma, emphysema), thus limiting their applicability.

Sometimes, when pain is surgically eliminated and complete anesthesia achieved, the ensuing numbness associated with sensory deprivation may become more intolerable than the original pain problem.[45] Even worse, pain may return within 6 months to a year. In such cases, patients generally feel that the short-term relief they obtained was hardly worth the emotional trauma and potentially dangerous side-effects of surgery.

The return of discomfort following surgical deafferentation may be related to the finding that approximately 27 per cent of the nerve fibers in the ventral (efferent) root are unmyelinated somatosensory afferents.[44] These fibers may become activated when dorsal root fibers are destroyed. Surgical ablation of these ventral root fibers would almost certainly produce profound motor paralysis.

Neuroablative procedures may also interfere with the effectiveness of other approaches to pain control. Recently, it has been discovered in animals that if certain descending pathways from the brain to spinal cord are destroyed, analgesia cannot be achieved in the somatic and visceral areas subserved by the dorsolateral funiculus (DLF).[10] If the DLF is sectioned and the animal then given morphine, analgesia to subsequent noxious stimuli will occur in all areas except those below the lesion on the ipsilateral side. Interestingly, the DLF consists of descending serotonin-containing fibers that originate in the *nucleus raphe magnus*.[52] Both morphine and stimulation-produced analgesia (SPA) are antagonized by prior administration of p-chlorophenylalanine, a potent inhibitor of serotonin synthesis.[1,2,127] Thus, it is possible that accidental destruction of descending serotonergic fibers in the DLF may prevent higher brain centers from inhibiting noxious stimulation at the level of the spinal cord. Therefore, it is generally recommended that neuroablative procedures be restricted to patients with certain terminal malignancies. They are clearly not applicable to the majority of patients with chronic benign pain.

Peripheral Neural Stimulation

The concept of pain relief through electrical stimulation rather than through ablation or anesthetization of an area is far from new. Attempts as early as the first century AD have been cited in which electric fish were used to combat headache and gout.[110] Nineteenth-century physicians subjected patients to galvanic therapy for a variety of ills, but these early stimulators brought with them the risk of electrocution or burns.

With more recent technological advances, a great number of investigators have attempted to alleviate pain by augmenting rather than reducing sensory input. For example, Wall reported that stimulation of large myelinated sensory fibers exerts a segmental inhibitory influence on the input to certain dorsal horn interneurones in the cat.[240] These same interneurones are activated by impulses in small-diameter afferents responsive to noxious stimuli. When peripheral nerves are selectively stimulated, pain is produced only when the threshold for small-diameter afferents is exceeded, while at lower levels of stimulation, only nonpainful paresthesias are produced.[45] These findings suggested that normal pain input could be inhibited by selective stimulation of large fibers, and it is now known that peripheral nerve stimulation in humans can in fact produce significant analgesia.[132,133,135,228,241]

The use of surgically implanted peripheral nerve stimulators has been largely obviated by the development of transcutaneous electrical nerve stimulation (TENS) devices. These will be discussed later in this chapter.

Central Neural Stimulation

Based on the results of early peripheral-nerve stimulation studies, stimulation of the dorsal column (which presumably is selective for the central projections of large-diameter afferent fibers) has also been utilized in an attempt to relieve pain.[69,210,212] Although initial enthusiasm was high with reports of success ranging from 50 to 80 per cent, more recent estimates have reported success rates of 25 per cent or below, a value even lower than can be attributed to the placebo effect.[134,176,210] In reporting the results of 6 years' experience with electrical stimulation for control of pain, Shealy concluded that dorsal column stimulation may be of some value in properly selected patients but should be considered only a last resort.[208]

A few studies have reported the effect of electrical stimulation of the brain itself in patients who suffer from intractable pain. Electrodes have been implanted into the septal area, caudate nucleus, ventral lateral posterior nucleus of the thalamus, ventral medial posterior nucleus, posterior limb of the internal capsule, and the mesencephalic peri aqueductal gray matter.[60,67,72,92,158,191,195] These investigations follow the classic animal studies of "reward" and "punishment" centers in the brain and the more recent reports of Mayer and others on central "analgesia" centers.[154,155,157,168,181]

The results of these attempts are highly variable because the number of patients involved is quite small. Although some positive results have been obtained, several disastrous failures have also been reported. In several cases, habituation to continued stimulation has developed, and effectiveness does not appear to be long-lasting. Clearly, implantation of electrodes into the brain is a technique of last resort and is not indicated for most patients with chronic pain.

ACUPUNCTURE

Traditional Concepts

For many years, occasional visitors from the West have returned from China with anecdotal reports of the successful use of acupuncture in the treatment of various medical problems. These reports remained largely curiosities in the United States until improvement of relations in the early 1970s brought new information that stimulated great interest in acupuncture.

Although acupuncture has been practiced in China for more than 3,000 years, its orgins are lost in antiquity. It is a complete and complex system of medicine, based upon the philosophy and world view of the culture from which it arose. Its endurance has been remarkable, in light of the many cultural and political changes that have swept China. It is quite possible that historically more people have been treated by acupuncture than by any other formalized system of medicine.

The classical Chinese conceptions of health and disease are intrinsically linked to the philosophical constructs of traditional Chinese thought. The ancient Chinese believed that the universe was permeated with a vital life-force or energy (called *Ch'i*) that circulated continuously through all living organisms. This energy was thought to follow specific pathways through the body (referred to as *meridians*), upon which the acupuncture *points* lie. Stimulation of specific acupuncture points was believed to affect the flow of Ch'i in specific organ systems of the body.

Originally, 12 bilaterally symmetrical meridians were described, with each meridian named for one of the 12 major internal organs conceptualized by traditional Chinese medicine. In addition to these 12 paired meridians, two nonpaired *control* meridians were described: the *governing vessel,* which followed the spine and ran along the midline on the dorsal surface of the body, and the *conception vessel,* which ran along the midline on the ventral surface of the body.

If the circulation of Ch'i became impeded or blocked in a given meridian as a result of external events (such as trauma, cold, dampness) or internal factors (such as fear, anger, sorrow), an abnormal surplus or deficit of Ch'i was thought to result. This imbalance affected the organism and was ultimately manifested by the presence of pain or disease. Utilizing a variety of diagnostic techniques, the traditional acupuncture practitioner first attempted to diagnose the nature of the imbalance of energy and then select the appropriate acupuncture points for treatment on the basis of this diagnosis. The points selected were stimulated by insertion of fine, solid needles (acupuncture), by heating with *moxa,* a traditional Chinese herb (moxibustion), or by massage (acupressure), depending upon the problem being treated. Modern technology has also made available a variety of new techniques including electrical stimulation of the needles, ultrasound stimulation, and even laser-beam stimulation.

The selection of specific points and the form of stimulation administered were determined by rather complex theoretical considerations.[25,146–148,184] Years of study were required for the traditional acupuncturist to master the theoretical basis of the art, as well as the precise location of each acupuncture point and the specific techniques of needle insertion.

Modern Concepts

Although the terminology of traditional Chinese medicine often appears strange and unfamiliar to Western physicians, scientists have now begun to document the physiologic, electrical, and chemical characteristics of the traditional acupuncture system. Many acupuncture points are anatomically identical to motor muscles, well known in electromyography, while others are identical to common trigger points, independently described by several Western investigators.[130,163,239] Still others lie along major nerve trunks.[153,205]

Also, it has been found that the electrical resistance of the skin that overlies acupuncture points is considerably lower than that of the surrounding area, although the significance of this observation has yet to be explained.[12,193,194]

Although basic research on acupuncture in the West has not been extensive, it has been shown that stimulation of various acupuncture points can affect a great variety of physiologic parameters. These include changes in red and white blood cell count, immunoglobulin levels, electroencephalogram (EEG) and electrocardiogram (ECG) recordings, bronchodilation, and vasodilation of the microcirculation, among others.[26,35,40,41,43,51,95,124,137,182,230,244,247]

Most theories of acupuncture have focused on the nervous system, and it seems clear that the phenomena of acupuncture are at least in part mediated through the nervous system, through mechanisms that are not as yet well understood. Neurophysiologic investigations of acupuncture have concentrated upon its analgesic effects, and various theories have been developed in an attempt to explain it. The existence of visceral–cutaneous reflexes and characteristic patterns of referred pain are well known, and it is possible that acupuncture may involve, in part, a complex manipulation of such reflexes.[38,98,136,149,219,234,235,242] Melzack and Wall have advanced the well known *gate theory* and others have amplified this with *multiple gate* theories.[144,160,164] Basically, these theories propose that needle insertion at acupuncture points stimulates large-diameter fibers in peripheral nerves, whose activity interferes at some level of the nervous system with the transmission of painful impulses mediated by small-diameter fibers. The impulses produced by acupuncture thus close the "gate" to impulses that mediate painful stimuli and prevent them from reaching the brain.

No single explanation of the phenomena has been generally accepted, and it is quite possible that a number of different factors may be involved, including peripheral neural stimulation, immune–inflammatory response to the needle insertion, and psychologic factors.[31] Quite recently, the discovery of endogenous polypeptides (endorphins) that bind to opiate receptors in the CNS has raised the intriguing possibility that release of these polypeptides may also be involved in mediating the analgesic effect of acupuncture.[49,96,115,189,218,232]

Endorphins are naturally occurring substances with opiatelike properties, whose analgesic actions can be reversed by opiate antagonists, such as naloxone. Preliminary investigations indicate that the analgesic effects of acupuncture may also be blocked by naloxone, which suggests the existence of a similar mechanism.[156,190]

Treatment

Many people are unnecessarily frightened by the prospect of receiving acupuncture, for they incorrectly equate acupuncture needles with the type of needles used for hypodermic injections. Hypodermic needles are large and hollow with a razor-sharp beveled point for piercing through tissue. Acupuncture needles, on the other hand, are extremely thin—often no thicker than a human hair. They are made of solid flexible stainless steel with a rounded pencil-tip point that pushes the tissue aside without cutting it. As a result, only a slight pin prick sensation is felt when they are inserted, and there is usually no bleeding during the entire treatment process.

The needles are inserted at a depth of from several millimeters to 3 to 6 cm, depending upon the particular point chosen and the physique of the individual patient. The number inserted at each treatment may range from two or three to 20 or 30 or even more, depending upon the problem under treatment, and the style of the individual acupuncturist. An average treatment involves the use of eight to twelve needles. Once the needle is properly in place, a characteristic tingling, heaviness, or paresthesia is experienced. Although this sometimes may feel strange and unusual, most patients report that it is not painful.

Following insertion, the needles may simply be left in place, or they may be stimulated in a variety of ways. For stronger stimulation, they may be gently manipulated by hand, or they may be connected to an *electroacupuncture* device, which delivers a mild, painless electrical current through the needles. They may also be heated by burning the Chinese herb moxa (the dried leaves of *Artemisia vulgaris*), which is traditionally used for this purpose. After about 20 to 30 minutes, the needles are removed without discomfort. A brief rest will then be recommended after the treatment is completed because some patients experience light-headedness and even euphoria. Most patients describe a characteristic feeling of contentment and relaxation.

The number of sessions required varies according to the individual and the problem being treated. For acute ailments, only a few treatments—sometimes just one—are necessary. Chronic problems usually require a greater number.

Some people are fortunate, experiencing improvement in their condition immediately. However, others may instead feel even worse after the initial treatments and then begin making profound improvement later. If acupuncture is capable of helping, progress is usually noticeable by the 10th treatment. But for certain chronic ailments, 15 to 20 treatments may be necessary. Typically, about two treatments are given per week.

Clinical Indications

Acupuncture was recognized long ago as an effective treatment in the management of chronic pain.[17,23,32,47,75,225,231] Subsequent studies have supported these early findings.[22,42,50,77,85,109,111–113,142,143,145,152,174,177,186,197,213,243] On the basis of our experiences with more than 4,000 pain patients over the past 8 years, we have found acupuncture to be of tremendous benefit in treating a wide variety of chronic pain problems.[30]

Slightly more than half of our patients, who were previously unresponsive to therapy, achieved significant pain relief, with decreased requirements for medications, improved sleep patterns, and increased ability to carry on daily activities.

Some types of pain problems appear to respond better than others to acupuncture. For example, it is effective in relieving many kinds of musculoskeletal pains, such as those of arthritis, bursitis, tenosynovitis, vertebrogenic pain, and other similar conditions. Patients with osteoarthritis generally respond much more favorably than those with rheumatoid arthritis. Perhaps this is related to the fact that rheumatoid arthritis is actually a multisystem disease while osteoarthritis is a local degenerative process. There also appears to be anatomical differences in the pattern of response, and problems of the large joints commonly respond better than those of the smaller joints. For example, the pain of bursitis or tenosynovitis of the shoulder is often relieved successfully and rapidly by acupuncture, while epicondylitis of the elbow responds more slowly.

Acupuncture appears to be particularly effective when there is a large component of muscle spasm involved. It can produce rapid and dramatic relief of spasm and can be quite useful in the treatment of acute musculoskeletal injuries. The application of acupuncture in sports medicine may prove to be especially successful. Headaches, both tension and migraine, can also be effectively treated by acupuncture. It can produce relief of acute headache pain and can eventually eliminate or markedly diminish the recurrence of headaches after completion of a full course of treatment.

The pain of various neurologic conditions may also respond to acupuncture. This includes disorders such as peripheral neuropathy, trigeminal neuralgia, postherpetic neuralgia, phantom limb pain, and causalgia. These are all conditions that may be extremely painful and for which no satisfactory form of treatment now exists.

While treatment with acupuncture is not always successful, many patients have been helped, and it certainly must be considered a possible form of treatment in these cases. Indeed, for disorders such as genuine trigeminal neuralgia, an agonizing condition unresponsive to most therapy, acupuncture may well be the treatment of choice. In many cases, the pain of trigeminal neuralgia can be considerably attenuated in intensity or frequency and in some cases entirely abolished.

One pain problem that deserves specific mention is temporomandibular joint (TMJ) pain-dysfunction syndrome. This is a problem usually treated by dentists, although it may also be seen by some physicians. It is not well understood by many members of both professions, and its management is somewhat controversial and often unsatisfactory. Acupuncture has been found to be particularly effective in the treatment of this problem, especially when it is used in conjunction with soft diet and other appropriate adjunctive measures. TMJ dysfunction often goes unrecognized or misdiagnosed but has a surprisingly high incidence, and acupuncture represents a very promising form of therapy.

We have also found acupuncture to be helpful in the treatment of anxiety and depression related to chronic pain. Most patients who receive acupuncture experience a profound feeling of relaxation and well-being and even occasionally a mild euphoria following their treatment. This seems to be a nonspecific effect of acupuncture unrelated to the particular problem being treated and may perhaps involve the release of endogenous opiates, as discussed earlier. However, certain kinds of treatment and certain acupuncture points appear to be more powerful in inducing this effect than others. Why this occurs is not known, but those who use acupuncture routinely recognize this as a typical response to therapy.

Many patients who begin treatment dreading the needles eventually come to regard their acupuncture treatment as a curiously pleasant experience. In addition, patients commonly report that they feel less anxious and more energetic or are sleeping better, in addition to changes in specific symptoms.

Some investigators who have explored the therapeutic efficacy of acupuncture have been unable to achieve positive results. A brief review of a few of the problems inherent in clinical evaluations of acupuncture therapy is, therefore, in order.

First of all, in order for any form of therapy to be effective it must be properly administered in the proper dosage according to the proper schedule, and for a sufficient period of time. The same is true with acupuncture. The proper points must be used, they must be stimulated correctly, and a sufficient number of treatments must be administered in order to achieve positive results.

Many studies of acupuncture have been conducted by researchers with no formal training, who simply followed instructions from a textbook. It is not surprising that their results are often disappointing. For example, when acupuncture is administered correctly, the patient experiences a characteristic mild paresthesia. The practiced acupuncturist has developed expertise in the proper placement of the needles and routinely obtains this sensation. A less experienced therapist may need to rely upon gently manipulating the needle and asking the patient to respond when the sensation is experienced. However, some studies performed by Western physicians without training in acupuncture have consisted of the placement of acupuncture needles at the approximate location and depth of points described in acupuncture texts. No attempt is made to elicit the sensation of paresthesia, which is the only assurance of proper needle placement. The acupuncture points must be located precisely. Slight variations do exist from one patient to the next. Needle insertion that only approximates the location cannot be expected to have a significant effect, and studies of this kind do not provide a valid appraisal of acupuncture.

Other studies by investigators inexperienced in acupuncture therapy have shown insufficient treatment either in the number of points stimulated or in the number of treatments administered, perhaps out of unfamiliarity with patterns of patient response to acupuncture. There is considerable variation in response. Some patients experience a gradual improvement in symptoms following each treatment, while others notice no change for several treatments before improvement begins to occur. Still others experience a transient exacerbation of symptoms after some of the initial treatments, which often precedes eventual improvement. Long-term aggravation of symptoms as a result of acupuncture does not seem to occur.

Because of this variability, it is quite difficult to generalize about the number of treatments that may be required for a particular patient. As a very rough estimate, we consider 10 treatments a fair trial of acupuncture for other than very acute problems. Most patients who will respond to acupuncture should begin to show improvement within this time, although there may be exceptions in particularly difficult cases. (Some patients find an occasional "booster" treatment helpful at intervals following a full course of treatment.)

An additional variable in acupuncture research is the kind of stimulation employed. An experienced acupuncturist will decide on an individual basis whether mild or vigorous stimulation is appropriate and whether manual stimulation of needles, massage, burning of moxa (moxibustion), or electrical current will produce the best results. Like other forms of medicine, acupuncture is an art, and its effectiveness cannot be adequately judged by investigators unfamiliar with its intricacy and who simply insert needles in the skin on the basis of a standardized protocol.

Thus, it would appear that some investigators have attempted to evaluate acupuncture without sufficient knowledge of the subject to perform their studies properly. Unfortunately, the poor results they have obtained have led portions of the medical community to adopt a negative, skeptical attitude toward acupuncture. While it is certainly important to protect the public against medical quackery, is it possible to believe that a medical system employed for thousands of years by a quarter of the world's population and now growing in acceptance throughout the world is really quackery? At any time in history, people tend to cling to accepted beliefs and resist the introduction of new ideas. We now reflect with amusement upon the narrowmindedness of past generations, but we must take care that we ourselves do not behave in the same way. Acupuncture represents an exciting opportunity for medical practitioners, and they should not reject it simply because it was not taught in medical school. Although we do not fully understand acupuncture, we must remember that we effectively use many drugs, such as aspirin or digitalis, whose mechanism of action is not completely understood.

Acupuncture is not without its limitations, however. First, it is not readily available in many parts of the world. Second, acupuncture is an invasive technique. It involves inserting a foreign object into the body, and, for that reason, the possibility of infection or nerve, vessel, or organ damage, though minimal, always exists.

Despite these shortcomings, acupuncture is an extremely safe technique when it is administered by a skillful, trained professional.[120]

PHYSICAL THERAPIES

Heat and Cold

The origin of the application of physical stimuli to the skin for the alleviation of pain is probably prehistoric. Although there are few controlled evaluations of the therapeutic effectiveness of physical therapy, the use of heat and cold is often helpful in the management of chronic pain.[48,55,61,165,175]

These stimuli may simply serve to produce counterirritation, which is known to attenuate pain.[70,180] For example, cold stimulation has been reported to have a potent analgesic effect when it is applied to a region other than the painful one, and causalgic hand pain reportedly can be suppressed by immersing the opposite hand in water.[18,21]

Nevertheless, the application of heat and cold represents one of the safest and simplest modalities available to patients with chronic pain and is often an extraordinarily useful adjunctive procedure.

Pressure and Touch

Pressure and touch are also important tools in the therapist's armamentarium. Therapeutic massage, for example, whether applied to a specific area of discomfort or throughout the body, can produce not only profound physical relaxation but psychological peace of mind as well.[11,56,203]

Unfortunately, the word *massage* has been discredited in recent years, for so-called massage parlors have offered just about every kind of physical stimulation imaginable except for authentic therapeutic massage. Consequently, patients who may well benefit from the treatment of a professional masseur are often reluctant to consider this worthwhile form of therapy.

The application of pressure can also be an effective approach to alleviation of pain. Many patients find that temporary relief can be quickly obtained by applying deep pressure to the acupuncture points associated with an area of discomfort (*acupressure*).[36,37,54,81,94,204]

There is increasing evidence that suggests that merely touching the patient can have profoundly positive therapeutic effects.[117–119,173] The use of *laying-on-of-hands* is one of the most rapid and effective ways to reduce acute anxiety and discomfort, and it is possible that the many beneficial effects of physical therapy may be directly related to this phenomenon.

Exercise and Movement

Therapeutic movement and exercise can also be used effectively as part of a pain management program. Today, exercise represents an important source of stress reduction for many people, but because of chronic pain, this outlet is no longer available to them. In such cases, therapeutic movement can be enormously beneficial.

Western researchers have only recently begun to explore the therapeutic value of ancient exercise techniques such as yoga, a 3000-year-old system that combines both physical and spiritual training. Many disciples of yoga claim that its various postures help to relax both the body and the mind.[24,53,90,91,169,170]

Two of the better known modern movement therapies are the Alexander and Feldenkrais techniques.[3,9,62,63] The Alexander technique is designed to help patients develop a "sensory appreciation" of movements that originate from the "primary control center" of the head and neck. With everyday movements such as walking, standing, and sitting, a new awareness of "natural" movement is facilitated, and old habitual patterns or "sets" are inhibited.

The Feldenkrais technique (also called Functional Integration) is a system of movements designed to eliminate chronic patterns of stress and tension. Using light touch and manipulation, the instructor helps to move muscles in more natural ways, thereby releasing mental and emotional tension, and restoring "harmony" to the "integrated self."

Electrical Stimulation

One of the most commonly utilized modern physical therapies is transcutaneous electrical nerve stimulation. As a result of the pioneering work of Shealy and Long, portable TENS units are now commercially available from at least a dozen manufacturers.[135,209] The majority of these units are battery-operated and produce a spike or rectangular waveform with variable controls for selecting frequency, voltage, and pulse width.[192]

The application of TENS is quite simple, and, with proper instruction, most patients have little difficulty in mastering self-administration. Pairs of rubber electrodes are coated with conductive jelly and attached to the skin above the area of discomfort or at distal sites. The electrodes are then attached to the TENS units, and mild electrical stimulation is applied.

The effectiveness of TENS is influenced by a large number of variables including repetition rate (frequency), amplitude (voltage), pulse width, site of electrode placement, duration of stimulation, and frequency of treatment sessions. Thus, optimal stimulation parameters must be established on an individualized basis, usually through trial and error. Of particular importance is the frequency of stimulation and site of electrode placement. For example, low-frequency stimulation (1–2 Hz) at distal acupuncture points associated with an area of musculoskeletal discomfort typically provides more positive results than higher-frequency stimulation directly above the affected area.

TENS has been used effectively in the management of postsurgical pain, athletic injuries, acute low back and cervical syndromes, and minor soft tissue trauma, as well as chronic pain.[97,129,131,196,226,233,238] It is extremely safe and has little in the way of adverse side-effects and no addictive potential. Thus, even if it does not provide relief, little is lost in trying it. Unlike many neurosurgical procedures, it does not disrupt normal neurologic function. Most important, TENS is easy to self-administer, permitting patients to assume a greater role in their own treatment program. As will be discussed later in this chapter, encouraging patient self-control is an effective way of alleviating the feelings of helplessness and depression that so typically accompany the chronic pain experience.

HYPNOSIS AND SUGGESTION

History

Hypnosis has progressed considerably since the 18th century, when Western scientists first began to consider its therapeutic potential. Friedrich Anton Mesmer, an Austrian physician, hypothesized that all men were "living magnets," and that some people ("magnetic animals") were able to affect the magnetic fluids of others. Sick people suffering from "an imbalance of magnetic fluid" were thought by Mesmer to be susceptible to help from these "magnetic animals."

For a time, Mesmer treated ill people from all over Europe in his Paris clinic. He wore flowing silk robes and held an iron wand in his hand as he cared for patients. But his work was cut short in 1784 when an investigating commission that included Benjamin Franklin, then ambassador to France, determined that therapeutic effects he obtained were due only to the imagination of his patients. Using appropriate scientific methodology, members of the commission concluded that the invisible fluid Mesmer postulated to account for his results did not exist. In many ways, the committee set the stage for later attitudes toward hypnosis by ignoring the obvious power of the effect when it could not establish its cause.

After the commission released its report, 115 case studies and testimonials were issued. Most of these came not from women (known to be of "submissive character and delicate minds"), but from male patients. Mesmerism spread to Britain, and numerous major surgical operations were performed using it as analgesic. John Elliotson, one of the first to employ the use of the stethoscope and advocate percussion in physical diagnosis, became fascinated with the technique. But his enthusiasm was a bit excessive for the times. He was severely castigated by the editor of *Lancet* and resigned when the practice of mesmerism in University Hospital was forbidden.

The name *hypnosis* was given by another British doctor, James Braid, who attempted to study its neurophysiologic basis. Braid made careful observations of his patients and their behavior while they were hypnotized, and he came under attack from Elliotson and the other "fluidists."

Meanwhile, mesmerism was being used for analgesia in surgery. An isolated mastectomy was performed as early as 1829, and another amputation in 1842, but rumors were circulated that the patients had lied about hypnosis as the sole anesthetic. Controversy continued about the role of hypnotism in surgery and with the development of chemical anesthetics, interest in the technique waned. Not until Charcot, Janet, Breuer, Bernheim, and Freud demonstrated and practiced hypnotism did the phenomenon assume scientific respectability.

Today, hypnosis is taught in several medical schools, with the sanction of the American Medical Association and the British Medical Association. However, because of the enormous clinical usefulness of the procedure (especially in the management of chronic pain), it is surprising that it has not gained widespread acceptance in the medical community. This may be due in part to the great mystery that continues to surround its mechanism of action.

It has become increasingly apparent that hypnosis is not placebo in itself; rather, the placebo effect may be a part of the total hypnotic experience.[139] The placebo effect results from the patient's belief that a sham procedure will be effective, and it can be utilized in both hypnotizable and nonhypnotizable subjects. Highly hypnotizable patients derive much more relief from hypnosis than from placebo alone. In fact, the degree of analgesia achieved with hypnosis may not even be correlated with the amount of pain relief obtained following placebo administration, but the two may be additive.

In addition, preliminary research indicates that the placebo effect may be based on release of endorphins, for the actions of placebos can be reversed by the narcotic antagonist naloxone.[66] Yet, naloxone does not affect hypnotically induced analgesia, thus suggesting that different mechanisms of action may be involved.[73]

Symptom Suppression and Substitution

In essence, hypnosis is a state of attentive, responsive concentration in which there is a heightened degree of suggestibility. Contrary to popular belief, it is not sleep. In fact, it is exactly the opposite of sleep, for attention is so highly focused that even minor distractions are minimized.

Medical hypnosis usually begins with an *induction* during which the patient is encouraged or allowed to develop a deep state of relaxation. While the patient's attention is focused on some object, image, or sound (*e.g.*, the therapist's voice), a suggestion about drowsiness or relaxation is given, and the patient may be asked to close his eyes. When he is apparently quite relaxed, the trance state is deepened, and he may be asked to raise his arms and keep them in front of him. This serves as a measure of depth of trance.

Suggestions that are relevant to the patient's complaint or problem may then be made. If the patient is seeking pain relief, he may be given an analgesic suggestion, instructed to notice his "feeling of comfort" and to realize that this is attainable any time he wishes. He may then be given a posthypnotic suggestion or a cue that can be used to reactivate this analgesic state. The trance state is a learned response and will become deeper with practice, and for this reason it is especially important at the beginning to maximize patient motivation. In our experience, few possible incentives are more motivating to patients with chronic pain than an acute demonstration of symptomatic relief.

A more thorough discussion of hypnosis in pain relief can be found elsewhere, as can detailed descriptions of hypnotic procedures.[39,86,121,122,201] However, there are a few hypnotic techniques that are particularly useful.

For example, while in a state of deep relaxation, a patient can be given the simple suggestion that "sensations typically interpreted as painful will now be experienced in a different, more positive way, perhaps as warm, tingly, itchy, or ticklish, whatever way is most comfortable for you." This kind of technique is called *symptom suppression*. And because the patient is in a state of focused attention and quite suggestible, he is highly receptive to the possibility that the part of his body that once felt "painful" now feels reasonably comfortable and relaxed. As J. A. Hadfield said, "suggestion does not consist of making an individual believe what is not true; suggestion consists of making something come true by making a person believe in its possibility."

Of course, symptom suppression is not a "cure" for the pain problem, for it does not deal with the cause of the pain nor the psychological trauma that may be associated with it. However, there are at least two reasons why it is useful.

Symptom suppression can "take the edge" from the pain. When a patient is in agonizing discomfort, it is difficult, if not impossible, for him to gain insight into his pain problem. But if some degree of relief can be provided, he may then be able to detach himself enough from his discomfort to try to understand its causes and effects.

As with other pain-management techniques, symptom suppression can sometimes be used to prove to a patient that it is possible for his pain to be controlled. Once he no longer feels completely helpless and hopeless, he can then begin to approach his pain problem more positively.

Symptom substitution is another hypnotic technique that has been applied successfully with patients with chronic pain. While not necessarily relieving pain, it involves moving the discomfort from one area of the body where it has been incapacitating to another where it is less disruptive. For example, most patients with migraine headaches prefer to experience them in the little finger instead of the head. Symptom substitution does not require the nervous system to inhibit pain or to mask the message it may be trying to communicate. The pain is still there, but it has moved to a part of the body where the patient can better overcome it.

The advantages of symptom substitution are similar to those of symptom suppression. It makes the pain more tolerable, thus allowing the patient to deal with it more effectively, and helps relieve oppressive feelings of helplessness and hopelessness. Once a patient recognizes that he can move his pain from, say, his head to his little finger or his big toe, he gains a profoundly clear sense of the extent to which his discomfort can be personally controlled.

Time Distortion and Age Regression

Another hypnotic technique for pain control is called *time distortion*. When patients report that "excruciating discomfort seems to drag on forever, while pain-free periods seem fleeting," time distortion may be helpful in reversing that situation.

Many patients can be hypnotized to experience time as being much slower or much faster than it is, objectively. For example, this technique has been used successfully with patients with advanced cancer for whom narcotics no longer provide relief. Under hypnosis, their painful times flash by so that hours seem like seconds. When they feel comfortable, however, the time moves so slowly that seconds seem like hours.

Age regression is also possible under hypnosis, and it can often be an indispensible therapeutic tool. Regression techniques can help a patient arrive at the basic causes of his pain by allowing him to remember traumatic events that may have been repressed or forgotten.

Frequently, when chronic pain is the outgrowth of an accident or injury, pain and suffering may primarily reflect the fears, anxieties, and threats of physical damage that accompanied the original trauma. By hypnotically regressing the patient to the time of the incident, and thus allowing him finally to confront and resolve it, discomfort can often be significantly alleviated.

Precautions and Limitations

In the hands of a well-trained, experienced therapist, hypnosis can be one of the most useful, safe, and successful modalities available for treatment of chronic pain. However, if it is used inappropriately, several problems may arise.[46,178,245] For example, hypnosis could lead to *traumatic insight*—that is, the sudden recollection of traumatic events that the patient is unable to deal with on a conscious level. If a patient is in a prepsychotic state, the inappropriate use of hypnosis could break down safeguards and defenses, thereby triggering a full-blown psychosis.

In addition, hypnosis may mask or transform the symptoms of an ailment without affecting its underlying cause. This should be kept in mind when patients who have experience with hypnosis are evaluated.

When age regression techniques are used, some patients react with panic. If, for example, a person regresses to the time of an automobile accident, he may experience the horror and terror of it all over again. Thus, regressive techniques must be used carefully, and if panic arises, competent psychotherapeutic support may be essential.

If conflicting or inappropriate posthypnotic suggestions are given, they can produce many disturbing effects, including anxiety, agitation, and increased physical discomfort. Even the most innocent suggestions can have traumatic consequences if, unknown to the therapist, they are associated with earlier traumatic events.

Most significant, when hypnosis is effective, the patient may credit the hypnotherapist for the improvement and become excessively dependent upon him for solving the problems associated with pain. A patient must be made aware that all hypnosis is essentially self-hypnosis and that his improvement is due to his own actions and responses, not those of the therapist's. In our opinion, a patient's best interests are served when he assumes responsibility for his own care, rather than being continually dependent on a therapist.

Guided Imagery

Many of the most successful hypnotic procedures—including symptom suppression and age regression—can be utilized more easily with the help of another technique called *guided imagery*. Through the creation of personalized mental images, guided imagery can be used to establish contact with the deepest levels of the subconscious mind.

Guided imagery does not require the formal, trancelike state characteristic of hypnosis to produce heightened suggestibility and its ensuing benefits. All that is needed is for the patient to become as relaxed and comfortable as possible. Thus, guided imagery is available to a larger number of people since it can be used effectively with patients who tend to be resistant to hypnosis.

Although guided imagery is a newer technique than hypnosis, both modalities probably operate through a similar mechanism—that is, guided imagery is in reality just a highly permissive, hypnotic procedure that utilizes the patient's images as the focus of its activity. Or, on the other hand, hypnosis is just a highly authoritative guided-imagery procedure, that utilizes the therapist's suggestions as the focus of its activity.

Despite guided imagery's recent emergence as a therapeutic tool, the importance of images and symbols has been known through history. The roots of this new technique may date to the ancient Hebrew mystics, who recognized the relationship of images to events that went far beyond normal experience. In more recent times, psychotherapists have utilized a variety of imagery techniques to tap the content of the subconscious mind. For example, Hermann Rorschach, the Swiss psychiatrist, employed standardized inkblot designs to assess the psychological relevance of various images and emotions to his patients' mental states.

Freud developed a technique he called *free association* as a way of reaching the subconscious. He believed that the subconscious was the storehouse of instinctual and forbidden desires and fears that were outside of conscious awareness, and through the images produced in free association, much of this rich information could be evaluated.

Carl Jung contended that the subconscious held more than just forbidden desires and fears and was also the repository of the deepest, most positive hopes for fulfillment and self-actualization. He developed several innovative imagery techniques designed to explore these aspects of the subconscious.[107]

As a growing number of therapists acknowledge the potential benefits of guided imagery, new techniques are constantly being developed.[6,102,140,151,183,198,199,214–217,220] One basic approach involves having the patient draw a symbolic picture of his or her discomfort. Such a picture can provide a more comprehensive perspective than can any verbal description.

For example, a patient may visualize facial pain as "a mouth on fire." With this image in mind, he can be asked to devise ways to extinguish the flames mentally. The innovative ways available for extinguishing a fire are limited only by the patient's imagination. One common approach is to visualize vividly the flames dissolving into cool, floating clouds of imaginary water that penetrate deeply into every cell of the area of discomfort.

One of the most powerful guided imagery approaches involves the creation of an "advisor," a "counselor," an "inner doctor," or a "spirit guide." The patient is first taught to relax and then is instructed on how to locate an imaginary living creature in his subconscious who thereafter serves as his advisor. These advisors have taken the form of everything from dogs and frogs to religious figures—but, of course, they are just a reflection of the person who is creating the image.

By definition, the advisor has access to the entire realm of the subconscious, that vast storehouse of insights, impulses, and desires. Through regular communication with his advisor, critically important information about a patient's inner world often emerges. Advisors frequently provide insights into past experiences that may have contributed to pain. They can offer advice on specific ways to relieve discomfort, and sometimes they can even produce instantaneous symptomatic pain relief.[29]

The advisor technique provides many advantages over traditional hypnotic approaches. When it is properly employed, for example, the problem of traumatic insight is easily avoided. If there is danger in breaking down a particular safeguard or defense, the advisor will usually refuse to pursue the matter until the patient is able to deal with it more effectively. In our experience, advisors never tell patients something they are not psychologically equipped to handle. Even more important, advisors can often tell exactly what must first be accomplished in order to make this information safely available.

Unlike hypnosis, guided imagery tends to decrease dependency on the therapist. After all, it is clearly the advisor, not the therapist, who is providing the insights that facilitate healing.

Although there are no proven complications resulting from guided imagery therapy, we do not recommend it for people who are emotionally hysterical, mentally unstable, schizophrenic, or prepsychotic. For these patients, guided imagery may some day prove to be as effective, or even more so, than conventional psychotherapy. But until more research has been conducted, it should be used with great discretion for such people.

PSYCHOTHERAPEUTIC APPROACHES

Psychiatric and Psychological Consultation

Because of the psychophysiologic nature of chronic pain, psychotherapy can often play a helpful role in a pain alleviation program.[108,167,188,222] Anxiety and depression are usually as much a part of the pain experience as the physical discomfort itself. In addition, each patient's reaction to painful stimuli may be related to personality factors and past experiences, which psychiatrists and psychologists are trained to investigate and identify.

A well-trained, competent psychotherapist can probably help all pain patients to some degree. He may, for example, be able to help someone deal with the everyday stresses that can profoundly exacerbate the pain experience. He may also help a patient through a "mourning" period that follows the death of a loved one. It is natural for a person to grieve after the loss of a loved one, but if mourning continues unabated for years, then psychotherapy may be indicated. Similarly, when an illness or injury has caused a person to be deprived of many of his pleasures, it is understandable that he might be depressed for awhile. But if depression continues for months or even years, then psychotherapy will be helpful, if not essential.

Secondary Gains

Some pain patients reap certain benefits or gains from their discomfort, and, on either a conscious or subconscious level, it becomes advantageous for them to maintain their pain. A typical gain occurs when a patient's pain helps him to manipulate others or to avoid various situations that he finds undesirable. If this benefit outweighs his discomfort, he may consciously or subconsciously decide that the gain is worth the pain.

For example, pain is one of the most effective ways to attract positive attention and sympathy. It can also provide financial rewards. Patients receiving workmen's compensation payments or other disability insurance payments related to their discomfort may be reluctant to relinquish the pain that provides a regular income for not working. Some patients may want to return to work, but they are too insecure about their prospects for obtaining well-paying or respectable employment. For them, the pain (and its accompanying insurance payments) becomes the lesser of two evils.

Patients may also cling to pain if they have litigation pending. When faced with an inability to work and large physician and hospital bills, most patients quickly recognize that a history of medical failures can be very advantageous when their case comes to court.

Pain can also be used to avoid human contact. It can provide the perfect excuse to postpone or cancel various social engagements or entanglements. Pain is also frequently a means of avoiding unwanted sexual encounters with a spouse or other person.

Pain fills other needs as well, including escape from existential problems such as "Why am I here?" or "Is there any meaning to life?"

Occasionally, a person's unwillingness to relinquish pain is based on fear of the unknown. Typically, such a patient will report, "I know what it's like to live with pain, but I've forgotten what it's like not to have it. I must admit that a part of me is afraid to see what would happen if my pain disappeared."

Finally, we have also observed patients who refuse to relinquish their pain because they believe it is a justified punishment for something they have done. It may be no mere coincidence that the word "pain" is derived from the Latin word *poena*, meaning punishment. In all of these situations, psychotherapy can be of enormous benefit.

Pain Games

As pain evolves from an acute phenomenon into chronic discomfort, a patient's personality often begins to reflect his medical dilemma significantly, and his entire life may start to become organized around his discomfort. He becomes, as Dr. Thomas Szasz has pointed out, an *homme douloureux* (*i.e.*, a pain person).[229] He literally makes a career of his pain for he does little else beside think and talk about it and consult doctors because of it. Without pain, his life would lose its focus for the pain experience has become as important as any profession.

Until the *homme douloureux* is extricated from his plight, he will usually avoid tackling the problem directly, often by playing "pain games" that sidestep any meaningful attempts at therapy.[20,211,222] One of the most familiar pain games might be called "The Addict" or "Cut Me." When it is played well, the dialogue between patient and physician might be like this:

Patient: Doctor, those pain pills you gave me last month just aren't helping me at all. Can't you cut a nerve or something?

Physician: Oh, let's not do anything that drastic. Why don't we try some stronger pills instead?"

In fact, the patient's sole intention from the outset is to obtain more potent medication, and the physician unknowingly satisfied that wish. If the physician had been more aware of this game, the dialogue might have proceeded quite differently.

Patient: Doctor, those pain pills you gave me last month haven't helped me at all. Can't you cut a nerve or something?

Physician: No, there's really no indication that cutting a nerve is appropriate. If the pain pills I've already given you haven't helped, I'm going to stop prescribing medication altogether. Why don't we try some other alternatives?

With this second approach, the game has been successfully frustrated, and, it is hoped, patient and physician can become more candid about both the pain problem and a possible dependence on drugs.

Another common pain game might be called "You Do It." Usually, it is played by a patient who has already been examined and treated by many physicians, some of whom are particularly well known and respected. Now, as the patient consults a new specialist, the scenerio may develop thus:

Physician: I see by your medical history that you've been to several other major medical centers throughout the nation. You've seen some very knowledgeable doctors, and none of them have been able to help you. How do you feel about that?

Patient: Yes, I've been to all those places, and not a single one of those so-called experts had a cure for my problem. What have you got for me?

The implicit message that the patient is attempting to communicate is, "It's up to you to heal me." This kind of patient is not willing to take any responsibility for his own treatment program for he expects someday to find a miracle worker to do it all for him.

Other common pain games include "Love Me or Leave Me." In this game, the patient with pain will be as unpleasant and uncooperative as possible with physicians as a way of testing to what extent they really care. Is the physician willing to tolerate brash and surly remarks by the patient? Or will he instead be so "insensitive" as to oust such an immature patient from his office?

A physician might be justified in feeling anger toward patients in pain who play such games, except that physicians also play games of their own. One of the games prevalent in the medical profession has been called "You're Just Too Dumb," which can be played in many situations. For instance, when a patient asks a question like "Why do I have arthritis?" some doctors refuse to spend the time on a lengthy explanation or are unwilling to admit that they simply do not know. Instead, they may respond, "The medical literature is too complex for a layman to understand. Trust me. I'm doing everything possible to make you feel better."

Some physicians also indulge in a game called "You're Imagining the Whole Thing," in which they are unwilling to work extensively with the patient, to spend the time needed to get to know him, or to empathize genuinely with his plight. Instead, they will briefly encourage him to deny his own experience and to accept the belief that the pain is not real. The patient knows otherwise, and, as a result, the credibility of all physicians is diminished in the patient's mind.

Certainly, pain games are inexcusable, whether engaged in by one or both parties in the doctor-patient relationship. A competent psychotherapist can often help pain patients to confront the games they may be playing and, eventually, to reverse such counterproductive behavior.

Of course, without a patient's full cooperation, the potential benefits of any type of psychotherapy are limited. Often, patients display strong resistance to psychotherapy because of fear. Some are frightened by the possibility that hidden, insidious mental factors may be involved in their chronic pain. Others fear that seeing a psychotherapist is a sign of "mental weakness." Still others are frightened to probe into the haunting guilt they might feel for some wrongdoing, having chosen instead to accept pain as a preferable form of punishment. Clearly, professional skills are needed to help such patients.

Operant Conditioning

One of the new psychological approaches for pain management is called *operant conditioning*, or *behavior modification*. With this technique, patients are rewarded for activities incompatible with pain behavior, and nonreinforced, or even punished for activities that perpetuate pain behavior. The administration of narcotic drugs, for example, is conducted on a *time-contingent* rather than a *symptom-contingent* basis—that is, medications are given, say, every 4 hours, regardless of a patient's pain level, rather than only when he hurts.

Under symptom-contingent conditions, the patient would receive narcotics every time he says, "I hurt," thus reinforcing each recurrence of his discomfort. Whenever he wants or needs more narcotics, his pain will flare up. But under time-contingency conditions, his receipt of medications does not depend in any way upon the intensity of his discomfort; thus, it reduces any drug-related incentive for him to hurt.

There are three major drawbacks to operant conditioning. First, the environment has to be very carefully controlled, which usually means that the patient must be hospitalized. Even if operant conditioning is successful in the hospital, once the patient moves back to his original, pain-reinforcing environment, his pain behavior can quickly return as if the operant conditioning had never even occurred.

Second, the goal of operant conditioning is to modify pain behavior, not necessarily the pain experience. As a result, it may produce changes in a patient's willingness to verbalize or demonstrate pain, but not necessarily any changes in his subjective amount of suffering and discomfort.

The third disadvantage to this approach is that the contingencies must be constantly and carefully scrutinized. We have seen some instances of operant conditioning in which it is unclear who is manipulating whom for what. Although a change in pain behavior has occurred, it merely reflects the patient's realization that he can achieve what he wants by pretending to be better. In a sense, the patient is conditioning the physician, not *vice versa*.

Counseling

Clearly, the family environment can significantly contribute to the pain problem, and to its resolution, as well. Thus, it is essential for the family to participate fully in the therapeutic process.

There are many ways in which family members can aggravate an illness.[67,78,100,101,116,171] For instance, the family can inadvertently reinforce pathologic behavior pattern, by giving love, affection, and attention to the patient only when he hurts. This conduct tends to reinforce pain because the discomfort then becomes the most effective means of ensuring that this positive emotional support will be continued.

In addition, various family conflicts, crises, and changes—whether related to the pain or not—can produce profound stress in the entire household, which will certainly tend to exacerbate the pain problem of the patient. The family can also sabotage patient compliance with prescribed therapy, simply by not offering encouragement for the program. Long-term change can be maintained only when the environment supports it.

Finally, other members of the family can actually profit firsthand from the patient's discomfort. By focusing so intently on his illness, they can justifiably divert attention away from other, more critical family issues, like a lack of love, the lack of communication, and excessive rivalries.

Although the family can significantly contribute to the pain problem, it may also be the key to overcoming it, with the help of appropriate family therapy. In essence, this counseling is a kind of psychotherapy in which the entire family unit is the patient, not just one person. The primary goal is not to change just one person but to alter the way the entire family interacts.

A skillful family therapist can help the family of the patient—and thus the patient himself—in many ways. For example, the family can be taught how to reinforce a healthy behavior pattern rather than a pathologic one. By giving love, affection, and attention to a patient when he doesn't hurt, the patient learns that feeling good is the most effective way of attaining this emotional support.

The therapist can help the family deal with its problem together, thus enhancing the likelihood of patient compliance with the recommended therapeutic program. Family camaraderie can also enhance the placebo effect of therapy, by elevating positive expectations and faith in the prescribed treatment.

Through counseling, the therapist can encourage families to cope more directly with other serious problems that have been overshadowed by pain. For instance, if the therapist assists the family in overcoming its communication barriers, pain will no longer be needed as the focus of family activity.

Family therapists can also serve as an educational resource for the family, teaching other members about the role that stress may have played in the patient's problems that may have been misunderstood. In addition, the therapist can encourage the family to develop personal health habits that can serve as a model for the patient.

Some therapists believe that family therapy is always beneficial, if not essential, for successful, long-term improvement for most patients with chronic pain. With the help of a sensitive and competent therapist, the family can become a critically important source of positive support.

Other kinds of counseling, such as nutritional, vocational, sexual, and even spiritual counseling, may be indicated in specific cases. It is the skilled pain therapist who knows how to utilize the diverse services of allied health professionals to achieve optimal therapeutic results. In many cases, this requires looking far beyond the physical symptoms that patients with chronic pain present.

SELF-CONTROL TECHNIQUES

The Importance of Self-Control

Recently, renewed interest has developed in the use of self-control techniques, which require the active participation of the patient in the therapeutic experience. These techniques include relaxation, biofeedback training, meditation, autogenic training, guided imagery, and other approaches. Their indications for pain control are described in detail elsewhere, but a few salient points can be noted here.[29]

Training in the use of self-control techniques may be one of the most effective ways to alleviate the feelings of helplessness that are so intimately related to the pain experience. Numerous laboratory studies with human subjects have shown that when people have the option of terminating an unpleasant situation, they are affected considerably less by it, even though they do not take the necessary steps to end it. Simply knowing that they have access to a solution makes their discomfort easier to bear. Furthermore, when subjects were allowed to administer shocks to themselves, they could endure stronger shocks and reported less pain than did other subjects who received the same shocks randomly.[126]

Unfortunately, very few studies have been conducted to explore self-control variables clinically, but it appears that the relationship among perceived control, pain tolerance, and the pain experience is complex.[76,236] Most modern treatment settings not only fail to encourage control by the patient but also actively discourage such participation by allowing little contribution from the patient or his family as the treatment plan is developed. Because the ability to control can be an important factor in the pain experience, clinicians should be attentive to their patients' need to control and should consider to what extent they are appropriate on a case-by-case basis.

Furthermore, treatments differ greatly in the amount of responsibility they demand from the patient, ranging from nerve blocks, which offer virtually no self-control possibilities, to relaxation training or biofeedback, in which success is almost exclusively the result of the patient's own efforts. We prefer to challenge patients with strategies that require degrees of self-control, in the belief that responsibility for personal care is an important step in relinquishing the chronic pain identity. Thus, we advocate therapeutic nerve blocks as the sole treatment only when it seems impossible for the patient to learn to take a more active role in his own life. We do not consider it reasonable to request a patient to surrender his identity as a dependent chronic pain patient while offering treatments that require only passive acquiescence at best.

An important part of the pain-control-unit program is a classroom in which patients and family members are instructed in the use of a variety of self-control procedures. Patients are asked to spend at least 30 minutes every day practicing self-management skills, and weekly class meetings focus on relaxation training, guided imagery, and ways to promote behavioral and attitudinal changes. Patients maintain personal journals and are required to turn in periodic homework assignments. Unlike group psychotherapy sessions in which patients confront their pressing problems, self-control classes represent an opportunity for patients to learn what to do about their problems.

Relaxation Training

For decades, researchers have suspected that there was an important link between stress and physical illness. Now this relationship has been well documented by hundreds of studies and thousands of individual medical histories.

Chronic psychosocial stress is an unfortunate aspect of 20th century life. Although stress has been a part of human existence since prehistoric times, the chief stresses for early man were acute or short-term environmental ones that could be effectively resolved with the "fight-or-flight" response. Today, man is faced with a far different situation for the significant contemporary stresses are chronic and are not usually resolved by the fight-or-flight response. As a result, anxiety, agitation, and a host of stress-related illnesses are epidemic.

More than 30 years ago, Beecher noted that the presence of anxiety, fear, and apprehension significantly influenced the perception of pain.[13,16] More recently, Evans has demonstrated that the reduction of anxiety (expressed either as a personality trait or as acute situational anxiety) potentiated the analgesic effects of a placebo.[58] Other investigators have found that if anxiety is dispelled and the subject is also given control over the pain-producing stimulus, the pain is perceived as significantly less painful than the same stimulus under conditions of high anxiety.[87–89,249]

One of the most effective ways to counteract anxiety in a self-control setting is through relaxation training.[27] Several research studies suggest that an integrated CNS reaction called the *relaxation response* may be associated with a significant reduction in both mental and physical suffering.[19] The response results in generalized decreased sympathetic nervous system activity and perhaps also increased parasympathetic activity. Its activation leads to hypo- or adynamic skeletal musculature, decreased blood pressure, decreased respiratory rate, and pupillary constriction. Daily elicitation of the response is of particular value when excessive sympathetic activity or anxiety is present.

One of the earliest approaches for eliciting the relaxation response was Jacobson's *progressive relaxation technique,* which utilized direct muscle manipulation.[99] Another early technique was *autogenic training,* a series of six basic exercises that were directed toward attaining specific physiologic responses characteristic of relaxation.[138,200,246] Exercise 1 focused on feelings of heaviness in the limbs; Exercise 2 on feelings of warmth; Exercise 3 on cardiac regulation; Exercise 4 on slow and regular breathing; Exercise 5 on warmth in the upper abdomen; and Exercise 6 on coolness in the forehead. After achieving mastery of these bodily relaxation exercises, the subject progressed to meditation exercises that utilized a variety of visual imagery techniques.

Relaxation training is almost universally beneficial to patients with pain, and those who diligently practice typically find that they can greatly decrease or modify their pain experience simply by entering a state of deep relaxation.

Biofeedback Training

For patients who have difficulty in learning to relax, a trial of biofeedback training may be beneficial. Biofeedback training is a technique whereby patients (with the aid of electronic devices) learn to regulate various physical functions once thought to be beyond voluntary control. For example, patients who suffer from muscular spasticity or tension can be taught to relax the muscles involved by monitoring their electromyographic (EMG) activity. When the correct mental strategy is discovered (by trial and error), EMG activity is decreased and an appropriate signal is instantaneously provided. Once the patient learns the relaxation response, the biofeedback training devices are no longer necessary.

Biofeedback has also been reported to be directly beneficial in the management of headaches, although this remains controversial.[34,159] What is clear, however, is that with proper training, patients can learn to achieve a remarkable degree of self-control. For example, some patients can learn to regulate finger temperature dramatically using a thermistor attached to a meter. If thermistors are placed on two fingers and the subject is asked to raise the temperature of one finger and to lower the other, a temperature differential between the two fingers of several degrees can be achieved. Differences as great as 13° have been reported.

Once a patient masters the biofeedback technique, he also acquires renewed self-confidence and self-control, which can help alleviate feelings of helplessness and depression. Biofeedback provides irrefutable, objective evidence that he can, in fact, control his own body.

Self-Therapy

Many of the procedures described above can also be utilized in a self-control setting. For example, when patients achieve positive results following acupuncture therapy, they are then taught how to locate the specific acupuncture points utilized and instructed to initiate acupressure or TENS therapy at home. The application of heat, cold, pressure, or touch is also appropriate on a self-therapy basis, as are regular movement and exercise programs.

One of the great advantages of guided imagery techniques is the ease with which patients can utilize them for self-therapy. Although they do not differ greatly in principle from self-hypnosis techniques, we find that patient compliance is much greater when formal induction can be avoided. In addition, patients report that their "inner advisors" are constant companions who are always available when needed.

The potential for transforming therapist-centered procedures into self-control techniques is a great creative challenge and one that most patients readily support. While clearly not indicated in the management of all chronic pain problems, we are impressed by how well our formerly dependent patients rise to the occasion and assume primary self-responsibility when the appropriate opportunity is presented.

New self-control techniques are constantly being developed, and soon, the primary role of the health-care practitioner may become that of diagnostician and teacher rather than therapist. In the area of pain control, the answer to man's greatest cry for help may soon be found inside man himself.

REFERENCES

1. Akil, H., and Liebeskind, J.C.: Monoaminergic mechanisms of stimulation-produced analgesia. Brain Res., *94*:279, 1975.
2. Akil, H., and Mayer, D.J.: Antagonism of stimulation-produced analgesia by p-CPA, a serotonin synthesis inhibitor. Brain Res., *44*:692, 1972.
3. Alexander, F.M.: The Resurrection of the Body. New York, Dell Publishing, 1971.
4. Amsterdam, E.A., Wolfson, S., and Gorlin, R.: New aspects of the placebo response in angina pectoris. Am. J. Cardiol., *24*:305, 1969.
5. Arthritis Foundation: Arthritis, The Basic Facts. Atlanta, The Arthritis Foundation, 1976.
6. Assagioli, R.: Psychosynthesis. New York, Viking Press, 1971.
7. Backman, H., Kalliola, H., and Ostling, G.: Placebo effect in peptic ulcer and other gastroduodenal disorders. Gastroenterologia, *94*:11, 1960.
8. Badaway, A.A.B., and Evans, M.: Tryptophan plus a pyrrolase inhibitor for depression. Lancet, *2*:869, 1975.
9. Barlow, W.: The Alexander Technique. New York, Alfred A. Knopf, 1973.
10. Basbaum, A.I., Marley, N., and O'Keefe, J.: Spinal cord pathways involved in the production of analgesia by brain stimulation. *In* Bonica, J.J., and Albe–Fessard, D.G. (eds.): Advances of Pain Research and Therapy, vol. I. Pp. 511–515. New York, Raven Press, 1976.
11. Beard, G., and Wood, E.: Massage: Principles and Techniques. Philadelphia, W.B. Saunders, 1964.
12. Becker, R.O., Reichmanis, M., Marino, A.A., and Spadaro, J.A.: Electrophysiological correlates of acupuncture points and meridians. Psychoenergetic Systems, *1*:105, 1976.
13. Beecher, H.K.: Pain in men wounded in battle. Ann. Surg., *123*:96, 1946.
14. ______: The powerful placebo. J.A.M.A., *159*:1602, 1955.
15. ______: Measurement of Subjective Responses. New York, Oxford University Press, 1959.
16. Beecher, H.K.: Surgery as a placebo. J.A.M.A., *176*:1102, 1961.
17. Belcombe, H.S.: Cases of sciatica and neuralgia, successfully treated by acupuncture. Medical Times and Gazette, *4*:85, 1852.
18. Bender, M.B.: Extinction and precipitation of cutaneous sensations. Arch. Neurol. Psychiatry, *54*:1, 1945.
19. Benson, H., Beary, J.F., and Carol, M.P.: The relaxation response. Psychiatry, *37*:37, 1974.
20. Berne, E.: Games People Play. New York, Grove Press, 1964.
21. Blitz, B., and Dinnerstein, A.J.: Effects of different types of instructions on pain parameters. J. Abnorm. Psychol., *73*:276, 1968.
22. Bowsher, D.: Treatment of intractable pain by acupuncture. Lancet, *2*:57, 1973.
23. Brav, E.A., and Sigmond, H.: Low back pain and acupuncture. Military Surgeon, *90*:545, 1942.
24. Brena, S.F.: Yoga and Medicine. Baltimore, Pelican Books, 1973.
25. Bresler, D.E.: Chinese medicine and holistic health. *In* Hastings, A., and Gordon, J. (eds.): Holistic Medicine: References for Health and Mental Health. Bethesda, National Institute of Mental Health, 1980.
26. ______: Electrophysiological and behavioral correlates of acupuncture therapy. *In* Reidak, Z. (ed.): Konference o Vyzkumu Psychotroniky. Prague, Sbornik Referatu, 1973.
27. ______: Conditioned relaxation: The pause that refreshes. *In* Gordon, J.S., Jaffe, D.T., and Bresler, D.E. (eds.): Mind, Body and Health: Toward an Integral Medicine. Bethesda, National Institute of Mental Health, 1980.

28. ______: Psychological Management of Pain: A Syllabus. Pacific Palisades, Center for Integral Medicine, 1976.
29. Bresler, D.E. with Trubo, R.: Free Yourself From Pain. New York, Simon and Schuster, 1979.
30. Bresler, D.E., Katz, R.L., Kroening, R.J., and Volen, M.P.: Acupuncture for Management of Chronic Pain: A Follow-Up Study. [Unpublished manuscript].
31. Bresler, D.E., and Kroening, R.J. Three essential factors in effective acupuncture therapy. American Journal of Chinese Medicine, *4*:81, 1976.
32. Bring, M.: Chinese acupuncture in sciatica therapy: Case report. Rev. Gen. Clin. Ther., *53*:486, 1939.
33. Bryan, G.T.: The role of urinary tryptophan metabolites in the etiology of bladder cancer. Am. J. Clin. Nutr., *24*:841, 1971.
34. Budzynski, T.H., and Stoyva, J.M.: An instrument for producing deep muscle relaxation by means of analog information feedback. J. Appl. Behav. Anal., *2*:231, 1969.
35. Calehr, H.: Acupuncture treatment of the asthmatic patient. Am. J. Med., *1*:41, 1973.
36. Cerney, J.V.: Acupuncture Without Needles. West Nyack, Parker Publishing, 1974.
37. Chan, P.: Finger Acupressure. Alhambra, Chan's Books, 1976.
38. Chang, H.T.: Integrative action of the thalamus in the process of acupuncture for analgesia. American Journal of Chinese Medicine, *2*:1, 1974.
39. Cheek, D.B., and LeCron, L.M.: Clinical Hypnotherapy. New York, Grune & Stratton, 1968.
40. Chen, K.C.: Effects of acupuncture and electroacupuncture on immunological reactions. Sansi Acupuncture Symposium, Sansi China Report, No. 102, 1959.
41. Chen, K.C.: Effects of electroacupuncture on the immunological reactions of rabbits to goat plasma anticoagulant facture. Sansi Acupuncture Symposium, Sansi China Report, No. 103, 1959.
42. Cheng, A.C.K.: The treatment of headaches employing acupuncture. American Journal of Chinese Medicine, *3*:181, 1975.
43. Chu, Y.M., and Affronti, L.F.: Preliminary observations on the effect of acupuncture on immune responses in sensitized rabbits and guinea pigs. American Journal of Chinese Medicine, *3*:151, 1975.
44. Coggeshall, R.E., Applebaum, M.L., Fazen, M., Stubbs, T.B., and Sykes, M.T.: Unmyelinated axons in human ventral roots, a possible explanation for the failure of dorsal rhizotomy to relieve pain. Brain, *98*:157, 1975.
45. Collens, W.F., Nulsen, F.E., and Randt, C.T.: Relation of peripheral nerve fiber size and sensation in man. Arch. Neurol., *3*:381, 1960.
46. Conn, J.H.: Is hypnosis really dangerous? Int. J. Clin. Exp. Hypn., *20*:61, 1972.
47. Copeman, W.S.C.: Fibrositis. J.A.M.A., *107*:1295, 1936.
48. Courage, G.R., and Huebsch, R.F.: Cold therapy revisited. J. Am. Dent. Assoc., *83*:1070, 1971.
49. Cox, B.M., Ophiem, K.E., Techmacher, H., and Goldstein, A.: A peptide-like substance from the pituitary that acts like morphine. Life Sc., *16*:1777, 1975.
50. Cracium, T.: Acupuncture treatment of vertebrogenic, cervical and lumbar syndromes. American Journal of Acupuncture, *2*:102, 1974.
51. Cracium, T., Toma, C., and Turdeanu, V.: Neurohumoral modifications after acupuncture. American Journal of Acupuncture, *1*:67, 1973.
52. Dahlstrom, A., and Fuxe, K.: Evidence for the existence of monamine-containing neurons in the central nervous system. Acta. Physiol. Scand., *247*:5, 1965.
53. Davis, M.: Understanding Body Movement. New York, Arno Press, 1972.
54. DeLangre, J.: Do-In. Magila, Happiness Press, 1972.
55. DeLateur, B.: The role of physical medicine in problems of pain. Adv. Neurol., *4*:495, 1974.
56. Downing, G.: The Massage Book. New York, Random House, 1970.
57. Duthie, A.M.: The use of phenothiazines and tricyclic antidepressants in the treatment of intractable pain. S. Afr. Med. J., *51*:246, 1977.
58. Evans, F.J.: The placebo response in pain reduction. Adv. Neurol., *4*:289, 1974.
59. Evans, W., and Hoyle, C.: The comparative value of drugs used in the continuous treatment of angina pectoris. Q. J. Med., *2*:311, 1933.
60. Ervin, F.R., Brown, C.E., and Mark, V.H.: Striatal influence on facial pain. Confin Neurol., *27*:75, 1966.
61. Faint, J.: Cold comfort—for alleviation of pain. Nursing Mirror, *132*:32, 1971.
62. Feldenkrais, M.: Body and Mature Behavior: A Study of Anxiety, Sex, Gravitation and Learning. New York, International Universities Press, 1949.
63. ______: Awareness Through Movement: Health Exercises for Personal Growth. New York, Harper Row, 1972.
64. Ferber, A., Mendelsohn, M., and Napier, A. (eds.): The Book of Family Therapy. New York, Science House, 1972.
65. Fernstrom, J.D.: Effects of the diet on brain neurotransmitters. Metabolism, *26*:207, 1977.
66. Fields, H.L: Secrets of the placebo. Psychology Today, *12*:172, 1978.
67. Fields, H.L., and Adams, J.E.: Pain after cortical injury relieved by electrical stimulation of the internal capsule. Brain, *97*:169, 1974.
68. Foer, W.H.: Percutaneous cervical radiofrequency cordotomy. J. Med. Soc. N. J., *68*:737, 1971.
69. Friedman, H., Nashold, B.S., and Somjen, G.: Physiological effects of dorsal column stimulation. *In* Bonica, J.J. (ed.): Advances in Neurology, vol. 4. New York, Raven Press, 1974.
70. Gammon, G.D., and Starr, I.: Studies on the relief of pain by counter-irritation. J. Clin. Invest., *20*:13, 1941.
71. Gebhardt, K.H., Beller, J., and Nischk, R.: Behandlung des Karzenomschmerzes mit Chlorimipramin (Anafranil). Med. Klin., *64*:751, 1969.
72. Gol, A.: Relief of pain by electrical stimulation of the septal area. J. Neurol. Sci., *5*:115, 1967.
73. Goldstein, A., and Hilgard, E.R.: Lack of influence of the morphine antagonist naloxone on hypnotic analgesia. Proc. Natl. Acad. Sci. U.S.A., *72*:2041, 1975.
74. Gonda, T.A.: The relationship between complaints of persistent pain & family size. J. Neurol. Neurosurg. and Psychiatry, *25*:277, 1962.
75. Goulden, E.A.: Treatment of sciatica by galvanic acupuncture. Br. Med. J., *1*:523, 1921.
76. Graig, K.D., and Best, J.A.: Perceived control over pain: Individual differences and situational determinants. Pain, *3*:127, 1977.
77. Gresser, E.: Successful treatment of trigeminal neuralgia by acupuncture following neurosurgery. American Journal of Acupuncture, *1*:101, 1973.
78. Haley, J.: Strategies of Psychotherapy. New York, Grune & Stratton, 1966.
79. Halpern, L.M.: Analgesics and other drugs for relief of pain. Postgrad. Med., *53*:91, 1973.
80. Hannington-Kiff, J.G.: Pain Relief. Philadelphia, J.B. Lippincott, 1974.

81. Hart, L.A.: Anybody Can Do It: Acupressure. New York, Lynn Mark Library, 1977.
82. Hartman, E.: Hypnotic effects of L-tryptophan. Arch. Gen. Psychiatry, *31*:394, 1974.
83. ______: L-Tryptophan: A rational hypnotic with clinical potential. Am. J. Psychiatry, *134*:366, 1977.
84. Herrington, R.N., Bruce, A., Johnstone, E.C., and Lader, M.H.: Comparative trial of L-tryptophan and amitriptyline in depressive illness. Psychol. Med., *6*:673, 1976.
85. Hiep, N., and Stallard, R.E.: Acupuncture—A valuable adjunct in the treatment of myofascial pain. J. Dent. Res., *53*:203, 1974.
86. Hilgard, E.R., and Hilgard, J.R.: Hypnosis in the Relief of Pain. Los Altos, Wm. Kaufmann, 1975.
87. Hill, H.E., Belleville, R.E., and Wikler, A.: Studies on anxiety associated with anticipation of pain. Arch. Neurol. Psychiatry, *73*:602, 1955.
88. Hill, H.E., Kornetsky, C.H., Flanary, H.G., and Wikler, A.: Effects of anxiety and morphine on discrimination of intensities of painful stimuli. J. Clin. Invest., *31*:473, 1952.
89. ______: Studies on anxiety associated with anticipation of pain. I. Effects of morphine. AMA Archives of Neurology and Psychiatry, *67*:612, 1952.
90. Hittleman, R.L.: Yoga for Physical Fitness. Englewood Cliffs, Prentice-Hall, 1964.
91. ______: Introduction to Yoga. New York, Bantam Books, 1969.
92. Hosobuchi, Y., Adams, J.E., and Rutkin, B.: Chronic thalamic stimulation for the control of facial anesthesia dolorosa. Arch. Neurol., *29*:158, 1973.
93. Houde, R.W.: The use and misuse of narcotics in the treatment of chronic pain. Adv. Neurol., *4*:527, 1974.
94. Houston, F.M.: The Healing Benefits of Acupressure. New Canaan, Keats Publishing, 1974.
95. Hu, H.H.: Therapeutic effects of acupuncture: A review. American Journal of Acupuncture, *2*:8, 1974.
96. Hughes, J., *et al.*: Identification of two related pentapeptides from the brain with potent opiate agonist activity. Nature, *258*:577, 1975.
97. Hymes, A.C., Roab, D.E., Yonehira, E.G., Nelson, G.D., and Printz, A.L.: Electrical surface stimulation for the control of acute post-operative pain and prevention of ileus. Surgical Forum, *25*:222, 1974.
98. Ionescu–Tirgoviste, C.: Theory of mechanism of action in acupuncture. American Journal of Acupuncture, *1*:193, 1973.
99. Jacobson, E.: Progressive Relaxation. Chicago, University of Chicago Press, 1938.
100. Jaffe, D.T.: Family therapy and physical illness. *In* Gordon, J., Jaffe, D., and Bresler, D. (eds.): Mind, Body and Health: Toward an Integral Medicine. Bethesda, National Institute of Mental Health, 1980.
101. ______: Healing from Within. New York, Alfred A. Knopf, 1979.
102. Jaffe, D.T., and Bresler, D.E.: Guided imagery: Healing through the mind's eye. *In* Gordon, J.S., Jaffe, D.T., and Bresler, D.E. (eds.): Mind, Body and Health: Toward an Integral Medicine. Bethesda, National Institute of Mental Health, 1980.
103. Jamison, K., Brechner, M.T., Brechner, V.L., and McCreary, C.P.: Correlation of personality profile with pain syndrome. *In* Bonica, J.J., and D. Albe–Fessard (eds.): Advances in Pain Research and Therapy, vol. 1. Pp. 317–321. New York, Raven Press, 1976.
104. Jellinek, E.M.: Clinical tests on comparative effectiveness of analgesic drugs. Biometrics Bull., *2*:87, 1946.
105. Jensen, K., *et al.*: Tryptophan/Imipramine in Depression. Lancet, *2*:920, 1975.
106. Joyce, C.R.B.: Consistent differences in individual reactions to drugs & dummies. Br. J. Pharmacol., *14*:512, 1959.
107. Jung, C.: Man and His Symbols. Garden City, Doubleday and Co., 1964.
108. Kahn, J.P.: How a psychiatrist looks at pain. Med. Times, *98*:127, 1970.
109. Kajdos, V.: Acupuncture therapy of secondary torticollis. American Journal of Acupuncture, *1*:183, 1973.
110. Kane, K., and Taub, A.: A history of local electrical analgesia. Pain, *1*:125, 1975.
111. Katz, R.L., Kao, L.Y., Spiegel, H., and Katz, G.J.: Pain, acupuncture, hypnosis. Adv. Neurol., *4*:819, 1974.
112. Kim, K.C., and Yount, R.A.: The effect of acupuncture on migraine headache. American Journal of Chinese Medicine, *2*:407, 1974.
113. ______: The effect of acupuncture on low back pain. American Journal of Chinese Medicine, *2*:421, 1974.
114. Kocher, R.: Use of psychotropic drugs for the treatment of chronic severe pain. *In* Bonica, J.J., and Albe–Fessard, D. (eds.): Advances in Pain Research and Therapy. vol. 1. Pp. 579–582. New York, Raven Press, 1976.
115. Kosterlitz, H.W., and Hughes, J.: Possible physiological significance of enkephalin, an endogenous ligand of opiate receptors. *In* Bonica, J.J., and Albe-Fessard, D. (eds.): Advances in Pain Research and Therapy, vol. 1. Pp. 641–645. New York, Raven Press, 1976.
116. Kovel, J.: A Complete Guide to Therapy. New York, Pantheon Books, 1976.
117. Krieger, D.: Therapeutic touch: The imprimatur of nursing. Am. J. Nurs., *75*:784, 1975.
118. ______: Healing by the laying-on-of-hands as a facilitator of bioenergetic change: The response of in-vivo hemoglobin. Psychoenergetic Systems, *1*:121–129, 1976.
119. ______: Therapeutic touch: A reality base for alternative health practices. *In* Gordon, J., Jaffe, D., and Bresler, D. (eds.): Mind, Body and Health: Toward an Integral Medicine. Bethesda, National Institute of Mental Health, 1980.
120. Kroening, R.J., Volen, M.P., and Bresler, D.E.: Acupuncture: Current status and clinical indications for American medicine. *In* Gordon, J., Jaffe, D., and Bresler, D. (eds.): Mind, Body and Health: Toward an Integral Medicine. Bethesda, National Institute of Mental Health, 1980.
121. Kroger, W.S.: Clinical and Experimental Hypnosis. Philadelphia, J.B. Lippincott, 1963.
122. Kroger, W.S., and Fezler, W.D.: Hypnósis and Behavior Modification: Imagery Conditioning. Philadelphia, J.B. Lippincott, 1976.
123. Lasagna, L., *et al.*: A study of the placebo response. Am. J. Med., *16*:770, 1954.
124. Lee, G.T.C.: A study of electrical stimulation of acupuncture locus Tsusanli (ST-36) on mesenteric microcirculation. American Journal of Chinese Medicine, *2*:1, 1974.
125. Lee, R., and Spencer, P.S.J.: Antidepressants and pain: A review of the pharmacological data supporting the use of certain tricyclics in chronic pain. J. Int. Med. Res., *5*:146, 1977.
126. Lefcourt, H.M.: Locus of Control. New York, John Wiley & Sons, 1976.
127. Liebeskind, J.C.: Pain modulation by central nervous system stimulation. *In* Bonica, J.J., and Albe–Fessard, D.G. (eds.): Advances in Pain Research and Therapy, vol. 1. Pp. 445–453. New York, Raven Press, 1976.
128. Liebeskind, J.C., and Paul, L.A: Psychological and physiological mechanisms of pain. Ann. Review. Psychol., *28*:41, 1977.

129. Linzer, M., and Long, D.M.: Transcutaneous neural stimulation for relief of pain. I.E.E.E. Trans. Biomed. Eng., *23*:341, 1976.
130. Liu, Y.K.: The correspondence between some motor points and acupuncture loci. American Journal of Chinese Medicine, *3*:347, 1975.
131. Loeser, J., Black, R., and Christman, A.: Relief of pain by transcutaneous stimulation. J. Neurosurg., *42*:308, 1975.
132. Long, D.M.: Cutaneous afferent stimulation for the relief of pain. Progress in Neurological Surgery, *7*:35, 1976.
133. Long, D.M., and Carolan, M.T.: Cutaneous afferent stimulation in the treatment of chronic pain. *In* Bonica, J.J., (ed.): Advances in Neurology. vol. 4. New York, Raven Press, 1974.
134. Long, D.M., and Erickson, D.E.: Stimulation of the posterior columns of the spinal cord for relief of intractable pain. Surg. Neurol., *4*:134, 1975.
135. Long, D.M., and Hagfors, N.: Electrical stimulation of the nervous system: The current status of electrical stimulation of the nervous system for relief of pain. Pain, *1*:109, 1975.
136. Looney, G.L.: Acupuncture study. J.A.M.A., *228*:1522, 1974.
137. Lung, C.H., Sun, A.C., Tsao, C.J., Chang, Y.L., and Fan, L.: An observation of the humoral factor in acupuncture analgesia in rats. American Journal of Chinese Medicine, *2*:203, 1974.
138. Luthe, W. (ed.): Autogenic Therapy. New York, Grune & Stratton, 1969.
139. McGlashan, T.H., Evans, F.J., and Orne, M.T.: The Nature of hypnotic analgesia and placebo response to experimental pain. Psychosom. Med., *31*:227, 1969.
140. McKim, R.H.: Experiences in Visual Thinking. Monterey, Brooks/Cole, 1972.
141. MacSweeney, D.A.: Treatment of Unipolar Depression. Lancet, *2*:510, 1975.
142. Man, P.L., and Chen, A.: Acupuncture analgesia for the treatment of trigeminal neuralgia: A series of 41 cases. Diseases of the Nervous System, *35*:520, 1974.
143. ———: Two year follow-up study on 182 chronic pain patients. American Journal of Acupuncture, *3*:143, 1975.
144. Man, P.L., and Chen, C.H.: Mechanisms of acupunctural anesthesia; Two gate theory. Diseases of the Nervous System, *33*:730, 1972.
145. ———: Acupuncture for pain relief: A double-blind, self-controlled study. Mich. Med., *73*:15, 1974.
146. Mann, F.: The Treatment of Disease by Acupuncture. London, Heinemann, 1963.
147. ———: The Meridians of Acupuncture. London, Heinemann, 1964.
148. ———: Acupuncture: Cure of Many Diseases. London, Heinemann, 1971.
149. ———: Acupuncture—The Ancient Chinese Art of Healing and How It Works Scientifically. New York, Random House, 1974.
150. Maroon, J.C., Holst, R.A., and Osgood, C.P.: Chymopapain in the treatment of ruptured lumbar discs. J. Neurolog. Neurosurg. Psychiatry, *39*:508, 1976.
151. Masters, R., and Houston, J.: Mind Games. New York, Viking Press, 1972.
152. Matsumoto, T., Levy, B., and Ambruso, V.: Clinical evaluation of acupuncture. Am. Surg., *40*:400, 1974.
153. Matsumoto, T., and Lyu, B.S.: Anatomical comparison between acupuncture and nerve block. Am. Surg. *41*:11, 1975.
154. Mayer, D.J., and Liebeskind, J.C.: Pain reduction by focal electrical stimulation of the brain: An anatomical and behavioral analysis. Brain Res., *68*:73, 1974.
155. Mayer, D.J., and Price, D.D.: Central nervous system mechanisms of analgesia. Pain, *2*:379, 1976.
156. Mayer, D.J., Price, D.D., and Rafii, A.: Antagonism of acupuncture analgesia in man by the narcotic antagonist naloxone. Brain Res., *121*:368, 1977.
157. Mayer, D.J., Wolfle, T.L., Akil, H., Carder, B., and Liebeskind, J.C.: Analgesia from electrical stimulation in the brainstem of the rat. Science, *174*:1351, 1971.
158. Mazars, G.J.: Intermittent stimulation of nucleus ventralis posterolateralis for intractable pain. Surg. Neurol., *4*:93, 1975.
159. Medina, J.L., Diamond, S., and Franklin, M.A.: Biofeedback therapy for migraine. Headache, *16*:115, 1976.
160. Melzack, R.: How acupuncture can block pain. Impact of Science on Society, *23*:65, 1973.
161. ———: The Puzzle of Pain. New York, Basic Books, 1973.
162. Melzack, R., and Scott, T.H.: The effects of early experience on the response to pain. J. Physiol. and Comp. Psychol., *50*:155, 1957.
163. Melzack, R., Stillwell, D.M., and Fox, E.J.: Trigger points and acupuncture points for pain: Correlations and implications. Pain, *3*:3, 1977.
164. Melzack, R., and Wall, P.: Pain mechanisms: A new theory. Science, *150*:971, 1965.
165. Mennell, J.M.: The therapeutic use of cold. J.A.O.A., *74*:1146, 1975.
166. Merskey, H.: Psychiatric aspects of the control of pain. *In* Bonica, J.J., and Albe–Fessard, D. (eds.): Advances in Pain Research and Therapy, vol. 1. Pp. 711–716. New York, Raven Press, 1976.
167. Merskey, H., and Spear, F.G.: Pain: Psychological and Psychiatric Aspects. London, Bailliere, Tindall and Cassell, 1967.
168. Miller, N.E.: Central stimulation and other new approaches to motivation and reward. Am. Psychol., *13*:100, 1958.
169. Mishra, R.: Yoga Sutras: The Textbook of Yoga Psychology. Garden City, Doubleday and Co., 1973.
170. ———: Fundamentals of Yoga. Garden City, Doubleday and Co., 1974.
171. Minuchin, S.: Families and Family Therapy. Cambridge, Howard University Press, 1974.
172. Moertel, G.G., Taylor, W.F., Roth, A., and Tyce, F.A.J.: Who responds to sugar pills? Mayo Clin. Proc., *51*:96, 1976.
173. Montagu, A.: Touching: The Human Significance of Human Skin. New York, Harper Row, 1972.
174. Moss, L.: Relief of Pain by Acupuncture. Lancet, *2*:320, 1973.
175. Murphy, A.J.: The physiological effects of cold application. Physical Therapy Review, *40*:112, 1960.
176. Nashold, B.S., Jr.: Dorsal column stimulation for control of pain: a three-year follow-up. Surg. Neurol., *4*:146, 1975.
177. Nemerof, H.: Clinical experiences with acupuncture. J.A.O.A., *71*:866, 1972.
178. Nesbitt, W.R.: The dangers of hypnotherapy. Med. Times, *92*:597, 1964.
179. Nissen, H.W., Chow, K.L., and Semmes, J.: Effects of restricted opportunity for tactual, kinesthetic & manipulative experience on the behavior of a chimpanzee. Am. J. Psychol., *64*:485, 1951.
180. Notermans, S.L.: Measurement of pain threshold determined by electrical stimulation and its clinical application: Methods and factors possibly influencing pain threshold. Neurology, *16*:1071, 1966.
181. Olds, J.: Self-stimulation of the brain. Science, *127*:315, 1958.
182. Omura, Y.: Effects of acupuncture on blood pressure, leu-

kocytes and serum lipids and lipoproteins in essential hypertension. Fed. Proc., *33*:430, 1974.

183. Oyle, I.: The Healing Mind. Millbrae, Celestial Arts, 1975.
184. Palos, S.: The Chinese Art of Healing. New York, Herder & Herder, 1971.
185. Paulley, J.W., and Haskell, D.J.: Treatment of migraine without drugs. J. Psychosom. Res., *19*:367, 1975.
186. Peng, A.T.C., Omura, Y., Cheng, H.C., and Blancato, L.S.: Acupuncture for relief of chronic pain and surgical anesthesia. Am. Surg., *40*:50, 1974.
187. Pepeu, G.: Involvement of central transmitters in narcotic analgesia. *In* Bonica, J.J., and Albe-Fessard, D. (eds.): Advances in Pain Research and Therapy, vol. 1. Pp. 595–600. New York, Raven Press, 1976.
188. Pilowsky, I.: The psychiatrist and the pain clinic. Am. J. Psychiatry, *133*:752, 1976.
189. Pomeranz, B.: Brain opiates at work in acupuncture? New Scientist, *73*:12, 1977.
190. Pomeranz, B., and Chiu, D.: Naloxone blockade of acupuncture analgesia: Endorphin implicated. Life Sci., *19*:1757, 1976.
191. Pool, J.L.: Psychosurgery in older people. J. Am. Geriatr. Soc., *2*:456, 1954.
192. Ray, C.D., and Maurer, D.D.: Electrical neurological stimulation systems: A review of contemporary methodology. Surgical Neurology, *4*:82, 1975.
193. Reichmanis, M., Marino, A.A., and Becker, R.O.: Electrical correlates of acupuncture points. I.E.E.E. Trans. Biomed. Eng., *22*:533, 1975.
194. ———: D.C. skin conductance variation at acupuncture loci. American Journal of Chinese Medicine, *4*:69, 1976.
195. Richardson, D.E.: Brain stimulation for pain control. I.E.E.E. Trans. Biomed. Eng., *23*:304, 1976.
196. Roeser, W.M., Meeks, L.W., Venis, R., and Strickland, E.: The use of transcutaneous nerve stimulation for pain control in athletic medicine. Am. J. Sports Med., *4*:210, 1976.
197. Rosenberg, R.P.: Acupuncture used in the treatment of arthralgias. American Journal of Acupuncture, *2*:283, 1974.
198. Samuels, M., and Bennett, H.: Spirit Guides. New York, Random House, and Berkeley, Bookworks, 1974.
199. Samuels, M., and Samuels, N.: Seeing with the Mind's Eye. New York, Random House, and Berkeley, Bookworks, 1975.
200. Schultz, J.H., and Luthe, W.: Autogenic Approach in Psychotherapy. New York, Grune & Stratton, 1959.
201. Scott, D.L.: Modern Hospital Hypnosis. Chicago, Year Book Medical Publishers, 1974.
202. Scott, W.A.M.: The relief of pain with an antidepressant in arthritis. Practitioner, *202*:802, 1969.
203. Serizawa, K.: Massage: The Oriental Method. Tokyo, Japan Publications, 1972.
204. ———: Tsubo: Vital Points for Oriental Therapy. Tokyo, Japan Publications, 1976.
205. Shanghai Medical Group Acupuncture Anesthesia Group: Study of relations between the acupuncture points and surrounding nervous structure by anatomical dissection, Liberation Daily News, January 5, 1972.
206. Shapiro, A.K.: Factors contributing to the placebo effect: their implications for psychotherapy. Am. J. Psychother., *18*:73, 1961.
207. ———: Psychological aspects of medication. *In* Lief, H.I., Lief, V.F., and Lief, N.R. (eds.): The Psychological Basis of Medical Practice. Pg. 167. New York, Harper & Row, 1963.
208. Shealy, C.N.: Six years' experience with electrical stimulation for control of pain. *In* Bonica, J.J. (ed.): Advances in Neurology, vol. 4. New York, Raven Press, 1974.
209. ———: Transcutaneous electrical stimulation for control of pain. Clin. Neurosurg., *21*:269, 1974.
210. ———: Dorsal column stimulation: optimization of application. Surg. Neurol., *4*:142, 1975.
211. ———: The Pain Game. Millbrae, Celestial Arts, 1976.
212. Shealy, C.N., Mortimer, J.T., and Hagfors, N.R.: Dorsal column electroanalgesia. J. Neurosurg., *32*:560, 1970.
213. Shen, A.C., Whitehouse, T.R., and Young, R.C.: A pilot study of the effects of acupuncture in rheumatoid arthritis. Arthritis Rheum., *16*:559, 1973.
214. Shorr, J.E.: Go See the Movie in Your Head. New York, Popular Library, 1977.
215. Simonton, O.C., Matthews-Simonton, S., and Creighton, J.: Getting Well Again, Los Angeles, J.P. Tarcher, 1978.
216. Singer, J.L.: Imagery and Daydream Methods in Psychotherapy and Behavior Modification. New York, Academic Press, 1974.
217. ———: The Inner World of Daydreaming. New York, Harper & Row, 1975.
218. Sjohund, B., Terenius, L., and Erikeson, M.: Increased cerebrospinal fluid levels of endorphins after electroacupuncture. Acta Physiol. Scand., *100*:382, 1977.
219. Small, T.J.: The neurophysiological basis for acupuncture. American Journal of Acupuncture, *2*:77, 1974.
220. Sommer, R.: The Mind's Eye. New York, Delta, 1978.
221. Sternbach, R.A.: Pain: A Psychophysiological Analysis. New York, Academic Press, 1968.
222. ———: Pain Patients: Traits and Treatment. New York, Academic Press, 1974.
223. ———: Psychological factor in pain. *In* Bonica, J.J., and Albe-Fessard, D. (eds.): Advances in Pain Research and Therapy, vol. 1. Pp. 293–299. New York, Raven Press, 1976.
224. Sternbach, R.A., Janowsky, D.S., Huey, L.Y., and Segal, D.S.: Effects of altering brain serotonin activity on human chronic pain. *In* Bonica, J.J., and Albe-Fessard, D. (eds.): Advances in Pain Research and Therapy, vol. 1. Pp. 601–606. New York, Raven Press, 1976.
225. Stevens, T.J.: Sciatica treatment by acupuncture. Boston Medical and Surgical Journal, *2*:392, 1869.
226. Stonnington, H.H., Stillwell, G.K., Ebersord, M.J., Thorsteinsson, G., and Laws, E.R.: Transcutaneous electrical stimulation for chronic pain relief. Minn. Med., *59*:681, 1976.
227. Sturdevant, R.A.L., Isenberg, J.I., Secrist, D., and Ansfield, J.: Antacid and placebo produced similar pain relief in duodenal ulcer patients. Gastroenterology, *72*:1, 1977.
228. Sweet, W.H., and Wepsic, J.G.: Treatment of chronic pain by stimulation of fibers of primary afferent neuron. Trans. Am. Neurol. Assoc., *93*:103, 1968.
229. Szasz, T.S.: The psychology of persistent pain: A portrait of l'homme douloureux. *In* Soulairac, A., Cahn, J., and Charpentier, J. (eds.): Pain. New York, Academic Press, 1968.
230. Tashkin, D.P., *et al.*: Comparison of real and simulated acupuncture and isoproterenol in methacholine-induced asthma. Ann. Allergy, *39*:379, 1977.
231. Teale, T.P.: On the relief of pain and muscular disability by acupuncture. Lancet, *1*:567, 1871.
232. Terenius, L., and Walhstrom, A.: Search for an endogenous ligand for the opiate receptor. Acta Physiol. Scand., *94*:74, 1975.
233. Thorsteinsson, G., Stonnington, H.H., Stillwell, G.K., and Elveback, L.R.: Transcutaneous electrical stimulation: A

double-blind trial of its efficacy for pain. Arch. Phys. Med. Rehab., *58*:8, 1977.

234. Tien, H.C.: Acupuncture anesthesia: neurogenic interference theory. World Journal of Psychosynthesis, *4*:36, 1972.
235. ______: Neurogenic interference theory of acupuncture anesthesia. American Journal of Chinese Medicine, *1*:105, 1973.
236. Toomey, T.C., Ghia, J.N., Mao, W., and Gregg, J.M.: Acupuncture and chronic pain mechanisms: The moderating effects of affect, personality, and stress on response to treatment. Pain, *3*:137, 1977.
237. Traut, E.F., and Passarelli, E.W.: Placebos in the treatment of rheumatoid arthritis and other rheumatic conditions. Ann. Rheum. Dis., *16*:18, 1957.
238. Van der Ark, G.D., and McGrath, K.: Transcutaneous electrical stimulation in treatment of postoperative pain. Am. J. Surg., *130*:338, 1975.
239. Vanderschot, L.: Trigger points vs. acupuncture points. American Journal of Acupuncture, *4*:233, 1976.
240. Wall, P.D.: Presynaptic control of impulses at the first central synapse in the cutaneous pathway. Prog. Brain Res., *12*:92, 1964.
241. Wall, P.D., and Sweet, W.H.: Temporary abolition of pain in man. Science, *155*:108, 1967.
242. Wancera, I., and Konig, G.: On the neurophysiological explanation of acupuncture analgesia. American Journal of Chinese Medicine, *2*:193, 1974.
243. Weintraub, M.: Acupuncture in musculoskeletal pain. Methodology and results in a double-blind, controlled clinical trial. Clin. Pharmacol. Therap., *17*:248, 1975.
244. Wen, H.L., and Chan, K.: Status asthmaticus treated by acupuncture and electrostimulation. Asian Journal of Medicine, *9*:191, 1973.
245. West, L.J., and Deckert, G.H.: Dangers of Hypnosis. J.A.M.A., *192*:9, 1965.
246. White, J., and Fadiman, J.: Relax. New York, Dell, 1976.
247. Yang, K.C., *et al.*: Relationship between acupuncture—moxibustion and infection and immunity. *In* Yu, H., and Hsieh, S. W. (eds.): Advances in Immunity. p. 140. Shanghai, Shanghai Science and Technology Press, 1962.
248. Zborowski, M.: People in Pain. San Francisco, Jossey-Bass, 1969.
249. Zenhausern, R., Moroney, W., and Lepanto, R.: Experimental pain. Science, *152*:1645, 1966.

29 Percutaneous Spinothalamic Tractotomy: The Prototype of Neurosurgical Pain Control

Sampson Lipton and
James E. McLennan

NEURAL BLOCKADE FOR RELIEF OF PAIN

. . . Every psychophysical motion rising above the threshold of consciousness is attended by pleasure in proportion as, beyond a certain limit, it approximates to complete stability, and is attended by unpleasure in proportion as, beyond a certain limit, it deviates from complete stability; while between the two limits, which may be described as qualitative thresholds of pleasure and unpleasure, there is a certain margin of aesthetic indifference . . .[12]

Pleasure and pain occupy polar positions in the continuum of human states of being; they define a necessary relationship to the outer world. These characteristics of humanity are consistent in higher mammals as well, and somewhere down the phylogenetic chain, they merge imperceptibly into a reflex response to a noxious stimulus. Human pain and suffering are not well defined either qualitatively or in quantity; C. S. Lewis, for example, explicates the complexities of behavioral aspects of suffering in a manner seldom discerned by physicians.[15,27] It is perhaps an axiom unique to the nervous system and akin to various uncertainty principles that in dealing with pain, the system that is "sick" is identical to that through which the organism reacts to the disorder—, for example, a reliable history or description of brain disease cannot be provided by a patient who harbors a lesion liable to alter function of that organ. A patient with pain may not report reliably on pain.

Countless maneuvers have been applied to the patient with pain. As neuroanatomists and neurophysiologists defined specific structures of the nervous system that subserve pain, many procedures naturally arose designed to alter or disrupt these pathways. Having a knife handy, neurosurgeons have no doubt been guilty of an egregious mixture of empathy and excessive enthusiasm on behalf of the suffering patient. Despite a number of striking results, this enthusiasm has slowly been diminished by the realization that the treatment of pain is not as straightforward as it once appeared. Short of total pain relief through general anesthesia, almost all pain treatment maneuvers have obvious shortcomings. What about the awake, ambulatory, rational patient with chronic pain, whose psychological profile has become altered in a predictable and well-studied manner?[46] What is the current perspective on appropriate selection from the multitude of possible modalities for relief? Who should take primary responsibility for the care or cure of these patients?

This chapter reviews the neurosurgeon's contribution to the problem of pain as background to detailing the surgical method for a prototype neural blockade, the radiofrequency percutaneous spinothalamic tractotomy. It is apparent that many of the possible procedures cited in Table 29-1 are seldom used at present; in particular, the rise of percutaneous needle and electrode techniques has vitiated a number of surgical pain-relieving operations. Almost without exception, patients with chronic pain are treated by local or regional transcutaneous blocking and electrical stimulation techniques prior to consideration for surgery. Chemical blockade may be repeated frequently, often in an outpatient setting. Surgery may often be postponed indefinitely.

Short of cutting or surgical manipulation of a pain-carrying or -modulating structure, neural blockade may be accomplished by several methods. Aside from the use of chemical agents, (discussed throughout most of the rest of this book), relief can also be achieved by the radiofrequency (thermal) lesion. The results of this technique do not depend upon electricity to alter the nervous system but rather utilize the by-product of heat to devitalize nerve fibers differentially. Variations in methodology for performance of the radiofrequency (RF) chordotomy are referenced in the literature; these articles should be consulted in detail before undertaking the procedure.

Table 29-1. Overview of Neurosurgical Control of Pain in Humans

Anatomic Level	*Specific Structures**	*Possible Procedures*
Cortex	Parietal; second sensory cortex	Corticectomy[2,6,31]
Hemisphere white matter tracts	Corona radiata	Leukotomy, RF[31]
	Intercortical U-fibers	Leukotomy
	Thalamofrontal fibers	Leukotomy, RF[16]
	Internal capsule	Stimulation[1]
Limbic system	Cingulate gyri	RF, surgical cingulotomy[9,44]
Thalamic nuclei	Primary sensory relay ventral posterior lateral nucleus, ventral posterior medial nucleus, dorsal medial nucleus	RF stereotactic, stimulation, chemical lesion[6,18,33,47]
Periventricular III gray matter	Periaqueductal gray, peri-third-ventricular	Stimulation[17,48]
Pituitary fossa	Pituitary gland; hypothalamus	Alcohol ablation[20,29,34]
Posterior fossa	Cranial nerves, 5,7,8,9, and 10 and nervus intermedius	Selective fiber stimulation, rhizotomy[65]
	Trigeminal root, ganglion	Crush, lysis[31]
	Root entry zone; cranial nerves 5,7,9	Move arterial loop (decompression)[8,19,26]
Middle fossa	Trigeminal root, ganglion	Temporal fossa root lysis, percutaneous RF lesion (by way of foramen ovale)[31,55]
Medulla oblongata	Trigeminal tract (at level of obex)	Tractotomy[11]
Spinal cord	C1–2	Chordotomy, RF or surgical; high cervical midline myelotomy[35,45,50]
	T1–2	Chordotomy, RF or surgical
	Cervical or thoracic (dorsal column)	Epidural electrode stimulation[32,40,58]
Sympathetic ganglia	Cervical, thoracic, or lumbar	Chemical block or surgical excision (reflex dystrophy, causalgia)[23,38,39,66]
Spinal root	Any (dorsal), lumbosacral (ventral), selective sacral	Sensory rhizotomy, RF or surgical; motor rhizotomy (spasticity; spastic bladder)[49,59,64,66]
Spinal ganglion	Ganglion, sympathetic nervous system rami of thoracic roots	Intercostal ganglionectomy[52,53]
Facet joint	Dorsal primary ramus of spinal root	Facet block, RF or surgical[43]
Subarachnoid space	Regional, entire axis	Neurolytic agents, steroids[66]
Epidural space	Regional or caudal canal	Neurolytic agents, steroids, electrode stimulation[66]
Peripheral nerve	Any	Decompression (entrapment), neurolysis, neurectomy, stimulation[24]
End organ	Muscle, ligament, joint, tendon, fascia, and so forth	Myofasciotomy, RF, and so forth[21]

RF = radiofrequency
* The anatomic structures involved may be those giving rise to pain, transmitting or modulating it, or interpreting it to consciousness.

Just which physician should perform a given pain procedure is not clear; tradition has involved interaction among neurosurgeons and anesthesiologists.The demarcation can, perhaps, be anatomic between the dorsal root and the spinal cord proper, with neurosurgeons creating lesions in or central to the latter structure. Either specialist may, of course, manage more peripheral problems. Obviously, this arrangement is somewhat artificial; subarachnoid chemicals introduced primarily to alter dorsal or ventral rootlet function also bathe the cord surface. Frequently, there is less than ideal specificity with any given procedure; although the precise side effects may not be manifested and probably involve vagaries of interaction between local chemical concentrations and tissue sensitivities.

Typically, anesthesiologists limit the neurosurgeon's task in pain problems to assessment of the nature of the pain, investigation into causation, and selection of a relatively few patients for specific surgical therapy. Recently an eminent group of anesthesiologists and their pain-clinic co-workers listed a neurosurgeon's role as performance of "rhizotomy, percutaneous chordotomy (for unilateral lower limb pain due to malignancy), cingulotomy (of limited value), and thalamotomy and leukotomy . . ." On the face of it, this is too simplistic. Pain therapy may be offered by any physician who has properly considered the anatomy, physiology, and behavioral aspects of the problem in light of current knowledge. It will be apparent that a multidisciplinary approach has important advantages. The neurosurgeon who treats a patient with pain with multiple radiographic contrast and operative procedures, without regard, for example, for the unavoidable psychological dimension is generally doomed to failure. A patient with chronic pain must not be viewed as a "disc" or an irritated "nerve root" or "nerve" that can be repaired by a specific procedure and then forgotten. Although temporary placebo effects are legion, the problem recurs or worsens, and the initial physician rapidly loses interest along with a little bit of his ego.

RADIOFREQUENCY SPINOTHALAMIC TRACTOTOMY

Several important features of radiofrequency spinothalamic tractotomy should be kept in mind.

First, anatomic localization of the lateral spinothalamic tract, away from the corticospinal tract and dorsal columns, allows specific lesions to be created in the human both surgically and percutaneously.

Second, the pertinent pathway is primarily unilateral and contralateral to the side of the pain; only a small percentage of pain fibers run on the same side as the pain. Prior to crossing in the anterior white commissure of the cord, fibers that will form the lateral spinothalamic tract may ascend or descend several spinal levels; this may result in contralateral sensory loss several levels below that of the created lesion.

Third, functional lamination of the fibers that subserve pain and temperature from various dermatomes allows a "graded" lesion to be achieved with (RF), both in density of anesthesia and in regionalization of relief. The surgical lesion is generally less specific.

Fourth, regional fibers associated with respiratory and bladder function may be injured, particularly in bilateral chordotomies.

Fifth, introduction of an electrode into the cervical cord of an awake, rational patient allows physiologic confirmation of lesion location by preliminary stimulation. Although the debilitated patient tolerates the RF procedure well, cooperation with the surgeon is imperative for success. In order to achieve a similar specificity with the surgical procedure, an arousal anesthesia technique is necessary with sensory testing of the usually drowsy patient and graduated creation of the lesion.

Sixth, in general, chordotomy should be reserved for patients with malignant disease and a life expectancy of less than a year. Long-term effects may become quite disabling. When life expectancy is a matter of only weeks, pharmacologic relief should probably be offered.

Anatomic Considerations

A review of anatomy is important to caution the overconfident practitioner that results may have little to do with detailed understanding of mechanism. Greater anatomic detail is available in other sections of this book and thoroughly reviewed in the literature.[22]

Spinothalamic tractotomy would appear to be one of the more rational procedures for pain interruption; the major bundle of fibers that carries noxious stimuli from the initiating periphery to the thalamus and ultimately to consciousness. Unaccountably, however, this may not always work. Only a partial explanation has been provided, but neurophysiologists are slowly adding to it. Perhaps the principal attribute of the human nervous system is the ability to remember a past experience. This essential quality of human evolution also serves to recall adverse (painful or unpleasurable) experience; for the most part, this memory may not be effectively eliminated or interrupted peripherally. The remaining portion of pain and pleasure is central and must be so treated.

The *gate-control* explanation for modulation of peripheral experience passing cephalad in the spinal cord, although updated and revised, has been a major factor in persuading neurophysiologists to discard the classically attractive idea of a neural chain that delivers messages to the brain free of lateral contributions and interferences.[5,41,61] The emphasis on servomechanism control by regional neural elements has provided more than a few explanations for surgical failure of nerve-cutting operations.

Rexed's laminations of the central gray matter of the cord, based on architectonic considerations, have proved to have specific neurophysiologic meaning.[4,42,62] Noxious stimuli from the periphery or viscera, which are assumed for the sake of simplicity to be pain and temperature, are projected onto cells of specific laminae of the posterior horn (and root entry zone) according to the topography of their origin in the dorsal root of specific body segments.[4,56,62] Allowing for species differences in various studies, laminae I, IV, and V appear to give rise to the majority of axons that carry pain in higher primates. Most of these fibers cross the midline in front of the central canal of the cord to form the lateral spinothalamic tract of the opposite anterior quadrant. Visceral stimulation is also recorded in lamina V neurons. It is of note that discovery of cells of origin for the human spinothalamic tract is difficult, based perforce on ill-controlled degeneration studies after tractotomy.[3,51,60] In higher primates, fibers that constitute the tract are increased topographically according to segmental origin. These fibers are conveniently spaced along the outer margin of the anterior quadrant with the sacral contribution lying at the horizontal meridian just under the dentate ligament, and the lumbar, thoracic, and cervical fibers lying progressively more anteriorly (see Fig. 29-1). Many of the fibers in this tract synapse directly in the posterior ventral thalamic primary relay nuclei, ventral posterior medial (VPM) and ventral posterior lateral (VPL). Numerous sites for influence over a particular noxious stimulus are available, from the complex physiology of the peripheral receptor to the major dorsal horn synapses. It is further apparent that modulation may occur prior to thalamic entry of the tracts. Many fibers, in fact, do not proceed to the thalamus, at least not to the primary sensory nuclei.[3,60] A painful peripheral stimulus interacts with the parasympathetic and sympathetic systems at various levels, ultimately activating appropriate regions of the hypothalamus to modify the pain experience. Multiple reticular system entries exist.[3] Information is co-distributed to thalamic VPL and VPM and also to the interlaminar nuclei, thus involving the limbic system in interpretation of the experience.[44] Intrathalamic interruptions may cause severe pain of the Dejerine-Roussy (thalamic) syndrome; in contrast, lesions in VPM and VPL nuclei cause significant loss of all kinds of peripheral sensibility but are not effective in relief of chronic pain.[2,18] Lesions of centrum medianum and the parafascicular group may relieve chronic pain without producing more than minor peripheral alterations. Between the thalamus and cortical consciousness, interpretation of the stimulus must occur to register pain. Psychobehavioral elements confuse the issue, and the omnipresent placebo effect arises. Recent discoveries of brain stem periaqueductal and peri-third-ventricular pain-control regions that contain morphine receptors, and active sites for endorphins and enkephalins, not only provide possible explanations for the placebo effect, the effect of acupuncture, and so forth, but also indicate a further complexity of pain determination at levels of the nervous system relatively distant from the assumed site of conscious experience.[13,14]

The only reasonable approach for the clinician, forced by the weight of evidence to surrender the notion of a neural chain for pain, is to accept the concerted overview of a pain system that may be adapted to explain almost any clinical situation or result. Many of the effective surgical procedures have evolved by trial and error; from this a practical anatomy—where and how to make the interruption or stimulation—has been learned. Spinothalamic tractotomy is perhaps the primary example of such utilitarian rationale.

Technique

The object of spinothalamic tractotomy is to interrupt some or all of the fibers of the lateral spinothalamic tract that conduct the sensations of pain and temperature to higher centers. The surgical lesion is generally less controlled than the RF lesion. Surgical section of the entire tract, at least acutely, stops all noxious input, both visceral and somatic. The level of pain relief may not correspond to the level of the cut in the cord because of variation in the cephalad and caudal movement of the fibers before crossing the midline. This is evidenced by a shape of sensory loss following midline dorsal myelotomy different from that following anterior quadrant tractotomy.[45] These are important considerations in determining the level of pain relief the patient requires. Classically, lesions are made at C1–2 to achieve a level on the thorax or upper extremity and

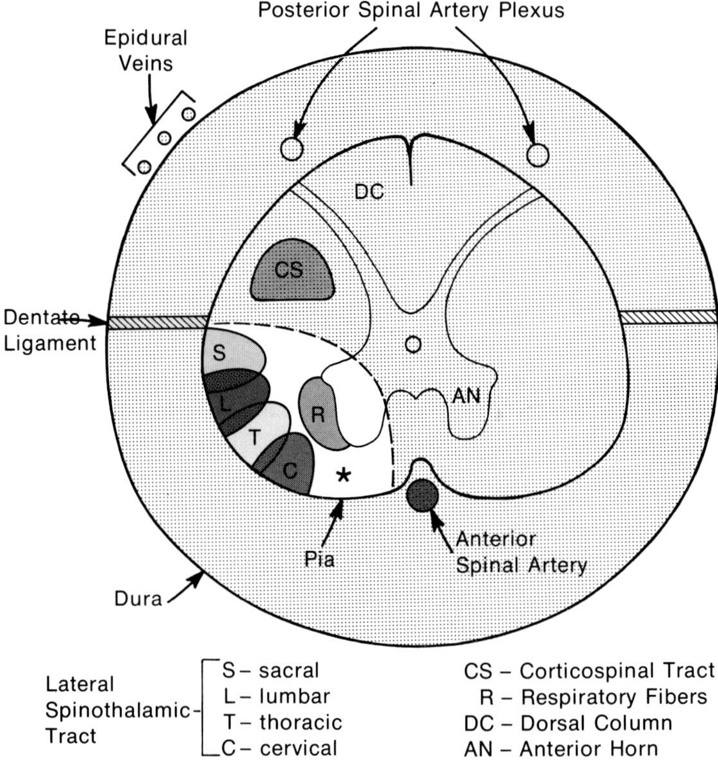

Fig. 29-1. Spinothalamic tract laminations and regional structures.

at T1–2 for pelvic or lower extremity pain. With RF control of lesion size and position, many of these problems are avoided, as is the painful surgical dissection that is above the level for which the chordotomy provides relief.[57]

Primary landmarks for either the surgical or RF lesion are the dentate ligament, which marks the equator of the cord roughly separating the motor and sensory regions, and the anterior spinal artery, which is to be avoided in the median sulcus of the ventral cord (Fig. 29-1). The surgical lesion is conceived as a single quadrant, usually cutting through the anterior horn and all other vertical fiber tracts in that region. Technically, open chordotomy involves grasping the dentate ligament with a hemostat, carefully rotating the cord about 30° to allow introduction of a small knife just anterior to the dentate ligament, and sweeping the blade ventrally to transect all intervening fibers. The blade is marked at a 5- or 6-mm length to avoid the median sulcus. Residual uncut fibers may effectively be crushed by compressing them against the anterior margin of the spinal canal. Generally, little hemorrhage occurs.

A chief advantage of the RF chordotomy is precise placement of the lesion through stimulation testing after an electrode has been positioned in the awake patient. The lesion may be enlarged by repetitive periods of heating the tissue at progressively increasing temperatures until frequent sensory testing indicates that the clinical result has been obtained (Fig. 29-2). Encroachment on the corticospinal system is discerned by motor (ipsilateral) testing during stimulation; the occasional problem with aberrant tract placement is discovered before a lesion is created.[51,54,57] These advantages are consistent for all methods of RF tractotomy; in addition, the reduced operative morbidity for the patient makes the RF procedure a widely accepted method of permanent neural blockade.

It is somewhat irrelevant just how the electrode is introduced into the cord, whether by the anterior (transinterspace) approach, posterolateral T1–2 ap-

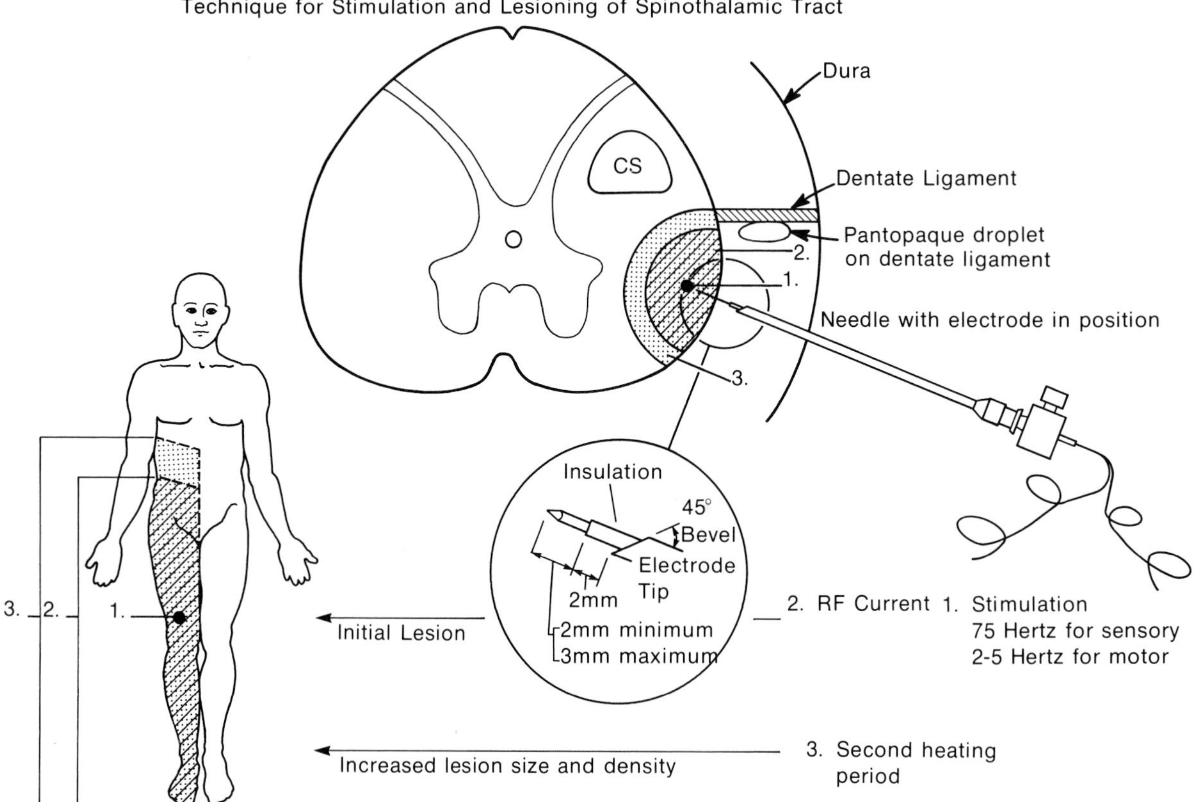

Fig. 29-2. Technique for stimulating and creating a lesion in spinothalamic tract.

proach, or the usual direct lateral placement at C1–2. The majority of neurosurgeons practice a variant of the methods advocated by Mullan or Rosomoff.[35,36,50] The principal difference between these methods is the amount of freehand manipulation of the electrode and the length of time spent in producing the lesion. It is a mistake to assume that this is a rapid, low morbidity technique that is uniformly successful. It is not unusual to spend up to 2 hours, perhaps even then without satisfactory results. A sloppy approach leads to spotty and incomplete anesthesia, analgesia in unwanted areas, or even major unexpected deficits.

Anesthetic Management. The patient should be admitted 24 hours prior to the planned procedure. History and current physical status should be recorded. Although many cancer patients are debilitated, abnormal values for serum chemistries, complete blood count, and so forth may not disqualify a patient since general anesthesia will not be used. Respiratory status should be tested if there is suspicion of inadequate reserve; this may be a contraindication.

A technique of intravenous *conscious sedation* is useful. The patient is premedicated with a psychosedative drug such as oral diazepam (or lorazepam). When the patient arrives in the procedure area (operating room or radiology suite), an intravenous line is established, and further psychosedative is administered by this route while positioning films are being taken. The surgeon uses local anesthetic infiltration in the skin, the needle tract, and the epidural space. During the procedure, the patient is given a small amount of intravenous analgesic such as fentanyl or meperidine. Methohexital, an ultra-short-acting barbiturate, is also used in 5- to 15-mg aliquots every 3 to 5 minutes, as needed. With this technique, the surgeon may converse with the patient and perform accurate sensory testing, but the patient will be largely amnesic for the experience. Vital signs should be monitored frequently; airway maintenance and resuscitation equipment and drugs should be available. Recovery from these medications is rapid.

Equipment. The RF percutaneous chordotomy is performed in the Radiology Department or in an operating theater equipped with radiographic capability for at least anteroposterior and lateral cervical spine studies; fluoroscopy with image intensification may be helpful but not essential, and polaroid imaging will reduce the time needed for each positioning step. Although some operators use a rigid head holder in the fashion of Rosomoff, the procedure may be performed equally well, in a cooperative patient, by placing the head on a rubber donut. The patient is supine with the head neutral and straight anteroposterior position; he should be comfortable enough to maintain the position indefinitely since head and neck movement with the electrode in position is potentially dangerous. This is particularly important if the fixed needle holder is used, for which the head should also be immobilized. The occiput and shoulders are on the same level, and the chin flexed slightly. Anteroposterior and lateral positioning films are taken and the adjustments made as necessary to have the upper cervical spine nearly horizontal.

A micromanipulator is commercially available and may be used to advance the needle. An advantage of freehand needle advancement is that the patient does not move against a rigid structure in the tissue. The surgeon's "feel" of the structures encountered is also enhanced, and needle position is easily maintained by the muscles and dura.

The electrodes are simple piano wire of about 0.02 inches in diameter of stainless steel, insulated with polyethylene. These can easily be cut to length or ordered commercially. The electrode is marked with an adjustable set-screw stop so that the bared tip extends the required number of millimeters beyond the tip of the short-bevel No. 18 spinal needle through which it is introduced. Appropriate leads are necessary for the electrode and the indifferent circuit (Fig. 29-3).

A number of models of the RF generator are available for various uses. Some incorporate stimulation circuits and impedance monitors. The operator must be thoroughly familiar with his particular model, especially its correlation of the current produced with electrode-tip temperatures in various tissues. It is useful to make a series of experimental lesions in egg albumin (egg white) prior to clinical work; this demonstrates the duration and geometry of expansion of the lesion for different currents and electrode-ground relationships.[10] A thermistor may be used in the electrode tip (this is standard for RF trigeminal lesions) but is not necessary and increases the complexity of the procedure. The power that the generator produces must be appropriate for the procedure; chordotomy requires rather low

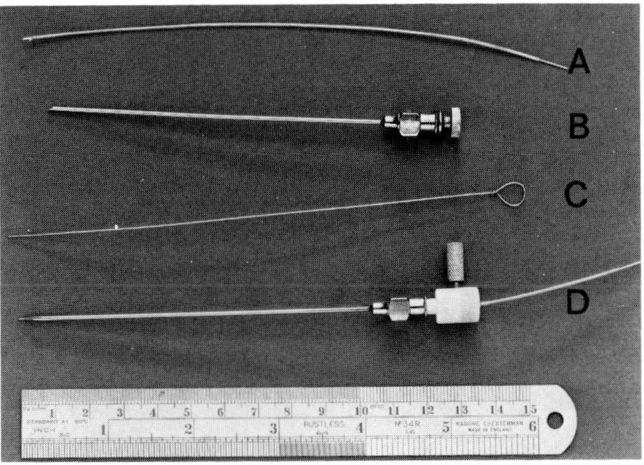

Fig. 29-3. Equipment for positioning electrode for radiofrequency chordotomy. (*A*) Wire electrode with polyethylene sheath, (*B*) No. 18 short-bevel spinal needle, (*C*) wire stylet, and (*D*) needle with electrode in position. Note set-screw stop, which has been attached to the electrode to allow the exposed tip to pierce the spinal cord.

power. An impedance monitor in the electrode circuit is helpful in positioning the needle. The circuit is grounded to the patient through a second large-gauge needle placed under the patient's skin. The impedance of the spinal fluid is low (100–200 ohms); when the electrode fully penetrates the cord tissue, impedance increases fivefold or so.

Electrode Positioning. After blocking the cutaneous tract with local anesthetic, a short beveled 18 gauge spinal needle is advanced horizontally to the epidural space at the C1–2 level; it is aimed toward the center of the spinal canal (roughly the center of the cord), and the initial trajectory documented radiographically. After the needle enters the epidural space, careful aspiration should be performed to avoid the needle tip from entering the vertebral artery or the cerebrospinal fluid (CSF) compartment. If positioning is adequate, the needle is advanced a few millimeters and penetrates the dura; the patient should be warned to expect a jolt of pain at this stage. The needle tip now lies immediately lateral to the cord surface. In the anteroposterior radiograph, the cord is about the width of the odontoid process of C2; the needle tip is viewed in relation to this structure (Fig. 29-4).

There are several variations in final electrode placement. Contrast material (air, pantopaque, or both) must be introduced to delineate the critical positions of the cord surface and the dentate ligament marking the equator (Fig. 29-5). The dentate lies 10 to 11 mm behind the anterior canal margin,

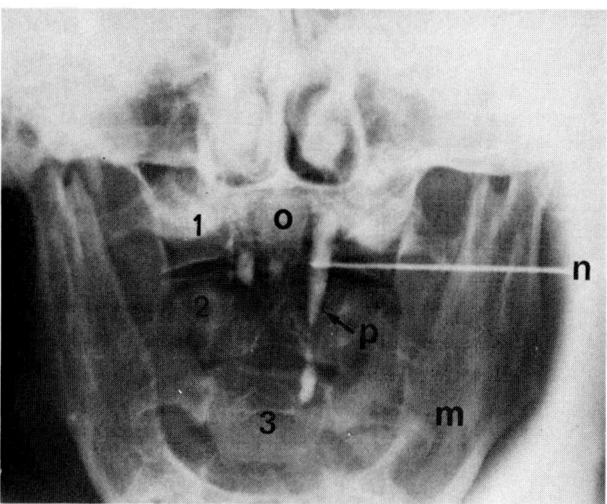

Fig. 29-4. Anteroposterior radiograph C1–2 junction, open mouth view. The needle is positioned just at the surface of the cord, which has been outlined by pantopaque. Note that the odontoid process roughly corresponds to width of cord. (*1*) C1, (*2*) C2, (*3*) C3, (*n*) needle, (*m*) mandible, (*p*) pantopaque, (*o*) odontoid process of C2.

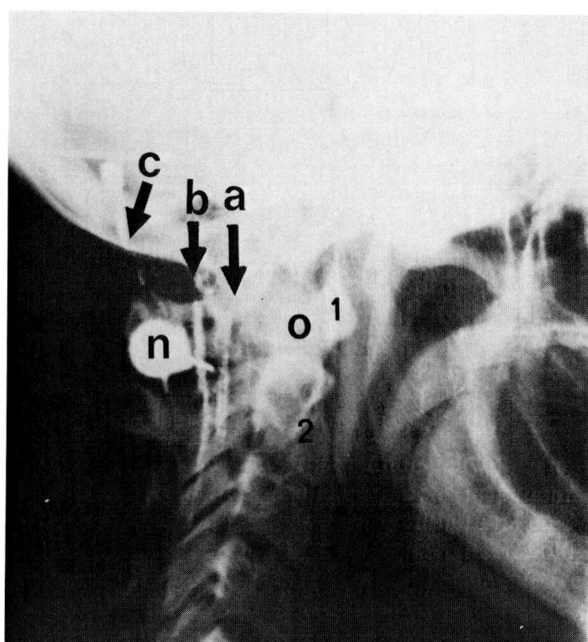

Fig. 29-5. Lateral radiograph, upper cervical region. Pantopaque outlines (*A*) the anterior margin or cord, (*B*) the dentate ligament, (*C*) posterior margin of cisterna magna. The needle tip is properly positioned just anterior to dentate ligament. (*1*) anterior ring of C1, (*2*) body of C2, (*n*) hub of needle, and (*o*) odontoid process of C2.

although it is clear that this relationship is not constant and related to the patient's position. By manipulating the hub of the needle externally, the electrode tip may be positioned to enter the cord a few millimeters anterior to the dentate, usually in the area of the lumbosacral fibers of the spinothalamic tract. Impedance monitoring will yield additional evidence of cord entry when the electrode is introduced through the needle so that its tip just penetrates the pial surface (see Fig. 29-2). The needle remains in the subarachnoid space and may be used as the indifferent electrode; CSF will often drip freely around the loose-fitting electrode during the operation. At the moment of pial penetration, the patient may again feel a sharp, poorly localized pain of brief duration. Sensory stimulation is then performed at 0.1 v, 75 Hz and motor testing at 2 to 5 Hz (Fig. 29-2); if contralateral sensory stimulation is appropriately placed and there is no ipsilateral motor deficit, the initial lesion may be attempted.

Creation of a Lesion. There are a number of factors pertinent to the interaction between the RF current and the tissue at the tip of the electrode (see references for details). CSF in contact with the tip may diffuse the heat sufficiently to prevent an adequate lesion. Rapid heating may cause the tissue to "boil," also limiting the controlled expansion. Tissue resistance changes as the lesion accrues, and the current flow will vary.

Generally, a heating period of 30 to 60 seconds at 35 to 50 ma current will achieve the required result. There should be periods of 5 to 10 seconds of heating, each followed by careful sensory and motor testing. The initial area of hypalgesia will indicate where in the spinothalamic fibers the electrode is placed; the lesion will advance in roughly spherical fashion by adding concentric shells with each additional period of current. The patient's grip should be tested as well as his ability to raise the arm and leg on the side of the lesion. If any compromise is noted, the electrode should be repositioned more ventrally or the procedure terminated. Persistently inexplicable stimulation results may indicate anatomic variation of the tract position or inability to separate the sensory fibers from other important modalities; this may also require cessation of the procedure. Various schedules of progressive heating periods or progressive power output at fixed intervals has been advocated. It is important to note, however, that the entire procedure should probably take at least an hour to perform properly, including a requisite final waiting period of at least 15 minutes to make certain that the expected lesion is stable. The sensory level is carried several dermatomes above the cephalad extent of the patient's pain. There may be a slight additional rise in level from perilesion edema over the next 24 hours, but ultimately the level will tend to fall below that initially achieved (this is also true of surgical chordotomy). Finally, it is critical to be in adequate communication with the patient and to be certain that he understands the nature of the sensory changes that he is being asked to differentiate. If sedation is too deep, or if cooperation wanes, the procedure is best rescheduled for completion a few days later.

Complications

Generally, if the technique outlined above is performed for unilateral pain of malignant origin in patients with several months of life expectancy and otherwise reasonably good health, it will be quite benign and overall about 80 per cent successful. The primary postoperative complications are respiratory depression, urinary retention, and occasionally hypotension. Fortunately, these are rare with a unilateral lesion, but it is nonetheless wise to monitor the patient in a recovery area overnight. Minor motor lesions will usually recede in a few days. With reasonable sterile precautions, sepsis is extremely rare. The only relative contraindication, in light of the nature of the indications for the procedure, is inadequate respiratory reserve. This should be tested preoperatively, when indicated. A review of the incidence of specific complications is given in the literature.[63]

Masked Pain. Tumors that involve midline structures may cause pain perceived to be principally unilateral until a chordotomy "unmasks" the contralateral pain. This is merely a reflection of the poor localization of deep pain and the inability of a patient to measure partial relief; he still hurts, although now the pain is on the other side. The patient is warned of this possibility and the question of bilateral lesions discussed. It is not infrequent that simultaneous bilateral surgical chordotomies have been made to avoid a second operation. Bilateral lesions increase the risk of all other complications significantly.

Bladder and Bowel Function. As with all neural blockade potentially involving sacral innervation or more central autonomic centers in the cord, excretory function may be influenced. Many patients with cancer have preexisting bowel and bladder diversions; without these, inclusion of autonomic fiber pathways in the RF lesion rises from a small percentage for unilateral lesions to nearly 50 per cent for bilateral procedures. This dysfunction may be rather transient or improve slowly over a period of weeks.

Respiratory Function. Severe respiratory depression occurs in about 4 per cent of patients with bilateral high cervical chordotomy, as reported by Rosomoff and others.[7,25,37,63] This often takes the form of sleep apnea and may be predicted by a 5-per-cent carbon-dioxide inhalation stimulus, which indicates a poor tidal-volume increase. This condition may not be manifested for 48 hours after the procedure. The syndrome may be accompanied by signs of other autonomic dysfunction. Endotracheal intubation and ventilatory support, particularly during drowsiness, may be necessary for several weeks.

Because of this potentially serious problem, planned bilateral chordotomies should be performed, if possible, at levels several dermatomes apart; surgically, this is common. The anterior approach has been developed for RF lesions to allow the procedure to be performed in the lower cervical spine on one side, below the level of the major respiratory pathways.[28,30] If high levels are required bilaterally, perhaps some other technique should be considered, such as pituitary alcohol ablation, which may provide relief for diffuse pain.[20,29,34] Generally, if a sensory level above C6 is not effected, the white matter immediately adjacent to the anterior horn, which contains the respiratory fibers, can be avoided.[35]

Dysesthesia. About 40 per cent of all patients who have had a chordotomy will admit they have experienced some abnormal, not necessarily uncomfortable, feeling in the anesthetic area at one time or another. Five per cent will find these sensations uncomfortable or otherwise disconcerting, and about 1 per cent will be very unhappy, perhaps wishing they had never had the procedure undertaken. It is this last group that limits the usefulness of the technique for long-term resolution of pain.[57] The same problem pertains to operations for trigeminal neuralgia.[18] Although refinements in technique have reduced the incidence of almost all other complications from the unilateral percutaneous RF procedure to nearly zero, this innate property of the nervous system has not been altered. The rate of dysesthesia increases with time after the chordotomy. It is the fear of this particular complication, and the lack of satisfactory methods to deal with it, that has stimulated a number of workers to investigate large series of alternatives such as dorsal rhizotomy for chronic pain of benign origin.[64] Unfortunately, the overall success rate of rhizotomy has also been disappointing. In the 6 per cent of patients who experience significant post-chordotomy discomfort, minor environmental stimuli tend to accentuate the problem; this includes emotional as well as sensory factors. Nature's apparent insistence on its primary mechanism of pain as protection of the organism from the environment has thwarted many an otherwise well-conceived pain operation—the diffuse pathways that may conduct noxious stimuli in the cord, and perhaps around the cord by way of the sympathetic nervous system, may lead to occasional disastrous results when one portion of the system, albeit the major pathway, is altered.

Motor deficit is not a problem if the procedure is carefully planned and performed. Most minor deficits will resolve in a few days. It is, of course, a coexistent problem with subarachnoid instillation of neurolytic drugs and a number of other pain relief procedures that involve roots or mixed nerves (see Chap. 27). By the nature of the disease, many cancer patients have preexisting weakness, either through direct involvement of motor structures or from the diffuse effects of debilitation, carcinomatous neuropathy, and so forth. When pain relief is preeminent, additional weakness may be acceptable, particularly if the patient is likely not to be ambulatory for other reasons.

The postoperative hospital confinement for a successful procedure averages 3 to 4 days if the patient is admitted only for chordotomy. This is sufficient time to define any problems that might arise from the procedure itself and to assess adequately the degree of pain relief and to taper the patient's previous narcotic dosage. Because most cancer patients are well known to their physicians and the chordotomy procedure adds little stress, the preoperative evaluation is limited (as previously mentioned, respiratory insufficiency is probably the only relative contraindication).

Results

Although the procedure of RF cordotomy is designed to remove all pain (superficial and deep) distal to the lesion without overlapping additional motor or proprioceptive deficits, it is clear from the discussion of the pain system that this is not always the outcome. As Freud indicated, it is not reasonable to expect to produce the polar extreme of pleasure by removing pain. The best that can be hoped, under circumstances of malignant pain, is an increase in the dying patient's ability to tolerate his last days. Other vigorous efforts to support the patient must also be continued.

As a result of the inability to measure pain, it is usual to find results of most pain procedures expressed in broad categories of general relief; frequently, examples of case histories are given to show how the patient's life has changed.[15] Thus, in Mullan's original report, "effective cordotomies [sic] with relief from pain have been achieved in 34 of our 42 patients," but "the type of results obtained might best be understood by giving several examples."[36] In one of the largest series in the literature, 789 patients underwent 1279 chordotomies; 25 per cent were available for follow-up beyond 1 year. Thirteen per cent of the patients had inadequate relief, even with repeated or bilateral procedures. Pain relief is excellent for 3 months in 90 per cent of cases—longer term follow-up finds 40 to 70 per cent with continued adequate relief. Many patients with terminal cancer will die before the placebo period has passed, and many others will have become semicomatose or otherwise impossible to evaluate objectively.

If the patient still focuses his attention on his pain, he has not genuinely been helped. It is for this reason that unmasked pain is an important problem. If the patient is able to proceed with other aspects of his life, relatively free from mind-disturbing medication, a salutory result has been achieved.

REFERENCES

1. Adams, J.E., Hosobuchi, Y., and Fields, H.L.: Stimulation of internal capsule for relief of chronic pain. J. Neurosurg. *41*:740, 1974.
2. Biemond, A.: The conduction of pain above the level of the thalamus opticus. Arch. Neurol. Psychiatry, *75*:231, 1956.
3. Bowsher, D.: Termination of the central pain pathway in man. The conscious appreciation of pain. Brain, *80*:606, 1957.
4. Brown, A.G., and Gordon, G.: Subcortical mechanisms concerned in somatic sensation. Br. Med. Bull., *33*:121, 1977.
5. Calvin, W.H., Loeser, J.D., and Howe, J.F.: A neurophysiological theory for the pain mechanism of tic douloureux. Pain, *3*:147, 1977.
6. Cassinari, V., and Pagni, C.A.: Central Pain, A Neurosurgical Survey. Cambridge, Harvard University Press, 1969.
7. Cohen, F.L.: Effects of various lesions on crossed and uncrossed descending inspiratory pathways in the cervical spinal cord of the cat. J. Neurosurg., *39*:589, 1973.
8. Dandy, W.: The Brain, A Classic Reprint. p.170. New York, Harper & Row, 1969.
9. Foltz, E.L., and White, L.E., Jr.: Pain "relief" by frontal cingulotomy. J. Neurosurg., *19*:89, 1962.
10. Fox, J.L.: Experimental relationship of radiofrequency electrical current and lesion size for application to percutaneous cordotomy. J. Neurosurg., *33*:415, 1970.
11. ———: Delineation of the obex by contrast radiography during percutaneous trigeminal tractotomy. J. Neurosurg., *36*:107, 1972.

12. Freud, S.: Beyond the pleasure principle. *In* The Complete Psychological Works of Sigmund Freud. vol. 18. London, Hogarth Press, 1975.
13. Goldstein, A: Opioid peptides (endorphins) in pituitary and brain. Science, *193*:1081, 1976.
14. ——: Enkephalins, opiate receptors and general anesthesia. Anesthesiology, *49*:1, 1978.
15. Gooddy, W.: On the nature of pain. Brain, *80*:118, 1957.
16. Gutterman, P., and Shenkin, H.A.: Saline frontal lobotomy in the treatment of intractable pain. J.A.M.A., *199*:123, 1967.
17. Hosobuchi, Y., Adams, J.E., and Linchitz, R.: Pain relief by electrical stimulation of the central gray matter in humans and its reversal by naloxone. Science, *197*:183, 1977.
18. Hosobuchi, Y., Adams, J.E., and Rutkin, B.: Chronic thalamic stimulation for the control of facial anesthesia dolorosa. Arch. Neurol., *29*:158, 1973.
19. Jannetta, P.J.: Arterial compression of the trigeminal nerve at the pons in patients with trigeminal neuralgia. J. Neurosurg., *26*:159, 1967.
20. Katz, J., and Levin, A.B.: Treatment of diffuse metastatic cancer pain by instillation of alcohol into the sella turcica. Anesthesiology, *46*:115, 1977.
21. Kennard, M.A., and Haugen, F.P.: The relation of subcutaneous focal sensitivity to referred pain of cardiac origin. Anesthesiology, *16*:297, 1955.
22. Kerr, F.W.L.: Neuroanatomical substrates of nociception in the spinal cord. Review Article. Pain, *1*:325, 1975.
23. Kirtley, J.A., Riddell, D.H., Stoney, W.S., and Wright, J.K.: Cervicothoracic sympathectomy in neurovascular abnormalities of the upper extremities: experience in 76 patients with 104 sympathectomies. Ann. Surg. *165*:869, 1967.
24. Kopell, H.P., and Thompson, W.A.L.: Peripheral Entrapment Neuropathies. Baltimore, Williams & Wilkins, 1963.
25. Krieger, A.J., and Rosomoff, H.L.: Sleep-induced apnea. Part 1: A respiratory and autonomic dysfunction syndrome following bilateral percutaneous cervical cordotomy. J. Neurosurg., *39*:168, 1973.
26. Laha, R.K., and Jannetta, P.J.: Glossopharyngeal neuralgia. J. Neurosurg., *47*:316, 1977.
27. Lewis, C.S.: The Problem of Pain. New York, Macmillan, 1945.
28. Lin, P.M., Gildenberg, P.L., and Polakoff, P.P.: An anterior approach to percutaneous lower cervical cordotomy. J. Neurosurg., *25*:553, 1966.
29. Lipton, S.: Percutaneous cervical cordotomy and the injection of the pituitary with alcohol. Anesthesia, *33*:953, 1978.
30. Lipton, S., Dervin, E., and Heywood, O.B.: A stereotactic approach to the anterior percutaneous electrical cordotomy. *In* Bonica, J.J. (ed.): Advances in Neurology, vol. 4. Pain. pp.689–697. New York, Raven Press, 1974.
31. Loeser, J.D.: The management of tic douloureux. Pain, *3*:155, 1977.
32. Long, D.M., and Hagfors, N.: Electrical stimulation in the nervous system. The current status of electrical stimulation of the nervous system for relief of pain. Pain, *1*:109, 1975.
33. Mark, V.H., and Tsutsumi, H.: The suppression of pain by intrathalamic lidocaine. *In* Bonica, J.J. (ed.): Advances in Neurology, vol. 4. Pain. pp. 715–721. New York, Raven Press, 1974.
34. Moricca, G.: Chemical hypophysectomy for cancer pain. *In* Bonica, J.J. (ed.): Advances in Neurology, vol. 4. Pain. pp. 707–714. New York, Raven Press, 1974.
35. Mullan, S.: Percutaneous cordotomy. *In* Bonica, J.J.(ed.): Advances in Neurology. vol. 4. Pain. pp. 677–682. New York, Raven Press, 1974.
36. Mullan, S., Harper, P.V., Hekmatpanah, J., Torres, H., and Dobbin, G: Percutaneous interruption of spinal-pain tracts by means of a strontium needle. J. Neurosurg., *20*:931, 1963.
37. Mullan, S., and Hosobuchi, Y.: Respiratory hazards of high cervical percutaneous cordotomy. J. Neurosurg., *28*:291, 1968.
38. Myers, K.A., and Irvine, W.T.: An objective study of lumbar sympathectomy. I. Intermittent claudication. Br. Med. J., *1*:879, 1966.
39. ——: An objective study of lumbar sympathectomy. II. Skin ischemia. Br. Med. J., *1*:943, 1966.
40. Nashold, B.S., and Friedman, H.: Dorsal column stimulation for control of pain. Preliminary report on 30 patients. J. Neurosurg., *36*:590, 1972.
41. Nathan, P.W.: The gate-control theory of pain. A critical review. Brain, *99*:123, 1976.
42. ——: Pain. Br. Med. Bull., *33(2)*:149, 1977.
43. Ogsbury, J.S., Simon, R.H., and Lehman, R.A.W.: Facet "denervation" in the treatment of low back syndrome. Pain, *3*:257, 1977.
44. Papez, J.W.: A proposed mechanism of emotion. Arch. Neurol. Psychiatry, *38*:725, 1937.
45. Papo, I., and Luongo, A.: High cervical commissural myelotomy in the treatment of pain. J. Neurol. Neurosurg. Psychiatry, *39*:705, 1976.
46. Pilowsky, I., and Spence, N.D.: Illness behavior syndromes associated with intractable pain. Pain, *2*:61, 1976.
47. Richardson, D.E.: Thalamotomy for intractable pain. Confin. Neurol., *29*:139, 1967.
48. Richardson, D.E., and Akil, H.: Pain reduction by electrical brain stimulation in man. Part 1: Acute administration in periaqueductal and periventricular sites. J. Neurosurg., *47*:178, 1977.
49. Rockswold, G.L., Bradley, W.E., and Chou, S.N.: Differential sacral rhizotomy in the treatment of neurogenic bladder dysfunction. J. Neurosurg., *38*:748, 1973.
50. Rosomoff, H.L.: Percutaneous radiofrequency cervical cordotomy for intractable pain. *In* Bonica, J.J. (ed.): Advances in Neurology. vol. 4. Pain. pp. 683–688. New York, Raven Press, 1974.
51. Smith, M.C.: Observations on the topography of the lateral column of the human cervical spinal cord. Brain, *80*:263, 1957.
52. Smith, F.P.: Trans-spinal ganglionectomy for relief of intercostal pain. J. Neurosurg., *32*:574, 1970.
53. ——: Pathological studies of spinal nerve ganglia in relation to intractable intercostal pain. Surg. Neurol., *10*:50, 1978.
54. Sweet, W.H.: Recent observations pertinent to improving anterolateral cordotomy. Clin. Neurosurg., *23*:80, 1976.
55. Sweet, W.H., and Wepsic, J.G.: Controlled thermocoagulation of trigeminal ganglion and rootlets for differenctial destruction of pain fibers. Part 1. Trigeminal neuralgia. J. Neurosurg., *39*:143, 1974.
56. Tasker, R.R.: Somatotopographic representation in the human thalamus, midbrain and spinal cord. The anatomical basis for the surgical relief of pain. *In* Morley, T.P. (ed.): Current Controversies in Neurosurgery. pp. 485–495. Philadelphia, W.B. Saunders, 1976.
57. ——: The merits of percutaneous cordotomy over the open operation. *In* Morley, T.P. (ed.): Current Controversies in Neurosurgery. pp. 496–501. Philadelphia, W.B. Saunders, 1976.
58. Taub, A.: Electrical stimulation for the relief of pain: two lessons in technological zealotry. Perspect. Biol. Med. *19*:125, 1975.

59. Uematsu, S., Udvarhelyi, G.B., Benson, D.W., and Siebens, A.A.: Percutaneous radiofrequency rhizotomy. Surg. Neurol., *2*:319, 1974.
60. Walker, E.A.: The spinothalamic tract in man. Arch. Neurol. Psychiatry, *43*:284, 1940.
61. Wall, P.D., and Sweet, W.H.: Temporary abolition of pain in man. Science, *155*:108, 1967.
62. Webster, K.E.: Somaesthetic pathways. Br. Med. Bull., *33(2)*:113, 1977.
63. Wepsic, J.G.: Complications of percutaneous surgery for pain. Clin. Neurosurg., *23*:454, 1976.
64. White, J.C., and Kjellberg, R.N.: Posterior spinal rhizotomy: a substitute for cordotomy in the relief of localized pain in patients with normal life-expectancy. Neurochirurgia (Stuttg.), *16*:141, 1973.
65. White, J.C., and Sweet, W.H.: Pain and the Neurosurgeon: A Forty-Year Experience. Springfield, Charles C Thomas, 1969.
66. Wood, K.M.: The use of phenol as a neurolytic agent: a review. Pain, *5*:205, 1978.

30 Neural Blockade and the Collaborative Concept of Pain Management

Terence M. Murphy

Neural blockade techniques can safely and effectively be used at the anesthesiologist's own initiative or at the request of a referring surgeon or physician for management of acute pain. However, extension of this approach to the management of chronic pain is both unsatisfactory and potentially dangerous. Chronic pain differs from acute pain in fundamental and important aspects that necessitate a very thorough evaluation of all possibly contributing factors before neural blockade may be considered.[1–3] The informed, rational, and safe use of neural blockade techniques requires a collaborative approach that involves the anesthesiologist beyond his role in performing the neural blockade procedure. The anesthesiologist should avoid acting as a block technician with no knowledge of the patient's often complex medical history. On the grounds of safe management of major local anesthetic blockade alone, a complete history is required. In order to contribute fully to diagnostic and therapeutic regimens, the anesthesiologist should participate in face-to-face collaboration. Decisions that concern procedures with serious complications, such as neurolytic neural blockade, should be reached only after vigorous discussion with all available members of the pain management group. To highlight the need for this approach to the use of neural blockade in chronic pain management, it is instructive to review the development of modern concepts of pain clinics or pain management units.[1–5,7]

COLLABORATIVE PAIN CONTROL

Lord Samuel wrote, "choose your specialist and you choose your disease," to which might be added: "and choose your treatment." Although the era of specialization in medicine has been responsible for great advancement of medical knowledge, it has produced a generation of doctors whose therapeutic repertoire, although becoming more skilled, has become narrower. The patient whose health problem falls completely within a narrow spectrum, will, of course, obtain optimal treatment from a specialist. However, patients with multisystem disease or complex disease processes that involve both mind and body will frequently need the attention of specialists from different fields. Although in theory the present system of health delivery makes this possible, the doctor all too often will attempt to treat the patient by his own special skills, perhaps inadequately attending to problems of the patient that are outside his own field of expertise. This is quite understandable since by and large physicians tend to do best what they have been trained to do. Therefore, when a difficult chronic pain problem is referred to, say, a neurosurgeon, it is most likely to be treated neurosurgically; if the same problem were to be referred to an orthopedic surgeon, it would most likely be treated orthopedically; and similarly, if it were to be referred to a psychiatrist it would most likely be treated psychiatrically. Only after the initial therapeutic attempt fails to produce the desired results would the patient be referred to a different specialist. Thus, patients with chronic pain, who often suffer from a complex potpourri of disease processes, will frequently be referred from specialist to specialist, each one exhausting his own field of endeavor before referring the patient to someone else. Such patients, therefore, frequently pass from doctor to doctor with each attending to perhaps part of the patient's problem but none dealing with the problem as a whole. Not only is the patient often denied the most appropriate treatment, but also if therapy such as unnecessary surgery or the use of harmful potent medications is undertaken along the way, iatrogenic problems may be added to the patient's preexisting disease.

There is, therefore, a group of patients who have become failures of the present health-care delivery system. In order to treat the problems of these and other patients with intractable pain, *pain clinics* were initially conceived.

Pain clinics or Pain-Relief or Pain-Management

Units have different connotations for different people; for example, the diagnostic nerve block clinic, in which an anesthesiologist or other physician skilled in regional anesthesia performs a specific nerve block and the referring physician determines the effect and interprets the results; the smaller one-man pain clinics, in which a physician who has experience with patients with pain—their problems and the appropriate treatments—, might attempt to treat them individually; the multidisciplinary approach, in which many physicians, each skilled in his own specialty as well as in the appropriate application of these specialities to the chronic pain problem, collaborate and coordinate their efforts to diagnose and treat a patient's disease. There is a fourth type of facility, a therapeutic pain clinic, in which patients are not treated from an individual diagnostic approach but are instead involved in a primarily rehabilitative effort, usually as a part of group therapy that combines physical therapy, medication control, and behavioral conditioning in an attempt to reverse pain behavior.

PAIN-MANAGEMENT UNIT

Role of the Anesthesiologist

The anesthesiologist's participation in the management of pain can run the gamut from informed technician who performs diagnostic blocks and leaves their interpretation to others, through managing physician in the administration and organization of a nerve block clinic, to practitioner who uses blocks both as diagnostic and therapeutic maneuvers in the management of pain. He may also affiliate with physicians of other specialities, with a common interest in pain and become a member of a multidisciplinary clinical approach to the management of pain, thereby gaining experience of what other therapies can and cannot contribute to the management of pain. The anesthesiologist experienced in regional anesthesia techniques and the management of pain problems is in an ideal position to coordinate such a multidisciplinary group. Thus, depending on his time, talents, and inclinations, the anesthesiologist can be as little or as greatly involved in the management of pain as he wishes.

Although such involvement with pain management is demanding of time and effort, it is eminently feasible to combine it with conventional anesthetic practice. Anesthesiologists who do so will find it a rewarding practice that provides clinical challenge and an interesting contrast to their primary commitment in the operating theater.

The anesthesiologist who acquires experience in managing pain problems can provide a very useful service to his community through his skills in neural blockade and medication management, even outside the optimal setting of a multidisciplinary pain clinic (which is the ideal) if such a facility is not feasible in the area. By setting aside one or two afternoons each week for seeing outpatients in either a private office or a hospital—and then scheduling the performance of any diagnostic and therapeutic blocks so as not to conflict with operating commitments on the other days of the week—he can provide a much appreciated service in the control of pain and related problems (such as the relief of spasticity with neurolytic blocks). The only limits imposed upon the anesthesiologist who wishes to extend his clinical repertoire along these lines is the amount of time and effort he is prepared to spend (and can spare from his other duties). The management of patients with chronic pain is time-consuming and does demand a considerable commitment. However, for anesthesiologists prepared to make this effort, the rewards of primary patient care with its satisfactions (and disappointments) are possible.

Function

The function of the Pain Unit is consultant service. It is primarily diagnostic, to provide the patient and the referring physician as accurate an opinion as possible on the most likely cause or causes for the pain complaint and also to advise the patient and the physician on what to do about this pain—both specific therapeutic suggestions (*e.g.*, chordotomy, neurolytic block, etc.), and also supportive, but noncurative, measures (*e.g.*, drug management, physical therapy, etc.). Another and very important function is often to provide advice to the patient and the referring physician on what not to do for the pain (*i.e.*, to avoid mutilating surgery and excessive use of depressant medications when there is no indication that their use will result in any benefit to the patient and when there is the possibility that the complications of such therapy might make the patient worse).

Organization

The rational use of neural blockade in chronic pain management depends upon adequate patient evaluation and objective criteria for assessment of the effects of blockade (see Chaps. 13 and 27). These entail the proper organization of a pain clinic.

Staff. *Administration.* In most enterprises, a good administrative assistant/secretary is invaluable.

This is especially important in a pain-management unit, primarily because patients with chronic pain are often difficult to handle, having become disillusioned with the health-care system and its ability to cope with their problem. Administrative workers also must frequently cope with the acquisition of voluminous data—and their organization—on patients who have had many detailed interactions with the medical profession during the course of their problems. It is especially important then that such administrative staff be very kind, understanding, and tactful in dealing with these often demanding patients and also that the staff be supportive of the general pain-unit philosophy on the management of these patients. Toward this end, the administrative supportive staff should be included in such pain unit activities as the unit conference so that staff members become familiar with the patterns of dealing with these patients. The administrative staff should be able to coordinate the different doctors from the different disciplines in the pain unit, and it will also require expertise and efficiency in collecting and compiling patient information, not only from the referral physician but also from many other doctors whom the patient will have seen in connection with his pain complaint. The pain unit must have highly sympathetic and tolerant nonmedical as well as medical staff.

Clinical coordinator of the Pain Unit may be any specialist medical practitioner with an interest in and commitment to patients with chronic pain. The particular field of specialization is of secondary importance to the ability and willingness to spend the time that is required for both the clinical and administrative demands of this position.

Consultants. Many different specialties can contribute constructively to the management of chronic pain, and perhaps more important than a physician's individual specialty field is his interest and knowledge in pain and how that relates to his field of expertise. In general, however, it is usually necessary, in a multidisciplinary Pain Unit, to have access to a behavioral scientist, such as a clinical psychologist or a psychiatrist. Neurosurgeons, physical therapist, and orthopedic surgeons will be very helpful in the physical assessment of these patients. Anesthesiologists usually make their major contribution in the use of diagnostic and therapeutic neural blockade and the management of analgesic medication (see Chap. 27). Because the pain can have such wide-spread repercussions upon a patient's life, occupation, and family relationships, an astute social worker can be invaluable in gathering relevant data. Many other personnel can and should be involved since patients will arrive with problems that demand expertise beyond the above-mentioned specialists, and, therefore, consultations with other specialties, both surgical and medical, will need to be obtained from time to time.

Trainees. Since the Pain Unit presents an ideal opportunity for the study of chronic pain and its effects on patients, it provides a suitable environment for instructing trainees in the management of pain. These can be students formally attached to the unit who have an interest in furthering their understanding of pain—that is, physicians from any specialty, who are interested in spending a 6- or 12-month fellowship for gaining experience with such patients. It also provides a sound opportunity to teach medical students and house staff, on a shorter term, the management of these patients, the applied anatomy of neural blockade, and the sequelae of blockade of various levels of the neuraxis.

Research. Because it brings together patients with various kinds of chronic pain, the Pain Unit could, and should, be used as a source of research into the causes and therapy of this major medical, health, and economic problem.

Facilities

The space and physical layout will obviously have to be tailored to the individual requirements of each institution. However, ideally, a Pain Unit should involve both outpatient and inpatient facilities.

Outpatient facilities can be those found in any hospital outpatient department or private clinic. However, there are special needs for performing diagnostic and therapeutic neural blockade. This requires particular facilities for the performance of the procedure and especially for the subsequent recovery period. Therefore, blockade can be performed in an operating room-recovery room area or in a special procedure room set aside for this purpose. The recovery room is ideal. It is convenient for anesthesiologists with operating room commitments, and post-block supervision, by the attending nurses is readily available. It is important to be able to observe the patient in this post-block period for variable periods of time, to note specifically the patient's symptoms to determine the quality, extent, and results of the diagnostic block. Optimally, a portable image-intensifier or radiographic system should be available for the nerve block room. Alternatively, blocks that require radiographic control should be performed in the radiographic department; thus, it would be necessary to transport there all the materials and facilities for nerve block and for coping with its complications (resuscitation equipment), as discussed in Chapter 6.

Inpatient facilities are needed for elective diagnostic admissions and also for emergency admissions that occur as complications of nerve blocks, drug toxicity problems, and so forth. Ideally, these beds should be on a single ward, with nursing personnel experienced in the observation and management of these patients. The Pain Unit's unique use of drug profiles (see below), time-contingency medication, and pain "cocktails" demands that the nurses have special knowledge and expertise, which is best accomplished by admitting such patients only to one special ward—thus, the nurses there will acquire the necessary experience.

There must be a "headquarters" where the coordination of the Pain Unit and the storage of its files and referral information can be consolidated and with the facility for holding the "Pain Management Conference." Headquarters can be as extensive as funds and space will allow, but at a minimum probably will require a desk and office space for the administrative secretary and occasional use of a meeting room, lecture hall, and so forth.

Patient Management

Referral and Screening. It is important that patients be seen on a referral basis. Since a Pain Unit is primarily a diagnostic facility, patients should be referred back to their private physician for long-term maintenance. Even if the clinic is willing to follow patients long-term, it is unlikely that it will have the resources to provide long-term care to all the patients referred to it, unless, of course, facilities and staff are in liberal supply.

Patients referred to Pain Units have diverse problems and some attempt should be made to screen them before acceptance. If facilities are limited, it is obviously more appropriate to devote time and effort to conditions that are more successfully treated by the therapies available, than to deploy resources on likely failures. It is usually not appropriate to refer a patient to a Pain Unit until conventional avenues of diagnosis and therapy have been tried and found wanting.

Each unit will probably determine its own criteria of acceptance. A sample of such criteria is as follows: all patients with cancer pain should be considered high-priority; priority should be given to patients with nonmalignant pain who can most successfully be managed, such as patients with drug intoxication problems, patients with reflex sympathetic dystrophies, patients whose behavioral analysis suggests that operant conditioning might correct the problem, patients with migraine and tension headache problems that biofeedback might relieve, and, of course, patients with intractable pain of unknown cause. Pain due to vascular occlusive disease should also receive high priority because it is often very successfully treated by temporary or permanent neural blockade (see Chap. 13).

The screening of applications to a pain clinic is a very important task. Unless unlimited facilities are available, it is unlikely that the Pain Unit can cope with the entire referral load. It is therefore important to attempt to assess which patients are most likely to benefit from a Pain Unit, and which are not. This will mean that the unit can be involved in more productive patient care and will not lead to unnecessary disappointments as a result of unfairly raising a patient's hopes. Thus, complete referral information must be obtained and assessed by the clinical coordinator prior to accepting the patient.

Diagnostic Assessment. When it is believed that a patient might benefit from the facilities the unit has to offer, it is important to collect as much information on medical history as possible. This will certainly include such information as old films, operative reports, and the results of previous medical consultations. With this information at hand, it is often possible to decide whether the patient will best be managed as an inpatient or an outpatient, and the appropriate arrangements can be made.

For outpatient management, an initial screening visit is scheduled. The patient sees the clinical coordinating physician; a comprehensive history and physical examination are undertaken; and, usually at this time, the patient will complete a psychological screening form (*e.g.*, Minnesota Multi-Phasic Personality Inventory). Depending on the results of the history and physical examination, the clinical coordinator may then suggest consultations with the representatives of other Pain Unit specialties, for example, behavioral analysis, neurosurgical assessment, social work evaluation, and so forth. Some further diagnostic tests may also be scheduled, such as radiographs before even a temporary diagnostic neural blockade is performed. The scheduling of these consultations, procedures, and tests often presents logistical problems. For patients from out-of-town, it is often more feasible to complete the more complex workup on an inpatient basis.

When completed, all this information is presented at the "Pain Management Conference." This assembles the consultants who have seen the patient with the Clinical Coordinator. There will often also

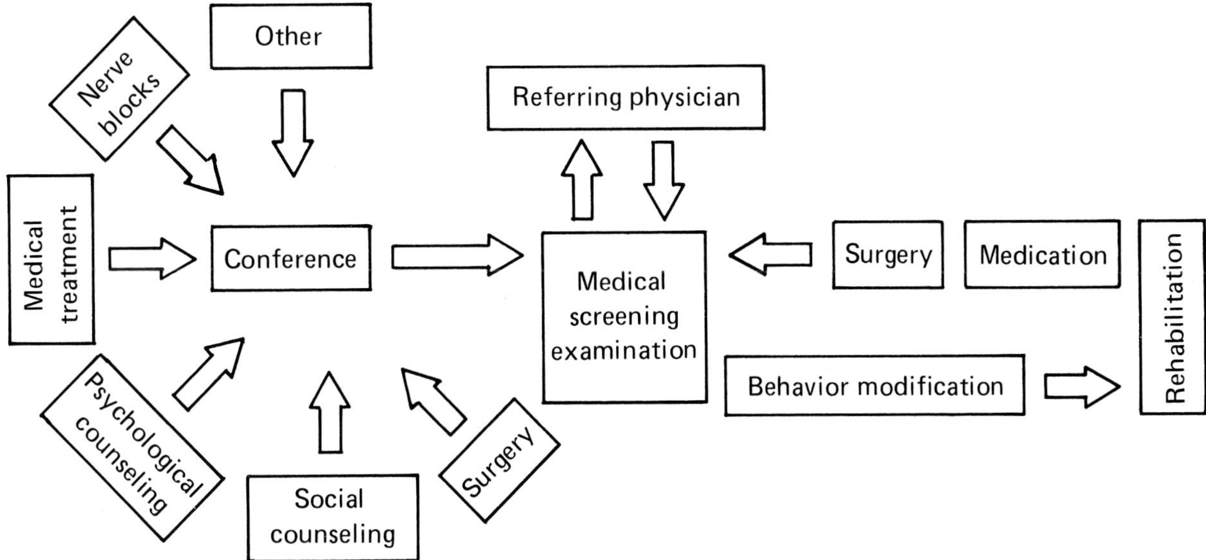

Fig. 30-1. This flowchart illustrates the options and program of diagnosis and treatment for patients in a multidisciplinary pain clinic. (*Left*) Multidisciplinary diagnosis, (*right*) therapy.

be other consultants present who, though not directly involved with the particular patient, can often contribute their expertise to the problem. The conference poses an excellent opportunity for teaching medical students, house staff, and others, and these should be welcome and encouraged to attend. At the conference, a synopsis of the patient's history and problem is distributed, and each of the consultants who have seen the patient contribute their own ideas and impressions from the results of various diagnostic tests, including neural blockade; the likely pathophysiology of the pain; and therapy suggestions. The patient and spouse are usually present at these conferences to permit members of the Pain Unit who have not directly been concerned with this patient to have an opportunity to question and examine the patient. The patient, too, is given an opportunity to describe his problem and its course to the conference, if appropriate. As a result of the presentations, a consensus on the most likely diagnosis for the patient's pain can be reached in addition to therapeutic suggestions. These are conveyed to the patient and the patient's referring physician by the coordinating clinical manager.

It will not infrequently happen that the therapeutic suggestions will be implemented within the framework of the Pain Unit by one or another of the consultants. However, the therapeutic suggestions may be administered by the patient's own referring physician, if he and the patient so choose.

The organization of diagnosis and treatment in a multidisciplinary pain clinic is shown in Figure 30-1.

The patient is referred to the clinic by his private physician. At the first screening visit, the coordinating physician in the pain clinic decides if the patient can be directed immediately into a treatment program in which he will undergo one or other of the therapeutic endeavors shown in the therapy pathway. If, however, the cause of the pain is still unclear after the screening visit, then the patient would enter the diagnosis pathway and see some or all of the specialists listed and undergo such further investigations as diagnostic nerve blocks, psychological screening, further films and so forth. At the conclusion of the testing, all the pain-unit specialists will decide at the conference what is the most likely diagnosis and suggest appropriate therapy. These findings are communicated to the patient and the referring doctor by the coordinating pain-unit physician. The patient may follow through with the clinic suggestions by the therapy pathway within the clinic, or, if mutually agreeable, will undergo therapy under the supervision of the referring doctor.

Two examples may help to clarify this procedure.

Case No. 1. An elderly woman with carcinoma of the pancreas has severe abdominal pain and is taking large doses of injectable morphine and many diazepam tablets. This treatment does not control the pain, and she is referred to the Pain Unit. On screening examination, it is decided that the patient probably has a dual problem: that of pain from her pancreatic cancer and a secondary problem of excessive and inappropriate medication. A decision is made to commence treatment: and she would then enter the therapy pathway, being stabilized on oral analgesics, probably methadone and phenobarbital "cocktail," and undergo diagnostic and probably neurolytic celiac plexus block. After the pain has been relieved by the block and the analgesic sedative-hypnotic medications have been reduced to a level that keeps the patient comfortable but not overmedicated, she would be referred back to her referring physician for maintenance therapy. This patient would not have required a multidisciplinary assessment because of her relatively straightforward problem.

CASE NO. 2. A 30-year-old unskilled laborer has injured his back, allegedly from the negligence of his employer, while working on a construction site. He has had a persistent low-back-pain problem since this incident, 3 years prior to his attending clinic. He has had two lumbar laminectomies in a so-far futile attempt to cure his back pain. He is now addicted to oxycodone and secobarbital. He is suing his employers for negligence, and his disability payments are being curtailed. Furthermore, his wife is threatening to leave him, and his teenaged son is in trouble with the police. On examination at the clinic, he shows unimpressive clinical signs of any physical defect in his back, yet he exhibits much pain behavior and many signs and symptoms of depression. This patient obviously needs a detailed multidisciplinary assessment of his physical and psychosocial status before any recommendations about diagnosis and treatment can be made. Therefore, the coordinating pain-unit physician embarks upon the diagnostic pathway, as shown in the diagram. After consultations and diagnostic nerve blocks, a Pain-Unit conference is held, and it might recommend the following: he would be advised against undergoing further surgery for his problems. Detoxification from his addicting medical regime would be undertaken on an inpatient basis, and, following this, long-term therapeutic suggestions would include a selective rehabilitation and physical therapy program and strong recommendations for marital and family counseling. He would be advised to settle his lawsuit expeditiously and to continue in a psychotherapeutic program for treatment of depression. Such an unfortunate patient not only needs a multidisciplinary diagnostic assessment but also a well-coordinated multidisciplinary therapeutic strategy.

Therapeutic Potential

It is important to place the use of neural blockade in the context of other approaches to pain management. Although some pain units tend to specialize in particular kind of therapy, a true multidisciplinary clinic would probably include the following modalities in its therapeutic repertoire.

Medication Control. Analgesics, tranquilizers, and hypnotics are frequently administered to patients with chronic pain. They are also much abused by such patients, and considerable effort is spent in pain units to stabilize patients on an appropriate medication regime. If the pain problem has genuine nociceptive elements, then analgesic medications will have a rightful place in management. Because of the potential for abuse, especially with the narcotic medications, adherence to a time-contingent pattern of administration (not an "as needed" schedule) is essential. For this reason and also to enable adjustments of dosage and content, a "pain cocktail" regime is frequently used. This means that the active ingredient is administered in a masking vehicle, for example, cherry syrup. This mixture is taken at set times during each day, and the active ingredients can be varied without the patient's knowledge. This is very useful for the acute detoxification process and also for long-term maintenance in patients who have shown a tendency to medication abuse. The psychoactive drugs (tranquilizers, hypnotics, etc.) are frequently used to help allay anxiety and sleeplessness. In most of the patients with chronic pain, long-term use of barbiturates is singularly disappointing, and such sedative tranquilizers as diphenhydramine (Benadryl) and hydroxyzine (Vistaril) are preferable for long-term use since they do not lead to an addiction with a withdrawal phenomenon, upon cessation of use. In deafferentation pain problems and central pain states, drugs such as diphenylhydantoin (Dilantin) and Carbamazepine (Tegretol) have proved very useful, and the more recently introduced combination of amitriptyline (Elavil) and fluphenazine (Prolixin) have proved useful in the treatment of postherpetic neuralgias. Much of the work in the pain unit is devoted to medication adjustment and administration, both on an inpatient and an outpatient basis.

Neural Blockade Procedures

Neural blockade techniques are frequently used by anesthesiologists in pain units. They fall into two broad categories.

Diagnostic neural blockade is used to determine

the afferent pathway of the nociceptive impulse (if any) and also to predict the effect of nerve-destroying procedures such as neurolytic blocks, neurectomy, sympathectomy, and so forth. Long-acting agents such as bupivacaine or etidocaine can give the patient some idea of the sequelae of a nerve-sectioning procedure. Such a prognostic experience is not entirely satisfactory for although the resulting numbness of these nerve blocks is often well tolerated on a short-term basis, the sensations that result from a prolonged denervation following neurectomy or neurolytic block are often less well tolerated. However, it is still useful to enable both the physician and the patient to decide on the wisdom of such radical procedures (see also Chap. 26).

Therapeutic neural blockade is often used in pain units, particularly of the autonomic nervous system, such as the stellate ganglion and lumbar sympathetic ganglia blockades for reflex sympathetic dystrophies of the arms and legs, respectively. Trigger-point injections are used in the myofascial syndromes. Neurolytic neural blockade has a limited, but very definite, application in pain-unit work. Because neurolytic blockade is rarely permanent (*i.e.*, it can last anywhere from 6 months to a year or so), it is more applicable for patients with terminal disease and, in cancer patients, can afford considerable welcome relief from pain. It is less useful in nonmalignant chronic pain states in which the sequelae of numbness and paralysis are less well tolerated in patients with a long life expectancy. An exception, however, is neurolytic lumbar sympathetic block for occlusive vascular disease and some of the reflex sympathetic disorders (see Chap. 13).

Other Procedures

Surgical Therapy. Surgical attempts to relieve chronic pain are infrequently successful; however, there is a very definite place for such neurosurgical procedures as chordotomy and neurectomy, especially in cancer patients. Like neurolytic blockade, these nerve-destroying procedures are well tolerated in patients with a limited life span and less successful in patients with a long life expectancy. A recently introduced technique of thermogangliolysis has proved very useful in the management of trigeminal neuralgia.[6] This procedure involves thermal coagulation of the gasserian ganglion with a heated stylus, and selective interruption of pain pathways can be achieved, leaving touch and sensation intact. This is an improvement over the total anesthesia produced by neurolytic block of the gasserian ganglion with its subsequent hemifacial numbness and its complicating eye problems secondary to the conjunctival anesthesia. The insertion of perineural and dorsal column nerve stimulators, either operatively or by more recently developed percutaneous techniques, appears to have some potential for controlling some chronic pain states.

Psychiatry. Few patients with chronic pain have exclusively pyschiatric causes of their problems; however, many suffer from depression. Chronic pain is viewed by some authorities as a depressive-equivalent, especially since many of the symptoms of depression and chronic pain are identical (*i.e.*, anorexia, sleep disturbances, decreased libido, decreased activity, etc.). Antidepressant medications are very useful in treating patients; with chronic pain, and psychotherapy may be required.

Psychological Therapy. Communication of pain is, in the final analysis, a behavioral phenomenon. Sometimes, many of the chronic complaints of pain can be treated by behavioral modification methods, especially in patients in whom there is no significant organic pathology and an abundance of pain behavior. These "operant conditioning" therapies usually involve prolonged hospitalization, and they demand the cooperation of the spouse and immediate family members. Although these therapies are often spectacularly successful in the hospital, if the patient returns to the environment that reinforces his pain behavior, then he is prone to relapse. Therefore, the domestic environment must be changed by the cooperation of the patient's family. Sternbach has suggested the term *pain patients* to distinguish from, for example, pain from cancer, which afflicts a *patient in pain*.[8]

Physiatry. Many patients lead very inactive lives and can benefit considerably from an active rehabilitation program—physiatry, or physical therapy. This is, in fact, an integral part of many of the therapeutic pain units and is certainly a very important factor in the operant conditioning program mentioned above.

Biofeedback. Muscle tension pains of the shoulder and neck region, along with migraine-type headaches, respond quite well to biofeedback therapy. This has proven to be a very useful adjunct for controlling pain in such patients.

The above should give some indication of the kinds of therapies available in a pain unit. Some patients with chronic pain will need more than one therapeutic modality and sometimes the combination of three or four in order to effect an improvement in their unfortunate state. This emphasizes the need for collaboration if neural blockade techniques are to be used safely and effectively.

Other Functions

In addition to its main multidisciplinary diagnostic function, the Pain Unit also is excellent for undertaking some other tasks. Because of the expertise acquired in managing both analgesic and sedative-hypnotic agents, patients who suffer from therapeutic (iatrogenic) drug addiction (as opposed to self-inflicted drug addiction), can often be helped immensely by the detoxifying regimen used in the Pain Unit. Such patients are admitted; all their medications are removed from them (by search if need be); and they are then put on a "drug profile" schedule, which permits the ingestion of medications of a nature and frequency of the patient's own choosing for a period of 24 to 48 hours. This permits a far better assessment of the patient's genuine medication consumption than that obtained by the report of either the patient or his family. The next step is the oral "pain cocktail" regime whereby all the narcotics are replaced by methadone and the sedative-hypnotics by phenobarbital, in equivalent dosages (administered in a masking vehicle—the "cocktail"), which are reduced over the course of the next 1 to 2 weeks. This effective method of stabilizing patients previously taking excessive medication is often necessary prior to attempting to assess their pain problem (and is often remarkably therapeutic as well).

The nerve block facilities of the Pain Unit can also be utilized in patients with paraplegia for treating problems of spasticity of voluntary muscles and problems of sphincteric control that are amenable to neurolytic blockade.

REFERENCES

1. Alexander, F.A.D., and Lewis, L.W.: The control of pain. *In* Hale, D.E. (ed.): Anesthesiology. Pp. 801–856. Philadelphia, F.A. Davis, 1954.
2. Bonica, J.J.: The Management of Pain. Philadelphia, Lea & Febiger, 1953.
3. Bonica, J.J., and Black, R.G.: The management of a pain clinic. *In* Swerdlow, M. (ed.): Relief of Intractable Pain. Pp. 116–129. Amsterdam, Elsevier, 1974.
4. McEwen, B.W., *et al.:* The pain clinic—A clinic for the management of intractable pain. Med. J. Aust., *1*:676, 1965.
5. Simpson, D.A., Saunders, J.M., Rischbieth, R.H.C., Burnell, A.W., and Cramond, W.A.: Experiences in a pain clinic. Med. J. Aust., *1*:671, 1965.
6. Sweet, W.T., and Wepsic, J.G.: Controlled thermocoagulation of trigeminal ganglion and rootlets for differential destruction of pain fibres, Part I: Trigeminal Neuralgia. J. Neurosurg., *39*:143, 1974.
7. Swerdlow, M.: The pain clinic. Br. J. Clin. Pract., *26*:403, 1972.
8. Sternbach, R.A.: Pain Patients. Traits and Treatment. New York, Academic Press, 1974.

31 New Horizons

Michael J. Cousins and
Christopher J. Glynn

Recent advances in the knowledge of neural blockade and pain indicate that the next decade will see a number of long-standing problems conquered. This chapter gives a few examples.

---

selective spinal analgesia
somatic neural blockade by cryoanalgesia
assessment of pain and its sequelae
pharmacokinetic-based techniques for improved supplementation of neural blockade in acute and chronic pain states
educational horizons

It should be recognized that these are but a small selection of science applied to acute and chronic pain management. The reader will appreciate this more fully by a perusal of the published abstracts of the International Pain Symposium, Seattle, 1974; the First World Congress on Pain in Florence, 1975; and the abstracts of the Second World Congress in Montreal, 1978.[6,7] Such is the range of interest in pain investigation and improved management of all forms of pain that the Second World Congress had participants from 30 disciplines and 50 countries.

SELECTIVE SPINAL ANALGESIA

The discussion of modern concepts of pain transmission in Chapter 24 makes it clear that this is the brink of an entirely new pharmacology of pain control, which manipulates not only the "facilitatory" primary afferent pain pathway but also inhibitory serotonergic and noradrenergic pathways.[10] It is quite likely that the options for pain control, at different levels, will become as wide-ranging as the current options for the treatment of hypertension. For example, experimental evidence presented in Chapter 24 already indicates that tricyclic antidepressant drugs with serotonergic and noradrenergic activity inhibit pain transmission in animals. In a completely different class of drugs, the spinal interneurone blocker lioresal (Baclofen) is also capable of an analgesic effect. Of even greater interest is the powerful effect of the antisubstance P agent capsaicin, which produces profound and prolonged analgesia of highly selective nature.* The possibilities for pharmacologic modification of pain at the spinal-cord level are only just coming into focus; however, they are extremely wide-ranging and exciting.

For the present, however, ethical and other considerations have limited studies in humans to direct administration of narcotics into the spinal fluid and epidural space. A series of cases of epidural administration of morphine providing excellent relief of chronic pain has been reported.[5] Subsequently, evidence was given of a selective spinal action of meperidine injected into the spinal subarachnoid and epidural space in humans.[10] In this study, data were obtained by pharmacokinetic studies of blood and cerebrospinal fluid (CSF) concentrations of meperidine and objective assessment of neural function, integrated with studies of analgesic effect and duration of analgesia. The stimulus to this work was the initial reports of Yaksh and co-workers and further studies from the Mayo Clinic of the analgesic effects of subarachnoid morphine.[43,46,48] Unlike the initial lumbar injections by Wang and colleagues, injections were made as close to the affected spinal segments as possible (*e.g.*, T_2–T_3 for pain due to advanced breast cancer.[43] Subarachnoid administration of 10 to 30 mg of meperidine or 1 to 3 mg of morphine in five patients with severe intractable cancer pain resulted in complete pain relief for up to 48 hours, compared with only 24 hours in the studies reported by Wang and colleagues. Although the analgesia obtained appeared to be selective if dilute solutions of morphine or meperidine were used, an initial local anesthetic effect was observed if the

---

* Current evidence indicates that capsaicin depletes substance P (see Chap. 24).

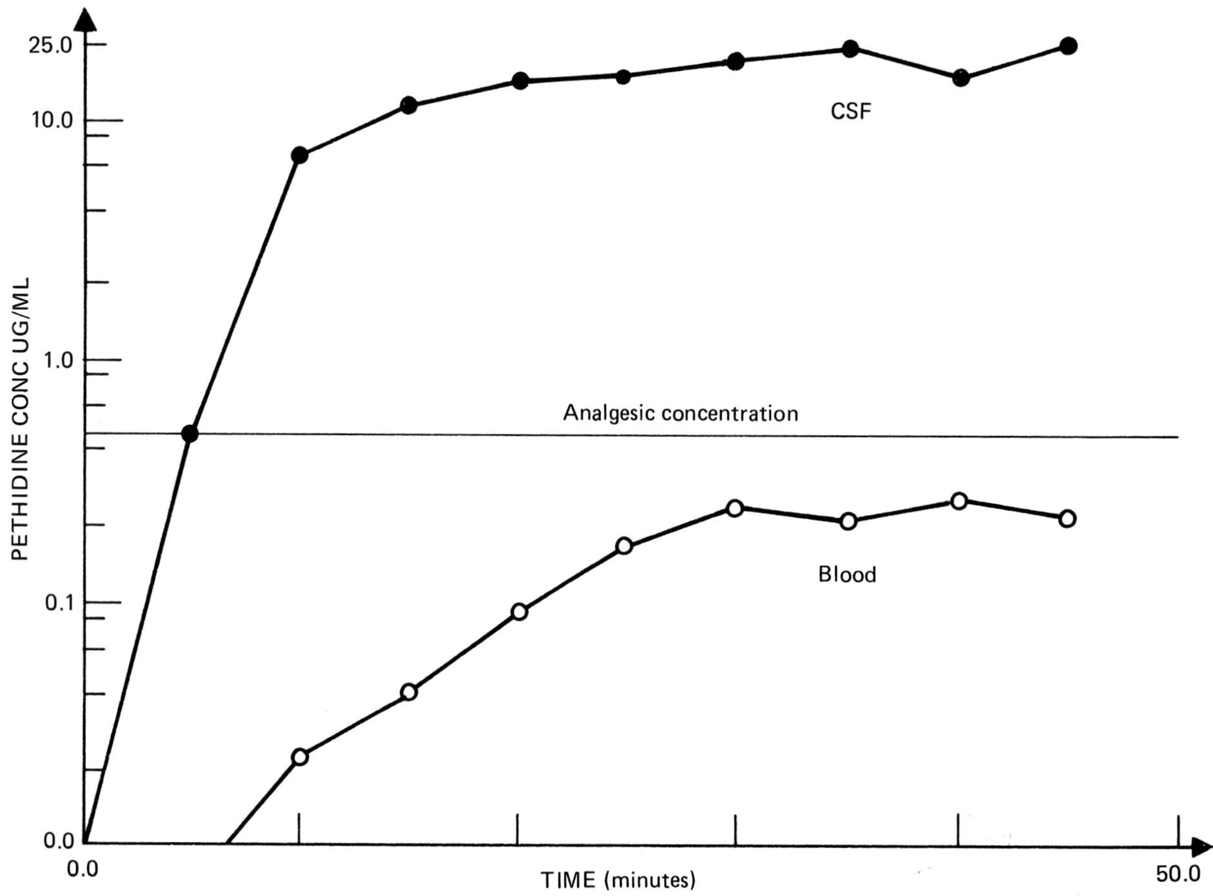

Fig. 31-1. Epidural meperidine (Pethidine). Simultaneous measurements of blood and CSF concentrations of meperidine are shown. The onset of analgesia coincided with very high CSF concentrations of meperidine at 5 minutes following epidural injection. (Cousins, M.J., *et al.:* Selective spinal analgesia. Lancet, *1*:1141, 1979)

meperidine concentration exceeded 2 per cent (20 mg of meperidine in 1 ml). This is not surprising since it has long been known that meperidine has local anesthetic properties, as, to a lesser extent, does morphine. Thus, the advantage of no sympathetic block may be lost if more concentrated solutions of narcotics are injected into the subarachnoid space.

Selective Epidural Blockade With Narcotics

Despite the success of subarachnoid narcotics in early studies, it has been clear that application was limited by the need to reinsert a subarachnoid needle every 2 days. Thus studies with an indwelling epidural catheter in patients with pain due to cancer or associated with surgery for cancer naturally followed. On the basis of its physicochemical properties, meperidine would be expected to enter the CSF more rapidly than morphine. Hence, pharmacokinetics and analgesic effects were initially studied after epidural administration of meperidine in eight patients with intractable cancer pain and in eight patients with severe pain after major surgery for cancer; pharmacokinetic studies were also performed after intravenous meperidine.[10] These combined data permitted calculations of the rate of absorption from the site of injection (*i.e.*, the epidural space).

Postoperative Pain

In patients with postoperative pain, preservative-free meperidine hydrochloride, 100 mg in 10 ml of physiologic saline, was injected by way of the epidural catheter. Onset of pain relief at 5 minutes coincided with the presence of high concentrations

(0.5–2 mg/L) of meperidine in CSF. Complete pain relief, as judged by the visual analogue scale, occurred within 12 to 20 minutes in all patients and corresponded to meperidine CSF concentrations of 10 to 20 mg/L. Typical beak blood concentrations occurred after approximately 40 minutes (Fig. 31-1). Mean absorption half-life after epidural administration of meperidine was 25 minutes. Over periods varying from 2 to 4 days, doses of meperidine as required gave a mean duration of analgesia of 6 hours (range 4.5–20 hours).

Subsequent studies indicate that 100 mg of meperidine or 10 mg of morphine epidurally is required for effective relief of severe post-operative pain. At this dosage level transient hypotension is seen in postoperative patients, and some patients develop an elevated $Paco_2$ in a range of 55 to 60 torr. By the second postoperative day, 30-mg doses of meperidine are quite adequate, and at this dosage there is neither hypotension nor hypercarbia.

Chronic Pain

In patients with chronic pain 30 mg of meperidine hydrochloride in 6 ml of physiologic saline, epidurally as required, provided complete pain relief. Blood concentrations after epidural injections were less than concentrations determined to be analgesic in each patient by previous studies with intravenous infusion of meperidine. The level from intravenous infusion corresponded closely to reported analgesic blood concentrations of meperidine (0.5 mg/L) determined in postoperative patients.[40] Over a period of 1 to 9 days, mean duration of analgesia was 8 hours (range 3.5–18 hours).

After 100-mg doses, meperidine blood concentrations did eventually approach analgesic levels in some patients by 30 to 40 minutes after injection. This resulted in no increase in analgesia and a transistory (10–15 minutes) mild sedation. In two patients, intravenous injection of naloxone, 0.4 mg, was followed by immediate reversal of sedation, with no change in level of analgesia; 30 minutes later there was a reduction but not a reversal of analgesic effect. These data strongly suggest that the initial analgesic effect of the high doses of epidural meperidine was due to a spinal action. At later stages (40–60 minutes after injection) analgesia may have resulted from a combination of a spinal action and the central nervous system (CNS) effects associated with blood-borne meperidine. However, the reversal of sedative effects of meperidine by intravenous naloxone with no immediate change in analgesic effect suggests that the predominant action is on the spinal cord. Yaksh and Rudy have shown that naloxone administered directly in the CSF rapidly antagonizes the analgesic effect of subarachnoid morphine in animals.[48] The lagtime between naloxone administration and antagonism of analgesia in our studies was probably due to the slow rate of naloxone delivery caused by the lower perfusion of the spinal cord than of the brain.

Selectivity of Block

Neurologic examination before and after epidural meperidine revealed no detectable change in sensory, motor, or sympathetic function. Lack of motor blockade was further illustrated by the ability of patients to ambulate within 30 minutes of injection. Lack of sympathetic block was confirmed by retention of a normal cobalt blue sweat test and no postural hypotension after epidural meperidine.[11] Venous occlusion skin plethysmography and ice response were used to assess reflex efferent sympathetic vasomotor activity; a normal ice response was retained (Fig. 31-2). In contrast, subsequent injection of 10 ml of local anesthetic (2% lidocaine) resulted in a large increase in foot blood flow and an abolition of the response to ice, indicating complete sympathetic blockade in lower limbs. Although the local anesthetic injection was effective in relieving pain, this was accompanied by sympathetic, sensory, and motor blockade. None of the patients with chronic pain obtained complete pain relief with a control injection of saline, whereas all obtained complete pain relief with epidural meperidine.

These pharmacokinetic and neurologic data provide strong support for a selective spinal analgesic action of epidural meperidine in humans. The lack of changes in sensory, sympathetic, and motor function indicates that this form of analgesia may have considerable advantages for relief of severe acute and chronic pain in humans; thus the term *selective spinal analgesia* was coined.[10]

It is now possible to provide the complete range of blockade of different neural modalities by selecting various concentrations of local anesthetic or the appropriate concentration of narcotic for epidural administration (Fig. 31-3). Diagnostic subarachnoid or epidural narcotic blockade has the advantage of avoiding the 'cues' to the patient that result from local anesthetic blockade (loss of skin sensation).

Adverse Effects of Spinal Narcotics

Epidural and subarachnoid narcotics have raised new possibilities for selective blockade of pain transmission at the spinal-cord level. However,

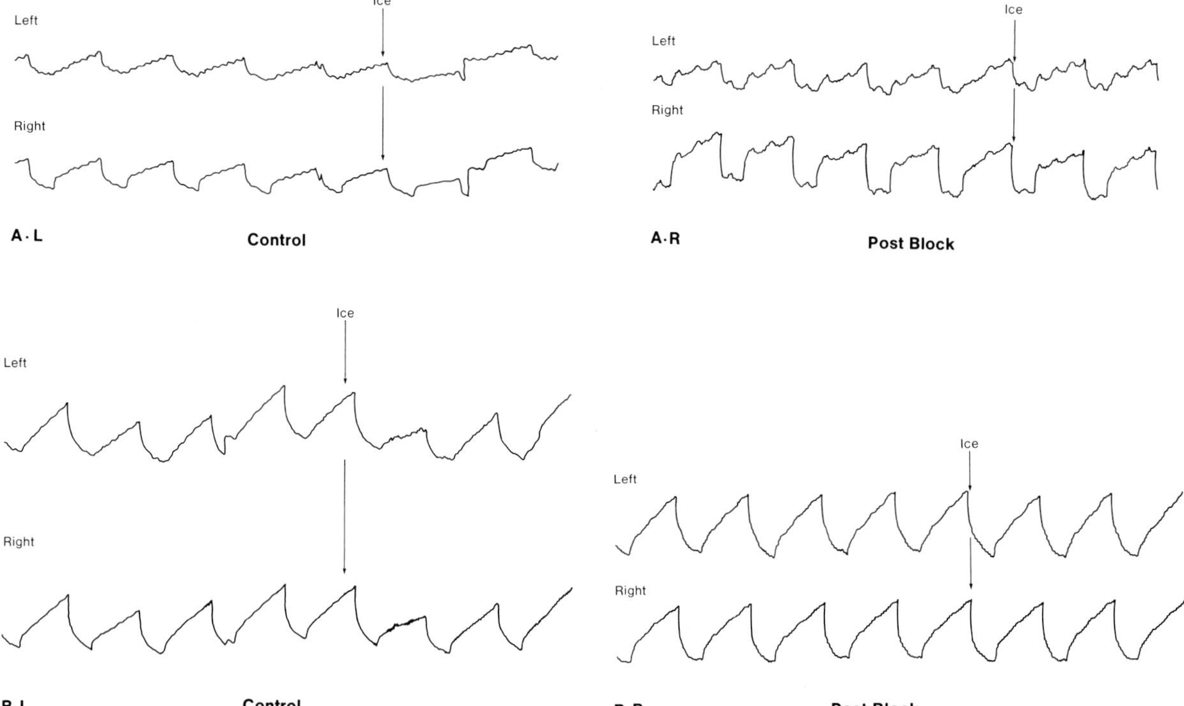

Fig. 31-2. Epidural meperidine: effect on sympathetic function. (*A*) Venous occlusion plethysmography (V.O.P.) of feet *before and following* epidural block with meperidine shows a moderate increase in foot blood flow after blockade (skin blood flow is 3.8 ml 100 ml/min compared to 1.0 ml/100 ml/min pre-block). However response to ice is the expected reduction in blood flow (−50 per cent, indicating normal efferent sympathetic function. (*B*) Same patient as above, V.O.P. of both feet *before and following* epidural block, 2 per cent lidocaine with 1/200,000 epinephrine. Note the marked increase in foot blood flow from 0.8 ml/100 ml/min to 5.0 ml/100 ml min, with clear evidence of marked vasodilatation. Also the response to ice has been abolished, indicating efferent sympathetic blockade.

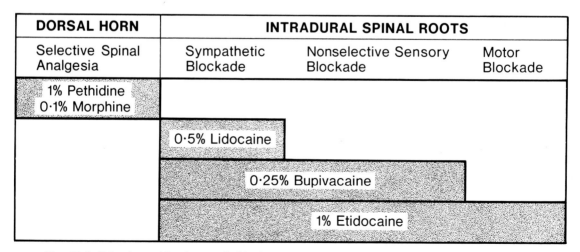

DORSAL HORN	INTRADURAL SPINAL ROOTS		
Selective Spinal Analgesia	Sympathetic Blockade	Nonselective Sensory Blockade	Motor Blockade
1% Pethidine 0·1% Morphine			
	0·5% Lidocaine		
	0·25% Bupivacaine	0·25% Bupivacaine	
	1% Etidocaine	1% Etidocaine	1% Etidocaine

Fig. 31-3. Selective epidural narcotic blockade compared to 'differential' local anesthetic blockade. A summary of current concepts of major sites of action and predominant modalities blocked.

these techniques must still be regarded as experimental until detailed pharmacologic data are available. It was noted in the original report of epidural meperidine that two patients at the higher dose level of epidural meperidine (100 mg) became sedated and required intravenous naloxone.[10] Respiratory depression has also been reported in patients who received narcotic premedication and then epidural meperidine for postoperative pain.[39] There are a number of possible reasons for this sedation and respiratory depression. Their onset approximately 30 minutes after epidural injection does coincide with high CSF meperidine concentrations. These may vary from 10 to 100 times the simultaneous blood concentrations. Also, the time course of blood concentrations of meperidine after epidural administration is similar to that following intramuscular injection.[10] Thus it is possible that either a combination of vascular absorption of narcotic premedication and postoperative epidural meperidine or excessive CSF concentrations caused the respiratory depression.

With regard to the subarachnoid administration of narcotics, high doses of hyperbaric morphine (20 mg in 15% dextrose) have been suggested by one group, compared to the initial report of Wang and colleagues, who used 1 mg in physiologic saline.[37,43]

Our experience with the larger doses of intrathecal hyperbaric morphine is limited to two patients. Both needed admission to an intensive-care unit because of respiratory depression and were given repeated doses of intravenous naloxone to maintain adequate ventilation.

Case One. The first patient (77-kg man aged 71 years) had meperidine (50 mg, and atropine (0.6 mg) premedication before a thoracotomy. Anesthesia consisted of thiopental, pancuronium, nitrous oxide with oxygen, and enflurane. On the patient's complaint of pain postoperatively, morphine (5 mg in 5% dextrose, 3 ml) was injected intrathecally at L2–3; 6 hours later the patient was comatose and Pa_{CO_2} had risen to 51 torr. He responded to intravenous naloxone (0.4 mg); over the next 12 hours he needed three more doses to maintain normal ventilation.

Case Two. The second patient (65-kg woman aged 74 years) was premedicated with diazepam (10 mg) and atropine (0.6 mg) before a laparotomy. Anesthesia consisted of thiopental, pancuronium, and nitrous oxide with oxygen including morphine (3 mg in 5% dextrose, 3 ml) injected intrathecally at L2–3. The operation (4.5 hours) was uneventful, and the patient was pain-free and could be roused for the 4 hours in the recovery ward. Eleven hours after the intrathecal morphine injection, the patient's respiratory rate was 6 per minute and Pa_{CO_2} was 55 torr. She was admitted to the intensive-care unit where she responded to an intravenous injection of naloxone (0.4 mg) by increasing respiratory rate to 16 per minute and Pa_{CO_2} improved to 45 torr. She required a further injection of naloxone (0.4 mg) 4 hours later.

In view of the time of onset, it is probable that these complications were a result of direct depression of respiratory centers in the brain stem mediated through high concentrations of narcotic in the CSF. Such depression is known to be specifically reversed by naloxone and was in fact reversed in these cases.[28] Respiratory depression was reversed but analgesia persisted.

Rate and Route of Removal. Scant attention seems to have been paid to the rate and route of removal of drugs from the CSF. There is no evidence that drugs undergo biotransformation in the spinal cord—hence the dynamics of CSF flow would seem to be extremely important. The mechanisms of CSF flow are unknown, but it is thought that pressure gradients brought about by fluid secretion, postural changes, and vascular pulsations are all involved.[47] The CSF is intimately related to the blood in three major areas: the choroid plexus, the arachnoid, and the arachnoid villi. It is generally believed that the major area for drug absorption from the CSF is the arachnoid villi, and it is noteworthy that the choroidal epithelium corresponds morphologically to that expected for an epithelium designed to absorb fluid rather than secrete (see Fig. 7-8).[47]

How and where epidurally or intrathecally administered narcotics are removed from the CSF is not known. If the choroid plexus is the major area for removal of these drugs, then it is not surprising that respiratory depression may be associated with larger doses. It is necessary for the drugs to pass through the fourth ventricle where the respiratory center is situated in order to reach the choroid plexus. Even if the three areas (the choroid plexus, the arachnoid, and the arachnoid villi) have equal absorptive potential, the amount of drug absorbed will be proportional to the rate of delivery of the drug to these areas (*i.e.*, the product of drug concentration in the CSF and CSF flow).

The group that used 20 mg of hyperbaric morphine has reported 27 hours of pain relief following intrathecal injection.[37] This is only 3 hours more than that reported by Wang and associates from 1 mg of morphine.[43] Hence, the hyperbaric technique with larger doses would appear to have no advantage over the original technique. Instead, there remains the distinct disadvantage that 20 times the dose may have 20 times the respiratory-depression effect.

Adverse cardiovascular effects could also theoretically result from high levels of narcotic in the CSF or from blood-borne narcotic absorbed from the epidural space. High CSF levels may have a brief local anesthetic effect with transitory blockade of efferent sympathetic vasomotor activity. Also, sympathetic reflexes could be reduced as a result of blockade of afferent nociceptive input to the spinal cord dorsal horn within the blocked area. It is conceivable that vasomotor center depression may result if large amounts of narcotic remain in the CSF and reach the brain stem. Blood-borne narcotic is more likely to result in direct effects on the peripheral vasculature since the blood levels achieved are unlikely to result in vasomotor center depression.

In the studies of Cousins and colleagues of low concentrations of meperidine ($<1\%$), V.O.P.† measurements of efferent sympathetic activity showed no change in reflex vasomotor activity (ice response); reflex efferent sympathetic activity, as assessed by application of ice outside the blocked area, was unchanged (see Fig. 31-2). The lack of changes in sudomotor activity (cobalt blue sweat test) also indicated normal efferent sympathetic activity in the blocked area. However, the higher doses of meperidine (100 mg) resulted in transitory hypotension when they were used to treat postoperative pain in the first 24 hours following surgery; this hypotension was short-lived (45 minutes) and did not persist for the period of analgesia. Neither was it seen when 100 mg was used for chronic pain. However, small increases in blood flow were measured in blocked limbs (Fig. 31-2).

Recently Bromage's group observed subtle changes in afferent neural activity when epidural hydromorphone was administered in the thoracic region; they could discern a sensory level as indicated by pin scratch, and also there was alteration in blood pressure response to immersing the blocked limb in ice water.*

Vasomotor Activity. Thus the question remains whether reduced afferent input to sympathetic responses poses a serious compromise to vasomotor activity even when sympathetic efferent activity is unblocked. It is possible that the transient hypotension seen in surgical patients following relief of severe pain in the early post-operative period is partly due to reduced afferent nociceptive input to the sympathetic nervous system. However, the persistence of analgesia after hypotension has subsided indicates that there may be a combination of factors. It seems likely that a peripheral vascular effect of absorbed narcotic may contribute, which is supported by the small increases in blood flow (Fig. 31-2).[10]

As noted in Chapter 24, the organization of the dorsal horn is still far from clear, and it is certain that much more remains to be learned about the spinal action of narcotics. Similar considerations apply to cerebral effects that may result from high CSF narcotic levels following spinal use of narcotics.

SOMATIC BLOCKADE BY CRYOANALGESIA

The term *cyroanalgesia* was coined by Lloyd, Barnard, and Glynn to describe the destruction of peripheral nerves by extreme cold to achieve pain relief.[27] The analgesic properties of extreme cold have been known for centuries. Indeed, the use of extreme cold constituted the earliest report of effective anesthesia, in an Anglo-Saxon manuscript of about 1050 A.D. Gratton and Singer translated this manuscript, which was attributed to a monk, Lacnunga. It says, in part, "Again, for eruptive rash, let him sit in cold water until it is deadened, then draw him up. Then cut four scarifications around the pocks and let them drip as long as he will."[20]

Refrigeration anesthesia was rediscovered over the succeeding centuries by such people as Bartholinus (1646) and Baron Larrey (1807). The latter, who was Napolean's Surgeon General, noticed that amputation was painless for soldiers who had been in the snow for some time. Armstrong Davidson states that "the discovery that cold, especially ice, would relieve pain must have been made time and again in the long history of man; Hippocrates himself knew of it, but never recommended its use for surgery. It was not until man's feelings in regard to pain had altered that general use could be made of this simple method of analgesia."[3]

Thus, Armstrong Davidson predicted the development of cryoanalgesia. It is a direct result of the increased interest in the assessment and treatment of patients with intractable pain and also the development of more powerful systems for the generation and maintenance of extreme cold.[2,6,7]

Cryoanalgesia was introduced to produce destruction of peripheral nerves for the relief of intractable pain which required somatic blockade. All other methods of peripheral nerve destruction, for

---

* Bromage, P.R.: Personal communication.

† Venous occlusion plethysmography.

example, cutting, crushing, or burning, are associated with an unacceptable incidence of neuralgia. Certainly, somatic blockade by the injection of chemical corrosives, such as phenol, has been shown, morphologically, to cause incomplete destruction of the nerve.[35] This may be the cause of the neuralgia that, not uncommonly, follows these injections or any other cause of incomplete destruction of a peripheral nerve.[32] Cryolesions are associated with less fibrous-tissue reaction than other forms of destruction.[44]

There is complete functional loss following a cryolesion in peripheral nerves of experimental animals; however, recovery can be expected over a period of weeks. This functional loss is associated with a second-degree nerve injury, according to Sunderland's (1968) classification; that is, there is Wallerian degeneration with axonal disintegration and breakup of the myelin sheaths, but with minimal disruption of the endoneurium and other connective tissue elements.[4,42]

The application and maintenance of extreme cold is achieved by using a 15-gauge cryoneedle. Blockade is based on the Joule Thompson effect with nitrous oxide as the refrigerant gas.[2] The Joule Thompson effect occurs when gas at about 700 pounds per inch is ejected through a nozzle, and, as it expands, cooling to around − 75°C occurs with nitrous oxide. The cold gas impinging on the inner surface of the needle tip absorbs heat from the surrounding tissue, and the warm gas is exhausted back up the needle and vented through a scavenging system. The Spembley-Lloyd cryoneedle incorporates a thermocouple to confirm the temperature achieved at the tip. In addition, there is an electrical connection at the tip of the probe connected to a peripheral nerve stimulator (Figs. 31-4 and 31-5).

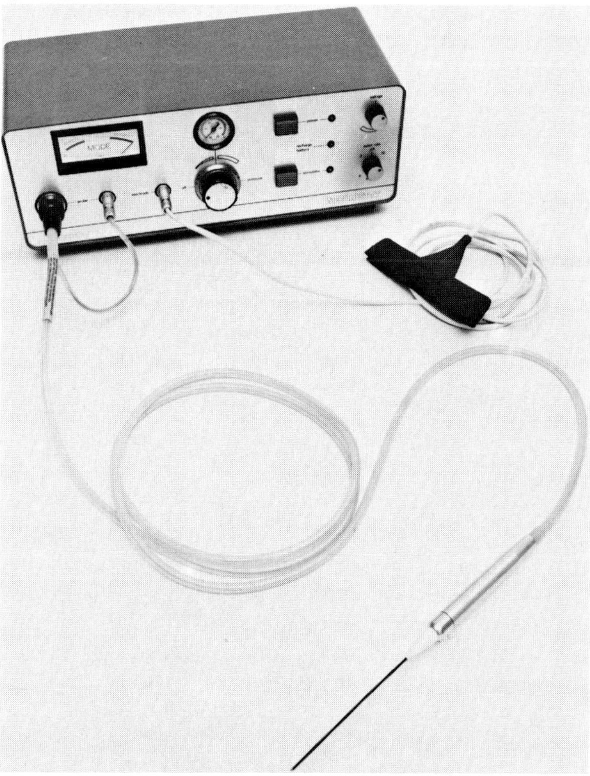

Fig. 31-4. Cryoanalgesia apparatus.

Clinical Applications

The use of cryoanalgesia has limitations in that the duration of analgesia is determined by the time taken for normal regeneration of the peripheral nerve. Thus, duration of pain relief is a function of the completeness of destruction of the peripheral nerve. The positioning of the needle is of paramount importance because the ice ball is of limited size and must incorporate the nerve to achieve complete destruction. Positioning of the needle is a function of the expertise of the clinician and the characteristics of the peripheral nerve to be frozen. The median duration of pain relief varies from about 2 weeks to about 5 months.[4,27] Cryoanalgesia should not be used on mixed nerves unless there are extenuating circumstances because it will result in complete loss of function in the nerve, including paralysis of the muscles supplied by that nerve.

The most fruitful uses for cryoprobe blockade appear to be special situations of postoperative and post-traumatic pain and medium-duration relief of chronic pain. Analgesia by intercostal block has been provided for patients undergoing thoracotomy; there was a significant reduction in the number of narcotic injections and the number of days narcotic was required compared to a control group.[18] The intercostal nerves can conveniently be blocked under direct vision at the end of the operative procedure. However if access from the chest is limited, an external approach can be used. This approach may also be used for analgesia for fractured ribs. Three important points should be noted.

First, the cryoprobe should not be withdrawn until it has fully thawed; otherwise the surrounding tissue may adhere to the probe, and it is possible to tear blood vessels and neural structures.

Second, great care should be exercised with cryoprobe blockade in the dural-cuff region. It is possible for the cold lesion to extend to the spinal

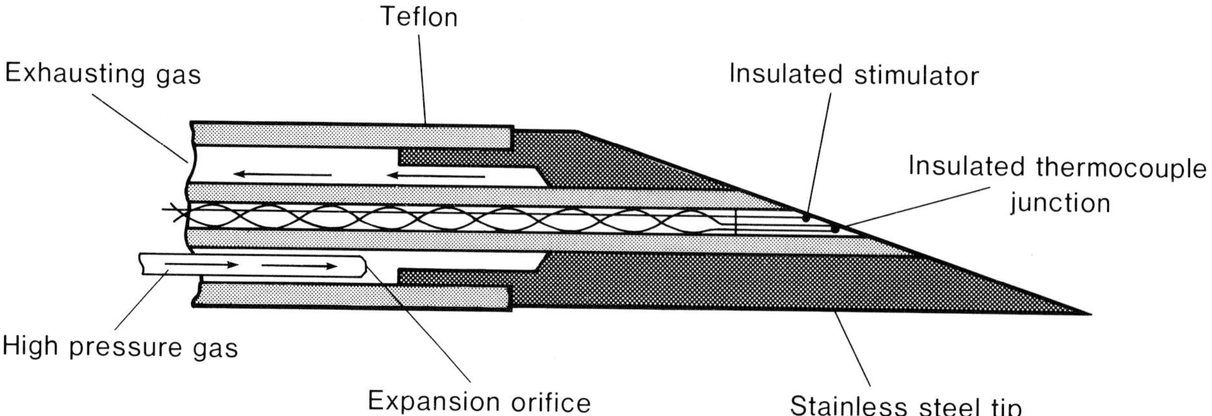

Fig. 31-5. Details of cryoprobe tip. (Lloyd, J.W., Barnard, J.D.W., and Glynn, C.J.: Cryoanalgesia. A new approach to pain relief. Lancet, *2*:933, 1976)

cord or for inadvertant thrombosis of a major "feeder artery" to result from the marked local reduction in temperature (see Fig. 8-11). Thus, in general, somatic blockade should be carried out lateral to the paravertebral muscles unless it is necessary to block the posterior primary ramus.

Third, a major disadvantage of percutaneous use is that the freezing that occurs along the needle may result in full thickness destruction of the skin. Following healing there is usually a depigmented scar. This can be prevented by heating the skin with an ordinary infrared lamp.

Applications in chronic-pain management include some of the difficult problems that require somatic blockade, for example, coccydynia and atypical facial pain in the distribution of the infraorbital nerve (with an intraoral approach).[4]

ASSESSMENT OF CHRONIC PAIN AND ITS SEQUELAE

It is generally agreed that, in a number of ways, the treatment of chronic pain differs from that of acute pain; therefore it is not surprising that the investigation of chronic pain should be different from that of acute pain (see Chap. 24). The cardinal rule of a pain clinic is that pain should not be treated symptomatically if there is a definitive treatment for the cause. This is one reason for the development of the multidisciplinary pain clinic (see Chap. 30). The investigation of chronic pain is made even more difficult by the lack of satisfactory animal models for chronic pain; indeed, there are ethical reasons for not developing such models.[41] As a result, the logical place for the investigation of chronic pain is within the pain clinic. It is possible that prevention may be the result of better understanding of the factors involved in the development of chronic pain. In order to achieve this knowledge, it is necessary to involve more basic scientists such as pharmacologists and physiologists in the clinical investigation of patients with chronic pain (Fig. 31-6).[19,29,31,40]

There are two other broad areas in which basic scientists can contribute enormously to the knowledge of chronic pain, namely psychology and anatomy. It is possible that the patients who are referred to pain clinics are from the 2.5 per cent of the population at each end of the gaussian curve on any one or any combination of the three parameters, pharmacology, psychology, and anatomy. For example, the gaussian variation within the Chinese population of 1,000 million, on any parameter, means that by definition 50 million people are abnormal (Fig. 31-7). To illustrate the point, pharmacologists have long been aware that there is a variation of response to any drug within the population. Indeed, as a direct result of these studies, a new discipline, pharmacogenetics, developed.[36] Some of this variability is known to be due to polygenic "normal" distribution while there are also marked differences in some persons owing to one abnormal pair of genes (*e.g.*, pseudocholinesterase abnormality). Differences in absorption, distribution, and clearance can be documented by appropriate pharmacokinetic studies. The role of the pharmacogenetist and the pharmacokinetist in the investigations of chronic pain must be identified. It is unrealistic to expect a standard dose of any drug to relieve pain in every patient. Thus, it is conceivable that pharmacogenetic or

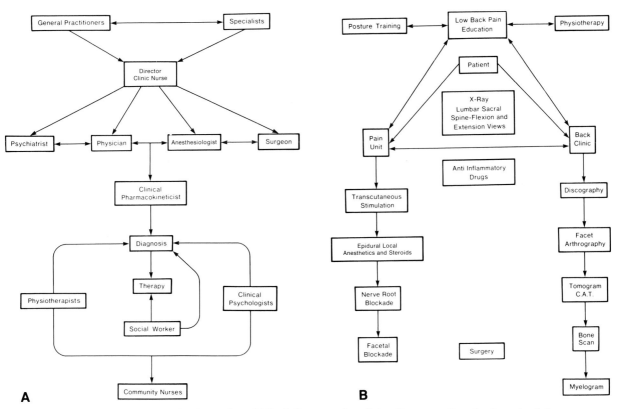

Fig. 31-6. (*A*) Organization of multidisciplinary pain clinic. Incorporating basic scientists. (*B*) Parallel activities of pain clinic and 'back' clinic.

pharmacokinetic variations contribute two very significant reasons for ineffective pain relief and the development of chronic-pain syndromes. However, it is unlikely that these differences alone would account for the chronicity of the pain.

Although much has been written about the psychology of pain, most of the information available pertains to acute and not chronic pain.[41] However, as basic scientists, psychologists have been involved in the clinical assessment and treatment of chronic pain for a number of years. Unfortunately, they have not yet been able to identify demonstrable differences between chronic pain patients as a group and the rest of the population. Once identified, it would then be necessary to determine if these differences antedate or postdate the onset of chronic pain. The identification of specific traits could predict a significant chance of acute pain becoming chronic, and it may be possible to decrease the incidence of development of chronic-pain syndromes.

Anatomical variation follows a gaussian distribution within a population and may render diagnosis of the cause of the pain difficult in some patients and the results of treatment of these patients less than ideal. There are unfortunately very few anatomists associated with pain clinics. For example, the anatomical variation of peripheral nerves can be identified by the anesthesiologist with the use of diagnostic neural blockade and confirmed by nerve-conduction studies. However, it is unlikely that by

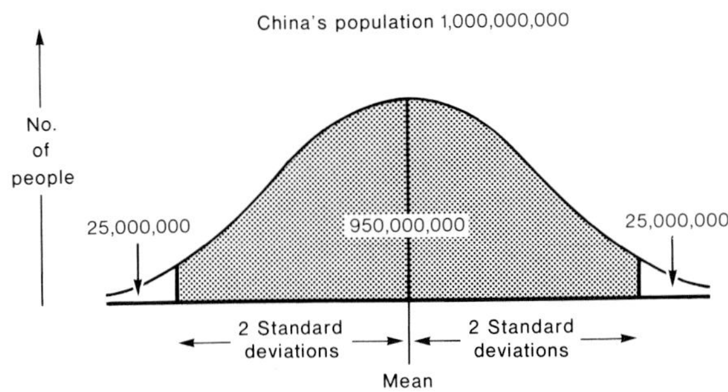

Fig. 31-7. Normal distribution of a population (*i.e.*, China) for any parameter.

the time a patient is referred to a pain clinic the etiology of chronic pain will be confined to one parameter. Thus all contributing factors must be investigated. Pain clinics, accordingly, should involve multiple clinical specialties and also should have associated with them basic scientists.

Because attitudes have changed toward acute pain, it is now possible to relieve almost all acute pain so that the same relief is expected for chronic pain. It is important to inform patients of the limitations of the treatment of chronic pain. For example, it is now well known that there are many more causes of low back pain than disk protrusion. It is important to educate patients about the possible reasons for their disability, the treatment available and its limitations, and their own role in decreasing their disability and coping with the pain (Fig. 31-6*B*).

Measurement of Physiologic Changes Associated With Pain

It is most unlikely that a reliable objective measurement of pain will ever be devised since by definition pain is a subjective experience (see Appendix). More attention should be directed to careful documentation of the patient's subjective report of pain; for example, only very recently have very basic data become available on diurnal variation in pain.[19] Although direct measurement of pain is unlikely to be a fruitful area of investigation, precise documentation of physiologic changes associated with pain offers great promise.

The discovery of endogenous opioid substances raised the possibility that measurement of these substances in the spinal fluid might provide a reliable indirect index for assessment of pain syndromes. However, to date there is no clear definition of the range of normal values nor of changes, if any, associated with various chronic-pain syndromes.

Terenius has developed a receptor binding assay to measure encephalinlike substances in the human CSF. Initial results from one group indicate low levels of CSF endorphins in patients with chronic pain of neurogenic origin, however, the diagnostic role of such measurements is yet to be defined.[1]

Various biochemical changes have been observed in patients with chronic pain. Chronic pain in patients with terminal cancer has been reported to be associated with metabolic alkalosis, and if this alkalosis is relieved, then the report of pain is less.[12]On the other hand, it has been suggested that metabolic acidosis is the cause or the result of chronic pain.[26] Some years earlier the same author described a condition he called *varalgia,* in which metabolic acidosis was the concomitant of chronic pain, and if these patients were treated with an acid-free diet, then the pain was relieved.[25]

In another study diurnal variation in plasma cortisol concentration was measured in two groups of patients with chronic pain, the cause of which in one group was believed to be organic and in the other psychogenic.[24] There were no significant differences in the plasma cortisol concentration between these two groups; indeed, the results were within the normal range throughout the day. In acute pain, plasma cholesterol and beta-lipoprotein concentrations have been reported to fall following upper abdominal surgery in parallel with a decrease in postoperative pain.[23] However, the plasma cholesterol and beta-lipoproteins were always within the normal range.

In an effort to clarify this confusing evidence about the biochemical changes associated with chronic pain, 52 patients with chronic pain had arterial blood gases (Pa_{O_2}, Pa_{CO_2}, and pH) and other biochemical parameters measured every 2 hours for 14 hours (diurnal variation). In addition, 12 of these patients had the same parameters measured over 24 hours (circadian variation).[16,17] There was no consistent alkalosis nor acidosis; the mean diurnal pH was 7.42 (range, 7.32–7.52). The only abnormal finding was chronic hyperventilation (low Pa_{CO_2} and normal pH).[8] The mean diurnal Pa_{CO_2} was 30.9 torr (range, 18.1–39.9 torr). The mean Pa_{CO_2} was outside the normal range (36–44 torr), and only one patient's mean diurnal Pa_{CO_2} was within the normal range.[2] The nocturnal Pa_{CO_2} (mean, 36.6 torr) in the 12 patients studied was below the normal range (38–49 torr), suggesting that this chronic hyperventilation continued during sleep (mean, 36.6 torr; range, 31.4–44.7 torr).[16] Only 10 of the patients who obtained pain relief were available for follow-up blood gas studies, and there was a significant increase in Pa_{CO_2} ($P < .001$; mean Pa_{CO_2}, 36.4 torr [range, 33.8–38.2 torr]), 1 week after pain relief.[17]

All the recognized respiratory stimuli, apart from chronic anxiety and plasma noradrenaline, were excluded as a cause of this hyperventilation.[16,17] Thus, it is possible that the chronic hyperventilation described is a concomitant of chronic pain and so might possibly be an objective measure of chronic pain. The most effective systemic analgesics, the narcotics, have concomitant respiratory depression, suggesting that there is some intimate association between pain and respiration. These results, however, must be confirmed by other studies.

The Pa_{O_2} found in this study was within the normal range, as were the levels of plasma cortisol and plasma cholesterol.

Pain relief may be confirmed in a number of ways, most commonly by a decrease in the demand for analgesia. If the chronic pain produces a decrease in function, for example, range of joint movement, then the return of this movement toward normal is used as an objective sign of pain relief.[22] However, not all patients complaining of chronic pain take analgesics nor do they all have decreased function. Consequently, other methods of assessment are needed. The most commonly used technique for the assessment of chronic pain is the Visual Analogue Scale, and the evidence suggests that this is the most sensitive test available. This technique relies on the patient's report of pain, and some of the factors that affect the reported pain have been identified.[14,19]

Diurnal Variation in Pain

The assessment of chronic pain should allow for the fact that many of these patients state that they are pain-free only when they are asleep. It is not surprising, therefore, that a significant diurnal variation of chronic pain has been described with the Visual Analogue Scale.[14,19] Patients with chronic pain reported significantly ($P < .001$) more pain at 22 hours that at 8 hours; indeed, there was consistent increase in the perception of pain throughout the day (Fig. 31-8). This diurnal variation differed significantly ($P < .001$) in men and women in that women reported three times as much pain throughout the day as did men. An assessment of personality was made by using the Eysenck Personality Inventory, which yields scores on extroversion and neuroticism.[13] There were significant differences found between the extroverts and introverts ($P < .05$) and also the neurotics and those with a stable profile ($P < .01$). The daily environment of these patients also significantly ($P < .005$) altered the diurnal variation of chronic pain in that patients who were at home reported more pain that those who were out to work. There was a diurnal variation in chronic pain that varied significantly according to sex, personality, and environment.[14,19] These three parameters are uncontaminated, that is, the significance of one does not effect the significance of another.

This reported diurnal variation of chronic pain was not affected by age, cause of pain, or the treatment, which was further divided into regular, irregular, or no treatment. There was no relationship among the diurnal variation and the mood factors, arousal and anxiety, and the diurnal variation of chronic pain.[16,19]

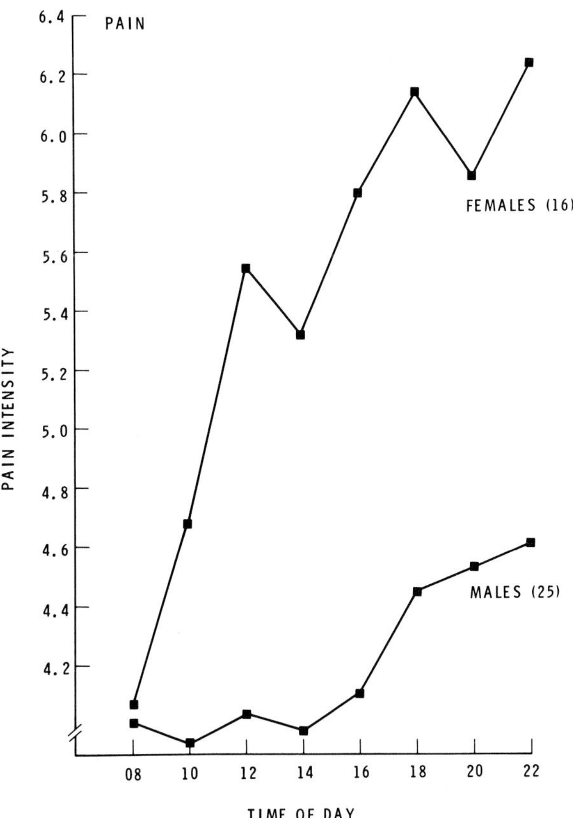

Fig. 31-8. Diurnal variation and intensity of reported pain. Note the gradual increase in pain during the day and the much higher level of pain reported by women. (Glynn, C.J., Lloyd, J.W., and Folkard, S.: The diurnal variation in perception of pain. Proc. R. Soc. Med., *69*:369, 1976)

However, the diurnal variation of chronic pain disappeared when the diurnal variation of the other two mood factors aggression and depression were included.* This suggests that there is some relationship between the diurnal variations of chronic pain and aggression and depression. The significance of this relationship remains to be identified.

Other Changes Associated With Chronic Pain

Several pain syndromes either result from or are associated with pathophysiologic changes amenable to objective measurement.

* Glynn, C.J.: Unpublished data.

Occlusive vascular disease results in readily measurable changes in blood flow, skin ulcers that can be measured, changes in skin temperature as indicated by telethermometry, and reduced capillary pulse amplitude (see Chap. 13). It is extremely helpful to document such parameters prior to beginning treatment for vascular pain and to continue such measurements in parallel with assessments of pain score.[11] If sympathetic blockade is employed in treatment, then an independent assessment of completeness of sympathetic denervation should be used, such as cobalt blue sweat test or the response to ice during skin plethysmography (see Chap. 13).

Reflex sympathetic dysfunction has remained difficult to define as a pain syndrome. It has been suggested that an attempt at objective evaluation should include the following:

- Measurement of active and passive joint range of all joints of normal and affected limb[22]
- Measurement of skin temperature of limbs
- Digital pulse amplitude as recorded by a digital plethysmograph
- Venous occlusion plethysmography with ice response (see Chap. 13)
- Thermography to demonstrate reduced blood flow due to increased sympathetic tone (Fig. 31-9)
- Sympathogalvanic response
- Radiographs of normal and affected limbs together to detect osteoporosis (Fig. 31-10)

Using such an approach Cousins was able to initiate a program for objective documentation of progress in patients with reflex sympathetic dysfunction.[22] The most important part of this program was the participation of a physical therapist who became familiar with the specific problems of this group of patients. The measurement of range of movement at each individual joint in the limb is by no means precise; however, repeated measurement by the same operator proved reliable. Also, it is extremely difficult for a patient to feign restriction of joint movement if individual joints in the hand are assessed. Although they are very simple, color photographs of both hands (or feet) can be a useful method of following progress and provide a visual record (Fig. 31-11). This record usually parallels measurable changes (*e.g.*, blood flow measurements by technique such as venous occlusion plethysmography). The importance of the use of objective criteria lies in early detection and early vigorous treatment. Unfortunately, as is with many chronic-pain syndromes, both psychological and physical changes may become essentially irreversible if diagnosis and treatment are delayed too long (Fig. 31-12). Further development of objective signs of disability associated with chronic pain should be an aim of every pain-management unit.

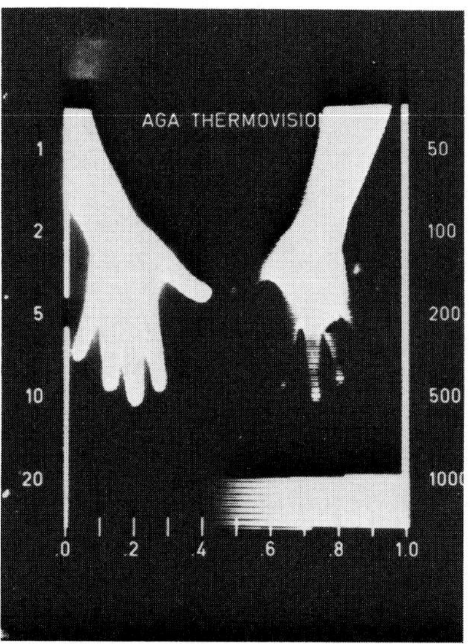

Fig. 31-9. Thermogram. Hands of a patient with a clinical syndrome suggesting reflex sympathetic dysfunction. Thermography revealed reduced blood flow (dark areas) in the left hand, indicating increased sympathetic activity. Right hand temperature was 29.1°C and left hand 26.5°C.

PHARMACOKINETIC-BASED TECHNIQUES AND NEURAL BLOCKADE

Use of Neural Blockade for Acute Pain

As presented in Chapters 3 and 4, application of pharmacokinetic techniques to the study of local anesthetic drugs has greatly increased their efficacy and safety. However, there has remained a longstanding drawback to the wide acceptance of neural blockade; it has been difficult to provide adequate supplementation without rendering the patient unconscious and adding the hazards of airway maintenance to the procedure. It seems very likely that the solution to this problem lies as much in the method of administration of narcotic and sedative drugs as in the drugs themselves. Thus, recent application of

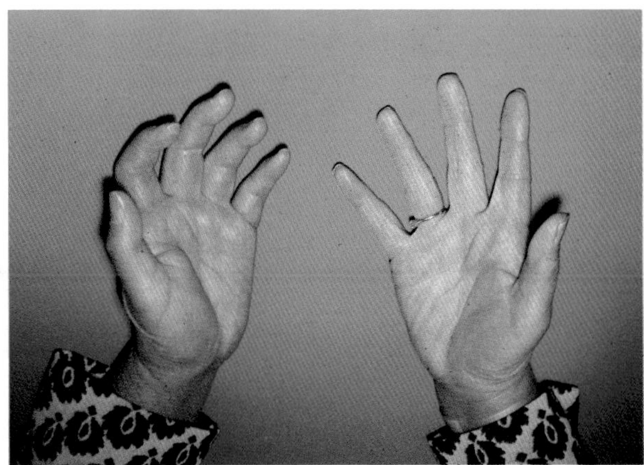

Fig. 31-11. Simultaneous color photograph of both hands of a woman with symptoms suggestive of reflex sympathetic dysfunction. The affected (left) hand shows clear evidence of swelling and is a mottled blue color, compared to the normal pink color of the right hand. Treatment by serial intravenous guanethidine (Ismelin) sympathetic blockade resulted in resolution of these changes and loss of pain.

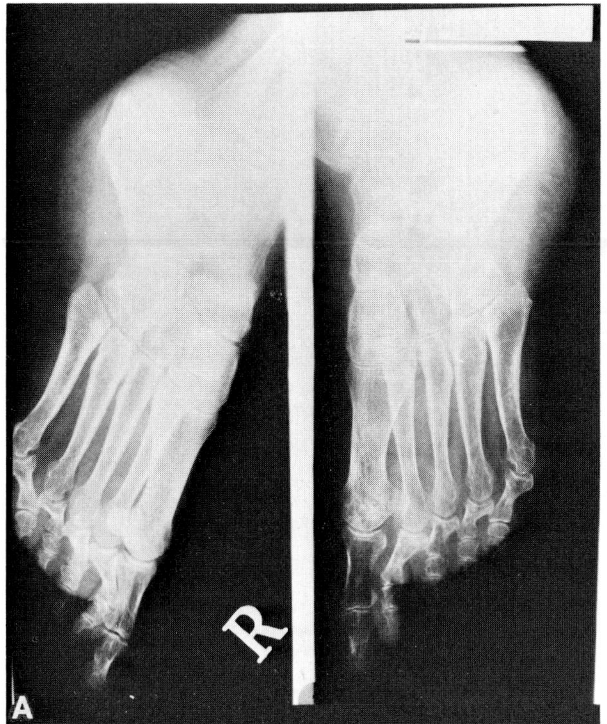

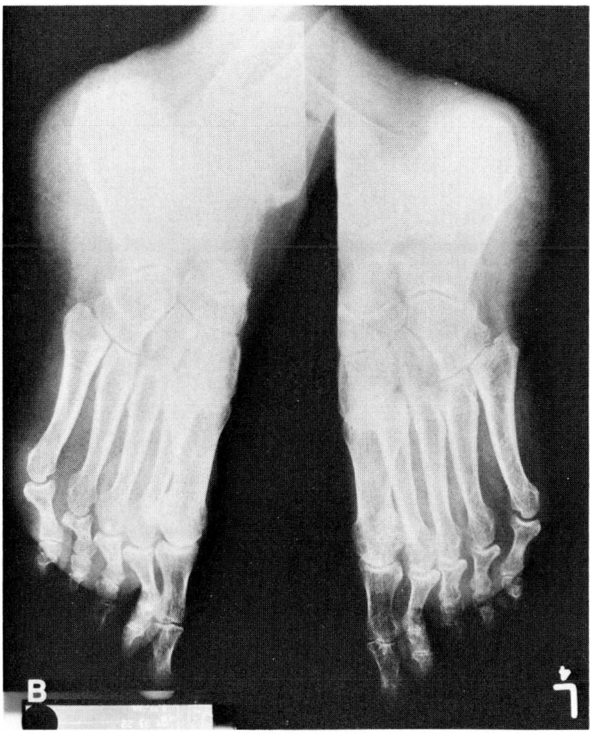

Fig. 31-10. (*A*) Simultaneous radiographs of both feet of a patient suspected of having reflex sympathetic dysfunction. Osteoporosis is seen in the affected (left) foot. (*B*) Radiographs following treatment, which included phenol lumbar sympathetic blocks, showed resolution of osteoporosis.

pharmacokinetic techniques to the analgesic and intravenous sedative agents has opened a range of options for much more satisfactory and controlled supplementation of neural blockade.[29–31] The need for such an approach was readily acknowledged by the early exponents of neural blockade who employ a drip of the short-acting barbiturate methohexitone. More recent reports have begun to appear of the use of morphine drips for postoperative pain.[9] However, the use of such techniques when there are no precise pharmacokinetic data fails to define the most efficient rate of drug delivery and also fails to highlight the margin between effective and dangerous blood concentrations, as well as the time course of any side-effects. Ideal intravenous supplementation involves a drug with a high clearance, which permits rapid changes in level of supplementation, if desired, and a rapid offset of action.

Narcotic Analgesic Supplementation. A prototype for precise pharmacokinetic control of supplementation for neural blockade can be considered by examining the data on low-dose continuous infusion of meperidine for postoperative pain control.[30,31,40] In a series of studies it has been clearly shown that analgesic effect is directly related to plasma narcotic concentration and that the wide fluctuations in blood concentration with oral, intramuscular, and intermittent intravenous bolus administration are associated with parallel fluctuations in pain control (Fig. 31-13). In contrast, consistent pain control can be achieved for long periods of time by use of a controlled continuous-infusion technique. This technique was developed by initial gathering of pharmacokinetic data by prolonged sampling during meperidine infusions and then extensive use of computer simulations to define the most efficient method of rapidly attaining and maintaining an analgesic plasma concentration (Fig. 31-14).[40]

It is now known that a steady-state plasma meperidine concentration of 0.5 mg/L (range, 0.2–0.6 mg/L) is required for effective analgesia. Continuous analgesia can now be provided intra- and postoperatively. An efficient method of achieving and maintaining analgesia is as follows:

No narcotic premedication is given. An intravenous infusion is commenced. Meperidine, 100 mg, is given by a constant-rate infusion pump over 30 minutes; then analgesia is maintained by infusing

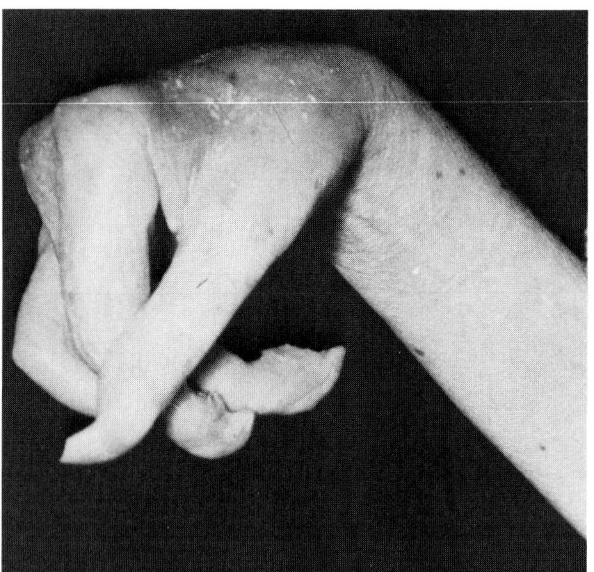

Fig. 31-12. Photograph of hand of woman who developed reflex sympathetic dysfunction following amputation of an infected finger. When first seen at the pain clinic the condition had been present for 15 years; it remained unresponsive to treatment.

meperidine at the rate of 30 mg per hour (Fig. 31-15). This regimen should be initiated only in the presence of an anesthesiologist and with close surveillance of vital signs, including respiratory rate. Adjustments must be made for patients with systemic disease and at the extremes of age. Precise predictions of resultant plasma concentrations are not yet available, but this is being investigated vigorously with a view to providing such data very shortly. Another important development involves the use of more complex *three-stage* sequential infusions, which more rapidly achieve an effective blood level with minimal "overshoot."

Supplementation With Sedative Agents. The ideal intravenous sedative with rapid clearance and rapid onset and termination of action is yet to be defined for constant-rate-infusion techniques. A number of groups throughout the world are examining drugs such as ketamine, methohexitone, alfathesin, and a water-soluble benzodiazepine. The problems still to be overcome are optimal airway maintenance with adequate sedation, avoidance of spontaneous movements, and rapid reversal of effects even after prolonged infusion. In addition to the agents noted above, interest has also been rekindled in the agent chlormethiazole (Hemineurin).

Chlormethiazole has been much maligned because of misinformed use of it in the treatment of alcoholism, largely as a result of failure of some clinicians to recognize that it has anesthetic properties. However, it has the great advantage that it produces a very tranquil state without significant cardiorespiratory depression and probably without affecting airway maintenance. Also, the drug is rapidly cleared by hepatic metabolism (and possibly metabolism at other sites in the body). We have used a regimen of a loading dose of 1500 mg of the ethane disulfonate salt solution over 30 minutes followed by a maintenance dose of 600 mg per hour, with adjustment on the basis of level of sedation and careful observation of airway maintenance in each patient.[29]

This regimen has proved extremely useful for supplementation of epidural block, particularly when uncomfortable positions such as prone are required. Onset of satisfactory sedation occurs in 5 to

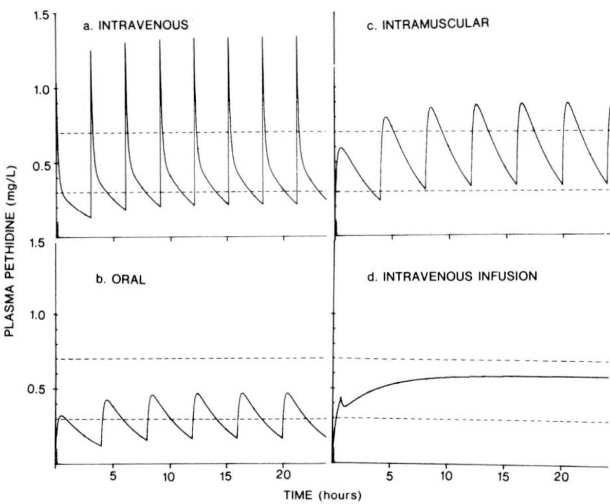

Fig. 31-13. Simulated plasma meperidine (Pethidine) concentrations based on data from surgical patients. (Data from Mather, L.E., Lindop, M.J., Tucker, G.T., and Pflug, A.E.: Pethidine revisited: Plasma concentrations and effects after intramuscular injection. Br. J. Anaesth., *47*:1269, 1975) Dotted lines indicate the limits of desirable plasma concentrations. Concentrations below the lower limit are unlikely to produce analgesia. Concentrations above the upper limit are likely to produce toxic effects. Panels (*a* to *c*) show three commonly used dosage regimens. (*a*) intravenous injections, 50 mg, 3 hourly; (*b*) oral 100 mg, 4 hourly; and (*c*) intramuscular 100 mg, 4 hourly. Panel *d* shows simulated plasma concentrations from an infusion of 50 mg given over 45 minutes followed by an infusion of 25 mg per hour. (Mather, L.E., and Meffin, P.J.: Clinical pharmacokinetic of pethidine. Clin. Pharmacokinet., *3*:352, 1978)

15 minutes, and recovery is usually complete within 3 to 5 minutes of discontinuing the infusion (Fig. 31-16). The drug is currently available in Europe and Australia as a 0.8-per-cent solution (8 mg/ml) so that an average 2-hour supplementation may involve a volume of solution of approximately 250 to 300 ml; such volumes are sometimes a concern in patients with incipient congestive cardiac failure. Initial problems with hemolysis caused by more concentrated solutions of chlormethiazole have been obviated by the 0.8-per-cent solution, and venous thrombosis is not a feature of 1- to 2-hour infusions.[29,38]

Although the clearance of the drug is significantly reduced in elderly patients during very prolonged infusion, the difference is not great enough to be of clinical significance during 1- to 2-hour infusion.[34] It is quite possible that new drugs with appeal similar to that of chlormethiazole may become available; however this agent fulfills many of the criteria for effective and safe supplementation of neural blockade.

- Rapid clearance (half-life of redistribution phase <0.5 hours)[29,34]
- Excellent sedation without spontaneous movement and with a state of great tranquility, particularly in elderly patients[15,29,38]
- Maintenance of jaw tone and respiration at effective sedative blood concentrations[29,38]
- Good cardiovascular stability with a tendency to mild tachycardia, which is useful during central neural blockade since it antagonizes parasympathetic dominance (see Fig. 8-21)[29,38,45]
- Patients readily aroused and obey commands but cannot recall the operative period afterward[28,39]
- Drug is a potent anticonvulsant[21,33]

Some patients experience itchiness around the nose but this rapidly passes as sedation ensues. The mild tachycardia, anticonvulsant activity, cardiorespiratory stability, and anxiolytic and amnesia properties provide an unusual number of the requirements for an ideal supplement to central neural blockade.[15,21,38,45] At this stage of investigation, the pharmacokinetics of the drug also indicate its suitability for highly controllable constant-rate infusion.[28]

Use of Neural Blockade for Chronic Pain

The use of pharmacokinetic techniques in association with the administration of narcotics can greatly enhance what is learned from diagnostic neural blockade for chronic pain and can supplement, if needed, therapeutic neural blockade.

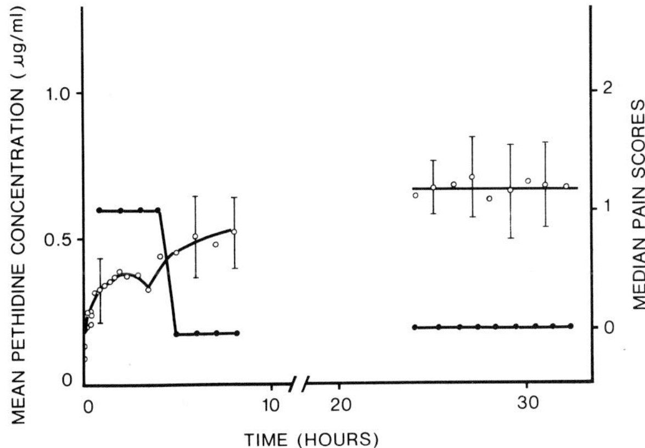

Fig. 31-14. Plasma meperidine (Pethidine) concentrations (○○) and median pain scores (●●) measured during two 8-hour sampling periods of intravenous infusion of meperidine, 1 mg per minute for 45 minutes then 0.53 mg per minute for 28 minutes, then 24 mg per hour. Concentrations were approximately 75 per cent of the final mean steady-state value (0.67 μg/ml) after 6 hours. Median pain scores were moderate for the first 4 hours of infusion and fell to 0 (pain-free) after a therapeutic plasma concentration of 0.46 μg per ml was reached. Median pain scores of 0 were recorded for the remainder of the 32-hour infusion. (Stapleton, J.V., Austin, K.L., and Mather, L.E.: A pharmacokinetic approach to postoperative pain. Continuous infusion of Pethidine. Anaesth. Intens. Care, *7*:25, 1979)

For diagnostic purposes, the information gained from selective epidural narcotic blockade can be refined by a pharmacokinetic profile of the narcotic in the blood and in the CSF, as a result of epidural absorption. This is important since it is necessary to establish that, at the time of pain assessment, there are adequate CSF concentrations at the appropriate spinal cord levels and that blood concentrations are below those known to produce blood borne analgesia in that patient (see Fig. 31-1). The analgesic plasma concentration is determined previously by constant infusion of narcotic and by measurement of the steady-state blood concentration associated with analgesia. Only with such data available is it possible to determine whether selective narcotic epidural blockade alone has relieved pain. Pain relief after selective blockade indicates the presence of a painful lesion at or distal to the spinal cord. Lack of relief indicates the likelihood that psychological factors are contributing to the pain.

The intravenous infusion data can also make

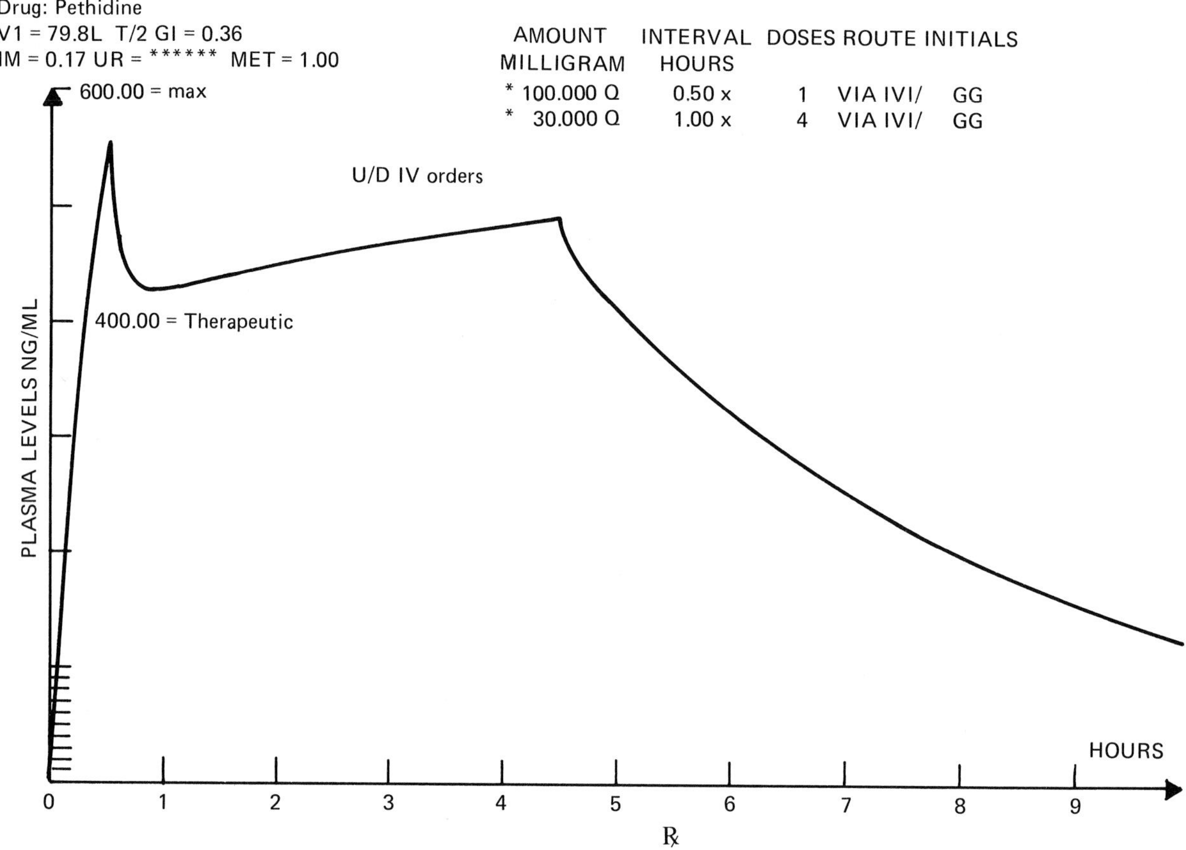

Fig. 31-15. Controlled intravenous meperidine infusion. Computer simulation of a simple regime to rapidly achieve and maintain an analgesic plasma concentration of meperidine; using a constant rate pump meperidine 100 mg is given over 30 min followed by 30 mg per hour. Lower loading and maintenance doses may be sufficient in patients with neural blockade who require lower plasma meperidine concentrations. Note rapid fall of plasma meperidine concentration when infusion is stopped.

possible the designing of narcotic analgesic regimens that will produce the appropriate analgesic blood level for each patient. This requires pharmacokinetic studies following oral or rectal or intramuscular administration. By appropriate adjustment of dosage and timing of doses, it is possible to design an analgesic regimen that achieves and maintains a minimum effective blood concentration for part or all of each day. Many patients with advanced cancer may obtain significant but incomplete analgesia with neurolytic neural blockade which can be converted to complete pain relief by the appropriate regimen, as outlined above. We have found rectal meperidine suppositories, 200 to 400 mg, with dose and timing determined by pharmacokinetics, to be an excellent supplement for neural blockade in cancer pain: nausea from oral administration is reduced, constipation is lessened, and duration of analgesia (6–10 hours) is much longer than after an oral or intramuscular narcotic.*

Similar pharmacokinetic approaches are much needed for other drugs used to supplement neural blockade, such as the tricyclic antidepressant drugs. These represent a particular problem since their rate of clearance can vary tenfold, thus making it impossible to achieve reliably a therapeutic blood concentration by prescribing a standard dose.

General Features of Intravenous Pharmacokinetic Technique in Chronic Pain. An intravenous infusion of narcotic is used to ascertain whether the patient can become pain-free at blood concentrations of the

* Mather, L.E., Glynn, C.J., Cousins, M.J.: Unpublished data.

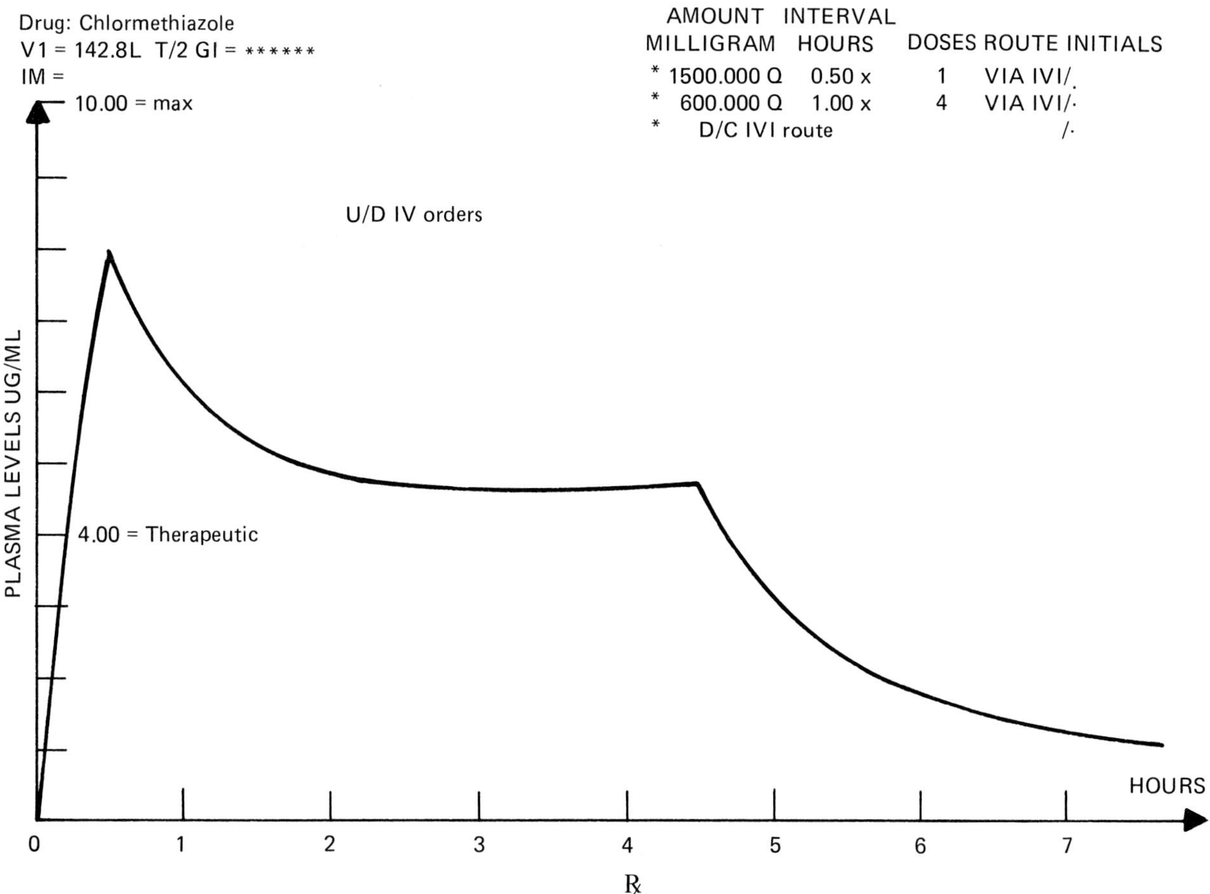

Fig. 31-16. Low-dose sedative infusion for supplementation of epidural block. Chlormethiazole is infused as a 0.8 per cent solution of the ethane disulfonate (Hemineurin): loading dose of 1500 mg over 30 minutes, maintenance dose, 600 mg per hour. Adjustments are required because of level of sedation desired and physical status of patient, particularly when there are changes in cardiac output and hepatic perfusion (the drug's clearance is flow-limited). Patients were all adequately sedated in this study but maintained their own airway. Note rapid fall of chlormethiazole concentration when infusion is ceased. (Data from Mather, L.E., and Cousins, M.J.: Low-dose chlormethiazole infusion as a supplement to epidural blockade. I: Pharmacokinetics. Anaesth. Intens. Care [*In press*])

analgesic that are tolerably free of adverse effects. If analgesia cannot be achieved, it is likely that the analgesic or systemic analgesic therapy in general is inappropriate. If an analgesic blood concentration is found, then a dosage regimen should be designed to produce this effect reliably. From serial blood samples taken throughout the infusion period and afterward, a model is constructed for the disposition of the analgesic in that patient. The model is made of the apparent volumes of distribution (relationship between dose and blood concentration), half-lives (how frequently multiple doses should be given), and clearances (how efficiently the body disposes of the drug). These data provide guidelines for designing future therapy and, in themselves, provide clues why previous therapy may have been unsuccessful. Once it is decided that systemic analgesia is appropriate, useful dosage forms and regimens of the analgesic are evaluated from the patient's response.

Studies in three selected patients illustrate their application to chronic pain therapy.†

† Mather, L.E., and Glynn, C.J.: Unpublished data.

Case One. The patient suffered post-traumatic neuralgia. Analgesia was consistently obtained over a 12-month period when a meperidine blood concentration of 0.3 mg per L was reached, irrespective of the route of administration. Multiple-dose oral administration gave blood concentrations in excess of the minimum for analgesia over many hours. Bioavailability of oral meperidine was 59 per cent in this patient, whereas rectal suppositories gave 100 per cent bioavailability but slower absorption.

Case Two. The patient had long-standing pancreatitis. Similar oral and rectal absorption profiles were obtained. In this patient, analgesia was obtained over a 12-month period at 0.25 mg per L and was readily produced after multiple oral doses. Supplementary narcotic analgesia was required following celiac plexus blockade.

Case Three. An intriguing problem was observed in patient #3. This patient with scleroderma and pain achieved complete pain relief at meperidine blood concentrations in excess of 0.25 mg per L. This corresponded to the first 90 minutes after a 100-mg intravenous bolus. Oral or rectal administration of 200 mg resulted in no analgesia at all. Each of these doses resulted in maximum blood concentrations of only 0.1 mg per L, corresponding to only 25 per cent bioavailability. In contrast, intramuscular injection of meperidine, 100 mg, produced rapid and complete absorption and provided excellent analgesia.

Sympathetic blockade with guanethidine in this patient improved perfusion but was not adequate for pain relief.

These three cases have been selected to illustrate the usefulness of pharmacokinetic techniques as an adjunct to the investigation and treatment of patients with chronic pain. Such techniques involve the construction and interpretation of mathematical models of blood drug concentration to time data and their integration with pharmacologic response data, which indicates how pharmacokinetics can supplement neural blockade in chronic pain.

It is of interest that these patients have shown no signs of pharmacokinetic tolerance. The absorption, distribution, and metabolism of meperidine remained unchanged during the period of the study, and analgesic blood concentrations remained the same.

Thus the diagnosis of chronic pain may be aided by obtaining a range of data from the following: (1) local anesthetic blockade at precise anatomical sites, (2) selective narcotic epidural blockade supplemented by CSF and blood pharmacokinetic data, and (3) intravenous infusion of narcotic analgetic with simultaneous recording of pain score and blood pharmacokinetic data. The use of placebos will assist in all of these but particularly in the second in which the patient does not know when a potent agent is given. The simultaneous recording of pain response and pharmacokinetic profile provides an excellent opportunity to determine if patient response consistently parallels the presence of effective blood or spinal fluid concentrations of the drug. These approaches lend much more certainty to the assignment of the relative contributions of neural and psychological factors. Such an approach has greatly reduced the inappropriate use of destructive neurolytic procedures or unnecessary surgery in patients whose pain is mainly a result of psychological factors.

EDUCATIONAL HORIZONS

Throughout this text it has been stressed that there is still a need for improved teaching of the techniques of neural blockade in the context of clinical anesthesia and also in the management of acute and chronic pain. It is hoped that both undergraduate and postgraduate educational institutions throughout the world are coming to an appreciation of this.

There is also considerable room for improvements in teaching of basic science and clinical management of acute and chronic pain. Major deficiencies in this area currently exist in the undergraduate curricula of many medical schools all over the world. The lamentable past record of the medical profession in the management of chronic pain will achieve widespread improvement only if undergraduate education directs serious attention to the subject of chronic pain. As one aspect of the educational potential of a pain unit, there is considerable potential to teach applied anatomy by using prosected anatomical specimens as a sequel to practical experience in neural blockade techniques. Also, the temporary neurologic deficit resulting from different neural blockade procedures can be an excellent aid to teaching neuroanatomy. Anatomical relationships pertinent to neural blockade can often be reinforced during surgery.

At the postgraduate level specialty areas must collaborate with the aim of educating one another on their possible contribution to pain management and with the objective of improved pain diagnosis and management. Such collaboration must extend to basic scientists so that research in pain management in the animal laboratory can be applied in the clinical pain-management unit. There seems little doubt that such collaboration will result in a contribution to humanity second only to the most dramatic development in the history of medicine—anesthesia. The rewards for basic scientists and clinicians who rise to this challenge will be the realization of a dream that began with the dramatic conquering of pain in surgery. There is a pressing need, based on both humanitarian and economic considerations, to ensure that Morton's epitaph does not remain unfulfilled for another hundred years: ". . . Since whom, science has control of pain . . ." (Epitaph for W. H. G. Morton, 1819–1868.)

APPENDIX: TAXONOMY OF PAIN*

PAIN

An unpleasant sensory and emotional experience associated with actual or potential tissue damage, or described in terms of such damage.

Note: Pain is always subjective. Each patient learns the application of the word through experiences related to injury in early life. Biologists recognize that stimuli that cause pain are liable to damage tissue. Accordingly, pain is the experience associated with actual or potential tissue damage. It is unquestionably a sensation in a part or parts of the body, but it is also always unpleasant and therefore also an emotional experience. Experiences that resemble pain (*e.g.*, pricking), but are not unpleasant, should not be called pain. Unpleasant abnormal experiences (dysaesthesias) may also be pain but are not necessarily so because, subjectively, they may not have the usual sensory qualities of pain.

Many people report pain in the absence of tissue damage or any likely pathophysiologic cause; usually this happens for psychological reasons. There is no way to distinguish their experience from that due to tissue damage based on the subjective report. If they regard their experience as pain and if they report it in the same ways as pain caused by tissue damage, it should be accepted as pain. This definition avoids tying pain to the stimulus. Activity induced in the nociceptor and nociceptive pathways by a noxious stimulus is not pain, which is always a psychological state, even though it may well be appreciated that pain most often has a proximate physical cause.

* Reprinted with permission of "Pain," The Journal of the International Association for the Study of Pain. From Pain 6:249–252, 1979.

ALLODYNIA

Pain due to a non-noxious stimulus to normal skin.

Note: This is a new term that is intended to refer to the situation where otherwise normal tissues that may have abnormal innervation or may be referral sites for other loci give rise to pain on stimulation by non-noxious means. "Allo" means "other" in Greek and is a common prefix for medical conditions that diverge from the expected. "Odynia" is derived from the Greek word "odune" or "odyne," which is used in "pleurodynia" and in "coccydynia," and is similar in meaning to the root from which words with -algia or -algesia in them are derived. Allodynia is suggested following discussions with Professor Paul Potter of the Department of the History of Medicine and Science at The University of Western Ontario.

ANALGESIA

Lack of pain on noxious stimulation.

ANESTHESIA DOLOROSA

Pain in an area or region that is anesthetic.

CAUSALGIA

A syndrome of sustained burning pain after a traumatic nerve lesion combined with vasomotor and sudomotor dysfunction and later trophic changes.

CENTRAL PAIN

Pain associated with a lesion of the CNS.

DYSESTHESIA

An unpleasant abnormal sensation.

Note: Compare with pain and with paresthesia.

HYPERALGESIA

Increased sensitivity to noxious stimulation.

Note: This represents a lowered threshold to noxious stimulation not an increased response to supra-threshold stimulation. It should not be used to refer to a response to non-noxious stimulation.

HYPERAESTHESIA

Increased sensitivity to stimulation, excluding special senses.

Note: The stimulus and locus should be specified. The word has often been used to indicate not only diminished threshold but also increased response to noxious stimulation and pain after non-noxious stimulation. For the former case, hyperpathia should be used. For the latter, the new term *allodynia* is suggested.

HYPERPATHIA

A painful syndrome, characterized by delay, overreaction, and aftersensation to a stimulus, especially a repetitive stimulus.

Note: It may occur with hypo- or hyperasthesia, or dysaesthesia. Faulty identification and localization of the stimulus, delay, radiating sensation, and aftersensation may be present, and the pain is often explosive in character.

HYPOALGESIA

Diminished sensitivity to noxious stimulation.

Note: Hypoalgesia is a particular case of hypoaesthesia.

HYPOAESTHESIA

Decreased sensitivity to stimulation, excluding special senses.

Note: Stimulation and locus to be specified.

NEURALGIA

Pain in the distribution of a nerve or nerves.

Note: Common usage often implies a paroxysmal quality. This is especially the case in Europe. More often neuralgia is used for nonparoxysmal pains. The technical usage is as given, and neuralgia should not be reserved for paroxysmal pains.

NEURITIS

Inflammation of a nerve or nerves.

Note: Not to be used unless inflammation is thought to be present.

NEUROPATHY

A disturbance of function or pathologic change in a nerve; in one nerve, mononeuropathy; in several nerves, mononeuropathy multiplex; symmetrical and bilateral, polyneuropathy.

Note: Neuritis is a special case of neuropathy and is now reserved for inflammatory processes affecting nerves. Neuropathy is not intended to cover cases like neurapraxia, neuronotmesis, or section of a nerve.

NOCICEPTOR

A receptor preferentially sensitive to a noxious or potentially noxious stimulus.

Note: Avoid use of terms like pain receptor, pain pathway, and so forth.

NOXIOUS

A noxious stimulus is a tissue-damaging stimulus.

PAIN THRESHOLD

The least stimulus intensity at which a subject perceives pain.

Note: This has been the common usage for most pain research workers. In psychophysics, thresholds are defined as the level at which 50 per cent of stimuli are recognized. In that case, the pain threshold would be the level at which 50 per cent of stimuli would be recognized as painful. Pain here serves as a measure of the stimulus. The stimulus is not pain and cannot be a measure of pain.

PAIN TOLERANCE LEVEL

The greatest intensity of stimulus that causes pain that a subject is prepared to tolerate.

REFERENCES

1. Akil, H., *et al.*: Enkephalin-like material in normal human CSF: Measurement and levels. Life Sci., *23*:121, 1978.
2. Amoils, S.P.: The Joule-Thomson cryoprobe. Arch. Ophthalmol., *78*:201, 1967.
3. Armstrong Davidson, M.H.: The history of anaesthesia. *In* Gray, T.C., and Nunn, J.F. (eds.): General Anaesthesia. p. 709. London, Butterworth, 1971.
4. Barnard, J.D.W., Lloyd, J.W., and Glynn, C.J.: Cryosurgery in the management of intractable facial pain. Br. J. Oral Surg., *16*:135, 1978–79.
5. Behar, M., Olswang, D., Magora, F., and Davidson, J.T.: Epidural morphine in treatment of pain. Lancet, *1*:527, 1979.
6. Bonica, J.J.: Advances in Neurology: International Symposium on Pain. New York, Raven Press, 1974.
7. Bonica, J.J., and Albe–Fessard, D.G.: Advances in Pain Research and Therapy. Proceedings of the First World Congress on Pain. New York, Raven Press, 1976.
8. Campbell, E.J.M., Dickinson, C.J., Slater, J.D.H.: Clinical Physiology. pp. 256–252, Oxford Blackwell Scientific, 1974.
9. Church, J.J.: Continuous narcotic infusions for relief of postoperative pain. Br. Med. J., *1*:977, 1979.
10. Cousins, M.J., *et al.*: Selective spinal analgesia. Lancet, *1*:1141, 1979.
11. Cousins, M.J., *et al.*: Neurolytic lumbar sympathetic blockade: Duration of denervation and relief of rest pain. Anaesth. Intens. Care., *7*:121, 1979.
12. Evans, R.J.: Acid–base changes in patients with intractable pain and malignancy. Can. J. Surg., *15*:37, 1972.
13. Eysenck, H.J., and Eysenck, S.B.G.: Manual of Eysenck Personality Inventory. London, Hodder and Stoughton, 1964.
14. Folkard, S., Glynn, C.J., and Lloyd, J.W.: Diurnal variation and individual differences in the perception of intractable pain. J. Psychosom. Res., *20*:289, 1976.
15. Galizia, E.J., Metrewell, C., and Prout, B.J.: A comparison of chlormethiazole and diazepam as intravenous sedatives for fibre-endoscopic examinations of the upper gastrointestinal tract. Br. J. Anaesth., *47*:402, 1975.
16. Glynn, C.J.: Ventilatory response to intractable pain. Unpublished M. Sc. Thesis. Oxford University, 1977.
17. Glynn, C.J., and Lloyd, J.W.: Biochemical changes associated with intractable pain. Br. Med. J., *1*:280, 1978.
18. Glynn, C.J., Lloyd, J.W., and Barnard, J.D.W.: Cryoanalgesia in the management of post thoracotomy pain. Thorax, In press, 1980.
19. Glynn, C.J., Lloyd, J.W., and Folkard, S.: The diurnal variation in perception of pain. Proc. R. Soc. Med., *69*:369, 1976.
20. Grattan, J.H.G., and Singer, C.: Anglo-Saxon Magic and Medicine (Lacnunga). p. 165. Oxford, Oxford University Press, 1952.
21. Harvey, P.K.P., Higgenbottom, T.W., and Loh, L.: Chlormethiazole in treatment of status epilepticus. Br. Med. J., *2*:603, 1975.
22. Hutcheson, A.: Physiotherapy, an adjunct to stellate ganglion and brachial plexus blocks for post-traumatic sympathetic dystrophy. Aust. J. Physiother., *23*:45, 1977.
23. Keele, K.D., and Stern, P.R.S.: Serum lipid changes in relation to pain. J.R. Coll. Physicians Lond., *7*:319, 1973.
24. Lascelles, P.T., Evans, P.R., Merskey, H., and Sabur, M.A.: Plasma cortisol in psychiatric and neurological patients with pain. Brain, *97*:533, 1974.
25. Lindahl, O.: Changes in the acid base balance in metabolic treatment for pain. Acta Orthop. Scand., *41*:8, 1970.
26. ______: Pain—A general chemical explanation. *In* Bonica, J.J. (ed.): Advances in Neurology. pp. 45–47. New York, Raven Press, 1974.
27. Lloyd, J.W., Barnard, J.D.W., and Glynn, C.J.: Cryoanalgesia. A new approach to pain relief. Lancet, *2*:932, 1976.
28. McGilhard, K.L., and Takemori, A.E.: Antagonism by naloxone of narcotic-induced respiratory depression and analgesia. J. Pharmacol. Exp. Ther., *207*:494, 1978.
29. Mather, L.E., and Cousins, M.J.: Low-dose chlormethiazole infusion as a supplement to epidural blockade. I: Pharmacokinetics. Anaesth. Intens. Care. In press, 1980.
30. Mather, L.E., Lindop, M.J., Tucker, G.T., and Pflug, A.E.: Pethidine revisited: Plasma concentrations and effects after intramuscular injection. Br. J. Anaesth., *47*:1269, 1975.
31. Mather, L.E., and Meffin, P.J.: Clinical pharmacokinetics of Pethidine. Clin. Pharmacokinet., *3*:352, 1978.
32. Melzack, R., and Wall, P.D.: Pain mechanisms: A new theory. Science, *150*:971, 1965.
33. Moir, D.D., Victor–Rodrigues, L., and Willocks, J.: Epidural analgesia during labour in patients with pre eclampsia. J. Obstet. Gynaecol., *79*:465, 1972.
34. Moore, R.G., *et al.*: Pharmacokinetics of chlormethiazole in humans. Eur. J. Clin. Pharmacol., *8*:353, 1975.
35. Nathan, P.W., Sears, T.A., and Smith, M.C.: Effects of phenol solutions on nerve roots of the cat: An electro-physiological and histological study. J. Neurol. Sci., *2*:7, 1965.
36. Propping, P.: Pharmacogenetics. Rev. Physiol. Biochem. Pharmacol., *83*:124, 1978.
37. Samii, K., Feret, J., Harari, A., and Uiars, P.: Intrathecal morphine. Lancet, *1*:1142, 1979.
38. Schweitzer, S.A.: Chlormethiazole (Hemineurin) infusion as supplemental sedation during epidural block. Anaesth. Intens. Care, *6*:248, 1978.
39. Scott, D.B., and McClure, J.M.: Selective epidural analgesia. Lancet, *1*:1410, 1979.
40. Stapleton, J.V., Austin, K.L., and Mather, L.E.: A pharmacokinetic approach to post operative pain: Continuous infusion of Pethidine. Anaesth. Intens. Care, *7*:25, 1979.
41. Sternbach, R.A.: The psychology of pain. p. 241. New York, Raven Press, 1978.
42. Sunderland, S.: Nerves and nerve injuries, ed. 2, pp. 131, 180. Edinburgh, Livingstone, 1978.
43. Wang, J.K., Nauss, L.A., and Thomas, J.E.: Pain relief by intrathecally applied morphine in man. Anesthesiology, *50*:149, 1979.
44. Whittaker, D.K.: An experimental study of the effects of cryosurgery on the oral mucous membrane. Unpublished Ph.D. Thesis. University of Wales, 1973.
45. Wilson, J., Stephen, G.W., and Scott, D.B.: A study of the cardiovascular effects of chlormethiazole. Br. J. Anaesth., *41*:840, 1969.
46. Yaksh, T.L., Wilson, P.R., Kaiko, R.F., Inturrisi, C.E.: Analgesia produced by a spinal action of morphine and effects upon parturition in rat and rabbit. Anesthesiology, *51*:386, 1979.
47. Wright, E.M.: Transport processes in the formation of the cerebrospinal fluid. Rev. Physiol. Biochem. Pharmacol., *83*: 26, 1978.
48. Yaksh, T.L., and Rudy, T.A.: Analgesia mediated by a direct final action of narcotics. Science, *192*:1357, 1976.

Index

Index